SECTION THREE: PRINCIPLES OF CANCER MANAGEMENT

SECTION FOUR: PRINCIPLES OF SYMPTOM MANAGEMENT

2ND EDITION

Mosby's
ONCOLO...
NURSING...
A Comprehensive Gu...

Susan Newt...
Vice President, Health Ma...
Quintiles
Oncology Advanced Pract...
Dayton, Ohio

Margaret Hi...
Sr. Director, Global Patient Relations
Novartis Oncology
East Hanover, New Jersey

Jeannine M. Brant, PhD, APRN, AOCN, FAAN
Oncology CNS/Nurse Scientist
Billings Clinic
Billings, Montana
Assistant Affiliate Professor
Montana State University, College of Nursing
Bozeman, Montana

ELSEVIER

ELSEVIER

3251 Riverport Lane
St. Louis, Missouri 63043

Library of Congress Cataloging-in-Publication Data

Names: Newton, Susan, 1967- editor. | Hickey, Margaret (Margaret M.), editor.
   | Brant, Jeannine M., editor.
Title: Mosby's oncology nursing advisor : a comprehensive guide to clinical
   practice / [edited by] Susan Newton, Margaret Hickey, Jeannine M. Brant.
Other titles: Oncology nursing advisor
Description: Second edition. | St. Louis, Missouri : Elsevier, Inc., [2017] |
   Includes bibliographical references and index.
Identifiers: LCCN 2016030251 | ISBN 9780323375634
Subjects: | MESH: Neoplasms--nursing | Oncology Nursing--methods
Classification: LCC RC266 | NLM WY 156 | DDC 616.99/40231--dc23 LC record
available at https://lccn.loc.gov/2016030251

Content Strategist: Lee Henderson
Content Development Manager: Jean Fornango
Senior Content Development Specialist: Laura Selkirk
Publishing Services Manager: Hemamalini Rajendrababu
Project Manager: Maria Luisa Ordonio
Design Direction: Paula Catalano

Printed in the United States of America

Last digit is the print number: 9   8   7   6   5   4   3   2   1

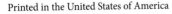

Acknowledgments

I am blessed to have the support of my loving husband Jack and my three sons: Alex, Casey, and Jackson. They are the joy of my life. My Mom is my biggest fan and has taught me about cancer through the eyes of a caregiver. I am inspired by my oncology nurse colleagues every day and dedicate this resource to helping them improve the lives of patients with cancer.

Susan (Susie)

This textbook is dedicated to patients and families who face a cancer diagnosis and the nurses who care for them. Special thanks and recognition are due the expert oncology nurses who contributed as authors because without their willingness to share their knowledge and experience, this book would not be possible. Lastly, I am sincerely grateful to my husband Kenny for his never-ending support and love.

Margaret (Margie)

Writing always takes a village. My heartfelt thanks go out to the nurses who contributed many hours of work to this book and for the dedication that went into each chapter. I hope and pray that it will be used to provide quality cancer care to patients and their families around the globe. I give special thanks to my family members who are always there for me—my husband Rich, my daughter Danielle and her husband Thomas, my granddaughter Annette, and my grandson Zach. You are the light of my life!

Jeannine

Authors

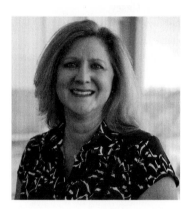

Susie Newton, RN, MS, AOCN, AOCNS, has worked as an Oncology Clinical Nurse Specialist in inpatient and outpatient centers during the past 21 years. She is currently the Vice President of Health Management Solutions at Quintiles, leading teams of clinical educators across the country. Susie is an international speaker and has published five oncology nursing textbooks and numerous articles and is finishing her term of office as Director-at-Large for the National Oncology Nursing Society.

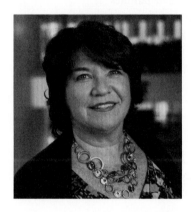

Margie Hickey, RN, MSN, MS, OCN, CORLN, has more than 30 years of oncology nursing experience and has worked in all oncology settings caring for inpatients and outpatients undergoing cancer surgery, radiation therapy, and medical treatments, including chemotherapy, biotherapy, and immunotherapy. Currently employed by Novartis Oncology, Margie has been an editor of five oncology nursing textbooks and has authored more than 25 publications.

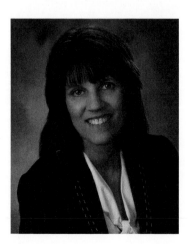

Jeannine M. Brant, PhD, APRN, AOCN, FAAN, has been an oncology nurse for more than 30 years and has worked as a staff nurse, infusion center nurse, and clinical nurse specialist in inpatient and ambulatory settings. She is currently an Oncology Clinical Nurse Specialist and Scientist at Billings Clinic in Montana. She has made more than 75 contributions to the literature and is an editor for the Standards of Oncology Nursing and the Core Curriculum for Oncology Nursing.

Contributors

Paula Anastasia, RN, MN, AOCN
Gyn-Oncology Clinical Nurse Specialist
Cedars-Sinai Medical Center, Women's Cancer Program
Los Angeles, California

Lisa Balster, BA, MA, MBA
Director, Patient and Family Support Services
Hospice of Dayton, Inc.
Dayton, Ohio

Laura Benson, RN, MS, ANP
Senior Vice President, Global Medical Affairs
Novocure
Portsmouth, New Hampshire

Karyl Blaseg, RN, MSN, OCN
Director of Cancer Services, Integrative Medicine, and
    Supportive Care
Clinic Administration
Billings Clinic
Billings, Montana

Carol S. Blecher, MS, RN, AOCN, APNC, CBCN
Advanced Practice Nurse/Clinical Educator
Trinitas Comprehensive Cancer Center
Trinitas Regional Medical Center
Adjunct Faculty, Trinitas School of Nursing Union County
    College
Elizabeth, New Jersey

Joshua L. Carter, RN, BSN, BS
Commercial Clinical Educator
Quintiles
San Diego, California

Kristin A. Cawley, RN, MSN, OCN
Nurse Leader
Memorial Sloan Kettering Cancer Center
New York, New York

Carrie H. Christiansen, RN, MSN, C-FNP
Certified Family Nurse Practitioner, Medical Oncology
City of Hope National Medical Center
Duarte, California

Anna Christofanelli, BSN, RN, OCN
Registered Nurse
Inpatient Cancer Care, Billings Clinic
Billings, Montana

Francisco A. Conde, PhD, APRN, AOCNS, FAAN
Advance Practice Registered Nurse, Oncology
Queen's Medical Center
Honolulu, Hawaii

Diane G. Cope, PhD, ARNP, BC, AOCNP
Oncology Nurse Practitioner
Florida Cancer Specialists and Research Institute
Fort Myers, Florida

Georgia Decker, MS, RN, ANP-BC, FAAN
Founder, Advanced Practice Nurse
Integrative Care
Albany, New York

Lorraine Drapek, FNP-BC, AOCNP
Nurse Practitioner, Radiation Oncology GI/GYN Services
Massachusetts General Hospital
Boston, Massachusetts

Denice Economou, RN, MN, CHPN
Senior Research Specialist
Department of Nursing Research & Education
City of Hope
Duarte, California

Pamela Gamier, RN, BSN, CHPN
Specialty Care Coordinator, Palliative Medicine
Cleveland Clinic
Cleveland, Ohio

Ruth Canty Gholz, RN, MS, AOCN
Oncology Clinical Nurse Specialist
Cincinnati, Ohio

Rupa Ghosh-Berkebile, MS, APRN-BC, AOCNP
Nurse Practitioner
Medical Oncology-Sarcoma
Arthur G. James Cancer Hospital and Richard J. Solove
    Research Institute
Columbus, Ohio

Amy Goodrich, BSN, MSN
Nurse Practitioner/Research Associate, Oncology
Johns Hopkins Kimmel Cancer Center
Baltimore, Maryland

Carolyn Grande, CRNP
Nurse Practitioner, Otorhinolaryngology
Hospital of the University of Pennsylvania
Philadelphia, Pennsylvania

Trechia Gross, RN, BS, CHPN
Director of Quality and Informatics
Quality and Compliance
Hospice of Dayton
Dayton, Ohio

Debra E. Heidrich, MSN
Nursing Consultant
West Chester, Ohio

Kristen Hurley, RN, DNP
Certified Nurse Practitioner
Hematology and Bone Marrow Transplant
Avera
Sioux Falls, South Dakota

Joanne Itano, RN, PhD, APRN
Associate Vice President for Academic Affairs
Academic Affairs/Policy and Planning
University of Hawaii System
Honolulu, Hawaii

Brenda Keith, MN, RN, AOCNS
Clinical Instructor, Nursing Yavapai College Prescott,
    Arizona
Sr. Oncology Clinical Coordinator II
HER2
Genentech USA, Inc.
South San Francisco, California

Nicole Korak, MSN, FNP-C
Senior Director, Health Management Services
Quintiles
Parsippany, New Jersey

Sandra Kurtin, RN, MS, AOCN, ANP
Nurse Practitioner, Hematology/Oncology
The University of Arizona Cancer Center
Clinical Assistant Professor of Medicine
Adjunct Clinical Professor of Nursing
The University of Arizona
Tucson, Arizona

Suzanne M. Mahon, DNSc, RN, AOCN, APNG
Professor, Internal Medicine, Division of Hematology/
    Oncology Adult Nursing, School of Nursing
Saint Louis University
St. Louis, Missouri

Kristen W. Maloney, MSN, RN, AOCNS
Nurse Manager, Oncology Nursing
Hospital of the University of Pennsylvania
Philadelphia, Pennsylvania

Mary Murphy, RN, MS, AOCN, ACHPN
Chief Nursing and Care Officer, Nursing
Hospice of Dayton
Dayton, Ohio

Susie Newton, RN, MS, AOCN, AOCNS
Vice President, Health Management Solutions
Quintiles
Oncology Advanced Practice Nurse
Dayton, Ohio

Colleen O'Leary, MSN
Clinical Nurse Specialist
The Ohio State University Comprehensive Cancer Center
Arthur James Cancer Hospital and Richard Solove
    Research Institute
Columbus, Ohio

Margaretta S. Page, RN, MS
Nurse Coordinator, Neurosurgery Neuro-Oncology
University of California–San Francisco
San Francisco, California

Lisa Parks, MS, BSN, CNP
Inpatient Hepato-Pancreas-Biliary Nurse Practitioner,
Division of Surgical Oncology
The Ohio State University Wexner Medical Center, The James
    Cancer Hospital and Solove Research Institute
Columbus, Ohio
Oncology Nursing Society Surgical Oncology Special Interest
    Group Coordinator
Pittsburgh, Pennsylvania

Jody Pelusi, PhD, FNP, AOCNP
Oncology Nurse Practitioner/Sub Investigator Clinical
    Research
Honor Health Research Institute, Honor Health
Scottsdale, Arizona

Carolee Polek, RN, PhD, AOCNS, BMTCN
Associate Professor
University of Delaware School of Nursing
Newark, Delaware

Julie Ponto, PhD
Professor, Graduate Programs in Nursing
Winona State University–Rochester
Rochester, Minnesota

Jane Rabbitt, BSN
Lead Nurse Coordinator, Neuro-Oncology
University of California–San Francisco
San Francisco, California

Sandra Remer, RN, BS, OCN
Neuro-Oncology Coordinator
Neurosurgery Hermelin Brain Tumor Center
Henry Ford Health System
Detroit, Michigan

Jeanene "Gigi" Robison, MSN, RN, AOCN
Oncology Clinical Nurse Specialist, Patient Care Services
The Christ Hospital
Cincinnati, Ohio

Marlon Garzo Saria, PhD(c), RN, AOCNS
Advanced Practice Nurse Researcher, Neuro-Oncology
University of California–San Diego
La Jolla, California

Leah A. Scaramuzzo, MSN, RN-BC, AOCN
Nurse Clinician II, Inpatient Cancer Care
Billings Clinic
Billings, Montana

Ray Scarpa, DNP, AOCN, APN-C
Clinical Assistant Professor Part Time Lecturer
Rutgers University, School of Nursing
Newark, New Jersey
Supervisory Advanced Practice Nurse
Otolaryngology Head and Neck Surgery
University Hospital
Adjunct Faculty University Hospital Medical Staff
Newark, New Jersey

Terry Wikle Shapiro, RN, MSN, CRNP
Instructor, Department of Pediatric Pennsylvania State
    College of Medicine
Nurse Practitioner, Pediatric Stem Cell Transplantation
    Program
Pediatric Hematology Oncology
Penn State Children's Hospital
Hershey, Pennsylvania

Lisa Kennedy Sheldon, PhD APRN, BC, AOCNP
Associate Professor
College of Nursing and Health Sciences
University of Massachusetts Boston
Boston, Massachusetts

Barbara Smelko, RN
Staff Nurse
Warren Cancer Care Center
Warren, Pennsylvania
Nurse on Call
AIM at Melanoma Foundation

Carrie Tompkins Stricker, PhD
Chief Clinical Officer
On Q Health, Inc.
Bay Harbor, Florida
Oncology Nurse Practitioner
University of Pennsylvania, Abramson Cancer Center
Philadelphia, Pennsylvania

Carrie Tilley, MS, RN, ANP-BC
Adult Nurse Practitioner, Survivorship Program
Tate Cancer Center at the University of Maryland
Baltimore, Maryland
Washington Medical Center
Glen Burnie, Maryland

Wendy H. Vogel, MSN, FNP, AOCNP
Oncology Nurse Practitioner
Wellmont Cancer Institute
Kingsport, Tennessee

Deborah Kirk Walker, DNP, FNP-BC, NP-C, AOCN
Assistant Professor
Coordinator of the Dual Adult-Gerentology Primary Care &
    Oncology Nurse Practitioner Specialty Track
School of Nursing, Acute, Chronic and Continuing Care
    Department
Scientist, Center for Palliative and Supportive Care
University of Alabama at Birmingham
Associate Scientist, Cancer Control and Populations Science
    Program
UAB Comprehensive Cancer Center
Birmingham, Alabama

Jennifer S. Webster, MN, MPH, RN, AOCNS
Oncology Clinical Specialist
Georgia Cancer Specialists, Affiliated with Northside
    Hospital Cancer Institute
Atlanta, Georgia

Debbie Winkeljohn, RN, MSN, AOCN, CNS
Clinical Nurse Specialist
Hematology Oncology Associates
Albuquerque, New Mexico

Laura S. Wood, RN, MSN, OCN
Renal Cancer Research Coordinator
Cleveland Clinic Taussig Cancer Institute
Cleveland, Ohio

Tyler Workman, BA, RN
Graduate Nursing Student
School of Nursing and Dental Hygiene
University of Hawaii at Manoa
Honolulu, Hawaii

Reviewers

Karen Abbas, MS, AOCN
Advanced Practice RN
University of Rochester Medical Center, Wilmot Cancer
    Institute
Rochester, New York

Ashley Leak Bryant, PhD, RN-BC, OCN
Assistant Professor, School of Nursing
The University of North Carolina at Chapel Hill, School
    of Nursing
Chapel Hill, North Carolina

Michele E. Gaguski, MSN, RN, AOCN, CHPN, APN-C
Clinical Director, Medical Oncology
Atlanticare Cancer Care Institute
Egg Harbor Township, New Jersey

Catherine Glennon, RN, MHS, NE-BC, OCN
Director, Cancer Center
University of Kansas Hospital
Kansas City, Kansas

Joyce Jackowski, MS, FNP-BC, AOCNP
Nurse Practitioner
Florida Cancer Specialists
Englewood, Florida

Marcelle Kaplan, RN, MS, AOCN, CBCN
Oncology Nurse Consultant; Adjunct Faculty
Adelphi University College of Nursing and Public Health
Garden City, New York

Denise Scott Korn, MSN, RN, OCN
Education Specialist II
Department of Learning and Organizational Effectiveness
High Point Regional Health UNC Healthcare
High Point, North Carolina

Sandra A. Mitchell, PhD, APRN-BC, FAAN
Research Scientist
National Cancer Institute
Bethesda, Maryland

Carol S. Viele, RN, MS, OCN
Associate Clinical Professor, Department of Physiological
    Nursing
University of California–San Francisco
San Francisco, California

Wendy H. Vogel, MSN, FNP, AOCNP
Oncology Nurse Practitioner
Kingsport, Tennessee

Michele Voss, RN, BSN, OCN
St. Louis, Missouri

Preface

Welcome to the second edition of *Mosby's Oncology Nursing Advisor*. This textbook is designed for the busy nurse who needs easy-to-access clinical information on a full range of oncology topics.

Mosby's Oncology Nursing Advisor provides nurses access to almost any oncology topic in a streamlined, concise format. The second edition provides updated, evidence-based information on sections such as major cancers, principles of cancer management, and symptom management. New additions to the second edition include a new nursing practice considerations section, information regarding oral adherence, navigation, clinical trials, and tumor treating fields, seven additional symptom management chapters, and a survivorship chapter. References are listed for further in-depth study.

Working on this text has provided a venue to allow us to contribute to the oncology nursing body of knowledge. It also enabled us to work with some of the brightest and best oncology nurses across the nation. We would like to thank the contributing authors whose expertise and willingness to share their knowledge made this book possible. The contributing authors are truly content experts in their topic areas, and they showed great patience and persistence through the entire writing and editing process. While we—Susie, Margie, and Jeannine—are oncology advanced practice nurses with varied clinical backgrounds, it is the expertise and diverse experiences of the many contributing authors that make this text a solid resource for nurses.

Susie Newton, RN, MS, AOCN, AOCNS

Margie Hickey, RN, MSN, MS, OCN, CORLN

Jeannine M. Brant, PhD, APRN, AOCN, FAAN

QR Codes for Patient Teaching Guides

Contents

SECTION THREE: PRINCIPLES OF CANCER MANAGEMENT

SECTION FOUR: PRINCIPLES OF SYMPTOM MANAGEMENT

SECTION FIVE: ONCOLOGIC EMERGENCIES

Cancer Epidemiology
Implications for Prevention, Early Detection, and Treatment

Suzanne M. Mahon

Overview

Cancer continues to be a significant public health problem in the United States and throughout the world. The American Cancer Society (ACS) annually estimates the number of new cancer cases and deaths expected in the United States in the current year and provides evidence-based recommendations for prevention and early detection (ACS, 2015a). The *Cancer Facts & Figures* documents, which are updated regularly, provide an epidemiologic report of cancer in the United States that offers insight into trends in cancer and its care (Brawley et al., 2011). Another major source of data is the Surveillance, Epidemiology, and End Results (SEER) program (http://seer.cancer.gov/) (Mariotto et al., 2014). An understanding of its epidemiology is important to achieve the long-term public health goal of decreasing the morbidity and mortality associated with a diagnosis of cancer.

Epidemiology is the study of how disease is distributed in a population, factors that influence its distribution, and trends over time. Although it often receives little attention in formal educational programs, an understanding of epidemiology is essential to comprehend cancer biology, identify its risk factors, and develop prevention and treatment strategies. Epidemiologic studies encompass the basis of disease and the impacts of treatment, screening, and preventive measures on the natural history of the disease (see box below).

Focus of Epidemiologic Studies

- Determine the extent of disease in a community, region, or defined area
- Identify potential etiologic sources and risk factors for a disease
- Study the natural history of the disease
- Study the prognosis of the disease with and without treatment or intervention
- Evaluate existing and new prevention and treatment measures and methods of health care delivery
- Examine the cost-effectiveness of various prevention and treatment strategies
- Provide the basis for public health policy and regulatory decisions about health care spending and environmental issues

Modified from Gordis L. (2013). *Epidemiology* (5th ed.). Philadelphia: Saunders.

Epidemiologists think that illness, disease, and poor health are not always random events. Some persons have risk factors that place them at risk for disease. Risk assessment is a critical component of epidemiology. Concepts and commonly used epidemiologic terms are shown in the box below and on page 2.

Terms Used in Cancer Epidemiology

Absolute risk: The occurrence of the cancer in the general population (i.e., incidence or mortality rate).

Asymptomatic: The person being screened and the examiner are unaware of signs or symptoms of cancer in the individual before the screening test is initiated.

Attributable risk: The number of cases of cancer that could be prevented with the manipulation of known risk factors.

Cancer prevention strategies:

Primary cancer prevention: Measures to avoid carcinogen exposure, to improve health practices, and, in some cases, to provide chemoprevention agents. Primary prevention may also include the use of prophylactic surgery to prevent or significantly reduce the development of a malignancy.

Secondary cancer prevention: Identification of persons at risk for malignancy and implementation of appropriate screening recommendations. Terms often used interchangeably in secondary cancer prevention are *early detection* and *cancer screening*.

Tertiary cancer prevention: Efforts that are aimed at persons with a history of malignancy, including monitoring for and preventing recurrence and screening for second primary cancers. In many cases, those who have had a diagnosis of cancer and who carry a mutation in a cancer susceptibility gene are at significantly higher risk for a second malignancy.

Cancer screening test: A method or strategy used to detect a specific cancer. It may be a single modality but often is a combination of tests. Laboratory tests of blood or body fluids, imaging tests, physical examination, and invasive procedures are sometimes used for screening tests.

Cost-effectiveness: A financial indicator that is achieved if the costs of the screening program are less than the costs in the unscreened group.

Diagnostic tests: Tests used in those with symptoms of cancer or abnormal screening test results to determine their cause.

Effectiveness: A measure derived by comparing the outcomes to determine whether the benefits outweigh the risks and harms and the actual costs of the benefits.

False negative: A test result indicating that the tested person does not have a particular characteristic when he or she actually does have it (e.g., a negative mammogram result for a woman with early breast cancer).

Terms Used in Cancer Epidemiology—cont'd

False positive: A test result indicating that the tested person has a particular characteristic when he or she actually does not have it (e.g., a very suspicious mammogram result for a woman who does not have breast cancer).

Incidence: The number of cancers that develop in a population during a defined period, such as 1 year.

Mortality rate: The number of persons who die of a particular cancer during a defined period, such as 1 year.

Outcomes: Health and economic results that occur related to screening. Outcomes may include the benefits, harms, and costs of screening or genetic testing and its incurred diagnostic evaluations. They may be short or long term in nature.

Prevalence: The number of cancers that exist in a defined population at a given point in time.

Relative risk: A statistical estimate that compares the likelihood of development of a cancer in a person who has a specific risk factor with the likelihood in a person who does not have the specific risk factor.

Sensitivity: Ability of a screening test to detect individuals with the characteristic being screened for. It is calculated by dividing the total number of true positives by the total number of individuals in the population.

Specificity: Ability of a screening test to correctly identify patients without the characteristic being screened for. It is calculated by dividing the total number of true negatives by the total number of individuals in the population.

Target population: Number of persons in a defined group who are capable of developing the disease and are therefore appropriate candidates for screening. *Population* may refer to the general population or to a specific group of people defined by geographic, physical, or social characteristics. For example, nurses who provide cancer genetics counseling need to assess whether a person is of Ashkenazi Jewish background. This special population of Jewish people is at higher risk for three specific mutations associated with hereditary breast cancer (Zhong et al., 2015).

True negative: Test result indicating that the tested person does not have a particular characteristic when the person indeed does not have it (e.g., a negative mammogram result for a woman in whom cancer does not develop during the next 12 to 24 months).

True positive: Test result indicating that the tested person has a particular characteristic that the person indeed does have (e.g., a suspicious mammogram for a woman in whom a subsequent biopsy demonstrates a breast malignancy).

Validity: Degree to which a test measures what it is supposed to measure.

Estimated Incidence and Mortality Statistics for Selected Cancers, United States, 2015

New Cases Men	Deaths Men	New Cases Women	Deaths Women
Prostate: 220,800	Lung: 86,380	Breast (invasive): 231,840	Lung: 71,660
Lung: 115,610	Prostate: 27,540	Lung: 105,590	Breast (invasive): 40,290
Colorectal: 69,090	Colorectal: 26,100	Colorectal: 63,610	Colorectal: 23,600
Bladder: 56,320	Pancreas: 20,710	Uterus: 54,870	Pancreas: 19,850
Melanoma: 42,670	Liver: 17,030	Thyroid: 47,230	Ovary: 14,180
Non-Hodgkin lymphoma: 39,850	Leukemia: 14,210	Non-Hodgkin lymphoma: 32,000	Leukemia: 10,240
Kidney: 38,270	Esophagus: 12,600	Melanoma: 31,200	Uterus: 10,170
Oral cavity: 32,670	Bladder: 11,510	Pancreas: 24,120	Non-Hodgkin lymphoma: 8310
Leukemia: 30,900	Non-Hodgkin lymphoma: 11,480	Leukemia: 23,370	Liver: 7520
Liver: 25,510	Kidney: 9070	Kidney: 23,290	Brain and nervous system: 6380
All sites: 848,200	All sites: 312,150	All sites: 810,170	All sites: 277,280

Data from American Cancer Society. (2015). *Cancer facts & figures 2015*. Atlanta, GA: American Cancer Society.

Types of Epidemiology

Two types of epidemiology are often applied in cancer: descriptive epidemiology and analytic epidemiology.

Descriptive Epidemiology

Descriptive epidemiology provides information about the occurrence of disease in a population or its subgroups and trends in the frequency of disease over time. The information includes incidence and mortality rates and survival data. Sources of data include death certificates, cancer registries, surveys, and population censuses (Greenlee et al., 2010). Descriptive measures are useful for identifying populations and subgroups at high and low risk for a disease and for monitoring time trends for specific diseases. They can be especially helpful in understanding the natural history of rare tumors. They provide the leads for analytic studies designed to investigate factors responsible for the disease profiles. Several common descriptive terms are used in epidemiology.

Incidence. *Incidence* refers to the number of new cases of disease that occur during a specified period of time in a defined population at risk for the disease. Incidence rates also provide information about the risk of a disease or condition one has by virtue of being a member of a specified population. The ACS publishes projected incidence rates annually for common cancers in its annual *Cancer Facts & Figures* publication (ACS, 2015a). The table above provides examples of the incidence of the most commonly diagnosed cancers in the United States. The ACS estimated that about 1,658,370 new cases of cancer would occur in the United States in 2015 (ACS, 2015a).

Introduction

1

Mortality Rates. The table on page 2 shows the projected number of deaths from cancer in the United States in 2015. The *mortality rate* is the number of persons who die of a particular cancer during a specified period. The ACS (2015a) estimated that approximately 589,430 Americans would die of cancer during 2015. This translates to about 1620 deaths per day.

Many epidemiologists consider the incidence and mortality rates together when making public health decisions. For example, breast cancer affects 1 in 8 women (i.e., 231,840 new cases) and results in 40,730 deaths annually (ACS, 2015a). It accounts for 29% of new cases of cancer among women and 15% of deaths annually (ACS, 2013a). In comparison, ovarian cancer affects approximately 1 in 66 women (21,290 new cases) and results in 14,180 deaths annually (ACS, 2015a). It accounts for 3% of new cases of cancer among women but 5% of deaths annually. Examination of these figures suggests either that ovarian cancer is diagnosed at a later stage on average than breast cancer or that treatment is less effective, or both.

Age-Specific Rates. Age-specific rates provide valuable insight and information about how disease risks vary among groups and populations (see figure below). This often is extremely helpful when conveying information about risk to an individual. It also helps when considering recommendations for initiating screening. For example, the median age for developing breast cancer is 62 years of age. Approximately 90% of breast cancer cases are diagnosed after the age of 40, and this is a consideration in screening recommendations. For example, mammography is often recommended to begin at age 40 because most cases occur at this age or older (ACS, 2013a).

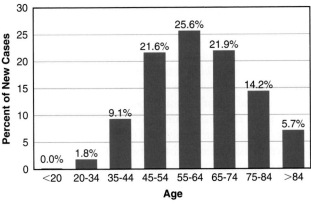

Percentage of New Cases of Breast Cancer over Selected Age Intervals. The percentage of new cases of breast cancer by age group demonstrates how the risk for breast cancer changes over time. (From SEER Stat Fact Sheets. [2014]. Female breast cancer. Available at http://seer.cancer.gov/statfacts/html/breast.html [accessed December 10, 2015]).

Prevalence. The *prevalence* of a disease or condition is the proportion of individuals in a specific population who have the disease or condition at a specific point or during a defined period of time. Prevalence includes both newly diagnosed and existing (i.e., previously diagnosed or current) cases of a particular disease. Cancer prevalence data provide information on the impact that cancer has on a population,

and they often have implications for the scope of cancer health services needed for a specific community or population. For example, in 2011, there were an estimated 2,899,726 women living with breast cancer in the United States (SEER Stat Fact Sheets, 2014). Breast cancer survivors often have an increased risk for osteoporosis due to chemotherapy, endocrine therapy, and premature menopause. Knowing that a large number of breast cancer survivors are at risk is useful for developing recommendations for screening and management to prevent long-term complications that may stem from osteoporosis (Kenyon, Mayer, & Owens, 2014).

Case-Fatality Rates. Cancer case-fatality rates are often an important indicator of the effectiveness of a particular cancer detection or treatment method and the impact of the cancer in a defined population. Cancer case-fatality rates provide information about the likelihood of dying from cancer among those diagnosed with the disease (Gordis, 2013). Case-fatality rates are different from mortality rates. The mortality rate represents an entire population at risk for cancer-related deaths and includes both those who do and those who do not have the cancer. Cancer case-fatality rates include only those who have the disease. For example, in a study of 562 women with ovarian cancer, the case-fatality rate was 13% for mucinous ovarian carcinoma and 62% for serous ovarian carcinoma (Seidman, Vang, Ronnett, Yemelyanova, & Cosin, 2015). Based on this information, the study authors recommended the development of new approaches to cancer prevention, detection, and treatment for serous carcinoma to ultimately decrease the mortality rate for ovarian cancer.

Risk Factor. A *risk factor* is a trait or characteristic that is associated with a statistically significant increased likelihood of developing a disease (Gordis, 2013). However, having a risk factor does not mean that a person will develop a disease or malignancy, nor does the absence of a risk factor mean that a person will not develop a disease or malignancy. Risk factors are becoming increasingly important because screening guidelines are often based on an individualized cancer risk assessment.

Absolute Risk. *Absolute risk* is a measure of the occurrence of cancer, in terms of incidence (i.e., new cases) or mortality rate (i.e., deaths), in the general population over a specific period of time. Absolute risk is helpful when a patient needs to understand what the chances are for all persons in a population having a particular disease. Absolute risk can be expressed as the number of cases for a specified denominator (e.g., 131 cases of breast cancer per 100,000 women annually) or as a cumulative risk up to a specified age (e.g., 1 in 8 women will develop breast cancer if they live to age 85 years) (ACS, 2013a). Another way to express absolute risk is to discuss the average risk of having breast cancer at a certain age. For example, 1 of every 43 women who are 50 years old will develop breast cancer by age 60. Another example is that a woman's risk of developing breast cancer may be 2% at age 50 years but 13% at age 85 years. Risk estimates are much different for a

50-year-old woman than for an 85-year-old woman because approximately 50% of the cases of breast cancer occur after the age of 61 years (see figure on pg. 3).

Certain assumptions are made to reach an absolute risk value for a particular cancer. For example, the 1-in-8 risk of breast cancer describes the average risk among white American women, and its calculation takes into consideration other causes of death over the life span. This figure overestimates breast cancer risk for some women with no risk factors and underestimates the risk for women with several risk factors.

The statistic means that the average woman's breast cancer risk is just 1.2% up to age 40 years, 3.7% from 40 to 60 years, 3.5% from age 60 to 69 years, and 3.9% from age 70 years on. The 12.3%, or 1-in-8, risk is obtained by adding the risk in each age category (1.2% + 3.7% + 3.5% + 3.9% = 12.3%). When a woman who has an average risk reaches age 40 years without a diagnosis of breast cancer, she has passed through 1.2% of her risk, so her lifetime risk is 12.3% − 1.2% = 11.1%. When she reaches age 70 years without a diagnosis of breast cancer, her risk is 12.3% − 1.2% − 3.7% − 3. 5% = 3.9%. Time must always be considered for the absolute risk figure to be meaningful. The 12.3% figure represents the lifetime risk of developing breast cancer (ACS, 2015b). Absolute risk is useful to help a patient understand how common a particular cancer is in the general population.

Relative Risk.   The term *relative risk* refers to a comparison of the incidence or mortality rate among those with a particular risk factor compared to those without the risk factor. By using relative risk factors, individuals can determine their risk factors and better understand their personal chances of developing a specific cancer compared to someone without the risk factors.

If the risk for a person who has no known risk factors for a disease is 1.0%, the risk for those with known risk factors can be evaluated in relation to this figure. This can be illustrated by considering several relative risk factors for breast cancer. A woman who has her first menstrual period before age 12 years has a 1.3% relative risk for development of breast cancer compared to a woman who has her first menstrual period after age 15 years (ACS, 2013a). For a woman with two first-degree relatives with premenopausal breast cancer, the relative risk is estimated to be 7.1% compared with a woman who has no relatives with premenopausal breast cancer. This means she is 7.1 times more likely to develop breast cancer than the woman without risk factors (Nelson et al., 2012). The table on this page provides examples of relative risk factors for the development of breast cancer.

Attributable Risk.   *Attributable risk* is the amount of disease within the population that could be prevented by alteration of a particular risk factor. Attributable risk has important implications for public health policy. More attention is being directed to assessment and management of attributable risk because it is a valuable means of primary cancer prevention.

A risk factor may be associated with a very large relative risk but be restricted to a few individuals; therefore, changing it would benefit only a small group. Conversely, some risk factors that can be altered may decrease the morbidity and mortality rates associated with malignancy in a large number of people. Smoking is a perfect example. The ACS estimates that 1 in 5 premature deaths (i.e., 443,000 deaths) in the United States each year can be attributed to smoking (ACS, 2013b). In 2015, almost 171,000 of the estimated 589,430 cancer deaths in the United States were forecast to be caused by tobacco use (ACS, 2015a). Altering this risk factor could significantly alter the morbidity and mortality associated with cancer in the future.

Odds Ratio.   The odds ratio is a measure of association that provides information similar to that found in relative risk calculations. *Odds ratios* are an estimate or measure of the chance of having a specific exposure (usually to an environmental agent) among those who have the disease compared to the chance among those who do not have the disease. It is most commonly used in cohort studies to address whether an association exists between the exposure and the disease (Gordis, 2013).

Analytic Epidemiology

Descriptive epidemiology helps to identify variations and trends in the distribution of cancer in a population. When analyzed, descriptive epidemiologic data provide information to formulate hypotheses about the health of a population. Analytic epidemiology provides strategies to test these hypotheses in an attempt to find the reasons or determinants that are associated with variations identified in descriptive epidemiology (Gordis, 2013). Analytic epidemiology strives to determine whether an association exists between a particular exposure or carcinogen and disease status.

Analytic epidemiologic studies can be observational or interventional in nature. Observational studies include cohort, case-control, and cross-sectional studies. Cohort studies

Relative Risk of Developing Breast Cancer

Risk Factors	Associated Relative Risk*
BRCA1 and BRCA2 or other inherited gene mutations	5-30
Two first-degree relatives diagnosed with breast cancer	3-7.1
Mother diagnosed before age 60	2-4
Mother diagnosed after age 60	1.5-2
High breast density	3-5
Atypical hyperplasia	4-5
Nulliparity	1.3-3
First pregnancy after age 30	1-3
First period before age 12	1.2-2.0
Last menstrual period after age 55	1.3
Drinking 2-4 drinks/day	1.2-1.4

*Adding relative risk scores does not give a total risk score.
Data from American Cancer Society. (2013a). *Breast cancer facts & figures 2013-2014*. Atlanta, GA: American Cancer Society; Amir, E., Freedman, O. C., Seruga, B., & Evans, D. G. (2010). Assessing women at high risk of breast cancer: A review of risk assessment models. *Journal of the National Cancer Institute, 102*(10), 680-691.

follow a group of people during a period of time. They can be retrospective or prospective in design. A case-control study is a retrospective study in which exposures and risk factors for persons with a disease are compared to those for persons who do not have the disease. In interventional studies, participants receive or do not receive a specific exposure (e.g., drug, treatment, lifestyle change), and changes in disease status are compared. Interventional studies are often referred to as clinical trials, and they may be randomized (randomly assigns participants into an experimental group or a control group) or blinded (the researchers but not the subjects know which subjects are receiving the active medication or treatment and which are not—i.e., single blinded—or neither the researchers nor the subjects know—i.e., double blinded).

Risk Assessment

A cancer risk assessment may include review of a person's medical history, history of exposures to carcinogens in daily living, and detailed family history. After the information is gathered, it must be interpreted for the patient in understandable terms. This often is accomplished by calculating absolute risk, relative risk, attributable risk, or specific risk values for various cancers.

Family History

A family history should focus on first- and second-degree relatives and should include at least three generations. It includes an assessment of both paternal and maternal sides of the family because many autosomal dominant syndromes can be passed through the father or the mother (Bennett, French, Resta, & Doyle, 2008). This lineage is typically displayed in a pedigree (see figure below).

First-degree relatives include parents, siblings, and children. Because first-degree relatives share 50% of their genes, these are the relatives most likely to inherit similar genetic

information. Information about second-degree relatives can also be helpful. Second-degree relatives include grandparents, aunts, and uncles.

Second-degree relatives have 25% of their genes in common. Older second-degree relatives can provide important information about genetic risk because an early-onset cancer would likely have manifested in the older person if a hereditary trait exists in the family. The pedigree should also include nieces and nephews because younger family members can provide information about childhood cancers that also has implications for the genetic risk assessment.

Third-degree relatives (i.e., cousins, great-aunts, great-uncles, and great grandparents) can be included in the family history, although reports about these relatives are not always accurate. Third-degree relatives share 12.5% of the same genes.

Ethnicity should be recorded. Some ethnicities are associated with an increased risk of malignancies. For example, persons of Ashkenazi Jewish ancestry have an increased risk for developing breast cancer (Stadler et al., 2010).

After all information is documented, it should be stored in a standard pedigree format (see figure on this page). The pedigree can be helpful in families with multiple cases of malignancy to help teach concepts of genetics, clarify relationships, provide a quick reference, and calculate the risk of having a cancer-causing mutation. The availability of software to generate these pedigrees has made updating the information simple.

The family history provides an organized way to document data such as whether a relative is alive or dead, age at death if applicable, significant medical diagnoses, and diagnosis of cancer. Space can be provided to describe in detail the specific type of cancer, age at diagnosis, and other characteristics (e.g., whether a breast cancer was premenopausal or bilateral). Specific information may influence recommendations for screening. Obtaining a detailed family history is useful for cancer risk assessment and is the first step in identifying families with a possible hereditary predisposition to malignancy and other illnesses. Health care providers should ask patients about specific relatives and their health individually rather than asking a general question such as, "Have any of your relatives been diagnosed with cancer?"

After gathering the family history, it is important to recheck whether any of the patient's relatives have been diagnosed with any type of cancer. Patients often forget to provide these details, and reiterating the question can prompt recall of valuable information. Those who have multiple family members diagnosed with cancer, especially at a younger age, should be referred to a health care provider with expertise in genetics, such as a board-certified physician in genetics, a master's-prepared genetic counselor, or a nurse with an Advance Practice Nurse in Genetics (APNG) credential. Genetics professionals assess genetic risk, provide counseling before and after genetic testing, and follow up to ensure that all at-risk family members are informed about their potential increased risk of developing cancer. Patients and family members can be offered the option of undergoing genetic testing to better clarify their risk.

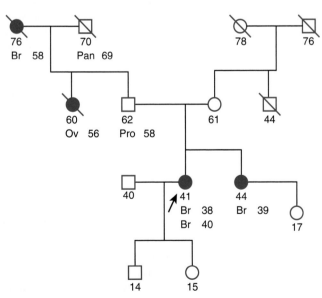

Pedigree. In a typical pedigree constructed to evaluate hereditary risk factors, the *squares* represent males and *circles* represent females. The *arrow* represents the proband or spokesperson for the family. *Slashes* represent deceased persons. *Solid circles* and *squares* represent persons with cancer. The age and anatomic site of diagnosis is recorded.

Genetic testing for hereditary cancer syndromes is an important component of cancer risk assessment. In persons with a documented hereditary cancer syndrome, the risk of cancer can be substantially increased. For example, a woman with a known mutation in the *BRCA1* gene has an estimated 90% lifetime chance of developing breast cancer and an estimated 50% lifetime risk of developing ovarian cancer. She may want to consider primary prevention measures to better manage her risk. Identification of persons with a suspected or known hereditary risk factor often results in substantial change in cancer prevention and early detection recommendations.

Medical History and Lifestyle Factors

Assessment of medical history and personal lifestyle factors that may increase the risk of cancer should be documented. The inventory can include information such as menstrual history, hormonal exposures, and exposure to carcinogens such as ultraviolet light or tobacco. Many risk factors are not within an individual's control (e.g., age at menarche) and are not amenable to primary prevention efforts. Some lifestyle factors are within the control of the individual and can be affected by providing education about primary prevention efforts.

After all risk data are collected, the clinician must assimilate the risk factors and provide information to the patient about their effect on each of the major cancers. For example, early menarche, nulliparity, and late menopause are risk factors for breast and endometrial cancer (ACS, 2015a). Communication of risk should include a discussion about the presence of these risk factors and the risk of developing both cancers. Risk can be communicated to patients in several different formats. Often it is best to explain the implications of a patent's medical history and lifestyle in terms of absolute risk, relative risk, and attributable risk.

For some cancers, it is possible to combine risk factors in well-tested models to calculate the risk of developing cancer at a specific age or over a lifetime. This is often done for breast cancer, colon cancer, and malignant melanoma.

The Gail model is an interactive tool designed by scientists at the National Cancer Institute and at the National Surgical Adjuvant Breast and Bowel Project to estimate a woman's risk of developing invasive breast cancer (Parmigiani et al., 2007). The risk factors used were age at menarche, age at first live birth, number of previous breast biopsies, and number of first-degree relatives with breast cancer. This model of relative risks for various combinations of these factors was developed with the use of case-control data from the Breast Cancer Detection Demonstration Project (Amir, 2010).

The Gail model estimates breast cancer risk and is most effectively used for women with a limited to moderate family history of breast cancer. It is often used to determine whether the patient should be enrolled in a chemoprevention trial or have breast magnetic resonance imaging (MRI). The Gail model is readily available for use on computers, and it is inexpensive and easy to use. However, it does not consider individuals on the paternal side of family with a diagnosis of breast or ovarian cancer, and it does not consider second-degree relatives with a diagnosis of breast or ovarian cancer. It has not been used extensively for many ethnic minorities, and this lack of data may limit its usefulness. It significantly underestimates risk in persons with a known genetic mutation.

The breast cancer risk assessment tool is available (http://www.cancer.gov/bcrisktool). Risk assessment tools are also available for colorectal cancer (http://www.cancer.gov/colorectalcancerrisk) and for melanoma (http://www.cancer.gov/melanomarisktool) (Fears et al., 2006; Park et al., 2009).

Oncology nurses can use these models to help individuals put their risk in perspective. The clinician is responsible for using the model that most accurately reflects the person's risk factors and for helping the individual to understand the strengths and limitations of the model in calculating risk and quickly stratifying risk to determine whether screening measures need to be modified.

Levels of Cancer Prevention

There are three levels of cancer prevention. *Primary prevention* refers to evading disease by methods such as immunization against childhood diseases, avoiding tobacco products, or reducing exposure to ultraviolet rays. Primary prevention measures can reduce the risk of cancer but do not guarantee that a person will not develop a malignancy. Primary prevention measures include adopting a healthier lifestyle, using chemoprevention (e.g., tamoxifen to prevent breast cancer), and undergoing prophylactic surgery if there is a genetic susceptibility to cancer (e.g., bilateral mastectomies in a woman without a diagnosis of breast cancer who has a known mutation in the *BRCA1* or *BRCA2* gene).

More attention is being directed to primary prevention by reducing attributable risk. In addition to eliminating tobacco use to reduce smoking-related deaths, efforts are being targeted at human papillomavirus (HPV) vaccination, reduction of exposure to ultraviolet light, improved nutrition, and increased physical activity (ACS, 2013b). One third of the more than 572,000 cancer deaths that occur annually can be attributed to the effects of diet and physical activity habits, including overweight and obesity, and another one third are caused by exposure to tobacco products (Kushi et al., 2012).

Secondary prevention refers to the early detection and treatment of subclinical, asymptomatic, or early disease in persons without signs or symptoms of cancer. Forms of secondary cancer prevention include the use of a Papanicolaou (Pap) smear to detect cervical cancer, a mammogram to detect a nonpalpable breast cancer, and colonoscopy to remove polyps and detect early colon cancers. Cancer screening is aimed at asymptomatic persons with the goal of finding disease when it is most easily treated.

Screening tests seek to decrease the morbidity and mortality associated with cancer. After a positive screening test result, further diagnostic testing is required to determine whether a malignancy exists. This is the traditional definition of cancer screening. Some also consider screening for genetic or molecular markers that put the individual at high risk for cancer as a specialized form of cancer screening.

Tertiary prevention refers to management of an illness such as cancer to prevent progression, recurrence, or other complications. In cancer care, examples of tertiary prevention include monitoring for early signs of recurrence by measuring levels of tumor markers or detecting second primary malignancies early in long-term survivors. An estimated 14.5 million persons are alive with a diagnosis of cancer (ACS, 2015a). Because of this ever-growing population, there has been push to develop cancer survivor care plans that include a component of tertiary prevention (Belansky & Mahon, 2012; Ligibel & Denlinger, 2013).

Accuracy of Screening Tests

In addition to communicating about cancer risks with patients, nurses must explain the accuracy of screening tests. It is not enough to recommend a screening test. Patients need to understand what the possibilities are regarding a truly positive or a truly negative test result.

Individuals often inquire about recommendations for a specific cancer screening test such as a mammogram or a Pap smear. Specific recommendations often vary among organizations such as the ACS, the United States Preventive Services Task Force (USPSTF), the National Comprehensive Cancer Network (NCCN), and the National Cancer Institute (NCI) (ACS, 2015a; NCCN, 2014a, 2014b, 2014c, 2015; USPSTF, 2014). These recommendations are readily available for comparison at www.guidelines.gov.

The specific criteria used by these organizations to make recommendations vary, which is why the recommendations are not universal and are very confusing for the general public. However, some requirements and characteristics of acceptable screening tests have consensus. When screening recommendations are presented, it is important to include the rationale, strengths, and limitations of the test and to present this information in light of the individual's risk of developing cancer (see box below).

Considerations for Cancer Screening Tests

- The disease should be an important health problem. There is little doubt that cancer is a significant health problem, but some types of cancers are more significant health problems than other types. For example, the estimated incidence of breast cancer is 231,840 new cases annually, and that of lung cancer is 221,200 new cases, making both cancers highly significant (Siegel, Miller, & Jemal, 2015). The mortality rate associated with these cancers is also high, with an estimated 40,290 deaths annually from breast cancer and an estimated 162,460 deaths annually from lung cancer.
- The disease should have a preclinical stage before symptoms become obvious. In breast cancer, mammography can detect the cancer before it is palpable. Although lung cancer has a high incidence, only 15% of lung cancers are diagnosed at a localized stage, for which the 5-year survival rate is 54% (ACS, 2015a).
- The disease should be treatable, and there should be a recognized treatment for lesions identified after screening. Breast cancer is clearly a disease that responds to surgery, chemotherapy, and radiation therapy, especially when it is detected early (ACS, 2013a). More importantly, when breast cancer is detected early, it can often be treated with less radical surgery, such as lumpectomy. The same is not true of lung cancer.
- The test must be clinically relevant. The test must be able to detect a condition for which intervention at a preclinical stage can improve outcome.
- The test must be accurate. The sensitivity and specificity must be acceptable.
- The test must be cost-effective.
- The test must be acceptable to individuals being screened. Highly invasive, painful, or risky procedures usually are unacceptable. The test must be widely available and easily accessible. Most women are willing to tolerate the discomfort and risks associated with mammography. Approximately 20% of individuals undergoing low-dose computed tomography screening for lung cancer had positive results requiring some degree of follow-up, including biopsy; only approximately 1% had lung cancer (Bach et al., 2012).

The accuracy of screening tests is described by several terms. A true-positive (TP) test result is anormal test result for cancer in an individual who actually has the disease. A true-negative (TN) test result is a normal or negative screening result for cancer in an individual who is subsequently found not to have the disease within a defined period after the last test. A false-negative (FN) test result is a normal test result for cancer in an individual who in fact has the cancer. A false-positive (FP) test result is an abnormal test result for cancer screening in an individual who does not have the disease.

Sensitivity

An understanding of true and false test results is necessary to calculate information about sensitivity and specificity. The sensitivity of a screening test is its ability to detect those individuals who have cancer. It is calculated by taking the number of TP results and dividing it by the total number of cancer cases (i.e., TP and FN cases). For example, a screening test given to 1000 persons resulting in 85 TPs and 15 FNs has a sensitivity of 0.85. This is calculated as $85/(85 + 15) = 0.85$. Most people are unwilling to accept a test with a high FN rate because many cancers will be missed.

Specificity

The specificity of a test is its ability to identify those individuals who do not have cancer. It is calculated by dividing the TN by the sum of the total number of individuals in the population who do not have cancer (i.e., TN and FP cases). For example, if a test is given to 1000 persons and there are 775 TNs and 225 FPs, the specificity is 0.78, which is calculated as $775/(775 + 225) = 0.78$. A high FP test rate can result in unnecessary follow-up testing and anxiety in persons who have a positive screening result.

Positive and Negative Predictive Values

The *positive predictive value* is the measure of the validity of a positive test. It is the proportion of positive tests that are TP cases. The predictive value of a test depends on the disease prevalence. As the prevalence of a cancer increases in the population, the positive predictive value of the screening tests increases, although its sensitivity and specificity remain unchanged.

The *negative predictive value* is the measure of the validity of a negative test. This refers to the proportion of negative tests that are TNs.

Bias

Bias affects screening tests. *Selection bias* occurs during clinical trials that evaluate the effectiveness of screening tests. Ideally, those screened should be similar to those not screened to determine the effectiveness of the tests. This problem is minimized with randomization. *Lead-time bias* refers to the bias that arises by adding the time gained as a result of early diagnosis to survival time. *Length bias* occurs because of the preferential diagnosis of more indolent cases of cancer through screening. This may be especially true with in situ cancers that never become a health threat (e.g., identification of early prostate cancers that may never progress enough to cause morbidity or mortality). There is a lack of consensus regarding the utility of prostate cancer screening (ACS, 2015a). Because of length bias, persons may have indolent cancers that are diagnosed early but take years to progress, resulting in the appearance of longer survival times. *Overdiagnosis bias* occurs with excess screening. FP rates and overzealous screeners may inflate the detection and diagnosis of early-stage cancers.

Outcomes

Outcomes of cancer screening are considered in epidemiologic studies. If there are no differences in outcome, particularly with respect to morbidity and mortality rates, it is often inappropriate to offer a screening maneuver. Similarly, some agencies consider cost-benefit analyses to determine purely on a financial basis whether years of life are saved and costs of treatment are reduced with early detection of cancer through a screening test. Quality of life can be another significant outcome.

Selection of a Screening Test

Understanding these principles is necessary to help patients comprehend the strengths and limitations of the test they are using to screen for a particular cancer. The perfect screening test does not exist. For example, screening mammograms, overall, miss about one in five breast cancers (ACS, 2015a). Other considerations drive screening recommendations. The cancer being screened for should have a high prevalence and incidence, significant mortality and morbidity rates and cost, and a hope for effective treatment if detected early.

Many individuals still choose to undergo a screening examination despite a lower sensitivity and specificity in the hope that it will be effective for them. Screening for ovarian cancer is an excellent example. Highly specific and sensitive screening tests are unavailable for the early detection of ovarian cancer. Many women, however, still want an annual pelvic examination to assess for ovarian masses. The test is relatively inexpensive to perform and is usually well tolerated. Some clinicians are better at detecting ovarian masses than others, but many ovarian cancers cannot be detected by this examination, even when it is performed by a skilled clinician. As long as a woman realizes the test may fail to detect ovarian cancer and is willing to accept this limitation, the pelvic examination may be considered to be effective by some.

Some steps can be taken by health care providers to improve the accuracy of screening tests. The establishment of certification and federal guidelines in the areas of radiology and laboratory services is an example. Guidelines are in place for mammography centers and laboratories providing cancer screening services to ensure that a minimum acceptable standard is met so that the screen is as accurate as possible.

The person conducting the examination or interpreting the laboratory or radiologic test result also affects the effectiveness of a cancer screening test. For example, some health care professionals are better at performing clinical examinations than others and are more likely to detect a subtle physical change. Monitoring the quality of clinical examinations is important. Monitoring and improving the quality of physical examinations in the clinical setting are far more challenging but important to improve the sensitivity and specificity of the examination.

Screening quality may be improved by developing standardized instructions for patient preparation. This may improve patient compliance and help obtain the best possible screening data. Examples include scheduling a breast screening 1 week after the menses begin, avoiding the use of deodorant before mammography, and instructing a patient to avoid douching for 24 hours before a Pap smear.

Cancer Screening Recommendations

A screening protocol or recommendation defines how cancer screening tests should be used. The table on page 9 illustrates the ACS recommendations for early detection of cancer in asymptomatic individuals. Screening protocols can vary among organizations and practitioners. A protocol usually describes the target population being served, the screening recommendation to be applied, and the interval at which the test should be applied.

Screening guidelines change over time. The ACS has been publishing guidelines for early cancer detection for more than 20 years (Brawley et al., 2011). Although the specific recommendations have changed over the years, the focus of the guidelines has changed very little. They mandate that health care providers use the guidelines to select the best screening tests for an individual of average risk and that modifications be made in some cases (e.g., for an individual who has a particularly high risk for a specific malignancy). For example, a woman with a known hereditary predisposition gene for hereditary nonpolyposis colorectal cancer (HNPCC) should begin having an annual colonoscopy at 25 years of age instead of following the population recommendation for a colonoscopy every 7 to 10 years beginning at 50 years of age. Her risk for development of colorectal cancer approaches 85% over a lifetime, and in individuals with this genetic mutation colon cancer develops in as little as 12 to 18 months after the development of a polyp. Polyps increase the risk of colorectal cancer in patients with HNPCC by at least 25% by age 50 years and up to 82% by age 70 years. Aggressive screening is imperative to decrease the morbidity and mortality rates associated with the disease (Kohlmann & Gruber, 2012). Similarly, the ACS recommends breast MRI in addition to mammography for any woman whose estimated lifetime risk of breast cancer is greater than 20% (ACS, 2013a).

Clinicians must remember that screening protocols are guidelines and that the recommendations vary across agencies (see table on page 9). Screening recommendations are not practice standards to be used with every individual. The goal of the ACS and NCCN standards is the detection of malignancy. The USPSTF uses very strict criteria for evidence of effectiveness. Cost-effectiveness of the screening recommendations is an important consideration for this group. When providing information on cancer screening recommendations, nurses need to inform the individual why a certain recommendation is being selected.

Comparison of Screening Guidelines for the Early Detection of Cancer in Asymptomatic People

Target Organ	American Cancer Society	United States Preventive Task Force	National Comprehensive Cancer Network
Breast	Women who choose not to do BSE regularly (monthly) or irregularly. Beginning in their early 20s, women should be told about the benefits and limitations of BSE. The importance of prompt reporting of new breast symptoms to a health professional should be emphasized (i.e., breast awareness). Women 20-39 yr of age should have a CBE at least every 3 yr and then CBE annually beginning at age 40 yr. Annual mammography to begin at age 40 yr. Women with a lifetime risk >20% should consider adding breast MRI.	Individualized decision to begin biennial mammography screening according to the patient's circumstances and values. Mammography screening is recommended for women every 2 yrs for ages 50-74.	For ages 20-39, breast awareness and CBE every 1 to 3 yr For ages 40+, annual CBE, breast awareness, and annual mammography Women with a lifetime risk >20% can consider breast MRI.
Cervix	For women ages 21-29, screening should be done every 3 yr with conventional or liquid-based Pap tests. For women ages 30-65, screening should be done every 5 yr with both the HPV test and the Pap test (preferred) or every 3 yr with the Pap test alone (acceptable). Women ages 65+ who have had ≥3 consecutive negative Pap tests or ≥2 consecutive negative HPV and Pap tests within the past 10 yr, with the most recent test occurring within the past 5 yr, and women who have had a total hysterectomy should stop cervical cancer screening.	Women ages 21-65 yr should be screened with cytology (Pap smear) every 3 yr. Women ages 30-65 yr can be screened with cytology every 3 yr or co-tested (cytology + HPV testing) every 5 yr. Women 65+ yr should not be screened	Same as American Cancer Society recommendations
Colon	FOBT with at least 50% test sensitivity for cancer, or FIT with at least 50% test sensitivity for cancer annually *or* Stool DNA test every 3 yr starting at age 50 yr *or* Flexible sigmoidoscopy every 5 yr, starting at age 50 yr performed alone or combined with FOBT or FIT annually *or* Double-contrast barium enema every 5 yr starting at age 50 yr *or* Colonoscopy every 10 yr starting at age 50 yr *or* CT colonography every 5 yr starting at age 50 yr	Adults age 50-75 yr can be screened with high-sensitivity FOBT annually, flexible sigmoidoscopy every 5 yr, or colonoscopy every 10 yr.	Colonoscopy every 10 yr *or* Annual FOBT or FIT *or* Flexible sigmoidoscopy with or without FOBT or FIT every 5 yr
Lung	Current or former smokers ages 55-74 and in good health with at least a 30 pack-year history can consider LDCT. This is not a substitute for smoking cessation.	Asymptomatic adults ages 55-80 who have a 30 pack-year smoking history and currently smoke or have quit smoking within the past 15 yr should screen annually with LDCT. Discontinue screening when the patient has not smoked for 15 yr.	Age 55-74 and >30 pack-year history with smoking cessation of <15 years, or age 50+ yr with a >20 pack-year history and one other risk factor other than secondhand smoke, annual LDCT every 2 yrs until the patient can no longer tolerate definitive treatment
Prostate	Men ages 50+ can consider DRE and PSA if they have at least a 10-yr life expectancy and have been fully informed of the risks and benefits.	Recommend against PSA screening for prostate cancer	For ages 50+, DRE and PSA every 1-2 yr

BSE, Breast self-examination; *CBE*, clinical breast examination; *CT*, computed tomography; *DRE*, digital rectal examination; *FIT*: fecal immunochemical test; *FOBT*, fecal occult blood test; *HPV*, human papillomavirus; *LDCT*, low-dose helical computed tomography; *MRI*, magnetic resonance imaging; *Pap*, Papanicolaou smear; *PSA*, prostate-specific antigen test.
Modified from American Cancer Society. (2015). *Cancer facts & figures 2015*. Atlanta, GA: American Cancer Society; National Comprehensive Cancer Network. (2015). *Lung cancer screening version 1.2015*. Available at http://www.cancer.org/acs/groups/content/@editorial/documents/document/acspc-044552.pdf (accessed from cancer.org on 1/11/2016); and United States Preventive Services Task Force (May 2014). *The guide to clinical preventive services 2014: Recommendations of the U.S. Preventive Services Task Force*. Rockville, MD: Agency for Healthcare Research and Quality. Available at http://www.ncbi.nlm.nih.gov/books/NBK235846 (accessed December 10, 2015).

Means to Express Cancer Prognosis and Outcomes

Patient survival is a primary means of assessing the effectiveness of screening tests and treatment. Because patients usually have had cancer for different lengths of time, survival rates are often expressed separately by stage. The figure on page 10 shows an example of relative survival rates by stage at diagnosis for breast cancer.

Percent of Cases by Stage

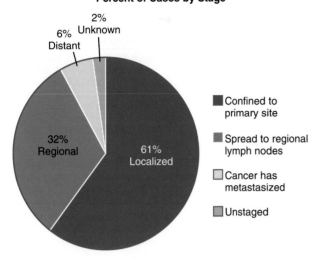

5-Year Relative Survival

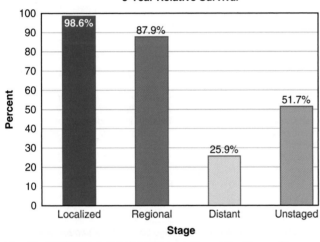

Five-Year Relative Survival for Breast Cancer by Stage. Five-year survival rates for persons with breast cancer by stage at diagnosis. (From SEER Stat Fact Sheets. Female breast cancer. Available at http://seer.cancer.gov/statfacts/html/breast.html [accessed December 10, 2015]).

a specific cancer relative to the survival rate that is expected for people of similar age, race, and sex in the general population during the same period of observation (see figure below).

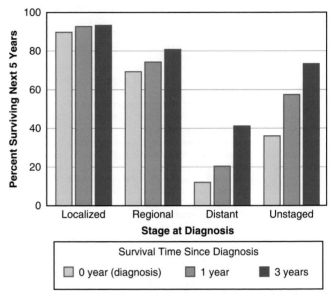

Five-Year Relative Survival for Colorectal Cancer by Stage. The graph represents the percentage of patients with a colorectal cancer who are alive 5 years after their disease is diagnosed. (From SEER Stat Fact Sheets. Colon and rectum cancer. Available at http://seer.cancer.gov/statfacts/html/colorect.html [accessed December 10, 2015]).

The 5-year survival rate represents the proportion of patients who did not experience a defined event (usually death) during the first 5 years after diagnosis. Selection of the 5-year mark is arbitrary (Siegel, Miller, & Jemal, 2015). Because a significant number of persons historically die during the first 5 years after diagnosis, health care providers use this period as an indicator of successful treatment and management of the disease.

Ethnic Differences

Knowledge of the overall trends in cancer incidence and mortality rates, particularly among individuals in certain age groups and racial or ethnic groups, can help oncology nurses identify populations at risk. These groups may require specialized prevention or early detection programs. If they live in identifiable communities, efforts can be made to provide more targeted prevention and early detection intervention strategies that are culturally acceptable.

Data on the differences in stage at diagnosis, prognosis, incidence, and mortality rates are readily available from the SEER program and from the ACS. The figures on page 11 illustrate differences in mortality rates and incidence among several ethnic groups. This information can be particularly helpful when screening programs that target populations at risk are developed.

The difference between living 6 months and living 10 years after diagnosis is important to patients and health care providers. Length of survival is often a function of disease stage at diagnosis, clinical characteristics of the disease, comorbidities, and treatments used to manage the disease.

The *observed survival rate*, which is also known as the *overall survival rate*, is a measure of the proportion of patients who survive all causes of death after a cancer diagnosis for a defined period of study. The cause- or disease-specific survival rate is a measure of the proportion of persons who do not die of the specific disease under study, such as cancer, during a defined period.

The *relative survival rate* is a ratio of the observed survival rate and the expected survival rate for a patient cohort. It is the observed survival rate for individuals with

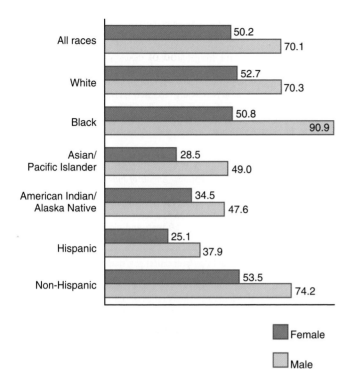

Number of New Cases of Lung Cancer per 100,000 Persons by Race or Ethnicity and Sex. The graph shows the distribution of lung cancer cases by race and ethnicity for men and women. (From SEER Stat Fact Sheets. *Lung and bronchus cancer.* Available at http://seer.cancer.gov/statfacts/html/lungb.html [accessed December 10, 2015]).

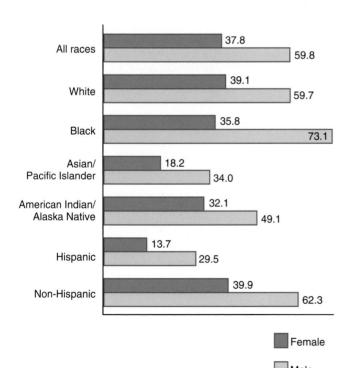

Number of Lung Cancer Deaths per 100,000 Persons by Race or Ethnicity and Sex. The graph shows the distribution of lung cancer deaths by race and ethnicity for men and women. (From SEER Stat Fact Sheets. *Lung and bronchus cancer.* Available at http://seer.cancer.gov/statfacts/html/lungb.html [accessed December 10, 2015]).

Epidemiology Resources

Each year, the ACS publishes *Cancer Facts and Figures*. It is an invaluable resource nurses can use to quickly gather estimated incidence data about cancer cases. The information is presented in several different formats, including the estimated projected number of new cases of specific cancers (i.e., incidence) and estimated mortality rates. The incidence rates are also given by state. Oncology nurses can obtain this publication free of charge from the local unit of the ACS or online (www.cancer.org) and may find it helpful to better understand the incidence of specific cancers in the geographic areas of the country in which they practice. The publication also offers detailed information about primary and secondary cancer prevention of major tumors and projected survival data by stage.

Similar resources are available for specific cancers such as breast or colon cancer, for which detailed information is provided (ACS, 2013a, 2014). Other resources detail cancer risks for specific racial or ethnic groups (ACS, 2012, 2013c). Resources are also available for prevention statistics and global cancer statistics (ACS, 2011, 2013b).

Another source of commonly cited data is the SEER program. Data have been collected by the SEER program for incidence, mortality rates, and survival rates from 1973 through 2011 (Mariotto et al., 2014). Data from the SEER geographic areas are used to represent an estimated 26% of the U.S. population. The database contains information on 8.2 million cases diagnosed since 1973. Approximately 250,000 new cases are added yearly. This information can be obtained easily at the National Cancer Institute's Web site (http://seer.cancer.gov).

Conclusion

Knowledge and integration of epidemiologic concepts are essential in oncology nursing practice. The concepts have implications for risk assessment, prevention recommendations, screening strategies, and monitoring of therapeutic effectiveness.

Epidemiologic data are presented in numerous formats. Nurses can use this information when educating patients, devising screening or prevention programs, conducting clinical research, and monitoring the effectiveness of therapy.

References

American Cancer Society. (2011). *Global cancer facts & figures* (2nd ed.). Atlanta, GA: American Cancer Society.

American Cancer Society. (2012). *Cancer facts & figures for Hispanics/Latinos 2012-2014.* Atlanta, GA: American Cancer Society.

American Cancer Society. (2013a). *Breast cancer facts & figures 2013-2014.* Atlanta, GA: American Cancer Society.

American Cancer Society. (2013b). *Cancer prevention and early detection facts & figures 2013.* Atlanta, GA: American Cancer Society.

American Cancer Society. (2013c). *Cancer facts & figures for African Americans 2013-2014.* Atlanta, GA: American Cancer Society.

American Cancer Society. (2014). *Colorectal cancer facts & figures 2014-2015.* Atlanta, GA: American Cancer Society.

American Cancer Society. (2015a). *Cancer facts & figures 2015.* Atlanta, GA: American Cancer Society.

American Cancer Society. (2015b). *Breast Cancer Facts & Figures 2015-2016*. Atlanta, GA: American Cancer Society.

Amir, E., Freedman, O. C., Seruga, B., & Evans, D. G. (2010). Assessing women at high risk of breast cancer: A review of risk assessment models. *Journal of the National Cancer Institute, 102*(10), 680–691.

Bach, P. B., Mirkin, J. N., Oliver, T. K., Azzoli, C. G., Berry, D., Brawley, O. W., & Detterbeck, F. C. (2012). Benefits and harms of CT screening for lung cancer: A systematic review. *JAMA: Journal of the American Medical Association, 307*(22), 2418–2429.

Belansky, H., & Mahon, S. M. (2012). Using care plans to enhance care throughout the cancer survivorship trajectory. *Clinical Journal of Oncology Nursing, 16*(1), 90–92.

Bennett, R., French, K., Resta, R., & Doyle, D. (2008). Standardized human pedigree nomenclature: Update and assessment of the recommendations of the National Society of Genetic Counselors. *Journal of Genetic Counseling, 17*(5), 424–433.

Brawley, O., Byers, T., Chen, A., Pignone, M., Ransohoff, D., Schenk, M., & Wender, R. (2011). New American Cancer Society process for creating trustworthy cancer screening guidelines. *JAMA: Journal of the American Medical Association, 306*(22), 2495–2499.

Fears, T. R., Guerry, D., Pfeiffer, R. M., Sagebiel, R. W., Elder, D. E., Halpern, A., & Tucker, M. A. (2006). Identifying individuals at high risk of melanoma: A practical predictor of absolute risk. *Journal of Clinical Oncology, 24*(22), 3590–3596.

Gordis, L. (2013). *Epidemiology* (5th ed.). Philadelphia: W. B. Saunders.

Greenlee, R. T., Goodman, M. T., Lynch, C. F., Platz, C. E., Havener, L. A., & Howe, H. L. (2010). The occurrence of rare cancers in U.S. adults, 1995-2004. *Public Health Reports, 125*(1), 28–43.

Kenyon, M., Mayer, D. K., & Owens, A. K. (2014). Late and long-term effects of breast cancer treatment and surveillance management for the general practitioner. *Journal of Obstetric, Gynecologic, & Neonatal Nursing, 43*(3), 382–398.

Kohlmann, W., & Gruber, S. B. (2012). *Lynch syndrome gene reviews*. Seattle, WA: University of Washington. Available at http://www.ncbi.nlm.nih.gov/books/NBK1211 (accessed December 10, 2015).

Kushi, L. H., Doyle, C., McCullough, M., Rock, C. L., Demark-Wahnefried, W., Bandera, E. V., & Physical Activity Guidelines Advisory Committee. (2012). American Cancer Society guidelines on nutrition and physical activity for cancer prevention. *CA: A Cancer Journal for Clinicians, 62*(1), 30–67.

Ligibel, J. A., & Denlinger, C. S. (2013). New NCCN guidelines® for survivorship care. *Journal of the National Comprehensive Cancer Network, 11*(5S), 640–644.

Mariotto, A. B., Noone, A. M., Howlader, N., Cho, H., Keel, G. E., Garshell, J., & Schwartz, L. M. (2014). Cancer survival: an overview of measures, uses, and interpretation. *JNCI Monographs, 2014*(49), 145–186.

National Comprehensive Cancer Network. (2014a). *Breast cancer screening and diagnosis version 1.2014*. Available at NCCN.org (accessed 1/11/2016).

National Comprehensive Cancer Network. (2014b). *Colorectal cancer screening version 1/2014*. Available at NCCN.org (accessed 1/11/2016).

National Comprehensive Cancer Network. (2014c). *Prostate cancer early detection version 1.2014*. Available at http://www.nccn.org/professionals/physician_gls/pdf/prostate.pdf (accessed December 10, 2015).

National Comprehensive Cancer Network. (2015). *Lung cancer screening version 1.2015*. Available at NCCN.org (accessed 1/11/2016).

Nelson, H. D., Zakher, B., Cantor, A., Fu, R., Griffin, J., O'Meara, E. S., & Miglioretti, D. L. (2012). Risk factors for breast cancer for women aged 40 to 49 years: A systematic review and meta-analysis. *Annals of Internal Medicine, 156*(9), 635–648.

Parmigiani, G., Chen, S., Iversen, J. E. S., Friebel, T. M., Finkelstein, D. M., Anton-Culver, H., & Euhus, D. M. (2007). Validity of models for predicting BRCA1 and BRCA2 mutations. *Annals of Internal Medicine, 147*(7), 441–450.

Park, Y., Freedman, A. N., Gail, M. H., Pee, D., Hollenbeck, A., Schatzkin, A., & Pfeiffer, R. M. (2009). Validation of a colorectal cancer risk prediction model among white patients age 50 years and older. *Journal of Clinical Oncology, 27*(5), 694–698.

SEER Stat Fact Sheets. (2014). *Surveillance research program*. National Cancer Institute. Available at http://seer.cancer.gov/statfacts/html/breast.html (accessed December 10, 2015).

Seidman, J. D., Vang, R., Ronnett, B. M., Yemelyanova, A., & Cosin, J. A. (2015). Distribution and case-fatality ratios by cell-type for ovarian carcinomas: A 22-year series of 562 patients with uniform current histological classification. *Gynecologic Oncology, 136*(2), 336–340.

Siegel, R. L., Miller, K. D., & Jemal, A. (2015). Cancer statistics, 2015. *CA: A Cancer Journal for Clinicians, 65*(1), 5–29.

Stadler, Z., Saloustros, E., Hansen, N. L., Schluger, A., Kauff, N., Offit, K., & Robson, M. (2010). Absence of genomic BRCA1 and BRCA2 rearrangements in Ashkenazi breast and ovarian cancer families. *Breast Cancer Research and Treatment, 123*(2), 581–585.

United States Preventive Services Task Force. (May 2014). *The guide to clinical preventive services 2014: Recommendations of the U.S. Preventive Services Task Force*. Rockville, MD: Agency for Healthcare Research and Quality. Available at http://www.ncbi.nlm.nih.gov/books/NBK235846 (accessed December 10, 2015).

Zhong, Q., Peng, H.-L., Zhao, X., Zhang, L., & Hwang, W.-T. (2015). Effects of *BRCA1*- and *BRCA2*-related mutations on ovarian and breast cancer survival: A meta-analysis. *Clinical Cancer Research: An Official Journal of the American Association for Cancer Research, 21*(1), 211–220. http://doi.org/10.1158/1078-0432.CCR-14-1816.

Cancer Pathophysiology

Carolee Polek

Cancer is a genetic disease in which the regulation, characteristics, and functions of normal cells are altered. Genes provide the instructions for making proteins and regulate their production. Proteins perform many functions essential for normal cellular operation. Deoxyribonucleic acid (DNA) encodes the amino acids used to form proteins. DNA mutations alter protein synthesis, allowing transformed cells to gain a selection advantage over normal cells and grow uncontrollably. Malignant transformation is influenced by oncogenes, growth factor overexpression, defective intracellular signal transducers, cell membrane changes, and other factors.

The development of cancer (i.e., carcinogenesis) is a multistep process governed by a series of genetic and epigenetic changes that take place over many years. This phenomenon is called the *multihit concept of tumor development*. Although some mutated genes that cause cancer are inherited (i.e., genetic predisposition), most malignancies result from a series of somatic mutations. Environmental and host factors such as diet, immune status, and exposures to chemicals, radiation, and viruses also affect cancer development.

Normal Cellular Biology

Cancer pathophysiology results from genetic and external factors that cause changes in normal cell biology. To provide insight into this process, the regulatory, anatomic, and functional characteristics of normal cells, embryonic cells, nonmalignant neoplastic cells (i.e., benign cells), and malignant cells are compared.

Normal Cells
Growth Characteristics. Cell division is a tightly regulated and orderly process. Cells capable of mitosis normally divide for only two reasons: development of normal tissue and replacement of lost or damaged tissues. Even when cell loss has occurred and tissue replacement is needed, normal cells undergo mitosis only under optimal conditions, which include specific cell growth factors, adequate nutrition, sufficient blood supply, molecules that control the cell cycle, and appropriate space. If one of these requirements is missing or deficient, cell division is diminished or does not occur.

After the cause for cell division is addressed (e.g., replacement of skin lost in a partial-thickness burn injury), cell division ceases so that redundant tissue does not form. This characteristic is demonstrated in vitro as *density-dependent contact inhibition* of cell growth in tissue culture. When a cell

is in direct contact on all sides with like cells, mitosis ceases, and normal cell division is halted.

Cell Cycle. The cell cycle is a sequence of events that leads to cell division and duplication of DNA to produce two identical cells (i.e., daughter cells). The cell cycle consists of four active phases: synthesis (S), mitosis (M), and the growth phases gap 1 (G_1) and gap 2 (G_2) (see figure below). The G_0 phase is the resting stage (i.e., quiescence).

During mitosis, which lasts about 1 hour, the chromatids (i.e., daughter strands of duplicated chromosomes) split and are segregated to form two daughter cells. Mitosis consists of five phases—prophase, prometaphase, metaphase, anaphase, and telophase—that lead to the final separation of all intracellular components and the formation of two daughter cells. Each daughter cell has a complete set of chromosomes and the essential components of the original cell. On completion of mitosis, the cell either begins a new cycle by entering the G_1 phase or proceeds to the G_0 phase.

In G_1, which lasts 4 to 6 hours, the nucleus enlarges and the cell performs the processes of transcription and translation, which are essential for the replication of DNA. During the S phase, cells perform DNA replication and produce a set of chromatids. On completion of DNA replication, the cells enter the G_2 phase, which lasts 2 to 8 hours. G_2 is characterized by intense synthesis of proteins and cellular organelles. During this phase, cells become committed to entering mitotic division (Yarbro, Wujcik, & Gobel, 2010).

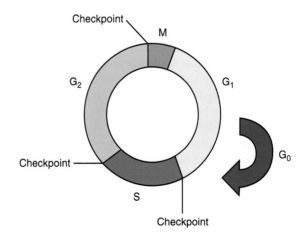

The cell cycle.

Cell Cycle Checkpoints. To move from one phase of the cell cycle to the next, the cell must pass through specific checkpoints. For example, normal cells must accurately complete the S phase before entering or exiting M phase. Checkpoints are control mechanisms to prevent potential errors in the replication of DNA (Yarbro, Wujcik, & Gobel, 2010).

The checkpoints are directed by a family of specialized proteins called *cyclins*. Three main checkpoints (G_1/S, S/G_2, and G_2/M) ensure that all processes have been completed successfully and that the cell and its environment are ready for the next stage.

Phenotypic Characteristics. Mature normal cells are functionally and morphologically differentiated, with a specific morphology and at least one specialized function. For example, neurons receive, process, and transmit information; erythrocytes deliver oxygen throughout the body; myocytes contract in response to nerve stimulation; and melanocytes produce pigment that determines eye, skin, and hair color.

Except for erythrocytes, leukocytes, and thrombocytes, which are supposed to be mobile, normal cells in a tissue tightly adhere to one another, preventing migration. This is accomplished by adhesion proteins located on cell surfaces that bind normal cells of one type firmly together. Each cell type remains within its organ of origin and does not migrate from one organ to another (Yarbro, Wujcik, & Gobel, 2010).

Genotypic Characteristics. Gene storage and activity occurs in the nucleus of cells. Each normal cell contains all the genetic material that is appropriate for the species. During the M phase of the cell cycle, DNA can be visualized as condensed matter called *chromosomes*. The term *euploid* signifies the normal number of chromosomes for a species. In humans, the euploid number of chromosomes is 46. The exceptions are the unfertilized egg and sperm, which each contain 23 chromosomes. Normal human cells contain 46 chromosomes: 22 pairs of (nonsex) autosomes and one pair of sex chromosomes. The sex cells are considered to be haploid cells because they contain only one half of the euploid number of chromosomes. Mature erythrocytes extrude their nuclei during the maturation process and therefore contain no chromosomes.

Although normal cells contain a full complement of human genes, not all genes in every cell are active. For example, only the β-cells of the pancreas synthesize insulin, although all cells have the gene for producing insulin. The insulin gene is suppressed or maintained in an inactive state in all cells except the pancreatic β-cells, where the insulin gene is expressed.

The nucleus, which contains most of a cell's genetic material, is relatively small compared with the cytoplasm, in which many intracellular activities are carried out. Normal differentiated cells therefore have a small nucleus-to-cytoplasm ratio (Yarbro, Wujcik, & Gobel, 2010).

Embryonic Cells

The concept of each normal mature cell having a specific morphology and function is astounding considering that all humans started life as a single cell. Although human embryonic cells (i.e., from conception until postconception day 8) are normal, for a short period of time, their behavior and characteristics are very different from those of mature, differentiated cells (Yarbro, Wujcik, & Gobel, 2010).

Growth Characteristics. Early embryonic cells undergo mitosis and expand the size and cell numbers of the embryo. Cell division for early embryonic cells is rapid but controlled.

Cell Cycle. Early embryonic cells move through each phase of the cell cycle in a specific sequence. Conditions surrounding the embryo are so favorable that as quickly as a cell completes mitosis, it is ready to reenter the cell cycle. Although these cells are under restriction point control (i.e., checkpoints), they do not spend a significant amount of time in G_0. It appears that early embryonic cells continue to enter the cell cycle even when contacted on all surfaces by other cells and do not exhibit density-dependent contact inhibition (Yarbro, Wujcik, & Gobel, 2010).

Phenotypic Characteristics. Early embryonic cells are functionally and morphologically undifferentiated. Anatomic features that distinguish the future neuron from the future myocyte are lacking. Early embryonic cells appear small and round (i.e., anaplastic morphology) and are unable to perform differentiated functions. They do not synthesize any of the intracellular or cell surface proteins found on mature differentiated cells. As a result, they loosely adhere to each other and continually reposition themselves within the growing embryonic cell mass.

At this developmental stage, embryonic cells have the potential to mature into any kind of differentiated cell. This flexible state is referred to as *pluripotent, multipotent*, or *totipotent*. Pluripotency coupled with rapid mitosis allows early embryonic cells to survive and progress even when conditions are unfavorable. If exposed to lethal conditions at this stage resulting in the destruction of 90% of the embryo, the remaining 10% of cells continue mitosis and replace the lost cells. Such a situation delays but does not disrupt cellular development (Yarbro, Wujcik, & Gobel, 2010).

Genotypic Characteristics. All normal human early embryonic cells are euploid, containing the normal diploid chromosome number. These cells are in an almost constant state of mitosis in which the DNA content must be duplicated; the nuclei of embryonic cells therefore appear larger than those of normal differentiated cells. Embryonic cells have no differentiated functions, and the cytoplasmic space of the cells is smaller than that of differentiated cells (i.e., large nucleus-to-cytoplasm ratio).

In the early embryonic cell, all genes are duplicated during cell division. Although these early embryonic cells contain the same genes that mature differentiated human cells contain, only a relatively few genes in the early embryo are expressed. The expressed genes are thought to regulate the growth and characteristics of the embryo at this stage while all other genes are suppressed (Eggert, 2010).

Commitment. At a predetermined point in early embryonic development, the cells initiate the steps to become differentiated.

This is thought to occur on or about postconception day 8 (National Institutes of Health, 2001). In response to unknown signals, each cell commits itself to a specific maturational outcome and positions itself within a group of cells that eventually take on a specific morphology and function.

Differentiation does not involve the loss of genes because all committed cells retain the same number of genes present in the fertilized egg. Differentiation is a function of the selective suppression and expression of individual genes. Commitment involves turning off the specific genes that regulated and directed the rapid growth of early embryonic cells and turning on other genes to initiate cellular differentiation of nerve, bone, muscle, and other cells. The genes that are selectively expressed determine the specific type of tissue that each embryonic cell will become.

Carcinogenesis

The process by which normal cells undergo malignant transformation to become cancer cells is called *carcinogenesis* (i.e., oncogenesis or tumorigenesis). Carcinogenesis is a multistep process that may take years to complete. It is governed by a series of genetic or epigenetic (i.e., nongenetic influence) changes. Genetic mutations may occur by deletion, duplication, inversion, insertion, or translocation (see figure in the next column).

Genetic mutations are not uncommon and are usually repaired by cellular mechanisms. Cancer arises when defects in the genes that regulate cellular proliferation and differentiation, suppress tumor growth, target irreparably damaged cells for apoptosis, or repair damaged DNA are not corrected. As a result of these defects, cancer cells are not governed by the signals that regulate cell growth and may exhibit uncontrolled proliferation.

Although cancer is sometimes caused by passing a defective gene to offspring, it is most often caused by mutations that occur over the course of a lifetime. These somatic mutations (acquired or sporadic) may result from physical, environmental, or chemical agents; ultraviolet (UV) or ionizing radiation; viruses; or errors in replication that can cause base changes or breaks in the DNA strands. Acquired mutations are not passed on to offspring because they are found only in the malignant neoplastic cell (Forbes et al., 2015).

Oncogenes

Two types of genes are responsible for the development of cancer: oncogenes and tumor suppressor genes (see the Selected Tumor Suppressor Genes table on page 16). Oncogenes are mutations of normal genes called proto-oncogenes that govern growth factors, growth factor receptors (GFRs), signal transducers, transcription factors, apoptosis regulators, and cell cycle regulators (see the Selected Oncogenes table on page 16).

Defects in any of these gene products can lead to a gain of function that causes a cell to grow out of control. For example, growth factors normally stimulate cellular growth and repair and act as signaling molecules between cells. They serve as ligands that bind to specific receptors on the plasma membrane cells and regulate cell proliferation. If a genetic mutation causes excessive amounts of a growth factor to be produced, the target cells can be overstimulated and proliferate in an uncontrolled

Types of mutations

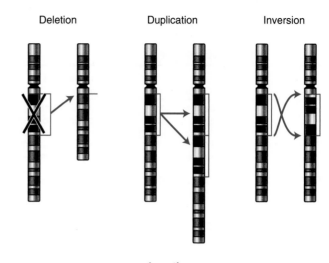

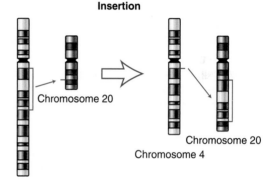

Gene mutations. (From the National Human Genome Research Institute: Gene mutations. Available at http://ghr.nlm.nih.gov/handbook/mutation sanddisorders [accessed February 21, 2016].)

manner. Other oncogenes can affect signal transduction in cells and activate a series of protein kinases, leading to uncontrolled cell proliferation. In these cases, the signal for cellular reproduction is constantly turned on (Yarbro, Wujcik, & Gobel, 2010).

The original mutation usually occurs in only one copy of a proto-oncogene, and subsequent mutations are required for cancer to develop. This phenomenon is referred to as the *multihit concept of tumor development*. Examples of proto-oncogenes that are altered in many types of cancers include *MYC* (e.g., leukemia, lymphoma, lung cancer), *RAS* (e.g., bladder, lung cancer, breast cancer, ovarian cancer), *PDGFB (SIS)* (e.g., glioma, dermatofibrosarcoma protuberans), and *HER2* (e.g., breast cancer, cervical cancer).

Selected Tumor Suppressor Genes

Gene	Major Functions	Mutation-Related Malignancies
APC	Controls specific transcription factors; inhibits cell division and mediates apoptosis	Familial adenomatous polyposis–associated colorectal adenomas, thyroid cancer, stomach cancer, pancreatic cancer
BRCA1, BRCA2	Repair damaged DNA	Breast cancer, ovarian cancer, prostate cancer, pancreatic cancer, melanoma

Growth Factor Receptors

Mutations in GFR genes cause multiple copies to be made (i.e., gene amplification), leading to overexpression of the encoded proteins. For example, amplification of *HER2* genes causes overexpression of the human epidermal growth factor receptor in some breast and other cancers. A greater degree of amplification is correlated with a poorer prognosis (Wolff et al., 2014).

Signal Transducers: Kinases and Transcription Factors

Kinases are enzymes that catalyze many critical processes, including signal transduction, transcription, and metabolism. Mutations in signal transducers such as kinases and other proteins can lead to uncontrolled cellular proliferation. Nuclear transcription factors are proteins that bind to specific DNA sequences and regulate the expression of genes that are involved in cellular growth, proliferation, metabolism, differentiation, and apoptosis. Overexpression of the transcription factor MYC is a common mutation found in people with cancer. It causes uncontrolled growth and a loss of apoptosis (Yu, Lee, Herrmann, Buettner, & Jove, 2014).

Tumor Suppressor Genes

Tumor suppressor genes (i.e., normal growth suppressor genes, or anti-oncogenes) encode proteins that limit cell division, promote apoptosis, and repair defective DNA. Defects in these functions contribute to uncontrolled proliferation of neoplastic cells. Defects in tumor suppressor genes are called *loss of function mutations*. A gain of function in an oncogene and a corresponding loss of function in tumor suppressor genes, repair enzymes, or activators of apoptosis are necessary to promote malignancy. When proto-oncogenes and tumor suppressor genes are mutated, there is little to prevent cancer cells from proliferating. The rate of tissue growth is increased because cancer cells spend very little time in G_0, before proceeding through the cell cycle.

The first tumor suppressor gene to be identified was the retinoblastoma gene *RB1*, which predisposes carriers to osteosarcoma and retinoblastoma. The best known mutated tumor

Selected Oncogenes

Oncogene	Major Functions	Examples of Malignancy
ABL1	Tyrosine kinase involved in cell division, adhesion, differentiation	Chronic myelogenous leukemia
AKT2	Mediates cell cycle progression, glucose transport, gene transcription, apoptosis	Ovarian, breast, and pancreatic cancers
ALK	Tyrosine kinase involved in signal transduction, nerve cell proliferation	Neuroblastoma, anaplastic large cell lymphoma, non–small cell lung cancer
BRAF	Transmits extracellular signals to the nucleus; regulates cellular growth, migration, apoptosis	Melanoma, colorectal cancer, ovarian cancer, thyroid cancer
BRC-ABL (fusion gene)	Formed by translocation of chromosomes 9 and 22; no known normal activity	Various leukemias
CD274 (PDL1)	Involved in cell proliferation, apoptosis, T-cell regulation	Lung cancer, melanoma, Hodgkin lymphoma, stomach cancer
EGFR (ERBB1)	Tyrosine kinase involved in signal transduction; promotes cell growth and proliferation	Squamous cell carcinoma, non–small cell lung cancer
ETS1	Transcription factor mediates differentiation of lymphoid cells	Various lymphomas; breast cancer, cervical cancer
FGF3	Growth factor	Breast cancer; squamous cell carcinoma
FGF4 (HST)	Growth factor involved in embryonic development, cell growth, tissue repair	Breast cancer; esophageal cancer, Kaposi sarcoma, bladder cancer
FOS	Transcription factor regulates cell proliferation, differentiation	Osteosarcoma, liver cancer, colorectal cancer, prostate cancer
HER2 (ERBB2)	Tyrosine kinase stabilizes ligand binding, activates signaling pathways, regulates DNA transcription	Breast, cervical, lung, gastric, and salivary gland cancers; glioma, neuroblastoma
JUN	Transcription factor involved in gene expression, cell cycle progression	Sarcoma, non–small cell lung cancer, breast cancer
KIT	Tyrosine kinase involved in many signaling pathways, cell growth, migration	Sarcoma, gastrointestinal stromal tumor, acute myeloid leukemia, seminoma
MDM2	Inhibits tumor suppressor proteins, cell cycle arrest, apoptosis	Soft tissue sarcomas, osteosarcoma, glioma
MYC	Transcription factor mediates DNA synthesis, cell cycle progression, apoptosis	Breast, cervical, colorectal, and lung cancers; Burkitt lymphoma, neuroblastoma, glioblastoma
MYCL	Regulates DNA synthesis	Lung cancer, neuroblastoma, medulloblastoma, colorectal cancer

suppressor gene in humans is *TP53*, which is found on chromosome 17. The encoded TP53 protein plays a role in blocking proliferation in G_1, apoptosis, and DNA repair and is referred to as the *guardian of the genome*. An individual who inherits only one working (normal) copy of the gene is predisposed to cancer. The lack of *TP53* allows cells with other genetic mutations to propagate, a situation found in many people with malignancies, including cancer of the lung, breast, esophagus, liver, bladder, ovary, and brain and sarcoma, lymphoma, and leukemia. More than 50% of cancers contain a missing or mutated *TP53* gene (Cancer.Net, 2015; Muller & Vousden, 2014).

Normal cell mitosis depends on accurate DNA transcription. Redundant molecular genetic mechanisms exist that examine newly transcribed DNA, check for damaged or mismatched base pairs, and ensure that accurate transcription has occurred. Damage to DNA can occur as a result of chemical toxins, exposure to radiation, and errors in replication. Some tumor suppressor genes encode DNA repair enzymes, which can restore damaged DNA before cell replication takes place.

DNA can be repaired by several mechanisms. Some damage to base pairs can be repaired by the DNA itself. When only one strand of DNA is damaged, the second strand can be used as a template to make the necessary restorations, including base excision repair, nucleotide excision repair, and mismatch repair. If both strands of DNA are damaged, nonhomologous end-joining and template-assisted repair (i.e., homologous recombination repair) mechanisms are used.

Examples of mutated tumor suppressor genes that predispose carriers to cancer are the *BRCA1* and *BRCA2* genes (breast and ovarian cancer), *TP53* gene (bladder, breast, liver, lung, prostate, and ovarian cancer), *APC* (familial adenomatous and noninherited colorectal cancer), and *RB1* (retinoblastoma, sarcoma, and bladder, breast, and lung cancer). Mutated *BRCA1* and *BRCA2* genes are identified in 20% to 25% of hereditary breast cancers and in 5% to 10% of all breast cancers (Gabai-Kapara et al., 2014; National Cancer Institute [NCI], 2015b).

Surface and Membrane Changes

Some of the acquired characteristics of cancer cells involve surface and membrane changes. The cells that make up a multicellular organism interact with each other and with the extracellular matrix (ECM). The structure of the ECM, a three-dimensional, noncellular medium, differs by tissue type, but it is essential for the growth and survival of normal cells. For example, ECM components interact and combine with growth factors, controlling their availability to the cells.

Without interactions with the ECM, normal cells undergo apoptosis. However, malignant neoplastic cells can survive and reproduce without the usual interactions with the ECM. Cancer cells produce plasminogen activator, which helps to break down plasminogen to plasmin. Plasmin can cause the release of growth factors in cancer cells, leading to greater proliferation of these mutant cells (i.e., gain of function) (Pickup, Mouw, & Weaver, 2014).

Matrix Metalloproteinases

Matrix metalloproteinases (MMPs) are a family of proteases (i.e., enzymes that degrade proteins) that regulate the microenvironment of cells by controlling growth factors and their receptors. They are active in cell adhesion and apoptosis, and

they can degrade the protein components of the ECM and basement membranes. Some MMPs generate specific signals that promote tumor development and the growth of new blood vessels (i.e., angiogenesis) to support tumor growth. Increased expression of MMPs correlates with a poor prognosis and more invasive disease (Kessenbrock, Wang, & Werb, 2015).

Cell Adhesion Molecules

Normal cells express a variety of cell adhesion molecules (CAMs) on their surface. Integrins span the plasma membrane of the cell, bind to specific ECM proteins, and play a vital role in cell-ECM interactions. Cadherins are CAMs that regulate signal transduction within the cell and interactions between similar cells. Some members of the immunoglobulin family play a role in cell adhesion. Changes in the expression of integrins and cadherins increase the ability of cancer cells to metastasize and foster more aggressive disease (Farahani et al., 2014).

Surface Antigens

Cancer cells express membrane surface components, particularly receptors and antigens, that are different from those of the normal differentiated cells from which they arose. Cancer antigens may be ordinary protein products that are synthesized by normal cells at an earlier developmental stage but are not expressed by mature cells or are expressed only in small quantities. Examples of normal cellular antigens include prostate-specific antigen (PSA), α-fetoprotein (AFP), carcinoembryonic antigen (CEA), human chorionic gonadotropin (hCG), lactate dehydrogenase (LD), and alkaline phosphatase (ALP). Elevated levels can indicate the malignancy.

Cancer cells may express surface antigens that are found only on malignant cells. These proteins are called *tumor-specific antigens* (TSAs). They can be used as markers to identify and quantify tumors. Examples include the HER2 protein (i.e., breast cancer) and CD20 (i.e., non-Hodgkin lymphoma).

Antibodies directed against TSAs are being used for cancer therapy and prevention. For example, trastuzumab (Herceptin) targets the HER2 protein that is overexpressed in about 20% of breast cancers. Rituximab (Rituxan) and ibritumomab tiuxetan (Zevalin) are used to treat non-Hodgkin lymphoma patients who overexpress the CD20 antigen (Coulie, van den Eynde, van der Bruggen, & Boon, 2014; NCI, 2015i).

Metastasis

A hallmark of malignant cells is their ability to metastasize to other parts of the body. Metastasis involves a complex progression of events. Cancer may spread by local invasion or through the lymphatic system or blood to distant sites. In hematogenous dissemination, malignant cells break away from the original tumor by a process called *intravasation*. They then enter blood vessels, travel through the circulatory system, exit the circulation (i.e., extravasation), migrate into interstitial spaces, and initiate new tumor growth.

Metastasis employs several mechanisms to penetrate the stroma surrounding the tumor, cancer cells express high levels of proteolytic enzymes, which break down cell membranes and ECM components. Altered gene expression patterns result in the breakdown of cell-cell junctions. After the basement membrane of the tumor is breached, tumor cells travel through the blood vessels or lymphatics. Malignant cells also can translocate because cellular growth factors, ECM molecules, and cytoskeleton regulators stimulate the formation of pseudopodia, allowing movement through adjacent tissues. Using these mechanisms, cancer cells switch from collective to individual migration patterns and navigate through the ECM and into the vasculature to reach distant sites.

After cancer cells have reached the target organ, they exit the circulation and initiate new growth. MMPs help to degrade the ECM that cancer cells must penetrate at the target site. Metastatic spread also depends on cell-cell and cell-matrix interactions between the circulating metastatic cells and the target organ.

One model of metastasis suggests that mutations in oncogenes or inactivation of tumor suppressor genes may result in a selective growth advantage for some cells in a tumor. As additional mutations occur, advantageous phenotypes develop and become dominant, conferring a growth advantage and metastatic competence on all cells in the tumor. Another model purports that aggressive tumor cells that are capable of metastasis comprise only a small percentage of the primary tumor's cells. Although tumors slough off many malignant cells that then travel through the circulatory system, only a few are capable of stimulating growth at a new site. The low metastatic potential of the shed tumor cells may be attributed to the fact that most of them are undergoing apoptosis as they disengage from the primary tumor.

Cancer cells vary in their metastatic potential. They are influenced by mutations in growth factors and their receptors, the products of tumor suppressor genes, and other proteins. Metastatic activity is also influenced by tumor-host interactions and the microenvironment of the target organ (Yarbro, Wujcik, & Gobel, 2010).

Cancer Stem Cells. Stem cells are undifferentiated cells that can differentiate into specialized cells to take the place of those that have been damaged or lost, or they have the ability to divide and renew themselves over long periods. The renewal of stem cells is highly regulated by chemical signals. Defects in signaling pathways allow cancer stem cells to produce tumor cells. Only a small percentage of tumor cells are thought to be derived from stem cells, but their clonal expansion may be responsible for disease recurrence after aggressive treatment (National Institutes of Health, 2005; Weissman, 2015).

Angiogenesis. Primary and metastatic tumors need an adequate blood supply to grow and survive. The process by which vascular networks are created to sustain malignant tumors is called *angiogenesis*. An independent vascular network provides malignant tumors with access to the circulatory system. In addition to supplying the tumor with nutrients, the blood supply facilitates metastasis to distant sites. Angiogenesis may be an important step in tumor initiation because there is evidence of angiogenesis in transformed tissue before the appearance of malignant tumor masses.

Angiogenesis differs from vasculogenesis, the formation of new blood vessels in developing embryos. Angiogenesis involves the formation of new blood vessels from preexisting ones. The budding vascular networks provide malignant cells with access to the circulatory system and facilitate tumor spread.

The development of new blood vessels depends on a variety of proangiogenic factors (e.g., interferons, tissue inhibitors of MMPs) and antiangiogenic factors (e.g., vascular endothelial growth factor [VEGF], epidermal growth factor). For example, early in the metastatic process, quiescent endothelial cells are activated and begin to proliferate and migrate. VEGF provides the stimulus for epithelial cells to proliferate and enhances vascular permeability. Tumor necrosis factor stimulates the migration of tumor cells. Basement membranes are degraded through the actions of MMPs. This is crucial to local invasion and distant metastasis (Pickup, Mouw, & Weaver, 2014).

Causes of Malignant Transformation

Carcinogenesis is the multistep process that transforms normal cells into malignant cells. Over time, malignant transformation can result from the effects of environmental and host factors, such as exposure to chemicals or radiation, viral infections, and lifestyle factors such as smoking and dietary practices (Yarbro, Wujcik, & Gobel, 2010).

Environmental Factors

Cancer development in the United States is usually the result of exposure to environmental or extrinsic factors (American Cancer Society [ACS], 2015b). Environmental carcinogens include chemicals, radiation, viruses, personal habits such as smoking, and dietary practices. Exposure to these agents can occur in the home, workplace, or elsewhere.

Chemical Carcinogenesis. Most instances of chemical carcinogenesis have been identified through clinical observations. In 1775, English physician Percival Pott noticed an unusually high incidence of scrotal cancer among men who were employed as chimney sweeps in childhood. He correctly surmised that the cancer was directly attributable to soot exposure and suggested that chimney sweeps bathe daily as a means of prevention. More than a century later, Japanese pathologists induced skin tumors in rabbits by the repeated application of coal tar to the ears. These early experiments supported the idea that environmental factors could be responsible for the development of cancer, especially with repeated exposures over time.

Chemically induced carcinogenesis has been demonstrated in comparisons of cancer rates in different parts of the world. Some cancers are more prevalent in certain geographic locations. For example, there are significantly higher rates of cervical cancer in developing countries (e.g., South America, Africa) but higher rates of prostate cancer in developed countries (ACS, 2015b). Gastric cancer is relatively rare in the United States but common in Japan. In populations of immigrants to Western nations, the initial patterns of cancer development change to became similar to those prevalent in the host country over several generations, implicating environmental factors (ACS, 2015b).

Other epidemiologic evidence supports the idea of chemically induced carcinogenesis. Chemical carcinogens react with the cell's DNA to induce mutations that alter the function of regulatory genes. The effects of some chemical agents increase cell proliferation. Chemical carcinogens can act directly or indirectly. Direct-acting chemicals do not require biotransformation to induce carcinogenesis. Indirect-acting chemicals, or procarcinogens, require metabolic conversion in the host to effect malignant transformation. Both direct-acting and metabolically converted chemicals have electron-deficient atoms that react with electron-rich substrates in the cell, including DNA and RNA. Tobacco and ethanol are examples of carcinogenic chemicals (Roberts, James, & Williams, 2015).

Smoking. Although evidence links cigarette use to the development of lung cancer, smoking remains the number one cause of the malignancy. Cigarettes contain at least 69 chemicals known to cause cancer (Centers for Disease Control and Prevention [CDC], 2015b; NCI, 2015e). Tobacco is a potent carcinogen, containing benzo(a)pyrene, dimethylnitrosamine, and nickel compounds, which can lead to malignant transformation of cells.

The prevalence of tobacco use in the form of cigarettes, pipes, cigars, and chewing tobacco persists despite warnings from the U.S. Surgeon General (U.S. Department of Health and Human Services, 2014). Smoking accounts for almost one third of cancer deaths (ACS, 2015b). Smoking has been linked to cancers of the lung, oral cavity, larynx, esophagus, kidney, pancreas, cervix, stomach, and bladder.

Lung cancer incidence has declined among men and women and now accounts for 13% of all cancer diagnoses (ACS, 2015b). However, cancer of the lung and bronchus accounts for approximately 27% of cancer-related deaths of men and women (ACS, 2015b). The latency period between the onset of smoking and the development of lung cancer can span 20 or more years. The risk of developing lung cancer depends largely on the quantity and duration of tobacco use. Passive smoking (i.e., secondhand smoke) is associated with an increased risk of lung cancer, and it is estimated that living with a smoker may increase a nonsmoker's chances of developing lung cancer by 20% to 30% (Jacobs et al., 2015; U.S. Department of Health and Human Services, 2014).

Alcohol. The mechanisms by which excessive alcohol intake affects cancer development have been identified (NCI, 2015a). Ethanol may potentiate the action of other carcinogens, and metabolism of alcohol turns it into a toxic chemical that can damage DNA. Alcohol is also an immunosuppressant. Ingestion of excessive ethanol has been linked to development of head and neck, esophageal, liver, colorectal, and breast cancers. Alcohol acts in conjunction with tobacco to greatly increase the risk of cancer. Combined tobacco and alcohol use can be attributed to a 30-fold increase in the risk of cancer of the oral cavity and pharynx (ACS, 2015; Bagnardi et al., 2015; Klatsky, Udaltsova, Li, Baer, Tran, & Friedman, 2015).

Radiation. Radiant energy can induce malignant transformation in experimental animals and humans. The two most common forms of radiant energy are ionizing radiation and UV radiation. *Ionizing Radiation.* Radiation is energy emitted and transferred through matter or space. Ionizing radiation creates enough energy to change a stable atom to an unstable one by ejecting orbital electrons (i.e., ionizing effect). Ionizing radiation consists of x-rays, gamma rays, and particles (e.g., protons, neutrons). Sources of exposure to ionizing radiation include nuclear accidents, occupational exposure, and medical treatments. Ionizing radiation can damage whole tissues, individual cells, and DNA.

After World War II, the effects of radiation exposure were seen in the survivors of the atomic bomb blasts who developed acute and chronic myelocytic leukemias. In the early part of the 20th century, radiologists who had frequent exposure to x-rays incurred a threefold to fourfold risk of leukemia. Marie Curie, two-time Nobel Prize winner whose work led to the discovery of radioactivity, died of aplastic anemia caused by prolonged radiation exposure.

Healthy tissues and tumors are affected by radiation. Some cells remain undamaged, some recover over time, and others die. Radiation therapy for malignancies, although one of the most common treatments for cancer, can promote secondary cancers (Casey et al., 2015; NCI, 2015g). Ionizing radiation exerts its effects directly on the double helix, damaging DNA by breaking the nucleotide and phosphate backbone of the molecule.

Before 1985, radiation dose was measured in radiation-absorbed doses (rads). The current dose unit of radiation therapy is the gray (Gy). One Gy is equal to 100 rads, and 1 centigray (cGy) is equal to 1 rad.

In living systems, radiation is absorbed randomly by atoms and molecules in cells. The risk of developing a radiation-associated cancer depends on the type, dose, and extent of exposure (NCI, 2015h). The effects of ionizing radiation exposure over time are cumulative.

Ultraviolet Radiation. Solar radiation is the primary source of UV radiation and is the major cause of skin cancer worldwide. UV rays can come from indoor tanning beds, booths, or sunlamps, and they also cause cancer (CDC, 2015a). UV rays affect the skin in several ways. UVA and UVB radiation can lead to carcinogenesis by damaging tumor suppressor genes, cell cycle control signaling pathways, cellular enzymes, and pyrimidine dimers in DNA molecules.

Epidemiologic evidence suggests that the risk of skin cancer depends on the intensity and type of exposure and the distribution of melanin (ACS, 2015b). The effects of UV exposure tend to be cumulative. Risk factors for skin cancer include fair skin, unprotected and repeated exposure to UV radiation, repeated severe sunburns as a child, certain types of moles, family history, immune suppression, sex, and age (ACS, 2015b; CDC, 2015a).

In 2015, more than 73,000 people were diagnosed with melanoma, the most serious form of skin cancer. Although basal cell carcinoma is fairly uncommon, it is an aggressive disease that accounts for most skin cancer–related deaths.

Chronic Inflammation. The role of chronic inflammation in the development of cancer was proposed as early as the mid-19th century, and it is now considered to be a causative factor in a variety of cancers. The longer the inflammation exists, the higher the risk of developing cancer. Mutations in some molecules involved in tissue repair (e.g., growth factors, ECM proteins, angiogenesis factors) have been shown to play a role in carcinogenesis. Several inflammatory conditions predispose individuals to malignancies, including chronic inflammatory bowel disease, hepatitis, osteomyelitis, and gastritis (Baniyash, Sade-Feldman, & Kanterman, 2014).

Viruses. Viruses play a role in the development of certain cancers. For example, the human papillomavirus (HPV) is linked to the development of cervical and vulvar cancers; the Epstein-Barr virus (EBV) is associated with nasopharyngeal and anal cancers; and the hepatitis B virus (HBV) and hepatitis C virus (HCV) increase the risk of liver cancer.

Viruses that cause cancer are known as *oncoviruses*. When they infect cells, they break the DNA chain and insert their own genetic material into it. Disruption of host DNA and viral gene insertion cause mutations that can activate an oncogene or inactivate a suppressor gene. Although any type of virus has the potential to enter a cell and mutate DNA, infection with retroviruses is more likely to be oncogenic.

Several vaccines are approved by the U.S. Food and Drug Administration to prevent the formation of cancer. One vaccine prevents infection with HBV, which can cause liver cancer. Gardasil and Cervarix vaccines prevent infection with several strains of HPV that can cause cervical, vaginal, vulvar, anal, penile, and oropharyngeal cancers (NCI, 2015c). The vaccines are produced from the purified proteins that are expressed by papillomaviruses. The body's immune response to the genetically engineered proteins protect against infection by the natural viruses (Morales-Sénchez & Fuentes-Pananá, 2014).

Dietary Influences. Dietary practices alone or in combination with environmental exposures are thought to be associated with carcinogenesis. However, the relationship between diet and carcinogenesis is poorly understood, and the understanding of the process by which carcinogenesis occurs is still evolving. Dietary influences are usually not independent of the effects of other possible carcinogenic agents and personal habits. Preservatives, contaminants, preparation methods, and additives (e.g., dyes, flavorings) can have carcinogenic effects. Studies suggest that a diet high in red and processed meats may increase the risk, whereas a diet high in vegetables and fruits may lower the risk of many cancers (ACS, 2015b).

Host Factors

Immune Function. The immune system provides protection against the development of cancer. Malignant cells are considered foreign (i.e., nonself) because they are no longer completely normal. The cells often express cell surface antigens that are different from those of normal cells, allowing recognition by macrophages, helper T lymphocytes, and natural killer cells. After malignant cells have been recognized as foreign, defensive and offensive actions are initiated by the immune system to eliminate them. This continuing protection, or *immunosurveillance*, is crucial in suppressing cancer development.

The vital role of the immune system in preventing cancer is supported by cancer incidence statistics for immunosuppressed people. Children younger than 2 years and adults older than 60 years of age have immune systems that function at less than optimal levels, and both groups have a higher incidence of cancer compared with that of the general population (ACS, 2015b). People receiving immunosuppressive therapy (e.g., organ transplant recipients) to reduce the risk of organ rejection and those with significant autoimmune disease for which chronic immunosuppression is the only means of controlling disease progression also have higher rates of cancer. Among people with human immunodeficiency virus (HIV) infection or acquired immunodeficiency syndrome (AIDS), the risk of developing cancer is substantial (NCI, 2015f).

Immune function can be compromised as a result of cytotoxic therapy, injury to marrow-forming areas of bones, surgical removal of primary or secondary lymphoid tissues (e.g., thymectomy, splenectomy), or exposure to chronic low-dose radiation. Research has shown that survivors of childhood cancer who were treated with chemotherapy are at higher risk for cancer later in life. Cancer patients treated with high-dose chemotherapy, which can cause immunosuppression, are at higher risk for a second malignancy (ACS, 2015b).

Advancing age is probably the most common risk factor for cancer. More than 78% of malignancies in the United States occur in people older than 55 years of age (ACS, 2015b). The higher incidence of cancer in this age group reflects the lifelong accumulation of DNA mutations resulting in malignant transformation and the diminishing immune response. The efficiency of DNA repair mechanisms can be compromised with age, and the body may not be able to repair even minor mutations (ACS, 2015b; Yarbro, Wujcik, & Gobel, 2010).

Surveillance Failure. An intact immune system provides the body with constant surveillance and detects the presence of foreign invaders and altered host cells, including malignant cells. Macrophages, T lymphocytes, and natural killer cells are actively involved in this protective function. However, even optimal performance cannot ensure complete protection.

Immune surveillance is most effective at identifying and attacking cancer cells that have been induced by viral and chemical agents. The system appears to have little protective value against tumors that are a result of inheritance or spontaneous DNA replication errors. A likely explanation for this selectivity is the difference in cell surface properties of malignant cells caused by different types of carcinogenic or mutational events. Malignancies arising from viral or chemical carcinogenesis have new cell surface proteins unique to the cancer cells and are more easily recognized by immunoreactive cells as foreign. Several mechanisms have been proposed for cancer surveillance failure in immunocompetent individuals, including those discussed in the next sections (Yarbro, Wujcik, & Gobel, 2010).

Malignant Cell Mimics. Some cancer cells may initially have a less malignant phenotype and more normal cell surface characteristics. These properties may not be sufficient to trigger an immune response. Cancer cells may go undetected by the immune system until significant proliferation has occurred (Weissman, 2015).

Decoy Jamming. Some cancer cells that synthesize specific surface proteins capable of triggering an immune response shed the TSAs. The immune response is directed toward the loose antigens rather than the malignant cell (Recondo, Díaz-Cantón, de la Vega, Greco, Recondo, & Valsecchi, 2014).

Bone Marrow Invasion. Invasion of bone marrow by cancer cells makes it less able to mount normal immune and inflammatory responses. The number of cells available to respond is decreased, resulting in lymphopenia and neutropenia (Shiozawa, Eber, Berry, & Taichman, 2015).

Enhanced Lymphocyte Suppression Activity. Some tumors release factors that selectively enhance the activity and number of regulatory T cells (Tregs), formerly known as suppressor T cells, so that they constitute a larger percentage of circulating leukocytes. Tregs can compromise the immune response and favor tumor growth by suppressing the proliferative response of other T lymphocytes, macrophages, and natural killer cells or by suppressing immunoglobulin production (Pae, Meydani, & Wu, 2012).

Immune Blockade. Some cancer cells release factors that specifically suppress natural killer cells, which normally can destroy tumor cells and cells infected with viruses. If natural killer cells are suppressed, the ability of cancer cells to reproduce is enhanced (Yarbro, Wujcik, & Gobel, 2010).

Subclinical Antigen Dose. The initial malignant colony contains so few cells that they are not capable of triggering the immune system. The delay allows the original cells to become well established and grow unnoticed until they reach a size that is detected by the immune system. At this point, the malignancy may be so large that the immune system cannot effectively destroy or inactivate the tumor cells (Weissman, 2015).

Increased Prostaglandin Production. Certain malignancies can increase the production and release prostaglandins by cancer cells or by normal tissue. Prostaglandins inhibit the ability of most lymphocytes to respond to lectins and other mitogenic agents so that the production of lymphocytes and the overall immunosuppressive effect are decreased (Manna, Wepy, Hsu, Chang, Cravatt, & Marnett, 2014).

Downregulation of Tumor-Specific Antigens. As cancer cells progress toward an increasingly malignant state, some undergo antigenic modulation, which may involve loss of TSAs, decreasing the likelihood of an immune response. Another type of modulation is to continually change the nature of the TSAs, requiring a corresponding change in immune surveillance before recognition and elimination can occur (Nielsen, Friis-Hansen, Poulsen, Federspiel, & Sorensen, 2014).

Immunoprivileged Sites. Malignant transformation occurs in areas of the body that have less active immune functions than other areas. These immunoprivileged sites (e.g., testis, brain) may differ with the developmental stage of the host. Cancer initiation or metastasis to an immunoprivileged site allows establishment of tumor cells and development of a relatively large tumor burden before recognition by the immune system (Corthay, 2014).

Genetic Predisposition

Although damage to a tumor suppressor gene or a change from a proto-oncogene to an oncogene can be caused by exposure to carcinogens, genetic predisposition also influences the process. In humans, the efficiency of DNA repair mechanisms is inherited and can decrease over time from aging, disease, toxins, and other genotoxic events. Mutations transform proto-oncogenes into oncogenes. In some people, the locations of specific proto-oncogenes within the genome are different and may increase susceptibility to mutation or activation. In others, the position of the oncogene may be normal, but the tumor suppressor gene that controls the oncogene's activity may be abnormal or translocated.

Although most mutations in cancer cells are somatic, about 5% to 10% of all cancers are inherited (i.e., germline cancers) (ACS, 2015a). In these cases, the mutation is carried in the genetic code of each cell in the body. Families with hereditary cancer syndromes usually demonstrate cancer in an autosomal dominant pattern in two or more generations. More than 50 types of inherited cancer syndromes have been identified (see box on page 22) (NCI, 2013, 2015d). Most of these tumors are caused by inactivation of tumor suppressor genes, although some are caused by oncogenes. Other tumors (e.g., hereditary breast cancer, hereditary nonpolyposis colorectal cancer) arise from mutations in DNA repair genes. Inheriting one mutated gene is usually not enough to cause cancer, although it is sufficient to transmit the trait (i.e., phenotype) to offspring. However, individuals with one mutated gene are at increased risk for cancer because one allele has already been compromised. A mutation in the second allele triggers the growth of a malignancy.

Gene activity depends on how well one or both genes of a pair function. For example, the *BCRA1* gene is a tumor suppressor gene. Faulty functioning of this gene is associated with the development of an inherited form of breast cancer. If both *BRCA1* genes are normal in structure and location, the woman is at normal risk for the developing breast cancer. However, if a woman inherits one mutated gene and one normal gene, her risk of developing breast cancer increases. If she inherits two faulty *BRCA1* genes, her risk of breast cancer increases substantially. For other types of cancers, a familial tendency may be identified, but no specific pattern of inheritance is evident.

Hereditary cancers may be limited to a particular type (e.g., colorectal cancer, breast cancer), or there may be a predisposition for different types of cancers. These are called *family cancer syndromes*. The ontogeny of the genetic predisposition can be difficult to elucidate and is often multifactorial in nature. Multiple small gene mutations may be responsible, and even normal exposure to carcinogenic agents can enhance the baseline level of genetic predisposition to cancer.

Race is a genetically determined characteristic that plays a role in cancer incidence. For example, African American men in the United States have a higher incidence of prostate cancer than white Americans. The incidence of breast cancer in the United States is highest among white women, followed by African American, American Indian or Alaskan native, Hispanic, and Asian American or Pacific Islander women (ACS, 2015a). Ashkenazi women are at increased risk for breast and ovarian cancer because of a higher incidence of *BRCA1* or *BRCA2* gene mutations (ACS, 2015a). Gastroesophageal cancer rates are higher among Asian Americans than among other Americans (ACS, 2015a).

Although race or ethnicity plays a role in the development of cancer, it should not be considered in isolation. Behaviors related to culture or ethnic group, geographic location, diet, and socioeconomic factors also must be considered. The ACS has reported that cancer incidence and survival are often related to socioeconomic factors, such as the availability of health care services or the belief that seeking early health care has a positive effect on the outcome of a cancer diagnosis (ACS, 2015b).

Hereditary Cancer Syndromes

- Beckwith-Wiedemann syndrome (Wilms tumor, liver cancer)
- Bloom syndrome (solid tumors)
- Cowden syndrome (breast, thyroid, head and neck cancer)
- Denys-Drash syndrome (Wilms tumor)
- Familial adenomatous polyposis (colon cancer)
- Familial breast cancer (breast, ovarian cancer)
- Familial melanoma (melanoma, pancreatic cancer)
- Familial retinoblastoma (retinoblastoma, osteogenic sarcoma)
- Fanconi anemia (acute myelogenous leukemia)
- Hereditary nonpolyposis colorectal cancer
- Hereditary papillary renal cancer (renal papillary cancer)
- Hereditary prostate cancer
- Li-Fraumeni syndrome (brain tumor, sarcoma, breast cancer, leukemia)
- Neurofibromatosis type 1 (neurofibroma, sarcoma, glioma)
- Peutz-Jeghers syndrome (colorectal, breast, ovarian cancer)
- Von Hippel–Lindau syndrome (renal cancer)
- Xeroderma pigmentosum (skin cancer)

Malignancy Quantification

Tumor Grade

A system of grading tumor cells was established to accurately describe the malignant characteristics of individual tumors diagnosed in humans. It compares cancer cells with their normal counterparts in terms of appearance and cellular activity. Cancer cells that retain more of their normal appearance and functions are considered low grade. Others are more aggressive

and treatment resistant and are classified as high-grade tumors (Yarbro, Wujcik, & Gobel, 2010). The table below provides an example of a grading system.

Grading System for Malignancy

Grade	Definition
GX	Grade cannot be determined
G1	Cells are well differentiated, closely resembling the tissue from which they arose, considered a low-grade tumor
G2	Cells are moderately differentiated, still resemble normal cells somewhat, but exhibit more malignant characteristics
G3	Cells are poorly differentiated, few normal cellular characteristics are retained, but the tissue of origin may still be established
G4	Cells are undifferentiated, no normal cellular characteristics can be found, and determining the tissue of origin is very difficult

From the National Cancer Institute (2015). Tumor grade fact sheet. Available at http://www.cancer.gov/about-cancer/diagnosis-staging/prognosis/tumor-grade-fact-sheet (accessed January 25, 2016).

Tumor Stage

Staging is a step-by-step process to determine the size and location of a tumor and the degree to which it has spread. The smaller the tumor at the time of diagnosis and the less it has spread, the greater the potential for cure or control. To select the best treatment options for a specific tumor, its stage must be determined. Three methods are used: clinical staging, pathologic staging, and restaging (Yarbro, Wujcik, & Gobel, 2010.)

Clinical Staging.   Clinical staging provides an estimate of the size and extent of the tumor. Stage is determined by physical examination and other diagnostic measures that may include laboratory tests (e.g., blood work), imaging tests (e.g., computed tomography, positron emission tomography, magnetic resonance imaging), biopsy, endoscopy, or laparoscopy. Some cancers may require surgery to determine their extent. The choice of diagnostic tests is based on the type of cancer that is being evaluated.

Pathologic Staging.   Tumor size, number of sites, and degree of metastasis are determined by pathologic examination of tissue obtained at surgery. Pathologic examination provides the clinician with information about the cellular characteristics of the tumor.

Restaging.   Although it is uncommon, surgery may be done for recurrent disease to help determine its extent and the best treatment options. The formal cancer stage usually does not change over time, even if the cancer recurs or spreads to other areas of the body (Yarbro, Wujcik, & Gobel, 2010). However, in certain cases after a period of remission, a physician may restage the cancer, using the same methods as for the initial diagnosis. The new stage is recorded with a lowercase *r* before the restaged designation.

Tumor-Node-Metastasis Staging System.   Survival rates are usually higher for individuals whose tumors are localized.

This observation gave rise to the notion that tumors progress over time, perhaps influenced by the type of cancer and other host factors. Although several systems for grading tumor cells are available, the tumor-node-metastasis (TNM) system is commonly used to stage malignancies and define prognostic variables such as their pattern of growth and spread. *T* signifies the extent or size of the tumor, *N* indicates the presence or absence of lymph node involvement, and *M* denotes the presence or absence of distant metastases. The numbers assigned to any of these components (e.g., T3, N2, M1) indicate the degree of tumor size, nodal involvement, and metastatic spread.

The TNM classification system serves several purposes: to stage a tumor at the time of diagnosis, to examine the progress of a cancer related to the natural course of the disease, to provide standardized data on which to base treatment options, and to specify prognosis. Other staging systems are used for some childhood cancers, lymphomas, leukemias, colorectal cancer, and cancers of the cervix, ovary, uterus, vagina, and vulva (Yarbro, Wujcik, & Gobel, 2010).

Conclusion

The process of carcinogenesis is multifactorial, with significant interactions between host and environmental factors. Not all people are at equal risk for cancer. The roles played by immune function, genetic predisposition, lifestyle, and exposure to mutagenic agents vary widely among individuals. Although most immune and genetic factors cannot be altered to prevent cancer, reduction of exposures to environmental carcinogenic agents can reduce the incidence of cancer significantly.

References

American Cancer Society (ACS). (2015a). *Family cancer syndromes*. Available at http://www.cancer.org/cancer/cancercauses/geneticsandcancer/heredity-and-cancer (inherited cancer) (accessed January 20, 2016).

American Cancer Society (ACS). (2015b). *Cancer facts & figures 2015*. Atlanta: American Cancer Society.

Bagnardi, V., Rota, M., Botteri, E., Tramacere, I., Islami, F., Fedirko, V., & La Vecchia, C. (2015). Alcohol consumption and site-specific cancer risk: A comprehensive dose-response meta-analysis. *British Journal of Cancer, 112*(3), 580–593.

Baniyash, M., Sade-Feldman, M., & Kanterman, J. (2014). Chronic inflammation and cancer: suppressing the suppressors. *Cancer Immunology Immunotherapy, 63*(1), 11–20.

Cancer.Net. (2015). *The genetics of cancer*. Available at http://www.cancer.net/navigating-cancer-care/cancer-basics/genetics/genetics-cancer (accessed January 20, 2016).

Casey, D. L., Friedman, D. N., Moskowitz, C. S., Hilden, P. D., Sklar, C. A., Wexler, L. H., & Wolden, S. L. (2015). Second cancer risk in childhood cancer survivors treated with intensity-modulated radiation therapy (IMRT). *Pediatric Blood & Cancer, 62*(2). http://onlinelibrary.wiley.com/doi/10.1002/pbc.v62.2/issuetoc311-316.

Centers for Disease Control (CDC). (2015a). *What are the risk factors for skin cancer?* Available at http://www.cdc.gov/cancer/skin/basic_info/risk_factors.htm (accessed January 20, 2016).

Centers for Disease Control and Prevention (CDC). (2015b). *Tobacco-related mortality*. Available at http://www.cdc.gov/tobacco/data_statistics/fact_sheets/health_effects/tobacco_related_mortality/ (accessed January 20, 2016).

Corthay, A. (2014). Does the immune system naturally protect against cancer? *Frontiers in Immunology, 5*, 197.

Coulie, P. G., van den Eynde, B. J., van der Bruggen, P., & Boon, T. (2014). Tumour antigens recognized by T lymphocytes: At the core of cancer immunotherapy. *Nature Reviews Cancer, 14*, 135–146.

Eggert, J. (Ed.). (2010). *Cancer Basics*. Pittsburgh: Oncology Nursing Society.

Farahani, E., Patra, H. K., Jangamreddy, J. R., Rashedi, I., Kawalec, M., Rao Pariti, R. K., & Wiechec, E. (2014). Cell adhesion molecules and their relation to (cancer) cell stemness. *Carcinogenesis, 35*(4), 747–579.

Forbes, S. A., Beare, D., Gunasekaran, P., Leung, K., Bindal, N., Boutselakis, H., & Campbell, P. J. (2015). COSMIC: Exploring the world's knowledge of somatic mutations in human cancer. *Nucleic Acids Research, 43*(D1), D805–D811.

Gabai-Kapara, E., Lahad, A., Kaufman, B., Friedman, E., Segev, S., Renbaum, P., & Levy-Lahad, E. (2014). Population-based screening for breast and ovarian cancer risk due to BRCA1 and BRCA2. *Proceedings of the National Academy of Sciences of the United States of America, 111*(39), 14205–14210.

Jacobs, E. J., Newton, C. C., Carter, B. D., Feskanich, D., Freedman, N. D., Prentice, R. L., & Flanders, W. D. (2015). What proportion of cancer deaths in the contemporary United States is attributable to cigarette smoking? *Annals of Epidemiology, 25*(3), 179–182.

Kessenbrock, K., Wang, C. Y., & Werb, Z. (2015). Matrix metalloproteinases in stem cell regulation and cancer. *Matrix Biology, 44-46*, 184–190.

Klatsky, A. L., Udaltsova, N., Li, Y., Baer, D., Tran, H. N., & Friedman, G. D. (2014). Moderate alcohol intake and cancer: The role of underreporting. *Cancer Causes & Control, 25*(6), 693–699.

Manna, J. D., Wepy, J. A., Hsu, K., Chang, J. W., Cravatt, B. F., & Marnett, L. J. (2014). Identification of the major prostaglandin glycerol ester hydrolase in human cancer cells. *Journal of Biological Chemistry, 289*, 33741–33753.

Morales-Sénchez, A., & Fuentes-Pananá, E. M. (2014). Human viruses and cancer. *Viruses, 6*(10), 4047–4079.

Muller, P. A. J., & Vousden, K. H. (2014). Mutant p53 in cancer: New functions and therapeutic opportunities. *Cancer Cell, 25*(3), 304–317.

National Cancer Institute (NCI). (2013). *Genetic testing for hereditary cancer syndromes*. Available at http://www.cancer.gov/about-cancer/causes-prevention/genetics/genetic-testing-fact-sheet (accessed January 20, 2016).

National Cancer Institute (NCI). (2015a). *Alcohol and cancer risk*. Available at http://www.cancer.gov/about-cancer/causes-prevention/risk/alcohol/alcohol-fact-sheet (accessed January 20, 2016).

National Cancer Institute (NCI). (2015b). *BRCA1 and BRCA2: Cancer risk and genetic testing*. Available at http://www.cancer.gov/about-cancer/causes-prevention/genetics/brca-fact-sheet (accessed January 20, 2016).

National Cancer Institute (NCI). (2015c). *Cancer vaccines*. Available at http://www.cancer.gov/about-cancer/causes-prevention/vaccines-fact-sheet (accessed January 20, 2016).

National Cancer Institute (NCI). (2015d). *Genetic testing for hereditary cancer syndromes*. Available at http://www.cancer.gov/about-cancer/causes-prevention/genetics/genetic-testing-fact-sheet (accessed January 20, 2016).

National Cancer Institute (NCI). (2015e). *Harms of cigarette smoking and health benefits of quitting*. Available at http://www.cancer.gov/about-cancer/causes-prevention/risk/tobacco/cessation-fact-sheet#q1 (accessed January 20, 2016).

National Cancer Institute (NCI). (2015f). *HIV infection and cancer risk*. Available at http://www.cancer.gov/about-cancer/causes-prevention/risk/infectious-agents/hiv-fact-sheet (accessed January 20, 2016).

National Cancer Institute (NCI). (2015g). *Late effects of treatment for childhood cancer (PDQ)*. Available at http://www.cancer.gov/types/childhood-cancers/late-effects-pdq (accessed January 20, 2016).

National Cancer Institute (NCI). (2015h). *Radiation risk assessment tool (RadRAT) for estimating lifetime risk of developing cancer from exposure to ionizing radiation*. Available at http://dceg.cancer.gov/tools/risk-assessment/radrat (for radiation exposure) (accessed January 20, 2016).

National Cancer Institute (NCI). (2015i). *Tumor markers*. Available at http://www.cancer.gov/about-cancer/diagnosis-staging/diagnosis/tumor-markers-fact-sheet (accessed January 20, 2016).

National Institutes of Health (NIH). (2001). *Stem cell information: Early development*. Available at http://stemcells.nih.gov/info/scireport/appendixa.asp#figure1 (accessed January 20, 2016).

National Institutes of Health (NIH). (2005). *Stem cell basics*. Available at http://stemcells.nih.gov/info/basics/basics2.asp (accessed January 20, 2016).

Nielsen, T. O., Friis-Hansen, L., Poulsen, S. S., Federspiel, B., & Sorensen, B. S. (2014). Expression of the EGF family in gastric cancer: Downregulation of HER4 and its activating ligand NRG4. *PLoS One, 9*(4), e94606.

Pae, M., Meydani, S. N., & Wu, D. (2012). The role of nutrition in enhancing immunity in aging. *Aging and Disease, 3*(1), 91–129.

Pickup, M. W., Mouw, J. K., & Weaver, V. M. (2014). The extracellular matrix modulates the hallmarks of cancer. *EMBO Reports, 15*(12), 1243–1253.

Recondo, G., Jr., Díaz-Cantón, E., de la Vega, M., Greco, M., Recondo, G., Sr., & Valsecchi, M. E. (2014). Advances and new perspectives in the treatment of metastatic colon cancer. *World Journal of Gastrointestinal Oncology*, 6(7), 211–224.

Roberts, S. M., James, R. C., & Williams, P. L. (2015). *Principles of toxicology: Environmental and industrial applications* (3rd ed.). Hoboken, New Jersey: John Wiley & Sons.

Shiozawa, Y., Eber, M. R., Berry, J. E., & Taichman, R. S. (2015). Bone marrow as a metastatic niche for disseminated tumor cells from solid tumors. *BoneKEy Reports*, 4, 689.

U.S. Department of Health and Human Services. (2014). *The health consequences of smoking: 50 years of progress. A report of the surgeon general.* Atlanta: U.S. Department of Health and Human Services, Centers for Disease Control and Prevention, National Center for Chronic Disease Prevention and Health Promotion, Office on Smoking and Health.

Weissman, I. L. (2015). Stem cells are units of natural selection for tissue formation, for germline development, and in cancer development. *Proceedings of the National Academy of Sciences of the United States of America*, 112(29), 8922–8928.

Wolff, A. C., Hammond, M. E., Hicks, D. G., Dowsett, M., McShane, L. M., & Hayes, D. F. (2014). Recommendations for human epidermal growth factor receptor 2 testing in breast cancer. *Archives of Pathology & Laboratory Medicine*, 138(2), 241–256.

Yarbro, C. H., Wujcik, D., & Gobel, B. H. (2010). *Cancer nursing: Principles and practice* (7th ed.). Burlington, MA: Jones & Bartlett Learning.

Yu, H., Lee, H., Herrmann, A., Buettner, R., & Jove, R. (2014). Revisiting STAT3 signaling in cancer: new and unexpected biological functions. *Nature Reviews Cancer*, 14, 736–746.

Cancer Genetics

Suzanne M. Mahon

Molecular Genetics

Genes, the smallest functional units of inherited information in living organisms, are the controlling factors for cellular development and function. Genes provide the instructions for making proteins by using different combinations of amino acids, and they regulate when and where a protein is produced (i.e., regulatory sequence). The process of making proteins is called *protein synthesis*.

Proteins are large, complex molecules that perform essential roles in cellular maintenance, growth, and function. Various types of proteins catalyze biochemical reactions (i.e., enzymes such as transferases), provide structure in the cytoskeleton and muscles (e.g., actin, tubulin), participate in immune responses (e.g., antibodies), act as messengers (e.g., hormones), and store or transport ligands (e.g., hemoglobin).

DNA Synthesis

Deoxyribonucleic acid (DNA) is a large, self-replicating molecule located in the nucleus and mitochondria of each cell. The condensed, coiled forms (i.e., chromosomes) contain smaller units (i.e., genes) that provide codes (i.e., instructions) for the construction of every protein in the body. Commonly used genetic terms are shown in the box on page 26.

The double-helix form of DNA is a pair of molecules consisting of polymers (i.e., long chains) of interlocking nucleotides, called *chromatin*. Nucleotides are the basic structural units of nucleic acids such as DNA and RNA. The chemical building blocks consist of a phosphate, a five-carbon sugar, and a base (i.e., adenine [A], guanine [G], thymine [T], or cytosine [C]). Arrangement of the bases can be likened to a genetic alphabet that is used to create the language of intercellular and intracellular communication (see figure below).

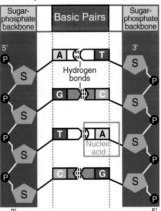

Deoxyribonucleic Acid (DNA)

Model of Deoxyribonucleic Acid (DNA). A base pair is two chemical bases bonded to one another, forming a rung of the DNA ladder. The DNA molecule consists of two strands that wind around each other like a twisted ladder. Each strand has a backbone made of alternating sugar (i.e., deoxyribose) and phosphate groups. Attached to each sugar is one of four bases: adenine (A), cytosine (C), guanine (G), or thymine (T). Adenine forms a base pair with thymine, and cytosine forms a base pair with guanine. The two strands are held together by hydrogen bonds between the bases. (From http://www.genome.gov/dmd/img.cfm?node=Photos/Graphics&id=85272 [accessed December 10, 2015]).

Terms Used in Genetics

Allele: One of several forms of a gene at a particular location on a chromosome.

Amino acid: Basic building block of all proteins. The genetic code encodes the 20 standard amino acids used by cells to build proteins and can produce nonstandard amino acids that are substituted for standard forms.

Aneuploidy: The gain or loss of chromosomes from the normal 46.

Anticipation: The signs and symptoms of some genetic conditions tend to become more severe and appear at an earlier age as the disorder is passed from one generation to the next.

Autosome: Chromosome that is not a sex chromosome. Humans have 22 pairs of autosomal chromosomes.

Autosomal dominant: Mendelian inheritance pattern in which an affected individual possesses one copy of a mutant allele and one normal copy, with a 50% chance that the allele and associated disorder or disease will be passed to offspring.

Autosomal recessive: A trait or disorder that appears only in people who have received two copies of a mutant or altered gene (i.e., one from each parent).

Base pairs: A nucleotide is composed of a molecule containing phosphoric acid, sugar, and a base. The bases are designated by the letters A, T, G, and C, representing adenine, thymine, guanine, and cytosine, respectively.

Biallelic: Both alleles of a gene are affected.

Chromosome: Threadlike structure of nucleic acids and proteins in the nucleus of the cell that contains genes. Humans have 23 pairs of chromosomes; 22 pairs are autosomes, and 1 pair is a set of sex chromosomes.

Codon: A group of three nucleotides that form a unit of genetic code in a DNA or RNA molecule.

Deletion: Type of chromosomal abnormality in which a piece of DNA is removed or omitted from a gene, which disrupts the normal structure and function of the gene.

DNA sequencing: Determination of the exact order of the base pairs (i.e., adenine, guanine, cytosine, and thymine) in a segment of DNA.

Duplication: Type of chromosomal abnormality in which a piece of DNA is abnormally copied one or more times.

Exon: Region of a gene that contains part of the code for producing a protein. Each exon codes for a specific portion of the complete protein.

Fluorescence in situ hybridization (FISH): Laboratory process that involves painting chromosomes or sections of chromosomes with fluorescent molecules. It is a useful technique for identifying chromosomal abnormalities and gene mapping.

Frameshift: Type of chromosomal abnormality in which there is an addition or loss of DNA bases that changes a gene's reading frame that codes for one amino acid.

Gene: Functional and physical unit of heredity that is passed from parent to offspring and contains information necessary for making a specific protein.

Genome: Entire set of chromosomes contained in each cell of an organism.

Genotype: Genetic identity that may or may not be physically manifested in outward characteristics.

Germline: Inherited material that comes from the egg or sperm and is passed to offspring.

Heterozygous: Possessing two different forms of a particular gene; one is inherited from each parent.

Homozygous: Possessing two identical forms of a particular gene; one is inherited from each parent.

Insertion: Type of chromosomal abnormality in which an extra piece of DNA is inserted into a gene, resulting in the disruption of the normal structure and function of that gene.

Intron: Segment of DNA or RNA that does not code for proteins and interrupts the sequence of genes; it is deleted during protein synthesis because it is not needed.

Karyotype: Visual presentation of the chromosomal complement of an individual, including all chromosomes and abnormalities.

Microsatellite: A repetitive, short sequence of DNA that is used as a genetic marker to track inheritance patterns in families.

Missense: Type of chromosomal abnormality in which one amino acid is substituted for another.

Monosomy: Form of aneuploidy in which there is only one copy of a particular chromosome instead of two.

Mutation: A permanent structural change in DNA.

Next-generation sequencing (NSG): Laboratory technique in which many strands of DNA are sequenced at the same time, generating far more data per instrument run than the Sanger method.

Nonsense: Point mutation in a sequence of DNA that results in a stop codon that prematurely ends the process of building a protein.

Oncogene: Mutated gene that leads to transformation of normal cells into cancer cells.

Penetrance: Portion of a population with a particular genotype or mutation that expresses the corresponding phenotype of disorder.

Phenotype: Set of observable characteristics or traits of an organism resulting from the interaction of its genotype with the environment.

Polymerase chain reaction (PCR): Laboratory technique that is a fast, relatively inexpensive means for making an unlimited number of copies of any piece of DNA.

Polymorphism: One or more variations in base pairs in a particular genetic sequence that do not affect protein function.

Proband: Person who serves as the starting point for the genetic study of a family; also called the *spokesperson*. Risks are calculated based on an individual's relation to the proband.

Promoter: DNA sequence that defines where transcription of a gene begins. Transcription is initiated in the promoter part of the gene by binding enzymes and proteins called transcription factors.

Sanger sequencing: Original sequencing technology that helped scientists to determine the human genetic code. Now automated, it is still used to sequence short pieces of DNA.

Single-nucleotide polymorphisms (SNPs): Each SNP (pronounced *snip*) represents a variation in a single nucleotide. SNPs normally occur about once in every 300 nucleotides in an individual's DNA. These variations usually are found in the DNA between genes functioning as biologic markers, helping scientists locate genes associated with disease. There are about 10 million SNPs in the human genome.

Somatic cells: All cells in the body except the reproductive cells.

Translocation: Breaking and removal of a large segment of DNA from one chromosome, followed by the segment's attachment to a different chromosome. This can alter gene expression.

Trisomy: The most common form of aneuploidy, it is the presence of an extra chromosome in each cell.

Tumor suppressor gene: A protective gene that usually limits the growth of tumor cells. If mutated, it may not be able to keep a cancer from growing (e.g., *BRCA* genes).

Variable expression: Many genetic disorders have a wide variety of signs and symptoms, but not all individuals with the same disorder express them to the same degree.

The two strands of DNA are aligned as two complementary threads and held together by hydrogen bonds. The bonds are disrupted when the cell undergoes DNA or protein synthesis. The bases in the two adjoining strands can pair with only one predetermined base. Two paired nucleotides are called a *base pair*. A pairs with T, and G pairs with C. The only possible combinations of the bases are A with T, T with A, C with G, and G with C. For example, an A on one strand of DNA can pair only with the T on the complementary strand. If the sequence of nucleotides on one DNA strand is known, the order of the complementary DNA strand can be predicted accurately. There are approximately 3 billion base pairs in the human genome. Base pairing ensures the structural integrity of DNA and is essential for the storage, retrieval, and transference of genetic information.

During mitosis, the DNA content of the dividing cell must first replicate through the process of DNA synthesis, which takes place in the nucleus of the cell. The original strands of DNA are the templates for the construction of new DNA. An enzyme, topoisomerase, is responsible for unwinding the double helix by cleaving a single strand of DNA. Other enzymes called *helicases* then disassociate the hydrogen bonds that connect the two strands. The unwinding of the two strands of DNA, with each one acting as a template for a new strand, is known as *semiconservative replication*. The DNA relaxes, unwinds, slightly straightens, and separates the two strands.

The intertwined double strands of DNA are antiparallel (i.e., run in opposite directions) with the asymmetric ends (referred to as *five prime* [5'] and *three prime* [3']) winding around a helix axis in a right-handed spiral. In a vertical double helix, 3' is designated as *ascending*, and 5' is designated as *descending*. The polymerase enzyme attaches itself to one strand and descends from the 5' to the 3' direction. As the enzyme moves along the strand, it reads the base sequence and forms a new string of DNA complementary to the template strand. After the strands of DNA are replicated, they condense into supercoiled chromosome sets that separate to become part of two new daughter cells.

Protein Synthesis

Protein synthesis is the process by which genes serve as codes for the production of amino acids and proteins. This activity occurs in the ribosomes, which are ribonucleoprotein complexes found in the cytoplasm of the cell. Proteins are formed by peptide bonds between individual amino acids in a linear strand. To accomplish protein synthesis, a particular DNA sequence (i.e., gene) for a specific protein is transcribed into a piece of ribonucleic acid (RNA). RNA consists of a sugar-phosphate backbone with a nucleotide attached. Although RNA is similar to DNA, it uses the nucleotide base U instead of T and has a hydroxyl group attached to its ribose sugar.

Protein synthesis consists of two phases: transcription and translation. The overall process arranges amino acids into proteins through the action of several types of RNA and various enzymes. Initially, the cells receive a message to produce a specific protein. Transcription begins when the enzyme RNA polymerase attaches to a segment of the DNA (i.e., gene)

and creates a transcription bubble, which separates ("unzips") the two strands of the DNA helix, as also occurs during cell division. RNA polymerase moves along the strand of exposed gene and transcribes the subunits of DNA by adding matching RNA nucleotides to the complementary nucleotides of the DNA strand. The new strand is called *messenger RNA* (mRNA). The previously exposed segment of DNA closes and remains in the nucleus of the cell. Before the transcribed mRNA moves from the nucleus into the cytoplasm, nuclear enzymes remove introns (i.e., noncoding sections, also called *junk DNA*) and splice together exons (i.e., sequences that code for proteins). This process is repeated as long as the signal to make the desired protein remains viable.

In the translation phase, the information contained in the mRNA is converted into a sequence of amino acids in proteins. The copies of mRNA enter the cytoplasm through channels (i.e., pores) in the nucleus, bind to ribosomal RNA (rRNA) found in the cytoplasm, and are decoded. The mRNA is encoded with information about the particular arrangement of amino acids that makes up the final protein. During translation, a molecule of transfer RNA (tRNA) matches the strand of mRNA and carries the correct amino acids to the ribosome. Three nucleotide bases (i.e., codons) are read at a time, and each codon represents a specific amino acid (see figure on page 28). As each codon is decoded, the corresponding amino acid is activated. The amino acids are brought into the proper sequence as the entire message is read, and the newly formed polypeptide chain then folds into its final three-dimensional shape based on chemical bonds formed between amino acids. The total number of amino acids in a specific protein and the exact code that links them together determine the nature and activity of the protein. Different sequences of amino acids change the shape of the proteins and therefore their function.

Neoplasia

The term *neoplasia* signifies a new growth of cells in the body. Although all neoplasms are considered abnormal, they are further designated as benign (i.e., noncancerous) or malignant (i.e., cancerous). All tumors, whether benign or malignant, have two things in common: a parenchyma (i.e., functional part) that contains proliferating neoplastic cells and a stroma (i.e., supportive structure) consisting of connective tissue and blood vessels.

Benign Neoplasia

Benign neoplastic cells enter and progress through the phases of the cell cycle in the same fashion as normal cells. Benign neoplastic cells arise from normal cells and tend to retain most of the properties of the cells from which they arose. At the microscopic level, benign cells are euploid, containing the normal chromosome complement. However, because their behavior is not completely normal, it is likely that some alteration in gene regulation exists.

Benign neoplastic cells are characterized by increased proliferation or decreased apoptosis (i.e., programmed cell death). Unlike normal cells, benign neoplastic cells have lost the characteristic of density-dependent contact inhibition. Benign neoplastic cells continue to grow by expansion into the surrounding tissue.

RNA codon table

1st Position	2nd Position				3rd Position
	U	**C**	**A**	**G**	
U	Phe Phe Leu Leu	Ser Ser Ser Ser	Tyr Tyr stop stop	Cys Cys stop Trp	U C A G
C	Leu Leu Leu Leu	Pro Pro Pro Pro	His His Gln Gln	Arg Arg Arg Arg	U C A G
A	Ile Ile Ile Met	Thr Thr Thr Thr	Asn Asn Lys Lys	Ser Ser Arg Arg	U C A G
G	Val Val Val Val	Ala Ala Ala Ala	Asp Asp Glu Glu	Gly Gly Gly Gly	U C A G

— Amino Acids —

Ala: Alanine
Arg: Arginine
Asn: Asparagine
Asp: Aspartic acid
Cys: Cysteine
Gln: Glutamine
Glu: Glutamic acid
Gly: Glycine
His: Histidine
Ile: Isoleucine
Leu: Leucine
Lys: Lysine
Met: Methionine
Phe: Phenylalanine
Pro: Proline
Ser: Serine
Thr: Threonine
Trp: Tryptophane
Tyr: Tyrosine
Val: Valine

Genetic Code. Instructions in a gene tell the cell how to make a specific protein. The chemicals adenine (A), cytosine (C), guanine (G), and thymine (T) are the nucleotide bases of the DNA code that are transcribed and translated by RNA to form a protein. In DNA transcription, thymine pairs with adenine, but in RNA, uracil is used instead of thymine. Each gene's code combines the four chemicals in various ways to spell out three-letter codons that specify which amino acid is needed at every step in making a protein. (From http://www.genome.gov/dmd/img.cfm ?node=Photos/Graphics&id=85173 [accessed December 10, 2015]).

Although benign neoplastic cells have lost some degree of growth control, they have not developed the ability to metastasize (i.e., spread to other organs), which is the hallmark of a malignant neoplasm. The suffix-*oma* is often assigned to designate a neoplasm on the basis of the cell of origin (e.g., fibroma [fibroblastic cell], osteoma [bone cell]). The type of pattern that it displays may be used to name a benign neoplasm. For example, an adenoma usually displays a glandular pattern, but it may arise from several different types of cells (e.g., epithelium, glandular).

Benign neoplastic tissues are typically well differentiated. They are morphologically and functionally similar to the normal tissues from which they arose. They retain a small nuclear-to-cytoplasmic ratio and continue to synthesize fibronectin, as do normal cells. Like normal cells, benign neoplastic cells adhere tightly and do not metastasize. Even so, benign neoplastic growth can cause physiologic dysfunction and death. For example, a benign tumor can exert pressure on nerves and blood vessels or obstruct lumens (e.g., trachea, brain, colon) (Hong & American Association for Cancer Research, 2010).

Malignant Neoplasia

Proteins play an important role in the development of malignant disease. The normal cell cycle is regulated by proteins called *cyclins, cyclin-dependent kinases,* and *cyclin-dependent kinase inhibitors.* The role of these proteins is to provide cell cycle checkpoints to control the signals that coordinate cell reproduction. Checkpoints occur in late G_1 before DNA synthesis, during the S phase when DNA content is duplicated, and in G_2 before cells become completely committed to mitosis. These checkpoints occur at times during the cell cycle when cells are most vulnerable to the harmful effects of DNA (genetic) damage. The checkpoints allow cells to make DNA repairs and remove damaged molecules before they threaten the survival of the organism (Hong & American Association for Cancer Research, 2010).

Normal cells have multiple copies of specific DNA sequences and proteins at the ends of their chromosomes called *telomeres.* Each time a cell divides, it loses a telomere, which shortens the chromosome. When the chromosome is shortened to a predetermined length, the cell is signaled to enter a resting stage, also known as *senescence.* The cell remains viable but stops reproducing. Normal cells in a culture plate have a limited life span and a specific number of doubling times before they enter senescence.

Normal cells display contact inhibition. After the cells reach the boundary of the culture dish, they stop proliferating. Malignant cells are immortal, and in a culture medium, their growth is not confined to the surface of the culture dish. When malignant cells reach the edges of the culture dish, they continue to grow on top of each other.

Normal cells are anchorage dependent. With the exception of hematopoietic cells, they must be attached to a surface (i.e., substratum) to proliferate. Malignant neoplastic cells are capable of growing without a supporting substratum. Because malignant cells have lost anchorage dependence, they grow easily in suspension in an agarose or other medium, whereas normal cells must adhere to the surface of the culture plate to grow.

Cancer cells range from well differentiated to anaplastic (i.e., undifferentiated). Anaplasia, or lack of differentiation, is a classic sign of malignant transformation. As cancer progresses, the cells become increasingly anaplastic until they no longer resemble the parent tissue, and most differentiated functions are lost. Cancer cells continually undergo mitosis and perform fewer and fewer differentiated functions. As a result, cancer cells have a large nucleus-to-cytoplasm ratio, whereas the reverse is true for normal cells.

The nomenclature for malignant neoplasms is the same as that used for benign tumors. Cancerous tumors of epithelial cell origin are called *carcinomas* (e.g., bronchogenic carcinoma [respiratory], renal cell carcinoma [kidney], hepatocellular carcinoma [liver]). *Adenocarcinoma* is a term reserved for tumors that display a glandular pattern. Cancers arising from smooth muscle are called *leiomyosarcomas*, whereas the term *leukemia* refers to a hematopoietic malignancy.

Germline and Somatic Mutations

Many different mutations occur in malignant cells (Fisher, Pusztai, & Swanton, 2013). Malignancies may develop as a result of the conversion of proto-oncogenes to oncogenes. Proto-oncogenes (i.e., normal genes before they are altered by mutations) regulate normal cell growth, whereas oncogenes (i.e., mutated genes) are associated with abnormal cell growth, leading to increased cellular proliferation and uncontrolled growth.

Some tumors arise because of the inactivation of both alleles of tumor suppressor genes, which play an important role in slowing or stopping abnormal cell growth. Tumor suppressor genes include caretaker genes, which maintain integrity of the genetic material, and gatekeeper genes, which regulate proliferation and cell life (Gunder & Martin, 2011).

Mismatch repair (MMR) genes repair mistakes that occur during DNA replication (Brown, 2009). When MMR genes are damaged, genetic stability is altered, and tumor cells replicate. Some mutations interfere with apoptosis.

Somatic mutations can spontaneously arise in any cell in the body except germ cells (i.e., eggs and sperm) at any time during the patient's life. This type of mutation is limited to the descendants of the original cell that developed the mutation, and it is not present in other cells in the patient's body (Gunder & Martin, 2011). Because it is not in the germ cells, the mutation cannot be passed from parent to child. Somatic mutations are responsible for most malignancies. Sporadic cancers occur from multiple somatic mutations in a cell. Acquired somatic mutations develop in DNA during a person's lifetime. Some somatic genetic mutations associated with a risk of developing cancer are shown in the table below.

The other type of mutation is a *germline mutation,* which occurs in the patient's germ cells and can be passed to future generations. A patient who inherits a germline mutation has that mutation in all of the cells of his or her body because the mutation was present at conception. Germline mutations are associated with hereditary cancer predisposition syndromes and account for approximately 10% of all malignancies (Gunder & Martin, 2011). Common germline mutations associated with the risk of developing cancer are shown in the table below and on page 30.

Selected Somatic Genetic Changes with Targeted Agent

Gene	Targeted Agent*	Clinical Situation
ALK	Crizotinib, ceritinib	Non–small cell lung cancer (NSCLC)
BRAF V600E	Vemurafenib, dabrafenib	Metastatic melanoma
BRCA1/2	Olaparib, veliparib, iniparib	Metastatic ovarian cancer and breast cancer with BRCA 1/2 mutations
EGFR	Erlotinib, gefitinib, cetuximab	Amplification in metastatic NSCLC
EGFR T790M	Erlotinib, gefitinib	Resistance to EGFR tyrosine kinase inhibitors in NSCLC
EGFR L858R	Erlotinib	Resistance to EGFR tyrosine kinase inhibitors in NSCLC
HER2 amplification	Trastuzumab, pertuzumab	HER2-positive breast cancer or metastatic gastric or gastroesophageal junction adenocarcinoma
KRAS	Cetuximab, panitumumab	Resistance to EGFR antibodies in metastatic colorectal cancer
PML/RAR	ATRA, arsenic trioxide	Acute promyelocytic leukemia

*These agents treat cancers driven by the mutated genes listed in the first column. For example, vemurafenib and dabrafenib are approved for the treatment of late-stage melanoma, a cancer driven by a BRAF mutation.
Data from Boyle, P. (2012). Triple-negative breast cancer: Epidemiological considerations and recommendations. *Annals of Oncology, 23*(Suppl 6), vi7-vi12; Unger, F., Witte, I., and David, K. (2015). Prediction of individual response to anticancer therapy: Historical and future perspectives. *Cellular and Molecular Life Sciences, 72*(4), 729-757; Walther, Z., and Sklar, J. (2011). Molecular tumor profiling for prediction of response to anticancer therapies. *The Cancer Journal, 17*(2), 71-79.

Common Germline Mutations Associated with Hereditary Cancer Syndromes

Gene (Syndrome)*	Associated Cancers
APC (familial adenomatous polyposis)	Colon, small bowel, thyroid
ATM	Breast, colon, pancreatic, ataxia telangiectasia
BARD1	Breast, ovarian
BMPR1A	Colon, gastric
BRCA1	Breast, ovarian, pancreatic, prostate, melanoma
BRCA2	Breast, ovarian, pancreatic, prostate, melanoma
BRIP1	Breast, ovarian
CDH1	Gastric, breast, colon
CDK4	Melanoma, pancreatic, breast
CDKN2A	Melanoma, pancreatic
CHEK2	Breast, prostate, colon
EPCAM (HNPCC)	Colon, endometrial, ovarian, gastric, pancreatic
MEN1 (multiple endocrine neoplasia type 1)	Pituitary, parathyroid, pancreatic adrenal
MLH1 (HNPCC)	Colon, endometrial, ovarian, gastric, pancreatic
MSH2 (HNPCC)	Colon, endometrial, ovarian, gastric, pancreatic
MSH6 (HNPCC)	Colon, endometrial, ovarian, gastric, pancreatic
MUTYH (polyposis syndrome)	Colon, small bowel, endometrial serous carcinoma, MUTYH-associated polyposis, a recessive syndrome
NF1 (neurofibromatosis type 1)	Neurofibromas, breast
NF2 (neurofibromatosis type 2)	Vestibular schwannomas

Continued

Management of Germline Mutations Associated with Hereditary Cancer Syndromes

Identification of a mutation in a family helps risk management and treatment planning for individuals with cancer and at-risk, unaffected family members. Genetic testing is not used in routine screening of a population because of the expense of testing and the complex counseling needs of families. It is best used to help selected individuals from high-risk families to make good decisions about cancer screening and prevention strategies. Key indicators of hereditary cancer syndromes are shown in the table below.

Genetic testing is best carried out by one of several types of credentialed genetics professionals. Geneticists are physicians with board certification in genetics from the American Board of Medical Genetics. Licensed genetics counselors are health care professionals with specialized graduate degrees in the areas of medical genetics and counseling who have been certified by the American Board of Genetic Counseling. Credentialed genetic nurses have specialized education and training in genetics and are credentialed by the American Nurses Credentialing Commission (ANCC) by portfolio and have the Advanced Genetics

Common Germline Mutations Associated with Hereditary Cancer Syndromes—cont'd

Gene (Syndrome)*	Associated Cancers
PALB2	Breast, pancreatic, colon
PMS2 (HNPCC)	Colon, endometrial, ovarian, gastric, pancreatic
PTEN (Cowden syndrome)	Breast, thyroid, endometrial, colon, gastric
RAD51D	Breast, ovarian
RET (multiple endocrine neoplasia type 2)	Thyroid cancer, pheochromocytoma, parathyroid
STK11	Breast, colon, pancreatic, gastric, small bowel, endometrial
TP53 (Li-Fraumeni syndrome)	Breast, sarcoma, brain, hematologic malignancies, adrenocortical malignancies
VHL (von Hippel–Lindau syndrome)	Renal, pancreatic neuroendocrine tumors, hemangioblastoma, pheochromocytoma
XRCC2	Breast, pancreatic

HNPCC, Hereditary nonpolyposis colorectal cancer (i.e., Lynch syndrome).
*All syndromes are autosomal dominant unless noted otherwise.
Modified from Lindor, N. M., McMaster, M. L., Lindor, C. J., & Greene, M. H. (2008). Concise handbook of familial cancer susceptibility syndromes—second edition. *Journal of the National Cancer Institute Monographs, 38*, 1-93.

Key Indicators of Hereditary Cancer Syndromes

Indicator	Examples
Cancer occurring at a younger age than expected in the general population	Breast cancer before age 50 Colon cancer before age 50 Ovarian cancer before 50 Endometrial cancer before age 50
More than one primary cancer	Breast and ovarian cancer Colon and endometrial cancer Synchronous colon cancer
Evidence of autosomal dominant inheritance pattern	Two or more generations affected Both men and women affected
Bilateral cancer in a paired organ	Breast cancer Ovarian cancer Thyroid cancer
Any pattern of cancer associated with a known cancer syndrome	Hereditary breast and ovarian cancer Lynch syndrome Li-Fraumeni syndrome Von Hippel–Lindau syndrome Multiple endocrine neoplasia types 1 and 2
Cancers occurring more frequently in a family than expected in the absence of known environmental and lifestyle risk factors	Cluster of the same cancers, especially in close relatives Breast cancer Colon cancer Pancreatic cancer Kidney cancer Melanoma
Presence of nonmalignant changes associated with a hereditary risk	More than 20 adenomatous polyps in a lifetime Hamartomas Dysplastic nevi

Data from Axilbund, J. E., & Wiley, E. A. (2012). Genetic testing by cancer site: Pancreas. *The Cancer Journal, 18*(4), 350-354; Chan-Smutko, G. (2012). Genetic testing by cancer site: Urinary tract. *The Cancer Journal, 18*(4), 343-349; Daniels, M. S. (2012). Genetic testing by cancer site: Uterus. *The Cancer Journal, 18*(4), 338-342; Gabree, M., & Seidel, M. (2012). Genetic testing by cancer site: Skin. *The Cancer Journal, 18*(4), 372-380; Jasperson, K. W. (2012). Genetic testing by cancer site: Colon (polyposis syndromes). *The Cancer Journal, 18*(4), 328-333; Pilarski, R., & Nagy, R. (2012). Genetic testing by cancer site: Endocrine system. *The Cancer Journal, 18*(4), 364-371; Shannon, K. M., & Chittenden, A. (2012). Genetic testing by cancer site: Breast. *The Cancer Journal, 18*(4), 310-319; Weissman, S. M., Weiss, S. M., & Newlin, A. C. (2012). Genetic testing by cancer site: Ovary. *The Cancer Journal, 18*(4), 320-327.

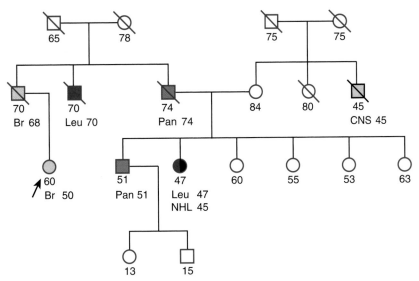

Components of a Pedigree. *Squares* represent males, and *circles* represent females. A *slash* represents a deceased person. *Solid circles* and *squares* represent diagnoses of cancer. The family member's current age or age at death is shown, as well as the age at a cancer diagnosis. The *arrow* represents the proband, or spokesperson, for the family. Three generations showing maternal and paternal sides are included. If information is known about ethnicity, it can be included. Ideally, all cancer diagnoses are verified by pathology reports or death certificates. *Br*, Breast cancer; *CNS*, central nervous system malignancy; *Leu*, leukemia; *Pan*, pancreatic cancer; *NHL*, non-Hodgkin lymphoma.

Mutation Probabilities

BRCA1		MLH1	
BRCAPRO	0.0141	MMRPRO	0.0002
BRCA2		**MSH2**	
BRCAPRO	0.0958	MMRPRO	0.0003
Any BRCA		**MSH6**	
BRCAPRO	0.1099	MMRPRO	0.0001
p16		**Any MMR**	
MELAPRO	0.0001	MMRPRO	0.0006
		Pancreas Gene	
		PANCPRO	0.1709

Cancer Risks	5-Year	Lifetime
Breast		
Gail	NA	NA
Chen	NA	NA
Claus	NA	NA
BRCAPRO	0.033	0.136
Ovarian	0.008	0.040
Colorectal	0.004	0.030
Endometrial	0.003	0.015
Melanoma	0.002	0.012
Pancreas	0.009	0.051

Risk Calculations. The risk calculations are for the proband in the previous figure. Multiple calculations are made using computer software to estimate the chance that an individual has one or more germline mutations. When the risk is greater than 10% (as in this example), offering genetic testing is a consideration. The risk of developing one or more cancers based on the family history is also calculated. In this example, no risks for breast cancer were calculated because the proband already has a diagnosis of breast cancer. *NA*, Not applicable.

Nursing–Board Certified (AGN-BC) credential (formerly the Advance Practice Nurse in Genetics credential). These professionals provide genetic risk assessment services, pedigree construction, and before and after genetic test counseling and coordinate follow-up for other at-risk family members.

Selection of the appropriate genetic test depends on risk factor assessment. This includes an assessment of the risk of developing the cancer and, in many cases, calculations of the risk of carrying a mutation. Genetic risk assessment begins with the construction of a pedigree as shown in the figure above and to the left. The pedigree is an excellent means to educate a family about autosomal dominant transmission, and if a mutation is detected in the family, the pedigree provides a useful tool to identify other family members at risk who should be offered genetic testing. It should be updated as the family history changes.

Ethnicity should be assessed and recorded because some groups (e.g., those of Ashkenazi Jewish ancestry) may be at increased risk for certain hereditary cancer syndromes. This is known as the *founder effect*, which is the accumulation of random genetic changes in an isolated population as a result of its proliferation from only a few parent colonizers (Gunder & Martin, 2011).

After the pedigree is constructed, risks for developing cancers are calculated based on the family history, personal history, and likelihood of having a mutation. If the family history suggests a germline mutation or the family meets designated criteria from a professional agency or Medicare criteria, the family can be offered the option of genetic testing (Berliner, Fay, Cummings, Burnett, & Tillmanns, 2013). Typical elements of genetic counseling before germline genetic testing are described in the box on page 32.

Counseling includes an extensive discussion about what recommendations will likely made based on each genetic testing outcome and about the implications of testing for germline mutations for the patient and the entire family. If a mutation is identified, the immediate family members should inform other relatives that they may be at increased risk. This is an extensive process; a typical pretest counseling session takes approximately 90 minutes (Mahon, 2013).

Typical Elements of Pretest Genetic Counseling

- Explore patient concerns, motivations, and expectations regarding the genetic testing process.
- Clarify misconceptions about the process or concepts.
- Construct a pedigree.
- Document lifestyle and medical history risk factors.
- Perform a targeted physical examination for features associated with hereditary syndromes.
- Discuss factors that limit interpretation and assessment, such as adoption, estrangement from the family, or a small family structure.
- Present basic risk information about developing cancers.
- Present basic information about suspected syndromes.
- Present calculations for the risk of having a mutation or discuss clinical criteria that suggest hereditary risk.
- Discuss principles of genetics such as autosomal transmission, penetrance, founder effect, and germline and somatic mutations.
- Identify and discuss who are the best individuals to test in the family. It is best to begin testing a person who is affected with the disease or cancer because there is a much higher probability of identifying the mutation.
- Discuss alternatives to testing, including not testing.
- Discuss specimen collection, which is usually done with a buccal (saliva) specimen or a blood specimen.
- Discuss potential test outcomes of testing, which can include
  - *True positive:* The person carries the mutation.
  - *True negative:* The person does not carry a mutation known to be in the family.
  - *Noninformative negative:* The person was the first one tested in a family and tested negative for a particular mutation. This means the person does not carry that particular mutation but could have another genetic mutation for which testing has not been completed.
  - *Variant of unknown significance:* The person has a change in genetic material, but it is not clear whether it is associated with a particular disease or malignancy.
- Discuss possible management strategies for each outcome.
- Discuss testing costs, insurance coverage, and preauthorization.
- Discuss possible discrimination issues, especially for life, disability, and long-term care insurance.
- Discuss the potential benefits, risks, and limitations of genetic testing.
- Assess psychosocial support, including resources from the family, community, and religious affiliation.
- Offer opportunities to ask questions for clarification.

Recommendations for cancer prevention and early detection are based on the test results. The results may or may not be informative, and several outcomes of testing are possible (see table on page 33). Recommendations may include increased surveillance, chemoprevention options, lifestyle strategies to decrease risk, and in some cases, prophylactic surgery. In cases of indeterminate results, participation in clinical trials may be an option. If a mutation is detected, other family members should be offered testing. In some cases, other family members may benefit from modified recommendations for cancer prevention and early detection.

Somatic Mutations in Cancer Treatment

Diagnosis. Somatic genetic testing is sometimes done on tumor specimens to clarify the diagnosis. For example, identification of the *BRAF* V600E mutation in a thyroid tumor specimen is diagnostic for papillary thyroid carcinoma (Dancey, Bedard, Onetto, & Hudson, 2012). The presence of a somatic *BRAF* mutation in a colorectal tumor showing high microsatellite instability suggests the tumor is sporadic and not a case of hereditary nonpolyposis colorectal cancer (HNPCC), which is sometimes referred to as *Lynch syndrome* (Schneider, Schneider, Kloor, Fürst, & Möslein, 2012).

Prognosis. Somatic mutation profiles can help clarify the prognosis for some malignancies. Patients who have activating mutations in *KRAS* who have adenocarcinomas of the lung, colon, and pancreas often have a poor prognosis (Unger, Witte, & David, 2015). For some women, the loss-of-function mutations in *PTEN* are associated with a poor prognosis in cases of breast cancer and oligodendroglioma but conversely are associated with a better prognosis in cases of endometrial cancer (Tan et al., 2012). Women diagnosed with breast cancer that is estrogen receptor negative, progesterone receptor negative, and nonamplified *HER2* (i.e., triple-negative breast cancer) may have a more aggressive form of breast cancer that can sometimes be more difficult to treat (Boyle, 2012).

Risk of Recurrence. Understanding what the risk of recurrence is for a cancer and the potential benefits of systemic therapy can help patients make treatment decisions. Systemic therapy can have toxic short-term and long-term effects. Genetic evaluation of breast, prostate, and colon malignant tumors can estimate the chance of recurrence and the potential benefit of systemic therapy. For example, the Oncotype DX test for stage I or II breast cancers that are estrogen receptor positive, progesterone receptor positive, and nonamplified *HER2* examines 21 genes in a tumor to determine a *recurrence score*. The recurrence score is a number between 0 and 100 that corresponds to the likelihood of breast cancer recurrence within 10 years of the initial diagnosis, and it is reported as low, intermediate, or high risk (Joh et al., 2011).

Treatment. Increasing numbers of somatic mutations have been identified that indicate whether a tumor will be susceptible or resistant to anticancer therapy. Activating mutations in kinase genes (e.g., *EGFR*, *KIT*, and *BRAF*) or translocations that lead to overexpression of kinases (e.g., *ALK*) often result in susceptibility of the tumor cells to small-molecule inhibitors that are selective for the affected kinase.

Tyrosine kinase inhibitors (TKIs) are a class of chemotherapy medications that block the enzyme tyrosine kinase. TKIs are a form of targeted therapy that lessens the risk of damage to healthy cells and increases the likelihood of treatment success. Unfortunately, treatment with these targeted agents often leads to acquired resistance as the result of selection for additional somatic mutations, such as the T790M missense mutation of *EGFR* (Walther & Sklar, 2011). The table on page 33 lists some selected somatic mutations and targeted therapy agents.

Pharmacogenomics

There is a growing body of knowledge about how some alleles in germline DNA contribute to therapeutic responses. Pharmacogenomics is the study of how gene variants affect a person's response to drugs. This relatively new field combines pharmacology and genomics to develop effective, safe medications and doses that

Possible Outcomes of Genetic Testing

Test Result	Implications for Individual	Implications for Family	Other Considerations
Positive for a deleterious mutation *or* Positive for a suspected deleterious mutation	At increased risk for developing cancers	First-degree relatives (siblings and offspring) have a 50% chance of having the mutation. Single-site testing can clarify whether the family member has the mutation and associated increased risk. Single-site testing is lower in cost.	Does not identify what type of cancer will develop or when, only that the risk is higher Enables individual to make decisions about prevention and early detection
True negative—no mutation detected in a person with known mutation in the family	Can follow population-based general recommendations for cancer prevention and early detection	Offspring from the individual are not at risk for autosomal dominant syndromes. Testing of offspring is unnecessary.	Provides a more accurate cancer risk assessment Provides psychological relief regarding risk for developing cancer and that offspring will not inherit the mutation Potential for a false sense of security, resulting in failure to get screening recommended for those of average risk May cause individuals to feel guilty that they "escaped" the mutation (i.e., survivor guilt)
Negative result—no mutation identified in the family	This noninformative result usually occurs when the first person in a family is tested. The cancer may be the result of a different mutation from the one tested, or the cancer seen in the family may occur because of nonhereditary reasons. Recommendations are based on personal and family risk factors. Individuals may consider participating in research studies or high-risk registries.	Testing is not appropriate for unaffected members in the family because they will also likely test negative.	Cancer prevention and early detection measures are based on personal and family history and risk factors.
Variant of indeterminate significance	Test identifies a mutation; it is not clear whether it is a polymorphism or deleterious. This indeterminate test result does not provide meaningful information. It may provoke anxiety and confusion. Cancer prevention and early detection measures are based on personal and family history and risk factors. Individuals may consider participation in a research study or hereditary cancer registry.	Meaningful testing will not be available to other family members.	Recommendations for cancer prevention and detection should be based on personal risk factors and family history with careful information about potential benefits and risks.

can be tailored to a person's genetic makeup. Response to drug therapy varies from person to person. It can be difficult to predict who will benefit from a medication, who will not respond at all, and who will experience negative side effects (i.e., adverse drug reactions). For example, a dihydropyrimidine dehydrogenase deficiency can limit dosages and sometimes lead to life-threatening toxicity in persons receiving 5-fluorouracil (Offer et al., 2014). Identification of patients who carry these variants can guide treatment selection to avoid unnecessary toxicity.

Conclusion

Knowledge of genetics is revolutionizing cancer care. Understanding these concepts is essential in oncology nursing practice. Nurses need to be able to identify patients and families with possible germline mutations and refer them to genetics professionals for evaluation. Patients should understand the difference between germline and somatic mutations.

More tests are being developed to analyze tumor specimens for somatic changes to provide information for diagnosis, prognosis, and effective treatment selection. Pharmacogenomics is an emerging field that offers a way to select the best treatment with the least toxicity.

References

Axilbund, J. E., & Wiley, E. A. (2012). Genetic testing by cancer site: Pancreas. *The Cancer Journal, 18*(4), 350–354.

Berliner, J., Fay, A., Cummings, S., Burnett, B., & Tillmanns, T. (2013). NSGC practice guideline: Risk assessment and genetic counseling for hereditary breast and ovarian cancer. *Journal of Genetic Counseling, 22*(2), 155–163.

Boyle, P. (2012). Triple-negative breast cancer: Epidemiological considerations and recommendations. *Annals of Oncology, 23*(Suppl. 6), vi7–vi12.

Brown, S. M. (2009). *Essentials of medical genetics* (2nd ed.). Hoboken, NJ: John Wiley & Sons.

Chan-Smutko, G. (2012). Genetic testing by cancer site: Urinary tract. *The Cancer Journal, 18*(4), 343–349.

Dancey, J. E., Bedard, P. ,L., Onetto, N., & Hudson, T. J. (2012). The genetic basis for cancer treatment decisions. *Cell, 148*(3), 409–420.

Daniels, M. S. (2012). Genetic testing by cancer site: Uterus. *The Cancer Journal*, *18*(4), 338–342.

Fisher, R., Pusztai, L., & Swanton, C. (2013). Cancer heterogeneity: Implications for targeted therapeutics. *British Journal of Cancer*, *108*(3), 479–485.

Gabree, M., & Seidel, M. (2012). Genetic testing by cancer site: Skin. *The Cancer Journal*, *18*(4), 372–380.

Gunder, L. M., & Martin, S. A. (2011). *Essentials of medical genetics for health professionals*. Sudbury, MA: Jones & Bartlett Learning.

Hong, W. K., & American Association for Cancer Research. (2010). *Holland-Frei cancer medicine 8* (8th ed.). Shelton, CT: People's Medical Publishing House.

Jasperson, K. W. (2012). Genetic testing by cancer site: Colon (polyposis syndromes). *The Cancer Journal*, *18*(4), 328–333.

Joh, J. E., Esposito, N. N., Kiluk, J. V., Laronga, C., Lee, M. C., Loftus, L., & Acs, G. (2011). The effect of Oncotype DX recurrence score on treatment recommendations for patients with estrogen receptor–positive early stage breast cancer and correlation with estimation of recurrence risk by breast cancer specialists. *The Oncologist*, *16*(11), 1520–1526.

Lindor, N. M., McMaster, M. L., Lindor, C. J., & Greene, M. H. (2008). Concise handbook of familial cancer susceptibility syndromes - second edition. *Journal of the National Cancer Institute, Monographs*, *38*, 1–93.

Mahon, S. (2013). Allocation of work activities in a comprehensive cancer genetics program. *Clinical Journal of Oncology Nursing*, *17*(4), 397–404.

Offer, S. M., Fossum, C. C., Wegner, N. J., Stuflesser, A. J., Butterfield, G. L., & Diasio, R. B. (2014). Comparative functional analysis of DPYD variants of potential clinical relevance to dihydropyrimidine dehydrogenase activity. *Cancer Research*, *74*(9), 2545–2554.

Pilarski, R., & Nagy, R. (2012). Genetic testing by cancer site: Endocrine system. *The Cancer Journal*, *18*(4), 364–371.

Schneider, R., Schneider, C., Kloor, M., Fürst, A., & Möslein, G. (2012). Lynch syndrome: Clinical, pathological, and genetic insights. *Langenbeck's Archives of Surgery*, *397*(4), 513–525.

Shannon, K. M., & Chittenden, A. (2012). Genetic testing by cancer site: Breast. *The Cancer Journal*, *18*(4), 310–319.

Tan, M.-H., Mester, J. L., Ngeow, J., Rybicki, L. A., Orloff, M. S., & Eng, C. (2012). Lifetime cancer risks in individuals with germline PTEN mutations. *Clinical Cancer Research*, *18*(2), 400–407.

Unger, F., Witte, I., & David, K. (2015). Prediction of individual response to anticancer therapy: Historical and future perspectives. *Cellular and Molecular Life Sciences*, *72*(4), 729–757.

Walther, Z., & Sklar, J. (2011). Molecular tumor profiling for prediction of response to anticancer therapies. *The Cancer Journal*, *17*(2), 71–79.

Weissman, S. M., Weiss, S. M., & Newlin, A. C. (2012). Genetic testing by cancer site: Ovary. *The Cancer Journal*, *18*(4), 320–327.

Breast Cancer

Nicole Korak

Invasive Breast Cancer

Definition

Invasive breast cancer, also referred to as infiltrating breast cancer, has spread beyond the basement membrane of the duct or lobule of the breast and into the surrounding tissue. Invasive breast cancer is considered a systemic disease because of its ability to spread to distant sites through the vascular or lymphatic systems. The breast includes the following anatomic areas (see figure below):

- Nipple
- Areola
- Duct and ductule
- Lactiferous Sinus and lactiferous duct
- Lobules
- Alveolus
- Adipose tissue
- Suspensory ligaments of Cooper
- Pectoralis major and minor muscles
- Associated lymph nodes

Incidence

- In the United States, breast cancer is the most common cancer and the second leading cause of cancer deaths among women.
- An estimated 231,840 new cases of invasive breast cancer were diagnosed in the United States in 2015. This represents 29% of all new cases of cancer in women.
- The incidence is highest among white women, followed by black women.
- The disease is most often diagnosed in women between 55 and 64 years of age (mean age, 61 years), and 89% of all cases between 2007 and 2011 occurred in women older than 45 years.
- The 5-year survival rate continues to improve, and death rates have fallen 1.9% each year between 2002 and 2011, with a projected death rate of 40,730 in 2015.
- Survival is lower for black than for white women at every stage of disease.
- Male breast cancer accounts for fewer than 1% of all breast cancers. An estimated 2350 new diagnoses and 440 deaths occurred in the United States in 2015.

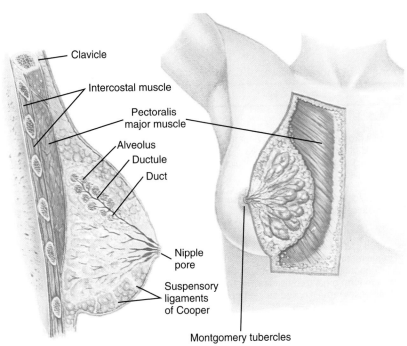

Clavicle
Intercostal muscle
Pectoralis major muscle
Alveolus
Ductule
Duct
Nipple pore
Suspensory ligaments of Cooper
Montgomery tubercles

Anatomy of the Breast (From Lowdermilk DL, Perry SE, Cashion MC, et al (2016). *Maternity and women's health care* (11th ed.) St. Louis: Elsevier Mosby.)

Etiology and Risk Factors

Breast cancer is a heterogeneous disease with no single cause. Several factors are commonly associated with an increased risk of breast cancer:

- Sex: More than 99% of cases occur in women
- Age: Risk increases with age, which is the strongest risk factor
- Personal history of breast cancer: threefold to fourfold increased risk of a second primary breast cancer
- Family history of breast cancer with a greater risk if:
  - One first-degree relative is affected doubles the risk.
  - Two first-degree relatives are affected increases the risk threefold.
  - The relative has bilateral breast cancer.
  - The relative with breast cancer is male.
  - The relative's breast cancer was diagnosed before menopause.
- Inherited genetic mutations account for up to 10% of all breast cancers:
  - *BRCA1* (17q21): Lifetime risk of developing breast cancer in some families is as high as 80%; average risk is 55% to 65%.
  - *BRCA2* (13q14): Lifetime breast cancer risk is approximately 45%.
  - Other rare genetic mutations may increase risk but far less than *BRCA* mutations (see table below).
- History of receiving ionizing radiation to the chest (e.g., patient with a history of Hodgkin lymphoma treated with mantle irradiation)
- Hormonal factors:
  - Menarche before age 12 or menopause after age 55
  - First term pregnancy after age 30
  - Nulliparity
  - Use of oral contraceptives before age 20 years, with use lasting 6 years or more

- Hormone replacement therapy with estrogen plus progestin for more than 5 years
- Use of diethylstilbestrol (DES) to prevent miscarriage from 1940 to 1971
- Overweight and obese women have a higher incidence of breast cancer.
  - Postmenopausal overweight (BMI >25 to 30) women are at 1.5 times higher risk for breast cancer than women with a BMI less than 25.
  - Postmenopausal obese (BMI >30) women are at two times higher risk for breast cancer than women with a BMI less than 25.
- Proliferative breast disease, atypical hyperplasia, or previous in situ disease
- Dense breast tissue on mammography
- Smoking and drinking 10 g (i.e., one drink) of alcohol per day increases the breast cancer risk 10% for each drink.
- Risks specific to men include radiation exposure, gene mutations, family history of breast cancer, obesity, testicular disorders, and Klinefelter syndrome (i.e., extra copy of the X chromosome in boys).

Signs and Symptoms

Breast cancer in its early stages is usually asymptomatic. Later signs and symptoms include the following:

- A firm, painless, possibly immobile lump
- Pain is uncommon in early disease
- Changes in the size or shape of the breast
- Swelling on all or part of the breast
- Spontaneous, unilateral nipple discharge that is clear, black, pink, or bloody
- Presence of enlarged, firm, nontender lymph nodes
- Skin changes such as dimpling, edema, erythema, ulceration, or thickening

Inherited Genetic Mutations That Increase Breast Cancer Risk

Gene	Normal Function	Mutation
ATM	Helps to repair damaged DNA	One mutated copy has been linked to a high rate of breast cancer in some families.
TP53	Encodes the TP53 (p53) protein, which acts as a tumor suppressor and stops growth of abnormal cells	Inherited mutations cause Li-Fraumeni syndrome, which carries an increased risk of cancer, including breast cancer.
CHEK2	Encodes the checkpoint kinase 2 (CHK2) protein, which act as a tumor suppressor	Mutations can lead to Li-Fraumeni syndrome. With or without the syndrome, CHEK2 mutations can lead to a twofold increase in breast cancer risk.
PTEN	Encodes a tumor suppressor enzyme found in most tissues, which helps to regulate cellular growth	Inherited mutation can cause Cowden syndrome, a rare disorder that increases the risk of benign and malignant breast tumors and growths in the gastrointestinal tract, thyroid, uterus, and ovaries.
CDH1	Encodes a protein called epithelial cadherin (E-cadherin), which is found in the membrane that surrounds epithelial cells and helps neighboring cells stick to one another (i.e., cell adhesion) to form organized tissues	Inherited mutations cause hereditary diffuse gastric cancer and, in women, an increased risk of invasive lobular breast cancer.
STK11	Encodes a tumor suppressor protein called serine/threonine kinase 11	Defects can lead to Peutz-Jeghers syndrome, which causes pigmented spots on the lips and in the mouth, gastrointestinal and urinary polyps, and an increased risk of cancer, including breast cancer.
PALB2	Encodes a protein that works with the BRCA2 protein to repair damaged DNA and stop tumor growth	Mutations can lead to an increased risk of breast cancer.

Modified from American Cancer Society. (2015). *What are the risk factors for breast cancer?* Available at http://www.cancer.org/cancer/breastcancer/detailedguide/breast-cancer-risk-factors (accessed December 5, 2015); U.S. National Library of Medicine. (2015). *Genetics home reference: your guide to understanding genetic conditions.* Available at http://ghr.nlm.nih.gov (accessed December 5, 2015).

- Nipple changes such as inversion, scaling, ulceration, pain, thickening, or color changes
- Symptoms of metastases to distant sites, include shortness of breath, cough, loss of appetite, abnormal liver function test results, headaches, and back pain

Diagnostic Work-up

A diagnostic mammogram is used for the detection of breast lesions. The diagnostic work-up is completed to stage the breast cancer and develop an appropriate treatment plan.

- Work-up may include ultrasonography, mammography with spot compression and magnification views, or magnetic resonance imaging.
- Clinical breast examination includes bilateral breasts, axillae, and supraclavicular and infraclavicular areas.
- Biopsy is done for a pathologic diagnosis using fine-needle aspiration (FNA) for a palpable lesion. Stereotactic core-needle biopsy with imaging guidance or surgical incisional or excisional biopsy is used for nonpalpable lesions. Biopsy techniques are reviewed in the table below.
- Imaging studies to assess the extent of disease may include a chest radiograph, bone scan, computed tomography (CT) of the chest and abdomen, and magnetic resonance imaging (MRI) of the brain.
- Laboratory tests include a complete blood count and chemistry panel.

Breast Biopsy Techniques

Type of Biopsy	Method of Analysis	Palpable Lesion	Nonpalpable Lesion
Needle	Cytology	Fine-needle aspiration	Stereotactic fine-needle aspiration
	Histology	Core biopsy	Stereotactic core biopsy
Open	Histology	Incisional or excisional biopsy	Needle localization breast biopsy

From Bernice, M. (2005). Nursing care of the client with breast cancer. In J. K. Itano & K. N. Taoka (Eds.). *Core curriculum for oncology nursing* (4th ed., p. 497). St. Louis: Elsevier Saunders.

Histology

Breast cancer is a heterogeneous disease with many histologic subtypes. The more common subtypes of invasive breast cancer include the following:

- Invasive ductal carcinoma: 70% to 80% of all breast cancers
- Invasive lobular carcinoma: 10% to 15% of all breast cancers
- Medullary carcinomas: 5% to 7% of malignant breast tumors

Less common subtypes include the following:

- Paget disease occurring in the nipple with intraductal or invasive ductal carcinoma
- Tubular, mucinous, and papillary carcinomas
- Angiosarcoma and phyllodes tumors of the breast (rare)
- Inflammatory breast cancer is not a subtype but a special manifestation that typically manifests with dramatic and diffuse skin edema, erythema, hyperemia, and induration of the underlying tissue.

Identification of prognostic factors is essential for determining the appropriate treatment of an individual woman's breast cancer:

- Axillary lymph node status: prognosis worsens with increased involvement
- Tumor size: increased risk of recurrence with increasing size
- Hormone receptor status: tumors without estrogen receptors (ER−) and progesterone receptors (PR−) are associated with a poorer prognosis.
- Deoxyribonucleic acid (DNA) ploidy: aneuploid tumors with an abnormal amount of DNA and an unorganized dividing pattern have a poorer prognosis.
- High S-phase fraction or higher division rate: predicts poorer outcome
- Histopathologic grading: takes into account the nuclear pattern, morphologic features, and mitotic activity; the higher the grade, the worse the prognosis
- Molecular subtypes that are being investigated and targeted for future therapies:
  - Luminal A type: 40% of all breast cancers; typically are slower growing and have a hormone profile of ER+/PR+/HER2−
  - Luminal B type: 10% to 20% of all breast cancers; are ER+/PR+ and have a high proliferation rate
  - Basal-like: 10% to 20% of breast cancers; are ER−/PR−/HER2− or triple negative
  - HER2 enriched: 10% of all breast cancers; are ER−/PR−/HER2+ and tend to be more aggressive

Therapies targeted against HER2 overexpression have led to improved survival. Molecular and biologic factors that may be associated with a poor prognosis include the following:

- Triple-negative breast cancer: ER−/PR−/HER2−
- Loss of functioning of tumor suppression genes such as *TP53* and *NME/NM23*
- Overexpression of oncogenes such as *HER2* and *EGFR*
- Roles of proteases such as cathepsin D and urokinase plasminogen activator in tumor cell invasion and metastasis

Clinical Staging

Clinical staging is based on the size of the primary tumor (T), the presence of palpable lymph nodes with cancer in the axilla (N), and distant metastases (M). The size, nodes, and location of the cancer determine the overall disease stage (I to IV). Pathologic staging can be more accurate and is recommended by the American Joint Committee on Cancer Staging (AJCC) and can be found in the AJCC manual (Edge, et al., 2010).

Treatment

There are a variety of therapies for breast cancer patients. Treatment is determined by the size of the tumor, the stage of the disease, menopausal and hormone receptor status, and the histology of the cancer, including tumor markers. Treatment goals depend on whether the breast cancer is localized, metastatic, or recurrent.

Surgery

- Surgical resection of the tumor with breast-conserving surgery includes a lumpectomy or partial mastectomy with a sentinel node biopsy. Evidence has shown that breast-conserving surgery with postoperative irradiation is as effective as a total mastectomy with lymph node dissection for early-stage breast cancer.

- Bilateral mastectomies with immediate reconstruction may be used in younger women with *BRCA*-associated early breast cancer in one breast.
- A summary of surgical procedures can be found in the table below.

Radiation Therapy

- Radiation therapy (RT) is the treatment of choice to achieve local control of cancer.
- To reduce the risk of recurrence and eradicate any remaining microscopic cancer cells, RT is given after surgery or chemotherapy.
- Accelerated partial breast irradiation (APBI) may be used. APBI delivers a higher concentrated dose of radiation to the tumor bed over a shorter period than other methods.
- APBI can be delivered intraoperatively with one treatment or postoperatively with an inserted balloon over 5 days. Clinical trials are being conducted in the United States before this can be recommended as the standard of care.
- In the setting of metastatic disease, irradiation is used to treat solitary bone metastasis and for emergency treatment of spinal cord compression.

Systemic Therapy

- The goal of systemic treatment is to destroy or control cancer cells throughout the body.
- Systemic treatment includes chemotherapy, hormonal therapy, and biologic therapy, which may be given in neoadjuvant, adjuvant, and metastatic settings.
- Treatments are chosen on the basis of factors such as age, health, size of tumor, nodal involvement, hormone receptor status, *HER2* status, and other factors.
- Hormonal therapies provide a response rate of 50% to 70% for women with ER+ and PR+ tumors.
- Hormonal therapies include anastrozole, exemestane, fulvestrant, and letrozole.

- Two agents have been approved to enhance the efficacy of hormonal therapies after disease progression.
  - Everolimus, an mTOR inhibitor, plus examustine is indicated for postmenopausal women with HER−/ER+/PR+ advanced breast cancer after progression on letrozole or anastrozole.
  - Palbocicib, a CDK inhibitor, plus letrozole is indicated for postmenopausal women with HER2−/ER+ advanced disease. The drug targets CDK4 and CDK6, which are involved in promoting the growth of cancer cells.
- Chemotherapy may be given to reduce the size of a tumor before surgery (i.e., neoadjuvant chemotherapy), to eliminate occult tumor cells after primary surgery, or for palliation in the setting of metastatic cancer.
  - Agents commonly combined and used in the adjuvant and neoadjuvant setting are doxorubicin, epirubicin, paclitaxel, docetaxel, cyclophosphamide, fluorouracil, and methotrexate.
  - For metastatic disease, the same agents may be used as single agents. Other frequently used agents are capecitabine, gemcitabine, and vinorelbine.

Prognosis

The prognosis for breast cancer depends on many factors, including stage of disease, histologic diagnosis and grade of the cancer, hormone receptor status, HER2 protein overexpression status, menopausal status, and overall health of the individual.

- Overall 5-year survival rate is 85% for those diagnosed before age 40 and 90% for patients diagnosed after 40, possibly due to increased aggressiveness of the disease in younger patients.
- Survival is lower for black than for white women at every stage of diagnosis. For all stages combined, the 5-year relative survival rate is 90% for white women and 79% for black women.
- Among the many known prognostic factors, stage of disease is one of the best indicators of prognosis. Five-year survival rates by stage for individuals with breast cancer who receive appropriate treatment are as follow:

Breast Cancer Surgical Procedures

Treatment	Procedure
Breast-conserving surgeries*	
• Lumpectomy	Excision of tumor with small margin of normal tissue around it
• Segmental resection (e.g., tylectomy, quadrantectomy, partial mastectomy)	Excision of tumor with a wider margin of surrounding tissue
Mastectomies	
• Subcutaneous mastectomy	Removes all breast tissue except overlying skin and nipple-areolar complex
• Skin sparing	Removes above plus limited overlying skin, at-risk biopsy scar, nipple-areolar complex
• Total (simple) mastectomy	Removes all breast tissue, including skin, gland, nipple-areolar complex
• Modified radical mastectomy	Removes above plus axillary node dissection
• Radical mastectomy	Removes above plus underlying pectoral muscles

*Usually done in conjunction with axillary node biopsy or dissection through a second incision.
From J. K. Itano & K. N. Taoka (Eds.). (2005). *Core curriculum for oncology nursing* (4th ed., p. 499). St. Louis: Elsevier Saunders.

- Stage I (localized disease): 99%
- Stage II to III (regional disease): 84%
- Stage IIIc to IV (distant disease): 24%

Prevention and Surveillance

- Breast cancer screening includes clinical examinations, self-evaluations, and mammograms:
  - Screening mammograms are obtained between the ages of 35 and 40 years, every 1 to 2 years between the ages of 40 and 49 years, and yearly for women 50 years of age or older.
  - The American Cancer Society (ACS) recommends providing information about the benefits and limitations of breast self-examination (BSE) to women beginning in their 20s.
  - The ACS recommends clinical breast examination by a health care professional at least every 3 years from ages 20 to 39 years and then annually.
- Several trials have been conducted to evaluate breast cancer prevention:
  - The Exemestane for Breast Cancer Prevention in Postmenopausal Women trial showed early positive results of a 65% decrease in developing invasive cancer versus placebo.
  - The Breast Cancer Prevention Trial (BCPT or National Surgical Adjuvant Breast and Bowel Project 1 [NSABP-1]) showed a 49% risk reduction in breast cancer for women with a known high risk of breast cancer who took 20 mg of tamoxifen daily compared with those taking a placebo.
  - The Study of Tamoxifen and Raloxifene (STAR) trial (i.e., NSABP-P2) was a randomized trial comparing two drugs for reducing the incidence of breast cancer among high-risk, postmenopausal women. The initial results of STAR showed that raloxifene and tamoxifen were equally effective in reducing invasive breast cancer risk, but after an average of 81 months (i.e., 5 years of medication and 21 months of follow-up), raloxifene had reduced the risk by about 38%, and tamoxifen had reduced the risk by about 50%.
  - The Multiple Outcomes of Raloxifene Evaluation (MORE) trial examined the effects of raloxifene versus placebo on the risk of osteoporosis and showed a reduced risk of osteoporosis and fractures. In a secondary end point of the trial, raloxifene also produced a 65% reduction in the risk of invasive breast cancer.
  - Prophylactic mastectomy accompanied by immediate reconstruction or oophorectomy may be appropriate for some women at high risk for breast cancer due to genetic profiles.

Noninvasive Breast Cancer

Definition

Noninvasive breast cancers, also referred to as in situ carcinomas, are precancerous lesions confined to the duct or lobule in the breast. The two types are ductal carcinoma in situ (DCIS) and lobular carcinoma in situ (LCIS).

- DCIS is a precancerous condition in which abnormal cells are found in the lining of a breast duct. DCIS may become invasive cancer and spread to other tissues.
- In LCIS, the abnormal cells are found only in the lobules of the breast. LCIS is 7 to 12 times more likely to progress to invasive breast cancer in the same or the opposite breast.

Incidence

- The incidence of noninvasive breast cancers is thought to be the same as invasive breast cancer (see Incidence section on page 35).
- DCIS accounts for about 20% of all new breast cancer cases and about 5% of male breast cancers.
- The incidence of LCIS is difficult to estimate because it is usually an incidental finding and is therefore likely to be underdiagnosed.

Etiology and Risk Factors

The cause of noninvasive breast cancers is thought to be the same as for invasive breast cancer (see Etiology and Risk Factors section on page 36).

Signs and Symptoms

- Most women with noninvasive breast cancer do not have palpable lesions or symptoms.
- Rarely, a woman with DCIS is seen for a lump, nipple discharge, or Paget disease of the breast.
- LCIS is asymptomatic and usually found by chance in tissue obtained during a breast biopsy or other surgical procedure.
- LCIS, although uncommon, occurs predominantly in premenopausal patients at an average age of about 45 years.

Diagnostic Work-up

- DCIS is typically diagnosed from routine mammograms.
- The mammogram shows an unusual cluster of microcalcifications.
- A needle-localization or needle-core biopsy may be required.
- Although not standard of care, some centers conduct sentinel node biopsies in cases of high-grade DCIS because there are reports of positive nodes in some cases.
- LCIS is usually diagnosed coincidently from tissue taken during a biopsy or breast surgery.

Histology

- DCIS is a precancerous condition in which abnormal cells are found in the lining of a breast duct.
- DCIS may become invasive cancer and spread to other tissues, although it is not known how to predict which lesions will become invasive.
- DCIS is further divided into noncomedo and comedo carcinomas and into low-, intermediate-, or high-grade lesions.
- LCIS is a precancerous condition in which abnormal cells are found in the lobules of the breast. It seldom progresses to an invasive cancer, but having LCIS in one breast increases the risk for breast cancer in both breasts.

Clinical Staging

On the basis of the AJCC staging classification system for breast cancer, a noninvasive cancer is stage 0.

Treatment

- Treatment for DCIS depends on the extent and grade of disease, the classification, the patient's health, and the medical history.
- Surgery, lumpectomy, or simple mastectomy is the standard treatment for DCIS and is intended to completely remove all cancer cells.
- Adjuvant treatments, such as radiation therapy and hormonal therapy, may be given to reduce the risk of DCIS recurring.
- Women with LCIS may be given the option of a lumpectomy or mastectomy.
- Many clinicians advocate local excision with close follow-up that includes mammography twice yearly and a clinical examination every 3 to 4 months.
- Women with LCIS may be given hormone therapy to reduce the risk of recurrence in the affected and bilateral breast.

Prognosis

- The prognosis for women with noninvasive beast cancer is almost 100% survival at 5 years after diagnosis.
- Women with DCIS or LCIS carry an 8-fold to10-fold risk for invasive breast cancer.
- DCIS classified as noncomedo, low-grade carcinoma carries a better prognosis than a high-grade, comedo carcinoma.
- LCIS is associated with a small but increased risk of invasive breast cancer.

Prevention and Surveillance

Information about the prevention of noninvasive breast cancers has not been specifically reported. It is thought to be the same as that for invasive breast cancer (see earlier Prevention and Surveillance section).

Bibliography

Allen, N. E., Beral, V., Casabonne, D., Kan, S. W., Reeves, G. K., Brown, A., et al. Moderate alcohol intake and cancer incidence in women: Million Women Study. *Journal of the National Cancer Institute, 101*(5), 296–305.

Afinitor (Everolimus) product information. (2015). *Novartis Oncology.* Available at http://www.afinitor.com/advanced-breast-cancer/hcp/index.jsp?usertrack.filter_applied=true&NovaId=4029462121354488946 (accessed December 10, 2015).

American Cancer Society. (2015). *Breast cancer facts and figures 2015-2016.* Available at http://www.cancer.org/acs/groups/content/@research/documents/document/acspc-042725.pdf (accessed December 10, 2015).

American Cancer Society. (2015). *Cancer facts & figures 2015.* Available at http://www.cancer.org/acs/groups/content/@editorial/documents/document/acspc-044552.pdf (accessed December 10, 2015).

American Cancer Society. (2015). *Signs and symptoms of breast cancer.* Available at http://www.cancer.org/cancer/breastcancer/detailedguide/breast-cancer-signs-symptoms (accessed December 10, 2015).

Bauer, E., & Lester, J. L. (2014). Accelerated partial breast irradiation: Efficacy and outcomes. *Clinical Journal of Oncology Nursing, 18*(5), 556–566.

Edge, S. B., Byrd, D. R., Compton, C. C., Fritz, A. G., Greene, F. L., & Trotti, A. (2010). *AJCC cancer staging manual* (7th ed.). New York, NY: Springer, 347–376.

Esserman, L. J., & Joe, B. N. (2015). *Up to date: Diagnostic evaluation of women with suspected breast cancer* (Topic 808, Version 28.0). Available at http://www.uptodate.com/contents/diagnostic-evaluation-of-women-with-suspected-breast-cancer (accessed December 10, 2015).

Itano, J. K., & Taoka, K. N. (2005). *Core curriculum for oncology nursing* (4th ed.). St. Louis: Elsevier Saunders, p. 499.

National Cancer Institute. (2012). *Breast cancer risk in American women.* Available at http://www.cancer.gov/cancertopics/factsheet/detection/probability-breast-cancer (accessed December 10, 2015).

National Cancer Institute. (2015). *Genetics of breast and gynecologic cancer—for health professionals.* Available at http://www.cancer.gov/cancertopics/pdq/genetics/breast-and-ovarian/HealthProfessional (accessed December 10, 2015).

National Cancer Institute. (2015). *Histopathologic classification of breast cancer.* Available at http://www.cancer.gov/cancertopics/pdq/treatment/breast/healthprofessional/page2 (accessed December 10, 2015).

National Cancer Institute, Surveillance, Epidemiology, and End Results Program. (2014). *SEER stat fact sheet: Breast cancer.* Available at http://seer.cancer.gov/statfacts/html/breast.html (accessed December 10, 2015).

U.S. Food and Drug Administration. (2015). *Palbociclib.* Available at http://www.fda.gov/Drugs/InformationOnDrugs/ApprovedDrugs/ucm432886.htm (accessed December 10, 2015).

Central Nervous System Cancers

Margaretta S. Page and Jane Rabbitt

Overview of Central Nervous System Malignancies

Definition

Central nervous system (CNS) malignancies are a heterogeneous group of cancers of the brain and spinal cord. They can originate in neural tissue (i.e., primary brain tumors) or nonneural tissue, or they can be metastatic tumors. The first section of this chapter provides an overview of these diseases, and later parts address specific CNS malignancies in more detail.

Incidence

- The Central Brain Tumor Registry of the United States (CBTRUS) estimates that 24,790 cases of primary malignant CNS tumors and 52,880 cases of nonmalignant tumors will be diagnosed in 2016.
  - Glioblastoma multiforme (GBM) is the most common malignant CNS tumor, accounting for 45.6% of malignant tumors.
  - The most prevalent nonmalignant tumor is meningioma, accounting for 53.7% of nonmalignant tumors.
- Age at onset and male and female incidence rates vary significantly on the basis of tumor type.
  - For example, the average age at onset is 62 years for both GBM and nonmalignant meningioma, but the incidence of GBMs is greater among males, and the incidence of nonmalignant meningioma is increased among females. The peak incidence of oligodendrogliomas occurs between the ages of 35 and 44 years.
- The figure in the next column shows the incidence of primary brain tumors by major histologic types.

Etiology and Risk Factors

The causes of brain tumors are unknown, but the following are considered risk factors:
- Therapeutic ionizing radiation to the head
- Genetic disorders, including neurofibromatosis types 1 and 2, tuberous sclerosis, von Hippel–Lindau syndrome, Li-Fraumeni syndrome, and Turcot syndrome
- Diet, vitamins, alcohol use, tobacco use, and environmental exposures have been studied, but little information has been produced about the causes of CNS tumors, especially gliomas.

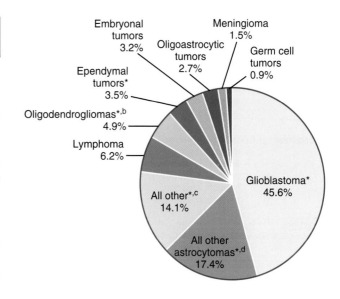

*All or some of this histology is included in the CBTRUS definition of gliomas, including ICD-O-3 histology codes 9380-9384, 9391-9460, 9480.
a. Percentages may not add up to 100% due to rounding.
b. Includes oligodendroglioma and anaplastic oligodendroglioma.
c. Includes glioma malignant, NOS, choroid plexus tumors, other neuroepithelial tumors, newronal and mixed neuronal-glial tumors, tumors of the pineal region, nerce sheath tumors of cranial and spinal nerves, mesenchymal tumors, primary melanocytic lesions, and other neoplasms related to the meninges, other hematopoietic neoplasms, hemangioma, neoplasm, unspecified, and all other.
d. Includes pilocytic astrocytoma, diffuse astrocytoma, anaplastic astrocytoma, and unique astrocytoma variants.

Distribution of Malignant Primary Brain and CNS Tumors by CBTRUS, 2007 to 2011 Histologic information is shown for 115,799 patients. (Modified from Ostrom, Q. T., Gittleman, H., Liao, P., Rouse, C., Chen, Y., Dowling, J., et al (2014). CBTRUS statistical report: Primary brain and central nervous system tumors diagnosed in the United States in 2007–2011. *Neuro-oncology, 16*(Suppl 4), iv1-iv63.)

Signs and Symptoms

Signs and symptoms related to increased mass in the cranial vault and increased intracranial pressure include headache, nausea, vomiting, altered level of consciousness, and seizures. Later sections of this chapter outline the specific signs and symptoms by tumor type. Focal signs and symptoms related to tumor location include seizures, weakness, sensory changes, personality changes, and endocrine abnormalities (see table below).

Brain Function and Symptoms Associated with Lesion Location

Lesion Location	Function	Associated Symptoms
Frontal lobe	Motor movement, thought, reasoning, behavior, executive functioning, memory, motor aspect of speech, and bowel and bladder control; dominant hemisphere controls language and writing	Personality changes, short-term memory loss, judgment, confusion, other mental changes, contralateral weakness, seizures, impaired speech or smell, visual field cuts, urinary frequency and urgency
Temporal lobe	Behavior, long-term memory, hearing and vision pathways, understanding of speech, emotion, sensation, abstract concepts	Receptive aphasia, seizures, vision impairment, poor memory
Parietal lobe	Sensory perceptions, spatial relations, reasoning, memory	Sensory deficits, seizures, inability to read, spatial disorders, difficulty with math, difficulty with complex reasoning, impaired memory
Occipital lobe	Vision, reading	Visual hallucinations, visual disturbances, blindness, inability to read
Cerebellum	Balance, coordination	Ataxia, slurred speech
Brainstem, midbrain, pons, medulla	Basic life functions, heart rate, breathing, consciousness, and attachment for all cranial nerves	Vomiting and headaches in the morning, ataxia, cranial nerve palsy, lethargy, weakness, double vision

Diagnostic Work-up

- Neurologic examination
- Magnetic resonance imaging (MRI) of the brain or spine
- Biopsy or craniotomy for a tissue diagnosis
- Optional or additional radiologic studies
  - Magnetic resonance spectroscopy (MRS)
  - Positron emission tomography (PET)

Histology

Brain tumors are classified according to the World Health Organization (WHO) classification of central nervous system tumors (see table in next column), which incorporates morphologic features, cytogenetics, molecular characterization, and immunologic markers. Malignancy is established on the basis of histologic features.

World Health Organization Grading of Tumors

WHO Grade	Description
I	Lesion with low proliferative potential. Cure is possible with surgical resection.
II	Infiltrating lesion with low mitotic activity that has a tendency to recur. Some tumors may progress to higher grades.
III	Lesions with evidence of malignancy usually seen in mitotic activity, infiltrative ability, and anaplasia. Usually treated aggressively with adjuvant therapy.
IV	Lesions with high mitotic activity that are prone to necrosis and usually are associated with a rapid disease progression seen preoperatively and postoperatively. Treatments are aggressive, and disease is usually fatal.

National Cancer Institute. (2015). *Adult central nervous system tumors treatment—for health professionals (PDQ)*. Available at http://www.cancer.gov/types/brain/hp/adult-brain-treatment-pdq#section/all (accessed December 11, 2015).

Clinical Staging

Because of the very low incidence of metastases, most CNS tumors do not require staging. If indicated, CNS staging involves imaging of the spine and obtaining cerebrospinal fluid (CSF) to identify evidence of metastasis.

Treatment

Treatment, which varies on the basis of tumor type, includes surgery, irradiation, and chemotherapy. Treatment options being studied in clinical trials include immunotherapy, targeted agents, and development of predictive biomarkers to assist in identifying patients who are likely to respond to a given agent. Clinical trials are looking at the efficacy of using the tumor characteristics of proliferation, angiogenesis, and invasion to select treatments. Concomitant medications used for brain tumors often include steroids, especially dexamethasone, for control of cerebral edema or symptom management and anticonvulsants for patients in the acute postoperative period and those who have seizures.

Prognosis

Prognosis depends on the tumor type and grade. Age, functional status, and neurocognitive status at diagnosis are strong prognostic indicators. The overall 5-year survival rate for primary malignant CNS tumors is 34.2%.

Prevention and Surveillance

- There are no known preventive measures to reduce the incidence of primary CNS tumors.
- Surveillance for CNS malignancies is discussed under the individual tumor types.

Bibliography

Fox, S. W., & Mitchell, S. A. (2006). Cognitive impairment in patients with brain tumors: Assessment in the clinical setting. *Clinical Journal of Oncology Nursing, 10,* 169–182.

Melin, B., & Bondy, M. (2011). Familial factors and inherited susceptibility to glioma. In M. Mehta, S. Chang, A. Guha, H. B. Newton, & M. A. Vogelbaum (Eds.), *Principles and practice of neuro-oncology: A multidisciplinary approach* (pp. 14–17). New York: Demos Medical.

National Comprehensive Cancer Network. (2015). *Central nervous system cancers.* Available at http://www.nccn.org/professionals/physician_gls/PDF/cns.pdf (accessed December 11, 2015).

Ostrom, Q. T., Gittleman, H., Liao, P., Rouse, C., Chen, Y., Dowling, J., et al (2014). CBTRUS statistical report: Primary brain and central nervous system tumors diagnosed in the United States in 2007–2011. *Neuro-oncology, 16*(Suppl 4), iv1–iv63.

Prados, M. (2006). Primary neoplasms of the central nervous system. In D. W. Kufe, R. C. Bast, W. N. Hait, W. K. Hong, R. E. Pollock, R. R. Weichselbaum, et al (Eds.), *Cancer Medicine* (7) (pp. 1037–1065). Hamilton, ON: BC Decker.

Astrocytoma

Definition

Astrocytomas, the most common type of glioma, arise from astrocytes, which are star-shaped cells that support neurons. Astrocytomas make up about one half of all primary brain tumors. Astrocytomas are classified by grade according to WHO criteria.

Incidence

- WHO grade I astrocytomas are most common in children and young adults. They include pilocytic astrocytomas and subependymal giant cell astrocytomas.
- WHO grade II astrocytomas, also known simply as *astrocytomas* or *low-grade astrocytomas,* make up 26% of primary glial tumors and account for 15% of brain tumors in adults. They most commonly occur between 20 and 50 years of age. In various reports, the median age at diagnosis is between 35 and 37 years.
- WHO grade III astrocytomas, also referred to as *anaplastic astrocytomas,* are faster growing than grade II astrocytomas and are considered malignant grade III astrocytomas or anaplastic astrocytomas. They commonly occur in patients between 30 and 50 years of age. The mean age at diagnosis is 45 years. They are slightly more common in men than women and make up 4% of all brain tumors.
- WHO grade IV astrocytoma, also known as *glioblastoma multiforme* (GBM), is a highly malignant astrocytic tumor that can evolve from a lower grade tumor by malignant degeneration to become a secondary glioblastoma, or it can be a GBM at the outset, known as a *primary* or *de novo glioblastoma.* The peak incidence occurs between 65 and 74 years of age. The mean age at diagnosis is 54 years. GBMs are slightly more common in men than women. They make up 23% of all brain tumors and 50% of astrocytomas.

Etiology and Risk Factors

There is no known cause for astrocytomas, but the following are considered risk factors:
- Therapeutic ionizing radiation to the head
- Genetic disorders, including neurofibromatosis type 1 and 2, tuberous sclerosis, von Hippel–Lindau syndrome, Li-Fraumeni syndrome, and Turcot syndrome

Signs and Symptoms

Signs and symptoms of astrocytomas depend on location (see Brain Function and Symptoms Associated with Lesion Location table on page 42), and severity is described by the WHO grade.
- WHO grade I: Symptoms may be subtle due to the slow-growing nature of these tumors.
- WHO grades II through IV: Symptoms depend on tumor size and location and may manifest as headaches, focal neurologic deficits, or impaired executive or cognitive function.
- Astrocytomas usually develop in the frontal lobes. Between 50% and 80% of patients have seizures as their initial symptom.

Diagnostic Work-up

- Neurologic examination
- MRI of the brain or spine
- Biopsy or craniotomy for a tissue diagnosis

Histology

- WHO grade I: Lesions have a low proliferative potential and are frequently discrete. Cure is possible with surgical resection alone.
- WHO grade II: Astrocytomas usually are infiltrating and have low mitotic activity but tend to recur. They consist of uniform cells showing increased cellularity and minimal pleomorphism. They are composed of well-differentiated fibrillary or gemistocytic neoplastic astrocytes. The three histologic variants are fibrillary astrocytoma, gemistocytic astrocytoma, and protoplasmic astrocytoma. Some of these tumor types tend to progress to higher grades of malignancy. The only consistent genetic alteration in low-grade gliomas is a mutation of *TP53*, which is a tumor suppressor gene. Altered genetic expression in these tumors is also thought to have a role in progression to GBM.
- WHO grade III: Anaplastic astrocytomas are highly cellular, with increased nuclear and cellular pleomorphism and mitoses. Increasing attention is being given to the molecular genetics of these tumors. O^6-Methylguanine-DNA methyltransferase (MGMT) is a DNA repair enzyme that confers resistance to alkylating chemotherapy agents. If a tumor has a methylated promoter region of the *MGMT* gene, the gene function is blocked, and there are decreased amounts of circulating repair enzyme. With less repair enzyme, the tumor is thought to have an increased sensitivity to alkylating chemotherapy agents. MGMT methylation status is included in the pathology report for astrocytomas and, in some cases, is used to assist with decisions about treatment with alkylating agents.
- WHO grade IV: GBM lesions have poorly differentiated, often pleomorphic astrocytic cells with brisk mitotic activity. The distinguishing features for GBMs are endothelial or microvascular proliferation and necrosis, which is the hallmark of this tumor. Two histologic variants are giant cell glioblastoma and gliosarcoma. The most frequent molecular characteristic of primary GBMs is amplification of the epidermal growth factor receptor (*EGFR*) gene, which occurs in 40% to 50% of patients.

Clinical Staging

Because of the very low incidence of metastasis, staging is not usually done for astrocytomas.

Treatment

Treatments depend on a number of factors, especially the WHO grade classification.

WHO Grade I

- Surgery may involve a craniotomy or biopsy, depending on tumor location. It is often curative alone.
- Radiation therapy may be administered if resection is suboptimal or the tumor recurs.

WHO Grade II

There is controversy about the best treatment option for WHO grade II tumors, including the extent of surgery, timing of radiation, and role of chemotherapy.

- Observation is not recommended because only limited data support it as an option.
- Surgery may involve a craniotomy or biopsy, depending on tumor location.
- Radiation therapy at diagnosis is controversial because of the slow-growing nature of the tumor and the potential for toxicity. If gross total resection has been obtained, irradiation may be deferred. Patients can be monitored with serial MRI scans. Radiation therapy is recommended, regardless of other factors, for patients 35 years of age or older. The recommended dose is 54 Gy in single fractions to the tumor volume and small surrounding margins.
- Chemotherapy may be administered at diagnosis in an effort to defer irradiation, but this strategy remains investigational. Temozolomide is the treatment of choice for low-grade gliomas. At recurrence, the treatment options of surgery, radiation therapy, and chemotherapy may be recommended.

WHO Grade III

- Surgery is done to establish a pathologic diagnosis and debulk as much tumor as possible.
- Irradiation is the single most effective therapy at this time. The recommended dose is 60 Gy given in single fractions to the tumor volume and small surrounding margins.
- Chemotherapy includes temozolomide at diagnosis and the use of nitrosoureas at recurrence.

WHO Grade IV

- Surgery is the initial therapy of choice. It is used to establish a pathologic diagnosis and debulk as much of the tumor as possible.
- Irradiation is the single most effective therapy for astrocytomas. The total dose given in single fractions is 60 Gy. Advances in technology have allowed treatment to focus on the tumor and minimize radiation delivered to critical structures near the tumor.
- Since 2005, treatment with concurrent temozolomide during irradiation followed by adjuvant temozolomide has been the standard of care. Adjuvant chemotherapy is recommended for patients younger than 40 years of age who have minimal disease and minimal dysfunction. At recurrence, approved therapies include implanting biodegradable wafers containing carmustine and using bevacizumab, a monoclonal antibody.
- Numerous clinical trials are investigating combinations of medications with different mechanisms of action. Investigational therapies may target growth factor receptors, platelet-derived growth factor receptors, EGFRs, vascular endothelial growth factor receptors, or various cell-signaling pathways. These treatment options may be considered at diagnosis or at recurrence. Immunotherapy and gene therapy are also being studied.

Prognosis

Astrocytoma prognosis depends on the WHO grade classification.

- WHO grade I: With complete resection, the prognosis is excellent.
- WHO grade II: Overall survival time is 6.5 to 8 years after diagnosis. Prognosis is better for patients younger than 40 years of age at diagnosis who have a positive seizure history and absence of additional neurologic deficits. Poor survival has been correlated with tumor size, degree of resection, contrast enhancement on MRI, and histopathologic factors. Mutation or deletion of the *TP53* gene is a negative prognostic indicator, and vascular endothelial growth factor expression correlates positively with survival.
- WHO grade III: Median time to tumor progression is 2 years, and median survival time is 2.5 to 4 years.
- WHO grade IV: Patients with grade IV astrocytomas (i.e., GBMs) have a very poor prognosis. Median survival time is 15 months with radiation therapy and temozolomide, although it may be almost 2 years for patients younger than 40 years of age who have undergone gross total resection and who have good performance status.

Prevention and Surveillance

- There are no known preventative measures to reduce the incidence of primary CNS tumors.
- After patients have completed the prescribed therapy, they should be monitored according to the National Comprehensive Cancer Network (NCCN) guidelines.
  - WHO grade I: Serial MRI scans are obtained every 3 to 6 months for 5 years after therapy and at least annually thereafter.
  - WHO grade II: Serial MRI scans are obtained every 3 to 6 months for 5 years after therapy and at least annually thereafter.
  - WHO grade III: Serial MRI scans are obtained at 2- to 4-month intervals for the first 2 to 3 years after therapy and then less frequently according to the physician's discretion.
  - WHO grade IV: Serial MRI scans are obtained at 2- to 4-month intervals for the first 2 to 3 years after therapy and then less frequently according to the physician's discretion.

Bibliography

Clarke, J., Ney, D. E., Shyu, C. C., & Lassman, A. B. (2011). Medical management of supratentorial gliomas in adults. In M. Mehta, S. Chang, A. Guha, H. B. Newton, & M. A. Vogelbaum (Eds.), *Principles and practice of neuro-oncology: A multidisciplinary approach* (pp. 562–578). New York: Demos Medical.

Fischer, I., Sulman, E., & Aldape, K. (2011). Molecular pathogenesis of glioma: Overview and therapeutic implications. In M. Mehta, S. Chang, A. Guha, H. B. Newton, & M. A. Vogelbaum (Eds.), *Principles and practice of neuro-oncology: A multidisciplinary approach* (p. 635). New York: Demos Medical.

Hou, L., & Harsh, G. R., IV (2012). Management of recurrent gliomas and meningiomas. In A. H. Kaye & E. R. Laws, Jr. (Eds.), *Brain tumors* (3rd ed.) (pp. 355–371). Edinburgh: Saunders.

Melin, B., & Bondy, M. (2011). Familial factors and inherited susceptibility to glioma. In M. Mehta, S. Chang, A. Guha, H. B. Newton, & M. A. Vogelbaum (Eds.), *Principles and practice of neuro-oncology: A multidisciplinary approach* (pp. 14–17). New York: Demos Medical.

National Comprehensive Cancer Network. (2015). *Central nervous system cancers.* Available at http://www.nccn.org/professionals/physician_gls/PDF/cns.pdf (accessed December 11, 2015).

Ostrom, Q. T., Gittleman, H., Liao, P., Rouse, C., Chen, Y., Dowling, J., et al (2014). CBTRUS statistical report: Primary brain and central nervous system tumors diagnosed in the United States in 2007–2011. *Neuro-oncology, 16*(Suppl 4), iv1–iv63.

Prados, M. (2006). Primary neoplasms of the central nervous system. In D. W. Kufe, R. C. Bast, W. N. Hait, W. K. Hong, R. E. Pollock, R. R. Weichselbaum, et al (Eds.), *Cancer medicine* (7) (pp. 1037–1065). Hamilton, ON: BC Decker.

Sanai, N., & Berger, M. (2012). Low-grade astrocytomas. In A. H. Kaye & E. R. Laws, Jr. (Eds.), *Brain tumors* (3rd ed.) (pp. 372–381). Edinburgh: Saunders.

Sarkar, A., & Chiocca, E. A. (2012). Glioblastoma and malignant astrocytoma. In A. H. Kaye & E. R. Laws, Jr. (Eds.), *Brain tumors* (3rd ed.) (pp. 384–407). Edinburgh: Saunders.

Wrensch, M. R., Minn, Y., & Bondy, M. (2000). Epidemiology. In M. Bernstein & M. Berger (Eds.), *Neuro-oncology: The essentials* (pp. 2–17). New York: Thieme Medical.

Benign Brain Tumors

Definition

Benign brain tumors are slow-growing brain tumors that can be removed or destroyed if in a surgically accessible location. The margins of a benign brain tumor can be clearly seen. Cells from benign tumors do not invade tissues around them or spread to other parts of the body. However, benign tumors can press on sensitive areas of the brain and cause serious health problems. Many of the tumors in this category grow inside the skull but outside the brain. Many histologic types of brain tumors are considered to be benign. They include meningiomas, craniopharyngiomas, acoustic neuromas, and pituitary adenomas.

Incidence

Meningiomas, pituitary adenomas, craniopharyngiomas, and nerve sheath tumors make up 45% of all primary brain tumors.

Etiology and Risk Factors

The causes of benign brain tumors remain unknown, but the following are considered risk factors:

- Prior radiation to the head predisposes patients to meningioma.
- Neurofibromatosis type 2 predisposes patients to bilateral acoustic neuromas and meningiomas.
- There is an increased incidence of meningioma for those with a history of breast cancer.

Signs and Symptoms

- Signs and symptoms are related to tumor location (see "Brain Function and Symptoms Associated with Lesion Location" table on page 42).
- Craniopharyngiomas and pituitary adenomas occur near the pituitary gland or axis, and patients may have hormonal abnormalities or visual disturbances.
- Acoustic neuromas occur along the acoustic nerve and can cause vertigo, dizziness, or loss of hearing.

Diagnostic Work-up

- Neurologic examination
- MRI of the brain or spine
- Biopsy or craniotomy for a tissue diagnosis

Histology

Histologic diagnosis depends on the tumor type. Typically, these tumors are well circumscribed and slow growing.

Clinical Staging

Staging is unnecessary because benign brain tumors do not tend to disseminate.

Treatment

- Surgical resection of a tumor is often curative.
- If incomplete resection is obtained or the tumor is in a surgically inaccessible area, stereotactic radiosurgery may be used. Radiation therapy may be recommended in rare cases of recurrence.
- Long-term follow-up with an endocrinologist is required if the pituitary gland or immediate area is involved.

Prognosis

The prognosis is usually very good. However, because these tumors develop in the brain, patients can have significant neurologic or endocrine sequelae from the tumor or treatments.

Prevention and Surveillance

- There are no known preventative measures to reduce the incidence of primary CNS tumors.
- After patients have completed the prescribed therapy, they are monitored according to the NCCN guidelines.
- For meningiomas, there are different opinions about the exact surveillance schedule. The typical recommendation is for serial MRI scans every 3 months for 1 year, every 6 to 12 months for the next 5 years, and less frequently thereafter.

Bibliography

Ostrom, Q. T., Gittleman, H., Liao, P., Rouse, C., Chen, Y., Dowling, J., et al (2014). CBTRUS statistical report: Primary brain and central nervous system tumors diagnosed in the United States in 2007–2011. *Neuro-oncology, 16*(Suppl 4), iv1–iv63.

Prados, M. (2006). Primary neoplasms of the central nervous system. In D. W. Kufe, R. C. Bast, W. N. Hait, W. K. Hong, R. E. Pollock, R. R. Weichselbaum, et al (Eds.), *Cancer medicine* (7) (pp. 1037–1065). Hamilton, ON: BC Decker.

Ependymoma

Definition

An ependymoma is a glial tumor that develops from the neuroepithelial lining of the cerebral ventricles and central canal of the spinal cord. Ependymomas are classified as WHO grade I through III tumors. Subtypes include myxopapillary ependymoma (WHO grade I), subependymoma (WHO grade I), ependymoma (WHO grade II), and anaplastic ependymoma (WHO grade III).

Incidence

- There are two incidence peaks occurring between the ages of 3 and 8 years and in the fourth and fifth decades of life.
- Ependymomas are more common in the pediatric population, comprising 5.6% of childhood CNS tumors diagnosed between the ages of 10 and 14 years and 4.5% of tumors found in those between the ages of 15 and 19.
- Ependymomas are the third most common brain tumor in children, with about 60% of these tumors occurring in the posterior fossa.
- In adults, 60% of ependymomas occur in the spine.
- In adults, ependymomas account for 1.9% of intracranial gliomas and 22% of spinal cord tumors.

Etiology and Risk Factors

The exact cause of ependymomas is not known. Spinal ependymomas can be associated with neurofibromatosis.

Signs and Symptoms

- Ependymomas often occur in an infratentorial location. Subsequently the signs and symptoms are those associated with increased intracranial pressure due to hydrocephalus, including morning headaches, vomiting, ataxia, cranial nerve deficits, and decreased level of consciousness.
- Because of their propensity to occur in the spinal cord, ependymomas can be associated with paresthesias, hemiplegias, and pain. Focal findings are related to tumor location (see Brain Function and Symptoms Associated with Lesion Location table on page 42).

Diagnostic Work-up

- Neurologic examination
- Cytologic examination of CSF
- MRI of the brain and spine
- Biopsy for a tissue diagnosis

Histology

- Ependymomas can be divided into supratentorial and infratentorial tumors.
- Most ependymomas are cellular tumors consisting of uniform polygonal cells in a collagenous background with well-defined cytoplasmic borders.
- May also contain areas of cysts, calcifications, and occasional hemorrhage.

- Anaplastic ependymomas have features that resemble GBMs, with high mitotic activity, endothelial proliferation, and necrosis.

Clinical Staging

Because of the location in or near CSF pathways, the staging process is essential to determine whether the ependymoma has metastasized. Staging includes a spinal MRI and obtaining a CSF sample for cytologic examination.

Treatment

- Surgery should be performed for maximal resection and relief of hydrocephalus. A ventriculoperitoneal shunt may be placed if needed. For patients older than 3 years of age with low-grade tumors of the brain or spine, gross total resection is considered complete therapy.
- Focal radiation therapy may be given for residual disease, unless it has disseminated along CSF pathways; craniospinal irradiation is then required.
- Adjuvant chemotherapy does not improve survival but may be used for a recurrence. It may be used on children younger than 3 years of age to defer radiation therapy.

Prognosis

- Prognosis depends on several factors, including age, tumor location, pathologic grade, and extent of surgical resection.
- Chromosomal abnormalities, genetic profiles, and biomarkers for the tumor may help to better specify the prognosis in the pediatric population.
- The overall 5-year survival rate for adults is 82%.

Prevention and Surveillance

- There are no known preventive measures to reduce the incidence of primary CNS tumors.
- After patients have completed the prescribed therapy, they are monitored according to the NCCN guidelines, which are based on the extent and location of disease.
- For localized disease, serial MRI scans are obtained every 3 to 4 months for 1 year after therapy, every 4 to 6 months in the second year, and every 6 to 12 months thereafter based on the disease status and according to the physician's discretion.

Bibliography

Beatriz, M., Lopes, S., & Scheithauer, B. W. (2012). Histopathology of brain tumors. In A. H. Kaye & E. R. Laws, Jr. (Eds.), *Brain tumors* (3rd ed.) (pp. 151–152). Edinburgh: Saunders.

CERN Foundation. (2014). *Ependymoma statistics.* Available at https://cern-foundation.org/?page_id=103 (accessed December 11, 2015).

King, J., & Kulkarni, A. V. (2012). Intracranial ependymomas. In A. H. Kaye & E. R. Laws, Jr. (Eds.), *Brain tumors* (3rd ed.) (pp. 435–449). Edinburgh: Saunders.

National Comprehensive Cancer Network. (2015). *Central nervous system cancers.* Available at http://www.nccn.org/professionals/physician_gls/PDF/cns.pdf (accessed December 11, 2015).

Michaud, K. (2011). Medical treatment of spinal cord tumors. In M. Mehta, S. Chang, A. Guha, H. B. Newton, & M. A. Vogelbaum (Eds.), *Principles and practices of neuro-oncology: A multidisciplinary approach* (p. 635). New York: Demos Medical.

National Cancer Institute. (2015). *Adult central nervous system tumors treatment—for health professionals (PDQ).* Available at http://www.cancer.gov/types/brain/hp/adult-brain-treatment-pdq#section/all (accessed December 11, 2015).

National Cancer Institute. (2014). *Childhood ependymoma treatment—for health professionals (PDQ).* Available at http://www.cancer.gov/types/brain/hp/child-ependymoma-treatment-pdq (accessed December 11, 2015).

Ostrom, Q. T., Gittleman, H., Liao, P., Rouse, C., Chen, Y., Dowling, J., et al (2014). CBTRUS statistical report: Primary brain and central nervous system tumors diagnosed in the United States in 2007–2011. *Neuro-oncology,* 16(Suppl 4), iv1–iv63.

Metastatic Brain Tumors

Definition

Metastatic brain tumors originate in other parts of the body and spread to the brain. They retain the microscopic appearance and characteristics of the original tumor cells.

Incidence

Metastatic brain tumors make up the greatest number of CNS tumors. They outnumber primary brain tumors by 10 to 1. An estimated 10% to 30% of cancer patients develop brain metastases. Although any solid tumor can metastasize to the brain, the most common metastatic tumors arise in the lung (50%), breast (10% to 30%), skin (melanoma, 5% to 21%), and colon and kidney (5% to 10%). Between 10% and 15% of metastatic brain tumors have an unknown primary site. The incidence of metastatic brain tumors is increasing, likely as a result of prolonged survival due to improved systemic therapies.

Etiology and Risk Factors

Metastatic brain tumors occur as a result of the spread of a primary cancer. Age and sex are risk factors, but they vary by the primary tumor type.

Signs and Symptoms

Signs and symptoms depend on tumor size and location, and they are often related to increased intracranial pressure (see Brain Function and Symptoms Associated with Lesion Location table on page 42).

Diagnostic Work-up

- Neurologic examination
- MRI of the brain or spine
- Biopsy or craniotomy for a tissue diagnosis

Histology

Biopsy or craniotomy is essential to obtain a tissue diagnosis. It can never be assumed that a brain lesion in the context of a prior cancer is a metastatic lesion.

Clinical Staging

Metastatic tumors to the brain are not graded according to the WHO system for primary brain tumors. Instead, they are evaluated based on the original tumor cell type, and all cancers with distant metastases are considered to be stage IV disease.

Treatment

Treatment depends on tumor size and histology. The status of a patient's primary disease is essential in determining treatment options for a metastatic brain lesion, and a patient with a newly diagnosed brain lesion must undergo a thorough work-up. If the primary disease is controlled, surgery and radiation therapy (e.g., whole brain, stereotactic radiosurgery) are the recommended treatments. Depending on the primary disease, chemotherapy may or may not be recommended.

Prognosis

Prognosis depends on the number, size, and location of metastases. Historically, many patients died of uncontrolled primary disease, not from metastatic brain lesions. However, with improved treatment of primary tumors and longer survival times, brain metastases have the potential to become a fatal complication of cancer.

Prevention and Surveillance

- There are no known preventive measures to reduce the incidence of primary CNS tumors, but some strategies are being considered to inhibit metastatic disease, including angiogenesis inhibitors that prevent blood vessel invasion and green tea polyphenols that interfere with signaling pathways.
- After patients have completed the prescribed therapy, they are monitored according to the NCCN guidelines.
- Serial MRI scans are obtained every 3 months for the first year after therapy and then according to the physician's discretion and status of systemic disease.

Bibliography

Melisko, M. (2011). Brain metastases and leptomeningeal disease. In M. Mehta, S. Chang, A. Guha, H. B. Newton, & M. A. Vogelbaum (Eds.), *Principles and practice of neuro-oncology: A multidisciplinary approach* (pp. 638–649). New York: Demos Medical.

National Cancer Institute. (2015). *Adult central nervous system tumors treatment—for health professionals (PDQ).* Available at http://www.cancer.gov/types/brain/hp/adult-brain-treatment-pdq#section/all (accessed December 11, 2015).

National Comprehensive Cancer Network. (2015). *Central nervous system cancers.* Available at http://www.nccn.org/professionals/physician_gls/PDF/cns.pdf (accessed December 11, 2015).

Sawaya, R., Bindal, R., Lang, F., & Suki, D. (2012). Metastatic brain tumors. In A. H. Kaye & E. R. Laws, Jr. (Eds.), *Brain tumors* (3rd ed.) (pp. 864–892). Edinburgh: Saunders.

Mixed Glioma

Definition

Mixed gliomas are malignant tumors that develop from a combination of glial cells, including astrocytes, oligodendrocytes, and ependymal cells. Glial cells normally maintain homeostasis, generate myelin, and protect neurons in the brain.

Incidence

Mixed glial cell tumors are most commonly found in adults 20 to 50 years of age. They are most common in men. About up 1% of primary brain tumors are mixed gliomas.

Etiology and Risk Factors

There is no known cause for brain tumors; however, the following are considered risk factors:

- Therapeutic ionizing radiation to the head
- Genetic disorders, including neurofibromatosis type 1 and 2, tuberous sclerosis, von Hippel–Lindau syndrome, Li-Fraumeni syndrome, and Turcot syndrome

Signs and Symptoms

Signs and symptoms depend on location (see Brain Function and Symptoms Associated with Lesion Location table on page 42).

Diagnostic Work-up

- Neurologic examination
- MRI of the brain or spine
- Biopsy or craniotomy for a tissue diagnosis
- Molecular characterization

Histology

The histologic features of mixed gliomas correlate with the grade and types of cells identified. The astrocytes, oligodendrocytes, and ependymal cells can have various degrees of malignant and nonmalignant features. The most aggressive type of cell found in the tumor specimen determines the tumor grade.

Cytogenetic analysis can provide molecular characterization of these tumors. Mixed tumors that have an oligodendroglioma-dominant component often have deletion of chromosome arms 1p and 19q. Astrocytoma-dominant tumors tend to have a *TP53* gene mutation with or without loss of chromosome 17p.

Clinical Staging

Because of the very low incidence of metastasis, staging is not usually done for mixed gliomas.

Treatment

Mixed gliomas are treated by using the recommended treatments (e.g., surgery, radiation therapy, chemotherapy, targeted therapy) for the most aggressive or anaplastic cell type found in the tumor.

Prognosis

The prognosis for mixed gliomas depends on the most aggressive or anaplastic part of the tumor and on factors such as number of recurrences, patient age and performance status, and molecular diagnostic results. Loss of chromosome arms 1p and 19q tends to confer longer progression-free survival.

Prevention and Surveillance

- There are no known preventive measures to reduce the incidence of primary CNS tumors.
- After patients have completed the prescribed therapy, they are monitored according to the NCCN guidelines for managing the most aggressive or anaplastic portion of the tumor.

- WHO grade I: Serial MRI scans are obtained every 3 to 6 months for 5 years after therapy and then at least annually thereafter.
- WHO grade II: Serial MRI scans are obtained every 3 to 6 months for 5 years after therapy and then at least annually thereafter.
- WHO grade III: Serial MRI scans are obtained at 2- to 4-month intervals for the first 2 to 3 years after therapy and then less frequently according to the physician's discretion.
- WHO grade IV: Serial MRI scans are obtained at 2- to 4-month intervals for the first 2 to 3 years after therapy and then less frequently according to the physician's discretion.

Bibliography

Beatriz, M., Lopes, S., & Scheithauer, B. W. (2012). Histopathology of brain tumors. In A. H. Kaye & E. R. Laws, Jr. (Eds.), *Brain tumors* (3rd ed.) (pp. 151–152). Edinburgh: Saunders.

National Comprehensive Cancer Network. (2015). *Central nervous system cancers.* Available at http://www.nccn.org/professionals/physician_gls/PDF/cns.pdf (accessed December 11, 2015).

National Cancer Institute. (2015). *Adult central nervous system tumors treatment—for health professionals (PDQ).* Available at http://www.cancer.gov/types/brain/hp/adult-brain-treatment-pdq#section/all (accessed December 11, 2015).

Ostrom, Q. T., Gittleman, H., Liao, P., Rouse, C., Chen, Y., Dowling, J., et al (2014). CBTRUS statistical report: Primary brain and central nervous system tumors diagnosed in the United States in 2007–2011. *Neuro-oncology, 16*(Suppl 4), iv1–iv63.

Oligodendroglioma

Definition

An oligodendroglioma is a tumor that develops from the oligodendrocytes, which are glial cells that support neurons in the brain.

Incidence

Oligodendrogliomas account for 6% of CNS gliomas. They are divided into WHO grade II and anaplastic grade III tumors. WHO grade II oligodendrogliomas are most common in patients between 20 and 40 years of age. The peak incidence occurs between 35 and 45 years, and they are more common in men than women. WHO grade III tumors are more common in older patients, with most occurring between the mid-30s and 60s. The peak incidence occurs between 55 and 64 years.

Etiology and Risk Factors

There is no known cause for brain tumors, but the following are considered risk factors:

- Therapeutic ionizing radiation to the head
- Genetic disorders, including neurofibromatosis type 1 and 2, tuberous sclerosis, von Hippel–Lindau syndrome, and Li-Fraumeni syndrome

Signs and Symptoms

Signs and symptoms of oligodendrogliomas depend on location (see Brain Function and Symptoms Associated with Lesion Location table on page 42).

Diagnostic Work-up

- Neurologic examination
- MRI of the brain and spine
- Biopsy or craniotomy for a tissue diagnosis
- Molecular characterization

Histology

The histology of oligodendrogliomas determines grade or type. They are classified as grade II or III using the WHO classification for CNS tumors (see World Health Organization Grading of Tumors table on page 42).

- Oligodendrogliomas are considered WHO grade II, and anaplastic oligodendrogliomas are WHO grade III. The grade III tumors are identified by increased cell density, increased number of mitoses, and thickened vascular endothelium due to cell hyperplasia. Because of the very low incidence of metastasis, staging is not usually done for oligodendrogliomas.

Cytogenetic analysis allows molecular characterization of these tumors.

- A hallmark of oligodendrogliomal tumors is deletion of chromosome arm 1p with or without deletion of chromosome 19q. Eighty percent of oligodendrogliomas have a loss of both chromosome arms.
- Grade II and III oligodendrogliomas also demonstrate a high frequency of *IDH1* gene mutations, which block the maturation of cells and result in overproduction of immature cells and tumor formation. *IDH1* mutations are commonly associated with the 1p and 19q deletions.

Treatment

Appropriate treatment depends on the grade of the tumor, extent of resection, and age of the patient.

- Surgery is recommended for all oligodendrogliomas to establish a diagnosis and minimize tumor burden. It may be the only therapy necessary for lower grade tumors if resection is complete.
- Radiation is used to treat aggressive grade III tumors and recurrence of lower grade tumors.
- Radiation therapy is highly recommended for patients who are older than 40 years of age with a subtotal resection and if chromosome arms 1p and 19q are intact.
- Chemotherapy is recommended for all oligodendrogliomas with the 1p/19q deletion.
- Depending on the patient's age and extent of resection, chemotherapy may be used instead of radiation therapy initially.
- For patients with WHO grade III oligodendrogliomas with 1p and 19q intact, chemotherapy may or may not be added to radiation therapy as part of the initial treatment.

Prognosis

- Prognosis depends on the grade of the oligodendroglioma, and it is usually better than for astrocytomas of similar grade.
- Median survival for low-grade oligodendroglioma patients is 9.8 years.
- 89% of patients survive 2 years, 79% survive 5 years, and 62% survive 10 years.

- Patients with WHO grade III tumors have a 68%, 52%, and 39% survival rate at 2, 5, and 10 years, respectively.
- For all grades of oligodendrogliomas, deletion of chromosome arms 1p and 19q is an additional prognostic factor, predicting responsiveness to alkylating chemotherapy agents and prolonged progression-free survival.
  - Low-grade oligodendroglioma patients with 1p and 19q deletions have a median survival of 13.0 years, compared with 9.1 years for those without the deletions.
  - Anaplastic oligodendroglioma patients with loss of chromosome arms 1p and 19q have a median survival of 6 to 7 years, compared with 2 to 3 years for those without the deletions.

Prevention and Surveillance

- There are no known preventive measures to reduce the incidence of primary CNS tumors.
- After oligodendroglioma patients have completed the prescribed therapy, they are monitored according to the NCCN guidelines, which are based on management of the most aggressive portion of the tumor.
  - WHO grade II: Serial MRI scans are obtained every 3 to 6 months for 5 years after therapy and at least annually thereafter.
  - WHO grade III: Serial MRI scans are obtained at 2- to 4-month intervals for the first 2 to 3 years after therapy and then less frequently according to the physician's discretion.

Bibliography

Beatriz, M., Lopes, S., & Scheithauer, B. W. (2012). Histopathology of brain tumors. In A. H. Kaye & E. R. Laws, Jr. (Eds.), *Brain tumors* (3rd ed.) (pp. 147–148). Edinburgh: Saunders.

Clarke, J., Ney, D. E., Shyu, C. C., & Lassman, A. B. (2011). Medical management of supratentorial gliomas in adults. In M. Mehta, S. Chang, A. Guha, H. B. Newton, & M. A. Vogelbaum (Eds.), *Principles and practice of neuro-oncology: A multidisciplinary approach* (pp. 562–578). New York: Demos Medical.

Fischer, I., Sulman, E., & Aldape, K. (2011). Molecular pathogenesis of glioma: Overview and therapeutic implications. In M. Mehta, S. Chang, A. Guha, H. B. Newton, & M. A. Vogelbaum (Eds.), *Principles and practice of neuro-oncology: A multidisciplinary approach* (p. 635). New York: Demos Medical.

McCarthy, B. (2011). Descriptive epidemiology of glioma. In M. Mehta, S. Chang, A. Guha, H. B. Newton, & M. A. Vogelbaum (Eds.), *Principles and practices of neuro-oncology: A multidisciplinary approach* (pp. 6–7). New York: Demos Medical.

National Cancer Institute. (2015). *Adult central nervous system tumors treatment—for health professionals (PDQ): Treatment of primary central nervous system tumors by tumor type.* Available at http://www.cancer.gov/types/brain/hp/adult-brain-treatment-pdq#link/_792 (accessed December 11, 2015).

National Comprehensive Cancer Network. (2015). *Central nervous system cancers.* Available at http://www.nccn.org/professionals/physician_gls/PDF/cns.pdf (accessed December 11, 2015).

Ostrom, Q. T., Gittleman, H., Liao, P., Rouse, C., Chen, Y., Dowling, J., et al (2014). CBTRUS statistical report: Primary brain and central nervous system tumors diagnosed in the United States in 2007–2011. *Neuro-oncology*, 16(Suppl 4), iv1–iv63.

Wu, A., & Lang, F. (2011). Insular tumors. In M. Mehta, S. Chang, A. Guha, H. B. Newton, & M. A. Vogelbaum (Eds.), *Principles and practices of neuro-oncology: A multidisciplinary approach* (p. 510). New York: Demos Medical.

Primitive Neuroectodermal Tumor

Definition

Primitive neuroectodermal tumor (pNET) is a WHO grade IV embryonal tumor that arises from the neural crest. Some pNETs occur in the brain, whereas peripheral pNETs occur in sites outside the brain such as in soft tissue, peripheral nerves, and solid organs. Only tumors of the CNS are discussed here; the peripheral pNETs are addressed with Ewing sarcomas in the Sarcoma chapter (see page 143). PNETs are further categorized by the predominant cell subtype, including CNS neuroblastoma and CNS ganglioneuroblastoma. Other subtypes include medulloepithelioma and ependymoblastoma, which are rare and occur only in neonates and children.

Incidence

PNETs are more common in children than adults. The tumors account for less than 1% of primary supratentorial brain tumors in adults. Most supratentorial pNETs diagnosed in adults occur between the ages of 21 and 30 years.

Etiology and Risk Factors

- Therapeutic ionizing radiation to the head
- Genetic disorders, including Turcot syndrome and Li-Fraumeni syndrome

Signs and Symptoms

- Usually related to increased intracranial pressure and tumor location (see Brain Function and Symptoms Associated with Lesion Location table on page 42).
- Cranial nerve palsies and spinal cord symptoms with tumors disseminated in the brain or spinal cord

Diagnostic Work-up

- Neurologic examination
- MRI of the brain or spine
- Biopsy or craniotomy for a tissue diagnosis

Histology

Supratentorial pNETs are derived from primitive neuroepithelial progenitors or stem cells distributed throughout the neuraxis. They demonstrate a high degree of cellularity, brisk mitotic activity, and a tendency for focal necrosis.

Clinical Staging

PNETs are fast growing, with a propensity to disseminate along CSF pathways. Staging is essential to detect whether the lesion has metastasized. Staging includes a spinal MRI scan and CSF cytologic examination before surgery or 2 to 3 weeks after surgery to look for evidence of dissemination.

Treatment

- Craniotomy or biopsy, depending on tumor location
- Irradiation of the entire neuraxis because of the high propensity of the tumor to disseminate through the CSF
- The advantage of adding chemotherapy to the treatment regimen remains unclear, but standard treatment includes regimens that use nitrosoureas and platinum-based regimens.

Prognosis

The mean survival time is 86 months, with a 3-year survival rate of 75%.

Prevention and Surveillance

- There are no known preventative measures to reduce the incidence of primary CNS tumors.
- After patients have completed the prescribed therapy, they are monitored according to the NCCN guidelines.
- Serial MRI scans are obtained every 3 months for the first 2 years after therapy, every 6 months for the next 3 years, and then annually thereafter.

Bibliography

Beatriz, M., Lopes, S., & Scheithauer, B. W. (2012). Histopathology of brain tumors. In A. H. Kaye & E. R. Laws, Jr. (Eds.), *Brain tumors* (3rd ed.) (pp. 163–165). Edinburgh: Saunders.

Gonzales, M. (2012). Classification and pathogenesis of brain tumors. In A. H. Kaye & E. R. Laws, Jr. (Eds.), *Brain tumors* (3rd ed.) (pp. 39, 47). Edinburgh: Saunders.

Grier, H. E. (1997). The Ewing family of tumors: Ewing sarcoma and primitive neuroectodermal tumors. *Pediatric Clinics of North America, 44*(4), 991–1004.

Kim, D. G., Lee, D. Y., Paek, S. H., Chi, J. G., Choe, G., & Jung, H. W. (2002). Supratentorial primitive neuroectodermal tumors in adults. *Journal of Neuro-Oncology, 60*, 43–52.

National Cancer Institute. (2015). *Adult central nervous system tumors treatment—for health professionals (PDQ): Treatment of primary central nervous system tumors by tumor type*. Available at http://www.cancer.gov/types/brain/hp/adult-brain-treatment-pdq#link/_792 (accessed December 11, 2015).

Ostrom, Q. T., Gittleman, H., Liao, P., Rouse, C., Chen, Y., Dowling, J., et al (2014). CBTRUS statistical report: Primary brain and central nervous system tumors diagnosed in the United States in 2007–2011. *Neuro-oncology, 16*(Suppl 4), iv1–iv63.

Pizer, B. L., Weston, C. L., Robinson, K. J., Ellison, D. W., Ironside, J., Saran, F., et al (2006). Analysis of patients with supratentorial primitive neuroectodermal tumors entered into the SIOP/UKCCSG PNET 3 study. *European Journal of Cancer, 42*(8), 1120–1128.

Recurrent Glial Tumor

Definition

A recurrent glioma is one that has recurred despite surgery, irradiation, or chemotherapy. Growth is demonstrated by changes in volume or enhancement on serial MRI scans and neurologic decline. It may require additional scanning (e.g., MRS) to differentiate among tumor, necrosis, and treatment effects.

Incidence

The incidence of recurrent gliomas is very high. High-grade gliomas recur in most patients.

Etiology and Risk Factors

There is no known cause for the development of a primary brain tumor. Recurrent glial tumors are gliomas that have continued to grow and accumulate genetic mutations despite treatment attempts.

Signs and Symptoms

Signs and symptoms depend on tumor size and location (see Brain Function and Symptoms Associated with Lesion Location table on page 42).

Diagnostic Work-up

- Neurologic examination
- MRI or MRS scans of the brain or spine
- Biopsy or craniotomy for a tissue diagnosis
- Molecular characterization

Histology

Recurrent gliomas usually have necrotic areas mixed with nuclear atypia, increased mitotic activity, and anaplasia. It is not uncommon for the tumor to recur as a more aggressive or malignant type of glioma (i.e., glioblastoma).

Clinical Staging

Staging is not usually done for recurrent gliomas.

Treatment

- Surgery is done to debulk the tumor, decreasing the tumor burden and alleviating symptoms.
- Radiation therapy depends on the location of the recurrence, prior radiation treatment, and type of radiation to be delivered. If the recurrence is in the same area as the original tumor, radiation therapy usually cannot be repeated. Stereotactic radiosurgery may be used in this context.
- Chemotherapy or other cytotoxic agents such as temozolomide or nitrosoureas may be administered if they were not used in the adjuvant setting. Other standard therapeutic agents include bevacizumab, etoposide, and carboplatin.
- Additional options include enrollment in clinical trials. The benefit of participating in a trial is that, although there is no guarantee, it is possible that the agent could improve survival. An example of such a trial is a test of a vaccine for patients with glial cell tumors who tested positive for the *EGFR* variant III mutation. Patients who received the vaccine had a longer time to progression (12 months) compared with those who did not (7.1 months). A patient must always weigh out the risks versus benefits to participation.

Prognosis

Median survival after recurrence is grim. It varies from 2 to 3 months for older, incapacitated patients to 1 year for younger, neurologically intact patients. Important factors when considering further therapy include age, performance status, and histologic diagnosis.

Prevention and Surveillance

- There are no known preventive measures to reduce the incidence of primary CNS tumors.
- The guidelines for using MRI for recurrent gliomas are based on the status of the disease and the prescribed treatment plan for the individual patient. After patients have completed the prescribed therapy, they are monitored according to the NCCN guidelines, which are based on management of the most aggressive portion of the tumor.
  - WHO grade I: Recurrent glioma scans are obtained every 2- to 4-month interval. Serial MRI scans are obtained at 2- to 4-month intervals for the first 2 to 3 years after therapy and then less frequently according to the physician's discretion.

Bibliography

Hou, L., & Harsh, G. R., IV (2012). Management of recurrent gliomas and meningiomas. In A. H. Kaye & E. R. Laws, Jr. (Eds.), *Brain tumors* (3rd ed.) (pp. 355–371). Edinburgh: Saunders.

National Cancer Institute. (2015). *Adult central nervous system tumors treatment—for health professionals (PDQ): Treatment of primary central nervous system tumors by tumor type.* Available at http://www.cancer.gov/types/brain/hp/adult-brain-treatment-pdq#link/_792 (accessed December 11, 2015).

Ostrom, Q. T., Gittleman, H., Liao, P., Rouse, C., Chen, Y., Dowling, J., et al (2014). CBTRUS statistical report: Primary brain and central nervous system tumors diagnosed in the United States in 2007–2011. *Neuro-oncology*, 16(Suppl 4), iv1–iv63.

Gastrointestinal System Cancers

Anal Cancer

Lisa Parks

Definition

The anus is the most distal part of the large intestine, and it connects the large intestine and the rectum. The anal canal is 1 to 2 inches long and allows stool to pass from the body as a bowel movement. Anal cancer arises from the squamous epithelial cells distal to the anal rim or from the squamous and cylindrical epithelial tissue of the anal canal. Eighty percent of anal cancers are squamous cell types. Cloacogenic carcinomas, which arise from the anal transition zone, are less common than squamous cell anal cancer. Uncommon types of anal cancers are adenocarcinoma, lymphoma, sarcoma, and melanoma.

Incidence

Anal cancer is rare, accounting for only 0.4% of all new cancer cases. The cause of anal cancer is uncertain, although it is often linked to human papillomavirus (HPV) infection. HPV infection can cause an anal intraepithelial neoplasia (AIN) to progress from low-grade to high-grade dysplasia and then to invasive carcinoma.

The incidence of anal cancer is higher among individuals with human immunodeficiency virus (HIV) infection, and 93% of them are men. Women with cervical intraepithelial neoplasia (CIN) have a three times greater risk of having a concurrent HPV infection of the anus.

Etiology and Risk Factors

- Infection with the HPV16 subtype is most frequently associated with anal cancer.
- HIV-positive persons are at increased risk for anal cancer, as are men and women who have receptive anal intercourse.
- Persons with a history of multiple sex partners and a history of smoking are at greater risk.
- Other risk factors include cervical, vulvar, or vaginal cancers; immunosuppression after solid organ transplantation; hematologic malignancies; and autoimmune disorders.

Signs and Symptoms

- Anal cancer is often asymptomatic.
- The most common symptom is rectal bleeding.
- Other symptoms include rectal itching, discomfort or pain in the anal area, changes in stool caliber, abnormal anal discharge, and swollen lymph nodes in the anal or inguinal area.

Diagnostic Work-up

Anal cancer can be diagnosed by several methods. Early detection carries a better prognosis, and examinations can be done in a health care provider's office:
- Digital rectal examination performed by a health care provider is the simplest technique.
- An anoscope may be inserted into the anal canal to visualize the anus and lower rectum.
- A rigid proctosigmoidoscopy requires patient preparation with a laxative or enema to visualize the anal canal and distal sigmoid colon.
- A biopsy is performed for further evaluation if anything suspicious is discovered.
  - Excisional biopsy may be performed.
  - Fine-needle aspiration (FNA) biopsy may be performed to sample surrounding lymph nodes in the groin or anal region to detect cancer spread.
- Anal Papanicolaou (Pap) tests can be used to obtain cell samples for evaluation of high-risk patients.
- Ultrasound can be used to assess cancer spread into surrounding structures.
- Computed tomography (CT) of the chest, abdomen, and pelvis is used to assess metastatic disease.
- Magnetic resonance imaging (MRI) is used to diagnose anal cancer. It uses no radiation and produces more detailed images than CT.
- Positron emission tomography (PET) is a specialized nuclear imaging test that uses a radioactive tracer. Cancer cells are highly metabolically active, and PET assesses the increased metabolic activity to diagnose metastatic changes.

Histology

The anus consists of three main histologic tissue types: glandular, transitional, and keratinized or nonkeratinized squamous.
- The proximal anus has glandular tissue consisting of irregular crypts and smooth muscle fibers in the underlying tissue (i.e., lamina propria).
- The transitional tissue of the anus is found between uninterrupted columnar mucosa above and uninterrupted squamous epithelia below. Transitional epithelia contain features of both urothelium (i.e., small basal cells) and squamous epithelium. It appears wrinkled and glistening and produces minimal mucin. The transitional tissue has anal glands in the submucosa and has endocrine cells and occasional melanocytes. The tissue expresses cytokeratin 7 positive (CK7+) and cytokeratin 20 negative (CK20-). The distal region of the anus consists of the dentate line to

the squamous mucocutaneous junction. It is composed of nonkeratinizing squamous epithelium without appendages or glands. This lower region contains melanocytes, keratin, hair, and apocrine glands.

Clinical Staging

Anal cancer is staged according to the tumor, node, and metastasis (TNM) system developed by the American Joint Committee on Cancer (AJCC) (Compton, et. al., 2012). Tumor staging describes the size of the primary tumor in centimeters. Nodal staging describes the extent of spread to nearby or local lymph nodes. Metastasis staging denotes spread to other body organs

Treatment

Treatment goals for anal cancer consist of removal of the primary tumor with preservation of the structure and function of anal sphincters.

- T1–T2N0 anal cancer: The primary treatment according to National Comprehensive Cancer Network (NCCN) guidelines is a regimen of 5-fluorouracil (5-FU) plus mitomycin and radiation therapy.
- T3–T4N0 or any T with positive nodes: The NCCN recommends the previously described therapy with irradiation of the original primary tumor site and affected lymph nodes over 6 to 7.5 weeks.
- Metastatic anal cancer: The NCCN recommends 6 to 7.5 weeks of irradiation plus chemotherapy with cisplatin and 5-FU.

Surgery is used for residual or recurrent anal cancer. Residual disease is defined as a tumor found within 6 months of treatment, and recurrent disease is a tumor that develops more than 6 months after a complete response.

Prognosis

Patients with a higher T category and positive nodal status have poorer survival and higher relapse rates. Patients with T0–T3N0 disease have the best survival and lowest relapse rates. T3-4N+ disease has the poorest survival rates and highest relapse rates. Patients with lower tumor burden and involved nodes have a better prognosis than those with node-negative disease but a high tumor burden.

Prevention and Surveillance

Strategies for prevention of anal cancer are public health issues. A quadrivalent HPV vaccine is available and approved for preventing AIN and anal cancer related to infection with HPV6, HPV11, HPV16, or HPV18 in men who have sex with men. Other recommendations include the following:

- Smoking or tobacco cessation
- Use of condoms during intercourse
- Avoidance of multiple sexual partners
- Avoidance of anal intercourse

Guidelines for routine screening for anal cancer have not been established. No studies have demonstrated the effectiveness or benefit of screening. The European Acquired Immunodeficiency Syndrome (AIDS) Clinical Society recommends screening high-risk groups such as HIV-infected men who have sex with men, patients with a history of anal condyloma, HIV-infected women, women with cervical or vulvar dysplasia, chronically immunosuppressed persons, organ transplant recipients, and women with a history of cervical or vulvar cancer. Digital rectal examinations annually can serve as simple screening method for high-risk individuals. Anal cytology may also be useful in screening high-risk persons.

Bibliography

Benson, A., Arnoletti, J., Kekaii-Saab, T., Chan, E., Chen, Y., Choti, M., & Freedman-Cass, D. (2012). Anal carcinoma, version 2.2012: Featured updates to the NCCN guidelines. *Journal of the National Comprehensive Cancer Network, 10,* 449–454.

Bown, E., Shah, V., Sridhar, T., Boyle, K., Hemingway, D., & Yeung, J. (2014). Cancers of the anal canal: Diagnosis, treatment, and future strategies. *Future Oncology, 10*(8), 1427–1441.

Coaker, M., & White, M. (2013). Anal cancer: Developments in treatment and patient management. *Gastrointestinal Nursing, 11*(1), 32–38.

Compton, C., Byrd, D., Garcia-Aguilar, J., Kurtzman, S., Olawaiye, A., & Washington, M. K. (2012). *AJCC cancer staging atlas.* New York: Springer, 165–174.

GattYoc, L., Flowers, L., & Ault, K. (2012). Anal intraepithelial neoplasia and anal cancer: Who should be screened? *Contemporary OB/GYN ONLINE* (April), 36–45.

Gunderson, L., Moughan, J., Ajani, J., Pedersen, J., Winter, K., Benson, A., & Willett, C. (2013). Anal carcinoma: Impact of TN category of disease on survival, disease relapse, and colostomy failure in US Gastrointestinal Intergroup RTOG 98-11 phase 3 trial. *International Journal of Radiation Oncology and Biological Physiology, 87*(4), 638–645.

Mallik, S., Benson, R., Julka, P., & Rath, G. (2015). Shifting paradigm in the management of anal canal carcinoma. *Journal of Gastrointestinal Cancer, 46*(1), 1–4.

National Comprehensive Cancer Network. (2015). *NCCN clinical practice guidelines in oncology: Anal carcinoma, version 2.2015.* Available at http://www.nccn.org/professionals/physician_gls/pdf/anal.pdf (accessed December 18, 2015).

Romanofski, D. (2014). Anal cancer. *Radiation Therapist, 23*(2), 165–193.

Smyczek, P., Singh, A., & Romanowski, B. (2013). Anal intraepithelial neoplasia: Review and recommendations for screening and management. *International Journal of STD & AIDS, 24*(11), 843–851.

Cholangiocarcinoma and Gallbladder Cancer

Lisa Parks

Definition

Cholangiocarcinoma (i.e., intrahepatic and extrahepatic bile duct cancer) is an epithelial cell malignancy of the biliary tract arising from the ductal epithelium in the liver (i.e., intrahepatic cancer) or outside the liver (i.e., extrahepatic cancer). Classification is based on the anatomic location and includes intrahepatic, perihilar, and distal cholangiocarcinoma.

- Intrahepatic cholangiocarcinoma is located proximally to the second-degree bile ducts. The term *proximal* refers to the direction of the bile flow, making the intrahepatic ducts proximal to the common bile duct.
- Perihilar cholangiocarcinoma is located between the second-degree bile ducts and where the cystic duct inserts into the common bile duct.
- Distal cholangiocarcinoma is located between the cystic duct origin and the ampulla of Vater.

Gallbladder cancer is an adenocarcinoma that arises from the biliary epithelium. It is the most common malignancy of the biliary tract and has the poorest prognosis.

Incidence

- The incidence of intrahepatic cholangiocarcinomas is increasing in many Western countries.
- In the United States in 2015, the incidence was 1 to 2 cases per 100,000 people in the general population, totaling approximately 10,910 new cases (with equal numbers of intrahepatic and extrahepatic disease) and 3700 deaths.
- Gallbladder cancer accounts for less than 40% of these malignancies. In 2014, the incidence of gallbladder cancer in the United States was 0.9 and 0.5 cases per 100,000 women and men, respectively.
- White women have a higher incidence of gallbladder cancer than other groups.
- Central and northern Europe, India, and Chile have a higher incidence of gallbladder cancer than the United States.

Etiology and Risk Factors

Most cholangiocarcinomas are not associated with risk factors. However, some risk factors are known:
- Intrahepatic cholangiocarcinoma: Risk factors include cirrhosis and viral hepatitis B and C.
- Cholangiocarcinoma: Risk factors include primary sclerosing cholangitis with chronic inflammation causing cholestasis and resulting in injury of the intrahepatic and extrahepatic biliary epithelium. Response to the injured epithelium leads to restructuring and destruction of the biliary tree.
- Bile duct cysts: The congenital disorder causes cystic dilation of a portion of the intrahepatic and extrahepatic biliary system, which dumps pancreatic enzymes into the biliary tree and causes bile stasis and malignant transformation of cells.
- Gallbladder cancer: Risk factors include chronic inflammation of the gallbladder mucosa due to gallstones, gallbladder polyps, typhoid infection, and anomalous junction of the pancreaticobiliary ductal system. In Asia, liver flukes are ingested along with raw fish. The worms infest the liver and produce eggs that are released in the biliary system, resulting in chronic inflammation that leads to malignant transformation.

Signs and Symptoms

Possible signs and symptoms of cholangiocarcinoma and gallbladder cancer are similar:
- Painless jaundice and pruritus
- Clay-colored stools and tea-colored urine
- Nausea
- Weight loss
- Fever due to cholangitis
- Right upper quadrant discomfort and a bloating sensation
- Elevated bilirubin, alkaline phosphatase, and transaminase levels

Diagnostic Work-up

- Right upper quadrant ultrasound is often the initial imaging study for the patient who is seen in primary care. Ultrasound can identify intrahepatic and extrahepatic ductal dilation, choledochal cysts, cholelithiasis, and choledocholithiasis.
- CT or MRI may follow ultrasound.
- The level of the CA 19-9 tumor marker may be obtained, but it is not a specific test for cholangiocarcinoma and gallbladder cancer.
- Endoscopic retrograde cholangiography (ERCP) is useful in making the diagnosis.
- FNA may be used to determine the pathology.
- Endoscopic ultrasound (EUS) is the gold standard for staging gallbladder cancer.

Histology

Most cholangiocarcinomas and gallbladder cancers are adenocarcinomas, which are malignant tumors formed from glandular structures in epithelial tissue.
- In gallbladder cancer, 98% of tumors are adenocarcinomas. Other histologic types are papillary, mucinous, squamous, and adenosquamous carcinomas.
- The three subtypes of extrahepatic bile duct adenocarcinomas are sclerosing, nodular, and papillary.
- Sclerosing adenocarcinoma is the most common subtype of bile duct tumor. Vascular and perineural invasions are frequently associated with sclerosing adenocarcinoma.
- Sclerosing and nodular adenocarcinomas extend along the mucosa and submucosa of the bile ducts, and there is often no evidence of extrabiliary tumor spread.
- Papillary cholangiocarcinomas are rare intraluminal masses with late transmural extension.

Intrahepatic cholangiocarcinoma is difficult to diagnose because there are no tumor markers. *IDH1* and *IDH2* gene mutations in a gland-forming tumor in the liver strongly suggest intrahepatic cholangiocarcinoma, although the mutations occur in only one third of these neoplasms.

Clinical Staging

Tumor size has no prognostic value for cholangiocarcinoma and gallbladder cancer, but vascular invasion, number of tumors, and extent of lymph node involvement determine the staging classification. TNM staging is determined differently for Gallbladder and extrahepatic bile duct cancers (Kwon, et. al., 2015).

Treatment

Gallbladder Cancer

Stage I and II gallbladder cancer is potentially curable with resection, but less than 10% of patients have resectable cancer at the time of surgery. Early-stage gallbladder cancer may be found incidentally during a routine laparoscopic cholecystectomy. Laparoscopic cholecystectomy is contraindicated in cholangiocarcinoma. If gallbladder cancer is suspected, the patient should undergo an exploratory laparotomy and open cholecystectomy. If the frozen section tissue sample is positive for cancer, a radical cholecystectomy should be performed. There is no effective adjuvant treatment for gallbladder cancer.

Most patients are diagnosed with late-stage disease and need systemic therapies. Combination regimens with gemcitabine, fluoropyrimidine, and platinum-based agents are used to treat gallbladder cancer. Combined gemcitabine and cisplatin offers a significant survival benefit for patients with advanced disease. Although radiation therapy may help in treating bony metastases, it is not useful in treating advanced gallbladder cancer.

Cholangiocarcinoma

Cholangiocarcinoma is often asymptomatic and is usually not diagnosed early. Few patients with cholangiocarcinoma have resectable disease at diagnosis. Surgery often involves a Whipple procedure, vascular reconstruction, bile duct resection, and hepaticojejunostomy. Biliary tract stenting before surgery is controversial. In the setting of inoperative disease, stenting and liver drainage can improve overall survival, but this approach predisposes the patient to cholangitis.

Chemotherapy with gemcitabine and cisplatin is used to treat advanced disease. Radiation therapy is not helpful in treating cholangiocarcinoma.

Prognosis

Gallbladder Cancer

The prognosis for gallbladder cancer is poor. The 5-year survival rate is 80% for early-stage cancer (stage 0), 50% for stage I, and 28% for stage II. Five-year survival rates for stages III and IV are 2% and 7%, respectively.

Cholangiocarcinoma

Cholangiocarcinomas are aggressive tumors, and the 5-year survival rate is 18%.

Prevention and Surveillance

Patients with primary sclerosing cholangitis should undergo surveillance to identify malignant transformation early. However, there is no standard screening for gallbladder cancer or cholangiocarcinoma.

Bibliography

Edge, S., Byrd, D. R., Compton, C. C., Fritz, A. G., Greene, F. L., & Trotti, A. (2010). *AJCC staging manual* (7th ed.). New York: Springer.

Augustine, M., & Fong, Y. (2014). Epidemiology and risk factors of biliary tract and primary liver tumors. *Surgical Oncology Clinics of North America*, 23, 171–188.

Benson, A., D'Angelica, M., Abrams, T., Are, C., Bloomston, M., Chang, D., & Sundar, H. (2014). Hepatobiliary cancers, version 2.2014. *Journal of the National Comprehensive Cancer Network*, 12(8), 1152–1182.

Brown, K., Parmar, A., & Geller, D. (2014). Intrahepatic cholangiocarcinoma. *Surgical Oncology Clinics of North America*, 23(2), 231–246.

Dickson, P., & Behrman, S. (2014). Distal cholangiocarcinoma. *Surgical Oncology Clinics of North America*, 94(2), 325–342.

Ercolani, G., Dazzi, A., Giovinamazzo, F., Ruzzenente, A., Bassi, C., Guglielmi, A., & Pinna, A. (2015). Intrahepatic, perihilar and distal cholangiocarcinoma: Three different locations of the same tumor or three different tumors? *European Journal of Surgical Oncology*, 41(2), 1162–1169.

He, X., Li, J., Liu, W., Qu, Q., Hong, T., Xu, X. Q., & Zhao, H. T. (2015). Surgical procedure determination based on tumor-node-metastasis staging of gallbladder cancer. *World Journal of Gastroenterology*, 21(15), 4620–4626.

Kwon, W., Jang, J., Chang, Y., Jung, W., Kang, M., & Kim, S. W. (2015). Suggestions for improving perihilar cholangiocarcinoma staging based on an evaluation of the seventh edition AJCC system. *Journal of Gastrointestinal Surgery*, 19(4), 666–674.

National Comprehensive Cancer Network. (2015). *NCCN clinical practice guidelines in oncology: Hepatobiliary Cancers, version 2.2015*. Available at http://www.nccn.org/professionals/physician_gls/pdf/hepatobiliary.pdf (accessed December 18, 2015).

Rakic, M., Patrlj, L., Koplijar, M., Klicek, R., Kolovrat, M., Loncar, B., & Busic, Z. (2014). Gallbladder cancer. *Hepatobiliary Surgery and Nutrition*, 3(5), 221–226.

Razumilava, N., & Gores, G. (2014). Cholangiocarcinoma. *The Lancet*, 383(9935), 2168–2179.

Siegel, R., Miller, K., & Jernal, A. (2015). Cancer statistics, 2015. *Cancer*, 65(1), 5–29.

Wernberg, J., & Lucarelli, D. (2014). Gallbladder cancer. *Surgical Clinics of North America*, 94(2), 343–360.

Zaydfudim, V., Rosen, C., & Nagorney, D. (2014). Hilar cholangiocarcinoma. *Surgical Oncology Clinics of North America*, 23(2), 247–263.

Colon and Rectal Cancer

Carolyn Grande

Definition

Colon cancer includes cancer of the ascending colon, transverse colon, descending colon, and sigmoid colon. Rectal cancer can develop anywhere between the rectosigmoid junction and the anal canal. Metastasis occurs when tumor invades through the bowel wall and travels to lymph nodes or distant organs, particularly the liver, lungs, and peritoneum.

Incidence

Colorectal cancer is the third most common cancer in men and women. In 2015, about 93,090 cases of colon cancer and 39,610 cases of rectal cancer occurred in the United States. Approxmately 49,700 Americans died of colon or rectal cancer.

Etiology and Risk Factors

- The risk of colorectal cancer increases with age. Ninety percent of cases are diagnosed in individuals older than 50 years of age.
- Risk is increased for individuals with a personal or family history of colon cancer or polyps and a personal history of inflammatory bowel disease or type 2 diabetes. Inherited genetic syndromes, including familial adenomatous polyposis (FAP) and hereditary nonpolyposis colon cancer (HNPCC), are associated with a significantly increased risk of colorectal cancer.
- Modifiable risk factors (e.g., personal lifestyle, environmental exposures) contribute to the risk of sporadic colorectal cancer. They include obesity; a diet high in red or processed meat; low calcium intake; low consumption of whole-grain fiber, fruits, and vegetables; moderate to heavy alcohol consumption; long-term smoking; and physical inactivity.

Signs and Symptoms

Early stages of colorectal cancer are typically not accompanied by symptoms, which emphasizes the importance of screening. Presenting symptoms depend on the location of the tumor.

- Right side of the colon (i.e., cecum and ascending colon)
  - Dull, vague abdominal pain
  - Palpable mass in right lower quadrant

- Melena
- Anemia
- Anorexia or weight loss
- Indigestion
- Transverse colon
  - Changes in bowel habits
  - Blood in the stool
- Left side of the colon (i.e., descending colon)
  - Change in bowel habits
  - Cramps or flatulence
  - Decreased stool caliber
  - Bright red blood in the stool
  - Incomplete evacuation
- Rectum
  - Gross bleeding
  - Pain
  - Tenesmus
  - Constipation
  - Incomplete evacuation
  - Decreased stool caliber

Diagnostic Work-up

- If colorectal cancer is suspected, a comprehensive history should be obtained. Individual and family risks, prior operations, medical history, and social factors are critical components. Family history of cancer, including type of cancer (especially colorectal, uterine, ovarian, ureter, or bladder cancer) and age at diagnosis, is important in identifying hereditary or familial syndromes. A thorough review of systems can provide insight to early or late signs of malignancy.
- A complete physical examination with an emphasis on lymph nodes, abdomen, breast, and rectum should be performed.
- Laboratory tests should include a complete blood count (CBC), liver function tests, coagulation profile, and carcinoembryonic antigen (CEA). CEA is a glycoprotein found in gastrointestinal mucosa cells. Overexpression of CEA can indicate malignancy. It is not a tumor marker but rather a tumor-associated marker.
- Endoscopic examination is performed to locate the tumor after the completion of the history and physical examination. Flexible sigmoidoscopy allows visualization to just above the rectosigmoid junction (20 cm), and a rigid sigmoidoscopy can visualize up to the proximal end of the sigmoid colon (60 cm). Colonoscopy visualizes the entire colon. Biopsy of the tumor can be obtained at this time.
- Transrectal ultrasonography can be used for staging rectal carcinomas.
- A noninvasive examination of the colon can be performed with a double-contrast barium enema.
- Diagnostic imaging studies are completed to ascertain the presence of metastatic disease. CT of the chest and CT of the abdomen and pelvis with intravenous and oral contrast can identify extracolonic disease. When CT with contrast is contraindicated, chest CT without contrast and MRI of the abdomen and pelvis are considered appropriate.

Histology

- Greater than 90% of colorectal carcinomas are adenocarcinomas that arise from epithelial cells of the colorectal mucosa.
- Adenocarcinoma is characterized by glandular formation, the percentage of which serves as the foundation for histologic grading.
- Approximately 70% of colorectal carcinomas are diagnosed as moderately differentiated, 10% well differentiated, and 20% poorly differentiated.
- Other rarer types of colorectal carcinomas include neuroendocrine, squamous cell, adenosquamous, spindle cell, and undifferentiated carcinomas.
- Histologic grade should be discussed using the terms *low grade* (G1-G2) and *high grade* (G3-G4), as data *suggest* that outcomes can be associated with grade independent of TNM staging for both colon and rectal adenocarcinoma.

Clinical Staging

Accurate staging is essential for deciding on adjuvant treatment and developing a prognosis. Staging is done according to the AJCC guidelines using the TNM classification system (Edge, et. al., 2010). In colorectal cancer, staging depends on the depth of tumor invasion through the bowel wall, involvement of regional lymph nodes, and the existence of distant metastasis. TNM staging can be preceded by a prefix, further delineating clinical, pathologic, and post- neoadjuvant treatment staging. Examples of prefixes used and their definitions are as follows: cTNM is the clinical classification, pTNM is the pathologic classification. The y prefix is used for those cancers that are classified after neoadjuvant pretreatment. Patients who have a complete pathologic response are ypT0N0cM0 that may be similar to Stage Group 0 or 1. The r prefix is used for those cancers that have recurred following a disease-free interval (rTNM).

Treatment

Colon Cancer

- Surgical removal of the primary tumor with lymph node resection is the initial therapy.
- Patients with stage IV disease at diagnosis should undergo evaluation by a multidisciplinary team to determine synchronous disease resectability at the time of primary tumor removal. Resection of synchronous disease should be attempted only if complete resection with negative tumor margins is achievable.
- For patients diagnosed with stage IV disease with synchronous metastasis deemed unresectable, a limited colon resection may be performed at any point along the cancer trajectory to relieve obstruction, followed by systemic therapy.
- Patients diagnosed with liver-limited, unresectable metastases may be converted to resectable status with neoadjuvant systemic therapy.
- Adjuvant chemotherapy depends on the stage of disease and the prognostic risk factors (see table on page 57).

- Patients with stage I disease do not require adjuvant therapy.
- Adjuvant chemotherapy for stage II disease is a topic of controversy and requires informed decision making on the part of the patient. For patients with low-risk or high-risk disease, observation is an option.
- Adjuvant chemotherapy for patients with stage III disease is given for a 6-month period.
- For patients with stage IV disease and with evidence of measurable disease, chemotherapy in combination with a biologic therapy is given indefinitely, with the potential for treatment breaks.
- Radiation therapy has a limited role in treating colon cancer. It may be recommended for patients who have had a bowel perforation in an attempt to improve local control. It may also be used for palliation of painful metastasis.

- A more invasive surgical procedure, transabdominal resection, should be considered for all other patients who are not appropriate candidates for local resection.
- Data on the use of the laparoscopic approach for rectal tumor resection are limited. Although the long-term outcomes seem similar to or better than an open procedure, it is recommended that this approach be used only in a clinical trial until more high-level evidence can be obtained.
- Combined-modality therapy is recommended for most patients with stage II (T3-4, node negative) or stage III (node positive without distant metastasis) disease. Neoadjuvant or adjuvant therapy should be given in one of the following sequences: chemotherapy plus radiation therapy preoperatively, resection, and chemotherapy postoperatively or chemotherapy followed by chemotherapy plus radiation therapy and then resection (see table below).
- Therapy for metastatic or recurrent rectal cancer includes regimens outlined in the treatment of colorectal cancer.

Treatment of Colorectal Cancer by Stage

Treatment Regimen	COLORECTAL CANCER STAGE					
	II*	II†	III	IV‡	IV§	IV¶¶
5-FU/leucovorin	x	x	X		x++	
Capecitabine	x	x	X		x++	
FOLFOX			x	X++	x++	x
CapeOx			x	X++	x++	x
FOLFIRI or FOLFOX or CapeOx ± bevacizumab				x+	x+	x
FOLFIRI + ramucirumab						x
FOLFIRI or FOLFOX ± panitumumab or cetuximab				x+	x+	x
FOLFOXIRI ± bevacizumab				x+	x+	x
Infusional 5-FU/leucovorin or capecitabine ± bevacizumab					x+	X⁻
Irinotecan + panitumumab or cetuximab¶ or bevacizumab						x
Panitumumab or cetuximab single agent¶						X⁻
FOLFIRI or irinotecan ± ziv- aflibercept						x
FLOX		x	X	x++	x++	
Irinotecan						x
Regorafenib						X⁻

CapeOx, Capecitabine and oxaliplatin; *FLOX*, folinic acid, leucovorin, and oxaliplatin; *FOLFIRI*, folinic acid, leucovorin, and irinotecan; *FOLFOX*, folinic acid, leucovorin, and oxaliplatin; *FOLFOXIRI*, folinic acid, leucovorin, oxaliplatin, and irinotecan; *x*, treatment option for this stage; *X⁻*, patients inappropriate for aggressive therapy; +, synchronous metastases, ++, metasynchronous metastases.
*Stage II with no high-risk features.
†Stage II with high-risk features.
‡Stage IV with neoadjuvant treatment.
§Stage IV with no evidence of metastatic disease after adjuvant therapy.
¶Only if positive for mutated *KRAS, NRAS, or APC* (WNT pathway) genes.
¶¶Unresectable stage IV cancer.
Modified from National Cancer Institute, National Institutes of Health. (2015). *Ramucirumab*. Available at http://www.cancer.gov/cancertopics/druginfo/ramucirumab (accessed December 18, 2015).

Rectal Cancer

- The type of surgical approach depends on the location and extent of disease. Surgical resection for T1 lesions in the low rectum within 8 cm of the anal verge may be accomplished by local procedures, including polypectomy, transanal excision, or transanal endoscopic microsurgery.

Combined-Modality Therapy for Stage II/III Rectal Cancer

Treatment Option 1*	Treatment Option 2*
Chemotherapy + radiation therapy • Capecitabine + radiation therapy • Infusional 5-FU + radiation therapy • Bolus 5-FU/leucovorin + radiation therapy	Chemotherapy • FOLFOX • CapeOx • FLOX • 5-FU + leucovorin • Capecitabine
Surgical resection	Chemotherapy + radiation therapy • Capecitabine + radiation therapy • Infusional 5-FU + radiation therapy • Bolus 5-FU/leucovorin + radiation therapy
Chemotherapy • FOLFOX • CapeOx • FLOX • 5-FU + leucovorin • Capecitabine	Surgical resection

CapeOx, Capecitabine and oxaliplatin; *5-FU*, 5-fluorouracil; *FOLFOX*, folinic acid, leucovorin, and oxaliplatin.
*Total duration of perioperative therapy should not exceed 6 months.
Modified from National Comprehensive Cancer Network. (2015). *NCCN clinical practice guidelines in oncology: Rectal cancer, version 2.2015*. Available at https://www.nccn.org/store/login/login.aspx?ReturnURL=http://www.nccn.org/professionals/physician_gls/pdf/rectal.pdf. Accessed December 18, 2015.

Prognosis

The overall 5-year survival rate for people with colorectal cancer is 65%. Survival decreases as the stage of disease worsens. For those with localized disease, the 5-year survival rate is 90%. For people whose cancer has spread to involve nearby organs or lymph nodes at diagnosis, the 5-year survival rate decreases to 71%. With spread of the disease to distant organs, the 5-year survival rate decreases to 13%. The overall death rate for people with colorectal cancer declined between the years 2007 and 2011 by 2.5% per year. This can be attributed to declining incidence rates and improvements in early detection and treatment.

Prevention and Surveillance

Prevention strategies include modifiable lifestyle risk factors:

- Eating more fruits and vegetables
- Reducing high-fat foods, particularly animal fat
- Minimizing alcohol intake and avoiding beer and beverages with a high percentage of alcohol that contain nitrosamines, which can be carcinogenic for the colon
- Maintaining weight within a healthy range
- Engaging in 30 minutes of exercise daily

The American Cancer Society recommends routine screenings for prevention through removal of polyps and early detection of colorectal cancer beginning at age 50 for men and women at average risk.

- Flexible sigmoidoscopy every 5 years; colonoscopy should follow if positive
- Colonoscopy every 10 years
- Double-contrast barium enema every 5 years
- CT colonography (i.e., virtual colonoscopy) every 5 years

Those who have a family history of colon cancer, a genetic predisposition to colorectal cancer, or abnormal findings or polyps during a previous evaluation should use routine screening practices as directed by their physicians.

Bibliography

American Cancer Society. (2015). *Cancer facts and figures 2015.* Available at http://www.cancer.org/acs/groups/content/@editorial/documents/document/acspc-044552.pdf (accessed December 18, 2015).

American Cancer Society. (2015). *American Cancer Society recommendations for colorectal cancer early detection.* Available at http://www.cancer.org/cancer/colonandrectumcancer/moreinformation/colonandrectumcancerearlydetection/colorectal-cancer-early-detection-acs-recommendations (accessed December 18, 2015).

Edge, S. B., Byrd, D. R., Compton, C. C., Fritz, A. G., Greene, F. L., & Trotti, A. (2010). *AJCC cancer staging handbook: From the cancer staging manual* (7th ed.). New York: Springer.

Fleming, M., Ravula, S., Tatishchev, S., & Wang, H. L. (2012). Colorectal carcinoma: Pathologic aspects. *J Gastrointest Oncol, 3*(3), 153–173.

National Comprehensive Cancer Network. (2015). *NCCN clinical practice guidelines in oncology: Colon cancer, version 2.2015.* Available at https://www.nccn.org/store/login/login.aspx?ReturnURL=http://www.nccn.org/professionals/physician_gls/pdf/colon.pdf (accessed December 18, 2015).

National Comprehensive Cancer Network. (2015). *NCCN clinical practice guidelines in oncology: Rectal cancer, version 2.2015.* Available at https://www.nccn.org/store/login/login.aspx?ReturnURL=http://www.nccn.org/professionals/physician_gls/pdf/rectal.pdf (accessed December 18, 2015).

National Cancer Institute, National Institutes of Health. (2015). *Ramucirumab.* Available at http://www.cancer.gov/cancertopics/druginfo/ramucirumab (accessed December 18, 2015).

Skibber, J. M., Minsky, B. D., & Hoff, P. M. (2001). Cancer of the colon. In V. T. DeVita, S. Hellman, & S. A. Rosenberg (Eds.), *Cancer principles and practice of oncology* (pp. 1216–1271). Philadelphia: Lippincott.

Sweede, M. R., & Meropol, N. J. (2001). Assessment, diagnosis and staging. In D. T. Berg (Ed.), *Contemporary issues in colorectal cancer: a nursing perspective* (pp. 65–80). Sudbury, MA: Jones & Bartlett.

Esophageal Cancer

Brenda Keith

Definition

Cancer that begins in the esophagus has two major histologic types. *Squamous cell carcinoma* arises in the squamous cells that line the esophagus. These cancers usually occur in the upper portion of the esophagus. *Adenocarcinoma* usually develops in the glandular tissue in the lower third of the esophagus. Other types, such as lymphomas and sarcomas, are rare and may occur anywhere along the esophagus.

At diagnosis, approximately 50% of patients with esophageal cancer have metastatic disease. Metastasis most frequently occurs through spread into local lymph nodes. The liver, lungs, and pleura are the most common sites of distant metastases.

Incidence

In the United States, about 16,980 people were diagnosed with esophageal cancer, and 15,590 died of the disease in 2015. It is the seventh leading cause of cancer deaths among men in the United States. Almost four times as many cases occur in men than women. Esophageal cancer is most frequently diagnosed in people between the ages of 65 and 74 years. Although esophageal cancer constitutes only 1.1% of the malignancies in the United States, it is the eighth most common malignancy worldwide, with most cases diagnosed in developing countries. Both squamous cell carcinoma and adenocarcinoma are more common among men.

- Squamous cell carcinomas
  - Worldwide, squamous cell carcinomas are the most common type, with high-prevalence areas in Asia, southern and eastern Africa, and northern France.
  - There has been a slight decline in squamous cell carcinomas in the United States and other industrialized Western countries over the past 3 decades, most likely due to decreased smoking.
  - Blacks and Asians are more at risk for squamous cell carcinoma than whites.
- Adenocarcinomas
  - In North America and Western Europe, adenocarcinomas are more common than squamous cell carcinomas.
  - The dramatic rise in adenocarcinoma of the distal esophagus, especially in some Western nations, is likely related to diet and increased obesity. The incidence of adenocarcinoma continues to rise each year in the United States.
  - The rate of increase exceeds that of all other cancers, including lung, breast, prostate, and melanoma.
  - Ninety percent of adenocarcinomas occur near the esophagogastric junction. Adenocarcinomas of the distal esophagus and gastroesophageal junction account for more than 70% of new cases of esophageal cancer in the United States.
  - Patients diagnosed with adenocarcinoma are predominantly white men.
  - Patients with esophageal cancer are also at increased risk of developing second primary cancers such as head, neck, and lung cancers.

Etiology and Risk Factors

The exact cause of esophageal cancer is unknown. Risk factors for squamous cell carcinoma include the following:

- Tobacco: Smoking cigarettes or using smokeless tobacco is a major risk factor for esophageal cancer.
- Alcohol: Long-term or heavy use of alcohol increases the risk of esophageal cancer. There is a synergistic effect when combined with tobacco.
- Diet: A diet that is low in fruits, vegetables, and vitamins A, B_{12}, and C increases the risk of esophageal cancer. Other factors include frequent ingestion of hot liquids or foods (thought to cause thermal injury to the esophagus); smoked, nitrate-cured, and salt-cured foods; pickled vegetables; processed meat; and betel nuts.
- Esophageal disease: Achalasia (i.e., spasms of the esophageal sphincter) increases the risk.
- Chemical irritation: Caustic injury to the esophagus (e.g., ingestion of lye) and radiation therapy are risk factors.
- Previous cancers of lung or head and neck: Other cancers associated with the risk factors of tobacco and alcohol use increase the risk of a secondary primary esophageal cancer.
- Viruses: HPV infection may be involved in a small subset of squamous cell carcinomas but does not appear to be an important risk factor.
- Hereditary cancer syndromes: For individuals with tylosis, also known as nonepidermolytic palmoplantar keratosis or Howel-Evans syndrome, the average age at diagnosis of squamous cell carcinoma of the esophagus is 45 years, and the risk of developing the disease is 40% to 90% by 70 years of age. People with Bloom syndrome, Fanconi anemia, or Plummer-Vinson syndrome are also at increased risk for squamous cell carcinoma of the esophagus.

Risk factors for adenocarcinoma of the esophagus include the following:

- Gastroesophageal reflux disease (GERD): Acid reflux is associated with an increased risk of adenocarcinoma of the esophagus. Long-standing GERD predisposes to Barrett esophagus, in which epithelial changes occur in the lower esophagus as a result of damage from acid reflux. The frequency, severity, and duration of reflux symptoms positively correlate with the increased risk of esophageal adenocarcinoma. Persons with Barrett esophagus have a 30 to 60 times greater risk of developing esophageal adenocarcinoma than the general population.
- Obesity: There is a strong relationship between body mass index and adenocarcinoma of the esophagus. Obesity is defined as a body mass index of 30 or greater.
- Smoking: Smoking, but not alcohol use, is associated with increased risk. It is a moderate established risk factor for esophageal cancer.
- *Helicobactor pylori* infection can cause stomach cancer, but it has not been associated with esophageal cancer.
- Familial Barrett esophagus

Signs and Symptoms

Early esophageal cancer usually does not cause symptoms. As the cancer grows, symptoms may include the following:

- Dysphagia (most common symptom, initially experienced with solids and then with liquids)
- Weight loss (second most common symptom)
- Heartburn
- Regurgitation of food
- Epigastric or retrosternal pain
- Hoarseness or chronic cough
- Vomiting
- Hemoptysis

Diagnostic Work-up

- Imaging studies include a chest radiograph, barium swallow, and esophagoscopy or esophagogastroduodenoscopy (EGD).
- Endoscopy and biopsy must follow to determine the invasiveness of the tumor, the integrity of the esophageal wall, and the tumor tissue type.
- CT or MRI is used to evaluate the extent of disease of the chest, abdomen, and pelvis after the diagnosis is confirmed.
- A PET scan is sometimes used to detect distant metastases in place of CT scans or as an additional study when the CT does not show metastatic disease.
- If CT and PET do not demonstrate distant disease, EUS should be performed to establish the extent of locoregional disease.
- A CBC and blood chemistry panel are part of diagnostic testing.
- Additional studies used to guide treatment decisions include the following:
  - Bronchoscopy may be considered for tumors in the upper and middle esophagus to rule out airway invasion.
  - Thoracoscopy and laparoscopy may be considered for selected patients such as those who may have a high risk of treatment-related complications.
  - Staging laparoscopy may have a role for patients with adenocarcinoma of the esophagus located at or near the esophagogastric junction.
  - Human epidermal growth factor receptor 2 (HER2) testing may be done for stage IV adenocarcinoma of the esophagogastric junction to determine whether targeted therapy with the monoclonal antibody trastuzumab is indicated.

Histology

The most common histologic types of esophageal cancers are squamous cell carcinoma and adenocarcinoma. Most adenocarcinomas are located in the distal esophagus. Most squamous cell carcinomas are located in the proximal or middle esophagus.

Clinical Staging

Staging of carcinoma of the esophagus is based on the TNM classification developed by the AJCC (Edge, et. al., 2010). Tumors with T4 status due to invasion of local structures are subdivided into those that are resectable or nonresectable. Staging includes groupings that consider the importance of histopathologic cell type, tumor grade, and tumor location. Stage groupings for adenocarcinoma and squamous cell carcinoma are different.

Treatment

Treatment goals (i.e., cure or palliation) are based on the clinical stage of the disease and the feasibility of surgical resection of the tumor. Primary treatment modalities include surgery alone or chemotherapy with radiation therapy. Combined-modality therapy (i.e., chemotherapy plus surgery or chemotherapy and radiation therapy plus surgery) is being evaluated clinically.

- Stage I: consideration of endoscopic therapy, especially for Tis and T1aN0 disease; consideration of initial surgery for T1b and any N
- Stages II and III: consideration of chemoradiation followed by surgery
- Stage IV: chemotherapy or symptomatic and supportive care

Surgery

- Surgery is the gold standard for the treatment of localized esophageal cancer. The goal of surgery is to provide a definitive cure or palliation of symptoms.
- Surgery alone is an accepted single-modality therapy for patients with localized disease or for patients who may not tolerate combined-modality treatment.
- Indications for surgical treatment include diagnosis of esophageal cancer in a patient who is a candidate for surgery and high-grade dysplasia in a patient with Barrett esophagus who cannot be adequately treated endoscopically.
- Surgical options include the following:
  - Open esophagectomy: transhiatal esophagectomy (THE) or transthoracic esophagectomy (TTE)
  - Minimally invasive esophagectomy
  - Endoscopic mucosal resection (EMR), which is used to treat very small tumors
- Contraindications to surgery include metastases to N2 nodes or solid organs, invasion of adjacent structures, severe associated comorbid conditions, and impaired cardiac or respiratory function.

Radiation Therapy

- Irradiation may be combined with surgery preoperatively or postoperatively.
- External beam radiation therapy or image-guided radiation therapy (IGRT) may be used.
- Irradiation may be combined with chemotherapy and surgery.
- Radiation therapy may be used to alleviate obstruction, control pain, or restore swallowing.

Chemotherapy

- Chemoradiation may be used.
  - 5-FU or capecitabine, or both, may be used before, during, or after radiation therapy.

- Cisplatin or oxaliplatin may be combined with a fluoropyrimidine (i.e., 5-FU or capecitabine) or a combination of paclitaxel with carboplatin.
- Preferred options for neoadjuvant (preoperative) chemoradiation include paclitaxel plus carboplatin and cisplatin or oxaliplatin with a fluoropyrimidine (i.e., 5-FU or capecitabine).
- Recurrent disease regimens include the use of 5-FU and cisplatin, irinotecan and cisplatin, paclitaxel and cisplatin, docetaxel and cisplatin, and paclitaxel or docetaxel with a fluoropyrimidine (i.e., 5-FU or capecitabine), all with irradiation if chemoradiation was not previously done.
- Metastatic disease may be treated with the following agents in various combinations: cisplatin, carboplatin, docetaxel, epirubicin, irinotecan, oxaliplatin, 5-FU, and capecitabine. Alternative therapies include gemcitabine, mitomycin, etoposide, and pegylated liposomal doxorubicin.

Ablation for Very Small Tumors

- Photodynamic therapy is used for superficial and mucosal lesions and to palliate dysphagia.
  - Principles from laser treatment are employed.
  - A light-sensitizing agent is administered intravenously. The chemical is taken up by the esophageal tumor, a laser light is administered at the tumor site, and tumor necrosis occurs.
- For cryoablation, liquid nitrogen is sprayed through an endoscope.
- For radiofrequency ablation, heat from electrodes is passed through an endoscope.

Symptom Management

- Esophageal dilation may be done to maintain esophageal patency and improve symptoms of dysphagia. A stent is inserted to maintain esophageal patency.
- Nutritional support is indicated for a patient undergoing treatment for esophageal cancer.
- Laser surgery or electrocoagulation (i.e., use of electric current) may be used to relieve symptoms and improve quality of life.
- Bleeding may be treated with surgery, irradiation, or endoscopy.
- Pain and nausea may require the use of medications and surgery.

Prognosis

Esophageal cancer is a treatable disease but is rarely curable. Survival of patients with esophageal cancer depends on the stage of disease. Lymph node or solid organ metastases are associated with low survival rates (see table on page 61). Esophageal squamous cell carcioma and adenocarcinoma appear to have equivalent survival rates. The 5-year survival rates have increased over time. The overall survival rate was 5% for 1975 to 1977, 9.5% for 1987 to 1989, 18.1% for 1999 to 2001, and 20.1% for 2005 to 2011.

Cases of Esophageal Cancer and 5-Year Relative Survival Rates by Stage at Diagnosis

Stage	Percent of Diagnosed Cases	5-Year Relative Survival (%)
Localized (confined to primary site)	21	40.4
Regional (spread to regional lymph nodes)	31	21.6
Distant (metastasized)	38	4.2
Unknown (unstaged)	11	12.0

Data from Surveillance, Epidemiology, and End Results (SEER). *Cancer Statistics Review 1975-2012. Cancer of the esophagus (invasive): 5-Year relative and period survival* (Table 8.8). Available at http://seer.cancer.gov/csr/1975_2012/results _merged/topic_survival.pdf#search=program+18+2004-2010 (accessed December 18, 2015).

Prevention and Surveillance

There are no recommendations for screening and early detection programs for esophageal cancer in the United States. High-risk candidates are those who use tobacco and alcohol, have poor dietary habits, have a history of GERD, or have a known genetic mutation. Measures to prevent esophageal cancer include avoidance or limited intake of alcohol, cessation of smoking and smokeless tobacco products, and weight control.

Prevention Measures for Squamous Cell Carcinomas

The evidence shows that avoidance of tobacco and alcohol can help decrease the risk of squamous cell cancer. Diets high in cruciferous vegetables (e.g., cabbage, broccoli, cauliflower), other green and yellow vegetables, and fruits are associated with a decreased risk of squamous cell esophageal cancer. Epidemiologic studies have found that aspirin or nonsteroidal antiinflammatory drug (NSAID) use may be associated with a decreased risk of developing or dying of squamous cell esophageal cancer. However, adverse effects of using NSAIDs include upper gastrointestinal bleeding and serious cardiovascular events such as myocardial infarction, heart failure, hemorrhagic stroke, and renal impairment. Screening may be recommended for those with a known hereditary predisposition (e.g., tylosis, Bloom syndrome, Fanconi anemia).

Prevention Measures for Adenocarcinomas

It is unknown whether elimination of gastroesophageal reflux by surgical or medical means can reduce the risk of adenocarcinoma of the esophagus. People diagnosed with Barrett esophagus should see a gastroenterologist (i.e., gastrointestinal system specialist) to determine a surveillance schedule. Controversy exists regarding endoscopic surveillance because of uncommon but serious side effects. The risk of developing cancer is low despite having Barrett esophagus.

Epidemiologic studies have found that aspirin or NSAID use may be associated with a decreased risk of developing or dying of esophageal cancer. However, harms associated with using NSAIDs include upper gastrointestinal bleeding and serious cardiovascular events such as myocardial infarction, heart failure, hemorrhagic stroke, and renal impairment.

Bibliography

Absi, A., Adelstein, D., & Rice, T. (2010). *Esophageal cancer.* Cleveland Clinic Center for Continuing Education. Available at http://www.clevelandclinicmeded.com/medicalpubs/diseasemanagement/hematology-oncology/esophageal-cancer/#treatment (accessed December 18, 2015).

American Cancer Society. (2015). *Cancer facts and figures 2015.* Available at http://www.cancer.org/acs/groups/content/@editorial/documents/document/acspc-044552.pdf (accessed December 18, 2015).

Baldwin, K., Patti, M., Espat, N., Herbella, F., & Harris, J. (2015). *Esophageal cancer.* Available at http://emedicine.medscape.com/article/277930-overview (accessed December 18, 2015).

Berry, M. (2014). Esophageal cancer: Staging system and guidelines for staging and treatment. *Journal of Thoracic Disease, 6*(Suppl 3), S289–S297.

Edge, S., Byrd, D. R., Compton, C. C., Fritz, A. G., Greene, F. L., & Trotti, A. (2010). *AJCC staging manual* (7th ed.). New York: Springer.

Ginex, P., Thom, B., Jingeleski, M., Vincent, A., Plourde, G., & Rizk, N. (2013). Patterns of symptoms following surgery for esophageal cancer. *Oncology Nursing Forum, 40*(3), E101–E107.

Howlader, N., Noone, A., Krapcho, M., Garshell, J., Miller, D., Altekruse, S., Cronin, K. (Eds.). *SEER Cancer Statistics Review, 1975-2012.* National Cancer Institute, Bethesda, MD. Available at http://seer.cancer.gov/csr/1975_2012/(based on November 2014 SEER data submission, posted to the SEER web site, April 2015) (accessed December 18, 2015).

Hur, C., Miller, M., Kong, C., Dowling, E., Nattinger, K., Dunn, M., & Feuer, E. (2013). Trends in esophageal adenocarcinoma incidence and mortality. *Cancer, 119,* 1149–1158.

Kleinberg, L., Kelly, R., Yang, S., Wang, J., & Forastiere, A. (2013). Cancer of the esophagus. In J. Niederhuber, J. Armitage, J. Doroshow, M. Kastan, & J. Tepper (Eds.), *Abeloff's clinical oncology* (5th ed.) (pp. 1207–1239). Philadelphia: Saunders.

National Cancer Institute. (2014). *Esophageal cancer: Health professional version.* Available at http://www.cancer.gov/types/esophageal/hp (accessed February 4, 2016).

National Cancer Institute. (2015). *SEER stat fact sheet: Esophageal cancer.* Available at http://seer/cancer.gov/statfacts/html/esoph.html (accessed December 18, 2015).

National Comprehensive Cancer Network. (2015). *NCCN clinical practice guidelines in oncology: Esophageal and esophagogastric junction cancers, version 2.2015.* Available at http://www.nccn.org/professionals/physician_gls/pdf/esophageal.pdf (accessed December 18, 2015).

Rice, T., Blackstone, E., & Rusch, V. (2010). Seventh edition of the AJCC cancer staging manual: Esophagus and esophageal junction. *Annals of Surgical Oncology, 17,* 1721–1724.

Siegel, R., Ma, J., Zhaohui, Z., & Jemal, A. (2014). Cancer statistics, 2014. *CA: A Cancer Journal for Clinicians, 64*(11), 9–29.

Gastric Cancer

Lisa Parks

Definition

Gastric cancer is classified by anatomic locations, which include the cardia, fundus, body, antrum, or pylorus. Tumors can manifest as malignant ulcers or polypoid lesions, or they can spread throughout the submucosal layers, producing a rigid, nondistensible stomach called *linitis plastica.*

Incidence

Gastric cancer is the fourth most common malignancy worldwide. In 2015, the United States had approximately 24,590 new cases of gastric cancer and 10,720 deaths from the disease. Gastric cancer occurs most often between the ages of 55 and 80 years and is rare among people younger than 30 years. The highest incidence is among men in Eastern Asia, Eastern

Europe, and Central America. The lowest incidence is found in Africa and North America. Cardial gastric cancer incidence during the past 40 years in Colombia, the United States, and Europe has increased among white men.

Etiology and Risk Factors

- Environmental, infectious, and familial factors may affect the development of gastric cancer.
- *Helicobacter pylori* are gram-negative bacteria that create an inflammatory reaction. Chronic inflammation can lead to malignant gastric epithelial transformation.
- Epstein-Barr virus infection is a risk factor for gastric cancer.
- A diet of processed foods high in nitrates and smoked foods high in sodium and deficient in vitamin A or C are risk factors for gastric cancer.
- Tobacco smoking and heavy alcohol use contribute to the development of gastric cancer.
- Gastric cancer is more common among whites, men, and those 60 years of age or older.
- Those with a mutated E-cadherin gene (*CDH1*) have a 70% risk of developing diffuse gastric cancer.
- A family with two documented cases of gastric cancer among their first- or second-degree relatives, with one family member younger than 50 years at diagnosis, or with three family members with documented gastric cancer are at a higher risk for gastric cancer.
- Other hereditary syndromes such as FAP and HNPCC are risk factors for gastric cancer.

Signs and Symptoms

- Symptoms of gastric cancer are often vague, and patients are often treated for other illnesses in response to their complaints, allowing the cancer to progress.
- Common symptoms of early gastric cancer include heartburn, bloating, appetite loss, and abdominal pain.
- As the cancer progresses, weight loss, anemia, melena, hematemesis, dysphagia, vomiting, an upper abdominal mass, and jaundice may occur.

Diagnostic Work-up

- EGD is the diagnostic method of choice.
- EUS is useful in staging.
- Gastric biopsies confirm the presence of cancer.
- After the diagnosis of gastric cancer, a CT scan of the chest, abdomen, and pelvis is performed to detect distant metastatic disease and to stage the gastric cancer.
- CT is superior to other imaging modalities for nodal staging.
- PET and MRI are superior to CT in detecting liver, bone, and peritoneal metastases.

Histology

- More than 95% of gastric cancers are adenocarcinomas, which are further classified as intestinal or diffuse types.
- Intestinal-type adenocarcinomas are preceded by progression from chronic nonatrophic gastritis by way of atrophic gastritis and intestinal metaplasia to dysplasia, known as the *Correa cascade*. Identification and treatment of these precancerous lesions,

which are caused by *H. pylori* infection, are associated with a decrease in the incidence and mortality rates for gastric cancer.
- Diffuse adenocarcinomas are aggressive and have a worse prognosis than other types. They develop in patients between the ages of 40 and 60 years and occur equally in men and women.
- A variant of diffuse gastric adenocarcinoma is the signet ring cell adenocarcinoma. The cells resemble signet rings when examined under a microscope because mucin displaces the cell nucleus from the center to the outer cell membrane.
- Mucinous subtypes may occur with intestinal and diffuse gastric adenocarcinomas.

Clinical Staging

Clinical staging is essential for determining the extent of disease and associated treatment strategies. Staging is performed using the AJCC guidelines for applying TNM data (Edge, et. al., 2010).

Treatment

Surgery

Gastric cancer can be cured by complete gastric resection with negative surgical margins, which is achieved in only 50% of patients with gastric cancer due to advanced disease at the time of surgery. Proximal and total gastrectomies are indicated for proximal gastric cancer. Subtotal gastrectomy is performed for distal gastric cancers.

Systemic Therapy

- There remains no consensus about the best systemic therapy for advanced gastric cancer.
- 5-FU is the most studied chemotherapy for gastric cancer. It has been used in combination with doxorubicin, methotrexate, etoposide, epirubicin, and cisplatin.
- Oxaliplatin has been studied in combination with docetaxel, 5-FU, irinotecan, and capecitabine.
- Irinotecan has been studied after failure of initial therapy and used in combination with platinum-based compounds, taxanes, 5-FU, and capecitabine.
- Capecitabine, an oral fluoropyrimidine that undergoes enzymatic conversion to 5-FU, can be used as single-agent therapy or in combination with other drugs.
- Targeted agents, including anti–epidermal growth factor receptor (anti-EGFR) and anti–vascular endothelial growth factor (anti-VEGF) agents, are being studied.

Prognosis

Despite surgical intervention in early-stage disease, patients with gastric cancer have a 40% to 65% recurrence rate. The 5-year survival rate for patients without lymph node involvement is 75%, and the 5-year survival rate for those with node-positive disease is 10% to 25%. At the time of diagnosis, two thirds of patients have advanced disease that is not curable, and survival time is less than 1 year.

Prevention and Surveillance

- Lifestyle changes are one strategy for prevention of gastric cancer, including tobacco cessation, alcohol avoidance, eating a diet rich in fruits and vegetables, and avoidance of salted, smoked foods, and foods processed with nitrites.

- Eradication of *H. pylori* bacteria can prevent gastric cancer.
- Patients with a family history (see earlier Etiology and Risk Factors section) and with a mutated E-cadherin gene (*CDH1*) may be offered a prophylactic gastrectomy. Other high-risk patients may undergo EGD surveillance with biopsies.
- A low serum pepsinogen I level and a low ratio of pepsinogen I to pepsinogen II have been proposed in Japan as a screening tool for gastric cancer. Screening is recommended starting at 30 years of age and continuing at 5-year intervals.

Bibliography

Ayyappan, S., Prabhaker, D., & Sharma, N. (2013). Epidermal growth factor receptor (EGFR)-targeted therapies in esophagogastric cancer. *Anticancer Research, 33*, 4139–4156.

Bailey, K. (2011). An overview of gastric cancer and its management. *Cancer Nursing Practice, 10*(6), 31–38.

Benson, A., D'Angelica, M., Abrams, T., Are, C., Bloomston, M., Chang, D., & Sundar, H. (2014). Hepatobiliary cancers, version 2.2014. *Journal of the National Comprehensive Cancer Network, 12*(8), 1152–1182.

El Abiad, R., & Gerke, H. (2012). Gastric cancer: Endoscopic diagnosis and staging. *Surgical Oncology Clinics of North America, 21*, 1–19.

Ercolani, G., Dazzi, A., Giovinazzo, F., Ruzzenente, A., Bassi, C., Guglielmi, A., & Pinna, A. (2015). Intrahepatic, perihilar and distal cholangiocarcinoma: Three different locations of the same tumor or three different tumors? *European Journal of Surgical Oncology, 41*(9), 1162–1169.

Gomez, J., & Young, A. (2014). Gastric intestinal metaplasia and early gastric cancer in the west: A changing paradigm. *Gastroenterology & Hepatology, 10*(6), 369–378.

He, X., Li, J., Liu, W., Qu, Q., Hong, T., Xu, X. Q., & Zhao, H. T. (2015). Surgical procedure determination based on tumor-node-metastasis staging of gallbladder cancer. *World Journal of Gastroenterology, 21*(15), 4620–4626.

Hu, B., El Hajj, N., Sittler, S., Lammert, N., Barnes, R., & Meloni-Ehriq, A. (2012). Gastric cancer: Classification, histology and application of molecular pathology. *Journal of Gastrointestinal Oncology, 3*(3), 251–261.

Li, B., Li, Y., Wang, W., Qui, H., Seeruttun, S., Fang, C., & Zhan, Y. (2015). Incorporation of N0 stage with insufficient numbers of lymph nodes into N1 stage in the seventh edition of the TNM classification improves prediction of prognosis in gastric cancer: Results of a single-institution study of 1258 Chinese patients. *Annals of Surgical Oncology.* Advance online publication http://dx.doi.org/10.1245/s10434-015-4578-0.

Won, W., Jang, J., Chang, Y., Jung, W., Kang, M., et al. (2015). Suggestions for improving perihilar cholangiocarcinoma staging based on an evaluation of the seventh edition of AJCC system. *Journal of Gastrointestinal Surgery, 19*, 666–674.

Malibari, N., Hickeson, M., & Lisbona, R. (2015). PET/computed tomography in the diagnosis and staging of gastric cancers. *PET Clinics, 10*, 311–326.

Massarrat, S., & Stolte, M. (2014). Development of gastric cancer and its prevention. *Archives of Iranian Medicine, 17*(7), 514–520.

Ouwerkerk, J., & Boers-Doets, C. (2010). Best practices in the management of toxicities related to anti-EGFR agents for metastatic colorectal cancer. *European Journal of Oncology Nursing, 14*, 337–349.

Piazuelo, M., & Correa, P. (2013). Gastric cancer: Overview. *Columbia Medica, 44*(3), 192–201.

Young, J., Mucheal, M., & Leong, T. (2011). Target therapies for gastric cancer. *Drugs, 71*(11), 1367–1384.

Siegel, R., Miller, K., & Jernal, A. (2015). Cancer statistics, 2015. *Cancer, 65*(1), 5–29.

Gastrointestinal Stromal Tumor

Lisa Parks

Definition

Gastrointestinal stromal tumors (GISTs) are the most common mesenchymal cancers of the gastrointestinal tract. GIST is a soft tissue sarcoma that originates in the interstitial cells of Cajal that are between smooth muscle and the autonomic nerve cells of the bowel wall. GISTs can occur anywhere in the gastrointestinal tract, but 60% to 70% occur in the stomach.

Incidence

GISTs account for less than 1% of gastrointestinal tumors; about 4000 new cases occurred in the United States in 2015. Thirty-five percent of GISTs occur in the colon and rectum, 5% occur in the appendix, and 2% to 3% occur in the esophagus. Before the discovery of the *KIT* proto-oncogene in 1998, smooth muscle neoplasms, leiomyomas, leiomyoblastomas, leiomyosarcomas, and schwannomas were thought to be GISTs.

Etiology and Risk Factors

- GISTs represent 0.1% to 3.0% of gastrointestinal malignancies.
- GISTs occur predominantly in adults older than 50 years (median age, 58 years).
- Tumors occur equally in men and women.
- Familial GIST has an autosomal dominant pattern.
- Five percent of GISTs occur in patients with neurofibromatosis type 1 syndrome, manifest in the small intestine, and are *KIT* negative.

Signs and Symptoms

- Only 70% of patients with GIST have symptoms, which reflect the location of the tumor.
- Following vague abdominal discomfort, bleeding is the most common symptom. Bleeding results from erosion into the GIST tumor lumen, and a ruptured tumor can lead to acute gastrointestinal or abdominal cavity bleeding. Hematemesis, melena, or anemia results from chronic gastrointestinal bleeding.
- Nausea, vomiting, weight loss, early satiety, and abdominal discomfort may also be symptoms of GIST.
- Depending on site of disease, symptoms can include dysphagia and intussusception of the small bowel.
- Pediatric GIST has a different pathogenesis and clinical behavior, and it is classified separately from the adult form.

Diagnostic Work-up

- CT with contrast is the diagnostic modality of choice. GISTs look like large, well-defined, soft tissue masses with heterogeneous enhancement. Various degrees of necrosis may be seen.
- EUS is used to assess the depth of invasion of the mass and to obtain a tissue sample for pathologic analysis.
- GISTs are PET positive because increased receptor tyrosine kinase levels amplify glucose transport protein signaling.

Histology

- Most GISTs express the KIT protein (CD 117), which is the most specific immunohistochemical marker for these tumors.
- The absence of KIT does not rule out a GIST diagnosis because 5% of GISTs are KIT negative or indeterminate.

- Between 60% and 70% of GISTS stain positive for CD34, 30% to 40% are positive for smooth muscle actin, and 5% are positive for S100.
- Mutations in the *KIT* gene are the most common genetic changes associated with GISTs. Most *KIT* mutations occur in exon 9, 11, 13, or 17.
- Platelet-derived growth factor receptor gene (*PDGFR*) mutations occur in exons 12, 14, or 18. Resistance to the agent imatinib is commonly seen in patients with a *PDGFR* exon 18 mutation.
- Loss-of-function mutations in the succinate dehydrogenase gene (*SDHB* or *SDHA*) subunits or loss of the SDH subunit B (SDHB) protein expression has been identified in wild-type GISTs lacking *KIT* and *PDGFR* mutations. These findings have led to the use of the term *SDH-deficient GIST*, which is preferred over the older term of *wild-type GIST*.
- Tumor mutation analysis is important to identify imatinib-resistant mutations.
- *KIT* exon 9 mutations may require a higher dose of imatinib (>400 mg/day).
- *KIT* exon 11 mutation is associated with improved response to imatinib, progression-free survival, and overall survival compared with *KIT* exon 9 or wild-type GIST.

Clinical Staging

The TNM classification system is not used for GISTs. These tumors do not metastasize through the lymphatic system but instead spread through the bloodstream and peritoneum. To characterize the tumor aggressiveness and malignant potential, the mitotic rate, tumor size, and tumor location are used as prognostic factors. Additional prognostic factors include resection margin status and tumor rupture.

Treatment

Surgery

Surgery is the first-line treatment for patients with localized and resectable GISTs. Patients with inconclusive immunohistochemistry results should be referred for surgery if the lesion is causing pain or bleeding. GISTs are fragile tumors and can rupture, causing tumor cell dissemination in the abdominal cavity. The NCCN treatment guidelines recommend surgical resection that leaves no residual microscopic disease (R0).

Medical Therapy

- Most GISTs have *KIT* mutations that result in increased enzymatic activity of tyrosine kinase.
- Imatinib (Gleevec) is an oral competitive inhibitor of mutated *KIT*- and *PDFGRA*-encoded tyrosine kinases. It works by blocking the action of the abnormal protein, which signals cancer cells to multiply.
- Ninety percent of tumors with a *KIT* exon 11 mutation benefit from imatinib. It is the standard first-line therapy for patients with unresectable or metastatic GISTs.
- Imatinib has been approved as adjuvant therapy for patients after resection of *KIT*-positive GISTs who are at high or intermediate risk for recurrence.

- The NCCN guidelines recommend 36 months of adjuvant imatinib therapy for patients with high-risk disease.
- Fifty percent of GISTS treated with imatinib develop resistance within the first 2 years.
- Secondary resistance is seen in patients who have been treated with imatinib for more than 6 months and is caused by tumor clones with secondary mutations of *KIT*. Sunitinib is a treatment option at this point.
- Regorafenib is a multikinase inhibitor with activity against abnormal *KIT*-, *PDGFR*-, and *VEGFR*-encoded tyrosine kinases. It has been approved for use in patients with imatinib- and sunitinib-resistant GISTs.
- Sorafenib, nilotinib, dasatinib, and pazopanib have shown activity in patients with GISTs resistant to imatinib and sunitinib.
- Dasatinib is used for the first-line treatment of GISTs and for advanced disease that has become refractory to imatinib and sunitinib. The oral multikinase inhibitor targets abnormal *KIT*- and *PDGFR*-encoded tyrosine kinases.

Prognosis

Mitotic index is the most important prognostic feature for GISTs. The higher the mitotic count, the worse the prognosis. Gastric GISTS have a better prognosis than those at other sites. Because larger GISTs usually exhibit aggressive behavior, the prognosis for these tumors is poorer than for smaller GISTs.

Prevention and Surveillance

- Germline mutations in *KIT* and *PDGFRA* are inherited in an autosomal dominant pattern.
- Individuals with familial mutations are at high risk for GIST and require close surveillance.
- The mean age at identification of these familial mutations is about 20 years.
- The Carney triad of extraadrenal paragangliomas, pulmonary chondromas, and GISTs occurs in young females.
- Carney-Stratakis syndrome is a familial disorder characterized by GISTs and paragangliomas.
- Some individuals with a germline *SDHB*-inactivating mutation may not be affected.
- Pediatric GIST patients often have *SDHB*-inactivating mutations, and their disease tends to follow an indolent course.
- Pediatric GISTs typically manifest between the ages of 13 and 14.5 years and have a female prevalence.
- There is no standard approach to treatment because of the evolving understanding of the biology and clinical features of pediatric GISTs. NCCN guidelines recommend that pediatric patients with GIST be treated in clinical trials or at specialty centers.
- No other risk factors have been identified that can be used to guide screening.

Bibliography

Antonopoulos, P., Leonardou, P., Barbagiannis, N., Alexiou, K., Demonakou, M., & Economou, N. (2014). Gastrointestinal and extragastrointestinal stromal tumors: Report of two cases and review of the literature. *Case Reports in Gastroenterology*, 8(1), 61–66.

Bellera, C., Penel, N., Ouali, M., Bonvalot, S., Casali, P., Nielsem, O., & Mathoulin-Pelissier, S. (2015). Guidelines for time-to-event end point definitions in sarcomas and gastrointestinal stromal tumors (GIST) trials: Results of the DATECAN initiative (Definition for the Assessment of Time-to-Event Endpoints in CANcer trials). *Annals of Oncology, 26*(5), 865–872.

Gheorghe, M., Predescu, D., Iosig, C., Ardeleanu, C., Banacanu, F., & Constantinoiu, S. (2014). Clinical and therapeutic considerations of GIST. *Journal of Medicine and Life, 7*(2), 139–149.

Janeway, K., & Weldon, C. (2012). Pediatric gastrointestinal stromal tumor. *Seminars in Pediatric Surgery, 21*, 31–43.

Joensuu, H., Rutkowski, P., NisYhida, T., Steigen, P., Brabec, P., Plank, L., & Emile, J. (2015). KIT and PDGRDA mutations and the risk of GI stromal tumor recurrence. *Journal of Clinical Oncology, 33*(6), 634–642.

Kang, W., Zhu, C., Yu, J., Ye, X., & Ma, Z. (2015). KIT gene mutations in gastrointestinal stromal tumor. *Frontiers in Bioscience (Landmark Edition), 20*, 919–926.

Mullady, D., & Tan, B. (2013). A multidisciplinary approach to the diagnosis and treatment of gastrointestinal stromal tumor. *Journal of Clinical Gastroenterology, 47*(7), 578–585.

Patil, D., & Rubin, B. (2011). Gastrointestinal stromal tumor: Advances in diagnosis and management. *Archives of Pathology and Laboratory Medicine, 135*(10), 1298–1310.

Rammohan, A., Sathyanesan, J., Rajendran, K., Pitchaimuthu, A., Perumal, A., Srinivasan, U., & Govindan, M. (2013). A gist of gastrointestinal stromal tumors: A review. *World Journal of Gastrointestinal Oncology, 5*(6), 102–112.

Von Mehren, M., Randall, R., Benjamin, R., Boles, S., Bui, M., Casper, E., & Sundar, H. (2014). Gastrointestinal stromal tumors, version 2.2014. *Journal of the National Comprehensive Cancer Network, 12*, 853–862.

Hepatocellular Carcinoma

Lisa Parks

Definition

Hepatocellular carcinoma (HCC) is a primary tumor of the liver. Hepatic tumors are categorized as HCC or intrahepatic bile duct cholangiocarcinoma.

Incidence

HCC is the fifth most commonly diagnosed cancer and the third most common cancer cause of death in the world. The incidence of HCC has rapidly risen in the United States and Europe due to hepatitis C virus (HCV) infection and non-alcoholic steatohepatitis (NASH). It is 4.9 cases per 100,000 people. The 5-year survival rate for HCC is less than 12%.

Etiology and Risk Factors

- Ninety percent of HCC cases occur in patients with chronic liver disease.
- Cirrhosis is the greatest risk factor for HCC.
- HCV cirrhosis is responsible for the rapid increase in HCC in the United States and Europe, and hepatitis B virus (HBV) infection is the most important risk factor in the rest of the world.
- Other risk factors include male gender, obesity, diabetes, alcohol abuse, tobacco abuse, and ingestion of aflatoxin, a mycotoxin produced by certain molds found in peanuts, soybeans, and corn.

Signs and Symptoms

- Patients with HCC usually have no symptoms other than those related to chronic liver disease.
- In the setting of cirrhosis, HCC manifests with hepatic decompensation such as hepatic encephalopathy, ascites, or jaundice.
- Without cirrhosis, symptoms are tumor related and may include dull abdominal pain, weight loss, weakness, anorexia, malaise, and an abdominal mass.
- Extrahepatic spread of HCC is found in 15% of cases at the time of diagnosis.
- The most common sites of spread are the lungs, intraabdominal lymph nodes, bones, and adrenal glands.

Diagnostic Work-up

- Abdominal CT or MRI is the standard for identifying HCC.
- Arterial hypervascularity and washout in the portal venous phase of CT imaging of a hyperenhancing lesion are classic diagnostic findings of HCC.
- For lesions less than 1 cm in diameter, these diagnostic criteria are controversial.
- For lesions for which CT or MRI findings are indeterminate, core-needle or FNA biopsy is indicated.
- A serum α-fetoprotein (AFP) level greater than 500 ng/mL is diagnostic of HCC.

Histology

HCCs are adenocarcinomas. Tumor grading for HCC is based on the Edmonson and Steiner classification. There is no grading classification for intrahepatic bile duct cholangiocarcinoma.

Clinical Staging

The goals of the clinical staging systems are to accurately predict prognosis and assist in developing a treatment plan. There is no consensus regarding which staging system for HCC is best. Four staging systems are commonly used:
- AJCC TNM system
- Okuda system
- Barcelona Clinic Liver Cancer (BCLC) system
- Cancer of the Italian Liver Program (CLIP) score

The consensus statement of the American Hepato-Pancreato-Biliary Association in 2010 recommends the use of the TNM system.

Treatment

Most patients with HCC have advanced disease and underlying liver dysfunction at diagnosis. Surgery is the only curative treatment for HCC, but only 15% of patients are eligible for surgical intervention. Management of HCC is based on the BCLC system, Milan criteria, and Child-Pugh score (see table on page 66). A liver resection for HCC depends on whether the tumor is confined to the liver, the tumor size and location, and whether an adequate remnant of normal liver can be obtained.

- HCC resection is limited to patients with early-stage disease with no cirrhosis (i.e., Child-Pugh class A).
- For patients with unresectable HCC, liver transplantation is the only viable surgical option. It is usually done in conjunction with transarterial chemoembolization (TACE) or percutaneous ablation. Liver transplantation is recommended for patients with moderate to severe cirrhosis (i.e., Child-Pugh class B and C).

Child-Pugh Score

Parameter	POINTS ASSIGNED FOR INCREASING ABNORMALITY*		
	1	2	3
Encephalopathy	None	Grade 1-2	Grade 3-4
Ascites	None	Mild	Moderate or severe
Albumin (g/dL)	>3.5	2.8-3.5	<2.8
Prothrombin INR	<1.7	1.71-2.30	>2.30
Bilirubin (mg/dL)	<2	2-3	>3

INR, International normalized ratio.
*The Child-Pugh score (i.e., Child-Turcotte-Pugh score) is used to assess the prognosis of chronic liver disease, mainly cirrhosis. Scores are interpreted as follows: class A (good operative risk) = 5-6 points; class B (moderate operative risk) = 7-9 points; and class C (poor operative risk) = 10-15 points.
Modified from Faria, S., Szklaruk, J., Kaseb, A., Hassabo, H., & Elsayes, K. (2014). TNM/Okuda/Barcelona/INOS/CLIP international multidisciplinary classification of hepatocellular, carcinoma: Concepts, perspectives, and radiologic implications. *Abdominal Imaging, 39*, 1070-1087.

Other treatment options include the following:
- Radiofrequency ablation
- Microwave ablation
- Percutaneous ethanol injection (PEI)
- TACE
- Radioembolization
- Cryoablation
- Conventional radiation therapy or stereotactic radiotherapy
- Systemic chemotherapy or molecularly targeted therapies

Prognosis

The 5-year survival rate for HCC patients is 47% to 53%, even for those with small, early-stage tumors who undergo surgical resection. After surgical resection, the 2-year recurrence rate is 55%. For patients with advanced disease, the prognosis is poor. The median survival time is less than 1 year.

Prevention and Surveillance

The American Association for the Study of Liver Diseases (AASLD) guidelines from 2010 recommend surveillance of high-risk patients:
- HBV carriers, especially Asian men age 40 years or older and Asian women age 50 years or older
- Patients with cirrhosis
- Africans and African Americans
- Persons with a family history of HCC

Surveillance using ultrasound imaging of the liver every 6 months is recommended. When a lesion is suspicious on ultrasound, CT of the abdomen is obtained. A lesion less than 1 cm in diameter should undergo surveillance imaging every 3 to 6 months.

Bibliography

Addissie, B., & Roberts, L. (2013). Classification and staging of hepatocellular carcinoma. *Clinics in Liver Disease, 19*(2), 277–294.
Bodzin, A., & Busutti, R. (2015). Hepatocellular carcinoma: Advances in diagnosis, management, and long term outcome. *World Journal of Hepatology, 7*(9), 1157–1167.
Crissien, A., & Frenette, C. (2014). Current management of hepatocellular carcinoma. *Gastroenterology & Hepatology, 10*(3), 153–161.
Faria, S., Szklaruk, J., Kaseb, A., Hassabo, H., & Elsayes, K. (2014). TMN/Okuda/Barcelona/UNOS/CLIP international multidisciplinary classification of hepatocellular carcinoma: Concepts, perspective, and radiologic implications. *Abdominal Imaging, 39*, 1070–1087.
Fong, A., & Tanabe, K. (2014). The clinical management of hepatocellular carcinoma in the United States, Europe, and Asia: A comprehensive and evidence-based comparison and review. *Cancer, 120*(18), 2824–2838.
National Comprehensive Cancer Center Network. (2015). *NCCN clinical practice guidelines in oncology: Hepatobiliary cancers, version 2.2015.* Available at http://www.nccn.org/professionals/physician_gls/pdf/hepatobiliary.pdf (accessed December 18, 2015).
Page, A., Cosgrove, D., Philosophe, B., & Pawlik, T. (2014). Hepatocellular carcinoma: Diagnosis, management, and prognosis. *Surgical Oncology Clinics of North America, 23*, 289–311.
Pirisi, M., Leutner, M., Pinato, D., Avellini, C., Carsana, L., Toniutto, P., & Boldorini, R. (2010). Reliability and reproducibility of the Edmondson grading of hepatocellular carcinoma using paired core biopsy and surgical resection specimens. *Archives in Pathology and Laboratory Medicine, 134*, 1818–1822.
Salgia, R., & Singal, A. (2014). Hepatocellular carcinoma and other liver lesions. *Medical Clinics of North America, 98*, 103–118.
Siegel, R., Miller, K., & Jernal, A. (2015). Cancer statistics, 2015. *Cancer, 65*(1), 5–29.

Pancreatic Cancer

Lisa Parks

Definition

More than 90% of pancreatic cancers are ductal adenocarcinomas. Pancreatic ductal adenocarcinomas evolve from precursor lesions such as pancreatic intraepithelial neoplasias, intraductal papillary mucinous neoplasms, and mucinous cystic neoplasms. Neuroendocrine tumors may also be found in the pancreas (see Neuroendocrine Cancers on page 141).

Incidence

Pancreatic cancer is the fourth leading cause of cancer-related death. The 5-year survival rate is 6% because 80% of cases are diagnosed at an advanced stage. Between 60% and 70% of pancreatic cancers involve the head of the pancreas. In 2015, approximately 49,000 new cases of pancreatic cancer were diagnosed, and 40,500 deaths occurred.

Etiology and Risk Factors

Pancreatic cancer results from an accumulation of acquired genetic mutations. Most patients with advanced pancreatic cancer carry one or more of four genetic defects. Other risk factors include the following:
- Tobacco exposure is a factor in 25% to 30% of cases.
- Eighty percent of patients are between 60 and 80 years of age.
- Incidence is higher among African American men.
- More than four drinks of alcohol per day
- Obesity and type 2 diabetes for more than 5 years
- Chronic pancreatitis and cystic fibrosis
- Familial syndromes such as FAP, familial atypical multiple mole melanoma (FAMMM), or HNPCC (i.e., Lynch syndrome)

- Genetic alterations contributing to pancreatic cancer susceptibility include mutated *BRCA1*, *BRCA2*, *PALB2*, *STK11* (i.e., Peutz-Jeghers syndrome), *CDKN2A*, *PRSS1*, and *SPINK1*.

Signs and Symptoms

- Symptoms of early-stage pancreatic cancers are often vague or absent. Symptoms vary with the location of the pancreatic mass.
- In 10% of patients, new-onset diabetes may be the first sign of pancreatic cancer.
- Tumors located in the head and body of the pancreas compress surrounding structures, such as the bile ducts, mesenteric vessels, celiac nerves, pancreatic duct, and duodenum, causing upper abdominal or back pain.
- Patients may experience early satiety.
- Patients may have obstructive jaundice.
- Pruritus, clay-colored stool, and amber-colored urine usually accompany jaundice.
- Patients may have fatigue and unintentional weight loss.
- Gastric outlet obstruction may occur with advanced disease.

Diagnostic Work-up

- Pancreas protocol CT is the standard for diagnosis and staging. It uses triphasic imaging (i.e., arterial, portal venous, and delayed phases) to detect pathology by enhancing the contrast between a cancerous lesion and the normal surrounding structures.
- After a pancreatic mass is identified on EUS, an FNA biopsy is obtained.
- If no mass is found, ERCP with MRI is obtained.
- The most common serum tumor marker used for pancreatic ductal adenocarcinoma is cancer antigen 19-9 (CA 19-9), which is expressed in pancreatic and hepatobiliary disease. CA 19-9 is not a sufficient screening tool because it is unable to distinguish among cancer, chronic pancreatitis, and other inflammatory processes.

Histology

The pancreas is composed of exocrine and endocrine glands. Exocrine glands release enzymes into the small intestine to aid in digestion. Exocrine glands account for more than 95% of cells in the pancreas. The endocrine function of the pancreas is carried out by the islets of Langerhans, which synthesize and release hormones into the bloodstream. The hormones regulate glucose, lipid, and protein metabolism. Ninety percent of pancreatic cancers are in the exocrine pancreas and manifest as infiltrating ductal adenocarcinomas.

Clinical Staging

Clinical staging is determined by tumor, regional lymph node involvement and the presence or absence of metastasis (TNM) using the AJCC criteria (Edge, et. al., 2010).

Treatment

Resectable Lesions

Surgery is the only curative treatment for pancreatic ductal adenocarcinoma. Between 15% and 20% of patients diagnosed with pancreatic cancer have resectable disease. The 5-year survival rate for patients with resected tumors is less than 20%. Patients with resectable disease have clear fat planes around the celiac axis, hepatic artery, and superior mesenteric artery (SMA) and no evidence of superior mesenteric vein (SMV) or portal vein (PV) distortion. The classic surgical procedure for resection of carcinoma of the pancreatic head is a pancreaticoduodenectomy or Whipple procedure.

Cancers that involve the body of the pancreas are usually locally advanced and rarely resectable. If resectable, a distal pancreatectomy with or without a splenectomy is performed.

Borderline Resectable Lesions

The absence of metastases is a criterion for classification of resectable and borderline resectable disease. Pancreatic metastasis is considered unresectable disease. Venous involvement of the SMV or PV with distortion or narrowing of the vein or occlusion of the vein with suitable vessel proximal and distal makes a tumor borderline resectable. Encasement of the short segment of the hepatic artery without tumor extending onto the celiac axis or tumor abutment of the SMA is also classified by the NCCN as borderline resectable.

The use of neoadjuvant therapy is a controversial. There is no evidence supporting its use; however, many NCCN institutions have been using neoadjuvant therapy before surgery. The theory is that chemotherapy can shrink the tumor away from the blood vessels so that the tumor can safely be removed without disrupting the blood supply to remaining tissues.

Locally Advanced Lesions and Metastasis

A histologic diagnosis is required for the treatment of locally advanced, unresectable, or metastatic disease. More than 80% of pancreatic cancer patients fall into this category. The primary goals of treatment for advanced pancreatic cancer are to palliate symptoms and improve overall survival.

- The NCCN recommends systemic chemotherapy followed by consolidation chemoradiation therapy.
- Gemcitabine or continuous 5-FU with radiation is a common regimen. Gemcitabine monotherapy may be used to treat the symptoms of pancreatic cancer.
- Irinotecan or the FOLFIRINOX regimen of 5-FU, leucovorin, irinotecan, and oxaliplatin is considered second-line therapy. The toxicity profile of irinotecan may limit its use in patients with pancreatic cancer.
- Intensity-modulated radiotherapy (IMRT) and stereotactic radiotherapy are used to treat pancreatic cancer. There is no established standard dose of radiation for either type of therapy.
- Because of the poor survival associated with pancreatic cancer, clinical trials should be considered.

Palliative Care

- A multidisciplinary team is essential to assess and reassess the goals of care and palliation.
- Palliative care should address symptoms from biliary obstruction, gastric outlet obstruction, malnutrition, thromboembolic disease, pain, and depression.
- Biliary obstruction occurs in 65% to 75% of pancreatic cancer patients. Endoscopic placement of a biliary stent is often required.
- Approximately 10% to 25% of pancreatic cancer patients have gastric outlet obstruction. An enteral stent or a gastrostomy tube with or without a jejunostomy tube may be placed surgically or endoscopically.

Prognosis

Patients with pancreatic cancer have a poor prognosis. Only 16% of patients survive 1 year, and only 6% survive 5 years. The median survival time for patients who do not qualify for chemotherapy is 3 to 4 months. Patients receiving chemotherapy have a median survival time of 6 to 7 months (see table below).

Prognosis by Stage at Diagnosis of Pancreatic Cancer

| Stage | MEDIAN SURVIVAL TIME (MO) | | |
	Patients with Resectable Disease	All Patients	Patients with Nonresectable Disease
IA	24.1	10	6.8
IB	20.6	9.1	6.1
IIA	15.4	8.1	6.2
IIB	12.7	9.7	6.7
III	10.6	7.7	7.2
IV	4.5	4.4	2.5

Modified from McIntyre, C., & Winter, J. (2015). Diagnostic evaluation and staging of pancreatic ductal adenocarcinoma. *Seminars in Oncology, 42*(1), 19-27.

Prevention and Surveillance

The U.S. Preventive Services Task Force (USPTF) recommends against routine screening of asymptomatic adults of average risk due to lack of mortality benefit. Persons from families with genetic defects and other high-risk factors may benefit from screening. Screening and surveillance can be performed with CT or EUS.

Bibliography

Appel, B., Tolat, P., Evans, D., & Tsai, S. (2012). Current staging systems for pancreatic cancer. *The Cancer Journal, 18*(6), 539–549.

De La Cruz, M., Young, A., & Ruffin, M. (2014). Diagnosis and management of pancreatic cancer. *American Family Physician, 89*(8), 626–632.

Edge, S., Byrd, D. R., Compton, C. C., Fritz, A. G., Greene, F. L., & Trotti, A. (2010). *AJCC staging manual* (7th ed.). New York: Springer.

Gee, C. (2011). Pancreatic cancer: A whistle-stop tour. *Gastrointestinal Nursing, 9*(7), 41–45.

MacIntyre, J. (2011). Metastatic pancreatic cancer: What can nurses do? *Clinical Journal of Oncology Nursing, 15*(4), 424–428.

McIntyre, C., & Winter, J. (2015). Diagnostic evaluation and staging of pancreatic ductal adenocarcinoma. *Seminars in Oncology, 42*(1), 19–27.

National Comprehensive Cancer Network. (2015). *NCCN Clinical practice in oncology guidelines: Pancreatic adenocarcinoma, version 2.2015.* Available from http://www.nccn.org/professionals/physician_gls/pdf/pancreatic.pdf (accessed December 18, 2015).

Siegel, R., Miller, K., & Jemal, A. (2012). Cancer Statistics, 2015. *Cancer, 65*(1), 5–29.

The Sol Goldman Pancreatic Cancer Research Center, Johns Hopkins Medicine. (2015). *NFPTR FAQs.* Available at http://pathology.jhu.edu/pc/nfptr/faq.php (accessed December 18, 2015).

Vincent, A., Herman, J., Schulick, R., Hruban, R., & Goggins, M. (2011). Pancreatic cancer. *The Lancet, 378*, 607–620.

Genitourinary Cancers

Francisco A. Conde and Tyler Workman

Bladder Cancer

Definition

Bladder cancer is the second most common urologic malignancy after prostate cancer and the fourth most common cancer in men. Most bladder cancers are transitional cell or urothelial carcinomas, and they are often discovered in the early stages of the disease. Bladder cancer can metastasize to the lymph nodes, bones, lung, liver, and peritoneum.

Incidence

- More than 74,000 Americans were diagnosed with bladder cancer in 2015, and more than 16,000 died of the disease.
- Incidence rates decreased by 1.6% per year for men from 2007 to 2011 and 1.1% per year for women.
- Incidence rates are high in the United States and Africa, especially in Egypt.

Etiology and Risk Factors

Risk factors include the following:

- Age: The median age at diagnosis is 65 years, and 9 of 10 people with bladder cancer are older than 55 years of age.
- Sex and race: The incidence is two times higher among white men than black men, and it is four times higher among men than women.
- Cigarette smoking
  - At least 50% of bladder cancer in men and women is attributed to cigarette smoking.
  - The risk is four times higher among smokers than nonsmokers.
- Industrial chemical exposures: Workers in the rubber, dye, paint, leather, aluminum, petroleum, and printing industries are at increased risk for bladder cancer.
- Arsenic: High levels of arsenic in drinking water increase the risk of bladder cancer.
- Cyclophosphamide: Long-term exposure to the chemotherapy drug is associated with an increased risk of bladder cancer.
- Radiation: Pelvic exposure increases the risk of bladder cancer.
- Parasitic infection: Chronic bladder irritation and infections, particularly by *Schistosoma hematobium* (causes schistosomiasis), increases risk.
- Genetics: The risk of bladder cancer is increased for people with Cowden disease, Lynch syndrome, or a mutation in the retinoblastoma gene (*RB1*).

Signs and Symptoms

- Patients with bladder cancer often have hematuria and other urinary symptoms:
  - Urinary frequency
  - Dysuria
  - Urgency
  - Altered stream
- Patients with advanced disease may have the following:
  - Palpable mass
  - Bone pain
  - Pelvic or rectal pain
  - Acute renal failure

Diagnostic Work-up

- Standard work-up
  - History and physical examination
  - Cystoscopy with biopsy and urine cytology
- Additional work-up for patients with noninvasive bladder cancer
  - Imaging of the upper tract collecting system
  - Pelvic computed tomography (CT) or magnetic resonance imaging (MRI) before performing transurethral resection of a bladder tumor (TURBT)
- Additional work-up for patients with invasive bladder cancer
  - Complete blood count and chemistry profile
  - Imaging of the chest and upper tract collecting system
  - CT or MRI of the abdomen and pelvis
  - Bone scan if the alkaline phosphatase level is elevated or the patient has bone pain

Histology

- Approximately 95% of bladder cancers are transitional cell or urothelial carcinomas.
- Squamous cell carcinoma accounts for 3%.
- Adenocarcinoma represents 1.4%.
- Small cell tumors make up 1% of bladder cancers.
- Bladder cancer is typically divided into two groups: superficial (i.e., nonmuscle invasive bladder cancer [NMIBC]) or muscle invasive.
  - Superficial bladder cancer (T1, Tis, or Ta) is usually low grade and noninvasive. Approximately 75% to 85% of patients have superficial or NMIBC bladder cancer.
  - Muscle-invasive disease (T2 to T4) tends to be more aggressive and invades the muscularis propria.

Clinical Staging

The American Joint Committee on Cancer (AJCC) tumor-node-metastasis (TNM) system is used for staging bladder cancer. The AJCC TNM system for bladder cancer describes the extent of the primary tumor (T), whether the cancer has spread to nearby lymph nodes (N), and the absence or presence of distant metastasis (M) (Edge et al., 2010).

Grading

For urothelial histologic types, the recommended grading system is based on low- and high-grade designations:

- Grade 0: papilloma
- Grade 1: low grade
- Grade 2: low grade or high grade
- Grade 3: high-grade urothelial carcinoma

Treatment

Surgery

- TURBT is the standard treatment for nonmuscle invasive tumors.
- For patients with muscle-invasive tumors, partial or radical cystectomy with pelvic lymph node dissection is performed.
  - In men, radical cystectomy involves removal of the bilateral pelvic lymph nodes, bladder, prostate gland, and seminal vesicles.
  - In women, radical cystectomy involves removal of the bilateral pelvic lymph nodes, uterus, fallopian tubes, ovaries, bladder, urethra, and segment of the interior vaginal wall.
- After surgical removal of the bladder, patients require an ileal conduit or a continent urinary diversion such as a Kock pouch or an Indiana pouch.

Radiation Therapy

Radiation therapy may be used for patients who are not surgical candidates as part of treatment for advanced bladder cancer or to treat symptoms caused by metastatic bladder cancer.

- Patients must have an empty bladder for simulation and treatment.
- The radiation dose to the whole bladder ranges from 40 to 45 Gy plus an additional boost of 9 to 11 Gy for a total of 49 to 66 Gy.
- Chemotherapy drugs such as cisplatin and 5-fluorouracil (5-FU) may be given concurrently with radiation therapy as radiosensitizers.

Chemotherapy

- Systemic chemotherapy may be given in several settings:
  - Neoadjuvant chemotherapy to downstage a tumor before surgery
  - Adjuvant therapy after cystectomy for muscle-invasive lesions
  - For metastatic disease
  - Concurrently with radiation therapy as a radiosensitizer
- Commonly prescribed chemotherapy regimens
  - Dose-dense methotrexate, vinblastine, doxorubicin, and cisplatin (DDMVAC)
  - Gemcitabine and cisplatin
  - Cisplatin, methotrexate, and vinblastine (CMV)

Intravesical Therapy

Intravesical therapy is used as prophylactic or adjuvant therapy to decrease recurrence, delay progression, and eradicate residual disease after transurethral resection.

- The most commonly used agent for intravesical therapy is bacillus Calmette-Guérin (BCG) vaccine.
  - Intravesical BCG is given weekly for 6 weeks.
  - Maintenance therapy is usually monthly or every 3 months for 1 to 3 years.
- Intravesical chemotherapy usually is given for patients at high risk for recurrence.
  - Mitomycin C and thiotepa are drugs commonly used for intravesical chemotherapy.
  - Intravesical chemotherapy should be administered within 24 hours of resection and may be followed by a 6-week induction regimen of intravesical chemotherapy.

Prognosis

- For all stages combined, the 5-year relative survival rate is 77%.
- The 5-year survival rate is 69% for patients with localized disease at diagnosis.
- For patients with regional and distant disease, the 5-year survival rates are 34% and 6%, respectively.

Prevention and Surveillance

- There are no known prevention measures, but risk reduction is possible by smoking cessation, avoiding exposure to industrial chemicals and arsenic, maintaining good hydration, and eating a healthy diet that is rich in fruits and vegetables.
- There are no screening recommendations.
- The National Comprehensive Cancer Network (NCCN) surveillance guidelines for bladder cancer are summarized in the table below.

National Comprehensive Cancer Network Surveillance Guidelines for Bladder Cancer	
Test or Procedure	**Frequency**
Urine cytology, liver function tests, creatinine and electrolyte levels	Every 6-12 months
Imaging of chest, abdomen, and pelvis	Every 3-6 months for 2 years, then as clinically indicated
For bladder preservation, cystoscopy and urine cytology with or without biopsy	Every 3-6 months for 2 years, then increasing intervals as appropriate
For radical cystectomy, urine cytology, liver function tests, creatinine and electrolyte levels	Every 3-6 months for 2 years, then as clinically indicated
For continent diversion	Monitor for vitamin B_{12} deficiency yearly

Modified from the National Comprehensive Cancer Network. (2015). Bladder cancer, v1.2015. Available at http://www.nccn.org/professionals/physician_gls/pdf/bladder.pdf (accessed January 17, 2016).

Bibliography

American Cancer Society (ACS). (2015a). *Cancer facts & figures, 2015.* Atlanta, GA: American Cancer Society.

American Cancer Society (ACS). (2015b). *What are the risk factors of bladder cancer?* Available at http://www.cancer.org/cancer/bladdercancer/detailed guide/bladder-cancer-risk-factors (accessed January 17, 2016).

Cheung, G., Sahai, A., Billia, M., Dasgupta, P., & Khan, M. S. (2013). Recent advances in the diagnosis and treatment of bladder cancer. *BMC Medicine, 11*(1), 1–8.

Goodison, S., Rosser, C. J., & Urquidi, V. (2013). Bladder cancer detection and monitoring: assessment of urine and blood-based marker tests. *Molecular Diagnosis & Therapy, 17,* 71–84.

National Comprehensive Cancer Network (NCCN). (2015). *Bladder cancer, version 1.2015.* Available at http://www.nccn.org/professionals/physician _gls/pdf/bladder.pdf (accessed January 17, 2016).

Raghavan, D., Stein, J. P., Cote, R., & Jones, J. S. (2010). Bladder cancer. In W. K. Hong, R. C. Bast, Jr., W. N. Hait, D. W. Kufe, R. E. Pollock, R. R. Weichselbaum, et al (Eds.), *Cancer medicine* (pp. 1219–1227). Shelton, CT: People's Medical Publishing House.

Kidney Cancer

Definition

Kidney cancer is among the 10 most common cancers in both men and women in the United States. Ninety percent of kidney cancers arise from the renal parenchyma and are referred to as *renal cell carcinomas* (RCC). Subtypes of RCC include clear cell, papillary, chromophobe, collecting duct, and renal medullary carcinomas. Other types of kidney cancers include urothelial carcinoma (UC), renal sarcoma, and Wilms' tumor. Kidney cancer can metastasize to the brain, lung, lymph nodes, liver, adrenal gland, and bone.

Incidence

- Kidney cancer accounts for approximately 4% of all adult malignancies.
- About 61,560 new cases of kidney cancer and 14,080 deaths occurred in the United States in 2015.
- Incidence rate has been rising on average 1.4% each year over the past 10 years, which may be due to the common use of high-resolution abdominal and pelvic imaging.
- Overall lifetime risk for developing kidney cancer is 1 in 63 (1.6%).
- The incidence is high in North America and Europe and is low in Asian and South American countries.

Etiology and Risk Factors

Risk factors include the following:

- Age: The average age at diagnosis is 64 years. Diagnosis is rare among people before 45 years of age.
- Sex: The incidence is higher among men than women.
- Race: African Americans have higher rates of kidney cancer.
- Cigarette smoking
  - Compared to nonsmokers, risk increased about 50% in male and 20% in female smokers.
- Obesity: Accounts for over 30% of kidney cancers.
- Genetics: The risk of kidney cancer is increased for people with von Hippel-Lindau (VHL) disease, hereditary papillary renal cell carcinoma, Birt-Hogg-Dubé (BHD) syndrome, and hereditary leiomyomatosis and renal cell cancer (HLRCC).
- Industrial chemical exposures: Workers exposed to cadmium, uranium, and trichloroethylene (TCE) are at increased risk for kidney cancer.
- Hypertension is a risk factor.
- Hemodialysis and renal transplantation: Increased risk of kidney cancer is seen in people who are on long-term hemodialysis for end-stage renal disease, as well as after renal transplantation.

Signs and Symptoms

- More than 50% of kidney cancers are discovered as an incidental finding on radiographic imaging tests in asymptomatic individuals.
- Hematuria, flank pain, and palpable flank mass are the classic triad of symptoms. Other symptoms may include fever, loss of appetite, unintentional weight loss, anemia, bone pain, adenopathy, and varicocele.

Diagnostic Work-up

- History and physical examination
- Complete blood count (CBC) and comprehensive metabolic panel
- Urinalysis
- Abdominal or pelvic CT
- Abdominal MRI: used if inferior vena caval involvement is suspected
- Chest imaging
- Bone scan if the alkaline phosphatase level is elevated or the patient has bone pain
- Brain MRI if the patient has signs and symptoms that suggest brain metastasis
- If urothelial carcinoma is suspected, urine cytology, ureteroscopy, and biopsy should be considered.
- Consider needle biopsy of small lesions to confirm a cancer diagnosis and guide treatment strategies.

Histology

- 90% of kidney cancers arise from the renal parenchyma and are referred to as *renal cell carcinomas* (RCC) or *renal adenocarcinomas*. Major subtypes of RCC include:
  - Clear cell carcinoma: 75% to 80% of RCC
  - Papillary: 10% to 15%
  - Chromophobe: 5% to10%
  - Medullary: Less than 1%
  - Collecting duct: Less than 1%
- About 10% of kidney cancers occur in the renal pelvis and ureter.
  - Urothelial carcinomas (UC), also known as *transitional cell carcinomas* (TCC), account for more than 90% of upper urinary tract tumors.
  - Squamous cell carcinomas: 8%
  - Tend to be more invasive at diagnosis and have a poorer prognosis than UCs
  - Adenocarcinomas: Below 2%

- Renal sarcoma: Less than1% of kidney cancers
  - Begins in the blood vessels or connective tissue of the kidneys
- Wilms' tumors: almost always found in children and very rarely in adults

Clinical Staging

The American Joint Committee on Cancer (AJCC) tumor-node-metastasis (TNM) system is used for staging kidney cancer (Edge et al., 2010).

Grading

- The Fuhrman grading system is used and has a scale of 1 (well differentiated) through 4 (undifferentiated).
- Grade 1 tumors are usually slow growing, less aggressive, and tend to have a good prognosis, whereas grade 4 tumors are most aggressive and have a worse prognosis.

Treatment

- Active surveillance: monitoring of tumors using abdominal imaging with delayed intervention when indicated
  - Should be considered for elderly patients with limited life expectancy or those with significant comorbidities that places them at excessive risk for invasive interventions
- Ablative therapy: include cryotherapy and radiofrequency ablation (RFA)
  - Option for patients with stage I disease who are not surgical candidates
- Surgery: mainstay of treatment for localized disease
  - Radical nephrectomy: involves removal of the kidney, perirenal fat, regional lymph nodes, and ipsilateral adrenal gland.
  - Preferred surgery if the tumor extends into the inferior vena cava
  - Techniques include open, laparoscopic, robotic-assisted surgeries.
- Partial nephrectomy or nephron-sparing surgery
  - Preferred surgery for stage I disease
  - Outcomes are comparable to radical nephrectomy.
  - Advantages over radical nephrectomy include preservation of renal function, reduction in overall mortality, and decreased frequency of cardiovascular events.
  - Contraindicated in patients with locally advanced disease or if the tumor is in an unfavorable location.
- Nephrectomy with surgical metastasectomy: used (1) in patients with RCC and a solitary site of metastasis in either the lung, bone, or brain or (2) in patients who were disease-free after nephrectomy and later developed a solitary recurrence.
- Lymph node dissection: recommended only for patients with enlarged regional lymph nodes detected on imaging tests prior to surgery (NCCN, 2016)
- Immunotherapy
  - High dose interleukin-2 (IL-2): used as first-line or subsequent therapy for patients with relapsed or unresectable stage IV clear cell renal carcinoma who have excellent performance status and normal organ function (NCCN, 2016)

- Targeted therapy: tyrosine kinase inhibitors (TKIs) and anti-VEGF antibodies commonly used in first- and second-line treatments
  - Agents approved by the U.S. Food and Drug administration (FDA): sunitinib, pazopanib, everolimus, axitinib, sorafenib, carbozantinib, temsirolimus, nivolumab, and bevacizumab
- Radiation therapy: may be used for palliation, such as bone metastasis
- Chemotherapy: not a standard treatment for kidney cancer. It may be used in patients who have failed immunotherapy and/or targeted therapy.

Prognosis

- Prognostic factors include disease stage, tumor size, histologic type and grade, histologic tumor necrosis, number and location of metastatic sites, prior nephrectomy, performance status, substantial weight loss, elevated serum calcium and lactate dehydrogenase (LDH) levels, low hemoglobin, and thrombocytosis.
- For all stages combined, the 5-year relative survival rate is 72%.
- The 5-year survival rate by stage at diagnosis:
  - Local: 92%
  - Regional: 65%
  - Distant: 12%

Prevention and Surveillance

- There are no screening recommendations and measures to prevent kidney cancer. However, increasing levels of physical activity, maintaining a healthy weight, tobacco-free or smoking cessation, and diets high in fruits and vegetables may reduce the risk of kidney cancer. A family history of RCC, particularly in individuals less than 50 years old, may indicate a hereditary predisposition to the disease. Patients with a family history or hereditary RCC (i.e., von Hippel-Lindau disease) should be closely monitored.
- Follow-up surveillance includes:
  - History and physical examination
  - Complete blood count and comprehensive metabolic panel
  - Abdominal CT or MRI
  - Chest CT or x-ray
  - Head CT, bone scan, MRI of spine: if metastasis is suspected

Bibliography

American Cancer Society (ACS). (2015). *Cancer facts & figures, 2015*. Atlanta, GA: American Cancer Society.

Chow, W., Dong, L. M., & Devesa, S. S. (2010). Epidemiology and risk factors for kidney cancer. *Nature Reviews Urology*, 7(5), 245–257.

Edge, S., Byrd, D. R., Compton, C. C., Fritz, A. G., Greene, F. L., & Trotti, A. (Eds.). (2010). *AJCC staging manual* (7th ed.) New York: Springer.

Lee, J. E., Mannisto, S., Spiegelman, D., Hunter, D. J., Bernstein, L., van den Brandt, P. A., et al. (2011). Intakes of fruit, vegetables, and carotenoids and renal cell cancer risk: A pooled analysis of 13 prospective studies. *Cancer Epidemiology Biomarkers and Prevention*, 18(6) 1739–1739.

National Comprehensive Cancer Network (NCCN). (2016). *Kidney cancer, version 2.2016*. Available at http://www.nccn.org/professionals/physician_gls/pdf/kidney.pdf (accessed February 15, 2016).

Rini, B. I., Heng, D. Y. C., Zhou, M., Novick, A., & Raghavan, D. (2010). Renal cell carcinoma. In W. K. Hong, R. C. Bast, Jr., W. N. Hait, D. W. Kufe, R. E. Pollock, R. R. Weichselbaum, et al (Eds.), *Cancer medicine* (pp. 1204–1211). Shelton, CT: People's Medical Publishing House.

Sun, M., Thuret, R., Abdollah, F., Lughezzani, G., Schmitges, J., Tian, Z., et al. (2011). Age-adjusted incidence, mortality, and survival rates of stage-specific renal cell carcinoma in North America: A trend analysis. *European Urology, 59*(1), 135–141.

Penile Cancer

Definition

Carcinoma of the penis is an uncommon malignancy in the United States. Ninety-five percent of cancers of the penis are squamous cell carcinomas that may evolve from the prepuce, glans, or shaft of the penis. Metastasis occurs primarily in regional lymph nodes (i.e., femoral, inguinal, pelvic, and iliac), and it rarely spreads to distant sites such as the lungs, liver, bones, and brain.

Incidence

- Carcinoma of the penis accounts for less than 1% of all malignancies in men.
- About 1820 new cases of penile cancer and 310 deaths occurred in the United States in 2015.
- The disease commonly affects men between the ages of 50 and 70 years.
- The incidence is low in North America and Europe; the rate of penile malignancies is higher in African, South American, and Asian countries.

Etiology and Risk Factors

- The exact cause of penile cancer is unknown.
- Risk factors include the following:
  - Risk increases with age, with a median age at diagnosis of 68 years.
  - The incidence is 3.2 times greater among men who have never been circumcised compared with men who were circumcised at birth.
  - Between 44% and 85% of men with penile cancer have a history of phimosis (i.e., tightness of the foreskin that prevents retraction).
  - Between 45% and 80% of penile cancer cases are related to human papillomavirus (HPV) infection.
  - Having multiple sex partners is a risk factor.
  - A history of sexually transmitted diseases, including HIV, increases the risk of penile cancer.
  - Tobacco use is a risk factor.
  - Patients with psoriasis treated with psoralens plus ultraviolet A (UVA) light are at increased risk for penile cancer.
- Premalignant lesions associated with squamous cell carcinoma of the penis include the following:
  - Balanitis xerotica obliterans
  - Cutaneous horn
  - Giant condyloma
  - Bowenoid papulosis

Signs and Symptoms

- Penile cancer at presentation ranges from a small papule or pustule that does not heal to a large, exophytic, fungating lesion.
- Lesions occur most commonly on the glans (48%) and prepuce (21%) and less commonly on the coronal sulcus and penile shaft.
- There may be penile pain, bleeding, discharge, or a foul odor.
- Patients with advanced disease may have palpable lymph nodes and constitutional symptoms such as weight loss.

Diagnostic Work-up

- The following tools are essential for the diagnosis and staging of penile cancer:
  - History and physical examination are important to assess risk factors and characteristics of the lesion, such as diameter, number and location, and relation to other structures, and to evaluate inguinal or pelvic lymphadenopathy.
  - A biopsy specimen is obtained from the penile lesion.
  - Imaging includes ultrasonography, CT, and MRI.

Histology

- Squamous cell carcinoma is the most common histologic form of penile cancer.
- Penile cancer can be classified as verrucous, papillary squamous, warty, or basaloid.
- The verrucous subtype has low malignant potential.

Clinical Staging

- The AJCC TNM system is used for staging penile cancer (Edge et al., 2010).
- Grading is based on the degree of anaplasia:
  - Grade 1: Well differentiated (no evidence of anaplasia)
  - Grade 2: Moderately differentiated (<50% anaplastic cells)
  - Grade 3: Poorly differentiated (>50% anaplastic cells)
  - Grade 4: Undifferentiated
- Higher grade is an important predictor of metastatic disease to the groin and even more powerful when combined with the depth of tumor invasion.

Treatment

- Treatment depends on the disease stage at diagnosis.
- The following treatments may be used:
  - Noninvasive or verrucous carcinomas: Mohs micrographic surgery, laser therapy, radiation therapy, and in some cases, topical imiquimod (5%) or 5-FU cream
  - Tumors involving only the prepuce: circumcision
  - Invasive tumors: partial or total penectomy with or without inguinal lymph node dissection
  - Advanced disease: single-agent or combination chemotherapy
- Preferred first-line combination chemotherapy regimens
  - Paclitaxel, ifosfamide, and cisplatin (TIP regimen)
  - Cisplatin plus 5-FU
  - Single-agent capecitabine, carboplatin, 5-FU, docetaxel, paclitaxel, or panitumumab.

Prognosis

- The extent of regional inguinal lymph node metastasis is the single most important predictor of long-term survival of men with penile cancer.
  - Untreated patients with inguinal metastases rarely survive 2 years.
  - In patients with clinically palpable adenopathy and histologically proven metastases, 20% to 50% are alive 5 years after inguinal lymphadenectomy.
  - An 82% to 88% 5-year survival rate has been reported when only one to three lymph nodes are involved.

Prevention and Surveillance

- Although there is no proven way to prevent penile cancer, measures can be taken to decrease risk.
  - Avoidance of HPV and HIV exposure
  - Smoking cessation
  - Good personal hygiene, especially completely cleaning under the foreskin
  - Circumcision
- There are no screening recommendations, but penile cancers usually start in the skin and can be detected early.
  - The area underneath the foreskin should be kept clean and regularly examined.
  - Any reddened or scaly lesion or sore should be reported promptly to the medical team.
- Follow-up surveillance for all patients includes clinical examination of the penis and inguinal nodes.
  - Imaging is not routinely recommended for those with early disease, but it may be used after an abnormal finding or if a recurrence is suspected.
  - CT of the chest, abdomen, and pelvis is recommended for those with inguinal or pelvic lymph node metastases.

Bibliography

American Cancer Society (ACS). (2015a). *Cancer facts & figures, 2015*. Atlanta, GA: American Cancer Society.

American Cancer Society (ACS). (2015b). *Penile cancer*. Available at http://www.cancer.org/cancer/penilecancer/detailedguide/penile-cancer-what-is-penile-cancer (accessed January 17, 2016).

Edge, S., Byrd, D. R., Compton, C. C., Fritz, A. G., Greene, F. L., & Trotti, A. (Eds.). (2010). *AJCC staging manual* (7th ed.). New York: Springer.

Lawindy, S. M., Rodriguez, A. R., Horenblas, S., & Spiess, P. E. (2011). Current and future strategies in the diagnosis and management of penile cancer. *Advances in Urology, 2011*, 1–9.

National Comprehensive Cancer Network (NCCN). (2015). *Penile cancer, version 2.2015*. Available at http://www.nccn.org/professionals/physician_gls/pdf/penile.pdf (accessed January 17, 2016).

Pow-Sang, M. R., Ferreira, U., Pow-Sang, J. M., Nardi, A. C., & Destefano, V. (2010). Epidemiology and natural history of penile cancer. *Urology, 76*(2), S2–S6.

Prostate Cancer

Definition

Prostate cancer is the second most common cancer in American men; skin cancer is the first. The cancer affects the prostate, a lobular gland that serves as a secondary male sex organ. The prostate is located in the pelvis, is surrounded by the rectum, and is responsible for erectile function and passive urinary sphincter control.

Six of 10 of men diagnosed with prostate cancer are older than 65 years. More than 90% of men are diagnosed with localized or regional disease. Metastasis can occur through direct extension into the seminal vesicles, urethral mucosa, bladder wall, and external sphincter. The cancer may also spread through the regional lymph nodes. Prostate vasculature is often the method of spread when the cancer invades the pelvic bones, lumbar spine, liver, or lungs.

Incidence

- About 220,800 new cases of prostate cancer and 27,540 deaths occurred in the United States in 2015.
- Overall, 1 in 7 men in the United States are diagnosed with prostate cancer, and 1 in 38 die of the disease.
- African American men have a higher incidence rate and an at least double mortality rate compared with men of other racial groups.

Etiology and Risk Factors

Several risk factors for prostate cancer have been identified.

- Age older than 50 years, with an average age at diagnosis of 66 years
- Ethnicity: African American men are at higher risk than all other ethnic groups, and Asian men who live in Asia have the lowest risk (2%).
- Geography: It is more common in North America, northwestern Europe, Australia, and the Caribbean Islands.
- Family history
  - The risk for prostate cancer is 2.1 to 2.4 times greater for men whose fathers had prostate cancer and 2.9 to 3.3 times higher for those whose brothers had the disease.
  - About 40% of early-onset prostate cancer and 5% to 10% of all prostate cancers are hereditary.
- Genetics
  - *BRCA1* or *BRCA2* genetic mutation
  - Lynch syndrome, which increases the risk of many cancers, including prostate cancer
- Diet: High intake of red meat and high-fat dairy products may increase the risk of prostate cancer.
- The degree to which factors such as obesity, recurring prostatitis, sexually transmitted infections, benign prostatic hypertrophy (BPH), prostatic intraepithelial neoplasia (PIN), and environmental exposures (e.g., herbicides such as Agent Orange) contribute to prostate cancer is inconclusive.

Signs and Symptoms

Because the signs and symptoms of prostate cancer can often be confused with normal signs of aging, BPH, or prostatitis, an accurate diagnosis is imperative. The most common signs and symptoms of prostate cancer include the following:

- Weak and interrupted urinary stream
- Frequent urination
- Nocturia
- Difficulty beginning urination
- Dysuria
- Hematuria

- Blood in semen
- Weakness or numbness in the legs or feet
- Unrelieved pain in the back, hips, or pelvis
- Shortness of breath
- Fatigue

Screening Recommendations

- The American Cancer Society recommends that men make an informed decision with their health care provider about whether to be tested for prostate cancer.
- Screening involves getting a prostate-specific antigen (PSA) blood test and a digital rectal examination (DRE) annually for men starting at the age of 50 years and for those who have a life expectancy of more than 10 years. However, for those at high risk (e.g., African Americans, men having a first-degree relative with the disease), screening should begin at 40 years of age.
- DRE
  - Palpation of the prostate can assess for tumors and can detect BPH and prostatitis.
  - The sensitivity of DRE is 59%, and the specificity is 94% (Hoffman, 2014).
- PSA blood test
  - The test measures a protein released by epithelial cells in the prostate.
  - The measurement is not prostate cancer specific, and the PSA level can be elevated in cases of advanced age, BPH, or prostatitis.
  - The PSA blood test has a sensitivity of 67.5% to 80%, which suggests that 20% to 30% of prostate cancers are misdiagnosed if only this test is used. Age-adjusted values are used to increase specificity.
  - Increasing PSA values often indicate the need for a prostate biopsy.
  - Other methods to increase PSA sensitivity include measuring PSA velocity, PSA density, and free PSA levels.

Diagnostic Work-up

A physical examination is the primary measure for diagnosing prostate cancer because men often seek treatment for urinary symptoms. Diagnostic measures of prostate cancer include the following:

- DRE
- PSA blood test
- Transrectal ultrasound (TRUS) allows the provider to visualize the prostate and confirm the diagnosis.
- Prostate biopsies usually require six specimens from both sides of the prostate and can enable a final pathologic diagnosis of the disease.
- Bone scans, CT, and MRI are used to evaluate metastatic disease.
- Newer tests for prostate cancer diagnostic markers include those for human glandular kallikrein 2, prostate-specific membrane antigen, cyclin-dependent kinase inhibitor 1B (CDKN1B, a cell cycle inhibitor formerly known as p27), and serum insulin-like growth factor. These tests are rarely used, and evidence for their effectiveness is limited.

Histology

More than 95% of prostate cancers are adenocarcinomas. The remaining 5% are squamous cell carcinomas, transitional cell tumors, and carcinosarcomas (rare).

Clinical Staging

- The AJCC TNM system for prostate cancer describes the extent of the primary tumor (T), whether the cancer has spread to nearby lymph nodes (N), and the absence or presence of distant metastasis (M).
- The Gleason score is a measurement of the tumor's grade, which describes its aggressiveness.
  - The score is derived from the two most common malignant histologic patterns in the tumor, and each is assigned a grade. Scores range from 1 to 5, and the more differentiated that a cell is, the higher the grade. The two scores are added together, giving a final score between 2 and 10.
  - Higher Gleason scores are associated with more aggressive tumors.
- The AJCC anatomic prognostic groups incorporate the TNM system, PSA values, and Gleason scores (Edge et al., 2010).

Treatment

Treatment options include active surveillance, surgery, radiation therapy, hormonal therapy or androgen-deprivation therapy, and chemotherapy.

- Choice of treatment is determined by several factors: presence of symptoms, stage of disease, life expectancy, comorbidities, effect on quality of life, and probability that the tumor can be cured by single-modality therapy.
- Because most prostate cancers are slow growing and older men often have other major health problems, active surveillance may be indicated because the individual is likely to die of other health concerns before succumbing to the cancer.
- If surgery is indicated, the most common option is a radical prostatectomy, in which the entire prostate is removed.
- If radiation therapy is recommended, two types are used.
  - External beam radiation therapy (EBRT) targets the prostate and regional lymph nodes. It requires the implantation of gold seed markers in the prostate to accurately deliver radiation to the desired treatment areas.
  - Brachytherapy uses small radioactive implants that are placed directly in the prostate to deliver localized radiation therapy to the gland. Brachytherapy can be delivered by an implanted catheter at a high dose, which uses iridium 192 photon energy, or a low dose, which uses iodine 121 photon energy.
- Androgen-deprivation therapy (ADT) can be achieved by surgery (i.e., orchiectomy) or by medical castration through the administration of pharmacologic agents.
  - The goal is to achieve a serum testosterone level below 0.5 ng/mL to decrease or inhibit prostate cancer cell proliferation.
  - The table on page 76 provides a list of commonly used pharmacologic agents for ADT.

- Chemotherapy is used when the disease becomes resistant to ADT.
- Commonly used chemotherapy agents include cisplatin, sipuleucel-T, mitoxantrone, cyclophosphamide, estramustine, vinblastine, vinorelbine, and cabazitaxel.
- New measures have been introduced for late-stage, castration-resistant metastatic disease that continues to spread or has recurred.
  - Adrenal inhibitors such as abiraterone acetate must be given in conjunction with prednisone.
  - Nonsteroidal antiandrogen enzalutamide is used in patients who were previously treated with docetaxel.

Common Pharmacologic Agents for Androgen-Deprivation Therapy

Generic Name	Drug Class	Dosage and Route
Abiraterone	Androgen Inhibitor	PO: 1000 mg /day with prednisone 5 mg twice daily
Goserelin acetate implant	GNRH analog	Implant: 10.8mg every 12 weeks
Degarelix	GNRH antagonist	Subcut: 240 mg; maintenance 80 mg subcut
Leuprolide acetate	LHRH agonist	IM: 5mg per day; 7.5 mg every mo; 22.5 mg every 3 mo; 30 mg every 4 mo; 45 mg every 6 mo
Triptorelin pamoate	LHRH agonist	IM: 3.75 mg every 4 wks; 11.25 mg every 12 wks; 22.5 mg every 24 wks
Enzalutamide	Nonsteroidal antiandrogen	PO: 160 mg daily
Bicalutamide	Nonsteroidal antiandrogen	PO: 50 mg daily
Flutamide	Nonsteroidal antiandrogen	PO: 250 mg every 8 hours
Nilutamide	Nonsteroidal antiandrogen	PO: 300 mg daily for 30 days, followed by 150 mg once a day

PO, by mouth; *subcut,* subcutaneous injection; *IM,* intramuscular injection; *mo,* monthly; *wks,* weeks.
Modified from Skidmore-Roth, L. (2017). *Mosby's 2017 Nursing Drug Reference. (30th ed.).* St. Louis: Elsevier

Prognosis

There about 2.8 million prostate cancer survivors in the United States, which represents 1 in 5 of all cancer survivors and 4 in 10 men. The prognosis for men with prostate cancer depends on disease stage.

- If the cancer is localized within the prostate and regional tissues, including seminal vesicles (stages I through III), the 5-year survival rate is 100%.
  - The rate drops to 31.9% for patients diagnosed with distant metastases.
  - The survival rate drops for African American patients who are diagnosed at younger ages with more advanced disease.
- Although the prognosis for survival is often good, most prostate cancer survivors have long-term effects of the disease.

- If the patient underwent prostatectomy or medical castration with ADT, late effects can include urinary incontinence, sexual dysfunction, bowel issues, gynecomastia, and osteoporosis.
- Psychological effects may include fear of recurrence and depression about sexual dysfunction. Worry about the loss of masculinity can lead to relationship issues with a partner.

Prevention and Surveillance

- There are no known medical measures to prevent prostate cancer. However, the risk may be reduced by maintaining a healthy weight, eating a low-fat diet that is rich in fruits (especially berries) and vegetables, and other dietary modifications.
- Surveillance recommendations for stages I through III prostate cancer include a PSA test every 6 to 12 months for 5 years and an annual DRE. The DRE may be omitted if the PSA value is undetectable.
- For metastatic disease, a history, physical examination, and PSA test every 3 to 6 months are recommended.

Bibliography

American Cancer Society (ACS). (2015). *Prostate cancer.* Available at http://www.cancer.org/cancer/prostatecancer/detailedguide/index (accessed January 17, 2016).

Brosman, S. (2012). *Prostate-specific antigen testing.* Available at http://emedicine.medscape.com/article/457394-overview#aw2aab6b8 (accessed January 17, 2016).

Crook, J., & Ots, A. (2013). Prognostic factors for new diagnosed prostate cancer and their role in treatment selection. *Seminars in Radiation Oncology, 23*(3), 165–172.

Dirksen, S. (2011). Male reproductive problems—testicular cancer. In S. Lewis, S. Dirksen, M. Heitkemper, L. Bucher, & I. Camera (Eds.). *Medical surgical nursing: Assessment and management of clinical problems* (8th ed., pp. 1396–1397). St. Louis: Elsevier Mosby.

Edge, S., Byrd, D. R., Compton, C. C., Fritz, A. G., Greene, F. L., & Trotti, A. (Eds.). (2010). *AJCC staging manual* (7th ed., pp. 457–468). New York: Springer.

Hoffman, R. (2015). *Screening for prostate cancer.* Available at http://www.uptodate.com/contents/screening-for-prostate-cancer (accessed January 17, 2016).

National Cancer Institute (NCI). (2015). *A snapshot of prostate cancer.* Available at http://www.cancer.gov/research/progress/snapshots/prostate (accessed January 17, 2016).

National Cancer Institute (NCI). (2014). *BRCA1 and BRCA2: Cancer risk and genetic testing.* Available at http://www.cancer.gov/cancertopics/factsheet/Risk/BRCA (accessed January 17, 2016).

National Comprehensive Cancer Network (NCCN). (2015). *Prostate cancer.* Available at http://www.nccn.org/professionals/physician_gls/pdf/prostate.pdf (accessed January 17, 2016).

Pollard, J. (2014). Prostate cancer and the practice nurse. *Practice Nurse, 44*(11), 41–45.

Prostate Cancer Foundation. (2015). *Prostate cancer risk factors.* Available at http://www.pcf.org/site/c.leJRIROrEpH/b.5802027/k.D271/Prostate_Cancer_Risk_Factors.htm (accessed January 17, 2016).

Scher, H. (2012). Benign and malignant disease of the prostate. In D. Longo, D. Kasper, J. Jameson, A. Fauci, S. Hauser, & J. Loscalzo (Eds.), *Harrison's principles of internal medicine* (18th ed., pp. 796–805). New York: McGraw-Hill Medical.

Skidmore-Roth, L. (2017). *Mosby's 2017 Nursing Drug Reference* (13th ed.). St. Louis: Elsevier.

Skidmore-Roth, L. (2017). *Evolve Resources for Mosby's 2017 Nursing Drug Reference* (30th ed.). St. Louis: Elsevier.

Skolarus, T., Wolf, A., Erb, N., Brooks, D., Rivers, B., Underwood, W., III, & Cowens-Alvarado, R. (2014). American Cancer Society prostate cancer survivorship care guidelines. *Cancer Journal for Clinicians, 64*(4), 225–249.

Turner, B., & Drudge-Coates, L. (2014). Pharmacological treatment of patients with advanced prostate cancer. *Nursing Standard, 28*(23), 44–48.

Wojcieszek, P., & Bialas, B. (2012). Prostate cancer brachytherapy: Guidelines overview. *Journal of Contemporary Brachytherapy, 4*(2), 116–120.

Testicular Cancer

Definition

Testicular cancer is an uncommon malignancy that forms in the tissues of one or both testes. It is the most common cancer in young men between the ages of 15 and 35 years.

Primary germ cell tumors (GCTs) constitute 95% of all testicular neoplasms. Testicular tumors are organized into the more common but slow-growing seminomas and the nonseminomas, which are rare but more aggressive than seminomas. The remaining 5% of neoplasms are stromal tumors, which develop in the stroma, the structural and hormone-producing tissue of organs. Although they account for only 5% of testicular malignancies, they make up 20% of childhood testicular tumors.

Testicular cancer metastasizes through the lymphatic system to the retroperitoneal lymph nodes. Distant metastasis sites include the lungs, liver, bones, and brain.

Incidence

- Testicular cancer accounts for 1% of all cancers in men each year and for 5% of all urologic tumors.
- About 8430 new cases of testicular cancer and 380 deaths occurred in the United States in 2015.
- In the United States, the chance for a man to develop testicular cancer is 1 in 270 (0.37%).
- Testicular malignancies have been on the rise in the United States and many other countries over the past few decades, increasing by 3% per year.
- The incidence is more than double the rate 40 years ago, but research has not identified the cause.
- The incidence is four to five times higher among white males than African American males and more than three times higher than among Asian American males. White males of Scandinavian descent are at highest risk.
- Neoplasms occur more often in the right testicle than in the left.
- Peak age of incidence is between 20 and 39 years of age, although it may occur at any age.
- Between 70% and 75% of patients have stage I, 20% have stage II, and 10% have stage III disease at diagnosis. There is no stage IV based on the AJCC staging system.

Etiology and Risk Factors

The exact cause of testicular cancer is unknown, but several risks factors have been identified:

- Cryptorchidism
  - Higher risk for patients with abdominal cryptorchid testes than inguinal cryptorchid testes
  - Boys who had orchiopexy performed after age 13 were at higher risk.
  - In 75% of this population, the malignancy occurs in the undescended testicle.
  - Researchers do not think cryptorchidism plays a direct role in testicular cancer. Instead, an unknown factor is thought to cause the malignancy and cryptorchidism.
- Men between the ages of 20 and 40 years have approximately one half of all testicular cancers.

- Two percent of men who develop a GCT in one testis eventually develop a GCT in the other testicle.
- Klinefelter syndrome
  - Genetic disorder manifested by testicular atrophy, gynecomastia, and absence of spermatogenesis
  - Increases the risk of a mediastinal GCT
- Testicular feminization syndrome increases the risk of a testicular GCT.
- HIV infection
- HPV infection
- Family history of testicular malignancies, particularly in a father or brother

Signs and Symptoms

- The most common symptoms of testicular malignancy are a palpable mass in the scrotum found on testicular self-examination and a feeling of heaviness in the scrotum or lower abdomen.
- The tumor or mass in the testicle can cause pain.
- Other signs include swelling in the scrotum similar to epididymitis or orchitis, gynecomastia (i.e., breast growth and tenderness), and early signs of puberty in young boys.
- Advanced-disease symptoms can include lower back pain (indicating the disease has spread to lymph nodes), urinary obstruction, bone pain, shortness of breath, headaches, seizures, and weight loss.

Diagnostic Work-up

- Physical examination, including testicular palpation
- Ultrasound of the testicles to help visualize inner structures and distinguish between cancer and benign conditions
- Increased blood levels of tumor markers
  - α-Fetoprotein (AFP), elevated only in cancers with a nonseminoma component
  - β-Human chorionic gonadotropin (β-hCG)
  - Lactate dehydrogenase (LDH), which can indicate widespread disease
- Transillumination of the scrotum to help establish the diagnosis
- Surgical intervention with a radical inguinal orchiectomy to remove the testicle and spermatic cord for pathologic evaluation
- Surgery can lead to a definitive diagnosis, stage the cancer, and provide curative treatment if the cancerous cells are removed.
- CT scan to evaluate regional lymph nodes
- Chest radiograph to evaluate possible metastasis
- Bone scan

Histology

- GCTs account for 95% of testicular malignancies.
- GCTs are classified as seminomas or nonseminomas.
  - Seminomas are considered only if the tumor is 100% within the sperm-producing cells.
  - Nonseminomas have four subtypes: embryonal carcinomas, yolk-sac tumors, teratomas, and choriocarcinomas.

Most nonseminoma tumors consist of a mixture of subtypes, but this does not affect how the cancer is treated.

- An embryonal carcinoma is identified in approximately 40% of all testicular neoplasms, and it increases levels of AFP.
- Yolk sac tumors, which get their name from their resemblance to an embryonic yolk sac, are the most common form of cancer in children and infants.
- Teratomas are further grouped as mature teratomas, immature teratomas, and those with elements of a somatic (non–germ cell) malignancy.
- Choriocarcinoma is rare, but it is the most aggressive form of testicular cancer.
- These cancers usually spread initially to the retroperitoneal lymph nodes.
- Non–germ cell tumors comprise the remaining 5% and include Leydig cell tumors and Sertoli cell tumors, which are often benign.

Clinical Staging

The two main staging systems for testicular cancer are the International Germ Cell Cancer Collaborative Group (IGCCCG) Risk Classification (see table below) and the AJCC TNM staging system (Edge et al., 2010). Based on the criteria developed by the IGCCCG, the prognosis can be good, intermediate, or poor. The prognosis helps to determine treatment options and has been incorporated into the AJCC anatomic prognostic groups.

International Germ Cell Cancer Consensus Group Risk Classification

Prognosis	Nonseminoma	Seminoma
Good	Gonadal or retroperitoneal primary site Absent nonpulmonary visceral metastases AFP <1000 ng/mL β-hCG <5000 mIU/ML LDH <1.5 × upper limit or normal	Any primary site Absent nonpulmonary visceral metastases Any LDH, β-hCG
Intermediate	Gonadal or retroperitoneal primary site Absent nonpulmonary visceral metastases AFP 1000-10,000 ng/mL β-hCG 5000-50,000 mIU/ML LDH 1.5-10 × upper limit or normal	Any primary site Presence of nonpulmonary visceral metastases Any LDH, β-hCG
Poor	Mediastinal primary site Presence of nonpulmonary visceral metastases AFP >10,000 ng/mL β-hCG >50,000 mIU/mL LDH >10 × upper limit or normal	No semimoma patients have a poor prognosis.

AFP, α-Fetoprotein; *β-hCG*, β-human chorionic gonadotropin; *LDH*, lactate dehydrogenase.
Modified from Motzer, R., & Bosl, G. (2012). Testicular cancer. In Longo, D., Kasper, D., Jameson, J., Fauci, A., Hauser, S., & Loscalzo, J. (Eds.). *Harrison's principles of internal medicine* (18th ed., pp. 806-810). New York: McGraw-Hill Medical.

Treatment

Treatment depends on tumor stage. Radical inguinal orchiectomy is often performed for diagnosis and treatment. Depending on the tumor type, staging, and degree of metastasis, further therapy may include additional surgery (e.g., regional lymph node dissection), radiation therapy, or chemotherapy.

- Seminomas are more responsive to radiation therapy, whereas nonseminomas are more sensitive to chemotherapy.
- Retroperitoneal radiation therapy cures almost 100% of patients with stage I seminoma; however, this approach may lead to overtreatment and higher rate of recurrence.
- The NCCN guidelines prefer active surveillance for pT1 to pT3 (i.e., stage IA and IB) seminomas and for clinical stage IA nonseminomas.
- Chemotherapy is used for patients with bulkier or metastatic disease.
  - The AJCC staging system and the IGCCCG risk assessment help to determine which chemotherapy regimens to use.
  - The most commonly used regimens include three cycles of etoposide and cisplatin (EP) or four cycles of bleomycin, etoposide, and cisplatin (BEP).
  - These combination therapies have cure rates of 70% to 80%, but their toxicity, especially the BEP regimen, is substantial.
  - Pulmonary fibrosis is the most severe toxicity, often manifesting as pneumonitis. This is common in elderly patients and those receiving high doses of BEP (e.g., 300 to 400 units), but it is also possible in young adults receiving lower doses.
  - The risk of toxicity increases when supplemental oxygen is given for other issues.
  - Other adverse effects include hypotension, mental confusion, fever, chills, and wheezing.

Prognosis

- Testicular cancer has an overall 5-year survival and cure rate of 95%.
- Eighty percent of patients with metastatic disease have a 95% survival rate.
- The rate is lower for the aggressive choriocarcinoma subtype of nonseminoma tumors, dropping below 80%.
- Survivors of testicular cancer are at a risk for late recurrence (i.e., relapse more than 2 years after remission).

Prevention and Surveillance

- There are no known prevention measures.
- The U.S. Preventive Services Task Force (USPSTF) and the ACS do not recommend testicular cancer surveillance for adolescent or adult males.
- The ACS recommends a testicular examination as part of the physical examination and routine cancer-related checkup by the health care team.
- Men with risk factors may consider doing a monthly testicular self-examination.

- Men should promptly report a lump on the testicle to the health care team.
- Testicular self-examination instructions can be found in the box in the next column.
- Surveillance of testicular cancer varies with clinical staging, treatment regimen, and tumor type. There are three main methods:
  - History and physical examinations
  - Abdominal and pelvic CT scans
  - Chest radiographs
- Surveillance guidelines for seminomas and nonseminomas are summarized in the tables below.

Instructions for Testicular Self-Examination

- Self-examination should be done during or after a bath or shower, when the skin of the scrotum is relaxed.
- Check one testicle at a time, holding it between the thumbs and fingers of both hands and rolling it gently between the fingers.
- Look and palpate for lumps (i.e., hard, rounded, and smooth) or a change in the testicle's size, shape, or consistency.
- It is normal for testicles to vary slightly in size or for one to hang lower than the other. Each testicle has an epididymis that can feel like a small bump on the upper or middle outer side. It may be confused with an abnormal lump. Concerns should be reported to the health care team.
- A testicle can increase in size for reasons other than cancer. Hydroceles and varicoceles can sometimes cause swelling or lumps around the scrotum. Concerns should be discussed with the health care team.

Modified from American Cancer Society. (2015). Testicular self-exam. Available at http://www.cancer.org/cancer/testicularcancer/moreinformation/ doihavetesticularcancer/do-i-have-testicular-cancer-self-exam (accessed January 17, 2016).

Follow-up Surveillance for Seminoma Testicular Cancer

Evaluation	Stage IA After Orchiectomy	Stage IA with Adjuvant Therapy	Stage IIA and Nonbulky Stage IIB After Radiotherapy	Bulky Stage IIB and Stage III
History and physical examination	*Year 1*: q4-6mo *Year 2-3*: q6-12mo *Year 4+*: annu	*Year 1-2*: q6-12mo *Year 3-5*: annu	*Year 1*: q3mo *Year 2-5*: q6mo	*Year 1*: q2mo* *Year 2*: q3mo *Year 3-4*: q6mo *Year 5*: annu
Abdominal or pelvic CT	*Year 1*: at 3, 6, and 12 mo *Year 2-3*: q6-12mo *Year 4+*: annu	*Year 1-3*: annu	*Year 1*: at 3, 6, and 12 mo *Year 2-3*: annu *Year 4+*: ACI	*Year 1*: at 3-6 mo† *Year 2-5*: ACI
Chest radiograph	ACI	ACI	*Year 1-2*: q6mo	*Year 1*: q2mo *Year 2*: q3mo *Year 3-5*: annu

ACI, As clinically indicated; *annu*, annually; *CT*, computed tomography; *mo*, month; *q*, every.
*Evaluation includes tumor markers.
†Includes PET when clinically indicated.
Modified from the National Comprehensive Cancer Network. (2015). Testicular cancer. Available at http://www.nccn.org/professionals/physician_gls/pdf/testicular.pdf (accessed January 17, 2016).

Follow-up Surveillance for Nonseminoma Testicular Cancer

Evaluation	Clinical Stage IA	Clinical Stage IB	Clinical Stage IB with Adjuvant Therapy	Clinical Stage II-II	Pathologic Stage IIA/B with Adjuvant Therapy and RPLND	Pathologic Stage IIA/B without Adjuvant Therapy and RPLND
History and physical examination with tumor markers	*Year 1*: q2mo *Year 2*: q3mo *Year 3-4*: q4-6mo *Year 5*: annu	*Year 1*: q2mo *Year 2*: q3mo *Year 3-4*: q4-6mo *Year 5*: annu	*Year 1-2*: q3mo *Year 3-4*: q6mo *Year 5*: annu	*Year 1*: q2mo *Year 2*: q3mo *Year 3-4*: q4-6mo *Year 5*: q6mo	*Year 1-2*: q6mo *Year 3-5*: annu	*Year 1*: q2mo *Year 2*: q3mo *Year 3*: q4mo *Year 4*: q6mo *Year 5*: annu
Abdominal or pelvic CT	*Year 1*: q4-6mo *Year 2*: q6-12mo *Year 3*: annu	*Year 1*: q4mo *Year 2-3*: q4-6mo *Year 4*: annu	*Year 1-2*: annu	*Year 1*: q6mo *Year 2*: annu	*Year 1*: after RPLND *Year 2+*: ACI	*Year 1*: at 3-4 mo *Year 2+*: ACI
Chest radiograph	*Year 1*: at 4 and 12 mo *Year 2-5*: annu	*Year 1*: q2mo *Year 2*: q3mo *Year 3-4*: q4-6mo *Year 5*: annu	*Year 1*: q6-12mo *Year 2*: annu	*Year 1-2*: q6mo *Year 3-4*: annu	*Year 1*: q6mo *Year 2-5*: annu	*Year 1*: q2-4mo *Year 2*: q3-6mo *Year 3-5*: annu

ACI, As clinically indicated; *annu*, annually; *CT*, computed tomography; *mo*, month; *q*, every; *RPLND*, retroperitoneal lymph node dissection.
Modified from the National Comprehensive Cancer Network (NCCN). (2015). Testicular cancer. Available at http://www.nccn.org/professionals/physician_gls/pdf/testicular .pdf (Accessed January 17, 2016).

Bibliography

American Cancer Society (ACS). (2013). *Testicular cancer*. Available at http://www.cancer.org/cancer/testicularcancer/detailedguide/index (accessed January 18, 2016).

American Cancer Society (ACS). (2015). *Testicular self-exam*. Available at http://www.cancer.org/cancer/testicularcancer/moreinformation/doihavetesticularcancer/do-i-have-testicular-cancer-self-exam (accessed January 18, 2016).

Dirksen, S. (2011). Male reproductive problems—testicular cancer. In S. Lewis, S. Dirksen, M. Heitkemper, L. Bucher, & I. Camera *Medical surgical nursing: Assessment and management of clinical problems* (8th ed., pp. 1396–1397). St. Louis: Elsevier Mosby.

Edge, S., Byrd, D. R., Compton, C. C., Fritz, A. G., Greene, F. L., & Trotti, A. (Eds.), (2010). *AJCC staging manual* (7th ed., 469–478). New York: Springer.

Hanna, N., & Einhorn, L. (2014a). Testicular cancer—discoveries and updates. *New England Journal of Medicine, 371*(21), 2005–2016.

Hanna, N., & Einhorn, L. (2014b). Testicular cancer: A reflection on 50 years of discovery. *Journal of Clinical Oncology, 32*(28), 3085–3092.

Lin, K., & Shrangpani, R. (2010). Screening for testicular cancer: An evidence review for the U.S. Preventive Services Task Force. *Annals of Internal Medicine, 153*, 396–399.

Motzer, R., & Bosl, G. (2012). Testicular cancer. In D. Longo, D. Kasper, J. Jameson, A. Fauci, S. Hauser, & J. Loscalzo (Eds.), *Harrison's principles of internal medicine* (18th ed., pp. 806–810). New York: McGraw-Hill Medical.

Nallu, A., Chimakurthi, R., Hussain, A., & Mannuel, H. (2014). Update on testicular germ cell tumors. *Current Opinion in Oncology, 26*(3), 294–298.

National Cancer Institute (NCI). (2014). *Testicular cancer*. Available at http://www.cancer.gov/types/testicular/hp (accessed January 18, 2016).

National Cancer Institute (NCI). (2015). *Testicular cancer treatment: Health professional*. Available at http://www.cancer.gov/types/testicular/hp/testicular-treatment-pdq#link/_453_toc (accessed January 18, 2016).

National Comprehensive Cancer Network (NCCN). (2015). *Testicular cancer*. Available at http://www.nccn.org/professionals/physician_gls/pdf/testicular.pdf (accessed January 18, 2016).

Nichols, C., Roth, B., Albers, P., Einhorn, L., Foster, R., Daneshmand, S., et al. (2013). Active surveillance is the preferred approach to clinical stage I testicular cancer. *Journal of Clinical Oncology, 31*(28), 3490–3493.

Reilley, M., & Pagliarro, L. (2015). Testicular choriocarcinoma: A rare variant that requires a unique treatment approach. *Current Oncology Reports: Genitourinary Cancers, 17*(2), 1–9.

Russell, S. (2014). Testicular cancer: Overview and implications for health care providers. *Urologic Nursing, 34*(4), 172–176.

Gynecologic Cancers

Paula Anastasia

Cervical Cancer

Definition

The cervix, the organ between the top of the vagina and the bottom of the uterus, can develop cancer due to human papillomavirus (HPV) infection. Cervical cancer arises at the squamous-columnar junction.

Precancerous lesions usually begin as cervical intraepithelial neoplasia (CIN) or adenocarcinoma in situ, which can become invasive. However, most cervical cancers are slow growing and progress over 10 years. Carcinoma of the cervix has three main routes of spread:

- Direct extension to the uterus, vagina, parametria, bladder, or rectum
- Lymphatic spread
- Hematogenous spread to the lungs, liver, or bowel

Incidence

- According to the American Cancer Society (ACS), about 12,900 new cases of cervical cancer and 4100 related deaths occurred in the United States in 2015.
- The mean age at diagnosis is 48 years.
- Minority and lower socioeconomic groups, including Hispanics, African Americans, American Indians, and Alaskan Natives, who do not have routine screening have a higher incidence of cervical cancer.
- Globally, cervical cancer is the fourth most common cancer, and it is the fourth most common cancer-related death among women.
- Underdeveloped countries have a greater incidence of cervical cancer than do developed countries.
- The incidence of cervical cancer is expected to decline among women who receive the HPV vaccine.

Etiology and Risk Factors

- HPV infection is responsible for 99% of cervical cancers.
  - Although it is estimated that up to 80% of sexually active adults are exposed to the virus, most individuals clear the virus.
  - More than 40 strains of genital HPV have been identified, but types 16 and 18 are identified in more than one half of cervical cancer cases.
- Many of the risk factors for cervical cancer are the same as those for sexually transmitted diseases
  - Early age at onset of sexual activity (<18 years)
  - Multiple sexual partners (>5)
- Sexual partners who have had multiple partners
- Cigarette smoking (squamous cell cancer risk)
- Immunosuppression
- Lower socioeconomic status
- Long-term use of oral contraceptives (>5 years)

Signs and Symptoms

- Presenting symptoms
  - New irregular or heavy bleeding
  - Bleeding after intercourse
  - Change in vaginal discharge to watery, mucous, purulent, or odorous fluid
- Late symptoms
  - Pain radiating to the flank or leg
  - Pelvic pressure and urinary changes such as hematuria
  - Vaginal hemorrhage and development of uremia

Diagnostic Work-up

- A pelvic examination should be performed for any woman with symptoms of cervical cancer.
- On speculum examination, the cervix may appear normal or have an obvious visible lesion.
- Cervical cytology or Papanicolaou testing (i.e., Pap smear) and HPV testing are used in combination for cervical cancer screening.
- Women with indications for cervical cancer undergo colposcopy of the cervix. A colposcope is a magnifying device for looking at the cervix.
- If the cervix appears abnormal, biopsies of the cervix or endocervical canal are obtained.
- If the biopsies confirm a malignancy, a more comprehensive procedure such as a conization with or without a hysterectomy may be indicated.
- A bimanual pelvic and rectovaginal examination is required to assess the tumor size and vaginal or parametrial involvement.
- Imaging methods such as magnetic resonance imaging (MRI), computed tomography (CT), and positron emission tomography (PET) are used for staging.

Histology

- Cervical cancer consists of mixed cell types, with squamous cell representing about 80% and adenocarcinoma representing 20% of cases.
- HPV types 16 and 18 are the most virulent strains causing cervical cancer.

- HPV16 and HPV18 are seen in 59% and 13%, respectively, of squamous cell carcinoma cases.
- HPV16 and HPV18 strains are identified in 36% and 37%, respectively, of adenocarcinoma cases.
- The incidence of squamous cell carcinoma of the cervix has declined due to effective screening, but the incidence of adenocarcinoma has increased over the past 30 years because the Pap smear is less effective for detecting this histologic type.

Clinical Staging

- Cervical cancer is staged clinically because surgical staging is not done in Third World countries, where there is an increased incidence but fewer resources.
- The 2010 International Federation of Gynecology and Obstetrics (FIGO) staging system is widely used for cervical cancer outlined in the table below, and a parallel tumor-node-metastasis (TNM) staging system is used by the American Joint Committee Commission on Cancer (AJCC).

International Federation of Gynecology and Obstetrics (FIGO) Staging for Cervical Cancer

Stage	Definition
I	Cervical carcinoma confined to uterus (extension to corpus should be disregarded)
IA	Invasive carcinoma diagnosed only by microscopy. Stromal invasion with a maximum depth of 5.0 mm from the base of the epithelium and a horizontal spread ≤7.0 mm
IA1	Measured stromal invasion ≤3.0 mm in depth and ≤7.0 mm in horizontal spread
IA2	Measured stromal invasion >3.0 mm but not >5.0 mm, with a horizontal spread ≤7.0 mm
IB	Clinically visible lesion confined to the cervix or microscopic lesion >T1a/IA2
IB1	Clinically visible lesion ≤4.0 cm in greatest dimension
IB2	Clinically visible lesion >4.0 cm in greatest dimension
II	Cervical carcinoma invades beyond uterus but not to pelvic wall or to lower third of vagina
IIA	Tumor without parametrial invasion
IIA1	Clinically visible lesion ≤4 cm
IIA2	Clinically visible lesion >4 cm
IIB	Tumor with parametrial invasion
III	Tumor extends to pelvic wall or involves lower third of vagina or causes hydronephrosis or nonfunctioning kidney
IIIA	Tumor involves lower third of vagina, no extension to pelvic wall
IIIB	Tumor extends to pelvic wall or causes hydronephrosis or nonfunctioning kidney
IVA	Tumor invades mucosa of bladder or rectum or extends beyond true pelvis (bullous edema is not sufficient to classify a tumor as stage IV)
IVB	Spread to distant organ

Modified from Pecorelli, S. (2009). Revised FIGO staging for carcinoma of the vulva, cervix, and endometrium. *International Journal of Gynecology Obstetrics, 105*(2), 103-104.

- Methods used for FIGO staging are limited to colposcopy, biopsy, conization, cystoscopy, and proctosigmoidoscopy.
- In the United States, imaging modalities and surgical staging are also used to select treatment options.

- Surgical staging for women with low-level disease and micro-invasive disease may include fertility-sparing approaches or radical trachelectomy.
- Sentinel lymph node mapping remains controversial but may be useful for early-stage disease.

Treatment

Early Disease

- Early-stage cervical cancer includes all stage I and stage IIA disease.
- Primary treatment is surgery or radiation therapy.
- In 2012, a fertility-sparing treatment algorithm was added.
  - For women who desire fertility preservation, a conservative approach is recommended with a cone biopsy and possible pelvic lymph node dissection and radical trachelectomy, depending on surgical margins and lymphovascular space involvement (LVSI).
  - A trachelectomy removes the cervix, parametrium, and upper 2 cm of the vagina. The uterus is left intact. A cerclage is placed to help maintain the pregnancy.
  - If a pregnancy goes to term, the baby is delivered by cesarean section.
- For women who no longer desire fertility, a hysterectomy is recommended. The choice of simple or modified radical hysterectomy with pelvic lymph node dissection depends on positive surgical margins and LVSI.
- Analysis of stage IB and IIA disease should be individualized to determine whether paraaortic nodes or sentinel lymph node mapping is suggested.
- No adjuvant therapy is indicated if lymph nodes, surgical margins, and parametria are negative.
- Treating bulky tumors with radiation therapy, brachytherapy, and cisplatin forms of chemotherapy instead of a hysterectomy is an approach for selected patients.
- Controversy remains about whether a complete hysterectomy is required after radiation therapy and chemotherapy. Studies show a decrease in the rate of pelvic recurrence but more morbidity and no overall survival benefit.

Advanced Disease

- Advanced cervical cancer is defined as stage IIB to IVA disease, although some clinicians categorize stage IB2 and IIA2 as advanced disease.
- Imaging studies such as PET and CT are recommended.
- If needed, a needle biopsy or laparoscopic surgical staging of lymph nodes is done.
- Radiation therapy and chemosensitization with cisplatin-containing regimens are the treatment of choice.
  - Patients usually receive pelvic irradiation with weekly cisplatin or cisplatin and 5-fluorouracil (5-FU) every 3 weeks during radiation therapy, followed by brachytherapy.
  - Additional treatment decisions, such as extended field radiation therapy, may be determined by lymph node status and paraaortic involvement.

Recurrent or Metastatic Disease

- Patients with recurrent disease may be candidates for radiation therapy, chemotherapy, or surgery, depending on the extent of spread and prior treatment.
- Local recurrence after chemoradiation therapy may involve surgical intervention with an exenteration.
- Patients with distant metastasis at presentation or a recurrence are usually given systemic chemotherapy.
  - Chemotherapy options include platinum-based chemotherapy with paclitaxel and bevacizumab.
  - Other combinations include topotecan, paclitaxel, and bevacizumab.
- Palliative radiation therapy may be indicated in situations such as bone metastasis or uncontrolled vaginal bleeding.

Radiation Therapy

- Adjuvant external beam radiation therapy is indicated for patients with stage IA to IIA disease who have tumor-negative lymph nodes after hysterectomy but have risk factors such as a large tumor (≥4 cm) and LVSI. The radiation dose is approximately 45 cG.
- Vaginal cuff brachytherapy is recommended if there are positive vaginal margins.
- For patients with positive common iliac or paraaortic lymph nodes or bulky tumors, extended field radiation therapy up to the renal vessels is suggested.
- Brachytherapy (i.e., internal intracavitary radiation therapy) may be used for patients after hysterectomy and for patients with an intact cervix.
- Patient selection and radiation dose are determined by patient risk factors such as positive surgical margins.

Chemotherapy

- Combined chemotherapy and radiation therapy has been shown to decrease the death rate for cervical cancer by up to 50% compared with radiation therapy alone.
- The National Cancer Institute issued an alert in 1999 recommending the use of chemotherapy with cisplatin in combination with 5-FU.
- Chemoradiation therapy is usually given weekly while the patient is receiving daily radiation therapy.

Prognosis

- The prognosis for patients with cervical cancers depends on the stage of disease, recurrence, and comorbid conditions.
- Race and socioeconomic characteristics are relevant because of greater exposure to other risk factors and more advanced disease at diagnosis, which reduces likelihood of undergoing curative therapy.
- The 5-year survival rate by stage is as follows:
  - Stage IA: 95%
  - Stage IB or IIA: 70% to 85%
  - Stage IIB, III, and IVA: 65%, 40%, and 20%, respectively
  - Stage IVB: 10%

Prevention and Surveillance

Prevention

- A healthy lifestyle
- Vaccination against HPV
  - Quadrivalent vaccine against HPV genotypes 6, 11, 16, and 18
  - Bivalent vaccine against HPV genotypes 16 and 18
- Screening for early diagnosis and identification of precancerous lesions

The ACS screening guidelines can be found in the table below.

American Cancer Society Screening Guidelines for Cervical Cancer

Age (Years) or Status	Recommendation
21	Screening should begin
21-29	Papanicolaou test (Pap smear) every 3 years
	Human papillomavirus (HPV) testing should not be used for screening in this age group. It may be used as a part of follow-up for an abnormal Pap test.
30-65	Pap smear and HPV test every 5 years and continuing until age 65. This should be done even for women who have had the HPV vaccine.
	Another option is a Pap smear every 3 years.
	Women at high risk (i.e., suppressed immune system or exposed to diethylstilbestrol (DES) should have more frequent screening according to the health care team.
>65	No Pap test needed if screening was regular in the previous 10 years and no cervical intraepithelial neoplasia (CIN) was found in the past 20 years.
	For a history of CIN2 or CIN3, testing should continue for 20 years after the abnormal finding.
After hysterectomy	After removal of uterus and cervix, stop screening (Pap smear and HPV) unless hysterectomy was done for cervical cancer.
	After supracervical hysterectomy (cervix is left intact), cervical cancer screening should be done according to guidelines.

Modified from American Cancer Society. (2014). The American Cancer Society guidelines for the prevention and early detection of cervical cancer. Available at http://www.cancer.org/cancer/cervicalcancer/moreinformation/cervicalcancerprev entionandearlydetection/cervical-cancer-prevention-and-early-detection-cervical-cancer-screening-guidelines (accessed January 13, 2016).

Surveillance

- Patients diagnosed with invasive cervical cancer should have a physical examination every 3 to 6 months by a gynecologic oncologist for 2 years and then yearly for the next 3 to 5 years.
- Imaging is usually indicated if patients have symptoms of recurrence (i.e., pelvic or back pain, vaginal discharge, persistent cough, or chest pain).
- Patient education includes lifestyle wellness tactics, including maintaining a healthy weight, proper nutrition, smoking cessation, and safe sexual practices.
- Patients who have had brachytherapy may have cervical stenosis and may benefit from a vaginal dilator.

Bibliography

American Cancer Society (ACS). (2015). *Cancer facts and figures 2015*. Atlanta, GA: American Cancer Society.

American Cancer Society (ACS). (2014). *The American Cancer Society guidelines for the prevention and early detection of cervical cancer*. Available at http://www.cancer.org/cancer/cervicalcancer/moreinformation/cervicalcancerpreventionandearlydetection/cervical-cancer-prevention-and-early-detection-cervical-cancer-screening-guidelines (accessed January 13, 2016).

Edge, S., Byrd, D. R., Compton, C. C., Fritz, A. G., Greene, F. L., & Trotti, A. (2010). *AJCC staging manual* (7th ed.,pp. 395–402). New York: Springer.

National Cancer Institute (NCI). (2015). *Cervical cancer treatment—for health professionals (PDQ)*. Available at http://www.cancer.gov/types/cervical/hp/cervical-treatment-pdq (accessed January 13, 2016).

National Comprehensive Cancer Network (NCCN). (2015). *Clinical practice guidelines in oncology: Cervical cancer, version 2015*. Available at https://www.nccn.org/store/login/login.aspx?ReturnURL=http://www.nccn.org/professionals/physician_gls/pdf/cervical.pdf (accessed January 13, 2016).

Pecorelli, S. (2009). Revised FIGO staging for carcinoma of the vulva, cervix, and endometrium. *International Journal of Gynecology Obstetrics*, 105(2), 103–104.

Salani, R., Backes, F. L., Fung, M. F., Holschneider, C. H., Parker, L. P., Bristow, R., & Goff, B. A. (2011). Posttreatment surveillance and diagnosis of recurrence in women with gynecologic malignancies: Society of Gynecologic Oncologists recommendations. *American Journal of Obstetrics & Gynecology*, 204(6), 466–478.

World Health Organization (WHO). (2015). *Cervical cancer risk factors and prevention*. Available at http://www.afro.who.int/en/clusters-a-programmes/dpc/non-communicable-diseases-managementndm/programme-components/cancer/cervical-cancer/2812-cervical-cancer-risk-factors-and-prevention.html (accessed January 13, 2016).

Ziebarth, A., Kim, K. H., & Huh, W. K. (2012). Cervical cancer. In B. Y. Karlan, R. E. Bristow, & A. Li (Eds.), *Gynecologic oncology clinical practices & surgical atlas* (pp. 85–103). New York: McGraw-Hill.

Ovarian Cancer

Definition

Ovarian cancer is the fifth leading cause of cancer-related death among women in the United States. Ovarian cancer is not a single disease. Epithelial ovarian cancer (EOC), which arises from cells that line or cover the ovaries, represents 90% of ovarian cancers. Less common histopathologic types include low-malignant-potential or borderline tumors, germ cell tumors, adenocarcinomas, sarcomas, and sex cord–stromal tumors. Fallopian tube carcinoma and primary peritoneal carcinoma are separate but similar diseases, and they are usually included in statistical and treatment data when referring to EOC.

Incidence

- According to the ACS, about 21,290 women were diagnosed with ovarian cancer and 14,180 died of their disease in the United States in 2015.
- Ovarian cancer is the most fatal of the gynecologic malignancies because it is typically diagnosed at a late stage.
- Most patients are diagnosed with stage III or IV disease. With primary surgical staging and combination platinum-based therapy, 80% can achieve a remission.
- The relative 5-year survival rate reported for 2004 through 2010 increased to 44.6% from 36% reported for 1975 through 1977.
- Although the rate of cure has not improved, survival times have increased as a result of better surgical and medical management and more effective adjuvant therapy.

Etiology and Risk Factors

- The most important risk factor for EOC is a family history of the disease, especially if two or more first-degree relatives have EOC.
- Epidemiologic studies have identified endocrine, environmental, and genetic factors as important in the development of ovarian cancer.
- Epidemiologically established risk factors include the following:
  - Nulliparity
  - Family history
  - Genetic mutations or syndromes, including *BRCA1*, *BRCA2*, *RAD51C*, *RAD51D*, *BRIP1*, and Lynch syndrome
  - Early menarche and late menopause
  - White race
  - Increasing age (average age at diagnosis of 63 years)
  - Residence in Western industrialized countries
- Women who are nulligravida and have used fertility medications have an increased risk of ovarian cancer.
- The use of hormone replacement therapy, especially with a combination of estrogen and progesterone, may increase a woman's risk.
- Hereditary ovarian cancer attributed to a mutation in the *BRCA1* and *BRCA2* genes accounts for up to 15% of ovarian cancer cases. These genes are normally involved in repair of mistakes in DNA that occur during cell division.
  - The risk of developing ovarian cancer in a *BRCA1* mutation carrier by age 70 is 39% and is 11% to 17% for carriers of the *BRCA2* mutation.
  - Other cancers associated with *BRCA1* mutations include breast cancer and prostate cancer.
  - *BRCA2* mutations are associated with breast cancer, melanoma, and pancreatic cancer in men and women and prostate cancer in men.
  - Members of the Ashkenazi Jewish community have a higher likelihood of mutations in the *BRCA1* or *BRCA2* gene than other groups.

Signs and Symptoms

Early-stage ovarian cancer rarely causes symptoms, and early-stage disease is less often detected because the symptoms are elusive. Later-stage ovarian cancer may cause nonspecific symptoms that may be mistaken for common benign conditions such as constipation or irritable bowel. Women usually do not recognize them as serious until disease has become far advanced.

- Bloating or increased abdominal girth
- Urinary changes such as urgency or frequency
- Abdominal or pelvic discomfort
- Difficulty eating or early satiety

Any of these symptoms that are persistent and occur for several weeks suggests a need for clinical assessment.

Diagnostic Work-up

- Because there are no effective screening modalities for early detection, educating clinical practitioners and women about the signs and symptoms of EOC is essential to prompt clinical assessment.
- A bimanual pelvic examination is necessary, but a pelvic examination may not be helpful in cases of early-stage disease or upper abdominal disease.
- Transvaginal ultrasound may show an abnormal pelvic mass or ascites, prompting further imaging with CT or MRI.
- The OVA1 blood test is used as a triage test for patients already known to need surgery. It helps gynecologic oncologists decide what type of surgery should be done.
- The cancer antigen 125 (CA 125) blood test is nonspecific. Because levels may be elevated in nongynecologic cancers, the test should not be used as a screening modality. However, a confirmed diagnosis of EOC and an elevated CA 125 test result may serve as useful markers to evaluate treatment response.
- Patients with advanced disease may have increased abdominal girth and ascites at presentation, prompting paracentesis and cytology to confirm the diagnosis.
- Symptoms such as shortness of breath consistent with a pleural effusion may also lead to diagnostic confirmation by thoracentesis and cytology.
- If a gynecologic malignancy is suspected, surgery should be performed by a gynecologic oncologist.

Histology

- EOC is a group of diseases (i.e., EOC, fallopian tube carcinoma, and peritoneal cancer) that have different molecular behaviors.
- Five main subtypes represent 98% of EOCs:
  - High-grade serous: 70%
  - Endometrioid: 10%
  - Clear cell: 10%
  - Mucinous: 3%
  - Low-grade serous: less than 5%
- Epithelial ovarian, fallopian tube, and primary peritoneal cancers are often found to be high-grade serous adenocarcinomas.
- Women with EOC who carry the *BRCA* germline mutation usually have high-grade serous carcinomas.
- The cancers may arise from lesions that originated in the fimbriae of the fallopian tubes rather than the surface of the ovary. They are often referred to as *extrauterine adenocarcinomas of müllerian epithelial origin.*
- Clear cell and endometrioid EOCs are often associated with endometriosis and have different molecular profiles from serous carcinomas.
- Endometrioid cell types can be seen in patients with Lynch syndrome.
- Synchronous uterine carcinoma and EOC are seen in 15% to 20% of patients with endometrioid-type tumors.
- Mucinous subtypes may account for up to 15% of EOCs, but 80% of them are benign or borderline tumors.

Clinical Staging

- The FIGO system is used for staging EOCs throughout the world (see table below).
- A revised staging system became effective in 2014, when it was approved by AJCC. The AJCC classification uses the TNM system for ovarian cancer and is scheduled to be updated in 2016.
- Epithelial ovarian, fallopian tube, and primary peritoneal cancers are categorized as one disease, although the recommendations call for designating the primary site when possible.

International Federation of Gynecology and Obstetrics (FIGO) Clinical Staging for Ovarian Cancer

Stage	Definition
I	Tumor limited to ovaries (one or both)
IA	Tumor limited to one ovary; capsule intact, no tumor on ovarian surface. Washings without malignant cells
IB	Tumor limited to both ovaries; capsules intact, no tumor on ovarian surface. Washings without malignant cells
IC	Tumor limited to one or both ovaries with any of the following:
	Capsule spill intraoperatively (IC1)
	Capsule rupture before surgery (IC2)
	Malignant cells in washings (IC3)
II	Tumor involves one or both ovaries with pelvic extension or implants
IIA	Extension or implants on uterus and/or tube(s)
IIB	Extension to or implants on other pelvic tissues (IIC) is excluded from staging)
III	Tumor involves one or both ovaries with microscopically confirmed peritoneal metastasis outside the pelvis or lymph nodes
IIIA	Spread to retroperitoneal lymph nodes with or without microscopic peritoneal involvement beyond pelvis
	IIIA (i) positive retroperitoneal lymph nodes only with positive cytology
	IIIA (ii) metastasis >10 mm
IIIA2	Microscopic extrapelvic peritoneal spread with or without positive retroperitoneal nodes
IIIB	Macroscopic peritoneal metastasis beyond pelvis ≤2 cm in greatest dimension with or without retroperitoneal node involvement
IIIC	Peritoneal metastasis beyond pelvis >2 cm in greatest dimension or regional lymph node metastasis
IV	Distant spread excludes peritoneal metastases
IVA	Pleural effusion with positive washings
IVB	Distant spread to extraabdominal organs and lymph nodes

Modified from Mutch, D. G., & Prat, J. (2014). FIGO staging for ovarian, fallopian tube and peritoneal cancer. *Gynecology Oncology, 133*, 401-404.

Treatment

- Primary treatment for stage II through IV ovarian cancer involves surgical cytoreductive staging, including hysterectomy, bilateral salpingo-oophorectomy, possible omentectomy, and pelvic and paraaortic lymph node dissection.
- Overall survival is improved for women who have surgery that optimally debulks disease (<1 cm remaining) by a gynecologic oncologist.

- Adjuvant chemotherapy with a taxane- and platinum-based drug is the standard of care.
- Among women with stage III ovarian cancer, an increased overall survival time of 16 months was demonstrated for those receiving intraperitoneal cisplatin and paclitaxel.
- Patients who are not candidates for intraperitoneal therapy should receive intravenous carboplatin and paclitaxel, which can be administered every 3 weeks or with dose-dense weekly paclitaxel.
- Neoadjuvant chemotherapy followed by interval cytoreductive surgery may be an alternative to primary surgery if the patient has comorbid illness.
- For women with stage I or early disease, surgery may remove only one ovary. Adjuvant chemotherapy with three to six cycles of a taxane- and platinum-based drug is indicated after surgery.
- Histology and grade are helpful prognostic indicators.

Recurrent Disease

- Even with cancer recurrence, long-term survival is achievable.
- EOC that recurs more than 6 months after primary chemotherapy is referred to as platinum-sensitive disease, for which there are many treatment options. These women have a better prognosis than patients who have recurrent disease less than 6 months after induction chemotherapy.
- There are several options for platinum-sensitive disease:
  - Chemotherapy retreatment with a platinum-based combination and a taxane
  - Platinum and gemcitabine, with or without bevacizumab
  - Carboplatin and pegylated liposomal doxorubicin (PLD)
- The choice of agent is determined by the patient's side effect profile during previous chemotherapy.
- Surgery is used if disease is localized and the disease-free interval is less than 1 year.
- Chemotherapy is indicated after surgery.
- Recurrence occurring less than 6 months after platinum-based chemotherapy is defined as platinum-resistant disease, whereas disease progression while on primary chemotherapy is defined as platinum refractory.
- For women with recurrent disease, switching to a nonplatinum-based chemotherapy is recommended. The average response rate is 20%.
- There are several options for platinum-resistant disease:
  - PLD with or without bevacizumab
  - Weekly paclitaxel, with or without bevacizumab
  - Topotecan
  - Docetaxel
  - Gemcitabine
  - Pemetrexed
  - Oral etoposide
- The choice of chemotherapy for patients with platinum-resistant or platinum-refractory disease is based on the side effect profile and the patient's toxicity experience from previous chemotherapy. The patient's performance status and renal and hepatic function are also considered.

- It is recommended that women with high-grade papillary ovarian, fallopian tube, or primary peritoneal cancer undergo genetic risk evaluation with a genetic counselor.
- Women with a mutation in the *BRCA1* or *BRCA2* genes may be candidates for olaparib (Lynparza), an oral poly(adenosine diphosphate–ribose) polymerase (PARP) inhibitor. It is given to women with advanced or recurrent cancer who have received three or more regimens of chemotherapy.
- The role of radiation therapy for women with recurrent ovarian cancer has not been established.
- Clinical trials should always be offered to patients with recurrent disease, regardless of the standard of care options.

Prognosis

- Survival outcomes are improved when a woman with ovarian cancer undergoes primary surgical staging by a gynecologic oncologist in a high-volume hospital rather than by a gynecologist or general surgeon.
- Favorable prognostic factors of EOC
  - Early stage
  - Younger age at diagnosis
  - Well-differentiated tumor
  - Serous histology
  - Optimally debulked tumor
- The 5-year survival rate for patients with EOC correlates with tumor stage. Five-year survival rates diminish greatly with advancing disease stage.
- Overall 1-year and 5-year survival rates for women diagnosed with EOC are 76% and 45%, respectively.
- Patients with early or local disease have a 5-year survival rate of 92.3%; however, only about 15% of ovarian cancers are diagnosed at a local stage.
- For regional and distant disease, the 5-year survival rates fall to 72% and 27.4%, respectively.
- Palliative care improves quality of life for patients with advanced disease.

Prevention and Surveillance

There are no methods to prevent ovarian cancer, but epidemiologically established factors that decrease the risk of EOC include the following:

- Younger age (<25 years) at first pregnancy and first birth
- Use of oral contraceptives for 5 or more years
- Breastfeeding
- Bilateral salpingo-oophorectomy

Surveillance

- Guidelines usually recommend follow-up for the first 2 years after a cancer diagnosis because recurrence is highest in the first 1 to 3 years after treatment.
- Coordination of care among health care providers can improve survival outcomes and cost-effective practices.
- Women who have completed primary therapy should be evaluated by their gynecologic oncologist or primary care physician every 3 months for 2 years and then every 6 months for up to 5 years.

- CA 125 blood tests are optional every 3 months, but they should be combined with CT if the patient has signs of recurrence.
- Pap smears are no longer indicated for ovarian cancer surveillance.

Bibliography

American Cancer Society (ACS). (2015). *Cancer facts and figures 2015.* Atlanta, GA: American Cancer Society.

American Cancer Society (ACS). (2014). *FDA approves Lynparza (olaparib) for some ovarian cancers.* Available at http://www.cancer.org/cancer/news/fda-approves-lynparza-olaparib-for-some-cancers (accessed January 13, 2016).

Armstrong, D. K., Bundy, B., Wenzel, L., Huang, H. Q., Baergen, R., Lele, et al. (2006). Intraperitoneal cisplatin and paclitaxel in ovarian cancer. *New England Journal of Medicine, 354,* 34–43.

Cliby, W., Powell, M., Al-Hammadi, N., Chen, L., Miller, J., Roland, P., & Bristow, R. (2015). Ovarian cancer in the United States: Contemporary patterns of care associated with improved survival. *Gynecology Oncology, 136,* 11–17.

Cohn, D. E., & Alvarez, R. D. (2012). High-grade serous carcinomas of the ovary, fallopian tube, and peritoneum. In B. Y. Karlan, R. E. Bristow, & A. Li (Eds.), *Gynecologic oncology clinical practices & surgical atlas* (pp. 217–236). New York: McGraw-Hill.

Dubeau, L., & Drapkin, R. (2013). Coming into focus: The nonovarian origins of ovarian cancer. *Annals of Oncology, 24*(suppl 8), viii28–viii35.

Goff, B. A., Mandel, L., Drescher, C. W., Urban, N., Gough, S., Schurman, K. M., & Andersen, M. R. (2007). Development of an ovarian cancer symptom index. *Cancer, 109,* 221–227.

Mutch, D. G., & Prat, J. (2014). FIGO staging for ovarian, fallopian tube and peritoneal cancer. *Gynecology Oncology, 133,* 401–404.

National Cancer Institute (NCI). (2015). *Ovarian epithelial, fallopian tube, and primary peritoneal cancer treatment—health professional version.* Available at http://www.cancer.gov/types/ovarian/hp/ovarian-epithelial-treatment-pdq (accessed January 13, 2016).

National Cancer Institute (NCI). (2014). *SEER cancer statistics review, 1975-2011.* Available at http://seer.cancer.gov/csr/1975_2011/ (accessed January 16, 2016).

National Comprehensive Cancer Network. (2015). *NCCN clinical practice guidelines in oncology: Ovarian cancer including fallopian tube cancer and primary peritoneal cancer, version 3.2014.* Available at https://intervalolibre.files.wordpress.com/2012/06/ovario-nccn-2014.pdf (accessed January 16, 2016).

Prat, J. (2012). New insights into ovarian cancer pathology. *Annals of Oncology, 23*(suppl 10), 111–117.

Prat, J. (2014). Staging classification for cancer of the ovary, fallopian tube, and peritoneum. *International Journal of Gynecologic Obstetrics, 124,* 1–5.

Salani, R., Backes, F. L., Fung, M. F., Holschneider, C. H., Parker, L. P., Bristow, R., & Goff, B. A. (2011). Posttreatment surveillance and diagnosis of recurrence in women with gynecologic malignancies: Society of Gynecologic Oncologists recommendations. *American Journal of Obstetrics & Gynecology, 204*(6), 466–478.

Uterine Cancer

Definition

Uterine carcinoma is often referred to as *endometrial cancer.* Endometrial cancer arises from the lining of the uterus and is most often confined to the body (corpus) of the uterus at the time of diagnosis. A small percentage of uterine carcinomas are sarcomas arising from endometrial glands and stroma or from the uterine muscle (i.e., leiomyosarcoma).

Carcinoma of the endometrium is easily diagnosed, but the well-differentiated cancers may be difficult to separate from advanced, atypical hyperplasia. In the past 10 years, criteria have been adopted for differentiating the two conditions as benign lesions (i.e., atypical hyperplasia) or neoplasms (i.e., well-differentiated carcinomas).

Incidence

- Endometrial carcinoma is the most common gynecologic malignancy, the fourth most common type of female cancer, and the seventh leading cause of female cancer–related death.
- According to the ACS, about 54,870 new cases of endometrial cancer and 10,170 deaths occurred in the United States in 2015.
- Endometrial adenocarcinomas are the most common type (90%), with endometrial sarcomas accounting for 6% of all endometrial cancer cases in the United States.
- Endometrial cancer occurs most commonly in postmenopausal women, although 25% of cases occur before menopause, and 5% occur in patients younger than 40 years.
- The rates for new endometrial cancer statistics have not changed significantly over the past 10 years.

Etiology and Risk Factors

- The incidence of endometrial cancer is higher in Western than Eastern countries.
- In the United States, white women have a twofold higher risk of this disease than African American women, and it is more common among urban than rural residents.
- Several factors increase the risk of endometrial carcinoma:
  - Unopposed estrogens
  - Obesity
  - Nulliparity
  - Menopause after age 52 years
  - Hypertension
  - Diabetes mellitus
  - Diet (possible relationship to high fat intake)
  - Complex endometrial hyperplasia
  - Use of tamoxifen
- Lynch syndrome (i.e., hereditary nonpolyposis colorectal cancer) is caused by inherited mutations in one or more of the DNA mismatch repair genes *MLH1, MSH2, MSH6,* and *PMS2.*
  - Patients with Lynch syndrome have a 40% to 60% lifetime risk of endometrial cancer compared with the general population.
  - The syndrome also predisposes people to colon, ovarian, stomach, small intestine, and hepatobiliary cancers.
  - Genetic counseling and testing for Lynch syndrome should be considered for women with endometrial cancer who are diagnosed earlier than age 50 or who have synchronous endometrial cancer and Lynch syndrome–associated cancers.
  - Relevant family history includes one or more first-degree relatives with Lynch syndrome–associated cancer and one member diagnosed before the age of 50 years.
  - Another risk factor is endometrial or colorectal cancer diagnosed at any age in two or more first- or second-degree relatives with Lynch syndrome.

Signs and Symptoms

- The most common sign of endometrial cancer is abnormal vaginal bleeding.
- Vaginal bleeding in a postmenopausal women or abnormal or prolonged menses in a premenopausal women is usually what prompts a visit to the gynecologist and explains why endometrial cancer is frequently diagnosed at an early stage.
- Signs and symptoms of advanced disease:
  - Pelvic pressure
  - Urinary changes
  - Leg swelling
  - Vaginal bleeding
  - Shortness of breath
  - Other symptoms indicating uterine enlargement or extrauterine tumor spread

Diagnostic Work-up

- Women with possible endometrial cancer should have a pelvic examination to evaluate the size and mobility of the uterus.
- Ultrasound may provide additional information such as thickness of the uterine lining or other causes of bleeding such as a uterine myoma.
- The standard method of assessing abnormal uterine bleeding and diagnosing uterine carcinoma is endometrial sampling, although there is a 10% false-negative rate. Assessment often can be done in the office setting.
- Patients who are symptomatic and have a negative office biopsy require fractional dilation and curettage (D&C).
- A hysteroscopy may be helpful in identifying a polyp as the cause of bleeding.
- Imaging such as CT or MRI may assist in determining extrauterine spread.

Histology

- Endometrial carcinomas are divided into two categories.
  - Type 1 is associated with unopposed estrogen stimulation and may arise from complex, atypical hyperplasia.
  - Type 2 is not associated with unopposed estrogen and most likely develops from atrophic endometrium.
- Endometrioid carcinoma, composed of malignant glandular epithelial components, represents 75% to 80% of endometrial carcinomas, including subtypes such as ciliated, secretory, villoglandular, and adenocarcinoma with squamous differentiation.
- Uterine papillary serous and clear cell histologic types represent 10% and 4%, respectively, of endometrial carcinomas and have a worse prognosis than other types.

Clinical Staging

- Disease stage is often the single strongest predictor of outcome for women with endometrial adenocarcinoma.
- FIGO staging guidelines were updated in 2009 (see table in the next column).

- Risk factors include older age, LVSI, size of tumor, and cervical and glandular involvement.
- Other unfavorable risk factors include high-grade tumors, more than 50% myometrial invasion, and clear cell or serous histology.

International Federation of Gynecology and Obstetrics (FIGO) Classification of Endometrial Carcinoma

Stage	Definition
I	Tumor limited to uterus
IA	Tumor limited to endometrium or invades <50% of myometrium
IB	Tumor invades ≥50% myometrium
II	Tumor invades stromal connective tissue of cervix and confined to uterus
IIIA	Tumor involves serosa and/or adnexa; positive cytology does not change stage
IIIB	Tumor involves the vagina or parametria
IIIC	Tumor metastases to pelvic and/or paraaortic lymph nodes
IV	Tumor invades bladder or bowel mucosa and/or distant metastases

Modified from Pecorelli, S. (2009). Revised FIGO staging for carcinoma of the vulva, cervix, and endometrium. *International Journal of Gynecology Obstetrics, 105*(2), 103-104.

Treatment

- The standard treatment is a total abdominal hysterectomy and bilateral salpingo-oophorectomy unless the patient is a candidate for fertility-sparing options.
- The hysterectomy can be performed vaginally or by exploratory laparotomy or laparoscopy, and the approach is determined by patient factors and physician preferences.
- Pelvic and paraaortic lymph nodes are assessed for nodal metastasis.
- Postoperative treatment, whether with chemotherapy or radiation therapy or both, is reserved for those who are found to have pathology-confirmed poor prognostic factors.
- Adjuvant treatment with radiation therapy is determined by risk and site of recurrence, such as the vaginal cuff or pelvis.
- Vaginal brachytherapy is often recommended for patients with tumors confined to the uterus.
- Tumor-directed radiation therapy refers to radiation targeted at sites of known tumor involvement, and methods may include external beam radiation therapy or brachytherapy, or both.
- Adjuvant chemotherapy is recommended for patients with high-grade histologic types or poor prognostic factors.
- Chemotherapy may include platinum compounds combined with paclitaxel or doxorubicin. Single agents may include topotecan and liposomal doxorubicin.

Recurrent Disease

- The treatment for recurrent endometrial cancer depends on the anatomic site and whether local or regional spread has occurred.

Major Cancers ②

- Individualized treatment usually includes some combination of surgery, radiation therapy, and chemotherapy.
- Carboplatin and paclitaxel are commonly combined and have a 40% to 62% response rate.
- Hormonal therapies, such as progestin, tamoxifen, or megestrol, are options for treating recurrent or metastatic disease.

Prognosis

- Prognosis and survival for most women with early-stage disease is excellent with appropriate intervention.
- The overall 5-year survival rate for women with endometrial cancer is 81.5%.
- More than 70% of cases are diagnosed at an early stage, for which the 5-year relative survival rate is 95%. For those with regional spread to lymph nodes, the 5-year relative survival rate is 68%.
- Grade of tumor and depth of invasion are important prognostic considerations.

Prevention and Surveillance

Prevention

- All women at menopause should be informed about the risks and symptoms of endometrial cancer.
- Women who have a history of breast cancer and are prescribed tamoxifen should be educated about their risk of endometrial cancer and should notify the physician if abnormal bleeding occurs.
- Patients who are on estrogen replacement therapy with an intact uterus should be counseled about using combination estrogen and progestin therapy.
- Women with Lynch syndrome should have an annual screening with an endometrial biopsy beginning at 30 to 35 years of age or 10 years before the age of the first family member diagnosed with endometrial cancer.

Surveillance

- Patients diagnosed with endometrial cancer should have physical examinations every 3 to 6 months by a gynecologic oncologist for 2 years and then yearly for the next 3 to 5 years.
- Pap smears are no longer performed unless an abnormality is visualized.
- Imaging is usually indicated if patients have symptoms of recurrence (e.g., pelvic or back pain, vaginal discharge, persistent cough, chest pain).
- Patient education includes lifestyle wellness tactics, including maintaining a healthy weight.
- Women with endometrial cancer should be counseled about the risks and benefits of hormone replacement.
- Women who are obese should be counseled about weight loss or referred to a weight loss management specialist.
- Patients who have had brachytherapy may have cervical stenosis and may benefit from use of a vaginal dilator.

Bibliography

American Cancer Society (ACS). (2015). *Cancer facts and figures 2015.* Atlanta, GA: American Cancer Society.

Burke, W., Orr, J., Leitao, M., Salom, E., Gehrig, P., Olawaiye, A., et al. (2014a). Endometrial cancer: A review and current management strategies: Part I. SGO Clinical Practice Endometrial Cancer Working Group for the Society of Gynecologic Oncology Clinical Practice Committee. *Gynecologic Oncology, 134,* 385–392.

Burke, W., Orr, J., Leitao, M., Salom, E., Gehrig, P., Olawaiye, A. B., & Shahin, F. A. (2014b). Endometrial cancer: A review and current management strategies: Part II. SGO Clinical Practice Endometrial Cancer Working Group for the Society of Gynecologic Oncology Clinical Practice Committee. *Gynecologic Oncology, 134,* 393–402.

Iglesias, D. A., Huang, M., Soliman, P. T., Djordjevic, B., & Lu, K. H. (2012). Endometrial hyperplasia and cancer. In B. Y. Karlan, R. E. Bristow, & A. Li (Eds.), *Gynecologic oncology clinical practices & surgical atlas* (pp. 105–137). New York: McGraw-Hill.

National Cancer Institute (NCI). (2015). *Endometrial cancer treatment—for health professionals (PDQ).* Available at http://www.cancer.gov/types/uterine/hp/endometrial-treatment-pdq (accessed January 16, 2016).

National Comprehensive Cancer Network (NCCN). (2015). *Clinical practice guidelines in oncology: Uterine neoplasms version 2.2015.* Available at https://www.nccn.org/store/login/login.aspx?ReturnURL=http://www.nccn.org/professionals/physician_gls/pdf/uterine.pdf (accessed January 16, 2016).

Pecorelli, S. (2009). Revised FIGO staging for carcinoma of the vulva, cervix, and endometrium. *International Journal of Gynecology Obstetrics, 105*(2), 103–104.

Salani, R., Backes, F. L., Fung, M. F., Holschneider, C. H., Parker, L. P., Bristow, R., & Goff, B. A. (2011). Posttreatment surveillance and diagnosis of recurrence in women with gynecologic malignancies: Society of Gynecologic Oncologists recommendations. *American Journal of Obstetrics & Gynecology, 204*(6), 466–478.

Vaginal Cancer

Definition

Primary vaginal cancer is rare. Metastatic disease to the vagina due to direct extension from the cervix or endometrium is seen more often. Because the vagina is adjacent to the cervix, vaginal cancer that originates at the apex but involves the cervix may be classified as cervical cancer, decreasing the number of vaginal cancers reported.

Incidence

- Vaginal cancer represents only 1% of all female genital tract malignancies.
- According to the ACS, about 4070 new cases of vaginal cancer and 910 deaths occurred in the United States in 2015.
- Squamous cell carcinoma represents 85% of cases, but melanoma, sarcoma, and adenocarcinoma histologic types also occur.
- The mean age at diagnosis is 60 years, although the disease can occur in women as young as 20 or 30 years of age.

Etiology and Risk Factors

- Most vaginal cancers are associated with HPV infection, and the risk factors are similar to those for cervical cancer (e.g., multiple sexual partners, cigarette smoking).
- Women who were exposed in utero to diethylstilbestrol (DES) have an increased risk of clear cell adenocarcinoma of the vagina.
  - The use of DES in pregnant women was common in 1950, explaining the peak incidence of clear cell vaginal malignancies in young women in the 1970s.

- Women with a known exposure to DES should be followed for this tumor.
- Women with a history of a gynecologic malignancy are at risk for a vaginal cancer metastasis.

Signs and Symptoms

- Many women with vaginal cancer have no symptoms, but the cancer may manifest as a mass or lesion on a routine gynecologic examination or be confirmed on a Pap smear.
- Vaginal bleeding is the most common patient-reported symptom.
- Postcoital spotting, irregular or postmenopausal bleeding, and dysuria also occur.
- Pelvic pain and enlarged inguinal nodes are late symptoms that are usually related to tumor extension beyond the vagina.

Diagnostic Work-up

- Patients with a suspected vaginal malignancy should undergo a thorough physical examination with speculum inspection.
- The posterior wall of the upper one third of the vagina is the most common site of primary vaginal carcinoma.
- The lesion may appear as a mass or an ulcer.
- An office biopsy often can be performed. When the vagina is stenosed, an examination and biopsy under anesthesia are warranted.
- Other physical assessments include palpating the groin for enlarged lymph nodes.

Histology

- Most primary vaginal carcinomas are squamous cell neoplasms and occur in women after menopause.
- Adenocarcinomas (e.g., clear cell) occur in women in their 20s.
- Melanoma is uncommon but occurs in women in the sixth decade of life.

Clinical Staging

- Primary malignancies of the vagina are staged clinically.
- A chest radiograph, bimanual and rectovaginal examination, cystoscopy, proctoscopy, and intravenous pyelogram are used by FIGO to determine the extent of disease (see table below).

International Federation of Gynecology and Obstetrics Staging System for Vaginal Cancer (and modified World Health Organization [WHO] prognostic scoring system)

Stage I	Limited to the vaginal wall.
Stage II	Involves the subvaginal tissue but has not extended to the pelvic wall.
Stage III	Extends to the pelvic wall.
Stage IV	Extends the true pelvis or has involved the mucosa of the bladder or rectum; bullous edemas as such does not permit a case to be allotted to stage IV.
Stage IVa	Invades bladder and/or rectal mucosa and/or direct extension beyond the true pelvis.
Stage IVb	Spread to distant organs.

Modified from FIGO Committee on Gynecologic Oncology. (2009). Current FIGO staging for cancer of the vagina, fallopian tube, ovary, and gestational trophoblastic neoplasia. *International Journal of Gynaecology and Obstetrics, 105(1), 3-4.*

Treatment

- Specific treatment plans are based on the stage and extent of disease.
- Early-stage disease with lesions less than 0.5 cm thick may be treated with wide local excision and upper vaginectomy. The treatment of choice often is vaginal brachytherapy or external beam radiation therapy, or both.
- For larger lesions, radical vaginectomy and pelvic lymphadenectomy are performed, followed by radiation therapy.
- For stage II disease and selected patients with advanced disease, radiation therapy may be the recommended treatment.
  - The type of radiation used is tailored to the stage and extent of disease.
  - Concomitant chemoradiotherapy agents such as 5-FU and cisplatin have shown promise for advanced disease.

Recurrent Disease

- Although the prognosis is usually poor for a vaginal recurrence, surgery or radiation therapy may be an option, depending on the foci of disease.
- Pelvic exenteration with or without vaginal reconstruction may be indicated for selected patients.
- There are no standard of care chemotherapy regimens recommended for recurrent disease.
- Ongoing clinical trials are being conducted.

Prognosis

- Prognosis depends on the disease stage and symptoms at the time of diagnosis.
- Early-stage tumors have an excellent prognosis.
- For patients who have metastatic disease or disease that has metastasized from another malignancy, the prognosis is poor.
- Reports have indicated survival rates are similar to those for patients with cervical cancer.
- Women with DES-associated cancers have a good prognosis with treatment.
- Women with non-DES adenocarcinoma have a less favorable prognosis.

Prevention and Surveillance

Prevention

- Many women have no known risk factors, precluding prevention.
- Women who smoke should be educated about smoking cessation programs.
- Healthy sexual practices with condoms and a monogamous relationship should be addressed to prevent the spread of HPV infection.
- Women who have had prior in utero DES exposure should have routine gynecologic examinations.

Surveillance

- Women with early-stage disease should be examined by a gynecologic oncologist every 6 months for 2 years and then annually.
- Patients with advanced disease should be examined by a gynecologic oncologist every 3 months.

- Imaging studies are not recommended for detecting recurrence unless patients are symptomatic.

Bibliography

American Cancer Society (ACS). (2015). *Cancer facts and figures, 2015*. Atlanta, GA: American Cancer Society.

FIGO Committee on Gynecologic Oncology. (2009). Current FIGO staging for cancer of the vagina, fallopian tube, ovary, and gestational trophoblastic neoplasia. *International Journal of Gynaecology and Obstetrics, 105*(1), 3–4.

Lowery, W. J., Chino, J., & Havrilesky, L. J. (2012). Vaginal cancer. In B. Y. Karlan, R. E. Bristow, & A. Li (Eds.), *Gynecologic oncology clinical practices & surgical atlas* (pp. 187–201). New York: McGraw-Hill.

National Cancer Institute (NCI). (2015). *Vaginal cancer treatment—for health professionals (PDQ)*. Available at http://www.cancer.gov/types/vaginal/hp/vaginal-treatment-pdq (accessed January 16, 2016).

Salani, R., Backes, F. L., Fung, M. F., Holschneider, C. H., Parker, L. P., Bristow, R., & Goff, B. A. (2011). Posttreatment surveillance and diagnosis of recurrence in women with gynecologic malignancies: Society of Gynecologic Oncologists recommendations. *American Journal of Obstetrics & Gynecology, 204*(6), 466–478.

Vulvar Cancer

Definition

- The vulva is the external female genitalia, which includes the labia minora and majora, introitus, clitoris, vaginal vestibule, perineal body, and their supporting subcutaneous tissues.
- Primary malignant tumors of the vulva account for 5% of all gynecologic cancers.

Incidence

- Most vulvar cancers occur in postmenopausal women, but reports show a trend toward younger age at diagnosis.
- According to the ACS, 5150 women were diagnosed with vulvar cancer and 1080 died of the disease in the United States in 2015.
- The rate of new cases of vulvar cancer has been rising by 0.5% and death rates by 0.7% each year for the past 10 years.

Etiology and Risk Factors

- The incidence for vulvar cancer remains low, but the risk increases in the older population.
- The peak incidence of invasive vulvar cancer occurs in the seventh decade of life.
- Cigarette smoking, infection with HPV types 16 and 18, and human immunodeficiency virus (HIV) infection are associated with the development of vulvar cancer.
- Preinvasive conditions such as vulvar intraepithelial neoplasia (VIN) and lichen sclerosis can increase the risk of developing vulvar cancer.

Signs and Symptoms

- Most women with vulvar cancer have pruritus and a recognizable lesion.
- Many women ignore or deny obvious symptoms and lesions for long periods and are diagnosed with advanced disease.
- The presentation in these cases usually is local pain, bleeding, and surface drainage from the tumor.
- The labia majora account for 50% of vulvar cancers, and the labia minora account for 15% to 20% of cases.

Diagnostic Work-up

- Initial evaluation includes the following:
  - Detailed physical examination with measurements of the primary tumor
  - Assessment for extension to adjacent mucosal or bony structures
  - Assessment for possible involvement of the inguinal lymph nodes
- Presentation with small cancers and clinically negative groin nodes requires few diagnostic studies other than those for preoperative clearance.
- Additional radiographic and endoscopic studies should be considered for those with large primary tumors or suspected metastases.
- Because neoplasia of the female genital tract is often multifocal, evaluation of the vagina and cervix, including cervical cytologic screening, should always be performed in women with vulvar neoplasms.

Histology

- The vulva is covered by keratinized squamous epithelium, and 85% of malignant vulvar tumors are squamous cell carcinomas.
- Melanoma is the second most common, accounting for 5% to 10% of cases.
- The remaining tumors are a diverse set of rare lesions that includes basal cell carcinoma, adenocarcinomas, Paget disease of the vulva, and sarcomas arising from connective tissue.

Clinical Staging

- FIGO uses a modified TNM and surgical staging scheme for vulvar carcinoma.
- The staging system incorporates the major identified prognostic factors of increasing primary tumor volume, lymph node metastasis, and distant spread (see table below).

International Federation of Gynecology and Obstetrics (FIGO) Staging for Vulvar Carcinoma

Stage	Definition
I	Tumor confined to the vulva
IA	Tumor confined to the vulva or vulva and perineum, 2 cm or less in greatest dimension, and with stromal invasion to greater than 1 mm
IB	Tumor confined to the vulva or vulva and perineum, 2 cm or less in greatest dimension, and with stromal invasion greater than 1 mm
II	Tumor with extension to perineal structure and negative nodes
III	Tumor of any size with or without extension to perineal structure; positive inguinal/femoral nodes
IIIA (i)	1 lymph node positive ≥5 mm
IIIA (ii)	1-2 lymph nodes positive (<5 mm)
IIIB (i)	≥2 lymph nodes positive (≥5 mm)
IIIB (ii)	≥3 lymph nodes positive (<5 mm)
IIIC	Positive lymph nodes and extracapsular spread
IVA (i)	Tumor invades any of the following: upper urethra, vaginal, bladder or rectal mucosa or fixed to pubic bone
IVA (ii)	Tumor involves inguinal/femoral lymph nodes
IVB	Distant metastases including pelvic lymph nodes

Modified from Pecorelli, S. (2009). Revised FIGO staging for carcinoma of the vulva, cervix, and endometrium. *International Journal of Gynecology Obstetrics, 105*(2), 103-104.

Treatment

- Surgery emphasizes an individualized approach for tumors.
- Smaller vulvar tumors can be managed by less radical surgical approaches than used in the past.
- Limited resections are proposed for certain subsets with early or low-risk disease.
- Most surgeons limit the initial procedure to radical vulvectomy and bilateral inguinal lymphadenectomy and do not proceed with pelvic node therapy unless metastasis is demonstrated in the inguinal node area.
- If tumor is documented in the inguinal nodes, pelvic lymphadenectomy is an option for therapy on the involved side only.
- Some gynecologists recommend pelvic lymph node irradiation for patients with positive inguinal nodes, but controversy still surrounds this approach.
- Combined radiation therapy and surgery, as well as radiation therapy alone and local surgery alone, have been used to treat this disease.
- No adequate prospective studies comparing therapies or their combinations are available for analysis.
- Chemotherapy has been used primarily as a salvage therapy.

Recurrent Disease

- Isolated or local recurrence is often treated with surgical re-excision and has a 5-year survival rate of up to 60%. If surgery is not an option, local radiation therapy may be an alternative.
- Inguinal and pelvic recurrences have a much worse prognosis, and depending on the patient's performance status and comorbidities, they are treated with chemotherapy.
- No standard of care chemotherapy regimens are recommended for recurrent vulvar disease, and data are extrapolated from those for metastatic or recurrent cervical cancer.
- The most common chemotherapy regimen recommended is carboplatin and paclitaxel.
- Palliative care should be initiated at the time of diagnosis.

Prognosis

- Survival in cancer of the vulva is directly related to the extent of disease at the time of diagnosis and when treatment is started.

- The 5-year relative survival rate is 70.5%.
- Localized disease is diagnosed in 59% of cases, and the 5-year relative survival rate is 86%.

Prevention and Surveillance

Prevention

- Prevention of vulvar cancer is predicated on a healthy lifestyle of smoking cessation and safe sexual practices.
- Women should be counseled at a young age about the relationship between HPV infection and vulvar cancer and about incidence reduction resulting from HPV vaccination.

Surveillance

- Follow-up and survival guidelines are extrapolated from cervical cancer guidelines because vulvar cancer is rare.
- Patients should have a physical examination and review of symptoms by their practitioner or gynecologic oncologist every 6 months for 2 years and then yearly thereafter.
- A Pap smear should be performed yearly, but no other blood tests or scans are indicated unless the patient has symptoms of recurrent disease.

Bibliography

American Cancer Society (ACS). (2015). *Cancer facts and figures 2015.* Atlanta, GA: American Cancer Society.

Milam, M., & Levenback, C. F. (2012). Vulvar cancer. In B. Y. Karlan, R. E. Bristow, & A. Li (Eds.), *Gynecologic Oncology Clinical Practices & Surgical Atlas* (pp. 173–186). New York: McGraw-Hill.

National Cancer Institute (NCI). (2014). *SEER cancer statistics review, 1975-2011.* Available at http://seer.cancer.gov/csr/1975_2011 (accessed January 16, 2016).

National Cancer Institute (NCI). (n.d.). (SEER stat fact sheets: Vulvar cancer. Available at from http://seer.cancer.gov/statfacts/html/vulva.html (accessed January 16, 2016).

Pecorelli, S. (2009). Revised FIGO staging for carcinoma of the vulva, cervix, and endometrium. *International Journal of Gynecology Obstetrics, 105*(2), 103–104.

Salani, R., Backes, F. L., Fung, M. F., Holschneider, C. H., Parker, L. P., Bristow, R., & Goff, B. A. (2011). Posttreatment surveillance and diagnosis of recurrence in women with gynecologic malignancies: Society of Gynecologic Oncologists recommendations. *American Journal of Obstetrics & Gynecology, 204*(6), 466–478.

Salom, E. M., & Penalver, M. (2002). Recurrent vulvar cancer. *Current Treatment Options in Oncology, 3,* 143–153.

Head and Neck Cancers

Ray Scarpa

Laryngeal Cancer

Definition

The larynx is an intricate neuromuscular organ located between the pharynx and trachea. It has three main functions. It prevents passage of food into the airway during swallowing, modulates air passing through the vocal cords to facilitate phonation, and regulates the flow of air into lungs during respiration. The larynx acts as a sphincter to prevent aspiration. The true and false cords, epiglottis, and aryepiglottic folds close, and the larynx moves slightly upward and forward to protect the trachea and prevent respiration during swallowing. A sound is created when the true vocal cords make contact with each other and air from the lungs passes between them. Phonation occurs when this sound is converted to recognizable speech by the contraction and relaxation of muscles in the oral cavity and tongue.

The larynx is divided into three anatomic regions.

- The supraglottic larynx includes the epiglottis, false vocal cords, laryngeal ventricles, aryepiglottic folds, and arytenoids. Approximately 34% of laryngeal cancers occur in this region.
- The glottis includes the true vocal cords and the anterior and posterior commissures. Approximately 65% of laryngeal cancers occur in this region.
- The subglottic region begins about 1 cm below the true vocal cords and extends to the lower border of the cricoid cartilage or the first tracheal ring. Approximately 1% to 8% of laryngeal cancers occur in this region.

Incidence

- About 13,560 new cases of laryngeal cancer and 3640 deaths from the disease occurred in 2015.
- Based on data for the 2008 to 2012 period, the annual age-adjusted rates of laryngeal cancer were 3.2 new cases and 1.1 deaths per 100,000 men and women.
- According to 2010 to 2012 data, approximately 0.4% of men and women are diagnosed with laryngeal cancer at some point during their lifetimes.
- In 2012, an estimated 88,852 people were living with laryngeal cancer in the United States.
- Men are almost six times more likely to be diagnosed with and die of the disease than women.
- The incidence increases with age.
- Laryngeal cancer deaths are highest among people between the ages of 65 and 74, accounting for 0.6% of all cancer deaths and 0.8% of all new cancer cases.

Etiology and Risk Factors

- More than three fourths of head and neck cancers in the United States are related to tobacco and alcohol use.
- Cigarette smoking is the single most important risk factor for head and neck cancer. The smoking-attributable risk for laryngeal cancer is 79% for men and 87% for women.
- Combined alcohol and tobacco use increases the risk of laryngeal cancer by about 50%. Alcohol and tobacco are thought to act synergistically. Although alcohol is not a carcinogen, it is thought to damage the mucosa and allow increased cellular permeability to known carcinogens.
- Exposure to wood dust, organic chemicals, coal products, cement, paint, varnish, and lacquer increase the risk of laryngeal cancer.
- Human papillomavirus (HPV) has been identified in some head and neck cancers.
- A personal history of laryngeal cancer is a risk factor; second primary tumors have been reported in up to 25% of patients whose initial lesion was controlled.

Signs and Symptoms

Supraglottic Cancers

- Sore throat
- Painful swallowing
- Referred ear pain
- Change in voice quality
- Enlarged neck nodes
- Weight loss
- Aspiration

Glottic Cancers

- Hoarseness
- Difficulty swallowing
- Dyspnea
- Stridor
- Irritation of throat

Subglottic Cancers

- Dyspnea
- Hemoptysis
- Stridor

Diagnostic Work-up

- Physical examination of the oral cavity and neck
- Thorough palpation of the neck for evidence of metastatic disease

- Mirror examination and endoscopy of the upper aerodigestive tract
- Imaging studies, including computed tomography (CT) with contrast and positron emission tomography (PET)
- Biopsy of suspicious lesions

Histology

Most malignant lesions found in the larynx are squamous cell carcinomas. Nonmalignant conditions such as vocal cord polyps or cysts and sarcoidosis can mimic the symptoms associated with malignant lesions.

Clinical Staging

Staging of laryngeal cancer is based on clinical and radiographic information obtained before treatment and uses the American Joint Committee on Cancer (AJCC) guidelines based on the tumor-node-metastasis (TNM) classification system (Crompton, et al., 2012).

Treatment

Early-stage lesions are treated with radiation therapy or surgery alone. Both approaches yield similar survival rates for early glottic and supraglottic lesions. Radiation therapy is confined to a small treatment area for T1 lesions of the glottis.

Treatment often involves a multimodal approach. The choice of treatment is determined by the anticipated functional and cosmetic results and by the availability of a multidisciplinary team with experience in treating this type of malignancy. Consideration is given to the efficacy of treatment and quality of life issues, such as preservation of the voice in cases of laryngeal tumors. Treatment for patients with recurrent disease depends on the tumor location and size and prior treatment in that area.

Surgery

- Surgical excision must encompass the gross tumor and microscopic disease.
- If positive regional nodes are identified, node dissection is usually done.
- Postoperative rehabilitation, including voice aids for patients who have undergone laryngectomy, is important to ensure the best quality of life.
- Surgical treatment of T1, T2, and selected T3 supraglottic lesions requires some form of supraglottic laryngectomy. Selective neck dissection is done with a tracheostomy to secure the airway in the postoperative period.
- Early glottic lesions can be managed surgically with a cordectomy to remove the affected vocal cord. This should be attempted only if the lesion does not extend to the anterior commissure or the arytenoid cartilage.
- Transoral robotic surgery (TORS) is a minimally invasive procedure used to resect small, well-circumscribed lesions in the glottic and supraglottic area.
- A carbon dioxide laser can be used transorally with ridged endoscopes to target small lesions in the supraglottic and glottic areas.

- Advanced-stage lesions that involve thyroid cartilage or other structures outside the larynx require a total laryngectomy.
  - Removal of the entire larynx may also involve removal of the thyroid gland, parathyroid glands, or other involved structures.
  - A permanent tracheostoma is created by suturing the trachea to the skin of the anterior neck. Postoperative adjuvant treatment is usually indicated.

Radiation Therapy

Although most early lesions can be cured by irradiation or surgery, radiation therapy may be a reasonable choice to preserve the voice, leaving surgery for salvage if needed.

- External beam radiation therapy is commonly used for treating the primary site and regional lymph nodes.
- Intensity-modulated radiation therapy (IMRT) lessens toxicity by limiting radiation exposure of the normal tissue surrounding the lesion.
- Side effects from irradiation of the area can lead to esophageal strictures, limited range of motion of the neck, and tracheostomy dependence.
- Treatment may cure disease but leave the patient with a nonfunctioning larynx.
- Patients who smoke while on radiation therapy may have lower response rates and shorter survival durations. They should be counseled to stop smoking before beginning radiation therapy.
- Research suggests that there is a significant loss of local control when radiation therapy was not delivered according to the planned schedule, and lengthening the radiation schedule should be avoided if possible.

Chemotherapy

Historically, surgery and radiation therapy have formed the foundation of therapy, with chemotherapy enhancing the effectiveness of irradiation.

- Platinum-based chemotherapy with concurrent radiation therapy is standard care for locally advanced nonresectable lesions and laryngeal lesions.
- Postoperative chemotherapy with radiation therapy is used for patients at high risk for recurrence, such as those with T3-4 lesions, positive nodes, or inadequate resection.
- Molecularly targeted therapies are available for head and neck cancers.
  - Epidermal growth factor receptor (EGFR) is expressed by most head and neck tumors. Its activation stimulates intracellular tyrosine kinase signaling and cell cycle progression.
  - Cetuximab, a monoclonal antibody that binds to EGFR and blocks cell proliferation, is used when conventional treatment is unsuccessful. It is used in combination with paclitaxel and carboplatin.
  - Neoadjuvant therapy for locally advanced disease is given before surgery. In some cases, it can facilitate organ preservation when combined with radiation therapy. Combined therapy with cisplatin and 5-fluorouracil (5-FU) is commonly used.

Prognosis

- Adverse prognostic factors for laryngeal cancers include advanced stage of disease and grade, unfavorable type of pathology, and metastases to lymph nodes.
- The finding of lymphatic invasion increases the risk of death by approximately 50%.
- Other prognostic factors include sex, age, performance status, and pathologic features of the tumor, including grade and depth of invasion.
- Metastasis to bone and other distant areas increases the risk of death.
- Comorbid conditions such as diabetes, hypertension, decreased pulmonary function, and malnutrition compromise successful treatment outcomes.
- Based on 2005 to 2011 data, the overall 5-year survival rate is 60.6%.
- The prognosis for early-stage laryngeal cancers that have not spread to lymph nodes is very good, with cure rates of 75% to 95%.
- Locally advanced lesions are better managed with surgery followed by adjuvant radiation therapy or combined irradiation and chemotherapy.
- Distant metastases can occur even if the primary tumor is controlled.
- Patients with distant disease are usually treated with palliative measures using chemotherapy and radiation therapy.
- Patients treated for laryngeal cancers are at the highest risk of recurrence in the first 2 to 3 years. Recurrences after 5 years are rare and usually represent new primary malignancies.

Prevention and Surveillance

The risk of developing laryngeal malignancies can be greatly reduced by avoiding certain risk factors.

- Use of tobacco in any form is the most significant cause of upper aerodigestive tract malignancies.
- Heavy alcohol abuse contributes to the increased risk, especially when used with tobacco.
- Exposure to known carcinogenic chemicals and wood dust must be eliminated by using proper ventilation and protective gear.
- The rate of HPV infection of the upper aerodigestive tract is increased among individuals who have oral sex and multiple sex partners.
  - Tobacco users are more prone to HPV infection as a result of a compromised immune system and because tobacco smoke injures respiratory cells.
  - Although HPV infection is linked to some cases of cancer of the larynx, most HPV-infected people do not develop cancers of the larynx, or the tumors do not contain HPV.
  - HPV vaccination may decrease the risk of cancers in the upper aerodigestive tract, but this has not been proved.
- Poor nutrition and the vitamin deficiencies associated with alcohol abuse and malnutrition contribute to the risk of developing laryngeal malignancies.
- Individuals with a history of head and neck cancer who cease using tobacco and alcohol retain a risk of developing a second primary at a rate of 3% to 7% per year.

Bibliography

American Cancer Society. (2014). *Can laryngeal and hypopharyngeal cancers be prevented?* Available at http://www.cancer.org/cancer/laryngeal andhypopharyngealcancer/detailedguide/laryngeal-and-hypopharyngeal-cancer-prevention (accessed December 20, 2015).

Compton, C., Byrd, D., Garcia-Aguilar, J., Kurtzman, S., Olawaiye, A., & Washington, M. K. (Eds.). (2012). *AJCC cancer staging atlas* (p. 129). New York: Springer.

National Cancer Institute. (2014). *Laryngeal cancer treatment: Stage information for laryngeal cancer.* Available at http://www.cancer.gov/cancertopics /pdq/treatment/laryngeal/HealthProfessional/page3 (accessed December 20, 2015).

National Cancer Institute. (2014). *SEER stat fact sheets: Larynx cancer.* Available at http://seer.cancer.gov/statfacts/html/laryn.html (accessed December 20, 2015).

Scarpa, R. (2009). Surgical management of head and neck carcinoma. *Seminars in Oncology Nursing, 25*(3), 172–182.

Scarpa, R. J. (2014). Surgical care of head and neck cancers. In G. W. Davidson, J. L. Lester, & M. Routt (Eds.). *Surgical oncology nursing* (pp. 65–78). Pittsburgh, PA: Oncology Nursing Society.

Titze, I. R. (2014). Bi-stable vocal fold adduction: A mechanism of modal-falsetto register shifts and mixed registration. *Journal of the Acoustical Society of America, 135*, 2091–2101.

Oral Cavity Cancer

Definition

Cancer of the oral cavity can occur in the following locations:

- Lips
- Mobile anterior two thirds of tongue
- Cheek or buccal mucosa
- Floor of the mouth
- Retromolar trigone
- Gingiva
- Hard palate
- Teeth

Incidence

The rates of new oral cavity and pharyngeal cancer cases have been stable over the past 10 years. About 45,780 new cases of oral cavity and pharyngeal cancer and 8650 deaths occurred in 2015.

- Based on 2007 to 2011 data, the annual age-adjusted incidence of oral cavity and pharyngeal cancer is 11 new cases per 100,000 men and women.
- Based on 2008 to 2012 data, the annual age-adjusted mortality rate is 2.5 deaths per 100,000 men and women.
- Based on 2009 to 2011 data, approximately 1.1% of men and women are diagnosed with oral cavity or pharyngeal cancer at some point during their lifetimes.
- In 2011, an estimated 281,591 people were living with oral cavity or pharyngeal cancer in the United States.
- The most common site for oral cancer is the tongue, accounting for 20% to 50% of cases.

Etiology and Risk Factors

- Oral carcinoma is the sixth most common type of malignancy worldwide.
- Oral cancers account for 30% of all new cancer diagnoses among men in India, Pakistan, and Sir Lanka.
- Oral cancers are six times more common among men than women.

- Oral carcinoma is more common in populations of lower socioeconomic status who abuse alcohol and tobacco. Individuals who abuse alcohol and smoke are 38 times more likely to develop oral malignancies than people who do not drink or smoke.
  - Cigarette smoking is the single most important risk factor for head and neck cancers.
  - Among men, 90% of the risk for oral cancer is attributed to tobacco use. The risk for women is 59%.
  - Use of smokeless tobacco causes a fourfold to sixfold increase in cancers of the alveolar ridge and buccal mucosa.
  - The carcinogens found in tobacco have a synergistic effect when combined with alcohol.
  - Alcohol is not a carcinogen; it damages the mucosa and allows increased cellular permeability to tobacco carcinogens.
- HPV infection (i.e., HPV16) increases the risk of oral carcinomas and may account for the increased incidence of these malignancies.
- Herpes simplex infection increases the risk of oral carcinomas.
- Exposures to wood dust, organic chemicals, coal products, cement, paint, varnish, and lacquer are risk factors.
- A personal history of head and neck cancer increases the chance of developing a second primary tumor.
- A diet low in fruits and vegetables is a risk factor for oral cancer.
- Sun exposure is a risk factor for cancer of the lip.

Signs and Symptoms

Presenting signs and symptoms may include the following:
- Leukoplakia
- Ulcer
- Lump or tissue thickening
- Feeling of fullness in the throat
- Dysphagia
- Voice changes (e.g., hot potato voice)
- Jaw swelling
- Unilateral otalgia without hearing loss
- Pain
- Bleeding

Diagnostic Work-up

- Physical examination of the oral cavity and neck includes thorough palpation of the neck, oral cavity, and tongue. Use of the mirror allows the examiner to view the base of the tongue and the supraglottis.
- Flexible fiberoptic endoscopy of the upper aerodigestive tract is used to look at areas that cannot easily be seen with mirrors.
- Imaging may be done with PET or CT with contrast. MRI may be indicated if the patient is allergic to contrast material or to determine the possibility of an intracranial extension.
- Biopsy is performed for suspicious lesions.
- Fine-needle aspiration (FNA) is performed for a suspicious lesion or lymphadenopathy.

Histology

- Approximately 95% of malignant tumors in the oral cavity are determined to be squamous cell carcinomas. The remaining 5% of malignancies arise from the salivary glands.
- Histologically, these tumors may be mucoepidermoid carcinomas or adenoid cystic carcinomas.
- Malignant tumors arising from bone, cartilage, fat, muscle, or fibrous tissue may be identified histologically as sarcomas.
- Malignant tumors arising from the pigmented areas may be melanomas.
  - Approximately 80% of melanomas in the oral cavity involve the palate and maxillary gingiva.
  - Less than 1% of melanomas involve the oral mucosa.
- Malignant buccal mucosa, mandibular gingiva, and tongue lesions have been identified.

Clinical Staging

Staging of oral cavity cancers employs the AJCC TNM classification system.

Treatment

Treatment often involves a multimodal approach. Depending on the site and extent of the primary tumor and the status of the lymph nodes, the treatment of lip and oral cavity cancer may be surgery alone, radiation therapy alone, the two modalities combined, or a combination of surgery, irradiation, and chemotherapy.

- Early cancers (i.e., stages I and II) are highly curable with surgery or radiation therapy. The choice of treatment is determined by the stage of disease, anticipated functional and cosmetic results of surgery, comorbid conditions, and recommendations of a multidisciplinary team.
- Most patients with stage III or IV tumors require a multimodality approach that includes surgery, irradiation, and chemotherapy.
- Treatment for patients with recurrent lesions depends on the location and size of the recurrent lesion and prior treatment.
- The risk of local recurrence or distant metastases is high and requires close monitoring. Patients should be considered for clinical trials.

Surgery

- Lesions of the oral cavity usually are surgically resected. Resection encompasses gross tumor and a 2-mm cuff of normal tissue surrounding the lesion.
- If positive regional nodes are identified, cervical node dissection is done.
- Postoperative swallowing, speech, and prosthodontic rehabilitation is important to ensure the best quality of life.

Radiation Therapy

- External beam radiation therapy or brachytherapy using interstitial implants may be used. Local implants can be successful in treating small, superficial cancers.

- Refinements in radiation therapy have led to techniques that spare more of the surrounding normal tissue and minimize side effects.
- IMRT is the latest technologic advancement in external beam radiation therapy.
  - Radiation is delivered conformally. Each x-ray beam is broken into many smaller beams. The intensity of the smaller beams can be adjusted to shape the beam and modulate the dose within the treatment area.
  - IMRT minimizes xerostomia and other side effects caused by radiation therapy.
  - IMRT has decreased the use of interstitial implants in the treatment of oral malignancies.
- Patients who smoke while on radiation therapy appear to have lower response rates and shorter survival durations than those who do not. Patients should be counseled to stop smoking before beginning radiation therapy.

Chemotherapy

- Chemotherapy (e.g., cisplatin) is typically combined with radiation therapy.
- In selected cases, chemotherapy can be used as the primary treatment.
- In patients who have advanced disease for which surgery would be too debilitating and compromise functional and cosmetic outcomes, chemotherapy plus radiation therapy may produce a better outcome than radiation alone.
- Adjuvant chemoradiation therapy may be given after surgery to enhance the chance of local tumor control.
- Neoadjuvant or induction chemoradiation may be used before surgery. Side effects can be severe and may make surgery more challenging.
- Chemotherapy with or without irradiation can be used for metastatic disease. The goal is to slow the growth of the cancer and provide symptom relief.
- Chemotherapy drugs may be used alone or combined with others.
  - Cisplatin and 5-FU is a common combination.
  - The triplet regimen of cisplatin, 5-FU, and docetaxel is often used.

The chemotherapy agents used for cancers of the oral cavity and oropharynx are listed in the box below.

Drugs Used Alone or in Combination to Treat Oral Cancers

Commonly Used Drugs
- Cisplatin
- Carboplatin
- 5-Fluorouracil (5-FU)
- Paclitaxel (Taxol)
- Docetaxel (Taxotere)
- Cetuximab

Less Commonly Used Drugs
- Methotrexate
- Ifosfamide (Ifex)
- Bleomycin

Prognosis

- Survival rates for oral and oropharyngeal cancers have risen slightly over the past 20 years.
- Based on 2005 to 2011 data, the overall 5-year survival rate is 63.2%.
- Approximately 40% of men and 43% of women survive oropharyngeal cancer at least 5 years after diagnosis.
- Survival rates are depend on tumor site and stage.
  - The 5-year survival rate for patients with cancer of the lip is 89%.
  - The 5-year survival rates for the tongue and all other sites are also gender specific; 55% of women and 44% of men with cancer of the tongue survive 5 years after diagnosis.
  - Survival rates for all other sites of the oral cavity are higher for women (55%) than men (48%).
- The earlier a malignancy is diagnosed and treated, the better the outcome. Survival rates for early-stage disease (i.e., stages 0, 1, and 2) are higher than for later stages (i.e., stage 3 and 4).
- People with oral cavity or oropharyngeal cancer who have tested positive for HPV may have a better prognosis than those who do not. Research is ongoing to determine how HPV can be used to predict the outcome and treatment modalities needed for patients with oral carcinoma.
- Prognostic factors include tumor size, local invasion, vascular invasion, margins of resection, mitotic index, tumor morphology, and lymph nodes metastases.
  - If nodes are positive, prognostic factors include the number of positive nodes, the size of the largest node, laterality of nodes, and extracapsular extension. Disease can metastasize to bones and lymph nodes.
  - The consequences of tumor extending beyond the limits of the primary site into adjacent tissues can be challenging to manage. Patients are prone to severe malnourishment, chronic pain, immobility, and depression.

Prevention and Surveillance

- Primary prevention of head and neck cancer requires cessation of alcohol and tobacco use.
  - Individuals who have had one cancer in a region are at an increased risk for other cancers with related risk factors, including other head and neck cancers, lung cancer, and esophageal cancer.
  - Patients should be referred for counseling and support to address issues related to tobacco and alcohol use.
- Individuals, with a history of head and neck cancer who cease tobacco and alcohol use, retain a risk of developing a second primary tumor at a rate of 3% to 7% per year.
- Ongoing clinical trials are seeking to determine the role of HPV vaccines in decreasing the incidence of HPV-related malignancies in the oral cavity.

Bibliography

American Cancer Society. (2014). *Chemotherapy for oral cavity and oropharyngeal cancer.* Available at http://www.cancer.org/cancer/oralcavityandoropharyngealcancer/detailedguide/oral-cavity-and-oropharyngeal-cancer-treating-chemotherapy (accessed December 20, 2015).

American Cancer Society. (2014). How are oral cavity and oropharyngeal cancers staged? Available at http://www.cancer.org/cancer/oralcavityand oropharyngealcancer/detailedguide/oral-cavity-and-oropharyngeal-cancer-staging (accessed December 20, 2015).

American Joint Committee on Cancer. (2010). Lip and oral cavity. In S. B. Edge, D. R. Byrd, C. C. Compton, A. G. Fritz, F. L. Greene, & A. Trotti (Eds.), *AJCC cancer staging manual* (7th ed.) (pp. 29–35). New York: Springer.

Brocklehurst, P., Kujan, O., O'Malley, L. A., Ogden, G., Shepherd, S., & Glenny, A. M. (2013). Screening programmes for the early detection and prevention of oral cancer. Cochrane Database of Systematic Reviews (11). CD004150. Available at http://onlinelibrary.wiley.com/doi/10.1002/14651858.CD004150.pub4/abstract (accessed December 20, 2015).

Christopoulos, A. (2013). Mouth anatomy. Available at http://emedicine.medscape.com/article/1899122-overview#a1 (accessed December 20, 2015).

Collins, B., Abernethy, J., & Barnes, L. (2014). Oral malignant melanoma. The Oral Cancer Foundation. Available at http://www.oralcancerfoundation.org/facts/rare/om/ (accessed December 20, 2015).

Howlader, N., Noone, A. M., Krapcho, M., Garshell, J., Miller, D., Altekruse, S. F., et al (Eds.). *SEER Cancer Statistics Review, 1975–2012.* Bethesda, MD: National Cancer Institute. Available at http://seer.cancer.gov/csr/1975_2012/ (based on November 2014 SEER data submission, posted to the SEER web site, April 2015).

Iwamoto, R. R., Haas, M. L., & Gooselin, T. K. (2012). Manual for radiation oncology nursing practice and education (4th ed.). Pittsburgh, PA: Oncology Nursing Society.

Khan, F. (2010). The physics of radiation therapy (4th ed.). Philadelphia PA: Lippincott Williams & Wilkins.

National Cancer Institute. (2014). SEER Stat fact sheets: Oral cavity and pharynx cancer. Available at http://seer.cancer.gov/statfacts/html/oralcav.html (accessed December 20, 2015).

Scarpa, R. (2009). Surgical management of head and neck carcinoma. *Seminars in Oncology Nursing, 25*(3), 172–182.

Pharyngeal Cancer

Definition

The pharynx is a muscular tube that connects the nasal cavity to the upper aerodigestive tract. This structure begins at the skull base and ends below the cricoid cartilage near the level of C6. It contains three distinct areas, the nasopharynx, oropharynx, and hypopharynx, any of which can develop malignancies.

- The nasopharynx, located between the base of the skull and the soft palate, is a continuation of the nasal cavity. It humidifies and filters inspired air and directs the air to the larynx. The eustachian tube openings are found on the left and right lateral walls of the nasopharynx and lead into the middle ear. It is innervated by the maxillary nerve, one of the three branches of the trigeminal nerve (cranial nerve [CN] V_2).

- The oropharynx is the middle part of the pharynx, located between the soft palate and the superior border of the epiglottis. It is innervated by the glossopharyngeal nerve (CN IX). It contains the base of the tongue, the lingual tonsils, and the palatine tonsils found in the oral cavity. The oropharynx is involved in the voluntary and involuntary phases of swallowing.

- The hypopharynx is the lower part of the pharynx, located between the upper part of the epiglottis and the upper border of the cricoid cartilage. It becomes part of the esophagus at the level of C6. It is located behind the larynx and communicates with it by the laryngeal inlet. The piriform sinuses are found on each side in this area. The hypopharynx contains the middle and inferior pharyngeal constrictor muscle.

Pharyngeal structures include the mucosa, lymphoid tissue, and longitudinal muscle layer that includes the stylopharyngeus muscle, palatopharyngeus muscle, and salpingopharyngeus muscle. These muscles elevate the larynx during swallowing. A circular muscle layer consists of the superior, middle, and inferior constrictor muscles. These muscles contract sequentially and propel a food bolus into the esophagus.

The pharyngeal plexus innervates the pharynx. It consists of branches of the glossopharyngeal nerve (CN IX), branches of the vagus nerve (CN X), and sympathetic fibers of the superior cervical ganglion.

Incidence

- Based on 2008 to 2012 data, the annual age-adjusted incidence of new oral cavity and pharyngeal cancers was 11 cases per 100,000 men and women. The associated mortality rate was 2.5 deaths per 100,000 men and women.

- In 2012, there were about 291,108 people living with oral cavity and pharyngeal cancers in the United States. In 2015, there were an estimated 45,780 new cases of pharyngeal cancer and 8650 deaths from the disease.

- Men are almost four times more likely to be diagnosed with pharyngeal cancer than women and almost three times more likely to die of the disease.

- The incidence of oropharyngeal cancer is higher among African Americans than whites.

- Incidence increases with age.

- The prevalence of HPV-associated oropharyngeal cancers increased by 225% from 1988 to 2004, and the numbers of HPV-negative cancers have declined by 50% according to the Surveillance, Epidemiology, and End Results (SEER) tissue repository data.

Etiology and Risk Factors

- The rising incidence of oropharyngeal cancer among younger individuals without a history of alcohol and tobacco use is associated with infection by HPV types 16, 18, 31, 33, and 35.

- Tobacco and heavy alcohol use are significant risk factors for oropharyngeal cancer. More than three fourths of head and neck cancers in the United States are related to tobacco and alcohol use.

- Cigarette smoking is the single most important risk factor for head and neck cancer.

- Alcohol and tobacco are thought to act synergistically. Alcohol is not a carcinogen, but it suppresses the immune system and damages the mucosa, increasing cellular permeability to known carcinogens such as tobacco.

- Other risk factors include the following:
  - A diet poor in fruits and vegetables
  - Consumption of a beverage called *mate,* a stimulant commonly drunk in South America
  - Chewing betel quid, a stimulant preparation commonly used in parts of Asia

- Defective elimination of acetaldehyde, a carcinogen generated by alcohol metabolism, because of an inactive mutant allele of alcohol dehydrogenase 2, which is found primarily in East Asians
- Occupational exposure to wood dust
- Exposure to organic chemicals, coal products, cement, paint, varnish, and lacquer
- Those with a personal history of head and neck cancers have an increased chance of developing a second primary tumor.
- Epstein-Barr virus infections have been linked to nasopharyngeal cancer.

Signs and Symptoms

Nasopharynx
- Neck mass
- Nasal obstruction
- Change in voice quality
- Unilateral serous otitis media
- Unilateral otalgia

Oropharynx
- May have no symptoms
- Sore throat
- Difficulty swallowing
- Foreign-body or globus sensation in the throat
- Altered voice
- Otalgia
- Neck adenopathy
- Weight loss

Hypopharynx and Cervical Esophagus
- Dysphagia
- Hoarseness
- Neck adenopathy
- Weight loss
- Aspiration

Diagnostic Work-up
- Physical examination of the oral cavity and neck
- Thorough palpation of the neck for evidence of metastatic disease
- Mirror examination
- Flexible fiberoptic examination of the upper aerodigestive tract
- CT and magnetic resonance imaging (MRI) with contrast
- Biopsy of suspicious lesions
- PET

Histology
- Most pharyngeal cancers are squamous cell carcinomas.
- Other types of oropharyngeal cancers are minor salivary gland tumors, lymphomas, and lymphoepitheliomas (i.e., Rigaud and Schmincke tumor types).
- A variety of malignant tumors may arise in the nasopharynx, but only squamous cell carcinoma is considered in this discussion because management of the others varies widely by histologic features.

- The histology of pharyngeal squamous cell carcinomas is divided into keratinizing and nonkeratinizing types, with nonkeratinizing forms further divided into differentiated and nondifferentiated subtypes.
- Terms such as type I (i.e., squamous cell carcinoma), type II (i.e., nonkeratinizing carcinoma), and type III (i.e., undifferentiated carcinoma) are no longer used.

Clinical Staging

Pharyngeal cancers are staged with the AJCC TNM classification system. Staging is the same for hypopharyngeal and oropharyngeal cancers, but nasopharyngeal cancer is staged differently (Edge, et al., 2010).

Treatment

The choice of treatment should be determined by the anticipated functional and cosmetic results and by the availability of the medical expertise required. Treatment plans for all disease stages should be discussed at a multidisciplinary tumor conference involving surgeons, radiation oncologists, medical oncologists, pathologists, and specialized nursing personnel.

Radiation therapy is the mainstay of treatment for all histologic types of nasopharyngeal carcinomas. Surgery at the primary disease site has a very limited role for nasopharyngeal carcinoma. Surgery is reserved for patients who fail to respond to radiation therapy. Patients with advanced or metastatic disease may receive additional therapy (i.e., irradiation or neck dissection), depending on the response to initial therapy.

Surgery
- Surgical excision must encompass the gross tumor and microscopic disease.
- If positive regional nodes are identified, node dissection is usually done.
- Postoperative rehabilitation is important to ensure the best quality of life.
- Postoperative chemotherapy is often used for patients with a high risk of recurrence (i.e., three or more lesions, positive nodes, or inadequate resection).

Radiation Therapy
- Radiation therapy alone is indicated for stage I nasopharyngeal carcinoma. A dose of 66 to 70 Gy is given over a 7-week period.
- Research suggests that there is a significant loss of local control when radiation therapy is not delivered according to the planned schedule. Lengthening the radiation schedule should be avoided whenever possible.
- IMRT has become more widely available. The technique limits radiation exposure of the normal tissue surrounding the lesion and reduces adverse tissue reactions, which can be considerable in the head and neck region.
- Patients who smoke during radiation therapy have lower response rates and shorter survival durations. Patients should be counseled to stop smoking before beginning radiation therapy.

Chemotherapy

- Chemotherapy with concurrent radiation therapy is the treatment of choice for locally advanced stage II to IVB nasopharyngeal cancers.
- Treatment for advanced nasopharyngeal cancers includes intravenous cisplatin at a dose of 100 mg/m^2 on days 1, 22, and 43 with irradiation, followed by a regimen of intravenous cisplatin at a dose of 80 mg/m^2 to 100 mg/m^2 on day 1 plus 5-FU at a dose of 1000 mg/m^2/day by continuous intravenous infusion on days 1 through 4 every 4 weeks for three cycles.
- The total radiation dose is 70 Gy.
- Recurrent or metastatic disease is treated with additional cisplatin, carboplatin, gemcitabine, methotrexate, paclitaxel, and docetaxel.
- EGFR is expressed by most head and neck tumors. Its stimulation results in activation of intracellular tyrosine kinase and cell cycle progression. Cetuximab, a monoclonal antibody that binds to EGFR and blocks cell proliferation, is used in combination with paclitaxel and carboplatin.

Prognosis

- Based on 2005 to 2011 data, the overall 5-year survival rate is 63.2%.
- Lymphatic spread is the single most inportant determinant of prognosis. If nodes are positive, the numbers of positive nodes, size of the largest node, laterality of nodes, and presence or absence of extracapsular extension alter the prognosis.
- Other prognostic factors are the size, thickness, local tissue and vascular invasion, margins of resection, mitotic index, and morphologic features of the tumor.
- The 5-year survival rate for nasopharyngeal carcinoma depends on the stage:
  - Stage I: 72%
  - Stage II: 64%
  - Stage III: 62%
  - Stage IV: 38%
- Although metastatic disease to bone and lymph nodes does occur, the consequences of locoregional disease, malnutrition, and cachexia remain the most difficult problems to manage.

Prevention and Surveillance

- Prevention measures are limited because there are no known avoidable risk factors for pharyngeal carcinoma.
- Although tobacco and heavy alcohol use are associated with other head and neck malignancies, the links are not as definitive in nasopharyngeal carcinoma. Primary prevention of head and neck malignancies requires limiting alcohol use and tobacco cessation.
- Close follow-up after treatment is essential for positive outcomes and early intervention in case of recurrence.
- Patients with pharyngeal cancer are at increased risk for second primaries.

Bibliography

American Cancer Society. (2015). *Can nasopharyngeal cancer be prevented?* Available at http://www.cancer.org/cancer/nasopharyngealcancer/detailed guide/nasopharyngeal-cancer-prevention (accessed December 20, 2015).

American Cancer Society. (2015). *Survival rates for nasopharyngeal cancer by stage.* Available at http://www.cancer.org/cancer/nasopharyngealcancer/detailedguide/nasopharyngeal-cancer-survival-rates (accessed December 20, 2015).

Cancer.Net Editorial Board. (2015). Nasopharyngeal cancer: Stages and grades. American Society of Clinical Oncology. Available at http://www.cancer.net/cancer-types/nasopharyngeal-cancer/stages-and-grades (accessed December 20, 2015).

Edge, S. B., Byrd, D. R., Compton, C. C., Fritz, A. G., Greene, F. L., & Trotti, A. (Eds.). (2010). *AJCC Cancer staging manual* (7th ed.). New York, NY: Springer.

Mannan, A. A. S. R. (2014). Nasal cavity: Nasopharyngeal carcinoma. Nonkeratinizing nasopharyngeal carcinoma—Undifferentiated. Available at PathologyOutlines.com. http://www.pathologyoutlines.com/topic/nasal nonkeratinizingundiff.html (accessed December 20, 2015).

National Cancer Institute. (2014). Oropharyngeal cancer treatment—For health professionals (PDQ). Available at http://www.cancer.gov/cancer-topics/pdq/treatment/oropharyngeal/healthprofessional#section1 (accessed December 20, 2015).

National Cancer Institute. (2014). SEER stat fact sheets: Oral cavity and pharynx cancer. Available at http://seer.cancer.gov/statfacts/html/oralcav.html (accessed December 20, 2015).

Pazhaniappan, N. (2014). The pharynx. Available at http://teachmeanatomy.info/neck/viscera/pharynx/ (accessed December 20, 2015).

Stevenson, M. M. (2013). Oropharyngeal and hypopharyngeal cancer staging. Available at http://emedicine.medscape.com/article/2048285-overview (accessed December 20, 2015).

Stevenson, M. M. (2013). Nasopharyngeal cancer staging. Available at http://emedicine.medscape.com/article/2048007-overview (accessed December 20, 2015).

Stevenson, M. M. (2013). Nasopharyngeal cancer treatment protocols. Available at http://emedicine.medscape.com/article/2047748-overview (accessed December 20, 2015).

Salivary Gland Cancer

Definition

Salivary glands are exocrine glands that are located in the upper aerodigestive tract. They release saliva, which contains enzymes such as amylase that predigest dietary starches and fats. Salivary glands also produce electrolytes, mucus, glycoproteins, and antibacterial compounds that protect the teeth from bacterial decay, moisten food, and shield mucosal surfaces from desiccation.

Salivary glands are divided into minor and major types. Between 800 and 1000 minor salivary glands are located in the upper aerodigestive tract and paranasal sinuses. They are found in the oral mucosa, palate, and uvula. They are also found in the floor of the mouth, posterior tongue, retromolar area, peritonsillar area, pharynx, and larynx. A minor salivary gland may have a common excretory duct with another gland or its own excretory duct.

The three types of major salivary glands are the parotid glands, submandibular glands, and sublingual glands, which occur in pairs. A parotid gland is located in front of and just below each ear. A submandibular gland is located just below the midline of the mandible on the right and left, and the sublingual glands are located under the tongue in the floor of the mouth and anterior to the submandibular glands.

More than 50% of tumors found in salivary glands are not cancerous. The parotid gland is the largest salivary gland and accounts for 70% to 80% of salivary gland abnormal growths. The palate is the most common site of minor salivary gland abnormalities. The frequency of salivary gland malignancies varies according to location:

- Parotid gland: 20% to 25%
- Submandibular gland: 35% to 40%
- Palate: 50%
- Sublingual gland: more than 90% of sublingual growths

Incidence

- Malignancies of the major salivary glands are rare, accounting for less than 1% of cancers in the United States.
- Salivary gland cancers account for 0.5% of all malignancies and 3% to 5% of all head and neck malignancies.
- Most are diagnosed in the sixth to seventh decades of life.

Etiology and Risk Factors

- Little information is available about the cause of malignant salivary gland tumors, but several factors are associated with increased risk:
  - Increased age
  - Exposure to ionizing radiation
  - Prior treatment for a head or neck malignancy
  - Tobacco use for squamous cell cancer but not for other salivary gland tumor types
  - Diet high in animal fat and low in vegetables
  - Occupational exposure to rubber products during manufacturing, asbestos mining, plumbing, and some types of woodworking

Signs and Symptoms

- Painless swelling of the parotid, submandibular, or sublingual glands
- Numbness or weakness in the face
- Persistent facial pain

Diagnostic Work-up

- Physical examination and medical history
- Imaging studies: MRI, CT, PET, or ultrasonography
- Flexible fiberoptic endoscopy of the upper aerodigestive tract
- Biopsy of suspicious lesions
- FNA of suspicious lesions or adenopathy

Histology

- Classification is complicated because there are more than 20 histologic subtypes of major and minor salivary gland malignancies, and similar histologic types can exist in the same tissue sample.
- Although salivary gland neoplasms are histologically diverse, the more common types of carcinomas include the following:
  - Mucoepidermoid carcinoma (i.e., most common malignant major and minor salivary gland tumor)
  - Adenoid cystic carcinoma
  - Adenocarcinoma
  - Malignant mixed tumors
  - Carcinoma ex pleomorphic adenoma (i.e., high-grade malignant epithelial neoplasm arising in a preexisting benign mixed tumor)

Histologic grading of salivary gland carcinomas aids in determining treatment. Grading is used primarily for mucoepidermoid carcinomas, adenocarcinomas not otherwise specified, adenoid cystic carcinomas, and squamous cell carcinomas. In most instances, the histologic type defines the grade (i.e., salivary duct carcinoma is high grade, and basal cell adenocarcinoma is low grade).

Clinical Staging

Various other salivary gland carcinomas can also be categorized according to histologic grade. Staging is done according to the AJCC TNM classification system (Edge, et al., 2010).

Treatment

- Salivary gland tumors may be cured with surgery alone.
- The cure rate depends on stage, histology, and grade of the tumor.
- Pathologic findings such as perineural invasion, vascular invasion, and extracapulslar spread dictate the need for adjuvant treatment.
- Surgical resection with postoperative adjuvant radiation therapy is done for the following:
  - Large, bulky tumors or high-grade tumors
  - Lymph node involvement
  - When adequate clear margins cannot be achieved by surgical resection
- Neutron beam radiation is more effective than conventional x-ray radiotherapy.
- Primary irradiation for palliative therapy may be given for inoperable, unresectable, or recurrent tumors.
- Fast neutron beam radiation therapy and accelerated hyperfractionated photon beam radiation therapy are more effective than conventional x-ray radiation therapy.
- Patients with stage IV salivary gland cancer should be considered for clinical trials. Their cancers may be responsive to aggressive combinations of chemotherapy and irradiation.
- Single-agent or combination chemotherapy with doxorubicin, cisplatin, cyclophosphamide, and 5-FU produces modest response rates.

Prognosis

Overall, about 72% of people diagnosed with salivary gland cancer are alive at least 5 years after diagnosis. Several factors impact prognosis:

- Salivary gland of origin
- Histologic features
- Grade
- Stage
- Involvement of the facial nerve
- Fixation to the skin or deep structures
- Spread to the lymph nodes or distant sites

Clinical stage, particularly tumor size, may be the crucial factor for determining treatment outcome, as it is for other head and neck cancers. Early-stage, low-grade malignant salivary gland tumors are usually curable with adequate surgical resection.

The prognosis is more favorable for major salivary gland tumors. Tumors of the parotid gland have the most favorable prognosis, followed by those of the submandibular gland. The least favorable sites are the sublingual and minor salivary glands.

Prevention and Surveillance

Because the cause of salivary gland malignancies is not understood, no specific recommendations for prevention are available. However, avoiding risk factors may have some effect.

Bibliography

American Cancer Society. (2014). *What is salivary gland cancer?* Available at http://www.cancer.org/cancer/salivaryglandcancer/detailedguide/salivary-gland-cancer-what-is-cancer (accessed December 20, 2015).

Boukheris, H., Curtis, R. E., Land, C. E., & Dores, G. M. (2009). Incidence of carcinoma of the major salivary glands according to the World Health Organization (WHO) classification, 1992–2006: A population-based study in the United States. *Cancer Epidemiology, Biomarkers & Prevention, 18*(11), 2899–2906.

Edge, S. B., Byrd, D. R., Compton, C. C., Fritz, A. G., Greene, F. L., & Trotti, A. (Eds.). (2010). *AJCC cancer staging manual* (7th ed., pp. 79–86). New York, NY: Springer.

National Cancer Institute. (2014). *Salivary gland cancer treatment—For health professionals (PDQ): Stage information for salivary gland cancer.* Available at http://www.cancer.gov/types/head-and-neck/hp/salivary-gland-treatment-pdq#link/_13 (accessed December 20, 2015).

Thyroid and Parathyroid Tumors

Definition

Thyroid carcinoma is the most common endocrine malignancy and the ninth most common carcinoma overall. The thyroid gland is located in the base of the neck on both sides of the lower part of the larynx and upper part of the trachea. The thyroid gland is a butterfly-shaped gland that consists of two lateral lobes connected by an isthmus composed of many follicles containing colloid, which contains an iodine-containing protein known as thyroglobulin. Thyroglobulin is converted into several active factors, including thyroxin.

The parathyroid glands secrete a substance known as *parathormone,* which regulates calcium and phosphorus metabolism. The four to six parathyroid glands are usually located on the inferior and superior poles of each thyroid lobe on the posterior surface. Each is about the size of a grain of rice (3 to 5 mm) and weighs between 30 and 60 mg.

Incidence

Thyroid Cancer

- In 2015, about 62,450 new cases of thyroid cancer and 1950 related deaths occurred in the United States.
- Based on 2008 to 2012 data, the annual incidence of thyroid cancer is 13.5 new cases per 100,000 men and women.
- It occurs three times more often among women than men.
- Most people are diagnosed between the ages of 45 and 54 years (median age, 50 years).

Parathyroid Cancer

Parathyroid carcinoma is rare. It occurs in 1% of individuals diagnosed with hyperparathyroidism.

Etiology and Risk Factors

Irradiation of the neck increases the risk of thyroid cancer. Historically, irradiation was used for the treatment of benign conditions such as tonsillitis, acne, and an enlarged thymus to a dose of 800 to 1200 cGy. Lower doses appear to cause more mutagenesis than the higher doses given for tumors.

Several other factors increase risk:
- Benign thyroid disease (e.g., goiter), which is more common in middle age
- Asian ancestry
- Female sex
- Multiple endocrine neoplasia (MEN)
  - A family history of medullary carcinoma of the thyroid increases the risk for patients with MEN type 1 or 2. A mutation in the *RET* proto-oncogene has been identified in the familial form of medullary thyroid cancer.
  - In families with cases of MEN, screening for this mutation can be done as early as 5 or 6 years of age, and those testing positive are considered candidates for a prophylactic total thyroidectomy.
  - MEN1 and MEN2 are disorders with an autosomal dominant pattern of inheritance. The genetic deficits produce hyperplasia or malignant tumors in several endocrine glands.
  - In MEN1, tumors occur in the parathyroids, pancreatic islet cells, adrenal cortex, and thyroid.
  - In MEN2, neoplasms include medullary thyroid cancer, pheochromocytoma, and parathyroid hyperplasia.

Signs and Symptoms

Thyroid Cancer
- Solitary thyroid mass
- Diffuse enlargement of the thyroid
- Voice changes
- Dysphagia
- Vocal cord immobility
- Enlarged neck node or mass

Parathyroid Cancer
- Hypercalcemia
- Fatigue
- Weight loss
- Forgetfulness
- Renal stones
- Low phosphorus levels
- High parathyroid hormone (PTH) serum levels

Diagnostic Work-up

Thyroid Cancer
- FNA of thyroid nodules
- Thyroid imaging: ultrasound, CT, MRI, or PET
- Laboratory tests: thyroid function, including triiodothyronine (T_3), thyroxine (T_4), thyroid-stimulating hormone (TSH), and thyroglobulin levels
- Flexible fiberoptic laryngoscopy to assess vocal cord function

Parathyroid Cancer

- Laboratory tests: calcium, parathyroid hormone, phosphorus, magnesium, and vitamin D levels
- Bone densitometry: Dual-energy x-ray absorptiometry is used to measure bone loss caused by conditions such as hyperparathyroidism.
- Sestamibi parathyroid scintigraphy: A small amount of radioactive material (technetium 99m) is given intravenously. If the parathyroid is overactive, ^{99m}Tc collects in the abnormal gland and is identified on the scan.
- Single-photon emission computed tomography (SPECT) imaging): In this type of CT scan, a small amount of radioactive material is injected, and a specialized scanner is used to obtain images of areas where the radioactive material is taken up by the cells. SPECT imaging can give information about blood flow to tissues and chemical reactions (e.g., metabolism) in the body.

Histology

Thyroid Cancer

There are four types of thyroid cancers: papillary, follicular, medullary, and anaplastic.

- *Papillary carcinoma* is the most common, accounting for 70% of thyroid cancers. The primary tumors are often multicentric and can metastasize to lymph nodes.
- *Follicular carcinoma*, which has a high likelihood of vascular spread and distant metastases, accounts for about 15% of thyroid cancers. Hürthle cell tumors are carcinomas consisting of oncocytic cells in the thyroid. Although considered a variant of follicular tumors, they carry a worse prognosis.
- *Medullary thyroid cancer* accounts for 5% to 8% of thyroid cancers. The tumors can manifest in a sporadic or familial form and arise from parafollicular (C) cells, which produce calcitonin.
- *Anaplastic (undifferentiated) thyroid cancer* accounts for only 0.5% to 1.5% of thyroid cancers, but the tumors are the most aggressive type and often are diagnosed with lymph node and distant metastases. The 5-year relative survival rate for anaplastic carcinoma is about 7%.

For clinical management, thyroid cancer usually is divided into two categories: well differentiated or poorly differentiated. The most common malignant tumors of the thyroid are well differentiated and include papillary, follicular, mixed, and Hürthle cell tumors.

Parathyroid Cancer

Histologic criteria for parathyroid carcinoma are difficult to define. The distinction between benign and malignant parathyroid tumors is rarely made on the initial histologic analysis.

- A malignant parathyroid gland tumor is firm, white-gray, and diffusely invasive.
- A nonmalignant lesion, such as a parathyroid adenoma, usually manifests as a red-brown mass that is soft, mobile, and noninvasive.

- Pathologic confirmation is determined by the frequency of mitoses, fibrosis, local invasion, vascular invasion, and nuclear pleomorphism.

Clinical Staging

Thyroid Cancer

The AJCC TNM classification system is used to stage thyroid cancer. Staging mostly depends on tumor type. For patients with papillary and follicular tumors, stage depends on age. Patients younger than 45 years of age at diagnosis are considered to have stage I or II disease, regardless of tumor size, nodal involvement, or metastatic disease. Clinical stage for patients 45 years of age or older and all those with medullary cancer is determined by the TNM classification system (Edge, et al., 2010).

Parathyroid Cancer

The staging system for parathyroid carcinoma was developed by Shaha and Shah in 1999 and uses TNM classification (Shaha & Shah, 1999).

Treatment

- The primary treatment for thyroid and parathyroid cancer is surgery. The parathyroid glands are not easily located, although the use of scan-guided surgery and quick PTH assays can aid surgery.
- Patients with poor prognostic factors may benefit from central neck dissection.
- The most common adjuvant therapy for thyroid cancer is radioactive iodine (^{131}I).
- External beam radiotherapy may be used for extensive nodal or mediastinal disease, for gross residual tumor after surgery, or for the management of bone or brain metastases.
- Chemotherapy has not played a significant role in treating well-differentiated tumors and is usually reserved for anaplastic tumors with metastatic disease.
- Targeted therapies for medullary thyroid cancer are being investigated.
  - Vandetanib (Caprelsa), a kinase inhibitor, is FDA approved for the treatment of metastatic medullary thyroid cancer in patients with symptomatic or progressive disease.
- In papillary thyroid cancer, the use of kinase inhibitors can help block the formation of new blood vessels and proteins that promote tumor growth.

Prognosis

Thyroid Cancer

- Overall survival depends on age at diagnosis and on tumor stage and histology. Age is the single most important prognostic factor in determining prognosis.
- Patients with localized, differentiated disease have a 5-year survival rate of 99.9%.
- Patients who are younger than 40 years old with differentiated carcinomas without extracapsular extension or vascular invasion have a more favorable prognosis.
- Lymph node status tends to be controversial in determining prognosis.

- Several factors contribute to a poorer prognosis for differentiated carcinomas:
  - Patients older than 45 years of age
  - Follicular histology
  - Primary tumor larger than 4 cm (T2 or T3)
  - Extrathyroidal extension (T4)
  - Distant metastases
- Some studies have shown that regional lymph node disease has no effect on survival rates.
- The 5-year relative survival rate for anaplastic (undifferentiated) carcinoma is about 7%.

Parathyroid Cancer

- Because parathyroid cancer is a rare disease, data are limited.
- Approximately 40% to 60% of patients with surgical excision of parathyroid malignancies have postsurgical recurrences, typically 2 to 5 years after the initial resection.
- The 5-year survival rate is 50% to 70%, but many patients die after 5 years. In one large series reporting results for a 43-year series, the median survival time was longer than 14 years.

Prevention and Surveillance

- There are no specific prevention measures.
- Genetic testing and counseling should be done for individuals with a family history of medullary cancer.
- Prophylactic thyroidectomy may be indicated for those with a family history of medullary cancer. Patients should be closely monitored to ensure an early diagnosis.

Bibliography

American Cancer Society. (2014). *Can thyroid cancer be prevented?* Available at http://www.cancer.org/cancer/thyroidcancer/detailedguide/thyroid-cancer-prevention (accessed December 20, 2015).

American Cancer Society. (2014). *Thyroid cancer survival by type and stage.* Available at http://www.cancer.org/cancer/thyroidcancer/detailedguide/thyroid-cancer-survival-rates (accessed December 20, 2015).

American Cancer Society. (2015). *Targeted therapy for thyroid cancer.* Available at http://www.cancer.org/cancer/thyroidcancer/detailedguide/thyroid-cancer-treating-targeted-therapy (accessed December 20, 2015).

Dadu, R., Ahn, P., Holsinger, C., & Hu, M. (2014). *Thyroid and parathyroid cancers.* Available at http://www.cancernetwork.com/cancer-management/thyroid-and-parathyroid-cancers (accessed December 20, 2015).

Edge, S. B., Byrd, D. R., Compton, C. C., Fritz, A. G., Greene, F. L., & Trotti, A. (Eds.). (2010). *AJCC cancer staging manual* (7th ed.). New York, NY: Springer.

Harari, A., Waring, A., Fernandez-Ranvier, G., Hwang, J., Suh, I., Mitmaker, E., et al, (2011). Parathyroid carcinoma: A 43-year outcome and survival analysis. *Journal of Clinical Endocrinology and Metabolism, 96*(12), 3679–3686.

Kim, L. (2013). Parathyroid carcinoma follow-up. In L. Kim. *Parathyroid carcinoma.* Available at http://emedicine.medscape.com/article/280908-followup#e7 (accessed December 20, 2015).

Marcocci, C., Cetani, F., Rubin, M. R., Silverberg, S. J., Pinchera, A., & Bilezikian, J. P. (2008). Review: Parathyroid carcinoma. *Journal of Bone and Mineral Research, 23*(12).

National Cancer Institute. SEER stat fact sheets. Larynx cancer. Available at http://seer.cancer.gov/statfacts/html/laryn.html (accessed December 20, 2015).

National Cancer Institute. (2013). *Thyroid cancer treatment—For health professionals (PDQ).* Available at http://www.cancer.gov/cancertopics/pdq/treatment/thyroid/HealthProfessional (accessed December 20, 2015).

Norton, J. A. (2001). Neoplasms of the endocrine system. In J. M. Bland, J. M. Daly, & C. P. Karakousis. *Surgical oncology: Contemporary principles and practice* (pp. 1055–1067). New York, NY: McGraw-Hill.

Shaha, A. R., & Shah, J. P. (1999). Parathyroid carcinoma: A diagnostic and therapeutic challenge. *Cancer, 86*(3), 378–380.

University of Michigan Health System. (2014). *Parathyroid surgery.* Available at http://www.uofmhealth.org/conditions-treatments/parathroid-surgery-0 (accessed December 20, 2015).

Leukemias

Kristen Hurley

Acute Lymphocytic Leukemia

Definition

Leukemias are malignant neoplasms that can occur across the life span. It is characterized by the production of increased numbers of immature leukocytes from the bone marrow and other blood-forming organs. These abnormal precursors proliferate and infiltrate the bone marrow, peripheral blood, and other organs suppressing the production of normal, mature cells.

Four types of leukemias are classified according to their cell type (i.e., lymphoid or myeloid) and whether they are acute or chronic. Acute leukemias are characterized by blocked lymphoid or myeloid progenitor cell differentiation, which results in massive accumulation of immature cells or blasts; onset is acute.

Acute lymphocytic leukemia (ALL), also called *acute lymphoblastic leukemia,* is a cancer of lymphoblasts. Eighty-five percent of ALL patients have the B-cell subtype, and 15% of patients are diagnosed with the T-cell subtype.

Incidence

- An estimated 6250 new cases of ALL (3100 males, 3150 females) and 1450 deaths (800 males, 650 females) occurred in 2015 in the United States.
- ALL is the most common form of leukemia in children younger than 19 years of age. The risk (1 in 750) is low for adults, but 80% of ALL-related deaths occur among adults.
- Children account for more than 30% of new cases of ALL.
- The incidence for children aged 1 to 4 years is more than nine times the rate for young adults between the ages of 20 and 24 years.
- More males than females have ALL.
- ALL is more common among whites and Hispanics compared with other racial or ethnic groups.

Etiology and Risk Factors

- Radiation exposure is linked to the development of ALL, although this has been demonstrated only in Japanese atomic bomb survivors.
- An increased risk of ALL is associated with some genetic conditions, including Down syndrome, Klinefelter syndrome, Fanconi anemia, Bloom syndrome, ataxia-telangiectasia, and neurofibromatosis.
- Cytogenetic abnormalities are found, indicating the involvement of oncogenes such as *RAS, BCR/ABL,* and *BCL2.*
- Prior treatment with intensive immunosuppressive therapies is a risk factor.

Signs and Symptoms

- Signs and symptoms (usually manifest abruptly)
  - Malaise
  - Fatigue
  - Bony pain (especially sternal)
  - Sweats
  - Bleeding, easy bruising
- Physical findings
  - Pallor
  - Petechiae
  - Ecchymoses
  - Lymphadenopathy
  - Splenomegaly
  - Hepatomegaly
  - Mediastinal mass (usually a T-cell subtype)
  - Abdominal adenopathy (Burkitt type)

Diagnostic Work-up

- Medical history and physical examination
- Complete blood cell count (CBC) with differential count
  - Pancytopenia resulting from marrow replacement by tumor may be identified.
  - Two thirds of patients have a white blood cell (WBC) count greater than $100,000/mm^3$.
  - Ten percent of ALL patients have a normal WBC count.
- Serum chemistry panel: elevated lactate dehydrogenase and uric acid levels correlate with a large tumor burden.
- Cytogenetic analysis
  - Analysis permits identification of chromosomal and genetic abnormalities.
  - The t(9;22) transposition, called the *Philadelphia (Ph) chromosome,* is the most common abnormality in adult ALL, occurring in 17% to 25% of cases.
  - The t(11q23) MLL is associated with poor prognosis found in adults and children <1 yr.
  - The t(12;21)(p12;q22) TEL/AML1 is associated with a good prognosis in children.
- Immunophenotyping enables the physician to determine the type of disease.
- Bone marrow aspiration to remove marrow fluid or a biopsy to remove a marrow sample is done to diagnose leukemic abnormalities.

- Lumbar puncture is done to identify malignant cells in the cerebrospinal fluid.
- A chest radiograph is obtained to determine whether leukemia cells have formed a mass in the chest. Plain film findings also help to distinguish early-stage ALL from other diseases such as juvenile idiopathic arthritis.

Histology

- Peripheral blood smear showing small lymphoblasts with scant cytoplasm, condensed nuclear chromatin, and indistinct nucleoli. Cytoplasmic granules may be present. There will not be Auer rods.
- In tissue sections, small to medium-sized tumor cells with scant cytoplasm; round, oval, or convoluted nuclei; fine chromatin; and indistinct small nucleoli. Antibody stains by flow cytometry are important. There will be expression of B-cell markers CD19, CD22, CD20, CD79a, CD45, and CD10.
- Additional antigens may define stages of differentiation from earliest to latest. Early precursors B$^-$ Membrane CD19$^+$, CD79a$^+$ and cytoplasmic CD22$^+$
- Common ALL-positive for CD10
- Late Pre B AA: positive for CD20.
- There may be coexpression of myeloid antigens in up to 30% of cases, most common are CD13 and CD33.

Clinical Staging

No clinical staging is performed for ALL.

Treatment

- The three phases of treatment for ALL usually require 1.5 to 3 years.
- Phase I is induction (i.e., remission induction) which typically requires hospitalization for approximately 4 weeks.
  - Many agents may be used.
    - Prednisone
    - Vincristine
    - Anthracycline
    - Asparaginase
    - Cyclophosphamide
    - Etoposide
    - Methotrexate
    - Cytarabine
    - Imatinib (for Ph chromosome–positive disease)
  - Complete response rates range from 60% to 90% with these induction regimens.
- Phase II is consolidation (i.e., intensification).
  - Patients must be in remission to begin the consolidation phase.
  - Typically lasts 1 to 3 months.
  - Many of the same agents administered during the induction phase are also used during consolidation.
  - High-risk patients may be considered for allogeneic stem cell or autologous stem cell transplantation.
- Phase III is maintenance.
  - It lasts approximately 2 years.
  - Several agents may be used.
    - Methotrexate
    - 6-Mercaptopurine (6-MP)
    - Vincristine
    - Prednisone
- Central nervous system prophylaxis is typically completed during the induction phase but may extend throughout therapy. Several agents are used.
  - Methotrexate
  - Hydrocortisone
  - Cytarabine
  - Cranial or spinal irradiation
  - High-dose intravenous methotrexate
- Patients who have relapsed after induction chemotherapy or maintenance therapy are unlikely to be cured by further chemotherapy alone.
  - Blinatumomab, which was approved in 2014, is a bispecific, CD19-directed, CD3 T-cell engager immunotherapy for use in relapsed and refractory Ph chromosome–negative B-cell ALL.
  - Reinduction chemotherapy followed by allogeneic bone marrow transplantation should be considered. For patients who do not have a human leukocyte antigen (HLA)-matched donor and may be considered for an unrelated stem cell or bone marrow transplantation.
  - Clinical trials should also be considered.

Prognosis

- Overall 5-year survival rates:
  - Adults: 67.5% according to the Surveillance, Epidemiology, and End Results (SEER) database for 2005 to 2011
  - Children and adolescents: 90.4% for 2000 to 2005 according to a report from the Children's Oncology Group
- Long-term follow-up of 30 patients with ALL in remission for at least 10 years identified 10 cases of secondary malignancies.
- Of 31 long-term, female survivors of ALL or acute myeloid leukemia younger than 40 years of age, 26 resumed normal menstruation after completion of therapy. Among 36 live offspring of survivors, two congenital problems occurred.

Prevention and Surveillance

There are no known preventive measures for ALL. The National Comprehensive Cancer Network (NCCN) guidelines for 2015 recommend close surveillance after completion of therapy.

- Year 1: every 1 to 2 months
  - Physical examination with CBC, differential count, and liver function tests
  - Bone marrow and cerebrospinal fluid evaluation and echocardiogram as indicated
- Year 2: every 3 months
  - Physical examination (including a testicular examination), CBC, and differential count
- Year 3: every 6 months
  - Physical examination (including a testicular examination), CBC, and differential count

- Survivorship recommendations
  - Human papillomavirus (HPV) vaccine for men and women 9 to 26 years old
  - Annual influenza vaccination
  - Dental examination and cleaning every 6 months
- Additional recommendations for children and young adults to screen for secondary malignancies are described in the table below.

Screening Recommendations for Children and Young Adults

Treatment Exposures	Recommendations
Cranial or spinal radiation	Neuroendocrine dysfunction screening
	Neuropsychological evaluation
Chest radiation	Females: breast cancer screening
	Thyroid screening
	Cardiovascular risk assessment and screening, including screening for cardiomyopathy and valvular heart disease
	Pulmonary screening
Abdominal or pelvic radiation	Colorectal cancer screening
	Gonadal function assessment
	Kidney and bladder function monitoring
Alkylating agents	Gonadal function assessment
	Pulmonary status monitoring
	Therapy-related acute myeloid leukemia (t-AML) or myelodysplasia screening
Anthracyclines	Cardiovascular function monitoring
	t-AML or myelodysplasia screening
Bleomycin	Pulmonary function monitoring
Cisplatin or carboplatin	Cardiovascular function monitoring
	Kidney and bladder function monitoring
	Hearing evaluation
	t-AML or myelodysplasia screening

Modified from National Comprehensive Cancer Network (2015). NCCN guidelines for adolescent and young adult, version 1.2016. Available at http://www.nccn.org/professionals/physician_gls/pdf/aya.pdf (accessed January 3, 2016).

Bibliography

American Cancer Society. (2014). *Leukemia—acute lymphocytic.* Available at http://www.cancer.org (accessed January 3, 2016).

Food and Drug Administration (FDA). (2014). *Blinatumomab.* Available at http://www.fda.gov/Drugs/InformationOnDrugs/ApprovedDrugs/ucm425597.htm (accessed January 3, 2016).

Hunger, S. P., Lu, X., Devidas, M., Camitta, B. M., Gaynon, P. S., Winick, N. J., Reaman, & Carrol, W. L. (2012). Improved survival for children and adolescents with acute lymphoblastic leukemia between 1990 and 2005: A report from the Children's Oncology Group. *Journal of Clinical Oncology, 30*(14), 1663–1669.

Leukemia and Lymphoma Society. (2015). *Acute lymphocytic leukemia.* Available at http://www.leukemia-lymphoma.org (accessed January 3, 2016).

National Cancer Institute. (2015). *Adult acute lymphoblastic leukemia (PDQ).* Available at http://www.cancer.gov/cancertopics/pdq/treatment/adultALL/HealthProfessional (accessed January 3, 2016).

National Cancer Institute. (2015). *SEER stat fact sheets: Acute lymphocytic leukemia (ALL).* Available at http://seer.cancer.gov/statfacts/html/alyl.html (accessed January 3, 2016).

National Comprehensive Cancer Network. (2015). *NCCN clinical practice guidelines for acute lymphocytic leukemia, version 2.2015.* Available at http://www.nccn.org/professionals/physician_gls/pdf/all.pdf (accessed January 3, 2016).

National Comprehensive Cancer Network. (2015). *NCCN guidelines for adolescent and young adult, version 1.2016.* Available at http://www.nccn.org/professionals/physician_gls/pdf/aya.pdf (accessed January 3, 2016).

Acute Myelogenous Leukemia

Definition

Acute myelogenous leukemia (AML), also called *acute myeloid leukemia,* is a disease in which there are too many myeloid progenitor cells (i.e., immature granulocytes or monocytes) in the blood and bone marrow. Most cases of AML are distinguished from other blood disorders such as myelodysplastic syndrome by the finding of more than 20% blasts in the blood and bone marrow.

AML results from the failure of the myeloid progenitor cells to mature. The mechanism causing arrest of cell maturation is not fully understood, but it involves the activation of abnormal genes through chromosomal translocations, deletions, duplications, or substitutions and genetic mutations leading to overexpression or underexpression of one or more proteins. Developmental arrest markedly decreases the production of normal blood cells, resulting in various degrees of anemia, thrombocytopenia, and neutropenia. The immature cells (i.e., blasts) accumulate in the blood, bone marrow, liver, and spleen as a result of their rapid proliferation and the reduction in apoptosis (i.e., programmed cell death).

Incidence

- An estimated 20,830 new cases of AML (more than 90% diagnosed in adults) and 10,460 deaths occurred in the United States in 2015.
- AML affects all age groups; the median age at diagnosis is 67 years.
- Prevalence increases with age. AML is the most common leukemia type in people between the ages of 75 and 84 years.
- AML is more common among whites than other groups.
- AML is more common in men than women, particularly among older patients.

Etiology and Risk Factors

- Compared with other leukemias, increased risk of AML has the strongest link to prior radiation, cytotoxic chemotherapy, and toxin exposure.
- Radiation exposure increases the risk, as seen in patients exposed to the atomic bomb explosion in Japan, in early radiologists (before appropriate shielding), and in patients irradiated for ankylosing spondylitis.
- Prior chemotherapy, particularly with alkylating agents and topoisomerase II inhibitors, increases the risk of AML.
- The period between an exposure and evidence of acute leukemia is approximately 3 to 5 years for alkylating agents or radiation exposure but only 9 to 12 months for topoisomerase II inhibitors.
- About 20% of AML cases are related to tobacco use.
- The most common risk factor is an antecedent hematologic disorder, usually high-risk myelodysplastic syndrome.
- Congenital disorders can result in AML during childhood, although some cases may develop in adulthood.

- Bloom syndrome, Down syndrome, congenital neutropenia, Fanconi anemia, and neurofibromatosis are risk factors.
- Risk increases tenfold between 30 and 70 years of age.

Signs and Symptoms

- Presenting symptoms are related to bone marrow failure, including anemia, neutropenia, thrombocytopenia, and organ infiltration with leukemic cells.
- Common sites include the spleen, liver, and gums. Organ infiltration occurs most commonly in patients with monocytic subtypes.
- Patient complaints
  - Fatigue
  - Weakness
  - Shortness of breath
  - Weight loss
  - Fever
  - Bleeding and easy bruising
  - Early satiety and fullness in right upper quadrant from splenomegaly
  - Bone pain resulting from a high leukemic cell burden and increased pressure in the marrow
  - Respiratory distress and altered mental status from leukostasis, which is a medical emergency that requires immediate treatment
- Physical findings
  - Pallor
  - Petechiae or ecchymoses
  - Hepatosplenomegaly
  - Signs of infection, including pneumonia
  - Gingivitis
  - Rash resulting from skin infiltration

Diagnostic Work-up

- Medical history and physical examination
- Laboratory tests
  - CBC with differential count
  - Serum chemistry panel; elevated lactate dehydrogenase and uric acid levels correlate with a large tumor burden.
  - Cytogenetics for identification of chromosomal or genetic abnormalities
- Additional studies
  - Bone marrow aspirate or biopsy
  - Immunophenotyping to determine the type of proteins (e.g., mutated FLT3 receptor) expressed by cells through identification of antigens on the cell surface and the corresponding antibodies produced by the body
  - Imaging studies such as chest radiography

Histology

- The AML subtype helps to determine the prognosis and suggests treatment implications. However, the treatment is similar for all subtypes.
- The older French-American-British (FAB) classification of AML was revised by the World Health Organization (WHO) to incorporate and interrelate morphology, cytogenetics, molecular genetics, and immunologic markers and

construct a classification system that is universally applicable and prognostically valid.
- Elements of the FAB classification that were specific to disease morphology have been retained. The WHO classification is outlined in the box below.

World Health Organization Classification of Acute Myelogenous Leukemia

- AML with characteristic genetic abnormalities
  - AML with t(8;21)(q22;q22) (AML/ETO)
  - AML with inv(16)(p13;q22) or t(16;16)(p13;q22) (CBFB/MYH11)
  - Acute promyelocytic leukemia–AML with t(15;17)(q22;q12) (PML/RARA) and variants
  - AML with 11q23 (MLL) abnormalities
  - AML with FLT3 mutations
- AML with multilineage dysplasia after myelodysplastic syndrome (>20% blasts in the blood or bone marrow), defined by the FAB MDS criterion as refractory anemia with excess blasts in transformation (RAEB-t)
- AML and MDS, therapy related
  - Alkylating agent–related AML and MDS
  - Topoisomerase II inhibitor–related AML
- AML not otherwise categorized (morphology reflects the older FAB morphology-based classification with a few changes)
  - Acute myeloblastic leukemia, minimally differentiated (FAB classification M0)
  - Acute myeloblastic leukemia, without maturation (FAB classification M1)
  - Acute myeloblastic leukemia with maturation (FAB classification M2)
  - Acute myelomonocytic leukemia (FAB classification M4)
  - Acute monoblastic leukemia and acute monocytic leukemia (FAB classifications M5a and M5b)
  - Acute erythroid leukemias (FAB classifications M6a and M6b)
  - Acute megakaryoblastic leukemia (FAB classification M7)
- AML/transient myeloproliferative disorder in Down syndrome
  - Acute basophilic leukemia
  - Acute panmyelosis with myelofibrosis
  - Myeloid sarcoma
- Acute leukemias of ambiguous lineage

AML, Acute myelogenous leukemia; *MDS,* myelodysplastic syndrome; *FAB,* French-American-British classification.
Modified from National Cancer Institute. (2015). Adult acute myeloid leukemias: Treatment—for health professionals (PDQ). Available at http://www.cancer.gov/cancertopics/pdq/treatment/adultAML/healthprofessional (accessed January 3, 2016).

Clinical Staging

Clinical staging is not done for AML.

Treatment

- Treatment is delivered in two phases: induction to attain remission and postremission therapy to maintain the remission.
- Intensive consolidation therapy is effective when given immediately after remission or when delayed.

Induction Therapy

- The most common induction therapy is called *7 and 3;* three days of an anthracycline are combined with cytarabine (i.e., cytosine arabinoside [ara-C]) as a 24-hour infusion for 7 days.
  - Approximately 50% of patients achieve a remission with one course of therapy, and another 10% to 15% enter remission after the second course.

- High-dose ara-C combined with an anthracycline may be used as induction therapy in younger patients.
- Remission is defined as a normal peripheral blood cell count and normocellular marrow with less than 5% blasts in the marrow and no signs or symptoms of the disease.
- Most patients with AML who meet the remission criteria have residual leukemia, which has led to modification of the definition of complete remission to include cytogenetic remission and molecular remission.
  - Cytogenic remission is determined when a previously abnormal karyotype reverts to normal.
  - Molecular remission is determined when interphase fluorescence in situ hybridization (FISH) or multiparameter flow cytometry is used to detect minimal residual disease.
- Combined immunophenotyping and interphase FISH have greater prognostic significance than the conventional criteria for remission.

Postremission Therapy

- Postremission therapy is indicated when curative intent is the goal.
- Current postremission therapy or consolidation therapy includes the following:
  - Short-term, relatively intensive chemotherapy with cytarabine-based regimens
  - High-dose chemotherapy or chemoradiation therapy with autologous bone marrow rescue
  - High-dose, marrow-ablative therapy with allogeneic bone marrow rescue

Prognosis

- The overall 5-year survival rate for AML is 25.9% for adults. The highest death rates are among those 75 to 84 years of age, and the median age at time of death is 72 years.
- Nontransplantation consolidation therapy with cytarabine-containing regimens has treatment-related death rates that are usually less than 10% to 20%, and they have yielded disease-free survival rates of 20% to 50%.
- Allogeneic bone marrow transplantation results in the lowest incidence of leukemic relapse.
  - Disease-free survival rates with allogeneic transplantation in the first complete remission have ranged from 45% to 60%.
  - Use of allogeneic bone marrow transplantation as primary postremission therapy is limited by the need for a human leukocyte antigen (HLA)-matched sibling donor and the increased mortality rate from allogeneic bone marrow transplantation for patients who are older than 50 years of age.
  - The mortality rate from allogeneic bone marrow transplantation that uses an HLA-matched sibling donor ranges from 20% to 40%.
- Autologous bone marrow transplantation results in disease-free survival rates between 35% and 50% for patients with AML in first remission. This approach is limited due to concerns about persistent leukemia cells in the collected marrow.

Prevention and Surveillance

- The cause of AML is not fully understood, and specific measures to prevent AML have not been identified.
- Exposure to controllable risk factors such as toxins, radiation, and tobacco should be limited. Individuals with known exposures should be monitored, but most people who have known risk factors do not get leukemia.
- Surveillance after consolidation includes a CBC and platelet evaluation every 1 to 2 months for 2 years and then every 3 to 6 months for up to 5 years.

Bibliography

National Cancer Institute. (2015). *Adult acute myeloid leukemia: Treatment—for health professionals (PDQ)*. Available at http://www.cancer.gov/cancertopics/pdq/treatment/adultAML/healthprofessional (accessed January 3, 2016).

National Comprehensive Cancer Network. (2015). *NCCN clinical practice guidelines for acute myeloid leukemia, version 1.2015*. Available at http://www.nccn.org/professionals/physician_gls/pdf/aya.pdf (accessed January 3, 2016).

Vardiman, J., Harris, N., & Brunning, R. (2002). The World Health Organization (WHO) classification of the myeloid neoplasms. *Blood, 100*, 2292–2302.

Chronic Lymphocytic Leukemia

Definition

Chronic lymphocytic leukemia (CLL), an indolent cancer of the B cells, is the most common type of leukemia. It is characterized by lymphocytosis, lymphadenopathy, and splenomegaly. It results from an acquired injury to the deoxyribonucleic acid (DNA) of a lymphocyte in the bone marrow, causing uncontrolled growth of CLL cells in the marrow and increasing their concentration in the blood. Lymphocyte counts are usually greater than 5000/mm³, and cells have a characteristic immunophenotype (i.e., CD5- and CD23-positive B cells).

CLL cells in the marrow do not impede normal blood cell production to the extent that ALL cells do. This important distinction from acute leukemia accounts for the less severe early course of the disease.

Incidence

- An estimated 14,620 new cases of CLL and 4650 deaths occurred in the United States in 2015.
- CLL affects middle-aged or elderly adults.
  - Median age at diagnosis is 71 years.
  - Most CLL patients are more than 55 years old.
  - CLL rarely affects children.
- CLL affects whites more often than African Americans and men more often than women.
- The lifetime risk for CLL is 1 in 200.

Etiology and Risk Factors

- It is not understood what induces the change in lymphocyte DNA.
- Risk factors include the following:
  - Smoking

- Long-term exposure to herbicides or pesticides (e.g., Agent Orange during the Vietnam War)
- Increasing age
- Family history of CLL or cancer of the lymphatic system
- Russian or Eastern European Jewish descent

Signs and Symptoms

- Symptoms usually exist with advanced disease.
- Diagnosis is typically made during routine blood work.
- Presenting symptoms
  - Fatigue
  - Shortness of breath with exertion
  - Weight loss
  - Night sweats
  - Frequent infections of the skin, lungs, kidneys, or other sites
- Physical findings
  - Ecchymosis
  - Lymphadenopathy
  - Splenomegaly

Diagnostic Work-up

- Medical history and physical examination
- Laboratory tests
  - CBC with differential count
    - Anemia is found in 35% of patients.
    - Thrombocytopenia is found in 25% of patients.
  - Serum chemistry panel shows elevated lactate dehydrogenase and uric acid levels that correlate with a large tumor burden.
  - Evaluation of immunoglobulins (i.e., γ-globulins); CLL patients may not have enough of these proteins, which may lead to repeated infections.
  - Cytogenetics for identification of chromosomal or genetic abnormalities
  - FISH to evaluate chromosome changes and to monitor response to treatment
  - Immunophenotyping (i.e., flow cytometry) to identify whether the CLL began with a B lymphocyte or T lymphocyte; B-cell CLL is the most common form.
- Additional studies
  - Bone marrow aspirate or biopsy
  - Histochemical staining on sample
- Imaging studies
  - Chest radiography
  - Computed tomography (CT)
  - Magnetic resonance imaging (MRI)

Histology

- The leukemic cell is a small lymphocyte with a round nucleus, clumped chromatin and discrete nucleolus.
- The majority of leukemic cells are B cell. The T-cell variant is difficult to identify in marrow morphology alone.
- Bone marrow is hypercellular with nodules of neoplastic cells; the bone marrow becomes more filled as the leukemia progresses.

Clinical Staging

- Staging is useful to predict prognosis and to stratify patients for treatment.
- Anemia and thrombocytopenia are the major adverse prognostic variables.

There is no standard staging system for CLL. The table below outlines the Rai staging system and the Binet classification.

Staging of Chronic Lymphocytic Leukemia

Rai Staging System

Stage 0	Absolute lymphocytosis ($>15,000/mm^3$) without adenopathy, hepatosplenomegaly, anemia, or thrombocytopenia
Stage I	Absolute lymphocytosis with lymphadenopathy without hepatosplenomegaly, anemia, or thrombocytopenia
Stage II	Absolute lymphocytosis with hepatomegaly or splenomegaly, with or without lymphadenopathy
Stage III	Absolute lymphocytosis and anemia (hemoglobin <11 g/dL) with or without lymphadenopathy, hepatomegaly, or splenomegaly
Stage IV	Absolute lymphocytosis and thrombocytopenia ($<100,000/mm^3$) with or without lymphadenopathy, hepatomegaly, splenomegaly, or anemia

Binet Classification

Clinical stage A	No anemia or thrombocytopenia and <3 areas of lymphoid involvement
Clinical stage B	No anemia or thrombocytopenia with ≥3 areas of lymphoid involvement
Clinical stage C	Anemia and/or thrombocytopenia regardless of the number of areas of lymphoid enlargement

Modified from National Cancer Institute. (2015). Chronic lymphocytic leukemia: Treatment—for health professionals (PDQ). Available at http://www.cancer.gov/cancertopics/pdq/treatment/CLL/healthprofessional (accessed January 3, 2016).

Treatment

- CLL typically occurs in elderly patients, progresses slowly, and usually is not curable; therefore, treatment is usually conservative.
- Treatment should be individualized and based on the clinical behavior of the disease.
- Treatment decisions depend on the patient's functional status, symptoms, prognostic factors, stage of disease, disease recurrence, and response to prior therapies.
- Treatment may range from watchful waiting to treatment for complications as needed with a variety of therapeutic options, including steroids; chemotherapy with alkylating agents, purine analogs, or combinations; monoclonal antibodies; radiation; or transplantation.
- In asymptomatic patients, treatment may be deferred until the patient becomes symptomatic.
- The rate of disease progression is patient specific, and there may be long periods of stable disease and sometimes spontaneous regressions; frequent and careful observation is required to monitor the clinical course.
- In 2014, newer agents targeting Bruton tyrosine kinase (BTK) and phosphatidylinositol 3-kinase (PI3K) showed improvements in treating relapsed CLL patients.
  - Clinical trials were able to demonstrate improvements in response rates in up to 95% and increased survival

with ibrutinib for BTK-related disease in combination with rituximab.

- In the clinical trial of idelalisib for PI3K-related disease, 93% of patients in the idelalisib plus rituximab arm had improvement in their cancers compared with 43% of patients in the placebo plus rituximab arm.
- Clinical trials should always be considered for patients with relapsed and refractory CLL. Trials are ongoing for newer agents, which may result in increased therapeutic efficacy and less toxicity.

Prognosis

- The overall 5-year survival rate for patients with CLL is 73%.
- Data from older trials in the 1970s and 1980s report median survival times for all patients of 8 to 12 years.
- There is a large variation in survival among individual patients, ranging from several months to a normal life expectancy.

Prevention and Surveillance

- There are no guidelines for preventing CLL.
- Although the NCCN has not published surveillance guidelines for CLL, close lifelong follow-up is needed.
  - People with CLL are at an increased risk for a second cancer, and the most common types are skin and lung cancers. Patients should be educated to notify their physician about any signs or symptoms.
  - In patients with an incomplete response, CLL is likely to recur.

Bibliography

Burger, J. (2013). Ibrutinib and rituximab trigger 95 percent response rates among chronic lymphocytic leukemia patients. *MD Anderson news release*. December 9, 2013. Available at http://www.mdanderson.org/news room/news-releases/2013/ibrutinib-and-rituximab-trigger.html (accessed January 3, 2016).

Byrd, J. C., Forman, R. R., Courte, S. E., Flinn, I. W., Burger, J. A., Blum, K. A., & O'Brien, S. (2013). Targeting BTK with ibrutinib in relapsed chronic lymphocytic leukemia. *New England Journal of Medicine, 369*(1), 32–42.

Furman, R. R., Sharman, J. P., Coutre, S. E., Cheson, B. D., Pagel, J. M., Hillmen, P., & O'Brien, S. M. (2014). Idelalisib and rituximab in relapsed chronic lymphocytic leukemia. *New England Journal of Medicine, 4*(370), 997–1007.

National Cancer Institute. (2015). *Chronic lymphocytic leukemia: Treatment—for health professionals (PDQ)*. Available at http://www.cancer.gov/cancer topics/pdq/treatment/CLL/healthprofessional (accessed January 3, 2016).

National Comprehensive Cancer Network. (2015). *NCCN clinical practice guidelines for non-Hodgkin's lymphoma, version 2.2015*. Available at http://www.nccn.org/professionals/physician_gls/pdf/nhl.pdf (accessed January 3, 2016).

Chronic Myelogenous Leukemia

Definition

Chronic myelogenous leukemia (CML), also called *chronic myeloid leukemia*, is a cancer of granulocytes or monocytes. It is considered a myeloproliferative neoplasm and causes the rapid growth of myeloid precursors in the bone marrow, peripheral blood, and body tissues.

The Philadelphia (Ph) chromosome is identified in more than 95% of patients diagnosed with CML. It results from a reciprocal translocation between chromosomes 9 and 22, which is designated t(9;22), in a myeloid stem cell in the bone marrow. The transfer of DNA results in one chromosome 9 that is longer than normal and one chromosome 22 that is shorter than normal. The DNA removed from chromosome 9 contains most of the Abelson gene (*ABL*). The break in chromosome 22 occurs in a gene in the middle of the breakpoint cluster region (*BCR*). Fusion of the two chromosome segments creates the *BCR/ABL* gene, which encodes an abnormal tyrosine kinase protein that causes CML.

Incidence

- In the United States, CML affects 1 to 2 of every 100,000 people and accounts for 7% to 20% of cases of leukemia.
- An estimated 6660 new cases of CML and 1140 deaths occurred in 2015 in the United States.
- The average age at diagnosis is 64 years; 80% of patients diagnosed are older than 65 years of age.
- CML accounts for 2.6% of leukemias in children between the ages of 0 to 19 years.

Etiology and Risk Factors

- According to SEER incidence rates from 2002 to 2004, 0.15% of men and women born in 2015 will be diagnosed with CML at some point in their lifetimes.
- High-dose radiation exposure may contribute to development of the Ph chromosome.
- Most patients with CML have not been exposed to radiation, and many who were exposed to high-dose radiation do not have CML.

Signs and Symptoms

- Symptoms typically develop gradually and are usually seen with advanced disease.
- The diagnosis is often made during a routine blood examination for other reasons.
- Patient complaints
  - Fatigue
  - Malaise
  - Fever
  - Weight loss
  - Night sweats
- Physical findings
  - Ecchymosis
  - Lymphadenopathy
  - Splenomegaly (about 50% of patients)

Diagnostic Work-up

- Medical history and physical examination
- Laboratory tests
  - CBC with differential count
  - Serum chemistry panel
  - Elevated lactate dehydrogenase and uric acid levels correlate with a large tumor burden.

- Cytogenetics to identify chromosomal or genetic abnormalities
- Polymerase chain reaction (PCR), a highly sensitive test to detect as little as one *BCR/ABL*-positive cell in a background of about 500,000 normal cells
- Additional studies
  - Bone marrow aspirate or biopsy
- Imaging studies
  - Chest radiography
  - CT
  - MRI

Histology

Peripheral Blood

- Leukocytosis with median WBC in the 100,000 range usually composed of neutrophilic series, from myeloblasts to mature neutrophils and an increased percent of myelocytes and segmented neutrophils. Blasts typically account for less than 2%.
- A greater proportion of myelocytes than metamyelocytes is a classic finding of CML, and dysplasia can develop in more advanced cases.
- Morphology will be normal but cytochemically abnormal. The cytochemical reaction called leukocyte alkaline phosphatase (LAP) will be low. This is useful in determining a differential diagnosis of CML from a reactive leukocytosis due to infection or polycythemia vera.
- Absolute basophilia is a universal finding in CML blood smears.
- The platelet count can be normal or elevated.

Bone Marrow

- Biopsy demonstrates granulocytic hyperplasia with maturation pattern that reflects the peripheral blood smear.
- Erythroid islands are reduced in number and size. Small hypolobulated megakaryocytes are present. Pseudo-Gaucher cells and sea-blue histiocytes are present. Iron-laden macrophages are reduced or absent.
- Although Ph chromosome translocation is the initiating event in CML, additional chromosomal or molecular changes are often found in accelerated or blast crisis phases of CML.
  - These can include trisomy 8, trisomy 19, duplication of the Ph chromosome, and isochromosome 17q (leading to loss of the P53 gene). When these occur, the prognosis is poorer.

Clinical Staging

- CML has three phases: chronic, accelerated, and blast.
  - Transition from the chronic phase to the accelerated and blast phases may occur gradually over 1 year or longer, or it may occur abruptly (i.e., blast crisis).
  - Chronic-phase CML: Most patients are in the chronic phase of CML at diagnosis. It is characterized by cytogenetic findings of less than 10% blasts and promyelocytes in the peripheral blood and bone marrow.

- Accelerated-phase CML: It is characterized by 10% to 19% blasts in the peripheral blood or bone marrow.
- Blastic-phase CML: A total of 20% or more blasts may be found in the peripheral blood or bone marrow. A patient with fever, malaise, and splenomegaly with 20% or more blasts is considered to be in blast crisis.
- The annual rate of progression from chronic phase to blast crisis is 5% to 10% in the first 2 years and 20% in subsequent years.

Treatment

- The goal of treatment in the chronic phase is to return hematologic values to normal and eliminate BCR/ABL positivity in laboratory test results.
- Treatment goals for the accelerated phase or blast crisis phase are to eliminate cells with the *BCR/ABL* gene and return the patient's disease to the chronic phase.
- Leukapheresis or hydroxyurea may be used initially to reduce WBC counts, but they are not considered to be long-term treatments. Interferon has also been used but does not demonstrate any overall survival advantage.
- The treatment of choice is a tyrosine kinase inhibitor (TKI). Imatinib mesylate, nilotinib, or dasatinib.
  - Analysis of marrow samples have been the preferred method for demonstrating complete responses (i.e., clearance of *BCR/ABL*-containing cells), but because peripheral blood tests with FISH and PCR are highly sensitive and specific, most testing now uses peripheral blood samples for ongoing monitoring. Marrow testing should still be completed at regular intervals.
  - FISH and PCR testing are often completed every 2 weeks until stable blood counts are achieved, and then testing is done every 3 months. If no hematologic response is seen (i.e., blood counts do not improve), the physician can consider switching agents.
  - Achievement of molecular remission requires ongoing testing to ensure that the response is maintained. Bone marrow biopsies are typically done at 3-, 6-, and 12-month intervals and then annually.
  - Those who achieve complete molecular remission (i.e., undetectable *BCR/ABL*) for at least 2 years of may be considered for TKI discontinuation. These patients must be monitored closely with frequent PCR peripheral blood and marrow testing. If they return positive results on two or more tests, the TKI should be resumed.

Transplantation

- Although allogeneic bone marrow or stem cell transplantation is the only potentially curative treatment, the use of transplantation is reserved for those who fail TKI therapy.
- Allogeneic transplantation is associated with significant morbidity and mortality rates, and because the typical age of CML patients is greater than 65 years, additional comorbidities should be considered.

- Nonmyeloablative stem cell transplantation (i.e., mini-transplantation) is being investigated, along with autologous stem cell transplantation, which may benefit patients not eligible for a traditional allogeneic transplantation.
- Cord blood stem cell transplantations are being investigated.

Donor Lymphocyte Infusion

- For patients who have a relapse after allogeneic stem cell transplantation, treatment alternatives include a second transplantation, a TKI, or a lymphocyte infusion from the original stem cell donor.

Prognosis

- The median age of patients at diagnosis with Ph chromosome–positive CML is 67 years.
- With the advent of TKI therapies, the median survival for most CML patients who are able to achieve complete molecular remission and stay on therapy for at least 2 years reaches the normal life expectancy of the general population.
- The life expectancy is typically much shorter for those who continue to have *BCR/ABL*-positive cells, develop resistance to TKI agents, or progress to accelerated-phase CML or blast crisis. Those in blast crisis may live only a few months.
- Ph chromosome–negative CML is a poorly defined entity that is less clearly distinguished from other myeloproliferative syndromes. The approximately 5% of patients with this form of CML usually have a poorer response to treatment and shorter survival than Ph chromosome–positive patients.

Prevention and Surveillance

- There are no prevention guidelines for CML.
- Patients in remission should receive lifelong follow-up to monitor for disease recurrence or late treatment effects.
- Care providers should encourage a healthy lifestyle, including influenza vaccinations, tobacco abstinence, maintenance of a healthy weight and diet, and recommended cancer screening for other malignancies.

Bibliography

Cancer.Net Editorial Board. (2014). *Leukemia—chronic myeloid—CML: After treatment*. Available at http://www.cancer.net/cancer-types/leukemia-chronic-myeloid-cml/after-treatment (accessed January 3, 2016).

Kantarjian, H., O'Brien, S., Jabbour, E., Garcia-Manero, G., Quintas-Cardama, A., Shan, J., & Cortes, J. (2012). Improved survival in chronic myeloid leukemia since the introduction of imatinib therapy: A single-institution historical experience. *Blood, 119*(9), 1981–1987.

National Cancer Institute. (2015). Chronic myelogenous leukemia: Treatment—for health professionals (PDQ). Available at http://www.cancer.gov/cancertopics/pdq/treatment/CML/HealthProfessional (accessed January 3, 2016).

National Comprehensive Cancer Network. (2015). *NCCN clinical practice guidelines for chronic myelogenous leukemia, version 1.2016*. Available at http://www.nccn.org/professionals/physician_gls/pdf/cml.pdf (accessed January 3, 2016).

Ross, D. M., Branford, S., Seymour, J. F., Schwaner, A. P., Arthur, C., Yeung, D. T., & Hughes, T. P. (2013). Safety and efficacy of imatinib cessation for CML patients with stable undetectable minimal residual disease results from the TWISTER study. *Blood, 122*, 515–522.

Myelodysplastic Syndromes

Definition

Myelodysplastic syndromes (MDSs) are a group of acquired bone marrow stem cell malignancies that result in ineffective hematopoiesis in one or more myeloid lineages. Although technically not cancer, MDS may transform over time into leukemia and is often referred to as *preleukemia*. In patients with MDS, the marrow produces too few red blood cells, WBCs, and platelets.

Incidence

- MDS is estimated to affect 200,000 persons in the United States.
- Between 10,000 and 15,000 new cases have been diagnosed per year during the past 2 years, and numbers are expected to increase as the population continues to age.
- The median age at diagnosis is between 60 and 70 years; 70% of patients are older than 50 years of age.
- MDS occurs in men more often than women and affects whites more often than other races.

Etiology and Risk Factors

- MDS can manifest de novo (i.e., primary MDS) or after treatment with chemotherapy or radiation therapy for other diseases and rarely after environmental exposures. Primary MDS accounts for 90% of cases.
- Risk factors include the following:
  - Age older than 60 years
  - Male sex
  - Alcohol use
  - Cigarette smoking
  - Exposure to ionizing radiation
  - Immunosuppressive therapy
  - Viral infection
  - Exposure to toxins:
    - Organic chemicals such as benzene, toluene, xylene, and chloramphenicol
    - Petroleum and diesel derivatives
    - Nitro-organic explosives
    - Exhaust gases
    - Stone and cereal dust
    - Heavy metals
    - Herbicides, pesticides, and fertilizers

Signs and Symptoms

- Symptoms typically develop gradually and are usually seen with advanced disease.
- Disease usually manifests as a result of marrow failure in one or more cell lines. The diagnosis is often made during routine blood examination.
- Symptoms
  - Fatigue
  - Malaise
  - Fever

- Shortness of breath with exertion
- Weight loss
- Physical findings
  - Pallor
  - Ecchymosis or bleeding
  - Infection
  - Anemia
  - Splenomegaly

Diagnostic Work-up

- Medical history and physical examination
- Laboratory tests
  - CBC with differential count
  - Cytogenetics for identification of chromosomal or genetic abnormalities; 50% of MDS patients have chromosomal abnormalities, commonly deletion of chromosome 5 or 7 or trisomy 8
- Bone marrow aspirate or biopsy is essential for the diagnosis.
  - The specimen is typically hypercellular.
  - Ten percent of cases are hypoplastic, manifesting as profound cytopenias, which may respond well to immunosuppressant therapy.
- Imaging studies
  - Chest radiography
  - CT
  - MRI

Histology

The marrow typically is normocellular or hypercellular.

Clinical Staging

- A variety of pathologic and risk classification systems have been developed to predict the overall survival of patients with MDS and the evolution from MDS to AML.
- Major prognostic classification systems include the International Prognostic Scoring System (IPSS), revised as the IPSS-R; the WHO Prognostic Scoring System (WPSS); and the MD Anderson Cancer Center Prognostic Scoring Systems.
- Clinical variables in these systems have included bone marrow and blood myeloblast percentage, specific cytopenias, transfusion requirements, age, performance status, and bone marrow cytogenetic abnormalities.
- IPSS incorporates bone marrow blast percentage, number of peripheral blood cytopenias, and cytogenetic risk group (see table in the next column).
- IPSS-R updates and gives greater weight to cytogenetic abnormalities and severity of cytopenias while reassigning the weighting for blast percentages.
- In contrast to the IPSS and IPSS-R, which should be applied only at the time of diagnosis, the WPSS is dynamic, meaning that patients can be reassigned to categories as their disease progresses.
- MD Anderson has published two prognostic scoring systems, one of which focuses on lower risk patients.

International Prognostic Scoring System for Assessing the Prognosis of Newly Diagnosed MDS Patients

Risk Sub-group	Score	Median Survival (Years)	Time to AML Transformation for 25% (Years)
Low risk	0	5.7	9.4
INT-1	0.5-1.0	3.5	3.3
INT-2	1.5-2.0	1.2	1.1
High risk	>2.5	0.4	0.2

Prognostic Variable	SCORE VALUE				
	0	0.5	1	1.5	2
BM blasts (%)	<5	5-10	—	11-20	21-30
Karyotype*	Good	Intermediate	Poor	—	—
Cytopenias†	0/1	2/3	—	—	—

AML, Acute myeloid leukemia; *BM*, bone marrow; *INT*, intermediate.
*Good: normal, −Y, del(5q), del(20q); poor: complex (≥3 abnormalities) or chromosome 7 anomalies; intermediate: other abnormalities.
†Cytopenias were defined as hemoglobin <10 g/dL, absolute neutrophil count <1500/μL, and platelets <100,000/μL.
Data from Greenberg, P., Cox, C., LeBeau, M. M., Fenaux, P., Morel, P., Sanz, G., et al (1997). International scoring system for evaluating prognosis in myelodysplastic syndromes. *Blood, 89*(6), 2079-2088.

Treatment

- MDS treatment individualizes therapy for each patient.
- Therapy for MDS has historically been supportive care for most patients.
- The only curative treatment is allogeneic stem cell transplantation, but intensive chemotherapy and transplantation are used only for the few MDS patients with available donors, higher risk disease, younger age, and adequate performance status.
- Supportive care
  - Transfusions to correct anemia and thrombocytopenia
  - Antibiotics
  - Hematopoietic growth factors such as recombinant erythropoietin, granulocyte colony-stimulating factor, or granulocyte-macrophage colony-stimulating factor
- Disease-modifying agents may be used.
  - Lenalidomide is an immunomodulatory agent approved for low-risk, transfusion-dependent patients with del (5q) MDS.
  - Immunosuppression therapy with antithymocyte globulin and cyclosporine is used in patients with hypoplastic marrow.
  - DNA methyltransferase inhibitors, which block the methylation of DNA and inhibit proliferation, include 5-azacitidine and decitabine.
  - AML induction-type chemotherapy may be tried but may be difficult for older patients to tolerate.

Prognosis

- Secondary myelodysplasia usually has a poorer prognosis than de novo myelodysplasia.
- Prognosis is directly related to the number of bone marrow blast cells, to certain cytogenetic abnormalities, and to the amount of peripheral blood cytopenia.

- MDS transforms to AML in about 30% of patients. By convention, the MDS is reclassified as AML with myelodysplastic features when blood or bone marrow blasts reach or exceed 20%.
- The time to AML transformation for the four IPSS risk groups (low, intermediate-1, intermediate-2, and high) was 9.4, 3.3, 1.1, and 0.2 years, respectively. Median survival for the four groups was 5.7, 3.5, 1.2, and 0.4 years, respectively.
- The acute leukemic phase is less responsive to chemotherapy than de novo AML.
- Many patients succumb to complications of cytopenias before progression to AML

Prevention and Surveillance

There are no recommended measures for the prevention of MDS.

Bibliography

Akhtari, M. (2011). When to treat myelodysplastic syndrome. *Oncology Journal*. Available at www.cancernetwork.com/myelodysplastic-syndromes/when-treat-myelodysplastic-syndromes (accessed January 3, 2016).

National Cancer Institute. (2015). *Myelodysplastic syndromes: Treatment—for health professionals (PDQ)*. Available at http://www.cancer.gov/cancertopics/pdq/treatment/myelodysplastic/HealthProfessional (accessed January 3, 2016).

National Comprehensive Cancer Network. (2015). *NCCN clinical practice guidelines for myelodysplastic syndrome, version 1.2016*. Available at http://www.nccn.org/professionals/physician_gls/pdf/mds.pdf (accessed January 3, 2016).

Samlev, D., Bhatt, V. R., Armitage, J. D., Maness, L. J., & Akhtari, M. (2014). A primary care approach to myelodysplastic syndromes. *Korean Journal of Family Medicine, 35*(3), 111–118.

Zhou, J., Orazi, A., & Czader, M. B. (2011). Myelodysplastic syndromes. *Seminars in Diagnostic Pathology, 28*(4), 258–272.

Major Cancers 2

Lung Cancers

Carrie H. Christiansen

Non–Small Cell Lung Cancer

Definition

Lung cancer can develop in any area of the lungs or bronchus. It usually arises from the bronchial endothelium.

Incidence

- Lung cancer remains the leading cause of cancer-related death in the United States, and it is the second most commonly diagnosed cancer in men and women. It accounts for about 13% of all cancer diagnoses.
- According to the American Cancer Society (ACS), 221,200 new cases of lung cancer and 158,040 deaths from the disease occurred in 2015.
- Since the mid-1980s, the incidence has been declining among men; a decline among women was not seen until the mid-2000s.
  - During the period from 2007 to 2011, the incidence of lung cancer decreased 3% and 2.2% annually for men and women, respectively.
  - Global initiatives encouraging smoking cessation and the ever-expanding public bans on smoking have played a large role in the drop in incidence.
- Although more than 80% of all lung cancers are thought to have been caused by smoking, more than 45,000 new cases occur annually among nonsmokers.
- Non–small cell lung cancer (NSCLC), the most common type, accounts for about 83% of all lung cancers.

Etiology and Risk Factors

- Exposure to cigarette, cigar, or pipe smoke is the major risk factor for lung cancer.
  - The risk increases with the number of years of smoking and number of cigarettes smoked.
  - Smoking cessation can significantly decrease the risk.
  - Secondhand smoke (i.e., smoke inhaled involuntarily when tobacco is smoked by others) exposure contributes to a lesser extent.
- Environmental and occupational exposures to arsenic, benzene, radon, asbestos (especially in smokers), copper, silica, lead, diesel exhaust, chromium, and air pollution increase the risk of lung cancer, as does radiation exposure from previous cancer treatment.
- A history of tuberculosis or chronic inflammatory diseases is a risk factor.
- Chronic obstructive pulmonary disease (COPD) is a risk factor for lung cancer.
- Genetic susceptibility contributes to the risk of lung cancer, although specific genetic abnormalities have yet to be identified.
- Mutations in oncogenes and tumor suppressor genes such as *MYC, RAS, TP53, ALK, EGFR, BRAF* and *HER2* are involved in lung cancers.

Signs and Symptoms

- There are few or no symptoms of early-stage lung cancer.
- Symptoms that occur as the cancer progresses include the following:
  - Persistent cough
  - Shortness of breath
  - Sputum streaked with blood
  - Chest pain
  - Hoarseness or voice changes
  - Recurrent pneumonia or bronchitis
- Late-stage symptoms include the following:
  - Pain from bone metastasis
  - Fatigue
  - Anorexia
  - Central nervous system changes from brain metastasis
  - Dysphagia
  - Weight loss
- Paraneoplastic syndromes, which are more common in lung cancer than in any other kind of cancer, may cause hypercalcemia of malignancy and hypercoagulable states.

Diagnostic Work-up

The purpose of the diagnostic work-up is to determine the location of the primary cancer, the best site for a biopsy to identify tumor histology and subtype (i.e., non–small cell, small cell, or malignant pleural mesothelioma), and whether there are sites of metastatic disease. Key elements of the work-up include the following:

- History and physical examination, including details of smoking and carcinogenic exposure
- Laboratory testing, including a complete blood cell count, kidney and liver function tests, and alkaline phosphatase (e.g., bone or liver disease), calcium (e.g., hypercalcemia), and sodium (e.g., hyponatremia) levels
- Computed tomography (CT) of the chest, abdomen, and pelvis with contrast to identify the location of the primary tumor and sites of metastatic disease (e.g., lymph nodes, liver, adrenal glands, bones), which may be followed by positron emission tomography (PET) or a bone scan.
- Biopsy under CT guidance or bronchoscopy

- Baseline brain magnetic resonance imaging (MRI) or CT
- If surgery is considered, pulmonary function tests should be obtained, and lymph node sampling by mediastinoscopy may be included in the initial work-up.

Histology

- There are three common histologic types:
  - Adenocarcinoma is the most common type (about 40%), and it is associated with irritated and scarred areas of lung tissue.
  - Squamous cell carcinomas make up about 30% of NSCLCs, and they are usually associated with smoking.
    - They tend to be slower growing than adenocarcinomas and stay localized for a longer period.
    - They typically arise in large bronchi with local extension that may result in atelectasis (i.e., collapse of the alveoli) and postobstructive pneumonia.
  - Large cell carcinoma represents about 10% to 15% of NSCLCs.
    - Because cells are typically undifferentiated, the cancer can be difficult to treat.
    - It usually arises as peripheral nodules within the lung and metastasizes early.

Clinical Staging

- NSCLC usually has a predictable pattern of growth.
  - It starts with localized lymphatic invasion and travels through the bloodstream to hilar, mediastinal, and supraclavicular lymph nodes; bronchial lumens; and the pleura and chest wall structures.
  - Eventually, distant metastases develop in bone, liver, adrenal glands, and the brain.
  - In rare cases, metastasis can be found in subcutaneous tissue, choroid of the eye, and the peritoneum.
- The purpose of staging is to determine how far the cancer has spread. This information dictates the appropriate treatment modalities and aids in establishing a prognosis.
- In most cases, only early stage NSCLC is considered resectable in most cases.
- NSCLC uses the tumor size, lymph nodes, and metastasis (TNM) system adopted by the American Joint Commission on Cancer (AJCC) (Edge et al., 2010).
- Histology is not a factor in clinical staging.

Treatment

Surgery

- Only about one fourth of cases can be surgically resected at diagnosis.
- When NSCLC cancer is localized and small (i.e., stages I, II, and some IIIA), surgery is usually the treatment of choice if the patient is a low surgical risk and expected to have a good quality of life after removal of part of the lung.
- Surgical procedures include a wedge resection that removes small peripheral nodules (most conservative), segmentectomy that removes part of a lobe of the lung, lobectomy that removes a lobe of the lung (most common), and pneumonectomy that removes the entire right or left lung.

- Depending on the clinical stage after surgery, adjuvant chemotherapy or radiation therapy, or both, can improve overall survival.
- Stage IIIB or IV NSCLC is considered to be inoperable. In some cases, however, solitary metastatic lesions in the lung and brain can be resected.

Radiation Therapy

- Patients who are not surgical candidates but whose cancer is stage I or II can receive radiation therapy, which can be curative in some cases.
- Adjuvant radiation therapy may be used after surgery for stage IIIA disease.
- Patients who cannot have surgery for a stage IIIA disease or those with stage IIIB disease usually receive a combination of definitive chemotherapy and radiation therapy.
- Neoadjuvant therapy (i.e., chemotherapy with or without radiation therapy before surgery) has been an area of intense study as a way of shrinking the tumor to improve the chances of a successful resection and prolong survival.
- Although the survival rates have improved for stages IB through IIIA with neoadjuvant therapy, it does carry a greater risk of complications.
- Palliative radiation therapy is reserved for the treatment of symptomatic bone pain, spinal cord compression, brain metastasis, and postobstructive pneumonia.

Chemotherapy

- Most patients with NSCLC receive chemotherapy because they are initially diagnosed with late-stage, unresectable disease, and about 80% of those with resectable disease will have cancer recurrence.
- Treatment with chemotherapy alone for metastatic disease produces only moderate response rates (up to 30%).
- First-line chemotherapy regimens of choice include a platinum-based doublet (i.e., cisplatin or carboplatin) in combination with paclitaxel, pemetrexed, nab-paclitaxel, docetaxel, gemcitabine, or vinorelbine.
- Evidence shows that maintenance therapy using pemetrexed can improve progression-free survival time after four to six cycles of a platinum-based doublet.
- Bevacizumab is approved for use in nonsquamous NSCLC concurrently with carboplatin and paclitaxel as first-line treatment. Contraindications are brain metastasis and hemoptysis.
- Patients with a poor performance status are usually treated with single agents or with supportive care.
- In the setting of metastatic disease the National Comprehensive Cancer Network (NCCN) guidelines recommend the introduction of palliative care at the time of diagnosis, regardless of patient performance status.
- Smoking cessation counseling should be offered during the initial visit, work-up, and throughout treatment.
- For disease progression, second-line therapy uses single-agent treatment such as docetaxel (with or without ramucirumab), gemcitabine, topotecan, vinorelbine, pemetrexed, or erlotinib.

- During treatment, patients are restaged with CT or PET every two to three cycles to assess response.
- Participation on clinical trials should be considered for patients with disease progression.

Targeted Therapies and Genetic Testing

- Genetic testing of lung cancer tissue is an exciting area of research.
  - Germline mutations can lead to cancer development, as in patients who harbor the *BRCA1* or *BRCA2* mutation.
  - Somatic mutations are found only in the malignant cells (i.e., not in healthy cells), and many have been identified in NSCLC.
- The NCCN guidelines recommend genetic testing at the time of diagnosis of any stage IV NSCLC patient whose histology includes adenocarcinoma or large cell carcinoma and recommend considering testing in cases of squamous cell carcinoma, especially if the patient is a nonsmoker.
- Second biopsies should be performed if the initial biopsy does not have enough tissue for testing.
- Targeted therapies have shifted the paradigm of NSCLC treatment for patients whose biopsy tissue has tested positive for certain oncogene mutations.
- The ability to target specific aspects of tumor development at the molecular level has improved patient survival and quality of life.
- The toxicities of targeted therapies can be more tolerable than those of chemotherapy, including less severe effects caused by bone marrow suppression.
- Several oral targeted therapies approved by the U.S. Food and Drug Administration (FDA) are commercially available. Many are being evaluated in clinical trials.
- Targeted therapies are indicated after certain genetic mutations are identified:
  - For those with the epidermal growth factor receptor (*EGFR*) mutation, afatinib, erlotinib, and gefitinib are approved as first-line treatment.
  - For those with the anaplastic lymphoma kinase (*ALK*) translocation and *ROS1* mutations, crizotinib is approved as first-line treatment.
  - For *ALK* translocation–positive patients who have disease progression or cannot tolerate crizotinib, ceritinib is approved as second-line treatment.
- Next-generation gene sequencing is gaining popularity as a way to identify rare genetic mutations.
  - Depending on the sophistication of the molecular laboratory, the number of mutations that can be tested for can range from 15 to more than 500.
  - Ongoing research is being performed to identify more actionable genetic mutations in lung cancer tissue.
- Despite the outstanding efficacy of targeted treatments, cancers ultimately develop resistance and resume growth. Continued research is needed to develop more treatments to combat disease resistance and improve overall survival of patients.

Prognosis

- Lung cancer remains the leading cause of cancer-related deaths in the United States, and most patients are diagnosed with late-stage disease.
- The overall 1-year and 5-year survival rates are 44% and 17%, respectively.
- The clinical stage of disease is the most important prognostic factor, with earlier stages having better responses to treatment and longer survival times. Survival rates based on clinical stage drop dramatically below stage I.
  - Stage I: 5-year survival rate of 60% to 80%
  - Stage II: 5-year survival rate of 25% to 50%
  - Stage IIIA: 5-year survival rate of 10% to 40%
  - Stage IIIB: 5-year survival rate of less than 5%
  - Stage IV: 5-year survival rate of less than 5%
- Poor prognostic factors include weight loss, poor performance status, alterations in serum hematology or chemistry results (including elevated lactate dehydrogenase levels), bone or liver metastases, and leptomeningeal disease (i.e., spreading to the cerebrospinal fluid and space).

Prevention and Surveillance

- The NCCN guidelines recommend screening CT scans for the early detection of lung cancer for specific populations. Use of the scans can reduce lung cancer deaths by 16% to 20% compared with standard chest radiographs.
- The NCCN recommended surveillance protocol includes the following:
  - A history, physical examination, and chest CT with contrast every 6 to 12 months for 2 years, decreasing to annual evaluations thereafter
  - Smoking cessation
  - Vaccinations, including influenza (annual), herpes zoster, and pneumococcal vaccines
  - Health promotion and wellness counseling

Bibliography

American Cancer Society (ACS). (2015). *Cancer facts and figures 2015*. Available at http://www.cancer.org/acs/groups/content/@editorial/documents/document/acspc-044552.pdf (accessed January 28, 2016).

American Cancer Society (ACS). (2015). *American Cancer Society estimated new cases for the four major cancers by sex and age group 2015*. Available at http://www.cancer.org/acs/groups/content/@editorial/documents/document/acspc-044511.pdf (accessed January 28, 2016).

Edge, S., Byrd, D. R., Compton, C. C., Fritz, A. G., Greene, F. L., & Trotti, A. (Eds.). (2010). *AJCC staging manual* (7th ed.). New York: Springer.

National Comprehensive Cancer Network. (2015). *NCCN national clinical practice guidelines in oncology: Non–small cell lung cancer, version 7.2015*. Available at http://www.nccn.org/professionals/physician_gls/pdf/nscl.pdf (accessed January 28, 2016).

Small Cell Lung Cancer

Definition

Lung cancer can develop in any area of the lungs or bronchus and usually arises from the bronchial endothelium. Small cell lung cancer (SCLC) is usually centrally located around a main bronchus. It is considered a more aggressive type of lung cancer than NSCLC due to its rapid tumor doubling time and tendency to metastasize early. It was formerly known as oat cell carcinoma.

Incidence

- See earlier information included in the NSCLC incidence.
- SCLC accounts for approximately 13% of all new lung cancer cases.

Etiology and Risk Factors

- See earlier information included in the NSCLC causes and risk factors.
- SCLC is closely associated with a history of smoking.

Signs and Symptoms

- See earlier information included in the NSCLC signs and symptoms.

Diagnostic Work-up

- See earlier information about the diagnostic work-up included in the NSCLC.

Histology

- SCLC is not usually categorized by histologic subtypes.
- The exception is neuroendocrine tumors of the lung (refer to Neuroendocrine Tumors Chapter, page 137), which typically use the same staging and treatment modalities as SCLC.

Clinical Staging

- Metastasis to distant sites occurs in more than 60% of patients at the time of diagnosis.
  - Typical sites include bone, bone marrow, liver, brain, lymph nodes, pleura, and adrenal glands.
  - The initial work-up is the same for SCLC as NSCLC, with the addition of a bone marrow biopsy and aspiration are sometimes included if metastasis is suspected.
- Although the AJCC has recommended a TNM staging system for SCLC, most clinicians use a limited-stage or extensive-stage determination.
  - Limited-stage tumor is confined to one hemithorax and regional lymph nodes that can be treated within a single radiation therapy port.
  - About 30% to 40% of patients at diagnosis have limited-stage disease.
  - The remaining 60% to 70% have extensive-stage disease, which means the tumor has spread beyond the hemithorax and regional lymph nodes.
- As with NSCLC, staging for SCLC is useful in determining treatment and prognosis.

Treatment

- Surgery is rarely indicated for limited-stage SCLC.
  - Patients must meet specific criteria, which include a small tumor and no metastases to regional lymph nodes.
  - Because the risk of recurrence is extremely high, patients undergoing surgery for SCLC usually have postoperative chemotherapy or radiation therapy.

- SCLC is very sensitive to chemotherapy and radiation therapy.
  - For patients with limited-stage disease, definitive chemoradiation therapy is indicated. Occasionally, a sequential approach of separate chemotherapy and radiation therapy may be used.
  - First-line chemotherapy regimens of choice usually contain a platinum-based doublet (i.e., cisplatin or carboplatin) in combination with etoposide.
  - Patients usually receive four to six cycles of chemotherapy and are followed with CT or PET scans every 8 to 10 weeks.
  - If the patient relapses more than 6 months after completing first-line chemotherapy, the original regimen can be used again.
  - When the disease progresses in less than 6 months after completing first-line therapy, single-agent chemotherapy, such as topotecan, paclitaxel, docetaxel, oral etoposide, gemcitabine, vinorelbine, or irinotecan, is used.
  - Eventually, the tumor becomes resistant to chemotherapy.
- Prophylactic cranial irradiation (PCI) continues to be controversial.
  - It may be done in patients with extensive-stage SCLC who have achieved a complete response to help decrease the chance of brain metastasis.
  - Potential toxicities include dementia, memory loss, and gait problems, which may be permanent.
- Palliative radiation therapy is done for treatment of bone pain, superior vena cava syndrome, spinal cord compression, brain metastasis, and postobstructive pneumonia.
- The initiation of palliative care for these patients is indicated at the time of diagnosis.
- Genetic testing is not indicated for patients with SCLC, and there are no approved targeted therapies to treat the disease.

Prognosis

- Very few patients are cured of SCLC.
- Despite high sensitivity to chemotherapy and response rates of up to 90% for limited-stage disease, the 5-year survival rate is less than 5%.
- The long-term survival rate for patients with extensive-stage SCLC is almost 0%.
- The median survival time for patients with limited-stage disease who complete definitive chemoradiation therapy is 15 to 26 months. For those with extensive-stage disease, it is 7 to 11 months. For untreated disease, the survival time is usually 6 to 12 weeks.
- Prognostic factors associated with improved outcomes include good performance status, female sex, and a normal lactate dehydrogenase level at diagnosis.

Prevention and Surveillance

- The NCCN guidelines recommend CT screening for the early detection of lung cancer for specific populations. Use of CT scans can reduce lung cancer deaths by 16% to 20% compared with standard chest radiographs.
- NCCN surveillance recommendations include the following:

- History, physical examination, chest imaging, and blood work at follow-up visits every 3 to 4 months for 2 years and then every 6 months through year 5
- A new pulmonary nodule should be evaluated as a potential new primary tumor.
- Smoking cessation
- Health promotion and wellness counseling

Bibliography

American Cancer Society (ACS). (2015). *Cancer facts and figures 2015.* Available at http://www.cancer.org/acs/groups/content/@editorial/documents/document/acspc-044552.pdf (accessed January 28, 2016).

American Cancer Society (ACS). (2015). *American Cancer Society estimated new cases for the four major cancers by sex and age group 2015.* Available at http://www.cancer.org/acs/groups/content/@editorial/documents/document/acspc-044511.pdf (accessed January 28, 2016).

National Comprehensive Cancer Network. (2015). *NCCN national clinical practice guidelines in oncology small cell lung cancer. version 1.2016.* Available at http://www.nccn.org/professionals/physician_gls/pdf/sclc.pdf (accessed January 28, 2016).

Malignant Pleural Mesothelioma

Definition

Malignant pleural mesothelioma (MPM) is a malignant tumor of the covering of the lung or the lining of the pleural and abdominal cavities. It is often associated with exposure to asbestos.

Incidence

- MPM is a rare cancer that is estimated to affect 2500 people each year.
- The incidence is higher among older men (>70 years).
- Although the most common site of mesothelioma is the pleural space, it can also be found in the lining of the pericardium, peritoneum, and testis.
- Although the incidence of MPM is leveling off due to decreased asbestos use, the United States continues to report more cases of MPM than anywhere else in the world.

Etiology and Risk Factors

- Unlike other lung cancers, smoking is not a risk factor for MPM.
- Asbestos exposure is the leading risk factor, but the exposure typically occurs 20 to 40 years before the cancer diagnosis.
- Radiotherapy, exposure to erionite (i.e., mineral found in gravel roads), and genetic factors may also increase the risk of developing MPM.

Signs and Symptoms

- Most patients have advanced disease by the time they are diagnosed.
- Significant symptoms include the following:
  - Chest pain
  - Dyspnea and cough
  - Palpable chest wall masses
  - Weight loss
  - Fever and sweating
- Pleural effusions may develop.

Diagnostic Work-up

- The purpose of the diagnostic work-up is to distinguish MPM from other pathologies, including benign pleural disease and primary lung cancer (compared with metastasis from another site), and to determine the extent of disease.
- MPM can metastasize to regional lymph nodes, the diaphragm, and the peritoneum. It much less commonly spreads outside of the thoracic anatomy to other visceral organs.
- The initial work-up includes the following:
  - History and physical examination, including details of asbestos exposures
  - Laboratory testing, including a complete blood cell count and kidney and liver function tests
  - CT scan of chest with contrast to identify the location of the primary tumor and sites of metastatic disease (e.g., lymph nodes, liver, adrenal glands, bones), which may then be followed by PET scans
- Pleural biopsy under CT guidance or using a thoracoscopic approach
- Thoracentesis is often required to diagnose and palliate pleural effusions, and it may need to be repeated several times.

Histology

- There are three histologic subtypes of MPM: epithelioid (most common), biphasic (i.e., mixed), and sarcomatoid.
- Epithelioid cell types usually have a better prognosis.

Clinical Staging

- The purpose of staging is to determine whether the patient is a surgical candidate.
- Histology is not a factor in staging.
- Clinical staging is based on the International Mesothelioma Interest Group (IMIG) staging system and uses the TNM system adopted by the AJCC (Edge et al., 2010).

Treatment

- Management of MPM uses a multidisciplinary team approach.
- Treatment options based on disease stage, performance status, and risk of morbidity include surgery, radiation therapy, and chemotherapy. The best outcomes result from the use of all three.
- Surgical approaches can be quite extensive and include pleurectomy with decortication (i.e., lung-sparing approach if possible), extrapleural pneumonectomy (i.e., removal of the entire lung, pleura, ipsilateral diaphragm, and often pericardium), and nodal dissection.
- Surgery can be considered for patients with stage I through III disease, although patients with sarcomatoid histology are often considered inoperable.
- Pemetrexed-based chemotherapy is the treatment of choice in combination with cisplatin or carboplatin before or after surgery and for patients who have stage IV or inoperable disease.

- On disease progression, patients can receive single-agent gemcitabine or vinorelbine.
- Radiation therapy alone is not recommended as the primary treatment for MPM.
  - Radiation therapy is typically used for adjuvant treatment after surgery.
  - Hemithoracic radiotherapy carries with it significant toxicity and is not recommended for patients with stage IV or unresected disease.
- Palliative radiation therapy is often used in smaller doses to treat painful chest wall or bone metastases.

Prognosis

- The median overall survival rate is approximately 1 year, and very few patients are cured.
- Those who are able to undergo surgery have a better chance of survival than those who are not surgical candidates.

Prevention and Surveillance

- There are no guidelines in place for screening of high-risk patients.

Bibliography

American Cancer Society (ACS). (2015). *Cancer facts and figures 2015.* Available at http://www.cancer.org/acs/groups/content/@editorial/documents/document/acspc-044552.pdf (accessed January 28, 2016).

American Cancer Society (ACS). (2015). *American Cancer Society estimated new cases for the four major cancers by sex and age group 2015.* Available at http://www.cancer.org/acs/groups/content/@editorial/documents/document/acspc-044511.pdf (accessed January 28, 2016).

Edge, S., Byrd, D. R., Compton, C. C., Fritz, A. G., Greene, F. L., & Trotti, A. (Eds.). (2010). *AJCC staging manual* (7th ed.). New York: Springer.

National Comprehensive Cancer Network. (2015). *NCCN national clinical practice guidelines in oncology: Malignant pleural mesothelioma, version 2.2015.* Available at http://www.nccn.org/professionals/physician_gls/pdf/mpm.pdf (accessed January 28, 2016).

Lymphomas

Amy Goodrich

Hodgkin Lymphoma

Definition

Lymphomas are cancers of the B or T lymphocytes or natural killer cells that originate in the lymphatic system. Lymphomas are divided into two major categories: Hodgkin lymphoma (HL) and all other lymphomas, called non-Hodgkin lymphomas (NHLs). HL, also referred to as *Hodgkin disease*, is an uncommon neoplasm arising from B lymphocytes and marked by a diagnostic tumor cell called the Reed-Sternberg cell. Two clinicopathologic entities are described: nodular lymphocyte–predominant HL (NLPHL) and classic HL (CHL).

Incidence

- HL represented about 11.2% of all lymphomas diagnosed in the United States in 2015.
- About 9050 new cases (5100 males, 3950 females) of HL and 1150 deaths from the disease occurred in the United States in 2015.
- The bimodal distribution of cases has one peak at 15 to 34 years of age and another at 50 years of age.
- In 2014, an estimated 177,526 people in the United States were living with HL, including those with active disease and those in remission.

Etiology and Risk Factors

- DNA mutations in B cells initiate HL, but not all risk factors or molecular pathways triggering these mutations have been identified. The abnormal B cells (i.e., multinucleated Reed-Sternberg cells) accumulate in the lymphatic system, where they crowd out healthy cells and cause the signs and symptoms of HL.
- Defective immune responses contribute to lymphoma progression. Evidence suggests that a dysregulated inflammatory response plays an important role in the pathogenesis of virus-associated HL.
  - A history of symptomatic infectious mononucleosis caused by the Epstein-Barr virus (EBV) is associated with almost one half of HL cases. The risk can persist for up to 20 years after EBV infection, which is more frequently associated with childhood and older adult HL cases.
  - EBV infection can cause direct DNA changes in B lymphocytes, leading to the development of Reed-Sternberg cells, which are the cancer cells in HL.
  - T-cell function is compromised in patients with HL, who do not demonstrate the normal immune response to particular antigens. Regulatory T cells inhibit antitumor immune responses by suppressing interferon-γ production by lymphocytes, including the T cells specific for EBV-positive HL.
- Having a compromised immune system, such as from human immunodeficiency virus (HIV) infection, predisposes to HL.
- Exposure to the measles virus, a lymphotropic virus, in childhood also increases the risk of HL in young adults.
- Some autoimmune conditions have been linked to an increased risk of HL.
- HL is most often diagnosed in people between the ages of 15 and 30 years and in those older than 55 years.
- Males are slightly more likely to develop HL than females.
- Having a first-degree relative with HL confers a threefold increased risk.
- Familial HL represents approximately 5% of new cases.

Signs and Symptoms

- Approximately one third of HL patients are symptomatic.
- Absence or presence of B symptoms is key in staging.
  - Unexplained loss of more than 10% of body weight in the 6 months before diagnosis
  - Unexplained fever with temperatures greater than 101.5° F (38° C) for longer than 3 days
  - Drenching night sweats
  - Pruritus
  - Pain in involved areas after ingestion of alcohol (less common)
- Physical findings
  - Painless adenopathy (commonly in the supraclavicular or cervical areas)
  - Splenomegaly

Diagnostic Work-up

- History and physical examination
- Laboratory tests
  - Complete blood cell count (CBC) with differential count
  - Erythrocyte sedimentation rate
  - Serum chemistries, including lactate dehydrogenase (LDH) levels
  - HIV test
  - Bone marrow aspirate and biopsy are indicated in the setting of stage IB, IIB, or III-IV disease; constitutional B symptoms or anemia; leukopenia; or thrombocytopenia. Bone marrow involvement occurs in 5% of patients.
- Imaging studies
  - Chest radiography

- Computed tomography (CT) of the neck, thorax, abdomen, and pelvis
- Positron emission tomography (PET) and CT, which have replaced gallium scans and lymphangiography for clinical staging

Histology

- The World Health Organization (WHO) modification of the Revised European-American Lymphoma (REAL) classification is used.
- Two distinct clinicopathologic entities are described: NLPHL and CHL.
  - The profile for NLPHL is CD15⁻, CD20⁺, CD30⁻, and CD45⁺.
  - The profile for CHL is CD15⁺, CD20⁻, CD30⁺, and CD45⁻.

Classic Hodgkin Lymphoma

- CHL accounts for 95% of cases.
- The typical immunophenotype is CD3⁻, CD15⁺, CD20⁻, CD30⁺, CD45⁻, CD79a⁻, PAX5⁺ B lymphocytes.
- There are four CHL subtypes.
  - Nodular sclerosis (grade I and II)
    - In the United States, 75% of HL cases
    - Equal distribution between sexes
    - More prominent in patients older than 50 years of age
    - Common anterior mediastinal involvement
    - Grade I: 75% of nodules contain scattered Reed-Sternberg cells
    - Grade 2: 25% contain numerous Reed-Sternberg cells surrounded by necrosis
  - Mixed cellularity
    - More prominent in males
    - Frequently associated with HIV and EBV infections
    - Classic Reed-Sternberg cells with inflammatory background rich in lymphocytes, plasma cells, and eosinophils
  - Lymphocyte rich
    - More common among males
    - Mostly stage I or II disease with rare B symptoms
    - Infrequent Reed-Sternberg cells in a background of small lymphocytes
  - Lymphocyte depleted
    - Least common subtype (<5% of cases)
    - More common in men
    - Typically advanced-stage disease and B symptoms are found at presentation
    - Reed-Sternberg cells predominant in a background of depleted lymphocytes

Nodular Lymphocyte–Predominant Hodgkin Lymphoma

- NLPHL accounts for approximately 5% of HL cases.
- It is typically diagnosed in asymptomatic young men with involved cervical or inguinal lymph nodes but without mediastinal involvement.
- Typical immunophenotype is CD3⁻, CD15⁻, CD20⁺, CD30⁻, CD45⁺, CD79a⁺, BCL6⁺, PAX5⁺ B lymphocytes.

- Patients are usually diagnosed with early-stage disease and have longer survival times and fewer treatment failures.

Clinical Staging

The staging system was originally adopted in 1971 at the Ann Arbor conference and modified at the Cotswolds meeting 18 years later (see table below).

- The Ann Arbor system characterizes disease by the number and location of involved lymph nodes and extranodal involvement.
- The Cotswolds modification maintains the original four-stage clinical and pathologic staging framework of the Ann Arbor system but adds information regarding the prognostic significance of bulky disease (denoted by an X) and regions of lymph node involvement (denoted by an E). The importance of imaging modalities (e.g., CT) is also underscored.
- Current practice is to assign a clinical stage based on the findings of the clinical evaluation and a pathologic stage based on the findings of invasive procedures. Pathologic confirmation of noncontiguous extralymphatic involvement is strongly suggested.

Ann Arbor Staging System for Hodgkin Lymphoma

Stage	Definition
I	Involvement of a single lymph node region (I) or localized involvement of a single extralymphatic organ or site (IE)
II	Involvement of more than two lymph node regions on the same side of the diaphragm (II) or localized involvement of a single associated extralymphatic organ or site and its regional lymph node(s) with or without involvement of other lymph node regions on the same side of the diaphragm (IIE)
III	Involvement of lymph node regions on both sides of the diaphragm (III), which may also be accompanied by localized involvement of an associated extralymphatic organ or site (IIIE)
IV	Disseminated (multifocal) involvement of one or more extralymphatic organs, with or without associated lymph node involvement, or isolated extralymphatic disease; organ involvement with distant (nonregional) nodal involvement
IVA	No systemic symptoms
IVB	Systemic B symptoms (unexplained fevers >38° C, drenching night sweats, or weight loss of >10% of body weight within 6 months before diagnosis)

Modified from Carbone, P. P., Kaplan, H. S., Musshoff, K., Smithers, D. W., & Tubiana, M. (1971). Report of the Committee on Hodgkin's Disease Staging Classification. *Cancer Research, 31*(11), 1860-1861.

- Letters are used in the various versions of the classification.
  - The A and B designations denote the absence or presence of B symptoms, respectively, which correlate with treatment response.
  - The letter E is used for stages I through III to denote extralymphatic disease resulting from direct extension of an involved lymph node region into other tissues or organs. It is not appropriate to use this designation for widespread disease or diffuse extralymphatic disease. Extranodal cancer that has spread to the spleen is indicated by the letter S.

A staging system that is particularly useful in clinical trials uses three major disease categories (early favorable, early unfavorable, and advanced) based on prognostic features. The European Organization for Research and Treatment of Cancer (EORTC) has defined favorable and unfavorable features for stage I and II disease, and the International Prognostic Factors Project has developed an International Prognostic Index with seven adverse factors for advanced stages (stage III and IV). They are described in the box below.

Risk-Based Staging System

Early Favorable Disease*

- <50 yr of age
- Clinical stage I and II
- No B symptoms or elevated erythrocyte sedimentation rate
- B symptoms + erythrocyte sedimentation rate <30 mm/hr
- Involvement of <3 lymph node areas
- Mediastinal involvement <33% of the thoracic width on the chest radiograph, <10 cm on CT

Early Unfavorable Disease*

- Age >50 yr
- Clinical stage II
- Elevated erythrocyte sedimentation rate >50 mm/hr or 30 mm/hr in the setting of B symptoms
- Involvement of >3 lymph node areas
- Mediastinal involvement >33% of the thoracic width on the chest radiograph, >10 cm on CT

Advanced Disease†

- Albumin level <4.0 g/dL
- Hemoglobin level <10.5 g/dL
- Male sex
- Age >45 yrs
- Stage IV disease
- White blood cell count at least 15,000/mm³
- Absolute lymphocytic count <600/mm³ or a lymphocyte count <8% of the total white blood cell count

*Definitions from the European Organization for Research and Treatment of Cancer.
†Definitions from the International Prognostic Index for patients with clinical stage *B symptoms*, Unexplained fevers greater than 38° C, drenching night sweats, or weight loss of more than 10% of body weight within 6 months before diagnosis; *CT*, computed tomography.
III or IV disease.
Modified from Mullen, E., & Zhong, Y. (2007). Hodgkin lymphoma: An update. *The Journal for Nurse Practitioners, 3,* 393-403.

Treatment

- Treatment is based on stage and prognostic factors.
- Standard treatment is intensive combination chemotherapy and involved-field radiation therapy, which yields a greater than 90% cure rate.
- First-line chemotherapy agents are usually given in combination and may include the following:
  - Bleomycin
  - Cyclophosphamide
  - Cytosine arabinoside
  - Dacarbazine
  - Doxorubicin
  - Etoposide
  - Mechlorethamine
  - Methotrexate
  - Prednisone or dexamethasone
  - Procarbazine
  - Vincristine or vinblastine
- Rituximab as monotherapy or in combination regimens may be given for patients with NLPHL (CD20⁺).
- Salvage treatments
  - The same regimen used for first-line therapy may be effective for late recurrences. Early recurrences should be treated with different agents.
  - Several chemotherapy drugs not used in initial treatment have demonstrated efficacy against recurrent disease:
    - Bendamustine (only for CHL)
    - Brentuximab vedotin (only for CHL)
    - Moderate- or high-dose cytarabine
    - Carboplatin or cisplatin
    - Carmustine
    - Etoposide
    - Everolimus (only for CHL)
    - Gemcitabine
    - Ifosfamide
    - Lenalidomide (only for CHL)
    - Liposomal doxorubicin
    - Melphalan
    - Mitoxantrone
    - Vinorelbine
    - Vinblastine
- Radiation therapy delivered to sites not previously irradiated

Prognosis

- HL is considered a curable disease, with an overall 5-year survival rate of 86%.
- The mortality rate in the United States has fallen more rapidly for adult HL than for any other malignancy.
- HL is the primary cause of death during the first 15 years after treatment. By 15 to 20 years after therapy, the cumulative mortality rate for a second malignancy exceeds that for HL.
- Patients with advanced favorable disease (i.e., zero to three adverse risk factors) have an 80% freedom-from-progression rate at 5 years with first-line chemotherapy.
- Patients with advanced unfavorable disease (i.e., stage II or IV disease and four to seven adverse factors) had a less than 70% freedom-from-progression rate at 5 years with first-line combination chemotherapy.

Prevention and Surveillance

There are no known preventive measures for HL. There are no specific screening tests, and regular physical examination is the best method for early diagnosis.

Bibliography

Carbone, P. P., Kaplan, H. S., Musshoff, K., Smithers, D. W., & Tubiana, M. (1971). Report of the Committee on Hodgkin's Disease Staging Classification. *Cancer Research, 31*(11), 1860–1861.

Cosset, J. M., Henry-Amar, M., Meerwaldt, J. H., Carde, P., Noordijk, E. M., Thomas, J., & Tubiana, M. (1992). The EORTC trials for limited stage Hodgkin's disease. The EORTC Lymphoma Cooperative Group. *Eur J Cancer, 28A*(11), 1847–1850.

Evens, A. M., Helenowski, I., Ramsdale, E., Nabhan, C., Karmali, R., Hanson, B., & Smith, S. M. (2012). A retrospective multicenter analysis of elderly Hodgkin lymphoma: Outcomes and prognostic factors in the modern era. *Blood, 119*(3), 692–695.

Leukemia and Lymphoma Society. (2014). *Hodgkin lymphoma facts and statistics.* Available at https://www.lls.org/content/nationalcontent/resourcecenter/freeeducationmaterials/generalcancer/pdf/facts.pdf (accessed January 7, 2016).

Mullen, E., & Zhong, Y. (2007). Hodgkin lymphoma: An update. *The Journal for Nurse Practitioners, 3,* 393–403.

National Cancer Institute. (2015). *Adult Hodgkin's lymphoma: Treatment—for health professionals (PDQ).* Available at http://www.cancer.gov/cancertopics/pdq/treatment/adulthodgkins/HealthProfessional (accessed January 7, 2016).

National Cancer Institute. (2015). *Childhood Hodgkin's lymphoma: Treatment—for health professionals (PDQ).* Available at http://www.cancer.gov/cancertopics/pdq/treatment/childhodgkins/HealthProfessional (accessed January 7, 2016).

National Comprehensive Cancer Network. (2014). *Hodgkin lymphoma, version 2.2014.* Available at http://www.nccn.org/professionals/physician_gls/pdf/hodgkins.pdf (accessed January 7, 2016).

Siegel, R. L., Miller, K. D., & Jemal, A. (2015). Cancer statistics, 2015. *CA: A Cancer Journal for Clinicians, 65,* 5–29.

Non-Hodgkin Lymphoma

Definition

NHLs are a diverse group of cancers of the immune system. NHLs are classified according to the cell of origin (i.e., B or T cell) and are further divided into aggressive and indolent types. B-cell NHLs include Burkitt lymphoma, diffuse large B-cell lymphoma, follicular lymphoma, immunoblastic large cell lymphoma, precursor B-lymphoblastic lymphoma, and mantle cell lymphoma. T-cell NHLs include mycosis fungoides, anaplastic large cell lymphoma, and precursor T-lymphoblastic lymphoma. The NHL subtype predicts the necessity of early treatment, the response to treatment, the type of treatment required, and the prognosis.

Incidence

- NHLs are the sixth most common cancer among men and women and the seventh most common cause of cancer-related deaths in the United States.
- About 71,850 (39,850 men, 32,000 women) new cases of NHL and 19,790 deaths occurred in the United States in 2015.
- Incidence increases with age; the median age at diagnosis is 67 years.
- NHL occurs more often in whites than blacks and is more common among men than women,
- In 2014, an estimated 584,133 people in the United States were living with NHL, including those with active disease and those in remission.

Etiology and Risk Factors

- Although the exact cause of NHL is unknown, an increased risk of developing the disease is associated with toxic exposures and many medical conditions, including infections, genetic syndromes, and immune deficiencies.

- The risk of NHL is increased by some viral and bacterial infections:
  - *Helicobacter pylori* (i.e., mucosa-associated lymphoid tissue [MALT] lymphoma)
  - Other bacteria such as *Borrelia burgdorferi, Campylobacter jejuni,* and *Chlamydia psittaci*
  - Epstein-Barr virus (associated with 30% of Burkitt lymphoma cases)
  - Human T-cell leukemia/lymphoma virus 1
  - Human herpes virus 8
  - Hepatitis C virus
  - Human immunodeficiency virus (HIV)
- Risk is increased by chronic suppression or derangement of the immune system by various medical conditions or their treatments:
  - HIV infection
  - Systemic lupus erythematosus
  - Celiac disease
  - Inflammatory bowel disease (e.g., Crohn disease)
  - Sjögren's syndrome
  - Psoriasis
  - Organ or bone marrow transplantation (i.e., required immune suppression medications)
  - Rheumatoid arthritis
  - Inherited disorders with adverse immune effects (e.g., Down syndrome, Klinefelter syndrome)
- There is a positive association between exposure to pesticides and herbicides and NHL.
- Age is a factor; rates are much higher among persons older than 65 years (68 cases for every 100,000 people).

Signs and Symptoms

- The most common early symptom is painless lymphadenopathy, usually in the neck, armpit, groin, or abdomen.
- The absence or presence of B symptoms is key in staging:
  - Unexplained loss of more than 10% of body weight in the 6 months before diagnosis
  - Unexplained fever with temperatures greater than 101.5° F (38° C) for more than 3 days
  - Drenching night sweats
  - Fatigue
  - Pruritus
- Given the heterogeneity of NHL, signs and symptoms can vary greatly depending on the areas of the body that are affected.
  - MALT lymphoma affects the stomach lining and can cause nausea, vomiting, and abdominal pain.
  - Cutaneous T-cell lymphoma affects the skin and can cause redness, itching, or raised patches on the skin.

Diagnostic Work-up

- Complete medical history and physical examination
- Laboratory tests
  - CBC with differential count
  - Erythrocyte sedimentation rate
  - Serum chemistries, including β_2-microglobulin

- Elevated LDH and uric acid levels that correlate with a large tumor burden
- HIV and hepatitis B screening
- Cytogenetics or fluorescence in situ hybridization (FISH) for identification of chromosomal or genetic abnormalities
- Immunophenotyping (for chronic lymphocytic leukemia [CLL], which is considered the same as small lymphocytic lymphoma [SLL], flow cytometry may be used to establish the diagnosis without tissue or bone marrow biopsy)
- Cerebrospinal fluid assessment for malignant cells
- Bone marrow aspirate and biopsy
- Imaging studies
  - Thoracic and abdominal-pelvic CT or magnetic resonance imaging (MRI); optional neck CT
  - PET, sometimes combined with CT, has replaced gallium scanning and lymphangiography for clinical staging.
- Biopsy of involved lymph nodes
  - Only definitive method to diagnose NHLs other than CLL/SLL
  - Necessary to determine presence of disease and type of lymphoma

Histology

- The World Health Organization (WHO) modification of the REAL classification system recognizes three major categories of lymphoid malignancies on the basis of morphology and cell lineage: B-cell neoplasms, T-cell/natural killer cell neoplasms, and HL.
- Lymphomas and lymphoid leukemias are included in the classification because solid and circulating phases occur for many lymphoid neoplasms, and the distinction between them is artificial.
- Within the B-cell and T-cell categories, two subdivisions are recognized: precursor neoplasms, which correspond to the earliest stages of differentiation, and the more mature differentiated neoplasms. These classifications are shown in the box at the top of the next column.
- The more than 20 clinicopathologic entities described by the WHO classification can be divided into more clinically useful indolent or aggressive lymphomas. They are listed in the box at the bottom of the next column and on page 131.
- Indolent or low-grade classifications account for approximately 35% of NHL diagnoses, and the remaining 65% are aggressive (i.e., intermediate- or high-grade NHL).
- In the United States, B-cell lymphomas account for about 90% of all NHL cases.

Clinical Staging

- Current practice assigns a clinical stage based on the findings of the clinical evaluation and a pathologic stage based on the findings of invasive procedures beyond that of the initial biopsy.
- The Ann Arbor staging system is most often used to describe the extent of NHL in adults.

WHO Modification of the REAL Classification of Lymphoid Tumors

B-Cell Neoplasms

I. Precursor B-cell neoplasm: precursor B-acute lymphoblastic leukemia/lymphoblastic lymphoma
II. Peripheral B-cell neoplasms
   A. B-cell chronic lymphocytic leukemia/small lymphocytic lymphoma
   B. B-cell prolymphocytic leukemia
   C. Lymphoplasmacytic lymphoma/immunocytoma
   D. Mantle cell lymphoma
   E. Follicular lymphoma
   F. Extranodal marginal zone B-cell lymphoma of mucosa-associated lymphatic tissue (MALT) type
   G. Nodal marginal zone B-cell lymphoma (± monocytoid B cells)
   H. Splenic marginal zone lymphoma (± villous lymphocytes)
   I. Hairy cell leukemia
   J. Plasmacytoma/plasma cell myeloma
   K. Diffuse large B-cell lymphoma
   L. Burkitt lymphoma

T-Cell Neoplasms

III. Precursor T-cell neoplasm: precursor T-acute lymphoblastic leukemia (LBL)
IV. Peripheral T-cell and natural killer cell neoplasms
   A. T-cell chronic lymphocytic leukemia/prolymphocytic leukemia
   B. T-cell granular lymphocytic leukemia
   C. Mycosis fungoides/Sézary syndrome
   D. Peripheral T-cell lymphoma, not otherwise characterized
   E. Hepatosplenic gamma/delta T-cell lymphoma
   F. Subcutaneous panniculitis-like T-cell lymphoma
   G. Angioimmunoblastic T-cell lymphoma
   H. Extranodal T-/natural killer cell lymphoma, nasal type
   I. Enteropathy-type intestinal T-cell lymphoma
   J. Adult T-cell lymphoma/leukemia (human T-lymphotropic virus type 1 [HTLV-1+])
   K. Anaplastic large cell lymphoma, primary systemic type
   L. Anaplastic large cell lymphoma, primary cutaneous type
   M. Aggressive natural killer cell leukemia

Modified from Pileri, S. A., Milani, M., Fraternali-Orcioni, G., et al. (1998). From the R.E.A.L. classification to the upcoming WHO scheme: A step toward universal categorization of lymphoma entities. *Annals of Oncology, 9*, 608; National Comprehensive Cancer Network. (2014). *Non-Hodgkin lymphoma, version 2.2015.* Available at http://www.nccn.org/professionals/physician_gls/pdf/nhl.pdf (accessed January 11, 2016).

Indolent and Aggressive Non-Hodgkin Lymphomas

I. Indolent lymphoma/leukemia
   A. Follicular lymphoma (follicular small-cleaved cell [grade 1], follicular mixed small-cleaved and large cell [grade 2], diffuse small-cleaved cell)
   B. Small lymphocytic lymphoma
   C. Lymphoplasmacytic lymphoma (Waldenström macroglobulinemia)
   D. Extranodal marginal zone B-cell lymphoma (mucosa-associated lymphoid tissue [MALT] lymphoma)
   E. Nodal marginal zone B-cell lymphoma (monocytoid B-cell lymphoma)
   F. Splenic marginal zone lymphoma (splenic lymphoma with villous lymphocytes)
   G. Mycosis fungoides/Sézary syndrome
   H. Primary cutaneous anaplastic large cell lymphoma/lymphomatoid papulosis (CD30+)
II. Aggressive lymphoma/leukemia
   A. Diffuse large cell lymphoma (includes diffuse mixed-cell, diffuse large cell, immunoblastic, T-cell–rich large B-cell lymphoma)
      1. Mediastinal large B-cell lymphoma
      2. Follicular large cell lymphoma (grade 3)

Continued

Indolent and Aggressive Non-Hodgkin Lymphomas—cont'd

3. Anaplastic large cell lymphoma (CD30+)
4. Extranodal natural killer cell/T-cell lymphoma, nasal type/ aggressive natural killer cell leukemia/blastic natural killer cell lymphoma
5. Lymphomatoid granulomatosis (angiocentric pulmonary B-cell lymphoma)
6. Angioimmunoblastic T-cell lymphoma
7. Peripheral T-cell lymphoma, unspecified
8. Subcutaneous panniculitis-like T-cell lymphoma
9. Hepatosplenic T-cell lymphoma
10. Enteropathy-type T-cell lymphoma
11. Intravascular large B-cell lymphoma
B. Burkitt lymphoma/Burkitt-like lymphoma
C. Precursor B-cell or T-cell lymphoblastic lymphoma
D. Primary central nervous system lymphoma
E. Adult T-cell lymphoma (HTLV-1+)
F. Mantle cell lymphoma
G. Polymorphic posttransplantation lymphoproliferative disorder
H. Acquired immunodeficiency syndrome–related lymphoma
I. True histiocytic lymphoma
J. Primary effusion lymphoma

Modified from National Cancer Institute. (2015). *Cellular classification: Adult non-Hodgkin's lymphoma: Treatment–health professional version (PDQ)*. Available at http://www.cancer.gov/cancertopics/pdq/treatment/adult-non-hodgkins/Health Professional; National Comprehensive Cancer Network. (2014). *Non-Hodgkin lymphoma, version 2.2015*. Available at http://www.nccn.org/professionals/physician_gls/pdf/nhl.pdf (accessed January 11, 2016).

- Stages I through IV (see table below) can be further categorized by the letters A, B, and E:
  - A indicates an absence of B symptoms.
  - B indicates the presence of B symptoms (see earlier Signs and Symptoms section).
  - E is also used in stages I through III.
    - E denotes the presence of extralymphatic disease resulting from direct extension of an involved lymph node region.
    - It is not appropriate to use the E designation in the setting of widespread disease or diffuse extralymphatic disease.

Ann Arbor Staging System for Non-Hodgkin Lymphoma*

Stage	Definition
I	Involvement of a single lymph node region (I) or localized involvement of a single extralymphatic organ or site (IE)
II	Involvement of more than two lymph node regions on the same side of the diaphragm (II) or localized involvement of a single associated extralymphatic organ or site and its regional lymph node(s) with or without involvement of other lymph node regions on the same side of the diaphragm (IIE)
III	Involvement of lymph node regions on both sides of the diaphragm (III), which may also be accompanied by localized involvement of an associated extralymphatic organ or site (IIIE)
IV	Disseminated (multifocal) involvement of one or more extralymphatic organs, with or without associated lymph node involvement, or isolated extralymphatic organ involvement with distant (nonregional) nodal involvement

*A different staging system is used for cutaneous T-cell lymphoma, mycosis fungoides, and chronic lymphocytic leukemia.

Treatment

- Treatment depends on the stage, histologic type, and indolent or aggressive nature of the disease.
- Chemotherapy is the most commonly used treatment.
- Other therapies include immunotherapy and radioimmunotherapy.
- Radiation therapy use is limited to treating localized disease or symptomatic areas.
- Surgery typically is used to establish the diagnosis; exceptions are early-stage gastrointestinal lymphomas and testicular lymphomas.

Indolent Stage I and Contiguous Stage II Disease

Localized disease is uncommon in patients with NHL, and any of the following treatments may be used:

- Watchful waiting for asymptomatic patients until disease progression or the patient becomes symptomatic
- Involved-site radiation therapy (ISRT)
- Extended (regional) radiation therapy to cover adjacent nodes
- Chemotherapy with radiation therapy
- Rituximab, an anti-CD20 monoclonal antibody, alone or in combination with chemotherapy or ISRT, or both
- Other therapies as designated for patients with advanced-stage disease

Aggressive Stage I and Contiguous Stage II Disease

- Chemotherapy with or without ISRT
- Rituximab plus cyclophosphamide, doxorubicin, vincristine, and prednisone (R-CHOP regimen)

Indolent, Noncontiguous Stage II, III, or IV Disease

- Optimal treatment of advanced stages of low-grade lymphoma is controversial because of the low cure rates with current therapies.
- Watchful waiting for asymptomatic patients until disease progression or until the patient becomes symptomatic
- Rituximab as single agent or in combination
- Chemotherapy, usually in a combination that includes purine nucleoside analogs and alkylating agents with or without steroids and bendamustine
- Radioimmunotherapy with yttrium 90–labeled ibritumomab tiuxetan and iodine 131–labeled tositumomab for patients with minimal (25%) or no marrow involvement
- Maintenance rituximab
- Intensive therapy with chemotherapy with or without total body radiation therapy or high-dose chemotherapy followed by autologous or allogeneic bone marrow transplantation or peripheral stem cell transplantation is being clinically evaluated.

Aggressive, Noncontiguous Stage II, III, or IV Disease

- Combination chemotherapy alone or with local-field radiation therapy
  - Doxorubicin-based combination chemotherapy produces long-term, disease-free survival for 35% to 45% of patients.
  - Rituximab may be used for CD20+ B-cell NHL.

- Bone marrow or stem cell transplantation for patients at high risk for relapse is being evaluated.
- Central nervous system (CNS) prophylaxis is recommended for patients with paranasal sinus involvement, testicular involvement, epidural involvement, bone marrow with large cell lymphoma, HIV-positive lymphoma, kidney or adrenal gland involvement, stage IE diffuse large B-cell lymphoma of the breast, concurrent *MYC* and *BCL2* gene expression, or 2+ extranodal sites and elevated LDH levels.

Adult Lymphoblastic Lymphoma

- Lymphoblastic lymphoma is an aggressive form of NHL that most often occurs in younger patients.
- It is commonly associated with large mediastinal masses and often disseminates to the bone marrow and CNS, much like acute lymphocytic leukemia (ALL).
- Treatment is usually patterned after that used for ALL.
- Intensive combination chemotherapy with CNS prophylaxis is the standard therapy.
- Radiation is sometimes used to treat bulky tumor areas.

Burkitt Lymphoma

- Patients with diffuse small Burkitt lymphoma have a 20% to 30% lifetime risk of CNS involvement.
- CNS prophylaxis is recommended for all patients.

Prognosis

- The overall survival rate at 5 years is more than 60%.
- Patients with indolent NHL have a relatively good prognosis, with a median survival time of up to 10 years, but advanced disease is usually not curable.
- Aggressive NHL has a shorter natural history, but more than 50% of patients can be cured.
- Most relapses occur in the first 2 years after therapy.
- Five significant risk factors of overall survival for patients with NHL have been identified. Patients with two or more risk factors have a less than 50% chance of relapse-free survival at 5 years:

- Age (<60 years versus >60 years)
- Performance status (0 or 1 versus 2 to 4)
- Serum LDH level (normal versus elevated)
- Stage (I or II versus III or IV)
- Extranodal site involvement (0 or 1 versus 2 to 4 areas)
- Increased risk for relapse is linked to specific sites of involvement, including bone marrow, CNS, liver, lung, and spleen.

Prevention and Surveillance

Because the specific cause of NHL is unknown, there are no guidelines for prevention. Some risk factors (e.g., infections) can be avoided, but most (e.g., genetic disorders) cannot.

Bibliography

Cabanillas, F., Velasquez, W. S., Hagemeister, F. B., McLaughlin, P., & Redman, J. R. (1992). Clinical, biologic, and histologic features of late relapses in diffuse large cell lymphoma. *Blood*, *79*(4), 1024–1028.

Leukemia and Lymphoma Society. (2014). *Non-Hodgkin lymphoma facts and statistics*. Available at https://www.lls.org/content/nationalcontent/re sourcecenter/freeeducationmaterials/generalcancer/pdf/facts.pdf (accessed January 12, 2016).

National Cancer Institute. (2015). *Adult non-Hodgkin's lymphoma: Treatment—for health professionals (PDQ)*. Available at http://www.cancer .gov/cancertopics/pdq/treatment/adult-non-hodgkins/HealthProfession al (accessed January 12, 2016).

National Cancer Institute. (2015). *AIDS-related lymphoma: Treatment—for health professionals (PDQ)*. Available at http://www.cancer.gov/cancertop ics/pdq/treatment/AIDS-related-lymphoma/HealthProfessional (accessed January 12, 2016).

National Comprehensive Cancer Network. *Non-Hodgkin lymphoma, version 2. 2015*. Available at http://www.nccn.org/professionals/physician_gls /pdf/nhl.pdf (accessed January 12, 2016).

Pileri, S. A., Milani, M., Fraternali-Orcioni, G., & Sabattini, E. (1998). From the R.E.A.L. classification to the upcoming WHO scheme: A step toward universal categorization of lymphoma entities? *Annals of Oncology*, *9*, 607–612.

Siegel, R. L., Miller, K. D., & Jemal, A. (2015). Cancer statistics, 2015. *CA: A Cancer Journal for Clinicians*, *65*, 5–29.

Skarin, A. T., & Dorfman, D. M. (1997). Non-Hodgkin's lymphomas: Current classification and management. *CA: A Cancer Journal for Clinicians*, *47*, 351–372.

Vachani, C. (2006). *Non-Hodgkin's lymphoma: The basics*. Available at http:/ /www.oncolink.org/types/article.cfm?c=359&id=9539 (accessed January 12, 2016).

Multiple Myeloma

Sandra Kurtin

Definition

Multiple myeloma (MM) is a plasma B-cell neoplasm characterized by secretion of excess paraproteins (i.e., monoclonal immunoglobulin molecules) with secondary organ effects, including renal, bone, bone marrow, neurologic, and immune dysfunction. MM is highly treatable but characterized by inevitable relapses.

- Myeloma cells are transformed plasma cells that continually produce abnormal immunoglobulins (i.e., monoclonal proteins), also referred to as M proteins.
- Three types of MM are based on the predominant type of abnormal protein secretion:
  - *Heavy chain:* Immunoglobulin (Ig) G is most common (60%) type, followed by IgA, and IgD (rare); abnormal IgM is most often associated with Waldenström macroglobulinemia.
  - *Light chain:* This type, which can be κ or λ light chain disease, represents about 20% of MM cases.
  - *Nonsecretory:* Although a high level of an M protein in the blood is the hallmark of myeloma, 1% to 2% of patients have nonsecretory myeloma, with no M protein detectable on serum or urine electrophoresis.

Incidence

- MM accounts for 1.4% of all cancers and 13% of hematologic malignancies; it is the second most prevalent hematologic cancer after non-Hodgkin lymphoma.
- About 26,850 new cases of MM and 11,240 related deaths occurred in the United States in 2015.

Etiology and Risk Factors

- Risk factors for MM include advanced age, male gender, obesity, and African American descent.
- There is a fourfold risk if a sibling or parent has the disease.
- Median age at diagnosis is 69 years; 62% of patients are older than 65 years, and 34% of patients are older than 75 years of age.
- In 2013 in the United States, the incidence of MM among African American men (14.4 cases/100,000) was more than double that among white men (6.6 cases/100,000). African American women are more likely to develop MM than white women (9.8 cases versus 4.1 cases per 100,000).
- Exposure to chemicals, including pesticides, arsenic, cadmium, lead, and various cleaning solutions, increases the risk of MM.
- Radiation exposure victims (e.g., survivors of atomic bomb explosions in Japan) have an increased risk, although the number is small.
- Obesity is a risk factor for many cancers, including MM.
- A history of other plasma cell diseases, including monoclonal gammopathy of undetermined significance and solitary plasmacytoma, increases the risk.

Signs and Symptoms

- The most common complaints at presentation are bone pain and fatigue.
- Signs and symptoms result from an overproduction of transformed plasma cells that make abnormal immunoglobulins and displace production of normal red blood cells, white blood cells, and platelets.
  - Plasma cell invasion of bone causes bone pain, fractures, and hypercalcemia and may cause spinal cord compression.
  - Bone marrow involvement causes fatigue, anemia, neutropenia, and thrombocytopenia.
  - Renal involvement causes fatigue, anemia, hematuria, frothy urine, elevated creatinine levels, hypercalcemia, urate nephropathy, and acute renal failure.
  - Abnormal immunoglobulin function causes fever, infections, hypogammaglobulinemia (i.e., paraprotein unaffected), and neurologic symptoms.
  - Hyperviscosity causes pain, paresthesia, immobility, peripheral neuropathy, and an increased risk for stroke.
  - Increased interleukin-6 secretion augments the risk of venous thromboembolism.

Diagnostic Work-up

- Laboratory, radiologic, and hematopathologic evaluations
- History and physical examination
- Complete blood cell, differential, and platelet counts
- Additional laboratory tests
  - Quantitative serum levels of immunoglobulins (IgG, IgM, IgA, IgD), serum protein electrophoresis (SPEP) with immunofixation, and assay of serum levels of free light chains (i.e., κ and λ)
  - Tests for blood urea nitrogen (BUN), creatinine, electrolytes, serum calcium (corrected value), serum albumin, β_2-microglobulin, lactate dehydrogenase, and C-reactive protein (i.e., surrogate for interleukin-6)
- A 24-hour urine test
  - Urine protein electrophoresis (UPEP) with immunofixation
  - Total protein
- Bone marrow biopsy and aspiration
  - Hematopathology
  - Percentage of plasma cells
  - Cellularity
  - Ploidy

- Cytogenetics
- Fluorescence in situ hybridization (FISH)
- Imaging
  - Skeletal survey
  - Positron emission tomography (PET) or computed tomography (CT)
  - MRI if vertebral compression fractures suspected
- After the diagnosis is made, determination of the stage and subtype of MM, including a prognostic evaluation, guides treatment selection.
- Identified problems requiring emergent intervention include severe hypercalcemia, acute renal failure, spinal cord compression, and severe pain or impending fractures.

Classification

MM has three categories:

- Monoclonal gammopathy of undetermined significance (MGUS)
- Asymptomatic multiple myeloma (ASMM) or smoldering multiple myeloma (SMM)
  - Increased M protein and more plasma cells in the bone marrow compared with MGUS
  - No evidence of symptoms or signs of MM or related organ disease
  - Diagnostic findings
    - IgG ≥3 g/dL and IgA >1 g/dL *or*
    - Bence Jones protein >1 g/24 hours *and/or*
    - Clonal plasma cells of 10% or more in bone marrow
- Symptomatic MM
  - The International Myeloma Working Group guidelines for the diagnosis of MM for 2014 are shown in the table below.

Diagnostic Criteria for Myeloma of Undetermined Significance, Smoldering Multiple Myeloma, and Symptomatic Myeloma

Condition	MGUS	SMM	Active Myeloma
Clonal BMPCs	<10%	10%-60%	≥10% or biopsy-proven bony or extramedullary plasmacytoma and one or more MDEs
MDEs	None	None	Yes
Monoclonal protein (M protein)	<30 g/L	≥30 g/L (IgG or IgA) serum protein; or ≥500 mg/24 hr urinary protein	No specific level required; active disease defined by MDEs

Myeloma-Related End-Organ Damage: Revised CRAB Criteria for MDEs

C: Calcium elevation : serum calcium >0.25 mmol/L (>1 mg/dL) higher than ULN *or* >2.75 mmol/L (>11 mg/dL)

R: Renal dysfunction: creatinine clearance <40 mL/min or serum creatinine >177 mcg/L (>2 mg/dL)

A: Anemia: hemoglobin >20 g/L below LLN or <100 g/L

B: Bone disease: one or more osteolytic lesions on skeletal radiography, CT, or PET and CT

Plus one or more biomarkers of malignancy:

BMPC >60%

Involved/uninvolved serum free light chain ratio ≥100

>1 focal lesion >5 mm on MRI studies

BMPC, bone marrow plasma cells; *CT,* computed tomography; *Ig,* immunoglobulin; *LLN,* lower limit of normal; *MDEs,* myeloma-defining events; *MGUS,* myeloma of undetermined significance; *MRI,* magnetic resonance imaging; *PET,* positron emission tomography; *SMM,* smoldering multiple myeloma; *ULN,* upper limit of normal.

Modified from Rajkumar, S. V., Dimopoulos, M. A., Palumbo, A., Blade, J., Merlini, G., Mateos, M. V. et al. (2014). International Myeloma Working Group updated criteria for the diagnosis of multiple myeloma. *Lancet Oncology, 15*(12), e538-e548

Clinical Staging

The Durie-Salmon system measures tumor burden by the number of myeloma-related bone lesions seen on a radiograph and the concentrations of serum calcium, serum M protein, and urine Bence Jones protein to classify patients as having stage I, II, or III disease. This staging system is most useful in comparing historical outcomes (see table below).

The International Staging System (ISS) provides a measure of proliferative tumor and prognostic information based on multivariate analysis of clinical features. Using β_2-microglobulin and serum albumin levels, MM is categorized as stage I (median survival, 62 months), stage II (median survival, 44 months), or stage III (median survival, 29 months).

Clinical Staging for Multiple Myeloma

Stage	Durie-Salmon Staging System	International Staging System
I	Hemoglobin >10 g/dL Calcium normal or ≥12 mg/dL Normal skeletal survey or solitary plasmacytoma Low M protein production • IgG <5 g/dL • IgA <3 g/dL Bence Jones protein <4 g/24 hr	β_2M ≤3.5 g/dL and albumin ≥3.5 g/dL
II	Neither stage I nor stage III	Neither stage I nor stage III
III	One of the following • Hemoglobin <8.5 g/dL • Calcium >12 mg/dL • Multiple lytic bone lesions • High M protein component • IgG >7 g/dL • IgA >5 g/dL Bence Jones protein >12 g/24 hr	β_2M ≥5.5 g/dL

β_2M, β_2-Microglobulin; *Ig,* immunoglobulin.

Treatment

- MM is a genetically heterogeneous disease with wide variations in response to treatment and no known cure.
- Treatment is based on risk stratification and transplantation eligibility.
- The treatment goal is an early and sustained complete response (CR) with no evidence of molecular disease (i.e., zero minimal residual disease [MRD])

- Risk-adapted therapy selection criteria are applied (see figure below).
  - Eligibility for hematopoietic stem cell transplantation (HSCT) is determined by several factors.
    - Age
    - Comorbidities
    - Performance status (i.e., fit versus frail)
  - Disease characteristics associated with increased risk are considered.
    - *High risk*: FISH shows del(17p), t(4;16), t(14;20), or high-risk gene expression profile.
    - *Intermediate risk*: FISH shows t(94;14), cytogenetic del(13), hypoploidy, or plasma cell labeling index (PCLI) of 3% or greater.
    - *Standard risk:* All other cases, including those with t(11;14) or t(6;14)
  - Personal choice
- Clinical trials have included successful use of a vaccine consisting of measles virus modified to make it selectively toxic to MM cells.

Supportive Care

- All patients with MM should receive supportive care.
- Common toxicities reported with agents used to treat MM are outlined in the table on page 132.
- Treatment of bone disease
  - All patients receiving anti-MM treatment for active disease should be given bisphosphonates (i.e., zoledronic acid or pamidronate) for up to 2 years to improve bone density.
  - The patient is monitored for renal function and osteonecrosis of the jaw.
  - Kyphoplasty or vertebroplasty may be beneficial for patients with vertebral compression fractures.

- Symptomatic hypercalcemia may be treated with hydration, furosemide, bisphosphonates, steroids, or calcitonin.
- Plasmapheresis may be helpful in treating symptomatic hyperviscosity. Concurrent anti-MM therapy is recommended.
- Treatment of anemia
  - Anti-MM treatment
  - Transfusion of packed red blood cells if indicated
  - Erythropoietin-stimulating agents may be used based on current safety guidelines.
- Treatment of infections
  - Pneumococcal infections are common in patients with MM, and pneumococcal vaccination should be completed at the time of diagnosis and repeated in 5 years to minimize preventable illness.
  - Shingles prophylaxis is recommended for all patients receiving bortezomib. Live shingles vaccines are not recommended.
- Renal compromise is common in patients with MM.
  - Less than 10% have severe renal failure at presentation.
  - Between 30% and 40% have elevated serum creatinine levels at presentation.
  - Between 25% and 50% have renal impairment during the disease course.
- Treatment of renal dysfunction
  - Treat the MM.
  - Treat hypercalcemia.
  - Treat hyperviscosity.
  - Avoid aggravating factors (e.g., dehydration, diabetes, hypertension).
  - Medications include nonsteroidal antiinflammatory drugs (NSAIDs) and loop diuretics.
  - Intravenous contrast for CT (incidence of contrast-induced nephropathy is low)

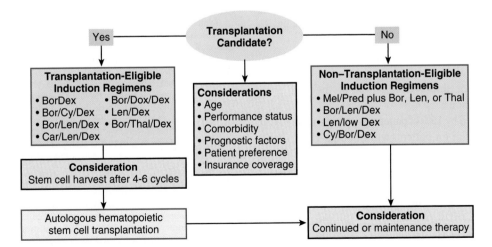

Bor, bortezomib; Car, carfilzomib; Cy, cyclophosphamide; Dex, dexamethasone; Dox, doxorubicin; Len, lenalidomide; Mel, melphalan; Pred, prednisone; Thal, thalidomide

Risk-adapted therapy selection is key. (Modified from Miceli, T., Lilleby, K., Noonan, K., Kurtin, S., Faiman, B., & Mangan, P. A. (2013). Autologous hematopoietic stem cell transplantation for patients with multiple myeloma: An overview for nurses in community practice. *Clinical Journal of Oncology Nursing, 17*[6 Suppl], 3-24.)

Common Toxicities of Agents Used to Treat Multiple Myeloma

Toxicity	Thalidomide	Lenalidomide	Pomalidomide	Bortezomib	Carfilzomib	Panobinostat
Neuropathy (PN)	Yes			Yes*	Yes	No
Thrombosis (DVT, PE)	Yes, more with Dex	Yes, more with Dex	Yes, more with Dex	No	No	No
Myelosuppression	Yes, neutropenia	Yes, anemia, thrombocytopenia, neutropenia	Yes, neutropenia	Yes, thrombocytopenia	Yes, neutropenia, thrombocytopenia	Yes, neutropenia, thrombocytopenia
Cardiopulmonary	Yes, slow heart rate		Yes, shortness of breath	Yes, hypotension	Yes, shortness of breath, other	Yes, prolongation of the QT interval
Fatigue, weakness	Yes	Yes	Yes	Yes	Yes	Yes
Sedation	Yes					
Rash	Yes	Yes	Yes			
Gastrointestinal disturbance	Yes, constipation	Yes, diarrhea, constipation	Yes, diarrhea, constipation	Yes, nausea, vomiting, diarrhea	Yes, nausea, vomiting, diarrhea, constipation	Yes, diarrhea; severe diarrhea in 25% of patients in registration trial

Dex, Dexamethasone; *DVT*, deep vein thrombosis; *PE*, pulmonary embolism; *PN*, peripheral neuropathy.
*Incidence is reduced with subcutaneous and weekly dosing

- Dose adjustment may be required for selected active agents.
- Prophylactic anticoagulation is recommended to prevent coagulopathies or thrombosis in patients treated with immunomodulatory drugs (IMiDs).
- Treatment of low-risk patients (i.e., no or one risk factor)
  - Thromboprophylaxis
  - Low-dose aspirin (81 to 100 mg/day) is effective if used consistently.
- Treatment of high-risk patients (i.e., two or more risk factors)
  - High-dose dexamethasone (≥480 mg/month)
  - Doxorubicin
  - Multiagent chemotherapy
  - Thromboprophylaxis with low-molecular-weight heparin or warfarin with therapeutic dosing (international ratio of 2 to 3)

Prognosis

- The 5-year relative survival rate has almost doubled since 1975, increasing from 26.3% in 1975 to about 44.9% in 2014.
- A CR is a key factor in improved progression-free survival and overall survival.
  - A CR does not imply elimination of the malignant plasma B-cell clone.
  - A CR is achieved by 15% of patients with high-risk disease.
  - Survival is similar for patients without high-risk features who have not achieved a CR.
- HSCT remains an important and potentially curative treatment option.
  - Patients with MRD confirmed by flow cytometry at day 100 after HSCT have inferior progression-free survival and overall survival times.
- Prolongation of overall survival time is always associated with prolonged progression-free survival; however, prolonged progression-free survival is not always associated with a longer survival time.

Prevention and Surveillance

- Risk factors for MM include advanced age, male gender, obesity, African American ethnicity, and exposure to chemicals and radiation. Some risk factors provide an opportunity for modification (e.g., obesity), and others are not modifiable (e.g., age, gender, ethnicity).
- The reason for the increased incidence of MM among the African Americans has not been determined, emphasizing the need for continued investigations into genetic predisposition.
- Survivorship planning for African American patients should incorporate genetic counseling and inclusion in epidemiologic studies if possible.
- After diagnosis, there are no clear data to suggest that continued exposure to pesticides, arsenic, cadmium, lead, or various cleaning solutions changes the course of the disease.

Bibliography

Center for Disease Control (CDC). (2015). *Vaccines and immunizations.* Available at http://www.cdc.gov/vaccines/vpd-vac/pneumo/default.htm (accessed January 28, 2016).

Colson, K. (2015). Treatment-related symptom management in patients with multiple myeloma: A review. *Supportive Care Cancer, 23*(5), 1431–1445.

Durie, B. G., Harousseau, J. L., Miguel, J. S., Blade, J., Barlogie, B., Anderson, K., & International Myeloma Working Group. (2006). International uniform response criteria for multiple myeloma. *Leukemia, 20*(9), 1467–1473.

Greipp, P. R., San Miguel, J., Durie, B. G., Crowley, J. J., Barlogie, B., Blade, J., & Westin, J. (2005). International staging system for multiple myeloma. *Journal of Clinical Oncology, 23*(15), 3412–3420.

Kurtin, S., & Faiman, B. (2013). The changing landscape of multiple myeloma: Implications for oncology nurses. *Clinical Journal of Oncology Nursing, 17*(Suppl 6), 7–11.

Miceli, T., Lilleby, K., Noonan, K., Kurtin, S., Faiman, B., & Mangan, P. A. (2013). Autologous hematopoietic stem cell transplantation for patients with multiple myeloma: An overview for nurses in community practice. *Clinical Journal of Oncology Nursing, 17*(Suppl), 13–24.

National Cancer Institute. (2014). SEER statistical fact sheets: Myeloma. Available at http://seer.cancer.gov/statfacts/html/mulmy.html (accessed January 28, 2016).

National Comprehensive Cancer Network. (2015). *NCCN clinical practice guidelines in oncology: Multiple myeloma, version 2.2016.* Available at http://www.nccn.org/professionals/physician_gls/pdf/myeloma.pdf (accessed January 28, 2016).

Palumbo, A., & Mina, R. (2013). Management of older adults with multiple myeloma. *Blood Review, 27*(3), 133–142.

Perrotta, C., Kleefeld, S., Staines, A., Tewari, P., De.Roos, A. J., Baris, D., & Cocco, P. (2013). Multiple myeloma and occupation: A pooled analysis by the International Multiple Myeloma Consortium. *Cancer Epidemiology, 37*(3), 300–305.

Rajkumar, S. V., Dimopoulos, M. A., Palumbo, A., Blade, J., Merlini, G., Mateos, M. V., & San Miguel, J. F. (2014). International Myeloma Working Group updated criteria for the diagnosis of multiple myeloma. *The Lancet Oncology, 15*(12), e538–e548.

Siegel, R. L., Fedewa, S. A., Miller, K. D., Goding-Sauer, A., Pinheiro, P. S., Martinez-Tyson, D., & Jemal, A. (2015). Cancer statistics for Hispanics/Latinos, 2015. *CA: A Cancer Journal for Clinicians, 65*(6), 457–480.

Siegel, R. L., Miller, K. D., & Jemal, A. (2015). Cancer statistics, 2015. *CA: A Cancer Journal for Clinicians, 65*(1), 5–29.

Terpos, E., Berenson, J., Cook, R. J., Lipton, A., & Coleman, R. E. (2010). Prognostic variables for survival and skeletal complications in patients with multiple myeloma osteolytic bone disease. *Leukemia, 24*(5), 1043–1049.

Vincent Rajkumar, S. (2014). Multiple myeloma: 2014 update on diagnosis, risk-stratification, and management. *American Journal of Hematology, 89*(10), 999–1009.

Wallin, A., & Larsson, S. C. (2011). Body mass index and risk of multiple myeloma: A meta-analysis of prospective studies. *European Journal of Cancer, 47*, 1606–1615.

Myelofibrosis

Kristen Hurley

Definition

Classified as a Philadelphia chromosome–negative myeloproliferative neoplasm, myelofibrosis (MF) can arise on its own (i.e., primary myelofibrosis [PMF]); or occur as a progression of polycythemia vera (post-PV-MF) or of essential thrombocythemia (post-ET-MF). The manifestations of PMF, post-PV-MF, and post-ET-MF are virtually identical, and treatment usually is the same for all three.

MF is a clonal disorder arising from the neoplastic transformation of early hematopoietic stem cells. The abnormal stem cells produce more mature cells that grow quickly and take over the bone marrow, causing fibrosis (i.e., scar tissue formation) and chronic inflammation. As a result, the bone marrow becomes less able to create normal blood cells, and blood cell production may move to the spleen, causing enlargement, or to other areas of the body. Many symptoms of MF are caused by insufficient numbers of normal blood cells or chronic inflammation.

Approximately 50% to 60% of patients with PMF have a gain in function in the Janus kinase 2 gene (*JAK2*), which normally encodes a protein that promotes the growth and proliferation of cells. The V617F *JAK 2* mutation leads to the overproduction of abnormal myeloid cells, which results in excess collagen production leading to scar tissue formation in PMF.

Incidence

- About 15,000 to 18,000 people are living with MF in the United States.
- Patients are typically middle-aged to elderly people. In published reports, the median age at diagnosis was 60 to 67 years, and 20% of patients were younger than 55 years at diagnosis.
- MF affects men and women equally.
- It is rare in children; young girls are twice as likely to be affected as boys.

Etiology and Risk Factors

- Between 50% and 60% of patients with PMF have the gain-of-function V617F *JAK2* mutation.
- Between 5% and 10% of patients have somatic mutations of *JAK2* exon 12 or activating mutations of the thrombopoietin receptor gene *MPL*.
- Mutations in the gene encoding calreticulin (*CALR*) were found in most patients who lacked mutations in *JAK2* or *MPL*.
- There are no known modifiable risk factors for PMF, but secondary MF can result from disease or damage to the bone marrow through exposure to radiation, Thorotrast and other contrast agents, industrial solvents (e.g., benzene, toluene), or viral infections.

Signs and Symptoms

- Patients at the time of diagnosis may have severe symptoms associated with advanced disease or may be asymptomatic.
- Between 15% and 30% of patients with early disease at diagnosis may be asymptomatic.
- Symptoms
  - Splenomegaly is the hallmark of the disease in 90% of patients, usually with accompanying symptoms of abdominal pain and early satiety. The diagnosis typically is made during the work-up for splenomegaly.
  - Fatigue (up to 70% of patients)
  - Weight loss
  - Low-grade fever
  - Bone and joint pain
  - Night sweats
  - Hepatomegaly (40% to 70% of patients)
  - Skin itching or burning sensation (due to increased circulating cytokines)

Diagnostic Work-up

- MF is typically diagnosed through a process of exclusion of other diseases that cause bone marrow fibrosis, such as leukemia, infection, metastatic cancer, lymphoma, myelodysplastic syndrome, and hairy cell leukemia.
- Medical history and physical examination
- Laboratory tests
  - Complete blood count (CBC) with differential count, with anemia (hemoglobin <10 g/dL) identified in 50% of patients
  - Compressive metabolic panel (CMP)
    - Aspartate transaminase (AST) and alanine transaminase (ALT)
    - Alkaline phosphatase (ALP)
    - Total bilirubin
    - Lactate dehydrogenase (LDH)
    - Uric acid
- *JAK2* quantitative assay
- *CALR* and *MPL* mutational analysis performed for prognostic purposes
- Bone marrow biopsy with cytogenetic testing may identify the following abnormalities that constitute an unfavorable karyotype: +8, −7/del(7q), i(17q), inv(3), −5/del(5q), del(12p), or 11q23 rearrangements.
- The marrow specimen can be difficult to obtain, and the biopsy often results in a dry tap.

Histology

- Typically, analysis shows abnormal megakaryocytes and neutrophils (i.e., hyperplasia) in the marrow, hyperlobulation of granulocytes, and normal or increased erythroid precursors.
- The patient may have fibrosis, but the biopsy specimen may not reveal extensive replacement of the marrow by fibrosis.
- The World Health Organization (WHO) established criteria for the diagnosis of MF in 2008 (see box below).

World Health Organization Myelofibrosis Diagnostic Criteria

Major Criteria*

1. Presence of megakaryocyte proliferation and atypia, usually accompanied by reticulin and/or collagen fibrosis; or, in the absence of significant reticulin fibrosis, the megakaryocyte changes must be accompanied by increased bone marrow cellularity characterized by granulocytic proliferation and often decreased erythropoiesis (so-called prefibrotic cellular-phase disease).
2. Not meeting criteria for polycythemia vera, chronic myeloid leukemia, myelodysplastic syndrome, or other myeloid neoplasm
3. Demonstration of JAK2 617V > F or other clonal marker; or, in the absence of a clonal marker, no evidence of bone marrow fibrosis caused by an underlying inflammatory disease or another neoplastic disease. About 60% of patients with primary myelofibrosis carry a JAK2 mutation, and about 5% to 10% of patients have activating mutations in the thrombopoietin receptor gene, MPL. Almost 90% of patients without JAK2 or MPL mutations carry a somatic mutation of the calreticulin gene, which is associated with a more indolent clinical course than is seen with JAK2 or MPL mutations.

Minor Criteria

1. Leukoerythroblastosis
2. Increased serum level of lactate dehydrogenase
3. Anemia
4. Palpable splenomegaly

*To make the diagnosis, all three major criteria plus two minor criteria must be met. From the National Cancer Institute. (2015). Chronic myeloproliferative neoplasms. Treatment—for health professionals (PDQ). Available at http://www.cancer.gov/cancertopics/pdq/treatment/myeloproliferative/HealthProfessional/page4 (accessed January 12, 2016).

Clinical Staging

No clinical staging is performed for MF.

Treatment

- A watch-and-wait approach is often used for patients who are symptom free and have no signs of disease (e.g., no anemia, no splenomegaly). Patients may remain symptom free for many years, but they must be followed routinely to detect disease progression.
- Only one U.S. Food and Drug Administration (FDA)-approved drug is available to treat intermediate-risk and high-risk MF patients.
  - Ruxolitinib, a JAK2 inhibitor, is an oral agent that demonstrated significant reduction in spleen size, relief of constitutional symptoms, improved anemia, and improved survival.
  - Ruxolitinib can be effective for patients with or without the JAK mutation.

- Side effects include dizziness, anemia, thrombocytopenia, neutropenia, diarrhea, and edema.
- Allogeneic stem cell transplantation (SCT) is the only cure for MF, but it is limited to patients younger than 60 years of age.
  - Patients who have two or more adverse features (e.g., hemoglobin < 10 g/dL, constitutional symptoms, an isolated cytogenetic abnormality, or circulating blasts >1%) should be considered for SCT. Other treatment options must be considered, especially for patients with lower risk disease.
  - Given the significant mortality and morbidity from allogeneic SCT along with the predicted overall survival with bone marrow transplantation (BMT) at less than 5 years, all other therapies should be exhausted or considered before committing a patient to BMT.
- Newer forms of nonmyeloablative transplantation using reduced-intensity conditioning have been used to reduce the mortality rates and increase the long-term survival times for these patients.
- A variety of other agents have been used with various degrees of success in the treatment of MF:
  - Alkylating agents such as busulfan have been used, but because they can cause prolonged, severe cytopenias even after discontinuation of therapy, they are rarely employed.
  - Hydroxyurea may assist in the reduction of spleen size, control of thrombocytosis and leukocytosis, and control of constitutional symptoms.
  - Immunomodulatory drugs (IMiDs) such as thalidomide, lenalidomide, and pomalidomide are oral agents that target cancer by affecting functions of the immune system. IMiDs can decrease spleen size, improve overall blood counts, and treat anemia.
  - Androgen therapy does not treat the disease but can be used as supportive care to help with the symptoms of anemia. For some patients, it promotes red blood cell production. Approximately 30% respond to this supportive therapy. It can be extremely toxic to the liver and requires close monitoring. It may also cause facial hair growth and masculinizing effects in women.
  - Recombinant erythropoietin is used for treating the anemia by stimulating red blood cell production, but it does not treat the underlying disease.
  - Anagrelide, an oral phospholipase A_2 inhibitor, has been used for MF patients with elevated platelet counts. Close monitoring is needed because it can cause significant pancytopenia.
- Radiation therapy is typically used to treat symptoms associated with an enlarged spleen. It can be difficult to get a long-standing response, and toxicity to underlying gastrointestinal structures is common in MF patients with advanced disease and marked splenomegaly.
- Splenectomy typically is not done late in the disease because spleen size and vascularity make surgical removal quite dangerous.
  - It may be considered if there is no response to other therapies.

- It should be considered only by an experienced surgeon.
- Close monitoring after surgery is required to ensure complications do not arise.
- Patients should be considered for clinical trials as appropriate.

Prognosis

- MF is a progressive disease with constitutional symptoms, splenomegaly, and cytopenias that worsen over time.
- Transformation to acute myeloid leukemia occurs in 8% to 23% of patients with MF during the first decade after diagnosis.
- The International Prognostic Scoring System (IPSS), which was developed by the International Working Group for Myelofibrosis Research and Treatment (IWG-MRT), is used to estimate prognosis based on risk factors identified at diagnosis (see table below).
- The Dynamic International Prognostic Scoring System (DIPSS) is used to reevaluate the prognosis as the disease advances over time. The DIPSS differs from the IPSS as it assigns a 2 point value to Hemoglobin <10g/dL. Survival is associated with the DIPSS score as follows:
  - Risk score of 0: median survival not yet reached
  - Risk score of 1-2: median survival is 14.2 years
  - Risk score of 3-4: median survival is 4 years
  - Risk score of 5-6: median survival is 1.5 years

International Prognostic Scoring System (IPSS) Risk Factors and Point Values

Risk Factor	Point Value*
Age >65 yr	1
Presence of constitutional symptoms	1
Hemoglobin <10 g/dL	1
White blood cell count >25 × 10⁹/L	1
Blood blasts ≥1%	1

*Applying the IPSS, subjects with zero (low risk), one (intermediate risk-1), two (intermediate risk-2), or ≥3 (high risk) of these variables at presentation had non overlapping median survival times of 135, 95, 48, and 27 months, respectively. Modified from Cervantes, R., Dupriez, G., Pereiral, A., Passamonti, F., Reilly, J. T., Morra, E. et al (2009). New prognostic scoring system for primary myelofibrosis based on a study of the International Working Group for Myelofibrosis Research and Treatment. *Blood, 113*(13), 2895-2901.

Prevention and Surveillance

- There is no known way to prevent PMF.
- Avoiding exposure to radiation, viruses, or industrial chemicals that damage the bone marrow may help to prevent secondary MF.

Bibliography

Ballen, K. (2012). How to manage the transplant question in myelofibrosis. *Blood Cancer Journal, 2*(3), e59. http://dx.doi.org/10.1038/bcj.2012.3.

Ballen, K. (Cancer Support Network. (n.d.). Myelofibrosis treatment. Available at http://www.cancersupportcommunity.org/MainMenu/About-Cancer/Types-of-Cancer/Myelofibrosis (accessed January 12, 2016).

Cervantes, R., Dupriez, G., Pereiral, A., Passamonti, F., Reilly, J. T., Morra, E., & Tefferi, A. (2009). New prognostic scoring system for primary myelofibrosis based on a study of the International Working Group for Myelofibrosis Research and Treatment. *Blood, 113*(13), 2895–2901.

Gangat, N., Caramazza, D., Vaidya, R., George, G., Begna, K., Schwager, S., & Tefferi, A. (2011). DIPSS plus: A refined dynamic international prognostic scoring system for primary myelofibrosis that incorporates prognostic information from karyotype, platelet count, and transfusion status. *Journal of Clinical Oncology, 29*(4), 392–397.

Lal, A. (2014). Primary myelofibrosis. *Medscape drug and diseases.* Available at http://emedicine.medscape.com/article/197954-overview#a5 (accessed January 12, 2016).

MPN Research Foundation. (n.d.). (Primary myelofibrosis (PMF). Available at http://www.mpnresearchfoundation.org/Primary-Myelofibrosis (accessed January 12, 2016).

National Cancer Institute. (2015). *Chronic myeloproliferative neoplasms treatment (PDQ): General information about chronic myeloproliferative neoplasms (MPN).* Available at http://www.cancer.gov/types/myeloproliferative/patient/chronic-treatment-pdq (accessed January 12, 2016).

Tefferi, A. (2011). How I treat myelofibrosis. *Blood, 117*(13), 3494.

Tefferi, A. (2013). Primary myelofibrosis: 2013 update on diagnosis, risk-stratification, and management. *American Journal of Hematology, 88,* 141.

Neuroendocrine Cancers

Nicole Korak*

Definition

Normal neuroendocrine cells have the characteristics of nerve and endocrine cells. The cells are diffusely spread throughout the body in various organs such as the gastrointestinal (GI) tract, pancreas, lung, and skin. They respond to neuronal stimuli by releasing peptide hormones that regulate normal function. The neuroendocrine system plays a specific role in each organ. For instance, the neuroendocrine cells in the GI tract regulate intestinal motility and the release of digestive enzymes. Islet cells in the pancreas release insulin.

Neuroendocrine tumors (NETs) are neoplasms that arise from cells of the endocrine (hormonal) and nervous systems. There are many types of NETs, but the neoplastic cells share common features such as morphology, special secretory granules, and the production of biogenic amines and polypeptide hormones.

In the United States, NETs, which most commonly occur in the intestine, have been traditionally referred to as *carcinoid tumors* and organized under the broad anatomic categories of foregut, midgut, and hindgut (see table in the next column). However, the nomenclature has changed to reflect the fact that the tumors are cancer, not cancer-like lesions. Use of the terms *neuroendocrine tumor* (NET) and *neuroendocrine carcinoma* (NEC) more accurately portrays the malignant nature of the disease, although some NETs are benign.

NETs also are described by the anatomic site of origin and the degree of differentiation. They may be further classified as symptomatic due to hormonal syndromes resulting from the release of peptides (i.e., functional tumors) or as asymptomatic (i.e., nonfunctional tumors) NETs.

In this chapter, the most common NETs are reviewed: gastrointestinal (GI NETs), pancreatic (pNETs), and bronchopulmonary NETs.

Incidence

- The annual incidence of NETs is approximately 5.76 cases per 100,000 people, and based on the SEER database (2003 to 2007), the estimated prevalence is 35 cases per 100,000 people.
- The increasing incidence and prevalence can be attributed to a growing body of knowledge over the past 2 decades, improved pathologic distinction by immunohistochemical properties

---

Classification of Neuroendocrine Tumors

Regional Categories

Foregut neuroendocrine tumors	Stomach, first portion of the duodenum, pancreas, bronchus, lung, ovaries, and thymus
Midgut neuroendocrine tumors	Second portion of the duodenum, jejunum, ileum, appendix, and ascending colon
Hindgut neuroendocrine tumors	Transverse colon, descending colon, and rectum

Neuroendocrine Tumors (Carcinoids) of the Gastrointestinal Tract, Lung, and Thymus

Appendiceal carcinoid
Atypical lung carcinoid
Bronchopulmonary or thymus carcinoid
Duodenal carcinoid
Gastric carcinoid
Jejunal, ileal, and colon carcinoid
Rectal carcinoid

Neuroendocrine Tumors of the Pancreas (pNETs)

Gastrinoma
Nonfunctioning pancreatic tumors
Vasoactive intestinal peptide (VIPoma)
Insulinoma
Glucagonoma
Somatostatinoma

Neuroendocrine Tumor of the Skin

Merkel cell carcinoma

---

from other tumor types, evolving diagnostic capabilities such as unique imaging for NETs, improved treatment modalities, and increased rates of reporting to cancer registries.

- GI NET detection is increasing over time. The SEER database reported a 520% increase between 1973 and 2003, reflecting an annual increase of approximately 5%.
- PNETs are diagnosed in approximately 1000 people per year, accounting for 3% to 5% of pancreatic malignancies. They encompass all neuroendocrine tumor anomalies in the pancreas, including insulinomas, glucagonomas, and VIPomas.
  - For bronchopulmonary NETs, 1.35 cases per 100,000 people occur each year. They account for only 1% to 2% of all lung cancers but account for 20% to 30% of all NETs.

Etiology and Risk Factors

Gastrointestinal Neuroendocrine Tumors

- The exact causes of GI NETs are unknown, but there is a higher incidence among patients who have a first-degree family member with colon or prostate cancer.

---

* Thanks to Nancy Roehnelt for her contribution to Neuroendocrine Cancer chapter.

- Most GI NETs are sporadic, but some cases are associated with familial syndromes. For example, there have been cases in which family members were diagnosed with midgut tumors.
- The risk of NETs is increased for the children of parents who have had a diagnosis of endometrial, kidney, or skin cancer or non-Hodgkin lymphoma.

Pancreatic Neuroendocrine Tumors

- When genetically linked, pNETs are most commonly associated with multiple endocrine neoplasia type 1 (MEN1) and MEN2 syndromes, von Hippel–Lindau (VHL) syndrome, and neurofibromatosis type 1.
  - MEN1 confers an 80% to 100% risk of pNET.
  - Patients with VHL syndrome have a 98% likelihood of developing a pNET and neurofibromatosis; however, only 10% to 17% of pNETs occur in patients with VHL.
- Insulinomas are associated with the MEN1 syndrome, and the tumors often express the mammalian target of rapamycin (mTOR), a protein kinase that is abnormally activated in a number of cancers.
- Glucagonomas, which result in overproduction of the peptide hormone glucagon, are associated with a family history of MEN1, but they also develop in people with no known risk factors.
- Gastrinoma is associated with MEN1 and Zollinger-Ellison syndromes.
- A meta-analysis found that diabetes and having a first-degree relative with cancer were associated with pNET.

Bronchopulmonary Neuroendocrine Tumors

- Although the exact causes of bronchopulmonary NETs are unknown, 10% of cases are associated with MEN1.
- MEN1-associated bronchopulmonary NETs occur five times more often in women than in men.

Signs and Symptoms

Gastrointestinal Neuroendocrine Tumors

- Carcinoid syndrome is a condition in which small tumors on the walls of the small intestine release excessive amounts of serotonin (5-HT), prostaglandins, or other neuropeptides. It occurs in about 30% of patients with GI NETs and most often in the setting of liver metastasis.
- Symptoms include the following:
  - Intermittent dry flushing occurs in 63% to 94% of patients with carcinoid syndrome.
    - Flushing can last minutes or hours and can be seen on the face, torso, and extremities.
    - It can be exacerbated by stress, exercise, or tyramine-containing foods such as cheese, wine, and chocolate.
  - Diarrhea affects 68% to 84% of patients with carcinoid syndrome.
    - It is described as urgent with watery stools and can be accompanied by colicky abdominal cramping.

- It differs from the symptoms of irritable bowel syndrome (IBS) in that patients with NETs are more often awakened in the middle of the night by the urge to have a bowel movement.
- Diarrhea can continue when fasting.
- Bronchoconstriction occurs in 3% to 19% of patients with carcinoid syndrome. The new-onset wheezing in adults is caused by overproduction of histamine, substance P, or 5-HT.
- Telangiectasia occurs in 25% of patients with carcinoid syndrome.
- Right heart disease occurs rarely after the introduction of somatostatin analogs. Cardiac valve fibrosis results from 5-HT overproduction. The tricuspid and pulmonary valves are most commonly affected, resulting in regurgitation, cardiac insufficiency, and dysrhythmias.

Pancreatic Neuroendocrine Tumors

- Signs and symptoms of a pNET are directly related to the cellular type and functional status of the tumor.
- If the pNET is nonfunctional, symptoms are related to the location of the metastasis.
- Most pNETs are diagnosed at an advanced stage, have metastasized to the liver, and produce symptoms such as jaundice, weight loss, and ascites.
- Functional pNETs have a variety of symptoms related to cell type and the hormone secreted.
- Insulinomas secrete insulin and are most often benign. Symptoms include the following:
  - Severe hypoglycemia (85% of patients)
  - Weakness
  - Sweating
  - Fainting
  - Confusion
  - Vision changes
- Gastrinomas secrete gastrin, and symptoms include the following:
  - Severe peptic ulcer disease (i.e., Zollinger-Ellison syndrome) with decreased response to medical interventions
  - Abdominal pain
  - Bleeding
  - Vomiting
  - Diarrhea
  - Chronic reflux leading to complications normally seen with reflux disease
  - Vitamin B_{12} deficiency
- Glucagonomas secrete glucagon, and symptoms include the following:
  - Glucose intolerance
  - Migratory necrolytic erythema (80% of cases), characterized by a raised erythematous patch beginning in the perineum and spreading to the trunk
  - Weight loss
  - Diabetes mellitus (80% to 90% of cases)
  - Anemia
  - Stomatitis
  - Higher rate of thromboembolic events (40% of cases)

- Symptoms are also known as the *four Ds*: dermatosis, depression, deep vein thrombosis, and diarrhea.
- VIPomas secrete excessive quantities of vasoactive intestinal peptide, and symptoms include the following:
  - Profound secretory diarrhea (>3 L/day)
  - Hypokalemia
  - Achlorhydria

Bronchopulmonary Neuroendocrine Tumors

- Carcinoid syndrome may occur in 6% to 8% of patients with bronchopulmonary NETs (described earlier for GI NETs), leading providers down the wrong path when looking for the primary tumor site.
- Presentation with hormonal fluctuations and paraneoplastic syndromes, such as those seen in small cell lung cancer, is possible.
- Up to 40% of patients with ectopic Cushing syndrome may be diagnosed with a bronchopulmonary NET.

Diagnostic Work-up

Gastrointestinal Neuroendocrine Tumors

- GI NETs are rare and understandably often mistaken for IBS.
- The subtle differences are outlined in the table below, and a thorough investigation may lead providers to an earlier diagnosis, especially if the patient is not responding to IBS therapy.
- Laboratory work-up
  - Test for 24-hour urinary 5-hydroxyindoleacetic acid (5-HIAA) level.
    - Foods to be avoided for 48 hours before testing include avocados, bananas or plantains, cantaloupe or honeydew melon, eggplant, pineapples, plums, tomatoes, kiwi, dates, grapefruit, and hickory nuts, pecans, or walnuts.
    - Coffee, alcohol, and smoking should be avoided.
  - Fasting serum 5-HIAA level (optional)
  - Chromogranin A (CGA) is elevated in 90% of patients with NETs.
    - Can be elevated in functioning and nonfunctioning tumors
    - Sensitivity of 78% to 84% and specificity of 71% to 85%, depending on tumor size
    - Proton pump inhibitors (PPIs) should be withheld because they can cause a false-positive result.

- Imaging studies
  - Octreotide scan or somatostatin receptor scintigraphy (SRS); the patient is injected with radiolabeled octreotide and evaluated for tumor uptake of the medication.
  - Magnetic resonance imaging (MRI)
  - Positron emission tomography (PET)
  - Bone scan if bone metastasis is suspected
  - Echocardiogram if carcinoid syndrome is identified
- Endoscopic procedures
  - Endoscopy
  - Bronchoscopy for the diagnosis of a lung carcinoid
  - Endoscopic ultrasound (EUS)

Pancreatic Neuroendocrine Tumors

- Insulinoma, for which a positive diagnosis is an inappropriately elevated level of insulin in the face of hypoglycemia during a 72-hour fast
  - Serum insulin level of more than 10 μU/mL (normal <6 μU/mL)
  - Glucose level of less than 40 mg/dL
  - C-peptide level of more than 2.5 ng/mL (normal <2 ng/mL)
  - Plasma proinsulin level of more than 25% (up to 90%) that of immunoreactive insulin levels
  - Screening result for sulfonylurea is negative.
- Gastrinoma
  - Positive fasting hypergastrinemia of more than 150 pg/mL (for levels >1000, consider Zollinger-Ellison syndrome)
  - Basal acid output of more than 10 mEq/hr
  - Intravenous secretin stimulation test result of more than 200 pg/mL in 2 minutes is positive for gastrinoma.
  - Gastric pH of less than 3.0
  - Elevated human chorionic gonadotropin (hCG) levels
- Glucagonoma
  - Plasma glucagon levels of 500 to 1000 pg/mL
  - Complete blood count (CBC) and chemistry panel, including fasting blood sugar and liver enzyme levels
- VIPoma
  - Elevated plasma VIP level that is 2 to 10 times the normal range; patient must be symptomatic at the time of testing
  - Secretory diarrhea volume of more than 700 mL/day
  - Hypokalemia
  - Achlorhydria

Comparison of Irritable Bowel Syndrome and Carcinoid Syndrome

Characteristic	Irritable Bowel Syndrome	Carcinoid Syndrome
Incidence	Most likely among white, female, 35-year-old patients	Most likely among 66-year-old patients
Sleep disturbances due to diarrhea	Rarely	Often
Bleeding	Rarely	Often
Weight loss	Rarely	Often
Persistent pain	Rarely	Often
Constipation alternating with diarrhea	Occasionally	Rarely
Diarrhea with fasting	Never	Often
Type of diarrhea	Malabsorptive	Secretory

Modified from Vinik, A. I., Woltering, E. A., Warner, R. R., Caplin, M., O'Dorisio, T. M., Wiseman, G. A., et al. (2010). NANETS consensus guidelines for the diagnosis of Neuroendocrine Tumors. *Pancreas, 39*(6), 713-734.

- Imaging studies of pNETs are useful for determining location, extent of metastatic disease, and surgical candidacy.
  - MRI with gadolinium contrast has been sensitive in finding insulinomas but not helpful for patients with glucagonomas.
  - Computed tomography (CT)
  - Octreotide scan or SRS
- EUS is sensitive for insulinoma and glucagonoma detection.
- Upper endoscopy for tumors that originate in the stomach and duodenum

Bronchopulmonary Neuroendocrine Tumors

- Laboratory work-up
  - CGA level
  - Neuron-specific enolase (NSE) level
  - Test of 24-hour urinary 5-HIAA level
- Imaging studies
  - CT
  - MRI
  - Octreotide scan or SRS; 70% to 80% of thoracic NETs have receptors for octreotide.
  - PET may be useful for detecting an undifferentiated tumor with a negative octreotide scan result.

Histology

Gastrointestinal Neuroendocrine Tumors

- Grading of GI NETs is done according to the 2010 World Health Organization (WHO) system.
  - G1: well-differentiated, low-grade NET with no necrosis
  - G2: well-differentiated, intermediate-grade NET
  - G3: poorly differentiated, high-grade NET (rare)
    - Appendix: 0.9%
    - Jejunum or ileum: 1.1%
    - Cecum: 14.2%
- Mixed adenoneuroendocrine carcinoma, a mixed-cell tumor that has neuroendocrine and glandular features, is rare, is seen mostly in tumors of the appendix and cecum, and has a poor prognosis.
- The Ki-67 labeling index is useful for diagnosing an unusual presentation of an aggressive NET.
- Size of tumor, multicentric disease, vascular or perineural invasion, and tissue margin status should be determined.

- Specific cell types and NET-secreted peptides are associated with certain areas of the GI tract (see table below).

Pancreatic Neuroendocrine Tumors

- Most pNETs are well-differentiated islet cell or carcinoid-type tumors but rarely can be anaplastic.
- The tumor cells can be arranged in lobular or acinar patterns.
- Tumors may be somatostatin positive, but gastrinomas are normally somatostatin negative.

Bronchopulmonary Neuroendocrine Tumors

- A well-differentiated, low-grade NET with fewer than 2 mitoses per 10 high-power fields (HPFs) and no necrosis is a typical carcinoid.
- A well-differentiated, intermediate-grade NET with 2 to 10 mitoses per 10 HPFs and a focus of necrosis is an atypical carcinoid.
- A poorly differentiated, high-grade NET with more than 10 mitoses per 10 HPFs is a small cell carcinoma or a large cell NEC.
- Pathology reports should include unusual histologic features, such as clear cell, glandular, or oncocytic characteristics.
- The Ki-67 labeling index is useful for diagnosing an unusual presentation of an aggressive NET.

Clinical Staging

- After histologic identification of a NET, staging is based on the location of the tumor and applying the tumor size, lymph nodes, and metastasis (TNM) system adopted by the American Joint Commission on Cancer (AJCC).

Treatment

Gastrointestinal Neuroendocrine Tumors

- Complete surgical resection is the preferred treatment for locally advanced disease because it yields a 70% to 90% cure rate.
- Cryotherapy or surgical debulking is recommended by the North American Neuroendocrine Tumor Society (NANETS) consensus guidelines if the patient is unable to have a complete resection.

Cell Types and Secretory Products Associated with Neuroendocrine Tumors According to Organ of Origin		
Location	**Cell Type**	**Peptides Secreted**
Entire gastrointestinal tract	Delta, EC, Gr, VIP	Somatostatin (delta cells); serotonin, substance P, guanylin, and melatonin (EC cells); ghrelin (Gr cells); vasoactive intestinal peptide (VIP cells)
Gastric fundus	ECL	Histamine
Gastric antrum and duodenum	Gastrin	Gastrin
Duodenum	I, motilin, secretin	CCK, motilin, secretin
Duodenum, jejunum	K	GIP
Small intestine	L, neurotensin	GLP1, PYY, NPY, neurotensin
Gastric fundus and antrum	Somatostatin	Amylin
Pancreas	Alpha, beta, delta, PP	Glucagon, insulin, somatostatin, PP

CCK, Cholecystokinin; *EC*, enterochromaffin; *ECL*, enterochromaffin-like; *GIP*, gastric inhibitory peptide; *GLP1*, glucagon-like peptide 1; *Gr*, ghrelin; *NPY*, neuropeptide Y (tyrosine); *PP*, pancreatic polypeptide; *PYY*, polypeptide YY (tyrosine, tyrosine); *VIP*, vasoactive intestinal peptide.
Modified from Modlin, et.al. (2008). Gastroenteropancreatic neuroendocrine tumours. *The Lancet Oncology, 9*(1): 61-72.

- Somatostatin analogs have been used for decades to control symptoms, and they have been shown to improve progression-free survival.
  - Sandostatin LAR and Somatuline Depot are injectable long-acting somatostatin analogs.
  - Subcutaneous octreotide may be used for breakthrough symptoms such as excessive flushing or diarrhea.
  - Somatostatin analogs may cause steatorrhea, diarrhea, and loose stools; malabsorption; gastrointestinal cramps; and occasional nausea. The drugs inhibit gallbladder contractions, which may result in gallbladder sludge or gallstones.
- The mTOR inhibitor, everolimus, is FDA approved for the treatment of progressive, well differentiated, non-functional GI NET patients with unresectable locally advanced or metastatic disease.
- Chemotherapy has not been proved to be effective for these tumors and is not usually recommended unless there are no other options.
- Peptide receptor radionuclide therapy (PRRT) is available outside of the United States. PRRT is radioisotope therapy that uses radiolabeled octreotide. When injected into the bloodstream, the radiopeptide travels to and binds to somatostatin receptors 2 and 5 on NET cells, delivering a high dose of radiation to the cancer cells.

Pancreatic Neuroendocrine Tumors

- When possible, complete surgical resection is the only curative treatment. However, it is limited to patients with local or locally advanced pNETs.
- Hepatic embolization can be used for palliation of patients with bulky liver disease who are not candidates for surgery. Embolization decreases hormone levels and side effects of the disease.
- Somatuline Depot, a somatostatin analog, is approved by the FDA for patients improves progression-free survival of patients with advanced pNETs.
- Targeted therapies can provide a progression-free survival benefit and have been approved by the U.S. Food and Drug Administration to treat progressive disease in patients with advanced advanced pNET.
  - Everolimus is an mTOR inhibitor.
  - Sunitinib is a tyrosine kinase inhibitor.
- Cytotoxic chemotherapy has not provided optimal results.
- Chemotherapy, including 5-fluorouracil (5-FU), capecitabine, dacarbazine, oxaliplatin, streptozocin, and temozolomide, may be used in patients with bulky, symptomatic, or progressive disease. Regimens include the following:
  - Temozolomide plus capecitabine
  - 5-FU, doxorubicin, and streptozocin (FAS)
  - Streptozocin plus doxorubicin
  - Streptozocin plus 5-FU

Bronchopulmonary Neuroendocrine Tumors

- Surgery is used for treating bronchopulmonary NETs.
  - For locally advanced disease, surgical resection is the treatment of choice.

- For metastatic disease that is not highly vascular, a sleeve resection is the surgery of choice, and intraoperative radiolabeled octreotide can be used to identify tumor tissue.
- Adjuvant therapy has not been beneficial. Radiation therapy, chemotherapy, and chemoradiation therapy do not prolong disease-free or median survival times.
- The mTOR inhibitor, everolimus, is FDA approved for the treatment of progressive, well differentiated, non-functional lung NET patients with unresectable locally advanced or metastatic disease.
- Bronchopulmonary NETs with a hormonal syndrome are treated with somatostatin analogs.
  - Somatostatin analogs (described earlier) are indicated for carcinoid syndrome.
  - Serotonin receptor antagonists include those for 5-HT1 and 5-HT2.

Prognosis

- NETs are known for their slowly progressive nature and well-differentiated histology, however, nearly half of NET patients are not diagnosed until the disease has become advanced. The earlier the diagnosis and intervention, the better the outcome.
- The stage of disease and tumor grade influence the prognosis (see table below).
- The location of the primary tumor affects the extent of metastatic disease. For instance, NETs that start in the ileum or jejunum are more likely to have distant metastasis at diagnosis than those that start in the rectum.
- The 5-year survival rate for GI NETs varies by site of origin: 95.6% for rectal and appendiceal tumors, 86.2% for small intestine tumors, 82.7% for stomach tumors, and 67.4% for colon tumors.
- PNETs have a better prognosis than pancreatic adenocarcinoma.
  - The overall 5-year survival rate for patients with pNETs is 42%.
  - Gastrinomas and insulinomas have favorable prognosis when the disease is localized (see table below).

Prognosis for Localized and Metastatic Disease

Neuroendocrine Tumor Type	Five-Year Survival Rate for Localized Disease	Five-Year Survival Rate for Metastatic Disease
Well-differentiated GI NET	82%	35%
Poorly differentiated GI NET	38%	4%
Gastrinoma	90%	20%-30%
Insulinoma (not surgically removed)	61%	16%

GI, Gastrointestinal; NET, neuroendocrine tumor.
Data from Yao, J. C., Hassan, M., Phan, A., Dagohoy, C., Leary, C., Mares, J. E., Abdalla, E. K., et al. (2008). One hundred years after "carcinoid": Epidemiology of and prognostic factors for neuroendocrine tumors in 35,825 cases in the United States. *Journal of Clinical Oncology, 26*(18), 3063-3072; Bonheur, J. L. (2014). Gastrinoma: Background, pathophysiology, epidemiology. Available at http://emedicine.medscape.com/article/184332-overview (accessed February 5, 2016); Ali, Z. A. (2015). Insulinoma: Practice essentials, background, pathophysiology. Available at http://emedicine.medscape.com/article/283039-overview (accessed February 5, 2016).

- Bronchopulmonary NETs that are locally advanced and resectable have a 5-year survival rate of 87% to 100% and a 10-year survival rate of 82% to 87%.

Prevention and Surveillance

- There are no preventative measures recommended by National Cancer Institute, American Cancer Society, or National Comprehensive Cancer Network for NETs.
- Surveillance recommendations for all NET diagnoses:
  - Postoperative patients with a low risk of recurrence should be evaluated every 3 to 6 months for the first year and then every 6 to 12 months for the next 7 years.
  - For patients with a higher risk of recurrence, follow-up evaluations every 3 to 6 months should include laboratory and imaging studies specific to the patient's disease in accordance with the NANETS consensus guidelines for the diagnosis and management of NETs.

Bibliography

Ali, Z. A. (2015, March 3). *Insulinoma: Practice essentials, background, pathophysiology.* Available at http://emedicine.medscape.com/article/283039-overview (accessed January 29, 2016).

The American Association of Endocrine Surgeons. (2013). *Pancreatic neuroendocrine tumors: Insulinoma.* Available at http://endocrinediseases.org/neuroendocrine/insulinoma.shtml (accessed January 29, 2016).

Bonheur, J. L. (2016). *Gastrinoma: Background, pathophysiology, epidemiology.* Available at http://emedicine.medscape.com/article/184332-overview (accessed January 29, 2016).

Boudreaux, J. P., Klimstra, D. S., Hassan, M. M., Woltering, E. A., Jensen, R. T., Goldsmith, S. J., et al (2010). The NANETS consensus guideline for the diagnosis and management of neuroendocrine tumors: Well-differentiated neuroendocrine tumors of the the jejunum, ileum, appendix and cecum. *Pancreas, 39*(6), 753–766.

Canadian Cancer Society. (2015). *Anatomy and physiology of the neuroendocrine system.* Available at http://www.cancer.ca/en/cancer-information/cancer-type/neuroendocrine/anatomy-and-physiology/?region=on (accessed January 29, 2016).

Caplin, M. E., Pavel, M., Cwikla, J. B., Phan, A. T., Raderer, M., Sedláčková, E., et al. (2014). Lanreotide in metastatic enteropancreatic neuroendocrine tumors. *New England Journal of Medicine, 371*(3), 224–233.

Carcinoid.com. *The symptoms of carcinoid syndrome: A Novartis oncology program.* (2014). Available at http://www.carcinoid.com/patient/understanding/carcinoid-syndrome-symptoms.jsp?usertrack.filter_applied=true&NovaId=4029462146185608202#flushing (accessed January 29, 2016).

Haugvik, S. P., Hedenström, P., Korsæth, E., Valente, R., Hayes, A., Siuka, D., et al. (2015). Diabetes, smoking, alcohol use, and family history of cancer as risk factors for pancreatic neuroendocrine tumors: A systematic review and meta-analysis. *Neuroendocrinology, 101*(2), 133–142.

Kulke, M. H., Anthony, L. B., Bushnell, D. K., De Herder, W. W., Goldsmith, S. J., Klimstra, D. S., & Jensen, R. T. (2010). NANETS treatment guidelines: Well-differentiated neuroendocrine tumors of the stomach and pancreas. *Pancreas, 39*(6), 735–753.

Modlin, I. M., Öberg, K. Chung, D.C., Jensens, R.T., de Herder, W.W., Thakker, R.V. Caplin, M., Delle Fave, G., Kaltsas, G., Krenning, E. Moss, S., Nilsson, O., Rindi, G., Salazar, R. Ruszniewski P., & Sundin, A (2008). Gastroenteropancreatic neuroendocrine tumours. *The Lancet Oncology, 9*(1), 61–72. doi://http://dx.doi.org/10.1016/S1470-2045(07)70410-2.

National Cancer Institute. (n.d.). (Dictionary of cancer terms. Available at http://www.cancer.gov/publications/dictionaries/cancer-terms?CdrID=44904 (accessed January 29, 2016).

National Cancer Institute. (2015). *Gastrointestinal carcinoid tumors treatment: Health professional version. PDQ cancer information summaries.* Available at http://www.ncbi.nlm.nih.gov/books/NBK65791 (accessed January 29, 2016).

National Cancer Institute. (2015). *Pancreatic neuroendocrine tumors (islet cell tumors) treatment (PDQ): For health professionals.* Available at http://www.cancer.gov/types/pancreatic/hp/pnet-treatment-pdq (accessed January 29, 2016).

National Comprehensive Cancer Network. (2015). *NCCN national clinical practice guidelines in oncology: Neuroendocrine tumors, version 1.2015.* Available at http://www.nccn.org/professionals/physician_gls/pdf/neuroendocrine.pdf (accessed January 29, 2016).

Phan, A. T., Oberg, K., Choi, J., Harrison, L. H., Hassam, M., Strosberg, J., et al. (2010). NANETS consensus guideline for the diagnosis and management of neuroendocrine tumors: Well-differentiated neuroendocrine tumors of the thorax. *Pancreas, 39*(6), 784–798.

Raymond, E., Dahan, L., Raoul, J. L., Bang, Y. J., Borbath, I., Lombard-Bohas, C., et al. (2011). Sunitinib malate for the treatment of pancreatic neuroendocrine tumors. *New England Journal of Medicine, 364*(6), 501–513.

Rindi, G., Arnold, R., & Bosman, F. T. (2010). Nomenclature and classification of neuroendocrine neoplasms of the digestive system. In T. F. Bosman, F. Carneiro, R. H. Hruban, & N. D. Theise (Eds.), *WHO classification of tumours of the digestive system* (4th ed.). Lyon: International Agency for Research on Cancer (IARC).

Rinke, A., Muller, H. H., Schade-Brittinger, C., Klose, K. J., Barth, P., Wied, M., et al. (2009). Placebo-controlled, double-blind, prospective, randomized study on the effect of octreotide LAR in the control of tumor growth in patients with metastatic neuroendocrine midgut tumors: A report from the PROMID Study Group. *Journal of Clinical Oncology, 27*(28), 4656–4663.

Santacroce, L. (2015). *Glucagonoma: Background, pathophysiology, epidemiology.* Available at http://emedicine.medscape.com/article/118899-overview (accessed January 29, 2016).

Tebbi, C. K. (2015). *Carcinoid tumor: Practice essentials, background, pathophysiology.* Available at http://emedicine.medscape.com/article/986050-overview (accessed January 29, 2016).

Tsikitis, V. L., Wertheim, B. C., & Guerrero, M. A. (2012). Trends of incidence and survival of gastrointestinal neuroendocrine tumors in the United States: A SEER analysis. *Journal of Cancer, 3*, 292–302.

Tsvetkova, E., Sud, S., Aucoin, N., Biagi, J., Burkes, R., Samson, B., et al. (2015). Eastern Canadian gastrointestinal cancer consensus conference 2014. *Current Oncology, 4*, e305–e315.

Vinik, A., Casellini, C., Perry, R. R., Feliberti, E., & Vingan, H. (2014). *Diagnosis and management of pancreatic neuroendocrine tumors (PNETS): Endotext.* Available at http://www.ncbi.nlm.nih.gov/books/NBK279074/ (accessed January 29, 2016).

Vinik, A. I., Woltering, E. A., Warner, R. R., Caplin, M., O'Dorisio, T. M., Wiseman, G. A., et al. (2010). NANETS consensus guidelines for the diagnosis of neuroendocrine tumors. *Pancreas, 39*(6), 713–734.

Yao, J. C., Shah, M. H., Ito, T., Bohas, C. L., Wolin, E. M., Van Cutsem, E., et al. (2011). Everolimus for advanced pancreatic neuroendocrine tumors. *New England Journal of Medicine, 364*(6), 514–523.

Yao, J. C., Hassan, M., Phan, A., Dagohoy, C., Leary, C., Mares, J. E., et al. (2008). One hundred years after "carcinoid": Epidemiology of and prognostic factors for neuroendocrine tumors in 35,825 cases in the United States. *Journal of Clinical Oncology, 26*(18), 3063–3072.

Yeung, S. J. (2014). *VIPomas workup: Approach considerations, laboratory studies, computed tomography.* Available at http://emedicine.medscape.com/article/125910-workup (accessed January 29, 2016).

Sarcomas

Rupa Ghosh-Berkebile

Chondrosarcoma

Definition

Chondrosarcomas are a group of malignant bone tumors that arise from the cartilage matrix. They are classified as primary or secondary lesions. They can range from low-grade tumors with a low risk of metastasis to high-grade tumors with a high risk of distant metastasis.

Incidence

- Primary bone cancers are extremely rare, accounting for fewer than 0.2% of all cancers.
- Chondrosarcoma is the second most common form of bone cancer, accounting for 30% of bone cancers in the United States.
- In 2015, an estimated 2970 new cases of bone cancer were diagnosed in the United States, and an estimated 1330 people died from the disease.
- Chondrosarcoma can occur at any age, but it is usually diagnosed in middle-aged and older adults (ages 40-75 years).
- There is a slightly increased occurrence in males compared with females.
- The most common primary sites of occurrence are the pelvis and the proximal femur.

Etiology and Risk Factors

- Chondrosarcomas characteristically produce cartilage matrices from neoplastic tissue.
  - Typically, no osteoid or bone-forming tissue is involved.
- Conventional chondrosarcomas account for about 85% of all chondrosarcomas and are divided into two groups:
  - Primary or central lesions, which arise from previously normal-appearing bone preformed from cartilage
  - Secondary or peripheral tumors, which arise or develop from previously benign cartilage lesions, such as enchondromas, or osteochondromas
    - Secondary tumors resulting from the malignant transformation of typically benign bone lesions have been reported in patients with
      - Ollier disease (enchondromatosis), a rare skeletal condition that results in abnormal bone development; increased growth of the long bone cartilage resulting in cartilage masses (enchondromas); and thinning of cortical bone, which is rendered thin and fragile.
      - Maffucci syndrome, which describes enchondromatosis accompanied by soft tissue hemangiomas

- Malignant hereditary exostoses, a genetic condition in which multiple benign bone tumors (exostoses) develop primarily at the end of long bones and on flat bones such as the scapula and pelvis
- Typically, these tumors are slower in onset and of low grade.
- In addition to conventional chondrosarcomas, there are other rare subtypes that account for 10% to 15% of all chondrosarcomas. These include clear cell, mesenchymal, juxtacortical, dedifferentiated, and myxoid types.
- Risk factors also include Paget disease and radiation injury to the area.
- Isocitrate dehydrogenase (IDH1 or IDH2) mutations are associated with approximately 50% of all chondrosarcomas and almost all cases of secondary chondrosarcoma from Ollier disease or Maffucci syndrome.
- Alterations in the retinoblastoma pathway are present in a significant number of clear cell, mesenchymal, and dedifferentiated chondrosarcomas.

Signs and Symptoms

Symptoms of chondrosarcoma depend on tumor size and location. Patients with pelvic or axial lesions are typically diagnosed later in the disease course because the associated pain has a more insidious onset and often occurs when the tumor has reached a significant size. The mean interval from pain to diagnosis is 15 to 19 months.

Clinical signs and symptoms of chondrosarcomas typically include the following:
- Pain: described as a deep, dull ache
- Night pain
- Decreased range of motion in the affected joint
- Paresthesias or nerve dysfunction if the tumor encroaches on the lumbosacral plexus or neurovascular bundle
- Pathologic fracture (primary symptom in 50% of dedifferentiated chondrosarcomas)

Diagnostic Work-up

- Computed tomography (CT) of the chest, abdomen, and pelvis; bone scan; and positron emission tomography (PET) may be used for staging of the tumor and evaluation for systemic disease.
- Imaging of the primary lesion includes the following:
  - Plain radiography
    - Typically reveals large (>5 cm), cartilaginous lesions with evidence of discrete calcification ("stippled" appearance).

- Lytic lesions are well defined, with endosteal scalloping and cortical thinning.
- Shows cortical destruction and loss of medullary bone trabeculations, especially in high-grade or dedifferentiated lesions.
- Serial radiography
  - Demonstrates a slow increase in size of the osteochondroma or enchondroma.
  - Demonstrates growth in a previously stable exostosis or enchondroma in an adult.
  - Reveals decreased calcification and increased lysis.
  - A cartilage "cap" measuring >2 cm on a preexisting lesion or documented growth after skeletal maturity should raise the suspicion of sarcomatous transformation.
- Magnetic resonance imaging (MRI)
  - Shows intramedullary involvement and extraosseous extension of the tumor.
  - Delineates extent of soft tissue involvement.
  - Is useful in preoperative planning.
- Biopsy of chondrosarcoma lesions is challenging because of the heterogeneity of the tumor. Considerations when performing a biopsy are as follows:
  - Have it done at a sarcoma center where definitive treatment can be given.
  - Biopsy should be directed at the most aggressive component of the tumor.
  - Core needle or open biopsy by an experienced sarcoma surgeon or sarcoma surgical pathologist is preferred to avoid seeding of the biopsy tract with tumor cells.
  - Appropriate communication with the surgeon, radiologist, and pathologist is crucial in obtaining a suitable biopsy specimen.
  - Usually an incisional (rather than excisional) biopsy specimen is obtained from soft tissue extension of the tumor. Definitive surgery should include removal of the entire biopsy tract.
  - Failure to follow appropriate biopsy procedures may result in adverse patient outcomes and higher morbidity.

Histology

The histologic grade and location of the chondrosarcoma are important in treatment decisions. There are three histologic grades, based on celluarity, atypia, and pleomorphism:
- Grade I (low grade): Intracompartmental, cytologically similar to enchondroma with higher cellularity
- Grade II (intermediate grade): Characterized by definitive increased cellularity, distinct nucleoli, possible foci of myxoid change. Often treated as a high-grade tumor.
- Grade III (high grade): Characterized by high cellularity, prominent atypical nuclei, increased mitotic rate.
  - Dedifferentiated chondrosarcomas are high-grade lesions and should be treated as osteosarcoma; they exhibit bimorphic histology, with a low-grade chondroid component and a high-grade spindle cell component.
  - Mesenchymal chondrosarcomas are treated as Ewing sarcoma according to their grade.

Clinical Staging

The American Joint Committee on Cancer (AJCC) TNM staging system for bone sarcomas is used for all bone sarcomas (Edge et al., 2010).

The Surgical Staging System (SSS) is also used for staging of musculoskeletal sarcomas. Like the AJCC system, the SSS determines stage on the basis of tumor, tumor grade, and the presence of metastasis (see table below).

Treatment

Surgery

- Surgery is the preferred primary treatment for chondrosarcoma.
- Patients with resectable low-grade lesions are treated with intralesional excision or wide excision with negative surgical margins (R0 resection). This may be achieved by limb salvage or amputation.
- High-grade lesions (grade II, III, or clear cell) are surgically treated with wide excision, obtaining negative surgical margins. This may be achieved by limb salvage or amputation.

Radiation Therapy

- High-dose photons are used to treat high-grade and low-grade lesions.
- Preoperative radiation therapy (RT) may be considered if microscopic residual disease (R1 resection) or positive margins (R2 resection) are likely, followed by postoperative RT.
- Postoperative RT may be considered after R1 or R2 resection for high-grade, dedifferentiated, or mesenchymal chondrosarcomas.
- For unresectable disease, consider high-dose therapy, with specialized techniques such as intensity-modulated RT, stereotactic radiosurgery, or fractionated stereotactic RT, to maximize tissue sparing and limit toxicities.
- Proton beam radiation therapy is used to treat unresectable or recurrent disease in a previously radiated site.

Chemotherapy

- Chemotherapy is considered for primary treatment in mesenchymal chondrosarcoma only.
- It has limited to no benefit in conventional and dedifferentiated chondrosarcomas.

Surgical Staging System

Stage	Grade	Site
IA	Low (G1)	Intracompartmental (T1)
IB	Low (G1)	Extracompartmental (T2)
IIA	High (G2)	Intracompartmental (T1)
IIB	High (G2)	Extracompartmental (T2)
III	Any (G) and regional or distant metastasis	Any (T)

From Enneking, W. F., Spanier, S. S., Goodman, M. A. (1980). A system for the surgical staging of musculoskeletal sarcoma. *Clinical Orthopaedics and Related Research*, (153), 106-120.

Recurrence

- Local recurrence (low and high grade)
  - Wide excision with surveillance if R0 resection.
  - Wide excision with RT if R1 or R2 resection.
  - Unresectable recurrences are treated with either conventional or proton beam radiation therapy.
- Systemic recurrence (high grade)
  - Patients should be considered for participation in a clinical trial.
  - Cyclophosphamide and sirolimus are used.
  - Surgical excision is an option for systemic relapse of a high-grade lesion.

Prognosis

- Late metastases and recurrences after 10 years are more common with chondrosarcoma than with other sarcomas.
- The higher the grade of chondrosarcoma, the worse the prognosis, with increased risk for early metastases.
- The 5-year survival rate is 80% to 90% for grade I and II tumors with a low potential for metastasis.
- The 5-year survival rate is reported to be 29% for grade III tumors, which have a 66% potential for metastasis.
- The most common site for metastasis is the lungs.
- Dedifferentiated chondrosarcomas have the greatest metastatic potential, with a survival rate of less than 10% at 1 year.

Prevention and Surveillance

Prevention

- Many of the risk factors, such as race, age, or certain bone diseases or inherited conditions, cannot be changed.
- Other than prior RT, there is no known lifestyle or environmental factor that causes chondrosarcoma, so there is no way to prevent chondrosarcoma at this time.
- For patients with Ollier disease, Maffucci syndrome, or multiple hereditary exostosis, close monitoring with serial images is indicated for earlier detection of secondary transformation into chondrosarcoma.

Surveillance

- Low-grade lesions
  - Physical examination
  - Imaging of the lesion and chest radiography every 6 to 12 months for 2 years, then yearly as appropriate
- High-grade lesions
  - Physical examination
  - Primary site or cross-sectional imaging as indicated
  - Chest imaging every 3 to 6 months for the first 5 years and yearly thereafter for a minimum of 10 years

Bibliography

Amary, M. F., Damato, S., Halai, D., Eskandarpour, M., Berisha, F., Bonar, F., & Flanagan, A. M. (2011). Ollier disease and Maffucci syndrome are caused by somatic mosaic mutations of IDH1 and IDH2. *Nature Genetics*, 43, 1262–1265.

American Cancer Society. (2015). *Cancer facts and figures, 2015*. Atlanta: American Cancer Society.

Andreou, D., Ruppin, S., Fehlberg, S., Pink, D., Werner, M., & Tunn, P. U. (2011). Survival and prognostic factors in chondrosarcoma. *Acta Orthopaedica*, 82, 749–755.

Bernstein-Molho, R., Kollender, Y., Issakov, J., Bickels, J., Dadia, S., Flusser, G., & Merimsky, O. (2012). Clinical activity of mTOR inhibition in combination with cyclophosphamide in the treatment of recurrent unresectable chondrosarcomas. *Cancer Chemotherapy and Pharmacology, 70*(6), 855–860.

Bovée, J. V., Cleton-Jansen, A. M., Taminiau, A. H., & Hogendoorn, P. C. (2005). Emerging pathways in the development of chondrosarcoma of bone and implications for targeted treatment. *Lancet Oncology*, 6, 599–607.

Chow, W., Haglund, K., & Randall, R. L. (2014). Bone sarcomas. In D. Haller, L. Wagman, K. Camphausen, & W. J. Hoskins (Eds.), *Cancer management: A multi-disciplinary approach* (14th ed.). Available at http://www.cancernetwork.com/cancer-management (accessed January 29, 2016).

Edge, S., Byrd, D. R., Compton, C. C., Fritz, A. G., Greene, F. L., & Trotti, A. (Eds.). (2010). *AJCC staging manual* (7th ed.) New York: Springer.

Enneking, W. F., Spanier, S. S., & Goodman, M. A. (1980). A system for the surgical staging of musculoskeletal sarcoma. *Clinical Orthopaedics and Related Research, 153*, 106–120.

Gelderblom, H., Hogendoorn, P. C. W., Dijkstra, S. D., van Rijswijk, C. C., Krol, A. D., Taminiau, A. H., & Bovée, J. V. (2008). The clinical approach towards chondrosarcoma. *Oncologist, 13*, 320–329.

Hug, E. B., & Slater, J. D. (2000). Proton radiation therapy for chordomas and chondrosarcomas of the skull base. *Neurosurgery Clinics of North America, 11*, 627–638.

Lakshmanan, P. (2014, April 21). *Chondrosarcoma*. Available at http://emedicine.medscape.com/article/1258236-overview (accessed January 29, 2016).

Liu, P. T., Valadez, D. Z., Chivers, F. S., Roberts, C. C., & Beauchamp, C. P. (2007). Anatomically based guidelines for core needle biopsy of bone tumors: Implications for limb sparing surgery. *Radiographics, 27*, 189–205.

Mankin, H. J., Cantley, K. D., Schiller, A. L., & Lippiello, L. (1980). The biology of human chondrosarcoma, II: Variation in chemical composite among types and subtypes of benign and malignant cartilage tumors. *Journal of Bone and Joint Surgery American, 62*, 176–188.

Meijer, D., de Jong, D., Pansuriya, T. C., van den Akker, B. E., Picci, P., Szuhai, K., & Bovée, J. V. (2012). Genetic characterization of mesenchymal, clear cell and dedifferentiated chondrosarcoma. *Genes, Chromosomes and Cancer, 51*, 899–909.

National Comprehensive Cancer Network. (2015). *NCCN clinical practice guidelines in oncology: Bone cancer, version 1.2015+*. Available at http://www.nccn.org/professionals/physician_gls/pdf/bone.pdf (accessed January 29, 2016).

Ollivier, L., Vanel, D., & Leclère, J. (2004). Imaging of chondrosarcomas. *Cancer Imaging, 4*(1), 36–38.

Riedel, R. F., Larrier, N., Dodd, L., Kirsch, D., Martinez, S., & Brigman, B. E. (2009). The clinical management of chondrosarcoma. *Current Treatment Options in Oncology, 10*(1-2), 94–106.

Ewing Sarcoma Family of Tumors

Definition

Ewing sarcoma is one type of primary bone cancer that has an uncertain histologic origin. The Ewing family of tumors are a group of small, blue, round-cell neoplasms that include Ewing sarcoma, primitive neuroectodermal tumor (pNET), Askin tumor (Ewing sarcoma of the chest wall), pNET of bone, and extraosseous Ewing sarcoma.

Incidence

- Primary bone cancers are extremely rare, accounting for fewer than 0.2% of all cancers.
- In 2015, an estimated 2970 new cases of bone cancer were diagnosed in the United States, and an estimated 1330 people died from the disease.
- Ewing sarcoma is the third most common form of bone cancer and accounts for 16% of all bone cancer cases.
- In 2014, the Surveillance, Epidemiology, and End Results (SEER) program reported an incidence of approximately

3 cases per 1 million persons per year. This incidence has remained unchanged for the past 30 years.

- Ewing sarcoma develops mainly in adolescents and young adults. The median age at diagnosis is 15 years, and 50% of patients are adolescents.
- The incidence among non-Hispanic whites is three times that among blacks, and the incidence is higher in males than females.
- Most common primary sites are diaphysis of the femur (41%), pelvis (26%), and bones of the chest wall (16%).
- For extraosseous Ewing sarcoma, the most common sites are the trunk (42%), extremities (26%), and head and neck (18%).

Etiology and Risk Factors

- There are no clear risk factors specific to Ewing sarcoma; risk factors are generally similar to those of other bone sarcomas.
- Ewing sarcoma is characterized by fusion of the EWS gene (*EWSR1*) on chromosome 22q12 with the ETS gene family, which includes *FLI1*, *ERG*, *ETV1*, *ETV4*, and *FEV*.

Signs and Symptoms

- There is localized pain or swelling, with a median duration of 2 to 5 months before diagnosis.
- It is sometimes accompanied by paresthesias or neuropathy.
- It is often mistaken for growing pains or a sports injury.
- Constitutional symptoms such as fever, weight loss, and fatigue are occasionally observed on presentation.
- Approximately 15% to 35% of patients have metastatic disease at the time of diagnosis.
- Common sites of metastatic disease are lung, bone, and bone marrow.

Diagnostic Work-up

- If a Ewing family tumor is suspected as a diagnosis, the patient should undergo a complete staging before biopsy.
- Imaging of the primary lesions includes the following modalities:
  - Plain radiographs of primary site
    - Destructive lesion with a "moth-eaten" appearance; may have reactive bone formation.
    - Periosteal reaction is classic and is referred to as "onion skin" by radiologists.
  - MRI of the entire involved bone or area
    - Identifies soft tissue extension and possible bone marrow involvement
    - Evaluates relationship of tumor to neurovascular structures and adjacent joints
  - CT of the chest
    - Identifies pulmonary metastasis
  - Bone scan
    - Evaluate for distant osseous metastasis
  - PET scan
    - Initial staging of disease
    - Identification of lymph node disease
    - The combination of PET or PET/CT with conventional imaging has 96% sensitivity and 92% specificity.

- MRI of the spine and pelvis should be considered to evaluate for distant metastasis if they are not the site of the primary tumor.
- Laboratory studies include the following:
  - Complete blood count: anemia, leukocytosis
  - Lactate dehydrogenase (LDH): elevated (prognostic value as a tumor marker)
  - Alkaline phosphatase (ALP): elevated
  - Erythrocyte sedimentation rate (ESR): elevated
- Cytogenetic analysis of the biopsy specimen to evaluate the t(11;22) translocation
- Bone marrow biopsy should be considered to complete the work-up.
- Biopsy of sarcoma lesions is challenging because of the heterogeneity of the tumor. Considerations when performing a biopsy are as follows:
  - Have it done at a sarcoma center where definitive treatment can be given.
  - Biopsy should be directed at the most aggressive component of the tumor.
  - Core needle or open biopsy by an experienced sarcoma surgeon or sarcoma surgical pathologist is preferred to avoid seeding of the biopsy tract with tumor cells.
  - Appropriate communication with the surgeon, radiologist, and pathologist is crucial in obtaining a suitable biopsy specimen.
  - Usually an incisional (rather than excisional) biopsy specimen is obtained from soft tissue extension of the tumor. Definitive surgery should include removal of the entire biopsy tract.
  - Failure to follow appropriate biopsy procedures may result in adverse patient outcomes and higher morbidity.

Histology

- The EWS-FLI1 fusion protein and its corresponding chromosomal translocation, t(11; 22)(q24;q12), are identified in 85% of patients with Ewing sarcoma by fluorescence in situ hybridization (FISH).
- Other fusion proteins also occur, including some with *FUS* substitutions for the *EWS* gene.
- There is strong expression of cell surface glycoprotein MIC2 (CD99).
- The tumor exhibits sheets of small round blue cells with prominent nuclei and minimal cytoplasm.
- "Rosettes" are present (tumor cells arranged in a circle around a necrotic center).

Clinical Staging

The American Joint Commission on Cancer (AJCC) staging system which is based on tumor size, nodal involvement and presence or absence of distant metastases is used for all bone sarcomas (Edge et al., 2010).

The Surgical Staging System (SSS) is also used for staging musculoskeletal sarcomas. The SSS determines stage on the basis of tumor, tumor grade, and the presence of metastasis (see the table on page 144).

Treatment

- Fertility preservation should be discussed at time of diagnosis because pelvic surgery, RT, and chemotherapy regimens can cause infertility.

Surgery

- Surgery is rarely considered at initial diagnosis; preoperative chemotherapy is recommended.
- Surgery is used for local control. The surgical procedure includes wide excision after 12 weeks of multiagent chemotherapy if the patient had a good response or if there was disease progression.
- Amputation may be required in some cases.

Radiation Therapy

- RT is recommended for R1 or R2 resections; it is usually given concurrently with chemotherapy.
- Definitive RT for treatment of primary tumor is given after 12 weeks of primary chemotherapy (see Chemotherapy, below).
- RT is given for unresponsive or progressive disease after 12 weeks of primary chemotherapy, with or without surgery for local control and palliation.

Chemotherapy

- Neoadjuvant and adjuvant chemotherapy are effective for localized disease at diagnosis and have improved outcomes for disease-free and progression-free survival.
- First-line chemotherapy for localized and metastatic disease typically includes a combination of the following drugs (known as VAC-IE): vincristine, doxorubicin, cyclophosphamide (usually alternating with ifosfamide), and etoposide.
  - Chemotherapy is administered over 49 weeks, including chemotherapy given before local therapy.
  - VAC-IE given every 2 weeks was found to be more effective than the traditional every-3-week schedule with no increase in toxicity in patients younger than 50 years of age.
    - Actinomycin-D may be substituted for doxorubicin after the patient's maximum lifetime anthracycline dose is reached ($450 \ mg/m^2$).
- Second-line therapy for relapsed, refractory, or metastatic disease includes a combination of the following drugs: docetaxel, gemcitabine, cyclophosphamide, topotecan, carboplatin, and etoposide, as well as ifosfamide.
- The dosing and drug combinations are typically myelosuppressive, and the use of myeloid growth factors is highly recommended.
- Patients are evaluated after 12 weeks of multiagent chemotherapy. If there is a good response to chemotherapy, the patient can proceed to one of the following:
  - Additional chemotherapy followed by definitive RT to the primary tumor and/or metastatic sites
  - Wide excision of the tumor with adjuvant chemotherapy for negative margins (R0 resection) or adjuvant chemotherapy and concurrent RT for microscopic or gross positive margins (R1 or R2 resection).
  - Amputation in selected cases, followed by adjuvant chemotherapy and concurrent RT, depending on margin status.

Recurrence

- The relapse rate without chemotherapy is 80% to 90%.
- For early relapse (<2 years), second-line chemotherapies are recommended. Consider RT after chemotherapy if there is lung involvement.
- For late relapse (>2 years), rechallenge with the original chemotherapy regimen if the patient had a good response previously.
- Patients with late relapse, lung-only metastasis, local recurrence that is surgically resectable have a more favorable prognosis than those who have early relapse with multiple metastatic sites and an elevated LDH level.
- Clinical trials should be considered for patients with recurrent and metastatic disease.

Prognosis

- Previously, Ewing sarcoma was associated with a poor prognosis.
- The development of multiagent chemotherapy regimens for both neoadjuvant and adjuvant treatment has improved the prognosis greatly for patients with Ewing sarcoma:
  - Between 60% and 75% progression-free survival has been observed in patients with localized Ewing sarcoma.
  - Even patients diagnosed with metastatic disease at presentation are able to achieve a cure.

Prevention and Surveillance

Prevention

- Many of the risk factors, such as race, age, or gender, cannot be changed.
- There is no known lifestyle or environmental factor that causes Ewing sarcoma, so there is no way to prevent Ewing sarcoma at this time.

Surveillance

- Physical examination and laboratory work
- Chest imaging (CT scan or radiographs) and MRI or plain films of the extremity
- Consider PET and/or bone scan.
- Evaluate every 3 months for the first 2 years, then every 4 months for the third year and every 6 months for the fourth and fifth years; then continue annually with chest radiographs and physical examination only.
- Long-term follow-up for late adverse effects is recommended. The most common late effects are cardiomyopathy, secondary cancers, permanent azoospermia, and renal impairment.

Bibliography

American Cancer Society. (2015). *Cancer facts and figures, 2015.* Atlanta: American Cancer Society.

Avigad, S., Cohen, I. J., Zilberstein, J., Liberzon, E., Goshen, Y., Ash, S., & Yaniv, I. (2004). The predictive potential of molecular detection in the nonmetastatic Ewing family of tumors. *Cancer, 100,* 1053–1058.

Bernstein, M., Kovar, H., Paulussen, M., Randall, R. L., Schuck, A., Teot, L. A., & Juergens, H. (2006). Ewing's sarcoma family of tumors: Current management. *Oncologist, 11,* 503–519.

Chow, W., Haglund, K., & Randall, R. L. (2014). Bone sarcomas. In D. Haller, L. Wagman, K. Camphausen, & W. J. Hoskins (Eds.), *Cancer management: A multi-disciplinary approach* (14th ed.). Available at. http://www.cancernetwork.com/cancer-management (accessed January 29, 2016).

Cotterill, S. J., Ahrens, S., Paulussen, M., Jürgens, H. F., Voûte, P. A., Gadner, H., & Craft, A. W. (2000). Prognostic factors in Ewing's tumor of bone: Analysis of 975 patients from the European Intergroup Cooperative Ewing's Sarcoma Study Group. *Journal of Clinical Oncology*, 18, 3108–3114.

de Alava, E., Kawai, A., Healey, J. H., Fligman, I., Meyers, P. A., Huvos, A. G., & Ladanyi, M. (1998). EWS-FLI1 fusion transcript structure is an independent determinant of prognosis in Ewing's sarcoma. *Journal of Clinical Oncology*, 16, 1248–1255.

Denny, C. T. (1996). Gene rearrangements in Ewing's sarcoma. *Cancer Investigation*, 14, 83–88.

Edge, S., Byrd, D. R., Compton, C. C., Fritz, A. G., Greene, F. L., & Trotti, A. (Eds.). (2010). *AJCC staging manual* (7th ed.) New York: Springer.

National Comprehensive Cancer Network. (2015). *NCCN clinical practice guidelines in oncology: Bone cancer, version 1.2015+*. Available at http://www.nccn.org/professionals/physician_gls/pdf/bone.pdf (accessed January 29, 2016).

SEER Program, National Cancer Institute. (2014). *SEER Stat Fact Sheets: Bone and Joint Cancer*. Available at http://www.seer.cancer.gov/statfacts/html/bones.html (accessed January 29, 2016).

Treglia, G., Salsano, M., Stefanelli, A., Mattoli, M. V., Giordano, A., & Bonomo, L. (2012). Diagnostic accuracy of ^{18}F-FDG-PET and PET/CT I patients with Ewing sarcoma family tumours: A systematic review and a meta-analysis. *Skeletal Radiology*, 41, 249–256.

Womer, R. B., West, D. C., Krailo, M. D., Dickman, P. S., Pawel, B. R., Grier, H. E., & Weiss, A. R. (2012). Randomized controlled trial of interval-compressed chemotherapy for the treatment of localized Ewing sarcoma: A report from the Children's Oncology Group. *Journal of Clinical Oncology*, 30, 4148–4154.

Zoubek, A., Dockhorn-Dworniczak, B., Delattre, O., Christiansen, H., Niggli, F., Gatterer-Menz, I., & Kovar, H. (1996). Does expression of different EWS chimeric transcripts define clinically distinct risk groups of Ewing's tumor patients? *Journal of Clinical Oncology*, 12, 1245–1251.

Osteosarcoma

Definition

Osteosarcoma is a malignant bone tumor that produces malignant osteoid cells; it is thought to originate from primitive mesenchymal bone-forming cells. Osteosarcomas can range from low-grade tumors with a low risk of metastasis to high-grade tumors with a high risk of distant metastasis.

Incidence

- Primary bone cancers are extremely rare, accounting for fewer than 0.2% of all cancers.
- In 2015, an estimated 2970 new cases of bone cancer will be diagnosed in the United States, and 1330 people will die from the disease.
- Osteosarcoma is the most common form of bone cancer, accounting for 35% of bone cancers in the United States. The SEER database reported in 2014 that the incidence of osteosarcoma was 400 cases per year.
- Osteosarcoma is the most common primary malignant bone tumor in children and young adults.
  - There is a bimodal age distribution pattern, with peaks in adolescence and after 65 years of age.
  - The median age for all osteosarcoma patients is 20 years.
- According to the SEER 2014 data, there is a higher incidence among males and blacks.

- The most common sites of osteosarcoma are metaphyseal areas of the distal femur (42%) or the proximal tibia (19%), which are the sites of maximum growth.
- Other common sites include the humerus (10%), the pelvis (8%), and the skull and jaw (8%).

Etiology and Risk Factors

There are 11 known variants of osteosarcoma. High-grade intramedullary osteosarcoma, otherwise known as classic or conventional osteosarcoma, comprises 80% of all osteosarcomas. It is a high-grade spindle cell tumor that overproduces osteoid or immature bone. Other types include low-grade intramedullary, periosteal, and parosteal osteosarcomas.

The exact cause of osteosarcoma is unknown. Several risk factors have been identified, including the following:

- Rapid bone growth, as evidenced by the common occurrence of osteosarcoma in the metaphyseal area adjacent to the growth plate in long bones and increased incidence during the adolescent growth spurt
- Trauma, which has been implicated in the development of sarcoma, although a cause-and-effect relationship has not been identified
- Genetic predisposition also plays a role:
  - Li-Fraumeni syndrome, a familial syndrome that results in a germline mutation of the *TP53* gene, causing a cluster of cancers, including soft tissue sarcoma, osteosarcoma, premenopausal breast cancer, brain tumor, adrenocortical carcinoma, leukemia, and bronchoalveolar lung cancer diagnosed before age 46 years
  - Retinoblastoma (*RB*) gene mutation (risk is higher in patients with retinoblastoma treated with RT)
  - Rothmund-Thomson syndrome, an autosomal recessive disorder associated with congenital bone defects, hair and skin dysplasias, hypogonadism, and cataracts
- Variants of osteosarcoma may be the result of the following:
  - Paget's disease
  - Prior RT (radiation-induced osteosarcoma can occur 5-15 years after primary treatment for cancer)

Signs and Symptoms

- Clinical signs and symptoms of osteosarcoma include the following:
  - Pain, particularly with activity (in the beginning, pain is often described as intermittent and is often associated with an injury or diagnosed as a sprain or as growing pains)
  - Localized soft tissue swelling, with or without warmth or edema
  - Joint effusions
  - Limited range of motion
  - Pathologic fracture, usually with telangiectatic osteosarcoma
  - Rarely, constitutional symptoms (fevers, chills, night sweats)
- Osteosarcomas spread hematogenously, with the lung being the most common metastatic site.

Diagnostic Work-up

Osteosarcoma usually manifests as a local lesion; however, there is concern for distant metastasis.

Imaging of the primary lesion includes the following modalities:

- Plain radiographs:
  - Show cortical destruction, periosteal reaction, and irregular reactive bone formation (appearing as a "sunburst")
- MRI
  - Best study to define the extent of the lesion in the bone and in the soft tissues
  - Detects "skip" metastasis
  - Used to evaluate anatomic relationships with surrounding neurovascular structures
  - Essential for preoperative planning
- Bone scan
  - Usually uniformly abnormal at the lesion
  - May be useful in identifying any additional synchronous lesions
- CT scans
  - Useful in evaluating for metastatic disease
- PET scan
  - Pretreatment staging
  - Evaluation of response to chemotherapy

Laboratory values most often elevated in osteosarcoma include ALP and LDH

Biopsy of osteosarcoma lesions are challenging because of the heterogeneity of the tumor. Considerations when performing a biopsy are as follows:

- Have it done at a sarcoma center where definitive treatment can be given.
- Biopsy should be directed at the most aggressive component of the tumor.
- Core needle or open biopsy by an experienced sarcoma surgeon or sarcoma surgical pathologist is preferred to avoid seeding of the biopsy tract with tumor cells.
- Appropriate communication with the surgeon, radiologist, and pathologist is crucial in obtaining a suitable biopsy specimen.
- Usually incisional (rather than excisional) biopsy specimen is obtained from soft tissue extension of the tumor. Definitive surgery should include removal of the entire biopsy tract.
- Failure to follow appropriate biopsy procedures may result in adverse patient outcomes and amputation of a potentially salvageable extremity.

Histology

- Osteosarcoma is classified into three histologic subtypes: intramedullary, surface, and extraskeletal.
- There are high-grade and low-grade intramedullary lesions.
- Surface, or juxtacortical, lesions include periosteal and parosteal variants.
  - Parosteal osteosarcomas are low-grade lesions and tend to metastasize later than the conventional form.
  - Transformation of low-grade to high-grade lesions has been documented in 24% to 43% of cases.
  - Periosteal osteosarcoma, a juxtacortical variant, is of intermediate grade in its severity.

- High-grade surface osteosarcomas occur in 10% of all cases of osteosarcoma and are considered very rare.
- Extraskeletal osteosarcomas are considered to be soft tissue tumors and are treated as such.

Clinical Staging

The American Joint Committee on Cancer (AJCC) TNM staging system for bone sarcomas is used for all bone sarcomas. (Edge et al., 2010).

The Surgical Staging System (SSS) is also used for staging musculoskeletal sarcomas. Like the AJCC system, the SSS determines stage on the basis of tumor, tumor grade, and the presence of metastasis (see the table on page 144).

Treatment

Fertility preservation should be discussed at time of diagnosis because pelvic surgery, RT, and chemotherapy regimens can cause infertility.

Surgery

- The goal of wide excision is to achieve histologically negative surgical margins (R0 resection) for optimal local tumor control and to decrease the risk of distant metastasis.
- Local tumor control may be achieved by limb-sparing surgery or limb amputation.
  - Limb-sparing surgery is preferred if reasonable nerve and motor function can be preserved.
  - Comparison of limb-sparing surgery versus amputation in patients with high-grade osteosarcoma has not shown a significant difference in overall survival or local recurrence rates.
  - However, there is a significant difference in functional outcomes, especially in patients who had a good histologic response to preoperative chemotherapy.
- Low-grade intramedullary and surface osteosarcomas, such as parosteal lesions, are treated with wide excision as primary treatment.
- For intermediate and high-grade lesions (intramedullary and surface types), preoperative chemotherapy is recommended before wide excision.

Radiation Therapy

- RT may be considered for high-grade osteosarcoma that remains unresectable after preoperative chemotherapy.
- RT may be considered for high-grade osteosarcoma that is resected with microscopic residual disease (R1 resection) or grossly positive surgical margins (R2 resection), followed by additional chemotherapy or surgical re-resection.

Chemotherapy

- Neoadjuvant and adjuvant chemotherapy are effective for localized disease at diagnosis and have improved outcomes in disease-free and progression-free survival.
  - Neoadjuvant chemotherapy is preferred for high-grade osteosarcoma and can be considered in periosteal lesions. Selected elderly patients may benefit from immediate surgery.

- Adjuvant chemotherapy should be used for patients with pathologic findings of high-grade disease after wide excision for suspected low-grade or periosteal sarcoma.
  - After wide excision, patients with high-grade osteosarcoma and a good histologic response (viable tumor is <10% of tumor area) should continue to receive several more cycles of the same chemotherapy.
  - Patients with a poor histologic response (viable tumor is ≥10% of tumor area) can be considered for adjuvant chemotherapy with a second-line regimen.
- First-line chemotherapy for primary, preoperative, adjuvant, and metastatic disease typically includes a combination of the following drugs: doxorubicin, cisplatin, ifosfamide, and high-dose methotrexate.
- Second-line therapy for relapsed, refractory, or metastatic disease includes a combination of the following drugs: docetaxel, gemcitabine, cyclophosphamide, topotecan, carboplatin, and etoposide, as well as ifosfamide and high-dose methotrexate.
- Sorafenib may also be considered, and other targeted therapies are being evaluated in clinical trials to improve outcomes in relapsed/refractory and metastatic disease.
- Dosing and drug combinations are typically myelosuppressive, and the use of myeloid growth factors is highly recommended.

Treatment for Metastatic Disease at Presentation

- Approximately 10% to 20% of patients present with metastatic disease at the time of diagnosis.
- The number of metastases and the complete surgical resection of these lesions are predictive of prognosis in this group of osteosarcoma patients.
- Preoperative chemotherapy followed by wide excision is recommended. Metastatectomy for lung lesions is included in the treatment plan.
- Management with chemotherapy and RT is recommended, as well as possible surgical resection of the primary lesion for local control.

Recurrence

- The goal is palliation of symptoms and maintenance of quality of life.
- Patients should be considered for participation in a clinical trial.
- Chemotherapy with either first-line or second-line therapy is used, followed by surgical resection.
- Manage relapse/progression or unresectable metastases with palliative RT, stereotactic radiosurgery, samarium-153 ethylene diamine tetramethylene phosphonate ([153]Sm-EDTMP) or best supportive care.

Prognosis

- In the past, osteosarcoma was associated with a poor prognosis.
  - All patients with extremity osteosarcomas were treated with amputation.

- Before the routine use of systemic chemotherapy, 80% to 90% of patients developed metastases despite local tumor control and died of their disease.
- The development of multiagent chemotherapy regimens for both neoadjuvant and adjuvant treatment has improved the prognosis greatly for patients with osteosarcoma.
  - Approximately 75% of osteosarcoma patients are cured.
  - Almost 90% of adult patients with osteosarcoma can be treated successfully with limb-sparing surgery instead of amputation.
- The 2-year disease-free survival rate is significantly higher in patients with fewer than three metastatic lesions (78% vs. 25%). However, the overall survival rate for patients who present with metastatic disease or develop metastasis is approximately 20%.

Prevention and Surveillance

Prevention

- Many of the risk factors, such as race, age, and certain bone diseases and inherited conditions, cannot be changed.
- Other than prior RT, there is no known lifestyle or environmental factor that causes osteosarcoma, so there is no way to prevent osteosarcoma at this time.

Surveillance

- Physical examination and laboratory work if patient received chemotherapy
- Chest imaging (CT scan or radiographs) and MRI or plain films of the extremity
- Consider PET and/or bone scan.
- Evaluate every 3 months for the first 2 years, then every 4 months for the third year and every 6 months for the fourth and fifth years; then continue annually with chest radiographs and physical examination only.
- Long-term follow-up for late adverse effects is recommended. The most common late effects are cardiomyopathy, secondary cancers, permanent azoospermia, renal impairment, and ototoxicity/hearing impairment.

Bibliography

American Cancer Society. (2015). *Cancer facts and figures, 2015.* Atlanta: American Cancer Society.

Anderson, P. M., Wiseman, G. A., Dispenzieri, A., Arndt, C. A. S., Hartmann, L. C., Smithson, W. A., & Bruland, O. S. (2002). High-dose samarium-153 ethylene diamine tetramethylene phosphonate: low toxicity of skeletal irradiation in patients with osteosarcoma and bone metastases. *Journal of Clinical Oncology, 20,* 189–196.

Bacci, G., Ferrari, S., Longhi, A., Forni, C., Bertoni, F., Fabbri, N., & Versari, M. (2001). Neoadjuvant chemotherapy for high-grade osteosarcoma of the extremities: Long-term results for patients treated according to Rizzoli IOR/OS-3b protocol. *Journal of Chemotherapy, 13,* 93–99.

Bacci, G., Briccoli, A., Rocca, M., Ferrari, S., Donati, D., Longhi, A., & Galletti, S. (2003). Neoadjuvant chemotherapy for osteosarcoma of the extremities with metastases at presentation: Recent experiences at the Rizzoli Institute in 57 patients treated with cisplatin, doxorubicin, and a high dose of methotrexate and ifosfamide. *Annals of Oncology, 14,* 1126–1134.

Bielack, S. S., Kempf-Bielack, B., Delling, G., Exner, G. U., Flege, S., Helmke, K., & Winkler, K. (2002). Prognostic factors in high-grade osteosarcoma of the extremities or trunk: An analysis of 1,702 patients treated on neoadjuvant cooperative osteosarcoma study group protocols. *Journal of Clinical Oncology, 20,* 776–790.

Chow, W., Haglund, K., & Randall, R. L. (2014). Bone sarcomas. In D. Haller, L. Wagman, K. Camphausen, & W. J. Hoskins (Eds.), *Cancer management: A multi-disciplinary approach* (14th ed.). Available at. http://www.cancer network.com/cancer-management (accessed January 29, 2016).

Edge, S., Byrd, D. R., Compton, C. C., Fritz, A. G., Greene, F. L., & Trotti, A. (Eds.). (2010). *AJCC staging manual* (7th ed.). New York: Springer.

Enneking, W. F., Spanier, S. S., & Goodman, M. A. (1980). A system for the surgical staging of musculoskeletal sarcoma. *Clinical Orthopaedics and Related Research, 153*, 106–120.

Geller, D. S., & Gorlick, R. G. (2010). Osteosarcoma: A review of diagnosis, management and treatment strategies. *Clinical Advances in Hematology and Oncology, 8*(10), 705–718.

Grigani, G., Palmerini, E., Dileo, P., Asaftei, S. D., D'Ambrosio, L., Pignochino, Y., & Aglietta, M. (2012). A phase II trial of sorafenib in relapsed and unresectable high-grade osteosarcoma after failure of standard multimodal therapy: An Italian Sarcoma Group study. *Annals of Oncology, 23*, 508–516.

Hawkins, D. S., Conrad, E. U., 3rd, Butrynski, J. E., Schuetze, S. M., & Eary, J. F. (2009). [F-18]-Fluorodeoxy-D-glucose-positron emission tomography response is associated with outcome for extremity osteosarcoma in children and young adults. *Cancer, 115*, 3519–3525.

Mavrogenis, A. F., Abati, C. N., Romangoli, C., & Ruggieri, P. (2012). Similar survival but better function for patients after limb salvage versus amputation for distal tibia osteosarcoma. *Clinical Orthopedics and Related Research, 470*, 1735–1748.

Mehlman, C. T. (2014, November 19). *Osteosarcoma*. Available at http://emedi cine.medscape.com/article/1256857-overview (accessed January 29, 2016).

National Comprehensive Cancer Network. (2015). *NCCN Clinical practice guidelines in oncology: Bone cancer, version 1.2015+*. Available at http://www.ncc n.org/professionals/physician_gls/pdf/bone.pdf (accessed January 29, 2016).

SEER Program, National Cancer Institute. (2014). *SEER Stat Fact Sheets: Bone and Joint Cancer*. Available at http://www.seer.cancer.gov/statfacts/html /bones.html (accessed January 29, 2016).

Soft Tissue Sarcoma

Definition

Soft tissue sarcomas are a diverse group of rare solid tumors. Adult soft tissue sarcoma occurs in the supporting structures and soft tissues of the body, including the following:

- Muscles
- Fat
- Blood vessels
- Lymph vessels
- Nerves
- Ligaments
- Tissues around joints
- Fibrous tissues

Soft tissue sarcomas can occur anywhere in the body:

- Extremities: 43%
- Viscera: 19%
- Internal organs or retroperitoneum: 15%
- Trunk: 10%
- Head and neck: 9%

There are more than 50 different subtypes of soft tissue sarcomas. Adult soft tissue sarcomas are classified by the types of tissue cells from which they arise.

Incidence

- Soft tissue sarcoma is a relatively rare cancer, accounting for about 1% of all adult cancers diagnosed and approximately 15% of pediatric malignancies.
- In 2015, an estimated 11,930 new cases of soft tissue sarcoma were diagnosed in adults and children in the United States, and an estimated 4870 patients died of the disease.
- There is an increased prevalence in males.
- From 2003 to 2007, the median age at diagnosis was 58 years.

Etiology and Risk Factors

- Exposure to ionizing radiation accounts for fewer than 5% of all soft tissue sarcomas.
  - The number of cases is expected to decline because RT techniques have steadily improved.
  - The most common form is RT for other primary cancers such as lymphoma, breast cancer, or cervical cancer.
  - The time between the exposure to radiation and diagnosis of soft tissue sarcoma is approximately 10 years.
- Family history: People with a family history of these inherited conditions or a strong family history of sarcomas may wish to discuss genetic testing with their health care providers. These genetic conditions are outlined in the table below.
- Impaired lymph drainage: Lymphangiosarcoma can occur rarely in parts of the body where lymph nodes have been removed or damaged by radiation.
- Chemical exposure:
  - Agent Orange has been linked to soft tissue sarcoma and is covered under Veteran's Administration (VA) benefits.
  - There is a moderately strong association between exposure to vinyl chloride, arsenic, anabolic steroids, or thorium and hepatic angiosarcoma.
- There is no evidence to date that injury causes soft tissue sarcoma.

Genetic Conditions Associated with Soft Tissue Sarcomas

Condition	Characteristics
Neurofibromatosis (NF1)	Autosomal dominant Clinical manifestations: café au lait spots, benign neurofibromas, optic gliomas One in 10 will develop into a malignant peripheral nerve sheath tumor.
Neurofibromatosis (NF2)	Autosomal dominant, less common Clinical manifestations: schwannomas, meningiomas, gliomas, neurofibromas Increased risk for radiation-induced cancers
Gardner syndrome	An inherited genetic disorder that leads to benign polyps, colon cancer, desmoid tumors in the abdomen, and benign bone tumors
Li-Fraumeni syndrome	Autosomal dominant syndrome that increases the risk for early-onset development of breast cancer, brain tumors, leukemias, adrenal cancer, and bone and soft tissue sarcoma Mutation in the *TP53* gene Carriers have an approximately 50% chance of developing cancer by the age of 30 years and an approximately 57% risk of developing a second primary cancer. Approximately 2-4% of sarcoma patients carry the *TP53* mutation. Patients with Li-Fraumeni syndrome who have received radiation therapy for cancer are at very high risk for development soft tissue sarcoma in the area of the body where they received the radiation.
Retinoblastoma syndrome	Autosomal dominant syndrome associated with mutation in the *RB* gene Children with the inherited form of retinoblastoma are at increased risk for development of both bone and soft tissue sarcomas.

Signs and Symptoms

Symptoms vary depending on what part of the body is affected.

- Sarcomas that develop in the extremities usually begin as a painless lump that may be stable in size or may grow rapidly over a period of weeks to months.
- Sarcomas that manifest elsewhere in the body (e.g., chest, abdomen) may also begin as painless lumps.
- Masses may become painful if they grow to >10 cm or compress neurologic structures.
- Retroperitoneal sarcomas or those that develop within the abdomen or chest begin with more vague symptoms, such as abdominal pain, bowel obstruction, or bleeding.
- About 50% of patients have lung metastasis on diagnosis. Respiratory symptoms vary depending on the extent of lung involvement.

Diagnostic Work-up

- A comprehensive cancer center specializing in sarcoma is recommended to complete the work-up.
  - The comprehensive, multidisciplinary team should include sarcoma-trained pathologists, radiologists, radiation oncologists, medical oncologists, and surgeons. If this is not possible, close consultation with a sarcoma center is strongly advised.
- Complete medical history and physical examination
- Imaging
  - General considerations
    - Initial imaging usually includes the site of the primary tumor and the lungs, which are the primary site of metastasis.
    - Consider CT of the abdomen and pelvis for myxoid/round cell liposarcoma, epithelioid sarcoma, angiosarcoma, and leiomyosarcoma.
    - Consider spine imaging for myxoid/round cell liposarcoma.
    - Consider brain MRI for alveolar soft part sarcoma and angiosarcoma.
  - Plain radiography
    - It is useful in assessment of bone tumors with associated soft tissue masses.
    - It can be useful in diagnosing lung metastasis with masses >1 cm in size.
    - It is not useful in the primary evaluation of retroperitoneal sarcomas but is helpful in diagnosing complications that result from the tumor, such as bowel obstruction or perforation.
  - CT scans
    - A three-dimensional view of the mass and surrounding structures is recommended.
    - CT is the preferred modality for primary evaluation of intraabdominal and intrathoracic lesions.
    - CT can determine the size of the tumor and nodal involvement.
    - CT detects the presence of early metastasis on presentation, particularly in the lung.
    - Use of contrast is preferred.

- MRI
  - MRI has better contrast resolution and a larger field of view than CT and is the preferred modality for extremity and trunk soft tissue lesions.
  - MRI is the best study to define the extent of the lesion in the bone and in the soft tissues.
  - MRI is used to evaluate anatomic relationships with surrounding neurovascular structures.
  - MRI is essential for preoperative planning.
  - Gadolinium contrast is essential to differentiate between soft tissue structures and tumor.
  - A magnetic field strength of 1.5 Tesla or greater is necessary for adequate imaging.
- ^{18}F-Fluorodeoxyglucose positron emission tomography (FDG PET)
  - Assess metabolic activity in conjunction with CT. Malignant tumors tend to have higher metabolic activity than normal soft tissue. Intensity is measured in standard uptake values (SUV).
  - FDG PET can distinguish between benign tumors and high-grade sarcomas, but it cannot reliably distinguish between benign tumors and low- to intermediate-grade sarcomas.
  - Imaging includes the entire body from skull base to feet.
  - FDG PET is useful in initial staging, detecting occult metastases, and evaluating the response to chemotherapy.
- Biopsy of soft tissue sarcomas is challenging because of the heterogeneity of the tumor. General considerations include the following:
  - Have it done at a sarcoma center where definitive treatment can be given.
  - Biopsy should be directed at the most aggressive component of the tumor.
  - Core needle or open biopsy by an experienced orthopedic surgeon, sarcoma surgeon, or sarcoma surgical pathologist is preferred to avoid seeding of the biopsy tract with tumor cells.
  - Appropriate communication with the surgeon, radiologist, and pathologist is crucial in obtaining a suitable biopsy specimen.
  - Usually an incisional (rather than excisional) biopsy specimen is obtained from soft tissue extension of the tumor. Definitive surgery should include removal of the entire biopsy tract.
  - Failure to follow appropriate biopsy procedures may result in adverse patient outcomes and amputation of a potentially salvageable extremity.
- Fine-needle aspiration (FNA)
  - FNA is used when the mass is palpable and superficial.
  - It can be done as an office procedure but is best performed in selected institutions by a sarcoma pathologist with clinical expertise.
  - The advantage of FNA is that a rapid preliminary diagnosis can be determined.
  - The disadvantage is that there may not be enough cells to determine the exact type and grade of a sarcoma, if one is present.

- FNA is useful in ruling out other conditions such as other types of cancers, benign tumors, and infection.
- If FNA leads to a diagnosis of sarcoma, usually another biopsy is needed to yield further information.
- Core needle biopsy
  - A larger tissue sample is obtained than with FNA.
  - The biopsy specimen usually contains enough tissue to adequately make a diagnosis of soft tissue sarcoma.
  - CT or ultrasound can be used to guide core needle biopsies when the mass cannot be palpated.
- Excisional biopsy
  - The entire tumor and a margin of surrounding normal tissue are removed, combining diagnostic biopsy and surgical treatment in one procedure.
  - Excisional biopsy is used when the tumor is small and not located next to any critical structures.
  - Excisional biopsy is used for a large mass that cannot be completely removed.

Histology

- Soft tissue sarcoma can occur anywhere in the body, and more than 50 subtypes have been identified. The most common ones are pleomorphic sarcoma (formerly malignant fibrous histiocytoma), leiomyosarcoma, liposarcoma, synovial sarcoma, and malignant peripheral nerve sheath tumor (MPNST).
- Cytogenetics, immunohistochemistry, and molecular genetic testing are useful in differentiating the subtype of soft tissue sarcoma, many of which have defined translocations, deletions, amplifications, and single-base-pair substitutions.
- Skeletal muscle tumors
  - Rhabdomyosarcoma
    - Most common subtype in children; also affects adults
    - Embryonal, alveolar, and pleomorphic forms
    - Occur most frequently in the arms and legs but may also be found in the head and neck area and in reproductive or urinary organs (i.e., vagina or bladder)
    - Chromosomal translocation results in a fusion gene transcript.
- Smooth muscle tumors
  - Leiomyosarcoma
    - Occurs primarily in older adults
    - Can occur anywhere in the body but is most commonly found in the retroperitoneum, internal organs, and blood vessels; may develop in the deep soft tissues of the arms and legs
    - Leiomyosarcoma of the uterus is common.
- Adipocytic tumors
  - Liposarcomas
    - Commonly found in the thigh, behind the knee, or in the retroperitoneum but may develop almost anywhere in the body
    - Most prevalent in middle-aged adults between 50 and 65 years of age
    - Range from slow-growing, atypical lipomatous tumors to very aggressive dedifferentiated liposarcomas

- Other forms include myxoid/round cell and pleomorphic types.
- The tumor can be heterogeneous, with areas of dedifferentiated liposarcoma arising from a well-differentiated tumor.
- Gene amplification of region 12q14-15 is involved.
- Peripheral nerve tumors
  - Malignant peripheral nerve sheath tumor includes the cells that surround the peripheral nervous system.
  - Neurofibrosarcomas involve degeneration of neurofibromatosis lesions.
- Connective tissue tumors
  - Fibrosarcomas
    - Affect adults, most commonly between the ages of 30 and 80 years
    - Musculoaponeurotic fibromatoses are closely attached to skeletal tissue.
    - Other types include low-grade myxofibrosarcoma, low-grade fibromyxoid sarcoma, sclerosing epithelioid fibrosarcoma, and dermatofibrosarcoma protuberans.
  - Chondro-osseous tumors
  - Extraskeletal chondrosarcoma (mesenchymal and other variants)
  - Extraskeletal osteosarcoma
  - Fibrohistiocytic tumors
  - Undifferentiated pleomorphic sarcoma (formerly malignant fibrous histiocytomas)
    - Tends to grow locally but can metastasize; typically considered a high-grade tumor
    - Most commonly found in the arms and legs, less commonly in the retroperitoneum
    - Occurs most frequently in older adults
    - Other types include giant cell, myxoid/high-grade myxofibrosarcoma, and inflammatory forms.
- Vascular tumors
  - Angiosarcoma
    - A rare, aggressive tumor arising from endothelium of blood vessels
    - Risk factors include chronic stasis, trauma, and previous site of irradiation.
    - Occurs more often in males and in the elderly
    - Tends to metastasize to lymph nodes and lungs
  - Other types include lymphangiosarcoma, cutaneous angiosarcoma, and epithelioid hemangioendothelioma.
- Tumors of uncertain differentiation: soft tissue sarcomas that cannot be linked to any specific type of soft tissue
  - Alveolar soft part sarcoma
    - Affects adolescents and young adults
    - Can metastasize to lung, liver, and brain
    - May resemble renal cell carcinoma or melanoma
  - Clear cell sarcoma
    - Develops primarily in the tendons of the arms or legs; can also develop in the gastrointestinal tract
    - Primarily affects young adults, ages 20 to 40 years
    - Chromosomal translocation of EWSR1/ATF1 or a EWSR1/CREB1 is involved.
    - It has some features of malignant melanoma.

- Desmoplastic small cell tumor
  - Characterized by small round blue cells surrounded by scar-like tissue
  - Found in the retroperitoneum and may metastasize to lung, liver, and lymph nodes; more than 40% of patients have distant metastasis at the time of presentation
  - Most often seen in adolescents and young adults of child-bearing age
  - Chromosomal translocation of t(11;22)(p13;q12) results in the EWS-WT1 fusion protein.
- Synovial sarcoma
  - Knees and ankles are the most common locations; may occur in shoulders or hips and may metastasize to lymph nodes, lung, and liver
  - Most common soft tissue sarcoma found in young adults, ages 15 to 40 years
  - Chromosomal translocation of t(x, 18) results in SYT-SSX1 fusion protein.
- Other types: epithelioid sarcoma, extraskeletal myxoid chondrosarcoma, primitive neuroectodermal tumor/extraskeletal Ewing tumor, extrarenal rhaboid tumor, undifferentiated sarcoma

Clinical Staging

- The AJCC TNM staging system based on tumor nodal involvement and presence or absence of metastasis is used for all soft tissue sarcomas. Staging has an important role in determining the most effective treatment of soft tissue sarcomas and estimating prognosis. (Edge et al., 2010).
- Nodal involvement is rare and occurs in fewer than 3% of soft tissue sarcomas.
- The SSS is also used for staging musculoskeletal sarcomas. Like the AJCC system, the SSS determines stage on the basis of tumor, tumor grade, and the presence of metastasis (see the table on page 144).
- Intracompartmental or extracompartmental extension of extremity sarcomas is also important for surgical decision making.
- For complete staging, a thorough physical examination, radiographs, laboratory studies, and careful review of all biopsy specimens (including those from the primary tumor, lymph nodes, and other suspicious lesions) are essential.

Treatment

General Principles

- It is essential that surgical/orthopedic oncologists, medical oncologists, and radiation oncologists have experience and expertise in sarcoma treatment and collaborate in the treatment plan.
- Treatment varies depending on the site and stage of the disease.
- Fertility preservation should be discussed at the time of diagnosis because pelvic surgery, RT, and chemotherapy regimens can cause infertility.

Surgery

- Surgery is standard primary treatment for most soft tissue sarcomas and stand-alone treatment for stage IA and stage IB tumors.
- Surgery is often preceded by RT and/or chemotherapy to downgrade and shrink large high-grade tumors to ensure negative surgical margins, avoid critical neurovascular structures, and preserve limb function.
- The biopsy site should be excised en bloc with the surgical specimen. Transverse incisions should be avoided because they can be considered areas that are contaminated with tumor.
- Hemostasis must be maintained; hematomas can contain tumor cells and can contaminate the site, increasing the risk of recurrence and the area of re-resection.
- Resection margins must be documented by the surgeon and the pathologist
  - R0 resection: no residual microscopic disease
  - R1 resection: microscopic residual disease
  - R2 resection: gross residual disease
- If surgical margins are positive on pathology (with the exception of bone, nerve, or major blood vessels), surgical re-resection should be considered if at all possible.
- Postoperative (adjuvant) radiation therapy should be considered for microscopically positive margin on a bone, nerve, or major blood vessel or for close surgical margins (<1 cm)
- Myxofibrosarcoma, dermatofibrosarcoma protuberans, and angiosarcoma are more infiltrative in nature, and it is more difficult to obtain an R0 resection.
- Abdominal surgery considerations:
  - If RT is to be considered, preoperative (neoadjuvant) radiation is preferred, with shielding of critical structures.
  - If R1 or R2 resection is anticipated, surgical clips should be left in place to identify high-risk areas for recurrence.
- Extremity surgery considerations:
  - Limb salvage surgery, with or without preoperative chemotherapy and RT, is the treatment of choice in more than 90% of sarcomas. Survival rates are 60% to 70%.
  - Reconstructive plastic surgery with split-thickness skin grafts or muscle flaps is often required.
  - Indications for amputation:
    - R0 resection would leave the patient with a nonfunctional limb and/or chronic pain
    - Infiltrative tumors of the hand or foot or regional (skip) metastasis
- Rehabilitation: Evaluate patient preoperatively for physical and occupational therapy, and continue rehabilitation therapy postoperatively until maximal function is achieved.

Radiation Therapy

- Can be administered as preoperative (neoadjuvant) and postoperative (adjuvant) treatment
- Indicated for stage II, III, and IV tumors and as palliative treatment
- Recommended for R1 and R2 resections
- Total dose delivered depends on tissue tolerance and toxicity
- Four types:

- External beam radiotherapy (EBRT), in which an external source of radiation is directed at the tumor bed using electron beams
- Brachytherapy: direct application of radioactive seeds into the tumor bed through surgically placed catheters; can be given as low dose or high dose
- Intensity-modulated radiotherapy (IMRT): conformal radiotherapy that shapes the radiation beams to closely fit the tumor or tumor bed
- Intraoperative radiotherapy (IORT): radiation delivered during surgery using brachytherapy or EBRT techniques
- Preoperative radiation therapy: typically delivered over 5 weeks
  - Advantages:
    - Direct visualization of tumor
    - Smaller treatment field with less exposure of normal tissues to radiation toxicity
    - Lower dose requirement and lower rate of late toxicity
    - Increased sensitivity of tumor due to intact blood supply
    - Creation of a pseudocapsule, allowing for ease of resection and lower risk of recurrence
  - Disadvantage: Wound healing complications, which can delay further treatment
- Postoperative radiation therapy: typically delivered over 6 to 7 weeks
  - Advantages:
    - Improves local control in patients with positive surgical margins
    - Allows for pathology review to determine whether postoperative RT is needed at all
    - Fewer wound complications, especially for thigh sarcomas
  - Disadvantages:
    - Larger treatment field required to include entire surgical bed and incision
    - Higher rate of treatment-related side effects

Chemotherapy

- Chemotherapy can be administered as preoperative (neoadjuvant) and postoperative (adjuvant) treatment.
- It is a treatment option for stage IIB, III, and IV tumors and as palliative treatment for disseminated metastatic disease.
- Patient selection and optimal drug selection are important criteria to decrease risk of short- and long-term toxicities.
- Reserve use for large, high-grade, chemosensitive tumors.
- Patients need to have good performance status to withstand potential toxicities, including myelosuppression.
- The most commonly used chemotherapeutic agents are ifosfamide and doxorubicin.
- Other chemotherapeutic agents include docetaxel, gemcitabine, cyclophosphamide, dacarbazine, temozolamide, trabectidin, pegylated liposomal doxorubicin, eribulin, methotrexate, irinotecan, vincristine, cisplatin, and paclitaxel.

- Chemotherapy agents can be given as monotherapy or combination therapy, depending on tumor histology and patient tolerance of regimen.
- Major side effects include myelosuppression, peripheral neuropathy, hepatic dysfunction, renal dysfunction, and cardiotoxicity.

Targeted Therapies

- Target angiogenesis of tumor cells by blocking growth factors that promote blood vessel formation, thus starving the tumor of nutrients and blood supply, leading to increased cell death
- Target the cell cycle signaling cascade at multiple sites by blocking nutrient, oxygen, and energy level sensing mechanisms that contribute to oncogenesis.
- Not used as first-line (primary) therapy but usually in cases of recurrent, advanced, or metastatic disease
- Best responses occur with specific histologic subtypes.
- Goal is stabilization of the tumor.
- Currently used agents:
  - Tyrosine kinase inhibitors: Pazopanib is approved by the U.S. Food and Drug Administration (FDA) for soft tissue sarcoma except liposarcoma; other agents include imatinib, sunitinib, and sorafenib.
  - Vascular endothelial growth factor (VEGF) inhibitors: bevacizumab used in combination with temozolamide
  - Mechanistic target of rapamycin (mTOR) inhibitors: everolimus, sirolimus, and temsirolimus
- Clinical trials studying targeted therapies for sarcoma are ongoing.

Recurrence

- The recurrence rate for high-grade tumors is about 50% during the first 3 years after diagnosis.
- Local recurrence is treated as a primary lesion
  - Brachytherapy may be used if the area has previously been irradiated.
- Treatment of metastatic disease depends on the extent of metastasis
  - Limited
    - Surgery with or without chemotherapy or RT
    - Single organ, limited bulk: consider metastatectomy, radiofrequency ablation, embolization
    - Metastasized to the lung: the site of the metastasis can be surgically removed
  - Disseminated
    - Watchful waiting if asymptomatic
    - Palliative chemotherapy and/or RT
    - Debulking surgery for symptom management
    - Radiofrequency ablation or embolization
  - Isolated regional disease or lymph node involvement
    - Regional node dissection with or without chemotherapy and/or RT
    - Metastatectomy

Prognosis

- Tumor stage and location are prognostic factors in predicting survival.

- Patients with extremity sarcomas have a higher survival rate than those with retroperitoneal or head and neck sarcomas.
- Re-resection of tumors to obtain negative surgical margins is a significant predictor of local control and good long-term outcome.
- Overall 5-year survival ranges from 60% to 80%, depending on age, tumor size, location and depth, histologic grade, and subtype.
- Estimated 5-year survival for localized sarcomas is 83% (54% if lymph node metastasis is present).
- Median overall survival time for patients with metastatic disease is 12 to 18 months.
- The 5-year survival rate with resectable metastasis is 25% to 40%; with unresectable distant metastasis, the estimated 5-year survival rate is 16%.
- Several predictive nomograms have been developed to help provide more accurate information to patients and providers. Future staging systems and nomograms are likely to include molecular markers and other biologic factors.

Prevention and Surveillance

Prevention

- Many of the risk factors, such as race, age, or gender, cannot be changed.
- Other risk factors and their associations with soft tissue sarcoma are still poorly understood.
- There are no current screening recommendations or effective preventative measures for soft tissue sarcoma.

Surveillance

- Low-grade lesions
  - Physical examination
  - Imaging of the lesion and chest radiography every 6 to 12 months for 2 years, then yearly as appropriate
- High-grade lesions
  - Physical examination
  - Primary site or cross-sectional imaging as indicated
  - Chest imaging every 3 to 6 months for the first 5 years and yearly thereafter for a minimum of 10 years

Bibliography

American Cancer Society. (2015). *Sarcoma: Adult soft tissue cancer.* Available at http://www.cancer.org/cancer/sarcoma-adultsofttissuecancer/detailed guide/sarcoma-adult-soft-tissue-cancer-soft-tissue-sarcoma (accessed January 29, 2016).

Amini, B., Jessop, A. C., Ganeshan, D. M., Tseng, W. W., & Madewell, J. E. (2015). Contemporary imaging of soft tissue sarcomas. *Journal of Surgical Oncology, 111,* 496–503.

Arnaldez, F., & Loeb, D. (2010). *Desmoplastic round cell tumor (DSRCT).* Available at http://sarcomahelp.org/dsrct.html (accessed January 29, 2016).

Barry, G., & Nielsen, T. (2012, October 1). *What is clear cell sarcoma?* Available at http://sarcomahelp.org/clear-cell-sarcoma.html (accessed January 29, 2016).

Burmingham, Z., Hashibe, M., Spector, L., et al. (2012). The epidemiology of sarcoma. *Clinical Sarcoma Research, 2*(1), 14. Available at http://www.clinicalsarcomaresearch.com/content/pdf/2045-3329-2-14.pdf (accessed January 29, 2016).

Chao, A., Mayerson, J., Chandawarkar, R., & Scharschmidt, T. (2015). Surgical management of soft tissue sarcomas: Extremity sarcomas. *Journal of Surgical Oncology, 111*(5), 540–545.

Edge, S., Byrd, D. R., Compton, C. C., Fritz, A. G., Greene, F. L., & Trotti, A. (Eds.). (2010). *AJCC staging manual* (7th ed.). New York: Springer.

Institute of Medicine. (1994). *Veterans and Agent Orange: Health effects of herbicides used in Vietnam.* Washington, DC: National Academies Press.

Kilpatrick, S. E., Cappellari, J. O., Bos, G. D., Gold, S. H., & Ward, W. G. (2001). Is fine-needle aspiration a practical alternative to open biopsy for the primary diagnosis of sarcoma? Experience with 140 patients. *American Journal of Clinical Pathology, 115,* 59–68.

Massarweh, N., Dickson, P., & Anaya, D. (2015). Soft tissue sarcomas: Staging principles and prognostic nomograms. *Journal of Surgical Oncology, 111*(5), 532–539.

Mayerson, J. L., Scharschmidt, T. J., Lewis, V. O., & Morris, C. D. (2014). Diagnosis and management of soft-tissue masses. *Journal of the American Academy of Orthopedic Surgeons, 22,* 742–750.

Mendenhall, W. M., Indelicato, D. J., Scarborough, M. T., Zlotecki, R. A., Gibbs, C. P., Mendenhall, N. P., & Enneking, W. F. (2009). The management of adult soft tissue sarcomas. *American Journal of Clinical Oncology, 32*(4), 436–442.

Miller, E., Xu-Welliver, M., & Haglund, K. (2015). The role of modern radiation therapy in the management of extremity sarcomas. *Journal of Surgical Oncology, 111*(5), 599–603.

National Comprehensive Cancer Network. (2015). *NCCN clinical practice guidelines in oncology: Soft tissue sarcoma, version 1.2015.* Available at http://www.nccn.org/professionals/physician_gls/pdf/sarcoma.pdf (accessed January 29, 2016).

National Cancer Institute. (2015). *Adult soft tissue sarcoma (PDQ): Treatment.* Available at http://www.meds.com/pdq/sarcoma_pro.html (accessed January 29, 2016).

National Cancer Institute. (2006). *General information about adult soft tissue sarcoma (PDQ).* Available at http://www.cancer.gov/cancertopics/pdq/treatment/adult-soft-tissue-sarcoma/HealthProfessional (accessed January 29, 2016).

Sborov, D., & Chen, J. (2015). Targeted therapy in sarcomas other than GIST tumors. *Journal of Surgical Oncology, 111*(5), 632–640.

Singer, S., Maki, R. G., & O'Sullivan, B. (2011). Soft tissue sarcoma. In V. Devita, T. Lawrence, & S. Rosenberg (Eds.), *Cancer principles and practice of oncology* (9th ed.) (pp. 1533–1577). Philadelphia: Lippincott Williams & Wilkins.

Thomas, D. M., & Ballinger, M. L. (2014). Etiologic, environmental and inherited risk factors in sarcomas. *Journal of Surgical Oncology, 111*(5), 490–495.

Tobias, K., & Gillis, T. (2015). Rehabilitation of the sarcoma patient: Enhancing the recovery and functioning of patients undergoing management for extremity soft tissue sarcomas. *Journal of Surgical Oncology, 111*(5), 615–621.

Torres, K., & Pollock, R. (2010, December). *Alveolar soft part sarcoma.* Available at http://sarcomahelp.org/asps.html (accessed January 29, 2016).

Von Mehren, M., Randall, R. L., Benjamin, R. S., Boles, S., Bui, M. M., Casper, E. S., & National Comprehensive Cancer Network. (2014). Soft tissue sarcoma, version 2.2014. *Journal of the National Comprehensive Cancer Network, 12,* 473–483.

Skin Cancers

Barbara Smelko

Melanoma

Definition

The epidermis, which is the outermost layer of skin, contains cells that help the skin protect the body, including squamous cells, basal cells, and melanocytes. Skin cancers are lesions that occur in these cells, including the less aggressive basal cell carcinomas (BCC) and squamous cell carcinomas (SCCs) and the more aggressive malignant melanoma, a malignant tumor of melanocytes. Melanocytes are the cells that make the pigment melanin, which gives skin its tan or brown color and helps protect the deeper layers of skin from damage due to exposure to ultraviolet (UV) light. Although most melanomas arise in the skin, they may develop on other parts of the body such as the eyes, mouth, anal area, or genitals.

Incidence

- The American Cancer Society estimates that 73,870 cases of melanoma were diagnosed in 2015.
- During the 1970s, the incidence of melanoma increased by about 6% per year. Since 1980, the rate of increase has slowed to slightly less than 3% per year, perhaps because of increased awareness and promotion of preventive measures.

Etiology and Risk Factors

- Skin cancers are generally associated with exposure to UV light: sunlight, tanning beds, and sun lamps.
  - They can be found anywhere on the skin, in the mucosal membranes, and in the eyes.
- Risk factors include the following:
  - Prior melanoma (occurs in 5% of melanoma population)
  - Family history of melanoma (first-degree relative)
  - Nevi (moles), particularly if numerous, large, or unusual (dysplastic nevus syndrome)
  - Fair complexion, light hair, and light eyes
  - History of unprotected or excessive sun exposure
  - Severe sunburns as a child
  - Use of tanning beds and sun lamps
  - Residence in the southern latitudes of the Northern Hemisphere
  - Exposure to coal tar, pitch, creosote, arsenic compounds, or radium
  - History of radiation therapy (RT) or UV treatments
  - Immune suppression from disease or medical treatment

Signs and Symptoms

- Suspicion of a skin cancer can arise with either a new lesion or a change in the shape, size, diameter, or color of an existing skin lesion.

- Melanoma most commonly occurs on sun-exposed areas but can occur anywhere.
- Melanoma signs are generally referred to as "ABCD":
  A: Asymmetry (one half of the mole does not match the other)
  B: Border (irregular)
  C: Color (blue, black, or variation in the same mole)
  D: Diameter (>6 mm)

Diagnostic Work-up

- Identification of any suspicious lesions starts with thorough self-examination of the skin and clinical examination. It is often difficult to distinguish a benign pigmented lesion from an early melanoma.
- A definitive diagnosis is made based on biopsy, preferably local excision of the entire lesion with clear margins.
- Any lesion, especially a suspicious lesion, whether pigmented or not, should never be shaved off or cauterized.
- Positron emission tomography/computed tomography PET/CT scanning and/or magnetic resonance imaging (MRI) are done to identify any potential sites of metastasis: brain, lung, liver, regional lymph nodes, or skin.

Histology

- Malignant melanoma is divided into clinicopathologic cellular subtypes. These subtypes are considered descriptive only; here they are listed in order of their diagnostic commonality:
  - *Superficial spreading*, the most common melanoma subtype, commonly arises in preexisting nevi and usually manifests with irregular borders; with a scaly, crusty surface; and in a variety of colors.
  - *Nodular melanoma* is raised, usually blue-black in color, and has a rapid vertical growth phase.
  - *Lentigo maligna* is a large, freckle-like lesion, tan to black in color, or a raised nodule with notched borders.
  - *Acral lentiginous* (palmar/plantar and nailbed subtype) is usually flat and irregular in shape and varies in color; it may be smooth or ulcerated, raised or flat.
  - Miscellaneous unusual types:
    - Mucosal lentiginous (oral and genital)
    - Desmoplastic
    - Verrucous (warty lesions)
    - Ocular
- A number of functional somatic mutations have been identified in malignant melanoma including BRAF, NRAS, PTEN, TP53, CDKN2A and MAP2K1.
  - The *BRAF* mutation is most common and occurs in 50% of patients and affects a single amino acid, valine that is replaced with glutamic acid at position 600 (BRAF V600E).

Clinical Staging

- The current method for staging melanoma involves a combination of pathologic findings, including vertical thickness, mitotic rate, and the presence or absence of ulceration, as well as lymph node involvement and distant metastasis. The following systems are used:
  - Breslow thickness: measures the actual vertical thickness of the lesion in millimeters
  - Clark level: scores the primary tumor as level I through level V to describe the penetration into the various layers of the skin.
  - The tumor size, lymph nodes, and metastasis (TNM) system: uses the Clark level and Breslow thickness measurements plus involvement of lymph nodes, mitotic rate, presence of ulceration, and distant metastasis to assign stages (Edge, et al., 2010).

Treatment

- Surgical excision with a wide margin if possible (depending on tumor thickness) is the primary treatment for melanoma.
  - Clear margins should be 1 cm in diameter.
  - Skin grafting may be needed to close the wound.
- Sentinel lymph node biopsy is done to identify nonpalpable lymph nodes that may contain micrometastases in patients with primary melanomas greater than 1 mm in depth.
  - Lymphoscintigraphy is the technique used to identify the "blue" (sentinel) node as the first lymph node encountered in drainage from the primary tumor.
  - This surgical procedure is used to determine the presence of the disease and allows the surgeon to remove as few as possible lymph nodes, leading to maximum benefit and decreasing the side effects and complications from lymph node dissection.
- Regional lymph node dissection is done when lymph nodes are palpable to identify regional spread. This allows increased control in diminishing the spread of melanoma through the lymph system.
- Surgery may also be done for palliation of painful or draining lesions.
- RT is not usually found to be of benefit for metastatic melanoma except in cases of palliative pain control or multiple brain metastases.
- Stereotactic radiosurgery (SRS) or gamma knife surgery is often used when there is a single metastatic lesion or several small brain metastases. This allows for increased amounts of radiation to be delivered to more precise areas with fewer side effects for the patient.
- Systemic therapy has come a long way in the past several years. In addition to chemotherapy, there are now several immunotherapies as well as targeted therapies for *BRAF*-mutated malignant melanoma that have proved to be of benefit to patients in both adjuvant and metastatic settings.
- Current adjuvant therapies are interferon alpha-2B and peginterferon alpha-2B. These are immunotherapies.

- Metastatic therapies fall into three categories: chemotherapy, immunotherapy, and targeted therapy. The table below provides a list of agents approved by the U.S. Food and Drug Administration (FDA).

FDA-Approved Systemic Therapies for Malignant Melanoma

Chemotherapy	Immunotherapy	Targeted Therapy
DTIC (Dacarbazine)	Pembrolizumab	Trametinib
	Nivolumab	Dabrafenib
	Interleukin 2 (IL-2)	Trametinib and dabrafenib in combination
	Ipilimumab	Vemurafenib

Prognosis

- The American Cancer Society estimated that approximately 9940 people died from melanoma in 2015.
- The 5-year survival rate for localized melanoma is 97%; for regional metastasis, it is 59%; and for distant metastatic stages, it is 15% to 20%.
- A number of factors affect the prognosis, including the location of the lesion and, more important, the histopathologic features of the tumor: thickness or level of invasion of the melanoma, mitotic rate, presence of tumor infiltrating lymphocytes, number of regional or distant lymph nodes involved, and ulceration or bleeding at the primary site.
- Women who have melanomas on the extremities generally have a better prognosis.

Prevention and Surveillance

- Skin screening, including monthly self-examination and examination of suspicious areas by a physician, should be done to identify lesions early.
- High-risk individuals (those with multiple nevi, dysplastic nevus syndrome, or a personal or family history of melanoma) should perform monthly self-examinations and have annual full-body skin examination by a dermatologist.
- The following guidelines help to prevent overexposure to UV rays:
  - Limit exposure to the sun during midday (10 AM to 4 PM).
  - Use protection with a wide-brimmed hat shading the face, neck, and ears; long sleeves and pants; and sunglasses.
  - Use sunscreen with a sun protection factor (SPF) of 15 or higher; more important, apply it liberally and reapply at least every 2 hours
  - Avoid tanning beds and sun lamps.
  - Protect children to minimize their sun exposure by using the Slip, Slop, Slap, and Wrap method: Slip on a shirt, Slop on sunscreen, Slap on a hat, and Wrap on sunglasses to protect from the sun.
- Common follow-up recommendations by the National Comprehensive Cancer Network (NCCN) include the following:
  - Skin examination at least annually for life
  - Educate patient about regular self-examination of the skin and lymph node examination.

- Regional lymph node ultrasonography may be considered for patients with a suspicious lymph node on clinical examination, those who did not have a sentinel lymph node biopsy (SLNB), and those with a positive SLNB who did not have a complete lymph node dissection.
- The follow-up schedule is determined by risk of recurrence, prior primary melanoma or a family history of melanoma, and other factors such as atypical moles, dysplastic nevi, and patient or physician concern.

Bibliography

Aim at Melanoma Foundation. (2015). *FDA approved agents for melanoma*. Available at http://www.aimatmelanoma.org/melanoma-treatment-options/fda-approved-drugs-for-melanoma/ (accessed January 29, 2016).

National Cancer Institute. (2015). *Melanoma: For health professionals (PDQ)*. Available at http://www.cancer.gov/cancertopics/pdq/treatment/Melanoma/HealthProfessional (accessed January 29, 2016).

National Comprehensive Cancer Network. (2015). *NCCN treatment guidelines for melanoma, version 3.2015*. Available at http://www.nccn.org/professionals/physician_gls/pdf/melanoma.pdf (accessed January 29, 2016).

Nonmelanoma Skin Cancer: Basal Cell Carcinoma and Squamous Cell Carcinoma

Definition

The vast majority of the cells in the epidermis are keratinocytes, so named because they make the protein keratin. They form as basal cells in the lowest layer of the epidermis and then gradually migrate upward, becoming flat squamous cells before reaching the surface of the skin. Nonmelanoma skin cancers are mostly BCCs or SCCs.

Incidence

- An estimated 3.5 million BCCs or SCCs of the skin were diagnosed in 2015 in about 2.2 million Americans (some people have more than one lesion).
- The American Cancer Society estimated that 2000 deaths occurred in 2015 from nonmelanoma skin cancer. This rate has been dropping in recent years.
- Nonmelanoma skin cancer is the most common type of cancer, yet it accounts for fewer than 0.1% of cancer deaths.

Etiology and Risk Factors

- BCC and SCC are generally associated with exposure to UV light from the sun and/or tanning beds.
- They are commonly found on sun-exposed areas of the skin, such as the face, ears, neck, lips, and backs of the hands. However, they can be found anywhere on the body, including the genitalia.
- Other risk factors
  - Fair complexion
  - Older age (possibly due to cumulative sun exposure over time)
  - History of unprotected or excessive sun exposure
  - Severe sunburns as a child
- Use of tanning beds
- Residence in the southern latitudes of the Northern Hemisphere
- Exposure to coal tar, large amounts of arsenic, paraffin, or radium
- History of RT or UV treatments for conditions such as psoriasis
- Immune suppression due to disease or medical treatment (e.g., organ transplantation)
- Family history of skin cancer
- Gender: Males are twice as likely to develop BCCs and three times more likely to develop SCCs than women
- Smoking increases the risk of SCC, especially on the lips.
- History of human papillomavirus (HPV) infection
- Prior history of skin cancer: Approximately 35% of people with BCC develop a second BCC within 5 years
- Basal cell nevus syndrome (also known as Gorlin syndrome, Gorlin-Goltz syndrome, or nevoid basal cell carcinoma syndrome) is a rare congenital condition in which people develop multiple basal cell lesions over their lifetime.

Signs and Symptoms

- A spot on the skin that is new or changing in size, shape, or color should be considered suspicious for skin cancer.
- Key signs are a new growth, a spot or bump that is getting larger over time, or a sore that fails to heal within several months.
- SCCs can occur anywhere, but they usually occur on sun-exposed areas that show evidence of sun damage (e.g., wrinkles, pigment changes, freckles, "age spots," loss of elasticity, broken blood vessels).
- SCCs that arise in areas of non–sun-exposed skin or that originate de novo on areas of sun-exposed skin have a worse prognosis because these have a greater tendency to metastasize.
  - SCCs usually manifest as a growing lump with a rough, scaly or crusted surface or as a flat, reddish patch that grows slowly. They can manifest as a sore that does not heal, and they can develop in scars or skin sores elsewhere.
- BCCs may be nodular to flat, firm, pale areas or small raised pink or red lesions. They are most commonly found on the head and neck.
  - They may also manifest as a nodular ulcerative lesion; a translucent, shiny, pearly area that bleeds easily after a minor injury; or a sore that does not heal. The nose is the most frequent site. Large basal cell lesions may also have oozing or crusted areas.

Diagnostic Work-up

- Skin cancer screening is the best tool for prevention and early detection of any type of skin cancer.
- Definitive diagnosis requires a biopsy of the suspicious lesion:
  - Excisional biopsy, in which the entire lesion is removed

- Punch biopsy, in which a small portion of the lesion is lifted
- Shave biopsy, in which a thin slice of the lesion is removed (not recommended if the lesion is suspicious for melanoma because it interferes with proper tumor depth measurement and staging)
- A metastatic work-up usually is not done for BCC because it rarely metastasizes.
- Patients with SCC primary sites in high-risk areas such as ears, lips, hands, or genitals should have a regional lymph node biopsy or dissection.
- If the BCC or SCC primary lesion is pathologically aggressive, is large, or was neglected, CT scans should be done to identify any sites of metastasis: brain, lung, liver, or regional lymph nodes.

Histology

- Both BCCs and SCCs are of epithelial origin.
- BCCs represent about 80% of all nonmelanoma skin cancers. Although they can be very destructive through local invasion, they have a low metastatic rate.
- SCCs represent about 20% of nonmelanoma skin cancers. The deeper (larger) the lesion, the more likely it is to grow into deeper layers of the skin and metastasize to distant sites, although this is uncommon.

Clinical Staging

- SCC is graded 1 to 4 on the basis of the proportion of differentiating cells present, the degree of atypical tumor cells, and the depth of tumor penetration.
- SCC and BCC are further defined by stage:
  - Stage I is any tumor ≤2 cm in greatest dimension.
  - Stage II is any tumor >2 cm in greatest dimension.
  - Stage III is a tumor of any size that invades cartilage, muscle, bone, or regional lymph nodes.
  - Stage IV is a tumor of any size with distant metastasis.
- Refer to the American Joint Committee on Cancer (AJCC) TNM staging system and in the next column.

High-risk features (used to distinguish between some T1 and T2 tumors):
- Tumor is thicker than 2 mm.
- Tumor has invaded down into the lower dermis or subcutis.
- Tumor has grown into tiny nerves in the skin.
- Tumor started on an ear or on non–hair-bearing lip.
- Tumor cells look very abnormal (poorly differentiated or undifferentiated) when seen under a microscope.

Treatment

- BCCs and SCCs that are localized have high cure rates.
- Mohs (pronounced "moes") micrographic surgery offers the highest cure rate for difficult-to-treat BCCs and SCCs. Factors such as size of the lesion, location, primary or recurrent tumor, possibility of penetration to local structures, prior treatment, and patient age and overall health are considered when the physician chooses the most effective treatment for a patient.
  - Mohs' micrographic surgery repeatedly removes thin layers of tissue. Each layer of tissue is examined for tumor cells. This procedure maximizes the greatest tumor control while maintaining cosmetic results.
- Simple excision is done with either frozen or permanent sectioning for evaluation and determination of clear margins ranging from 3 to 10 mm, depending on the diameter of the original tumor. Clear margins allow for the greatest chance of cure.
- Electrodesiccation and curettage should be limited to very small tumors. In this method, the tumor is scraped away, and electricity is used to destroy the remaining tumor cells; the process is then repeated. This method limits the visualization of the depth of tumor invasion.
- Cryosurgery may be used for clinically well-defined or in situ tumors. This procedure uses liquid nitrogen to freeze cancer cells, causing cell death.
- External beam radiation therapy (15-30 treatments) may be used on lesions that cannot be excised or when surgery is not recommended due to comorbidities.
- Photodynamic therapy (PDT) is a two-step process in which light is used to destroy cancer cells. A chemical is applied to the area and given time to absorb, after which a special light is used to promote cancer cell death.
- Topical chemotherapy with 5-fluorouracil can be used for premalignant lesions (actinic keratoses), recurrences, or cases in which surgery and RT cannot be done.
- Systemic chemotherapy with cisplatin or doxorubicin may be used for metastatic disease.
- Smoothened receptors have been identified as genetic drivers of BCC development and a treatment target for BCC. There are two FDA-approved smoothened inhibitors, sonidegib and vismodegib. Both are oral agents approved for treatment of advanced BCC.

Prognosis

- Early diagnosis allows for the best outcomes in patients with BCC or SCC.
- The overall cure rate is directly related to the stage of disease and the treatment used for the primary lesion.
- Precise disease-free survival rates are not known because neither BCC nor SCC of the skin is a reportable disease.
  - However, it is estimated that the 5-year disease-free survival rate for BCC ranges from 85% to 95%.
  - Disease-free survival rates for SCC are dependent on the size and aggressiveness of the primary lesion.
    - For small lesions, it is about 90%.
    - For squamous cell lesions of the lip, ears, and palms of the hands or soles of the feet, there is an increased incidence of metastatic disease to regional lymph nodes and distant sites.
    - In 2012, an estimated 2% of U.S. patients with SCC died of the disease.

Prevention and Surveillance

- The most important preventative measure is self-examination of the skin. Monthly skin examination allows patients to identify new or changing skin lesions, leading to early diagnosis and treatment.

- Patients who are at a higher risk of developing these skin cancers should have annual skin examinations by a dermatologist as part of their routine care.
- Guidelines help to prevent overexposure to UV rays include the following:
  - Limit exposure to the sun during midday (10 AM to 4 PM).
  - Use protection with a wide-brimmed hat shading the face, neck, and ears; long sleeves and pants; and sunglasses.
  - Apply sunscreen containing an SPF of 15 or higher generously, and reapply it at least every 2 hours.
  - Do not use tanning beds or sun lamps.
  - Protect children to minimize their sun exposure by using the Slip, Slop, Slap, and Wrap method: Slip on a shirt, Slop on sunscreen, Slap on a hat, and Wrap on sunglasses.
- NCCN follow-up recommendations for patients with BCC include the following:
  - History and physical examination, including a complete skin examination, every 6 to 12 months for life.
  - Patient education about sun protection and self-examination of the skin.
- Follow-up for patients with localized SCC includes the following:
  - A complete history and physical examination, including skin and lymph node examination, every 3 to 12 months (depending on risk) for 2 years, then every 6 to 12 months for 3 years, and then annually for life.
  - Patient education on sun protection and self-examination of the skin.

- Follow-up for patients with regional SCC includes the following:
  - A complete history and physical examination, including skin and lymph node examination for 1 year, then every 2 to 4 months for 1 year, then every 46 months for 3 years, then every 6 to 12 months for life.
  - Patient education on sun protection and self-examination of the skin.

Bibliography

Aim at Melanoma Foundation. (2015). *Other skin cancers*. Available at http://www.aimatmelanoma.org/about-melanoma/other-skin-cancers (accessed January 29, 2016).

American Cancer Society. (2015). *Skin cancer: Basal and squamous cell*. Available at http://cancer.org/acs/groups/cid/documents/webcontent/003139-pdf.pdf

Edge, S. B., Byrd, D. R., Compton, C. C., Fritz, A. G., Greene, F. L., & Trotti, A. (Eds.). (2010). *AJCC cancer staging handbook* (7th ed.). New York: Springer.

Jemal, A., Siegel, R., Ward, E., Murray, T., Xu, J., & Thun, M. J. (2007). Cancer statistics, 2007. *CA: A Cancer Journal for Clinicians, 57*, 43–66.

Karia, P. S., Han, J., & Schmults, C. D. (2013). Cutaneous squamous cell carcinoma: Estimated incidence of disease, nodal metastasis, and deaths from disease in the United States, 2012. *Journal of the American Academy of Dermatology, 68*(6), 957–966.

National Cancer Institute. (2014). *Skin cancer treatment: For health professionals (PDQ)*. Available at http://cancer.gov/types/skin/hp/skintreatment-pdq (accessed January 29, 2016).

National Comprehensive Cancer Network. (2015). *NCCN clinical practice guidelines for basal cell carcinoma, version 1.2015*. Available at http://www.nccn.org/professionals/physician_gls/pdf/nmsc.pdf (accessed January 29, 2016).

National Comprehensive Cancer Network. (2015). *NCCN clinical practice guidelines for squamous cell skin cancer, version 1.2015*. Available at http://www.nccn.org/professionals/physician_gls/pdf/squamous.pdf (accessed January 29, 2016).

Surgical Therapy

Lisa Parks

Surgery is the oldest form of oncology treatment and the only curative therapy for solid tumors (Choh & Madura, 2009). Cancer surgery can have many goals of therapy, such as prevention, cure, reconstruction, and palliation. Care of the surgical oncology patient requires knowledge of both oncology care and surgical care.

Goals of Surgical Procedures

Prevention

Gene mutations within families have been identified that predispose patients to a higher risk of developing cancer. Establishing a personal and/or family history of cancer is essential for identification of these gene mutations. Once the mutations are detected through genetic testing, patients and their family members should be monitored closely and may undergo surgery for precancerous lesions. Some patients undergo prophylactic surgery, such as mastectomy or oophorectomy, because of positive genetic testing or a positive family history. Routine screening with colonoscopy or mammography may lead to discovery of precancerous lesions that should be removed to prevent the development of cancer. Patients with a prior history of cancer also may undergo prophylactic surgery, such as prophylactic mastectomy to eliminate the chance of developing contralateral breast cancer.

Diagnosis

The diagnostic role of surgery is the removal of tissue for histologic examination. Incisional biopsy of tissue or lymph nodes is performed, and the specimen is examined for pathology with additional stains and markers specific for the type of cancer identified. It is important to obtain and prepare tissue to allow for molecular testing for known oncogene targets. Additional staining allows for determination of specific adjuvant chemotherapy agents. Diagnostic laparoscopy is another surgical therapy that is often used to collect tissue for diagnosis. This procedure is less invasive than an open incision because port sites are used to insert a camera and instruments.

Staging

Staging is essential in determining appropriate treatment options: systemic therapies, radiation therapy, and/or surgery. All cancers are staged at diagnosis (National Cancer Institute, 2015). This is typically called *clinical staging*; further staging may be done after surgery, or additional biopsies provide further information about the extent of the disease. For example, sentinel lymph node biopsy is a surgical technique that is used in several cancers to evaluate disease spread via the lymphatics. This staging designation is referred to as *pathologic staging*; it combines clinical staging and surgical results and helps to further refine therapy.

Common elements in staging include tumor size and extension, regional lymph node involvement, presence of distant metastasis, and tumor grade or differentiation. Carcinoma in situ can be referred to as stage 0. Stages I, II, and III represent successive increases in the extent of the disease, indicating larger tumor size or spread beyond the primary site to nearby tissues or lymph nodes. Stage IV represents the presence of distant metastasis.

Treatment

Surgery involves removal of the entire primary cancer, including a margin of normal tissue surrounding the cancer, and offers the patient a chance for cure. A margin of at least 1 cm of normal tissue is considered adequate. Adequate clear margins are critical in oncologic surgery. If there is a positive margin—that is, if cancer cells remain within the margin—the resection is considered incomplete or noncurative. Re-resection or adjuvant chemoradiation may be required. In addition to tumor removal, the surgical resection may include removal of lymph nodes, blood vessels, or organs that abut the cancer.

Since the 1980s, there has been a substantial increase in minimally invasive surgery. The development of laparoscopic procedures has led to other techniques such as transanal endoscopic microsurgery (TEM), robotic surgery, and natural orifice transluminal endoscopic surgery (NOTES). Use of these surgical techniques has progressed more slowly in oncology than in other fields because of the concern of ensuring an adequate resection and lymphadenectomy (Choh & Madura, 2009). However, these therapies may be used by skilled and experienced surgeons, for example, to access areas that are deep in the pelvis where there is little room to maneuver.

Surgical Preoperative Evaluation

Cardiac System

Patients who have previously undergone chemotherapy may require additional cardiac evaluation because of the potential side effects of chemotherapy. Chemotherapy-induced myocardial ischemia is more likely to develop in patients with existing coronary artery disease (CAD) because of decreased coronary flow reserve (Khawaja, Cafferkey, Rajani, Redwood, & Cunningham, 2014). The American College of Cardiology Foundation/American Heart Association (ACCF/AHA) suggests that all patients receiving chemotherapy should be considered to be at risk for heart failure (Jacobs et al., 2013). These patients may require evaluation with echocardiography and nuclear medicine evaluation.

Pulmonary System

Patients with both hematologic and oncologic malignancies are at increased risk for pneumonia because of impaired immunity (Neumann, Krause, Maschmeyer, Schiel, & von Lilienfeld-Toal, 2013). There is an increasing incidence of unsuspected pulmonary embolism in cancer patients. Detection of pulmonary embolism is common in patients undergoing computed tomography (CT) for routine cancer staging (Donadini, Dentali, Squizzato, Guasti, & Ageno, 2014). Patients with mesothelioma or other cancers who develop malignant pleural effusions may undergo preoperative thoracentesis to optimize pulmonary function before surgery (Myatt, 2014). Chest radiography and pulmonary function testing may be used to evaluate patients preoperatively.

Hematologic System

Patients with cancer are at increased risk for perioperative bleeding due to chemotherapy, malnutrition, anticoagulation therapy, or malignant spread to the liver or bone marrow compromising coagulation. Patients with cancer need to be screened for coagulation factor deficiencies with measurements of the prothrombin time and partial prothromboplastin time (Clevenger & Mallett, 2014). Patients with malnutrition or cirrhosis may need to be treated with vitamin K and fresh frozen plasma before surgery because of coagulopathies.

Blood transfusions are given for patients with severe anemia (hemoglobin level <7 g/dL) or symptomatic anemia. Elective surgery should be postponed until chemotherapy is completed and the patient's absolute neutrophil count is greater than 1000 cells/mm². A platelet count of at least 50,000/mm² is required for most surgical procedures; otherwise, platelet transfusions may need to be administered.

Gastrointestinal System

Gastrointestinal complications may develop in cancer patients. Hydration and nutrition can be impaired by pain, nausea, stomatitis, or tumors involving the oropharynx or the gastrointestinal system. Intravenous fluids with corrective electrolytes or total parenteral nutrition (TPN) may be used to promote wound healing after surgery (Evans, Martindale, Kiraly, & Jones, 2013). Severely malnourished patients are those with loss of greater than 15% of body weight, a low body mass index, and a serum albumin level of less than 2.5 mg/dL. These patients may benefit from preoperative TPN or enteral feedings through a nasoduodenal tube.

Renal System

Patients requiring hemodialysis should be dialyzed on the day before surgery to correct hyperkalemia and fluid overload. Heparin used during dialysis has a residual anticoagulant effect that can last for 2 to 3 hours after dialysis (Renew & Sher-Lu, 2014). Uremia can cause platelet dysfunction resulting in increased bleeding potential.

Endocrine System: Glycemic Control

The stress of surgery can cause a rise in the glucose level, which should be closely monitored; this is particularly important in patients with diabetes. Glycemic control is important to decrease the risk of infection and promote wound healing. Uncontrolled diabetes can lead to increased surgical site infections, volume depletion, and electrolyte imbalance due to osmotic diuresis, ketoacidosis, and nonketotic hyperosmolality. Glucose levels of less than 71 mg/dL may induce cognitive changes or arrhythmias (Chow et al., 2014). A glucose management protocol should be used to keep the serum glucose level lower than 140 mg/dL throughout the perioperative and postoperative course (Engoren, Schwann, & Habib, 2014). This may require an insulin drip and consultation with an endocrinologist to control the hyperglycemia.

Pregnancy

Surgery can be performed in each trimester of pregnancy without increasing the risk to the mother or fetus (Juhasz-Boss, Solomayer, Strik, & Raspe, 2014). There is no increase in fetal malformations with the use of general anesthesia; however, there is a slight increase in the rate of spontaneous abortion (Juhasz-Boss et al., 2014). Fetal monitoring should be performed beginning at week 16 of gestation. When the mother is anesthetized, the fetus is also anesthetized, and the half-life of anesthesia may be prolonged (Juhasz-Boss et al., 2014). Ideally, surgery during pregnancy should be performed in centers with expertise in surgical management of the pregnant woman and where an obstetrician and a neonatologist are readily available.

Preoperative Medication Guidelines

Patients are advised to continue their medications unless instructed to stop because of potential interaction with anesthesia. Cardiovascular medications including antiarrhythmics, β-blockers, statins, calcium channel blockers, digoxin, and clonidine should be continued (Vetter, Downing, Vanlandingham, Noles, & Boudreaux, 2014).

Use of warfarin is based on the patient's condition and the risk of hemorrhage versus the risk of thromboembolism. For low-risk patients, warfarin is withheld for 4 to 5 days before surgery. In high-risk patients, warfarin may be stopped 3 to 5 days before surgery and the patient placed on intravenous unfractionated heparin (IV UFH) or low-molecular-weight heparin (LMWH). Postoperatively, the patient is restarted on IV UFH or LMWH while oral anticoagulation reaches therapeutic levels (Perrin et al., 2010).

A number of other agents can increase the risk of bleeding, including prescription drugs, over-the-counter drugs (e.g., aspirin, nonsteroidal antiinflammatory drugs [NSAIDs]), vitamins (e.g., high doses of vitamin E, omega fatty acids), and natural supplements (e.g., ginger, *Ginkgo biloba*). The table on page 165 provides an overview of a variety of medications, vitamins, and herbs that affect bleeding and recommended stopping times developed by the Nursing Department at the University of Wisconsin Hospitals and Clinics (2015).

Stopping Schedule Before Surgery or Invasive Procedure of Medications, Vitamins, and Herbs That Affect Bleeding (Not All Inclusive)

ANTICOAGULENTS	
Heparin	Discontinue IV 6 hours pre-op and check PTT
Low Molecular Weight Heparin	Discontinue 12 hours before surgery
Warfarin (Coumadin)	Discontinue 3-5 days preoperatively (5 days if INR <1.5); Check INR or PR before surgery
FIBRINOLYTIC DRUGS	
Streptokinase, urokinase, tissue plasminogen activator	Discontinuation may not be an option when prescribed for life-threatening conditions
ANTI-PLATELET AGENTS	
Aspirin or aspirin containing agents	Usually discontinued 7 days before surgery; cardiology consult may be needed if patient is high risk or recently underwent cardiac surgery (<1 year).
Nonsteroidal anti-inflammatory (NSAIDs)	Usually discontinued 4 days before surgery
Clopidogrel (Plavix)	Usually discontinued 5-7 days preoperatively; aspirin if used concurrently may be continued peri-operatively. Cardiology consult indicated if patient is high risk or had recent cardiac surgery or event (<1 year)
Ticlopidine (Ticlid)*	Usually discontinued 7-10 days preoperatively; aspirin if used concurrently may be continued peri-operatively. Cardiology consult indicated for high risk patients particularly if patient had recent cardiac surgery or event (<1 year)
Cilostazol (Pletal)	Discontinue 1 -2 days before procedure
Dipyridamole (Persantine)	Discontinue 1-2 days before procedure
Prasugrel (Effient)	Discontinue 5-7 days before surgery
Ticagrelor (Brilinta)	Discontinue 5 days before surgery

*This agent has been discontinued in the United States.
From Rothrock, J. (2015). Alexander's care of the patient in surgery (15th ed.). St. Louis: Elsevier; Nagelhout, J.J. & Plaus, K. L. (2014). Nurse anesthesia (5th ed.). St. Louis: Elsevier; University of Wisconsin Hospitals and Clinics, Department of Nursing. (2015). Health facts for you: Medicines, herbs, and vitamins which affect bleeding. Available at https://www.uwhealth.org/healthfacts/cardiology/6404.pdf#toolbar=1&statusbar=1&messages=1&navpanes=1 (accessed February 1, 2016).

Pulmonary drugs such as inhaled β-agonists, anticholinergics, leukotriene inhibitors, and glucocorticoids are generally given on the day of surgery. Theophylline should be discontinued the evening before surgery (Barnes, 2013). Histamine 2 blockers and proton pump inhibitors should be taken preoperatively to reduce stress-related mucosal damage (Alaniz & Hyzy, 2014).

Patients with type 2 diabetes mellitus should discontinue oral hyperglycemic drugs or noninsulin injectables on the morning of surgery. Metformin should be withheld for 24 to 48 hours before surgery (Levesque, 2013). Patients with type diabetes (and some patients with type 2) will need some basal insulin despite their presurgery fast to prevent ketoacidosis (Levesque, 2013).

Perioperative Nursing Care

Many areas of the skin are colonized by *Staphylococcus aureus,* which is one of the pathogens most commonly associated with surgical site infections. Patients are instructed to bathe using antibacterial soap and chlorhexidine gluconate (CHG)-impregnated cloths. CHG has the property that, once applied, it weakens and kills bacteria and fungi. Best practice is to use CHG the evening before and again on the morning of surgery (McCarron, 2014).

Proper hair removal at the surgical site is imperative. Hair should be removed with the use of electric clippers. Shaving results in microabrasions and hair follicle disruption, altering the skin barrier against organisms and creating a portal of entry for bacteria and fungi (McCarron, 2014).

Preoperative administration of appropriate antibiotics is essential to prevent surgical site infections. A prophylactic antibiotic should be administered 1 hour before surgical incision. The 1-hour window ensures maximum tissue distribution. Vancomycin and fluoroquinolones may be administered 2 hours before incision (McCarron, 2014). The standard antibiotic stop time is 24 hours after surgery; there is no benefit for infection prophylaxis after the incision has been closed (McCarron, 2014).

Postoperative Nursing Care

Pain Management

The severity of pain experienced by a patient depends on preexisting conditions, current use of narcotics to treat cancer pain, and the type of surgery performed. Opioids are used in postsurgical management. Patient-controlled analgesia (PCA) is commonly used in the immediate postoperative period. Physiologic, sensory, cognitive, and sociocultural components that are unique for each individual should also be considered in pain management (Glowacki, 2015).

Dysfunction of the liver and kidneys affects the distribution, clearance, and excretion of opioids (Ward, 2015). Liver failure causes decreased metabolism, decreased elimination, and increased bioavailability of opioids. This may lead to respiratory depression and sedation (Ward, 2015). Renal insufficiency decreases drug elimination, leading to increased accumulation of active drug metabolites.

In cancer patients already using opioids for cancer pain, the postoperative dose may be two to four times higher than that in patients who are opioid naïve. In older adults, the lowest effective opioid dose should be used at first and increased slowly for pain control. Elderly opioid-naïve patients should be started at half the recommended low dose. The presence of pain can cause delirium, and opioids should still be administered to delirious patients for pain control (Ward, 2015). The potential of depression and anxiety occurs with uncontrolled pain, or pain may exacerbate current depression and anxiety.

Adequate pain control leads to improved postoperative mobility, decreasing the chance of muscle atrophy and respiratory complications. When pain is controlled, patients and their families are able to respond to the stress of surgery and cope with the patient's situation (Hayes & Gordon, 2015). Assessment of the patient's pain should include the patient's perception of pain, previous experiences with pain, current knowledge of pain, spiritual and religious beliefs, and sociocultural components. The American Board of Family Medicine and the Institute of Medicine use a numeric rating scale for pain screening (Glowacki, 2015).

Nurses need to educate their patients to use pain medication before activities and before the pain becomes too intense. Often once the pain is out of control, it is difficult to gain pain control with the medications. It is important for nurses to assess the level of a patient's pain before administering medications. The same numeric scale can be used to assess pain relief after administration of medications and to evaluate the adequacy of pain control. Health care providers should be notified of medication regimens that do not adequately control the patient's pain.

Nonopioid drugs include NSAIDs, opioid-sparing therapies, and local anesthetics. Nonopioid therapies may be used in conjunction with opioid therapy for postoperative pain management. For instance, a patient may have a PCA with scheduled intravenous toradol or may alternate Percocet and an NSAID.

Laparoscopic procedures are associated with quicker recovery and less pain. Open procedures result in a larger incision and are associated with longer recovery time and more pain (Quidley, Bland, Bookstaver, & Kuper, 2014).

Respiratory Care

Incentive spirometry should be performed every hour while the patient is awake to provoke coughing and deep breathing. Several bedside devices may be used to increase inspiratory effort. These can be personalized according to the specific needs of the patient. Patients may also require nebulizer treatments to prevent atelectasis and pneumonia. Postoperative ambulation assists with ventilation and should be encouraged in the immediate postoperative period (Guyette et al., 2012).

Nausea and Vomiting

Nausea and vomiting are expected complications of surgery because of the side effects of anesthesia, opioids, and withdrawal of medications. Antiemetics are used to control nausea. Nasogastric tubes may be used for decompression until the return of bowel function. Some surgeries, such as the Whipple procedure, may prolong delayed gastric emptying for months postoperatively. Avoiding narcotics on an empty stomach and eating small, frequent meals may help prevent nausea and vomiting.

Venous Thromboembolism

The rate of venous thromboembolism (VTE) ranges from 0.3 to 3%, with mortality from pulmonary embolism as high as 30%. Cancer activates the coagulation cascade, increasing coagulability and putting oncology patients at higher risk of developing VTE. Immobility, a history of VTE, obesity, and a smoking history are also risk factors for VTE. Subcutaneous UFH or LMWH may be used for VTE prevention. Nonpharmacologic options include sequential stockings, inferior vena cava filters, and early ambulation (Kushnir & Diaz-Montes, 2013).

Reconstruction

Disfigurement can be a side effect of oncologic surgery. Reconstructive surgeons are important members of the multidisciplinary surgical team because of their expertise in microsurgery, reconstruction, restoration of function, and repair of defects resulting from cancer surgery. A major source of anxiety in patients who are coping with a cancer diagnosis is the potential for altered body image with surgical intervention (Snobohm, Friedrichien, & Heine, 2009). Some distress can be alleviated by performing the reconstruction at the time of the initial surgery with implants, muscle flaps, skin grafts, tissue transfers, or free flaps with bone grafts. Other reconstruction may require a series of surgeries over time. The overall goal of reconstructive surgery is rehabilitation of the patient through return of form and function with the goal of improving quality of life.

Palliation

Tumor progression may cause compression of structures, leading to pain, nausea, vomiting, constipation, or other symptoms. The goal of palliative surgery is to alleviate symptoms and facilitate comfort. This may involve debulking, decompression, and diversion. Debulking refers to removal of large tumor even if some tumor is left behind due to inaccessibility because of vascular structures. Decompression relieves pressure on structures; an example is placement of a gastrostomy tube for gastric outlet obstruction. Diversion is done for obstructed structures—for example, placement of a diverting ostomy to relieve a bowel obstruction. Nurses, patients, and families need to understand the intent and long-term outcomes of palliative surgery and that the goal of surgery is not cure (Mois, Reiter-Theil, Oertil, & Viehl, 2013).

Conclusion

Surgical oncology nursing combines oncology and surgical nursing skills. From prevention and early detection to surgery, rehabilitation, palliation, and survivorship, nurses are essential for support, education, and physical care of surgical oncology patients and their support systems. Collaboration with all aspects of a patient's cancer journey is essential for optimal patient outcomes.

References

Alaniz, C., & Hyzy, R. (2014). Time to declare moratorium on stress ulcer prophylaxis in critically ill. *Critical Care Medicine, 42*(9), e636–e637.

Barnes, P. (2013). Theophylline. *American Journal of Respiratory Critical Care Medicine, 1188*(8), 901–906.

Choh, M., & Madura, J. (2009). The role of minimally invasive treatments in surgical oncology. *Surgical Clinics of North America, 89*(1), 53–77.

Chow, E., Bernjak, A., Williams, S., Fawdry, R., Hibbert, S., Freeman, J., & Heller, S. (2014). Risk of cardiac arrhythmias during hypoglycemia in patients with type 2 diabetes and cardiovascular risk. *Diabetes, 63*, 1738–1747.

Clevenger, B., & Mallett, S. (2014). Preoperative assessment of coagulation and bleeding risk. *British Journal of Hospital Medicine, 75*(5), C71–C74.

Donadini, M. P., Dentali, F., Squizzato, A., Guasti, L., & Ageno, W. (2014). Unsuspected pulmonary embolism in cancer patients: A narrative review with pooled data. *Internal and Emergency Medicine, 9*(4), 375–384.

Engoren, M., Schwann, T., & Habib, R. (2014). Hyperglycemia, hypoglycemia and glycemic complexity are associated with worse outcomes after surgery. *Journal of Critical Care, 29*, 611–617.

Evans, D., Martindale, R., Kiraly, L., & Jones, C. (2013). Nutrition optimization prior to surgery. *Nutrition in Clinical Practice, 29*(1), 1–18.

Glowacki, D. (2015). Effective pain management and improvements in patients' outcomes and satisfaction. *Critical Care Nurse, 35*(3), 33–42.

Guyette, F., Gomez, H., Suffoletto, B., Quintero, J., Mesquida, J., Kim, H., & Pinsky, M. (2012). Prehospital dynamic tissue oxygen saturation response predicts lifesaving interventions in trauma patients. *Journal of Trauma and Acute Care Surgery, 72*(4), 930–935.

Hayes, K., & Gordon, D. (2015). Delivering quality pain management: The challenge for nurses. *AORN Journal, 101*(3), 327–337.

Jacobs, A., Kushner, F., Ettinger, S., Guyton, R., Anderson, J., Ohman, E., & Somerfield, M. (2013). ACCF/AHA clinical practice guideline methodology summit report: A report of the American College of Cardiology Foundation/American Heart Association Task Force on Practice Guidelines. *Journal of the American College of Cardiology, 61*(2), 213–265.

Juhasz-Boss, I., Solomayer, E., Strik, M., & Raspe, C. (2014). Abdominal surgery in pregnancy: An interdisciplinary challenge. *Deutsches Arzteblatt International, 111*, 465–472.

Khawaja, M., Cafferkey, C., Rajani, R., Redwood, S., & Cunningham, D. (2014). Cardiac complications and manifestations of chemotherapy for cancer. *Heart, 100*, 1133–1140.

Kushnir, C., & Diaz-Montes, T. (2013). Perioperative care in gynecologic oncology. *Current Opinion in Obstetrics and Gynecology, 23*, 23–28.

Levesque, C. (2013). Perioperative care of patients with diabetes. *Critical Care Nursing Clinics of North America, 25*, 21–29.

McCarron, K. (2014). Don't skip the SCIP. *Nursing Made Incredibly Easy, 12*(5), 15–18.

Mois, A., Reiter-Theil, S., Oertil, O., & Viehl, T. (2013). Palliative surgery in cancer patients: What do we know about it? *European Journal of Palliative Care, 20*(1), 1352–2779.

Myatt, R. (2014). Diagnosis and management of patients with pleural effusions. *Nursing Standard, 28*(41), 51–58.

National Cancer Institute. (2015). *What is staging?* Available at http://www.cancer.gov/about-cancer/diagnosis-staging/staging/staging-fact-sheet#q1 (accessed February 1, 2016).

Neumann, S., Krause, W., Maschmeyer, G., Schiel, X., & von Lilienfeld-Toal, M. (2013). Primary prophylaxis of bacterial infections and *Pneumocystis jirovecii* pneumonia in patients with hematological malignancies and solid tumors: Guidelines of the Infectious Diseases Working Party AGIHO) of the German Society of Hematology and Oncology (DGHO). *Annals of Hematology, 92*, 433–442.

Perrin, M., Vezi, B., Ha, A., Keren, A., Nery, P., & Birnie, D. (2012). Anticoagulation bridging around device surgery: Compliance with guidelines. *Pacing & Clinical Electrophysiology, 35*, 1480–1486.

Quidley, A., Bland, C., Bookstaver, P., & Kuper, K. (2014). Perioperative management of bariatric surgery patients. *American Journal of Health-System Pharmacy, 71*, 1253–1264.

Renew, R., & Sher-Lu, P. (2014). A simple protocol to improve safety and reduce cost of hemodialysis patients undergoing elective surgery. *Middle East Journal of Anesthesiology, 22*(5), 487–492.

Snobohm, C., Friedrichien, M., & Heine, S. (2009). Experiencing one's body after a diagnosis of cancer: A phenomenological study of young adults. *Psych-Oncology, 19*, 863–869.

University of Wisconsin Hospitals and Clinics, Department of Nursing. (2015). *Health facts for you: Medicines, herbs and vitamins which affect bleeding*. Available at https://www.uwhealth.org/healthfacts/cardiology/6404.pdf#toolbar=1&statusbar=1&messages=1&navpanes=1 (accessed February 1, 2016).

Vetter, T., Downing, M., Vanlandingham, S., Noles, K., & Boudreaux, A. (2014). Predictors of patient medication compliance on the day of surgery and the effects of providing patients with standardized yet simplified medication instructions. *Anesthesiology, 121*, 29–35.

Ward, C. (2015). A decision tree model for postoperative pain management. *Medical Surgical Nursing, 24*(2), 77–88.

Radiation Therapy

Lorraine Drapek

Definition

Radiation therapy involves the use of high-energy x-rays to treat local or regional areas of disease. Ionizing radiation, which is radiation with high enough energy to disrupt atoms by ejecting orbital electrons, is the form of therapeutic radiation used in treatment. In standard radiation therapy, photons or x-rays are administered from a machine called a *linear accelerator*. Particles such as electrons, protons, and neutrons, which are emitted from a linear accelerator or from a proton cyclotron, and gamma rays, which are emitted from a radioactive source, are often used in brachytherapy. In radiopharmaceutical therapy, a liquid radioactive source is ingested, instilled, or injected. Radiopharmaceuticals are engineered to concentrate in specific areas of the body.

Radiobiology

The term *radiobiology* refers to the process of events experienced by a living organism once ionizing radiation is administered. Radiation damage is caused by breakage of chemical bonds, which creates biologic changes.

There is evidence indicating that many solid cancers contain a small population of cancer stem cells, and a cancer cure may be unlikely unless this population of radiation-resistant cells is eliminated. The success or failure of radiation therapy depends on the four R's of radiobiology: (1) reoxygenation of hypoxic areas of tumor, (2) repair of DNA damage, (3) redistribution of cells in the cell cycle, and (4) repopulation of cells (Pajonk, Vlashi, & McBride, 2010). Factors affecting radiobiology include the type of radiation, the radiation dose administered, the dose absorbed, and the rate of administration. DNA is the primary and critical target of radiation therapy. DNA damage can lead to cell alteration or cell death. Both normal and cancerous cells are susceptible to radiation and may be injured or destroyed. Apoptosis, or programmed cell death, is often enhanced by radiation therapy (Iwamoto, Haas, & Gosselin, 2012).

There are three stages of radiobiology leading to cell destruction: (1) the *physical stage*, which includes the ionization of atoms; (2) the *radiochemical stage*, which includes formation of free radicals; and (3) the *biologic stage*, when DNA damage occurs. Such damage occurs during cell division. Cells are most sensitive to radiation damage during the late G_2 and M phases of the cell cycle and most resistant during the late S phase. Cells that have a more rapid rate of mitosis are more radiation sensitive. Double chromosomal strand breaks are likely the most important type of damage produced in chromosomes as a result of radiation therapy. Such breaks may result in cell death, cell mutation, or carcinogenesis. They can possibly activate an oncogene or inactivate a tumor suppressor gene (Iwamoto et al., 2012).

Although normal cells are better able to repair radiation damage than cancer cells, there is a maximum tolerated dose that can be administered without causing permanent, irreparable damage. The radiation dose given must be the maximum amount needed to treat the particular tumor cell line while also being safely tolerated by the surrounding normal tissues. Dose per fraction and dose per time period are factors in delivering effective doses of radiation with adequate tissue tolerance so as to limit toxicities experienced by the patient.

Radiation Delivery

Radiation Planning

Radiation planning and technology have evolved. Individualized treatment planning is aimed at delivering the maximum tolerated radiation dose with minimal toxicity or side effects. Planning enables the goals of the prescribed radiation therapy to be reached. Radiation simulation uses computed tomography or magnetic resonance imaging to formulate a multidimensional treatment plan, taking into consideration external landmarks and any shielding of critical organs. It also allows for optimal patient positioning for treatment with consideration of the patient's comfort and safety. This planning process usually requires 60 to 90 minutes.

External Beam Radiation Therapy

External beam radiation therapy (EBRT) is the most common form of delivery of radiation treatment. It is important for patients to understand that they will not become radioactive as a result of EBRT. A linear accelerator is a treatment machine that generates ionizing radiation by accelerating electrons along a tube. In this form of radiation therapy, the patient is positioned on a treatment couch. The total dose of radiation required is achieved through administering equal daily fractions of radiation, typically once a day on 5 days each week, until the total dose is reached. There are many types of EBRT:

- Three-dimensional conformal radiation therapy (3D CRT) is a planning system wherein the beams of radiation used in treatment are shaped to match the tumor, based on three-dimensional patient data.
- Intensity-modulated radiation therapy (IMRT) involves the use of multiple small beam arrangements to customize delivery of the optimal dose distribution.
- Image-guided radiation therapy (IGRT) uses imaging obtained during treatment to ensure tumor location and accurate beam delivery.
- Volumetric modulated arc therapy (VMAT) is a type of IMRT in which intensity modulation is created by overlapping arcs produced by the rotating linear accelerator. It is a

newer technology focused on treatment precision with less time per treatment fraction (Cao, 2012).

- Intraoperative radiation therapy (IORT) involves the use of x-rays or photons in an operating room setting. A linear accelerator is present in the operating room, and radiation can be delivered to an area of tumor while the area is opened for surgery. It is used primarily for abdominal, pelvic, and soft tissue cancers.

Brachytherapy

Brachytherapy is the temporary or permanent placement of a radioactive source within a body cavity, interstitially, or on the surface of the body. For example, small catheters can be inserted directly into tumors such as oral or breast tumors. Brachytherapy can be used alone or in conjunction with EBRT, as in treatment of cervical or endometrial cancers. The primary advantage of brachytherapy is its ability to deliver high doses of radiation directly to the tumor while sparing normal surrounding tissues, thus decreasing toxicity to the patient.

There are two types of brachytherapy: low dose rate (LDR) brachytherapy and high dose rate (HDR) brachytherapy. LDR brachytherapy provides enhanced radiation effect through the repair, redistribution, and repopulation principles. It is effective even in poorly oxygenated tissue. Treatment times can range from 24 to 144 hours (Gosselin, 2011). HDR brachytherapy is delivered quickly, which enables patient comfort and decreases radiation exposure to ancillary personnel. It is usually completed in the outpatient setting. Common diseases treated with either LDR or HDR brachytherapy include cancers of the prostate, cervix, vulva, endometrium, and vagina, cancers of the head and neck, and choroidal melanoma.

Because the radioactive sources are housed in shielded units, there is no exposure risk to staff when the sources are inserted remotely into patients. The implants may be left in the patient's body for a prescribed period of time. During this time, the patient is radioactive, and precautions are necessary until the implants are removed. Because the radiation source is sealed, there is no contamination of body fluids.

Patients receiving LDR brachytherapy are admitted as inpatients. Nurses caring for these individuals are instructed to observe the important precautions of time, distance, and shielding to protect themselves from radiation exposure. This means spending a defined amount of time at a defined distance from the source and using shielding as available. Radiation dosimetry monitors are worn by any staff members who enter the patient's room during this time. After the radiation source has been removed and returned to storage and the area shows no radiation contamination when surveyed, no further radiation protection is needed.

Permanent implants may be used; the radioactive materials are inserted and not removed. The sources used are weak emitters of gamma radiation and yield low surface doses. The most common application is implanted "seeds" of iodine 125 or palladium 103 in patients with prostate cancer. Patients are given discharge instructions on how to minimize exposure to others (e.g., not having small children sit on their lap, not coming into close contact with pregnant women, reducing use of public transportation) for a finite period as directed by radiation safety personnel.

Radioisotope Therapy

Radioisotope therapy uses unsealed sources of radiation in liquid or capsule form that are ingested by mouth. The patient's body fluids are radioactive, and hospitalization is required for a length of time that is calculated based on the activity of the isotope. Radioactive iodine 131 for thyroid cancer is the most common application of isotope therapy. Precautions are necessary when handling body fluids and items that have come into contact with the patient. With isotope therapy as well as inpatient brachytherapy, staff members are provided with education, written instructions, protocol references, and resources. Radiation safety personnel are always available to answer questions.

Stereotactic Radiosurgery

Despite the name, stereotactic radiosurgery (SRS) is a nonsurgical procedure. It is a technique that delivers a high dose of radiation by means of precise beams to a small volume of tissue in order to completely destroy the tumor with minimal radiation exposure to surrounding normal tissue. It requires three-dimensional guidance to maximize precision. Treatment is completed in one session or in up to five sessions. The high dose per fraction facilitates direct cytotoxic damage, similar to the DNA damage seen in a course of low-dose fractionated radiation therapy. It is also effective in damaging the microvasculature of tumors. It may be more effective than other forms of radiation therapy against radioresistant tumor stem cells. An advantage of using SRS to eradicate a small volume of metastatic brain cancer, when compared with whole-brain radiation therapy, is that SRS causes less cognitive damage.

Gamma knife radiation therapy, used in the management of brain tumors, is an example of this treatment. SRS can also be administered using protons, particularly for brain or eye tumors. SRS is also used to treat arterial venous malformations, meningiomas, spinal metastases, and pituitary adenomas.

Stereotactic Body Radiation Therapy

In stereotactic body radiation therapy (SBRT), high radiation doses are delivered to tumors using a hypofractionated schedule. Doses often range from 10 to 20 Gy per fraction. SBRT uses image guidance to facilitate treatment precision. It is a definitive treatment option for patients with early-stage non–small cell lung cancer, with an estimated 88% control rate for early-stage inoperable tumors (Timmerman, 2010). Treatment courses are usually very short; five or fewer fractions may be used. SBRT can also be used to treat lung metastases, primary hepatocellular cancers, liver metastases, and pancreatic cancers. Response rates and local control have been shown to be improved with SBRT.

Measuring Radiation Dose

The radiation absorbed dose (rad) has been used to measure the dose of radiation delivered. The preferred measure is the gray (Gy). One rad is equal to 1 Gy or 100 centigrays (cGy).

The Role of Radiation in Cancer Care

Approximately 60% of patients with cancer receive radiation therapy at some point during the treatment of their disease. Radiation therapy may be used as a single treatment modality, but it is often combined with surgery or chemotherapy. The following terms describe the use of radiation therapy as a treatment modality:

- *Definitive therapy* can be used with curative intent, as in early head and neck, cervical, anal, and prostate cancers. In some of these cancers, chemotherapy is given concurrently with radiation therapy. In other cases, radiation therapy is used as definitive therapy for local disease control when a patient has comorbid conditions that prevent surgical resection.
- *Neoadjuvant radiation* is given before primary therapy (e.g., surgery). For example, in esophageal or rectal cancer, it is given preoperatively with the goal of debulking the tumor to render it more operable. In these situations, radiation therapy is given concurrently with chemotherapy, which acts as a radiation sensitizer.
- *Adjuvant therapy* is given after primary surgical therapy, as in breast or lung cancer. It may be given after surgery and/or chemotherapy to keep the cancer from returning.
- *Prophylactic therapy* is given when there is no evidence of disease but the risk is high. An example is cranial radiation therapy in a patient with small cell lung cancer. It may also be given when a positive surgical margin is present after surgical resection.
- *Palliative therapy* is used to alleviate symptoms.

Side Effects

The side effects of radiation therapy are related to the specific area being treated. One common treatment-related side effect is fatigue. Another is skin reactions in the irradiated area, which manifest as erythema and can progress to desquamation, depending on the dose and the amount of radiation received by the skin as well as the specific area of treatment.

Acute or early side effects occur during or immediately after a course of radiation therapy. Late side effects occur from 2 months to years after radiation therapy and are usually a result of damage to the microcirculation. In traditional EBRT, late effects are typically more severe with a higher dose per fraction of treatment. Late treatment effects (e.g., vaginal stenosis) can occur several years after treatment completion. Both the severity and the percentage of patients experiencing late effects can increase over time.

Hypofractionization schedules, in which patients are given higher doses of radiation in fewer fractions, are becoming more common. As a result of this abbreviated schedule, side effects may be experienced after completion and not during the course of radiation therapy. Patients need to know when and how to call to report symptoms. Patient education (e.g., about self-care measures) can be a challenge because the daily visits to the treatment center may end before the onset of side effects. The implementation of a telephone call-back system to patients who have completed treatment could help patients manage radiation side effects. A follow-up nursing appointment within 1 week after completion of radiation therapy may be necessary to assist patients in their recovery.

Oncology nurses have an instrumental role in educating patients to anticipate side effects and understand measures to minimize them and in alerting patients to "red flags" and symptoms that need to be reported to the physician. Teaching should include information about what side effects to expect, when to expect the onset of symptoms, and their anticipated duration. Preventive and self-care measures at the start of treatment are also important aspects of patient education:

- Light exercise, such as walking, can help patients manage fatigue, enhance sleep, and maintain their appetite for food.
- A diet that is high in protein with adequate oral hydration can help patients tolerate the challenges of completing their course of treatment.
- Complementary therapies such as acupuncture, massage, or Reiki can assist patients in managing symptoms such as pain, anxiety, fatigue, hot flashes, and nausea.

Printed information regarding these interventions should be provided and discussed.

It is imperative to provide physician and nurse contact information with telephone numbers to call during business hours, evenings, or weekends and to review this information at each visit. Nursing assessment of the need for additional resources such as a support group, social worker, dietitian, community agency, or spiritual or pastoral care is also important. Nursing staff can routinely assist with referrals for any of these services.

Survivorship care plans after treatment completion are an important element of follow-up care to assist patients in living with cancer as a chronic disease. These care plans should include the following information: treatments received for their cancer, potential late effects of treatment and any self-care measures to minimize these effects, primary cancer prevention measures (e.g., smoking cessation, diet, exercise), and measures to enhance quality of life. Secondary health prevention measures, such as reminding patients of a colonoscopy, mammogram, or gynecologic examination, are also important, along with instructing patients to follow up with their primary care provider for general health maintenance.

The table on page 171 provides a general list of side effects based on site-specific areas of radiation treatment and the associated interventions to help manage these problems.

Site-Specific Side Effects and Management

Site	Radiation Effect	Management
Brain	Alopecia, late cognitive changes, occasional nausea, fatigue	• Mild moisturizing skin products • Sun protection measures such as sunscreen and wearing a hat • Assess neurocognitive function. • Teach energy conservation measures. • Antiemetics as needed
Head and neck	Xerostomia, mucositis, dental caries, dysphagia, odynophagia	• Soft bland food • Sucking on hard candy • Saliva substitutes • Analgesics • Prophylactic dental care • These patients often need G-tube placement for nutrition; provide nursing assessment and education regarding tube feedings and G-tube care.
Chest	Cough, pneumonitis, late fibrosis	• Expectorants • Corticosteroids • Watch for signs and symptoms of pneumonitis; dry, nagging cough; shortness of breath.
Abdomen	Nausea and vomiting; symptoms of gastroesophageal reflux disease (GERD)	• Antiemetics • Diet modification • Maintain oral hydration. • Histamine 2 blockers or proton pump inhibitors as needed for GERD symptoms • Avoid acidic foods.
Pelvis	Diarrhea, cystitis, infertility; menopause; sexual dysfunction	• Maintain oral hydration. • Antidiarrheal medications • Fertility counseling • Teach signs and symptoms of menopause. • Diet modification: low-fiber diet. • Ask patients about sexual function.
Skin	Erythema, dry and moist desquamation	• Loose, comfortable clothing • Avoid friction to skin. • Washing skin is a priority during radiation therapy; use a mild moisturizing soap. • Use creams and lotions that are fragrance free and hypoallergenic. Steroid creams may be used.

References

Cao, D. (2012). *Volumetric modulated arc therapy (VMAT): The future of IMRT*. Seattle, WA: Swedish Cancer Institute.

Gosselin, T. K. (2011). Principles of radiation therapy. In C. H. Yarbro, D. Wujcik, & B. H. Gobel (eds.), *Cancer nursing: Principles and pratice* (7th ed., pp. 250–255). Sudbury, MA: Jones and Bartlett.

Iwamoto, R. R., Haas, M. L., & Gosselin, T. K. (2012). *Manual for radiation oncology nursing practice and education*. Pittsburgh, PA: Oncology Nursing Society.

Pajonk, F., Vlashi, E., & McBride, W. H. (2010). Radiation resistance of cancer stem cells: The 4 R's of radiobiology revisited. *Stem Cells, 28*(4), 639–648.

Timmerman, R., Paulus, R., Galvin, J., Michalski, J., Straube, W., & Bradley, J. (2010). Stereotactic body radiation for inoperable early stage lung cancer. *JAMA, 303*(11), 1070–1076. http://dx.doi.org/10.1001/jama.2010.261.

Tumor Treating Fields

Laura Benson

This chapter provides an understanding of the science of Tumor Treating Fields (TTFields), an innovative antimitotic therapy used to treat solid tumors. The mechanism of action, the delivery system, and the use of TTFields are addressed, as are the prevention and management of side effects and the importance of patient adherence to optimize outcomes when using this therapeutic device.

Definition of TTFields

TTFields are low-intensity alternating electric fields within the intermediate frequency range. TTFields disrupt cell division through physical interactions with key molecules during mitosis. This mechanism is grounded in the properties of physics that exploit the inherent attributes of cellular components (Kirson et al., 2004). Specifically, TTFields take advantage of the electrical characteristics, geometrical shape, and replication rate of dividing cancer cells, all of which make them susceptible to the effects of frequency-tuned alternating electric fields. TTFields therapy is unlike any other previous applications of electricity in medicine. TTFields therapy does not deliver electric current to tissue, stimulate nerves or muscles, or heat tissue (Kirson et al., 2009).

Mechanism of Action

TTFields exert an anticancer effect through a multipronged mechanism of action. TTFields therapy creates an alternating electric field within the tumor that attracts and repels the charged components of the cells during mitosis at intermediate frequencies of 100 to 300 kHz and at an intensity of approximately 1 V/cm, TTFields. This alternating field acts at multiple phases of the cell cycle (see figure below):

- It disrupts normal mitotic spindle assembly during metaphase, which leads to mitotic arrest and subsequent apoptosis (Giladi et al., 2014a).
- It produces nonuniform electric fields within dividing cells that exerts a force known as *dielectrophoresis*. This force within the electric fields affects intracellular components such as organelles and macromolecules. During mitosis, the effect of dielectrophoresis pushes the cell parts toward the cell cleavage furrow and interferes with normal cell division cytokinesis.
- It disrupts normal cell division, causing abnormal chromosomal segregation and multinucleation and thereby reducing the clonogenic potential in cellular progeny (see figure below).

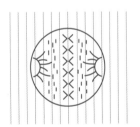 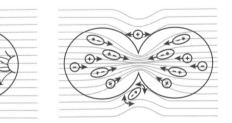

Metaphase   Anaphase   Telophase

Mechanism of action of TTFields. (© 2015 Novocure. All rights reserved.)

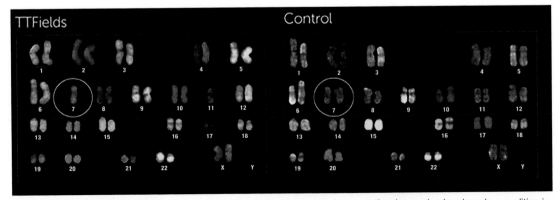

TTFields impair normal cell nuclear division. This causes abnormal chromosomal segregation (example showing abnormalities in chromosome 7). (© 2015 Novocure. All rights reserved.)

- It induces mitotic catastrophe (i.e., a major cell disruption during mitosis), which eventually leads to apoptotic cell death.
- It induces endoplasmic reticulum (ER) stress pathways and increases the expression of proteins known to activate immunogenic cell death.
- It impair a cell's ability to repair DNA damage caused by exposure to radiation.

TTFields therapy is a regional anticancer modality with no half-life or impediment posed by the blood-brain barrier, thus sparing off-target systemic adverse effects. TTFields are frequency tuned to exert a maximal cytotoxic effect on specific cancer cell types, sparing normal healthy cells. Different cell lines exhibit maximal proliferation reduction at different frequencies (Kirson et al., 2007). For example, glioma cells exhibit the greatest reduction in proliferation at a frequency of 200 kHz (Kirson et al., 2007), whereas for non–small cell lung cancer (NSCLC) cells, the greatest reduction in cell proliferation is at 150 kHz (see table below) (Giladi et al., 2014b). Efficacy is dose dependent; cytotoxic effects increase when the electric field intensity increases. Threshold value, below which cells are largely unaffected, is approximately 1 V/cm. Unlike drug therapy, TTFields deliver therapy only while activated.

Efficacy of TTFields Is Frequency Dependent

Tumor Cell Line	TTFields Frequency for Greatest Reduction in Cell Proliferation (kHz)
Glioma	200
Meningioma	200
Non–small cell lung cancer	150
Ovarian	200
Pancreatic	150

From Benson, L. (2015). Technology meets oncology: Understanding the science of tumor treating fields, a novel antimitotic therapy for solid tumors. Presented at the Oncology Nursing Society 40th Annual Congress, April 23-26, Orlando, Florida. Poster session #35. *Oncology Nursing Forum, 42*(2), E154; Davies, A. M., Weinberg, U., Palti, Y. (2013). Tumor treating fields: A new frontier in cancer therapy. *Annals of the New York Academy of Sciences, 1291,* 86-95.

TTFields Therapy System

Optune (Novocure Inc., Porstmouth, NH), formerly called the NovoTTF-100A System, is a medical device approved in the United States and Japan for use as monotherapy for the treatment of recurrent glioblastoma (GBM). Optune is a CE Marked device that is cleared for sale in the European Union, Switzerland, Australia, and Israel for glioblastoma and NSCLC. The complete TTFields therapy delivery system includes an electric field generator; insulated transducer arrays; portable, rechargeable batteries; battery charger; plug-in power supply; connection cable; and carrying case (see figure in next column) (Optune, 2014). Ongoing therapy is patient administered in the home after prescription by a certified health care provider. The U.S. Food and Drug Administration (FDA) mandates that prescribers of

this therapy successfully complete a certification course provided by the manufacturer. The patient is monitored in the outpatient setting by the oncology team on a regular basis. During the course of therapy, patients receive replacement system parts, most often the transducer arrays, from the manufacturer. When the therapy is discontinued, the system is returned to the manufacturer.

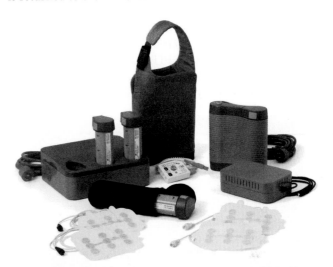

Optune medical device.

Cell response to TTFields is direction dependent. The cells that divide parallel to the electric field show higher rates of damage than those dividing perpendicular to the field (Kirson et al., 2004). Therefore, to maximize the clinical effects, TTFields are delivered noninvasively via two pairs of transducer arrays that produce two perpendicular electric fields. These arrays are applied directly on the surface of the skin in the region surrounding the tumor. TTFields are frequency-tuned to the targeted histology, and during treatment, generation of the electric field switches between the two pairs of arrays at a rate of approximately once per second.

Each array comprises nine insulated ceramic discs (see lower left part of figure on page 172) which have a high dielectric constant, are biocompatible, and are soldered to a flexible circuit board. These discs are separated from the skin by a layer of conductive hydrogel. To keep the arrays in place on the scalp and in continuous direct contact with the skin, the ceramic discs, hydrogel, and circuitry are attached to a hypoallergenic medical adhesive bandage (Lacouture et al., 2014). TTFields therapy should not be used in patients with GBM who have an active implanted medical device, a skull defect, or bullet fragments (Optune, 2014).

A wire from each array plugs into the connection cable, which then plugs into the portion of the device that generates TTFields. Patients may describe a "warm sensation" under the transducer arrays. Each array has eight temperature sensors that monitor temperature; the device will shut off and sound an alarm if array temperature exceeds 41° C (105.8° F), well below the threshold for a thermal skin burn (Lacouture et al., 2014).

In patients with GBM, transducer array placement is based on the results of magnetic resonance imaging. The array locations on a patient's shaved scalp are calculated with the use of FDA-approved simulation software (Novo-TAL, Novocure) that optimizes field intensity within the tumor, based on head size and tumor location (see figure below) (Lacouture et al., 2014). Treatment parameters are preset at 200 kHz and a minimal field intensity of 0.7 V/cm in the brain. Neither the health care provider nor the patient needs to make electrical adjustments (Lacouture et al., 2014). Responses to TTFields therapy are typically observed on radiographic evaluations 3 to 5 months after treatment initiation (Vymazal et al., 2014).

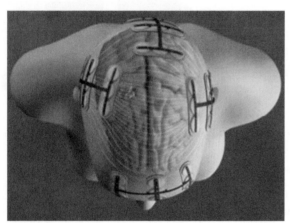

Transducer array placement is guided by a patient's MRI results. (© 2016 Novocure. All rights reserved.)

TTFields Therapy for Recurrent Glioblastoma

In 2011, TTFields therapy was approved by the FDA for use in adults (22 years of age or older) who have recurrent GBM in the supratentorial region of the brain after receiving chemotherapy and whose disease is refractory to surgical and radiation treatment options. The pivotal phase III trial that led to FDA approval in recurrent GBM demonstrated comparable median overall survival time with TTFields therapy compared with chemotherapy, including bevacizumab (Stupp et al., 2012). TTFields therapy was found to be as effective as chemotherapy, with fewer side effects. In addition, patients reported a better quality of life, including improved cognitive and emotional functioning, compared with patients receiving chemotherapy (Stupp et al., 2012). Treatment adherence, or time on therapy, has proved to be an important factor in treatment outcomes. Analysis of the pivotal phase III trial for recurrent GBM showed that an adherence rate of at least 75%, or approximately 18 hours/day, was a clear predictor of survival (Gutin & Wong, 2012; Mrugala et al., 2014; Optune, 2014).

In the Patient Registry Dataset (PRiDe), a postmarketing registry of all commercially treated patients with recurrent GBM receiving TTFields, median overall survival significantly exceeded that observed in the pivotal trial. Favorable prognostic factors included use in first recurrence, no prior exposure to bevacizumab, and high performance status (Mrugala et al., 2014).

The National Comprehensive Cancer Network (NCCN) Clinical Practice Guidelines in Oncology for Central Nervous System Cancers indicate that physicians should consider TTFields therapy for patients with GBM who experience recurrence or progression after initial treatment (category 2B) (NCCN, 2015).

Newly Diagnosed GBM

When combined with temozolomide in human glioma cell line studies, TTFields were found to exert additive cytotoxic effects. This provided the rationale for a phase III trial in patients with newly diagnosed GBM who had completed standard-of-care concomitant chemoradiotherapy. Patients were randomly assigned in a 2:1 ratio to receive either adjuvant temozolomide chemotherapy alone or temozolomide in combination with TTFields therapy (200 kHz). The primary end point was progression-free survival; secondary end points were overall survival, safety, cognitive function, and quality of life. Based on a prespecified interim analysis of 315 patients, the trial was closed early. The first analysis of the full dataset of 700 patients randomized in the trial found progression-free survival to be 7.1 months for the combined therapy versus 4.0 months for temozolomide alone. Overall survival was 20.5 versus 15.6 months, respectively. This translated into 2-year survival rates of 43% for combined therapy with temozolomide and TTFields, compared with 29% for temozolomide alone. No significant added toxicity was observed with the addition of TTFields. Quality of life and gross cognitive function were comparable in both study arms (Stupp et al., 2014; Stupp et al., 2015). Based on these results U.S. FDA has approved Optune in combination with temozolomide for the treatment of adult patients with newly diagnosed GBM.

Patient and Caregiver Education Before TTFields Therapy

Because TTFields is a continuous, at-home therapy, patient and caregiver education is important. Patients and caregivers should have a basic understanding of the mechanism of action, the system parts and functions, proper use of the equipment, and the importance of compliance with therapy. TTFields therapy is delivered only when the system is in place and activated; therefore, the device is portable and designed to be worn continuously, around the clock. Patient adherence is critical because greater time on therapy is linked to better outcomes (Mrugala et al., 2014). Therefore, patient teaching, ongoing assessments, and continued motivation of patients and their caregivers are key to maximizing the potential benefits received from TTFields therapy. Education on skin preparation and care, prevention and management of side effects, and what to expect during treatment is essential.

Patient Teaching

Patients should use TTFields only after being trained by qualified personnel who have completed a training course (Optune, 2014). This includes instruction about caring for the system components, how best to prevent and manage skin irritation, and the importance of treatment adherence.

It is important for the family to understand that electric field therapy is not hazardous to those in close proximity to the patient. The electric fields do not contain radiation or pose a hazard to others.

Patients are instructed to remove the transducer array portion of the system every 4 to 7 days to re-shave the head and reapply the transducer arrays. The four transducer arrays that are placed on the scalp need to be replaced every 4 to 7 days and are for single use only. Used system parts (e.g., transducer arrays) are returned to the manufacturer for disposal. Practical tips on how to complete activities of daily living are taught. For example, the patient is taught how to shower without removing the transducer arrays by using a shower cap for bathing.

The delivery system is portable, allowing patients to go about their daily activities while receiving treatment (see figure below). Patients can spend time with family, work, travel, and generally engage in their usual activities, including showering or bathing.

arrays must be changed one or two times per week (i.e., every 4 to 7 days). The time between changes varies based on factors such as sweating, hair growth, and weather. The patient and caregiver are taught this procedure at the start of therapy.

Side-Effect Profile

Device-related adverse events can impact a patient's quality of life, affect adherence to therapy, and contribute to medical costs (Lacouture et al., 2014). The most commonly occurring adverse event associated with the use of TTFields therapy is skin irritation, largely grade 2 (mild to moderate), under the transducer arrays (see figure below). The types and potential causes of dermatologic adverse events are summarized in the table below, and the signs of skin events based on underlying pathogenesis in the table on page 176.

Prophylactic strategies to prevent skin irritation include proper shaving with an electric razor and avoiding the placement of ceramic discs directly over postsurgical screws or plates (Lacouture et al., 2014). Patients are taught how to properly shave and how to adjust the placement of the transducer arrays; they are advised to assess skin condition every 4 to 7 days. The table on page 176 highlights what the patient and caregiver can do to prevent dermatologic adverse events.

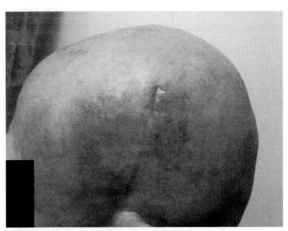

Skin irritation. Dermatologic erosions and skin infection (folliculitis) in a 60-year-old man who had been receiving temozolomide and NovoTTF Therapy for 3 months. (© 2016 Novocure. All rights reserved.)

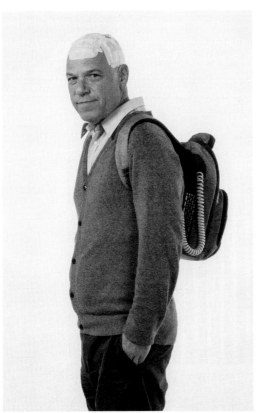

Simulation of patient receiving TTFields therapy for GBM. (© 2016 Novocure. All rights reserved.)

Because treatment is delivered via a visible, constantly present device, support and dedication by both the patient and caregiver are critical to a successful outcome. The transducer

Types and Potential Causes of Dermatologic Adverse Events

Adverse Event	Potential Cause
Irritant contact dermatitis	Chemical irritation from hydrogel, moisture, alcohol
Allergic contact dermatitis	Allergy to tape, hydrogel
Erosion	Mechanical trauma from shaving, array pressure/removal
Ulcer	Decreased perfusion from array pressure (especially in areas overlying scars, hardware, or prior radiation fields)
Skin infection/pustules	Secondary bacterial infection

From Lacouture, M. E., Davis, M. E., Elzinga, G., Butowski, N., Tran, D., Villano, J. L., et al (2014). Characterization and management of dermatologic adverse events with the NovoTTF-100A System, a novel anti-mitotic electric field device for the treatment of recurrent glioblastoma. *Seminars in Oncology, 41*(Suppl 4), S1-S14.

Signs of Skin Events Based on Underlying Pathogenesis

Dermatitis	Skin Infection	Mechanical	Ischemia
Erythema	Erythema	Erosions	Ulcers
Scaling	Discharge	Abrasions	Pain
Erosions	Pustules	Lacerations	
Edema	Pain	Pain/burning	
Pruritus	Yellow/green crusting		

From Lacouture, M. E., Davis, M. E., Elzinga, G., Butowski, N., Tran, D., Villano, J. L., et al (2014). Characterization and management of dermatologic adverse events with the NovoTTF-100A System, a novel anti-mitotic electric field device for the treatment of recurrent glioblastoma. *Seminars in Oncology*, *41*(Suppl 4), S1-S14.

Preventive Strategies for Dermatologic Adverse Events

Category	Guidelines for Patient or Caregiver
Shaving and preparation of the scalp	Perform proper handwashing before preparation of the scalp for array application. Take time shaving the scalp, using gentle but firm circular motions. Ensure a close shave before applying the arrays. Cleaning the electric razor *after* every shave is important to lessen the risk of skin infection. Wash scalp with fragrance-free, mild shampoo (e.g., baby shampoo); seborrheic dermatitis shampoo may be used because it has antibacterial properties (e.g., pyrithione zinc 2%, ciclopirox 1%, ketoconazole 2%) Ensure that scalp is completely dry before applying a new set of arrays.
Use of 70% isopropyl alcohol	Use of first aid antiseptic rubbing alcohol before array application is a necessary step to remove naturally occurring scalp oils, resulting in better adherence of the arrays to the scalp. After shaving and before placing the arrays, wipe the scalp with a gauze or cotton ball soaked in the rubbing alcohol. Avoid areas of skin irritation, because the rubbing alcohol may further irritate the skin.
Transducer array exchanges	Change arrays on a regular basis (at least every 3-4 days). When removing the arrays, avoid "pulling" on the skin; take approximately 60 sec to remove each array. Use of mineral (baby) oil on the edges of the array may make removal of the adhesive tape easier and less irritating to the skin. To remove leftover array adhesive, use gauze or a cotton ball soaked in mineral (baby) oil or pour oil into hands and gently rub scalp in areas of remaining adhesive. Pay close attention to the scalp at each array exchange, and notify the doctor or nurse if there are signs of skin irritation or open areas, to receive information on how to treat them; taking a picture of the affected areas on the scalp and sharing it with the doctor or nurse is advised.

From Lacouture, M. E., Davis, M .E., Elzinga, G., Butowski, N., Tran, D., Villano, J. L., et al (2014). Characterization and management of dermatologic adverse events with the NovoTTF-100A System, a novel anti-mitotic electric field device for the treatment of recurrent glioblastoma. *Seminars in Oncology*, *41*(Suppl 4), S1-S14.

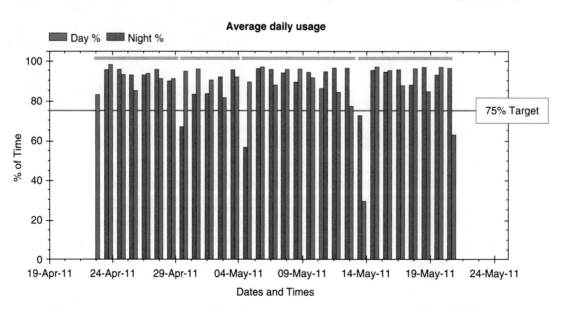

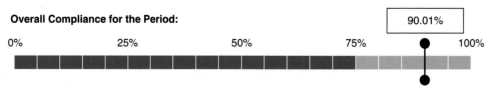

Sample of a patient-specific adherence report. (© 2016 Novocure. All rights reserved.)

Specific treatments for dermatologic adverse events may include topical or oral antibiotics, topical corticosteroids (high potency as needed), and isolation of the affected skin areas from adhesives and pressure. If patients have intolerable grade 2 or 3 dermatologic adverse events, treatment should be interrupted and topical therapies applied. When the arrays are reapplied, they may be relocated (Lacouture et al., 2014). Other side effects reported by patients include headaches, weakness, falls, fatigue, and muscle twitching (Optune, 2014).

Adherence

Patient adherence is recorded by the device onto internal log files. A patient-specific report is generated monthly and provided to the treating health care team (see figure on page 176) (Greifzu, Kuchinka, DiMeglio, Shackelford, & Benson, 2015). Patients may take short treatment breaks of 1 to 2 hours for personal care activities but are otherwise encouraged to continue normal activities of daily living while on therapy. Adherence can be maximized by having patients and caregivers adopt skin care strategies described in the previous section, minimizing the need for any treatment breaks. Use of properly ventilated hats and wigs may also improve adherence to TTFields therapy (Greifzu et al., 2015). Tightly woven wigs and hats made of material that traps heat can cause the device to alarm. The use of lighter materials, such as loosely woven wigs or ventilated wigs, permits heat to escape while providing a cosmetic effect.

Ongoing Research with TTFields

A substantial body of evidence exists that supports the anticancer activity of TTFields across multiple cancer cell lines—including glioma, small cell lung cancer, breast cancer, melanoma, NSCLC, ovarian cancer, and pancreatic cancer—as well as in multiple animal tumor models and in patients with a variety of solid tumors. TTFields therapy has safely been combined with chemotherapy in clinical trials (Munster et al., 2015; Pless, Droege, von Moos, Salzberg, & Betticher, 2013).

Additional Information

Optune is classified as durable medical equipment and it is approved for use within the home without continuous medical supervision. The therapy is covered by most major insurance carriers, either through published medical policy or on case-by-case review. Patient coinsurance varies by plan, and patients who cannot afford their coinsurance may be eligible for assistance from the manufacturer and third-party foundations. At completion of therapy, the device and system parts are returned to the manufacturer.

Other Solid Tumors

TTFields are being studied at therapeutic intensities to treat solid tumors in the thorax (NSCLC, mesothelioma, squamous cell lung cancer), abdomen (pancreatic cancer), central nervous system (brain metastases from NSCLC), and pelvis (ovarian cancer). This novel treatment provides an opportunity for tumor response with potentially fewer side effects than with other treatments.

References

Benson, L. (2015). Technology meets oncology: Understanding the science of tumor treating fields, a novel antimitotic therapy for solid tumors. Presented at the Oncology Nursing Society 40th Annual Congress, April 23-26, Orlando, Florida. Poster session #35. *Oncology Nursing Forum*, 42(2), E154.

Davies, A. M., Weinberg, U., & Palti, Y. (2013). Tumor treating fields: A new frontier in cancer therapy. *Annals of the New York Academy of Sciences*, 1291, 86–95.

Giladi, M., Schneiderman, R. S., Porat, Y., Munster, M., Itzhaki, A., Mordechovich, D., & Palti, Y. (2014a). Mitotic disruption and reduced clonogenicity of pancreatic cancer cells in vitro and in vivo by tumor treating fields. *Pancreatology*, 14(1), 54–63.

Giladi, M., Weinberg, U., Schneiderman, R. S., Porat, Y., Munster, M., Voloshin, T., & Palti, Y. (2014b). Alternating electric fields (tumor-treating fields therapy) can improve chemotherapy treatment efficacy in non-small cell lung cancer both in vitro and in vivo. *Seminars in Oncology*, 41(Suppl 6), S35S41.

Greifzu, S., Kuchinka, B., DiMeglio, L., Shackelford, M., & Benson, L. (2015). Compliance as a predictor of outcome in recurrent glioblastoma multiforme utilizing Optune (*formerly NovoTTF-100A System*). Presented at the Oncology Nursing Society 40th Annual Congress, April 23-26, Orlando, Florida. Poster session #80. *Oncology Nursing Forum*, 42(2), E171.

Gutin, P. H., & Wong, E. T. (2012). Noninvasive application of alternating electric fields in glioblastoma: A fourth cancer treatment modality. *American Society of Clinical Oncology Educational Book*, 32, 126–131.

Kirson, E. D., Gurvich, Z., Schneiderman, R., Dekel, E., Itzhaki, A., Wasserman, Y., & Palti, Y. (2004). Disruption of cancer cell replication by alternating electric fields. *Cancer Research*, 64, 3288–3295.

Kirson, E. D., Dbalý, V., Tovaryš, F., Vymazal, J., Soustiel, J. F., Itzhaki, A., & Palti, Y. (2007). Alternating electric fields arrest cell proliferation in animal tumor models and human brain tumors. *Proceedings of the National Academy of Sciences of the United States of America*, 104, 10152–10157.

Kirson, E. D., Giladi, M., Gurvich, Z., Itzhaki, A., Mordechovich, D., Schneiderman, R. S., & Palti, Y. (2009). Alternating electric fields (TTFields) inhibit metastatic spread of solid tumors to the lungs. *Clinical & Experimental Metastasis*, 26(7), 633–640.

Lacouture, M. E., Davis, M. E., Elzinga, G., Butowski, N., Tran, D., Villano, J. L., & Wong, E. T. (2014). Characterization and management of dermatologic adverse events with the NovoTTF-100A System, a novel anti-mitotic electric field device for the treatment of recurrent glioblastoma. *Seminars in Oncology*, 41(Suppl 4), S1–S14.

Mrugala, M. M., Engelhard, H. H., Dinh Tran, D., Kew, Y., Cavaliere, R., Villano, J. L., & Butowski, N. (2014). Clinical practice experience with NovoTTF-100A System for glioblastoma: The Patient Registry Dataset (PRiDe). *Seminars in Oncology*, 41(Suppl 6), S4–S13.

Munster, M., Roberts, C. P., Schmeiz, E. M., Giladi, M., Blat, R., Schneiderman, R. S., & Palti, Y. (2015). Alternating electric fields (TTFields) in combination with paclitaxel are therapeutically effective against ovarian cancer cells in vitro and in vivo. Presented at the 2015 annual meeting of the American Association for Cancer Research, Philadelphia, PA, April 18-22. Abstract #5365. *Cancer Research*, 75, 5365.

The National Comprehensive Cancer Network. (2015). *NCCN clinical practice guidelines in oncology (NCCN Guidelines): Central nervous system cancers*. version 1.2015. Available at http://www.nccn.org/professionals/physician_gls/pdf/f_guidelines.asp (accessed February 1, 2016).

Optune. (2014). *Instructions for use*. Portsmouth, NH: Novocure Inc. Available at www.optune.com/hcp/instructions-for-use.aspx (accessed February 1, 2016).

Pless, M., Droege, C., von Moos, R., Salzberg, M., & Betticher, D. (2013). A phase I/II trial of Tumor Treating Fields (TTFields) therapy in combination with pemetrexed for advanced non-small cell lung cancer. *Lung Cancer*, 81, 445–450.

Stupp, R., Wong, E. T., Kanner, A. A., Steinberg, D., Engelhard, H., Heidecke, V., & Gutin, P. H. (2012). NovoTTF-100A versus physician's choice of chemotherapy in recurrent glioblastoma: A randomised phase III trial of a novel treatment modality. *European Journal of Cancer*, 48, 2192–2202.

Stupp, R., Wong, E. T., Scott, C. B., Taillibert, S., Kanner, A., Kesari, S., & Ram, Z. (2014). NT-40. Interim analysis of the EF-14 trial: A prospective, multi-center trial of NovoTTF-100A together with temozolomide compared to temozolomide alone in patients with newly diagnosed GBM. *Neuro-Oncology*, 16(Suppl 5), v167. http://dx.doi.org/10.1093/neuonc/nou265.40.

Stupp, R., Taillibert, S., Kanner, A., Kesari, S., Steinberg, D., et al (2015). Maintenance Therapy With Tumor Treating Fields Plus Temozolomide vs Temozolomide Alone for Gliobalstoma A Randomized Clinical Trial. *Journal of the American Medical Association*, *314*(23), 2535–2543. [DOI:10.1001/jama.2015.16669].

Vymazal, J., & Wong, E. T. (2014). Response patterns of recurrent glioblastomas treated with tumor-treating fields. *Seminars in Oncology*, *41*(Suppl 6), S14–S24.

Hematopoietic Stem Cell Transplantation

Terry Wikle Shapiro

Introduction

Five decades ago, the concept of using bone marrow (i.e., hematopoietic stem cell transplantation [HSCT]) to treat humans with inherited diseases of immune function, marrow failure syndromes, and leukemia was met with much skepticism and varying degrees of enthusiasm. Transferring what was known from experimental animal models to humans was fraught with many challenges and disappointments. Suitable candidates for HSCT were patients whose primary disease meant certain death (de la Morena & Gatti, 2010). Considered radicals in the early 1970s, HSCT pioneers E. Donall Thomas and Robert Goode were able to demonstrate in humans that diseased or poorly functioning bone marrow could be replaced by a central venous infusion of bone marrow from a healthy donor after cytotoxic doses of chemoradiotherapy (Appelbaum, Forman, Negrin, & Blume, 2009).

HSCT is no longer a treatment modality only for lethal diseases such as primary immunodeficiency diseases or hematologic malignancies. It is also a valid approach of cellular engineering for treating solid tumors, hemoglobinopathies, marrow failure syndromes, autoimmune diseases, inherited disorders of metabolism, histiocytic disorders, and other nonmalignancies.

Advances in histocompatibility matching; reduced-intensity conditioning (RIC) regimens; improvements in stem cell collection and cryopreservation techniques; development of pharmacologic agents to accelerate the recovery of hematopoiesis; advances in infectious disease monitoring and detection; development of effective antimicrobial agents; refinements in the prevention, diagnosis, and management of acute and chronic graft-versus-host disease (GVHD); and a better understanding of the biology of the graft-versus-tumor (GVT) effect have contributed to the evolving success of HSCT (Neiss, 2013). In addition to these medical advances, astute nursing care of transplant recipients continues to be the cornerstone for the prevention and treatment of HSCT-related complications and death (Wikle Shapiro, 2015). This chapter reviews the principles of caring for patients undergoing autologous and allogeneic HSCT.

Rationale for High-Dose Therapy with Stem Cell Transplantation

HSCT involves replacing diseased, destroyed, or nonfunctioning hematopoietic cells with healthy hematopoietic progenitor cells (i.e., stem cells). Stem cells are primitive hematopoietic cells that are capable of self-renewal, and they are pluripotent, meaning that they can mature into a red blood cell (RBC), white blood cell (WBC), or platelet. Stem cells may be collected directly from the bone marrow spaces by a bone marrow harvest procedure, from the peripheral blood by apheresis, or from the umbilical cord of newborns by cannulation of the large vessels of the umbilical cord and placenta after delivery.

For adult allogeneic HSCT, peripheral blood stem cells (PBSCs) have become the preferred source for grafting. Collection of PBSCs through apheresis is easier and less costly and may also result in more rapid recovery of neutrophil and platelet counts (Schmit-Pokorny, 2013; Wikle Shapiro, 2015). For pediatric allogeneic HSCT, bone marrow remains the preferred source of stem cells due to the long-term risk of chronic GVHD. In unrelated donor allogeneic HSCT, the source of stem cells may be bone marrow, PBSCs, or umbilical cord blood (UCB). PBSCs are used almost exclusively in autologous HSCT.

Types of Hematopoietic Stem Cell Transplantations

The various types of HSCTs can be differentiated in terms of the hematopoietic stem cell donor, the method used to collect the cells, and the intensity of the conditioning regimen. Each source of stem cells has advantages and disadvantages, as summarized in the table on page 180. In autologous HSCT, the patient serves as his or her own donor of stem cells, whereas for allogeneic HSCT, the donor is related (typically a sibling) or unrelated. If an identical twin donor is available, the procedure is called *syngeneic transplantation*. Stem cells may be collected from the peripheral bloodstream (i.e., PBSCs), from the bone marrow spaces (i.e., bone marrow stem cells), or from the umbilical cord and placenta of newborns (i.e., UBC stem cells). HSCTs can also be differentiated on the basis of the intensity of the conditioning regimen.

Myeloablative transplantation involves the use of high doses of chemotherapy with or without total body irradiation (TBI) to treat the underlying disease, ablate the bone marrow, and cause myelosuppression that would be irreversible without the infusion of hematopoietic stem cells.

RIC during allogeneic HSCT reduces transplantation-related mortality (TRM) and morbidity by relying more on the GVT effect than the conditioning regimen to eradicate disease. RIC regimens can provide a curative option for patients who may otherwise not be candidates for myeloablative (intensive) transplantation because of age or poor performance status (Koreth et al., 2013). RIC transplants are often used when there is increased concern about fatal or debilitating TRM and morbidity.

Indications for and Outcomes of Hematopoietic Stem Cell Transplantation

HSCT represents an important advance in restoring or replacing hematopoietic or immune function in patients whose bone marrow has been destroyed by the cytotoxic effects of radiation therapy and high-dose chemotherapy to treat an underlying disease. Many factors influence the indications and patient eligibility for transplantation. HSCT is used when the bone marrow or immune system is diseased, defective, or destroyed as a result of prior treatment. The second table below lists the diseases treated with autologous or allogeneic HSCT (Perumbeti, 2014; Wikle Shapiro, 2015).

Factors that may affect the outcomes of HSCT include the type and stage of disease at the time of transplantation, type of procedure (i.e., allogeneic or autologous), degree of human leukocyte antigen (HLA) matching for allogeneic transplants, intensity of the conditioning regimen, ages of the donor and recipient, cytomegalovirus (CMV) status compatibility of the donor and recipient, and experience of the transplantation center (Appelbaum, 2012). The TRM risk for allogeneic HSCT improved from 30%

to 50% in the 1990s to about 5% to 10% in 2012 (Appelbaum, 2012; de la Morena & Gatti, 2011). The improved rate most likely resulted from the increasing use of RIC regimens, agents that avoid hepatic and renal toxicity, and better infection control methods (Appelbaum, 2012). At most transplantation centers, the acceptable TRM rate for autologous HSCT is less than 5%.

Disease-free survival at 5 years can range from 10% to 75% after HSCT, depending on the age of the recipient, underlying disease, disease status at the time of transplantation, type of HSCT procedure, and extent of prior treatment. The table on page 181 lists 5-year disease-free survival rates for the most common malignant diseases treated with HSCT (Center for International Blood and Marrow Transplant Research [CIBMTR] & National Marrow Donor Program [NMDP], 2015).

Overview of the Process and Implications for Nursing Care

Pretransplantation Evaluation of the Recipient and Donor

The pretransplantation evaluation of the recipient includes a thorough physical and psychosocial evaluation, assessment of the adequacy of insurance coverage, and evaluation of the adequacy of family and caregiver support. Before transplantation, the patient and family should receive extensive education about the risks, benefits, and process of transplantation to permit informed consent for the procedure. For allogeneic HSCT, selection of an appropriate donor includes confirmatory high-resolution tissue typing, an assessment of specific viral serologies, a donor health assessment, and a physical examination.

Donors must be carefully evaluated and fully informed before the donation of PBSCs or bone marrow (Schmit-Pokorny, 2013). Legal and ethical aspects should be considered, especially when using minors as donors. Although the selection of an appropriate donor should be performed by the HSCT team, the donor evaluation should be performed by a provider who is not directly involved in the recipient's care during the transplantation process (Foundation for the Accreditation of Cellular Therapy, 2014). Evaluation for autologous and allogeneic HSCT includes an assessment of the patient's overall performance status, disease status, and organ function; evaluation of specific viral serologies; and exclusion of active infection. Components of the evaluation of recipient and donor are summarized in the box on page 181.

Comparison of Hematopoietic Stem Cell Sources

Technique	Advantages and Disadvantages
Bone marrow harvest	Harvest-related pain
	General anesthesia required
	May be more cost-effective and more convenient for donors
	No growth factor mobilization required
	Lower incidence of chronic GVHD
Peripheral blood stem cells (PBSCs)	Less invasive
	Higher cell procurement for autologous procedures
	Incidence of GVHD may be higher
	Improved graft-versus-tumor effect
	More than 1 day of collection may be required
	Requires mobilization with chemotherapy or hematopoietic growth factors, or both
Cord blood	Inexpensive to collect
	Excellent source to increase pool of unrelated donors
	Associated with less GVHD
	More than one cord blood unit may be necessary in adults
	Increased risk of graft rejection
	Delayed posttransplantation immune recovery
	No donor available for posttransplantation DLI, boost, or CTLs

CTLs, Cytotoxic T lymphocytes; *DLI*, donor lymphocyte infusion; *GVHD*, graft-versus-host disease.

Diseases Treated with Hematopoietic Stem Cell Transplantation

AUTOLOGOUS TRANSPLANTATION		ALLOGENEIC TRANSPLANTATION	
Malignant Disorders	**Nonmalignant Disorders**	**Malignant Disorders**	**Nonmalignant Disorders**
Neuroblastoma		Acute myeloid leukemia (AML)	Aplastic anemia
Non-Hodgkin lymphoma		Non-Hodgkin lymphoma	Fanconi anemia
Hodgkin disease		Hodgkin disease	Severe combined immunodeficiency
Acute myeloid leukemia (AML)	Autoimmune disorders	Acute lymphoblastic leukemia (ALL)	Thalassemia major
Medulloblastoma	Amyloidosis	Chronic myeloid leukemia (CML)	Diamond-Blackfan anemia
Germ cell tumors		Myelodysplastic syndromes	Sickle cell anemia
Multiple myeloma*		Multiple myeloma*	Wiskott-Aldrich syndrome
		Chronic lymphocytic leukemia (CLL)*	Osteopetrosis
			Inborn errors of metabolism
			Autoimmune disorders

*Uncommon in children but a common reason for transplantation in adults.
Data from Copelan, E. A. (2006). Hematopoietic stem-cell transplantation. *New England Journal of Medicine, 354*(17), 1813-1826.

Five-Year Disease-Free Survival Rates

Disease	Stage	Autologous Transplantation	SURVIVAL RATE (%) ALLOGENEIC TRANSPLANTATION Sibling Donor	Unrelated Donor
Acute lymphoblastic leukemia (ALL)	CR 1	NA	65	45
	CR2	NA	55	35
Acute myeloid leukemia (AML)	CR1	60	65	30
	CR2	40	45	50
	No remission	20	NA	25
Chronic myeloid leukemia (CML)	Chronic phase <1 yr	NA	70	55
	Chronic phase >1 yr	NA	60	50
Hodgkin disease	CR1	80	NA	NA
	CR2	70	NA	NA
	No remission	45	NA	NA
Diffuse large cell lymphoma	CR1	65	25	30
		50	25	NA
		45	20	NA
Neuroblastoma		40	NA	NA

CR, Complete response; NA, not applicable.
Data from Center for International Blood and Marrow Transplant Research (CIBMTR) & National Marrow Donor Program (NMDP). (2015). Data. Available at www.CIMBTR.org (accessed February 18, 2016).

Pretransplantation Evaluation of Recipient and Donor

Evaluation of the Autologous and Allogeneic Hematopoietic Stem Cell Transplant Recipient

Pretreatment testing and evaluation of the patient undergoing hematopoietic stem cell transplantation includes the following:
- History of current illness, including presenting signs and symptoms, previous therapies, initial diagnosis, pathology and staging, complications, relapses or progressions, current disease status, and transfusion history
- Medical history, including major illnesses, chronic illnesses, recurring illnesses, surgical history, childhood illnesses, and infectious disease exposure. For women, the medical history should also include menarche, onset of menopause or date of last menstrual period, pregnancies, and outcomes.
- Current medications
- Allergies
- Social and family history, including identified caregiver and alternate
- Performance status
- Complete blood cell count (CBC), which must be obtained within a 24-hour period before the first peripheral blood stem cell collection and within 24 hours of each subsequent collection
- Current laboratory studies, including liver and renal function studies; 24-hour urine test for creatinine clearance if there is a history of renal dysfunction or nephrotoxins; prothrombin time (PT), partial prothrombin time (PTT), or international normalized ratio (INR); blood grouping and Rh typing (ABO and Rh)
- Infectious disease serologies, including human immunodeficiency virus type 1 (HIV-1) antibody, HIV-2 antibody, HIV antigen, human T-cell lymphotrophic virus (HTLV), hepatitis B surface antigen, hepatitis B core antigen, hepatitis C antibodies, human T-cell leukemia/lymphoma virus type 1 (HTLV-1), West Nile virus, and Trypanosoma cruzi (Chagas disease) within 30 days of collection
- Infectious disease serologies specific to allogeneic recipients, such as cytomegalovirus (CMV) antibodies (immunoglobulin G [IgG] and immunoglobulin [IgM]), herpes simplex virus (HSV), antibodies (IgG and IgM), toxoplasmosis IgG and IgM antibodies, and Epstein-Barr virus (EBV) nuclear antibodies
- Human leukocyte antigen typing (allogeneic)
- Pretransplantation chimerism studies (by polymerase chain reaction [PCR] if the donor and recipient are the same sex or XY DNA analysis if the donor and recipient are different sexes)
- Chest radiograph
- Electrocardiogram and echocardiogram
- Multiple gated acquisition (MUGA) scan for adult patients or echocardiogram for children
- Pulmonary function tests, including single-breath diffusing capacity

- A 24-hour urine test for creatinine clearance
- Computed tomography (CT) of chest and sinuses for pretransplantation infection surveillance if there are symptoms, a history of repeated infections, or periods of prolonged neutropenia
- Disease restaging, including radiographic studies (e.g., CT), nuclear medicine studies, bone marrow aspirate and biopsy (hematologic malignancies), cytogenetics, molecular diagnostics, and measures of minimal residual disease
- Dental evaluation, including full-mouth x-ray record and cleaning
- Sperm or fertilized embryo banking
- Informed consent for treatment, transfusion support, clinical trials
- Nutritional evaluation, if appropriate
- Consultations with radiation therapy, infectious disease, pulmonary, cardiology, or renal services if clinically indicated
- Financial screening
- Psychosocial evaluation
- *The following must be documented:*
  - Suitability to undergo transplantation
  - Abnormal findings and rationale for proceeding to transplantation
  - Counseling of patient regarding abnormal findings
  - Patient informed of tests performed to protect the health of the patient
  - Patient informed of right to review test results

Evaluation of the Hematopoietic Stem Cell Donor

Pretreatment testing and evaluation of the hematopoietic stem cell donor usually includes the following:
- Human leukocyte antigen A (HLA-A), HLA-B, HLA-DR, and HLA-DQ typing
- History and physical examination, documenting serious or chronic illnesses, hematologic problems (including bleeding tendencies), cancer history, prior transfusions, current medications, allergies, and pregnancy history for females
- Presence of risk factors for HIV or viral hepatitis infection and other communicable diseases
- Physical examination for abnormalities and assessment of the adequacy of peripheral veins
- CBC with differential count, chemistry panel, liver and renal function tests, coagulation studies, pregnancy test (within 7 days of starting growth factors)
- ABO group and Rh type (red cell phenotype, RBC crossmatch between donor and recipient, and anti-A and anti-B titers as appropriate)
- Hemoglobinopathy assessment
- Confirmatory HLA typing

Continued

Pretransplantation Evaluation of Recipient and Donor—cont'd

- Pretransplantation chimerism studies (by PCR if the donor and recipient are the same sex or XY DNA analysis if the donor and recipient are different sexes)
- Infectious disease serologies, including human HIV-1 antibody, HIV-2 antibody, HIV antigen, HTLV, hepatitis B surface antigen, hepatitis B core antigen, hepatitis C antibodies, HTLV-1, cytomegalovirus (CMV) antibodies (IgG and IgM), EBV nuclear antibodies, West Nile virus, and *Trypanosoma cruzi* (Chagas disease) within 30 days of collection
- Electrocardiogram based on age and history if undergoing general anesthesia for bone marrow harvest
- *The following must be documented:*
  - Suitability of the donor to undergo stem cell or bone marrow collection

- Vaccination history
- Travel history
- Blood transfusion history
- Risk of disease transmission, including a targeted screening history, physical examination, and laboratory testing (as previously described)
- Abnormal findings and rationale for proceeding to transplantation
- Counseling of donor regarding abnormal findings and planned follow-up
- Recipient informed of abnormal findings and findings documented in his or her chart
- Patient informed of tests performed to protect the health of the patient
- Patient informed of the right to review test results

Data from Foundation for the Accreditation of Cellular Therapy (FACT). (2015). Patient care and laboratory procedures. Available at http://www.factwebsite.org/ (accessed February 17, 2016); Schmit-Pokorny, K. (2013). Stem cell collection. In S. A Ezzone (Ed.). *Hematopoietic stem cell transplantation: A manual for nursing practice* (2nd ed., pp. 23-46). Pittsburgh, PA: Oncology Nursing Society.

In selecting an individual to serve as an allogeneic HSCT donor, histocompatibility testing (i.e., tissue typing) is performed to evaluate the HLA match between the tissue antigens of the donor and those of the recipient. HLAs are expressed on the surface of various cells, particularly WBCs. The genes that encode these antigens are known as the major histocompatibility complex (MHC) in nonhuman vertebrates. Most HLA genes occupy the short arm of chromosome 6. This genetic region has been subdivided into chromosomal regions called classes I, II, and III. The role of class III antigens in HSCT remains unclear.

Class I antigens are encoded by *HLA-A*, *HLA-B*, and *HLA-C* genes, as well as genes that are less frequently discussed (e.g., *HLA-E, HLA-F, HLA-G*). Class II antigens are encoded by *HLA-DR, HLA-DP,* and *HLA-DQ* genes, as well as variations of these genes. Traditionally, the loci critical for matching in HSCT are *HLA-A, HLA-B,* and *HLA-DR. HLA-C* and *HLA-DQ* are also sometimes considered when determining the appropriateness of a donor (Fürst et al., 2013). A person's tissue type is determined by these genes, which contain information for cell surface antigens that all T lymphocytes use to differentiate self from nonself. To ensure the best possible acceptance of donor stem cells and to prevent significant GVHD, it is best to match all HLA sites.

Each person has two *HLA-A, HLA-B, HLA-C, HLA-DR,* and *HLA-DQ* genes that are inherited as a haplotype (i.e., DNA segment containing closely linked gene variations that are inherited as a single unit) from each parent. Many genetic variations can occur at each locus, resulting in a large number of HLA combinations. The higher the number of antigens that match between donor and transplant recipient, the higher the likelihood of compatibility and the lower the risk of severe acute and chronic GVHD and graft rejection.

Donor selection is critical to the success of allogeneic HSCT (Schmidt & Porkorny, 2013; Tay, Allan, Tinmouth, Coyle, & Hébert, 2013). Selection of an appropriate HLA-matched donor for allogeneic HSCT is based on a number of factors, the most important of which is the degree of HLA matching between the donor and recipient. Other factors are the CMV serologic status of the donor and recipient, type and stage of the recipient's underlying disease, urgency to move ahead with transplantation, speed of engraftment, need for a subsequent graft or donor lymphocyte infusion (DLI), donor and recipient ages, and recipient comorbidities.

Related donors are usually siblings because they have the greatest chance of matching HLA major and minor antigens. Because one half of an HLA type is inherited from each parent, patients statistically have a one in four chance of having a sibling that is a full HLA match. If more than one donor is HLA identical to the patient, donor selection is based on sex of the donor, CMV serologic status of recipient and the donor, ABO compatibility, donor age, recipient-donor body size difference, and donor (if female) parity. All of these factors are associated with improved outcomes of HSCT (Tay et al., 2013).

A mismatch in ABO blood group between patient and donor does not preclude successful HSCT. Depending on the direction of the incompatibility (i.e., major or minor incompatibility), the hematopoietic stem cell product may have to be depleted of RBCs to prevent a hemolytic reaction at the time of infusion caused by ABO antibodies. After engraftment of the donor cells and approximately 100 days after transplantation, the recipient of an ABO-mismatched transplant seroconverts to the ABO type of the donor.

Alternative Donor Sources of Hematopoietic Stem Cells

Matched Unrelated Donor. The average patient in the United States in need of an allogeneic HSCT has about a 30% chance of finding an HLA-matched family donor (Forman & Nakamura, 2011). For the 70% of patients who do not have an HLA-compatible donor, an unrelated donor is sought through the bone marrow donor registries and placental cord blood registries, the largest of which is the National Marrow Donor Program (NMDP, 2015). The NMDP was established in 1986 to allow patients without a related donor to find an HLA-matched unrelated donor or a matched unrelated source of UCB.

The same factors that are considered when choosing a matched sibling donor apply when choosing among multiple matched unrelated donors (MUDs). Eleven million potential bone marrow or PBSC donors and 193,000 UCB units have been typed for the NMDP, giving a patient in need of allogeneic HSCT transplantation a 91% to 99% chance of finding an appropriate donor (NMDP, 2015). Minority patients (i.e., non-white groups) have a significantly lower chance of finding a well-matched donor due to the limited donor pool. Finding an appropriate, well-matched, healthy adult volunteer donor may take weeks to months. The recipient's transplantation physician may request PBSC or bone marrow collection. The overall risk of GVHD, graft rejection, and TRM are higher with MUD transplantation (CIBMTR & NMDP, 2015; Perumbeti, 2014) than with matched sibling donor transplants.

Umbilical Cord Blood. UCB transplantation refers to the use of hematopoietic stem cells collected from the umbilical cord and placenta at the time of birth. About 40 to 70 mL of fetal cord blood is collected immediately after the cord is clamped and cut. Worldwide, these units are cryopreserved and then stored in a public or private cord blood bank for future use. This type of collection has no risk to the donor if the cord is appropriately clamped. Recipients of UCB stem cells may be related (i.e., cells from a family member) or unrelated (i.e., cells donated to a UCB registry) (Tiercy, 2014).

Because of the relative immaturity of the immune system in cord samples, stem cells from UCB allow crossing of immunologic barriers that would otherwise be prohibitive. The degree of tolerable HLA disparity is much greater in cord blood transplants. A match of four to six of the six HLA-A, HLA-B, and HLA-DRB1 antigens is sufficient for transplantation because the degree and severity of GVHD are lower after cord blood transplantation (Ballen, Gluckman, & Broxmeyer, 2013; Forman & Nakamura, 2011). Unfortunately, the lack of GVHD may also result in a diminished GVT effect and higher rates of posttransplantation relapse compared with MUD transplantations using PBSCs or bone marrow.

Advantages of a UCB transplant are that it is readily available and can be shipped to the recipient's transplantation center immediately on request; it carries less risk of viral contamination (e.g., CMV, EBV); and it is transplantable across HLA barriers with diminished risk of GVHD compared with similarly mismatched stem cells from peripheral blood or bone marrow (Schmit-Pokorny, 2013). UCB stem cells have historically been thought of as immunologically naïve and are typed and matched for HLA-A, HLA-B, and HLA-DRB1 only, without consideration of HLA-C. Some data suggest that mismatch of HLA-C is an independent risk factor for TRM, and it is being further reviewed (Tiercy, 2014).

A major limitation of UCB HSCT is the relatively small number of stem cells obtained from each collection. This approach is difficult for transplantation in older (larger) children and adults because the small stem cell volume may result in delayed engraftment and increased risk of infections and TRM. Many adult patients require more than one cord blood unit to achieve adequate engraftment (Ballen, Gluckman, & Broxmeyer, 2013). Other limitations include a decreased GVT

effect and an inability to obtain additional cells from the donor if a DLI or graft boost is needed (Ooi, 2009).

Haploidentical Hematopoietic Stem Cell Transplantation. Haploidentical (i.e., four-antigen or half-matched family member) HSCT may provide an opportunity for most patients to benefit from HSCT when an HLA genotypically matched sibling is not available. Early, mismatched allograft results from the late 1980s and 1990s were disappointing because of unacceptable TRM and morbidity such as fatal GVHD and infectious complications.

Haploidentical stem cell grafts require the removal of T lymphocytes because they are responsible for the immunologic response of GVHD. Advances with effective T-cell depletion (TCD), including the use of posttransplantation cyclophosphamide for in vivo depletion and the use of megadoses of stem cells, has lowered the risk of acute and chronic GVHD, produced acceptable TRM rates, and improved overall survival (Alpdogan, Grosso, & Flomenberg, 2013; Di Bartolomeo et al., 2013; Wang, Wang, Sun, & Huang, 2013). However, the problems related to delayed immune reconstitution causing posttransplantation infectious complications and posttransplantation relapse remain.

Ongoing studies are comparing the effectiveness of haploidentical bone marrow donated from family members with two partially matched unrelated donor UCB units in adult patients with high-risk leukemia or lymphoma (National Cancer Institute, 2015). Studies such as these offer HSCT to selected patients who lack a well-matched HLA sibling or unrelated donor.

Stem Cell Harvesting, Mobilization, and Collection

Although the bone marrow spaces contain more pluripotent stem cells than blood, a significant number of them circulate in the peripheral blood and are used in autologous and allogeneic HSCT. The process of harvesting and collecting hematopoietic stem cells depends on the type of transplantation. Progenitor (pluripotent) stem cells may be obtained by bone marrow harvest or collected from the peripheral blood by apheresis. The third option for obtaining pluripotent stem cells is the use of umbilical cord and placental blood. These cells are harvested immediately after delivery and cryopreserved for subsequent use.

Bone Marrow Harvest

Bone marrow is the most common stem cell source in pediatric allogeneic transplantation because of the long term-risk of chronic GVHD associated with PBSCs. When stem cells are obtained from the donor's bone marrow, the harvesting procedure is performed in the operating room under spinal or general anesthesia. The figure on page 184 shows a bone marrow harvest procedure. Multiple aspirations are obtained from each posterior iliac crest with large-bore bone marrow harvest needles until a total of 1 to 4×10^8 nucleated cells per kilogram of the recipient's body weight or ideal body weight is achieved (Forman & Nakamura, 2011). The total volume of bone marrow harvested usually is 10 mL/kg of the recipient's actual or ideal body weight.

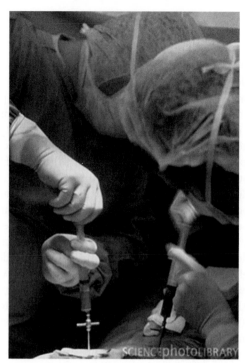

Bone marrow harvest procedure. (Courtesy BSIP Boucharlat/Science Photo Library.)

The marrow is placed in a heparinized tissue culture medium and filtered for the removal of fat and bone particles and then is infused at the recipient's bedside. Marrow is ideally harvested from the donor on the same day it is infused into the patient. Rarely, the bone marrow may be cryopreserved until the recipient is ready for transplantation. The bone marrow harvest procedure usually takes 1 to 2 hours, and most donors are discharged the same day. Postoperative pain after a bone marrow harvest is mild to moderate and usually lasts 2 to 7 days after the procedure.

Complications of bone marrow harvest are rare, but donors may experience infection, hypovolemia, hematoma, and general anesthesia side effects. Bone marrow donors may also become anemic and require an RBC transfusion. The bone marrow donor may elect to bank his or her blood for autotransfusion after the bone marrow harvest. It is recommended that bone marrow donors take 5 to 7 days off from work or school. Typically, the bone marrow cells removed from the donor are replaced within a few weeks after harvest (Schmit-Pokorny, 2013).

Peripheral Blood Stem Cell Collection

Hematopoietic stem cells may be collected from the peripheral blood for autologous and allogeneic HSCT. Collecting stem cells from the blood compared with harvesting them from the bone marrow has demonstrated several advantages for the transplant recipient. The greatest advantage is that PBSCs provide a more rapid hematopoietic recovery (CIBMTR & NMDP, 2015; Forman & Nakamura, 2011; Schmit-Pokony, 2013).

Because stem cells are not abundant in the peripheral blood, chemotherapy (for autologous transplant recipients providing their own stem cells) or colony-stimulating factors

(for autologous transplant recipients and healthy donors providing an allogeneic stem cell transplant) must be given before collecting PBSCs. Chemotherapy, granulocyte colony-stimulating factor (G-CSF), and granulocyte-macrophage colony-stimulating factor (GM-CSF) are commonly used before collection because they stimulate the stem cells that originate in the bone marrow to move into the peripheral blood circulation. This process is called *mobilization*. Chemotherapy given before autologous stem cell collection stimulates stem cell mobilization and provides an antitumor effect. Chemokine antagonists such as plerixafor have been used in combination with G-CSF to mobilize stem cells into the bloodstream of patients who have difficulty mobilizing cells with CSFs alone or with chemotherapy (Shaughnessy et al., 2013). Stem cell collection usually begins after 4 or 5 days of daily G-CSF or GM-CSF injections, depending on the donor's WBC count.

After stem cell mobilization, hematopoietic progenitor cells are collected from the peripheral blood by a method called *apheresis*. The patient's (autologous) or donor's (allogeneic) blood is withdrawn through a wide-bore, double-lumen central venous catheter or large-bore, antecubital Angiocath intravenous catheter. An apheresis machine, a commercial cell separator, is used to centrifuge the blood and separate the components by density into various layers (Schmit-Pokorny, 2013). The WBC and platelet layer is located between the RBC and plasma layers. Pluripotent stem cells are located in the WBC layer. The stem cell layer is transferred into a collection bag, and the remaining blood components are returned to the patient. The figure below shows a donor undergoing PBSC collection. The procedure takes approximately 3 to 6 hours, and the number of leukapheresis procedures required is determined by the number of stem cells harvested at each session. The goal is to collect 5×10^6 CD34$^+$ cells per kilogram of the recipient's body weight (Forman & Nakamura, 2011). The CD34$^+$ antigen is expressed on the surface of early progenitor cells.

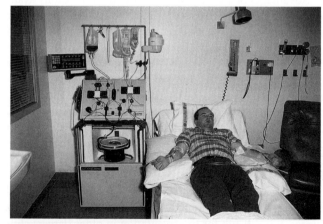

Patient undergoing peripheral blood stem cell collection. (From Hoffbrand A. V., Pettit J.E., Vyas P. (2010). *Color atlas of clinical hematology* (4th ed.). Philadelphia: Mosby.)

Side effects during and immediately after PBSC collection are usually minimal but include transient headache, hypocalcemia, chills, fatigue, vertigo, and tingling in the lips and extremities. Hypocalcemia is relatively common and is caused by the sodium citrate solution that is used to prevent blood clotting in the machine during the collection procedure. Symptoms may be averted by administering an oral calcium carbonate supplement during the collection. Intravenous calcium supplementation may be required if the serum calcium level is low or hypocalcemia symptoms are severe.

Conditioning Therapy and Preparative Regimen

The treatment course begins with the preparative or conditioning regimen. The combination of chemotherapy, radiotherapy, and biologic therapy in preparation for HSCT is referred to as the *preparative regimen*. Because evidence has not shown that one conditioning regimen is superior to another, the choice is often based on the transplantation team's experience and preference. Selection of the ideal regimen for the patient should take into account stem cell source (i.e., autologous or allogeneic), diagnosis, disease stage at the time of transplantation, prior therapies, and comorbidities (Alousi & de Lima, 2008; de Lima, Alousi, & Giralt, 2015; Gyurkocza & Sandmaier, 2014; McAdams & Burgunder, 2013).

The preparative regimen usually includes high doses of chemotherapy with or without TBI, which is administered over the days preceding stem cell infusion. The doses and schedule of the preparative regimen depend on the patient's disease, type of transplantation (i.e., autologous or allogeneic), and goal of therapy (Gyurkocza & Sandmaier, 2014; Harris, 2010; McAdams & Burgunder, 2013; Wikle Shapiro, 2015). In allogeneic transplantation, the purpose of the preparative regimen is to eradicate malignant disease, ablate the existing bone marrow to create space for the donor stem cells to engraft, and provide sufficient immunosuppression to allow the recipient to accept the transplanted stem cells. The goal of the preparative regimen in autologous transplantation is to deliver high-dose, intensive myeloablative therapy. Subsequent infusion of autologous stem cells rescues the patient from myeloablation. Posttransplantation immunosuppression is not required for autologous transplantation because the patient receives his or her own hematopoietic stem cells, avoiding the risk of graft rejection and GVHD.

Myeloablative Preparative Regimen

The rationale for selecting agents for a myeloablative preparative regimen is that a greater degree of tumor cell death can provide improved disease response and overall survival. High-dose chemotherapy preparative regimens are combinations of the most effective agents for a particular disease given at high doses with the goal of myeloablation. Drugs with different (i.e., nonoverlapping) nonhematologic dose-limiting toxicities are typically combined and given at maximal doses. Alkylating agents such as cyclophosphamide, carboplatin, busulfan, thiotepa, cisplatin, melphalan, and carmustine are used in combination with other agents such as etoposide, fludarabine, and cytarabine and sometimes with TBI to destroy the bone marrow and eradicate disease.

The tables in the next column and on page 186 list common preparative regimens and their indications (Childs, 2011; de Lima, Alousi, & Giralt, 2015; Forman & Nakamura, 2011; McAdams &

Burgunder, 2013) and the adverse effects of individual drugs used in combination in the preparative regimen for transplantation.

Common Preparative Regimens and Indications

Regimen	Indication
Total body irradiation, etoposide, cyclophosphamide (TBI/CY/VP)	Lymphoid malignancies
Cyclophosphamide, total body irradiation (CY/TBI)	Hematologic malignancies, non-Hodgkin lymphoma, myelodysplastic syndromes
Busulfan, cyclophosphamide (BU/CY)	Myeloid leukemias, metabolic disorders, myelodysplastic syndromes
Busulfan, fludarabine (Bu/Flu)	Hematologic malignancies, myelodysplastic syndromes, nonmalignant allogeneic hematopoietic stem cell transplantation
Carmustin, etoposide, cytarabine, melphalan ± rituximab (BEAM ± R)	Hodgkin lymphoma, non-Hodgkin lymphoma
Cyclophosphamide, carmustine, etoposide ± rituximab (CBV ± R)	Hodgkin lymphoma, non-Hodgkin lymphoma
Cyclophosphamide, antithymocyte globulin (CY/ATG)	Marrow failure syndromes (severe aplastic anemia), hemoglobinopathies
Carboplatin, thiotepa (Carbo/Thio)	Brain tumors
Melphalan ± bortezomib	Multiple myeloma
Reduced-Intensity Regimens	
Fludarabine, melphalan (Flu/Mel)	Multiple myeloma
Low-dose total body irradiation, fludarabine	Multiple myeloma

From Childs, R. W. (2011). Allogeneic stem cell transplantation. In T. S. Lawrence & S. A. Rosenberg (Eds.). *Cancer: Principles and practice of oncology* (9th ed., pp. 2244-2263). Philadelphia: Lippincott, Williams & Wilkins; de Lima, M., Alousi, A., & Giralt, S., S. (2015). Preparative regimens for hematopoietic cell transplantation. In R. Hoffman, B. Furie, E. J. Benz, Jr., P. McGlave, L. E. Silberstein, & S. J. Shattil (Eds.). *Hematology: Basic principles and practice*. Philadelphia: Elsevier; Gyurkocza, B., & Sandmaier, B. M. (2014). Conditioning regimens for hematopoietic cell transplantation: One size does not fit all. *Blood, 124*(3), 344-353.

Monoclonal and polyclonal agents such as antithymocyte globulin (ATG) or alemtuzumab are added to the preparative regimen to provide the additional immunosuppression needed to prevent graft rejection and acute GVHD when an unrelated adult donor, an unrelated cord blood unit, or a haploidentical donor is used.

Reduced-Intensity Conditioning Regimens

GVHD can be a serious complication (described later), but it also controls the underlying malignancy by causing a GVT effect. The immunologic response is mediated by donor immunocompetent T cells that recognize the host tumor cells as foreign and destroy them. The GVT effect was recognized over time as contributing to the success of allogeneic HSCT.

In an effort to exploit the benefit of GVT, many investigators lowered the dose of radiation and chemotherapeutic agents in the conditioning regimen. This approach caused a major paradigm shift, and the pool of eligible patients for allogeneic HSCT was greatly expanded. However, not all malignancies are equally susceptible to the GVT effect. Myeloid leukemias, chronic lymphocytic leukemia, Hodgkin lymphoma, neuroblastoma, and low-grade indolent lymphomas (i.e., follicular

Nonhematologic Side Effects of Agents Used in Preparative Regimens and Conditioning Therapy

Therapeutic Agent	Side Effects
Antithymocyte globulin (ATG) and alemtuzumab	Fever, chills, and hypersensitivity during infusion (reaction may worsen with each subsequent dose), prolonged immunosuppression
Busulfan	Seizures, interstitial pulmonary fibrosis, hepatic dysfunction (including veno-occlusive disease), acute cholecystitis, mucositis, skin hyperpigmentation, desquamation, and acral erythema
Carmustine	Hepatic, pulmonary, central nervous system (with BCNU), cardiac effects (arrhythmias and hypotension), nausea, and vomiting
Carboplatin	Nausea and vomiting, nephrotoxicity, liver function abnormalities (including veno-occlusive disease), ototoxicity
Cisplatin	Nausea and vomiting, neurotoxicity (peripheral neuropathy, ataxia, visual disturbances), ototoxicity, renal dysfunction
Cyclophosphamide	Cardiac effects (cardiomyopathy, congestive heart failure, hemorrhagic cardiac necrosis, pericardial effusion, electrocardiographic abnormalities), interstitial pulmonary fibrosis, hemorrhagic cystitis, elevated liver enzyme values, nausea and vomiting, metabolic (syndrome of inappropriate antidiuretic hormone secretion [SIADH])
Cytosine arabinoside (Ara-C)	Cerebellar toxicity, encephalopathy, seizures, conjunctivitis, skin (rash, acral erythema), nausea and vomiting, diarrhea, renal insufficiency, liver function abnormalities, pancreatitis, noncardiogenic pulmonary edema, fever, arthralgias
Etoposide (Etopophos)	Hypersensitivity reactions, hypotension, liver function abnormalities and chemical hepatitis, renal dysfunction, nausea and vomiting, metabolic acidosis, mucositis, stomatitis, painful rash on the palms, soles, and periorbital area
Fludarabine	Mucositis, diarrhea, pulmonary fibrosis, pneumonitis, hypersensitivity reaction during infusion, neuropathy, central nervous system toxicity, coma
Ifosfamide	Hemorrhagic cystitis at high doses, encephalopathy, coma, hallucinations, confusion, mental status changes
Melphalan	Acute hypersensitivity, renal toxicity, mucositis, nausea and vomiting, hepatic toxicity (including veno-occlusive disease)
Thiotepa	Hyperpigmentation, acute erythroderma, dry desquamation, liver function abnormalities (including veno-occlusive disease), mucositis, esophagitis, dysuria, hypersensitivity reaction during infusion
Total body irradiation	Nausea, vomiting, diarrhea, parotiditis, xerostomia, stomatitis, erythema, pneumonitis, veno-occlusive disease

From Alousi, A., &, de Lima, M. (2008). Ablative preparative regimens for hematopoietic stem cell transplantation. In R. Soiffer (Ed.). *Hematopoietic stem cell transplantation* (2nd ed., pp. 321-347). New York: Humana Press; de Lima, M., Alousi, A., & Giralt, S. (2015). Preparative regimens for hematopoietic cell transplantation. In R. Hoffman, B. Furie, E. J. Benz, Jr., P. McGlave, L. E. Silberstein, & S. J. Shattil (Eds.). *Hematology: Basic principles and practice.* Philadelphia: Elsevier; Gyurkocza, B., & Sandmaier, B. M. (2014). Conditioning regimens for hematopoietic cell transplantation: One size does not fit all. *Blood, 124*(3), 344-353.

lymphoma and mantle cell lymphoma) appear to be particularly responsive to the GVT effect.

An RIC regimen followed by allogeneic HSCT provides treatment options for older patients and those who have undergone a prior transplantation or have comorbidities such as heart, lung, kidney, or liver disease and would therefore not tolerate a high-dose conditioning regimen. RIC regimens typically use combinations of chemotherapy drugs, such as fludarabine, busulfan, and melphalan at reduced doses with or without low-dose TBI. Combinations of potent immunosuppressive medications such as ATG or alemtuzumab are also commonly added to the RIC chemoradiotherapy regimen.

The RIC regimens are not without risk. Patients undergoing transplantation after an RIC regimen experience many of the same complications as those undergoing conventional, fully myeloablative allogeneic transplantation regimens. Problems encountered in the early posttransplantation period, such as infection, bleeding, and regimen-related toxicities, may be less after an RIC regimen for HSCT, but the risk of GVHD and the long-term risk of infection continue to be problems.

Stem Cell Infusion

The infusion of stem cells is a relatively simple procedure, much like a blood transfusion. In allogeneic HSCT, the stem cells (i.e., bone marrow or PBSCs) are usually infused immediately after they are collected. Autologous stem cells are cryopreserved with dimethylsulfoxide (DMSO) and must be thawed in a warm solution bath at the bedside just before reinfusion.

The cells are typically infused through a central venous catheter over 30 to 90 minutes, depending on the total volume of the product and the size of the recipient. Cryopreserved stem cells (i.e., autologous PBSCs and UCB cells) are usually preserved in smaller volumes and are usually aspirated from the cryopreservation bag into a large syringe and are slowly pushed through the central venous catheter. A leukocyte-depleting (leukopoor) filter should never be used when infusing HSCTs. An infusion pump should not be used to administer stem cells, and only normal saline solution is used to prime and flush the tubing.

Premedication with acetaminophen and diphenhydramine is often recommended, and patients should receive hydration before and after the procedure to maintain renal perfusion. Patients who receive a cryopreserved product should be premedicated with an antiemetic to combat nausea from the DMSO or residual nausea from the chemotherapeutic preparatory regimen. Vital signs and pulse oximetry are monitored closely before, during, and at intervals after stem cell infusion.

Complications of stem cell infusion are rare but may include pulmonary edema, hemolysis, infection, and anaphylaxis. Infrequently, DMSO can cause an infusion reaction that may include bradycardia (and rarely heart block) or hypertension, and an acute hypersensitivity reaction may occur. DMSO-associated RBC hemolysis may require vigorous hydration to prevent renal toxicity. Throughout the infusion, patients should be monitored for volume overload and complaints suggesting pulmonary embolism, such as chest pain, dyspnea, and cough.

Early Complications of Stem Cell Transplantation

After stem cell infusion, the hematopoietic stem cells migrate to the bone marrow spaces, where they are attracted by chemotactic factors. Engraftment occurs when the transplanted progenitor cells begin to grow and manufacture new hematopoietic cells in the bone marrow. After stem cell infusion but before complete hematopoietic cell engraftment, patients have severe pancytopenia that results in a heightened risk of infection and bleeding. Other early toxicities include mucositis, skin breakdown, renal dysfunction, and veno-occlusive disease of the liver. Examples of early and late complications arising from autologous and allogeneic stem cell transplantation can be found in the box below.

Nonhematologic adverse effects depend on the agents used for the preparative regimen. The nonhematologic adverse effects that are associated with the agents that typically comprise stem cell transplant conditioning regimens are outlined in the table on page 186.

Early and Late Complications of Autologous and Allogeneic Stem Cell Transplantation

Early (Before Day 100)
- Regimen-related toxicity
  - Hemorrhagic cystitis
  - Pulmonary complications
  - Renal complications
  - Neurologic complications
  - Severe immunosuppression
- Nutritional deficiencies
- Idiopathic pneumonitis
- Graft failure
- Infection
  - Viral
  - Bacterial
  - Fungal
- Acute graft-versus-host disease
- Relapse

Late (After Day 100)
- Regimen-related toxicity
  - Cataracts
  - Neurologic conditions (peripheral and autonomic neuropathies)
  - Gonadal dysfunction
  - Endocrine dysfunction
- Immunodeficiency
- Infection
  - Encapsulated bacteria
  - Viruses (cytomegalovirus, varicella-zoster virus)
  - Fungal (*Aspergillus* spores)
- Epstein-Barr virus posttransplantation lymphoproliferative disorder (PTLD)
- Musculoskeletal problems
  - Osteoporosis
  - Avascular necrosis
- Chronic graft-versus-host disease
- Relapse of malignancy
- Secondary relapse

Pancytopenia

Hematopoietic growth factors (e.g., G-CSF, GM-CSF) are given after transplantation to accelerate neutrophil recovery, reducing the period of neutropenia and decreasing the risk of early infection. Transfusion support is provided by platelets and packed RBCs.

Except for hematopoietic stem cell grafts and donor lymphocytes, all blood products given to HSCT recipients should be leukoreduced to remove WBCs, which may transmit CMV, and irradiated with 2500 cGy to prevent transfusion-associated GVHD. Most centers recommend that allogeneic stem cell recipients receive irradiated blood products for the rest of their lives, and they are encouraged to purchase a Medic-Alert bracelet that specifies their need for irradiated blood products.

Infection

Infections have constituted a major threat since the introduction of HSCT. They remain a significant obstacle to the success of HSCT, along with relapsed malignancy and GVHD.

Most posttransplantation infections are divided into three phases. Phase I is the pre-engraftment phase, phase II is the postengraftment phase, and phase III is the late infection phase.

During phase I (day 0 to 15), prolonged neutropenia and breaks in the mucocutaneous barrier result in a substantial risk of bacteremia and fungal infections, including those by *Candida* species and, as neutropenia continues, *Aspergillus* species. Herpes simplex virus (HSV) reactivation occurs during this phase.

During phase II (day 15 to 100), infections are primarily associated with impaired cell-mediated immunity. The scope and impact of this defect is determined by the extent of GVHD and the immunosuppressive therapy used to control it. Herpesviruses, particularly CMV, are common infectious agents during this period. Other dominant pathogens include *Pneumocystis jiroveci* and *Aspergillus* species.

During phase III (day 100+), persons with chronic GVHD and recipients of alternative-donor allogeneic transplants remain most at risk for infection due to delayed or prolonged immunosuppression. Common pathogens include CMV, varicella-zoster virus (VZV), and encapsulated bacteria (e.g., *Streptococcus pneumoniae*).

The risk of disease from community-acquired respiratory viruses is elevated during all three phases. In phase III, the outpatient status of hematopoietic stem cell recipients can complicate efforts to reduce exposure and provide timely intervention. The figure on page 188 shows the three posttransplantation phases of infections and contributory factors (Tomblyn et al., 2009).

The risk of infection is primarily determined by the time from transplantation, degree of immune reconstitution, and presence or absence of GVHD. Other factors include donor-/host histocompatibility, disease status, type of transplantation (e.g., PBSCs), marrow conditioning intensity, and neutrophil engraftment. The table on page 188 outlines the factors affecting the HSCT patient's risk of infection (Chawala & Greenstein,

2013; McAdams and Burgunder, 2013; Tomblyn et al., 2009). Strategies to limit exposure to infectious organisms are essential for transplant recipients who are neutropenic and those receiving immunosuppressive medications.

Infection Prophylaxis and Treatment. Most post-HSCT infections are predictable and surmountable with the use of tailored preventative and early-detection strategies. Infectious disease prophylaxis and vaccinations can be used to prevent infections. Changes in the transplantation procedures and the implementation of effective supportive care strategies have decreased the incidence and severity of infectious complications in each posttransplantation phase (Tomblyn et al., 2009).

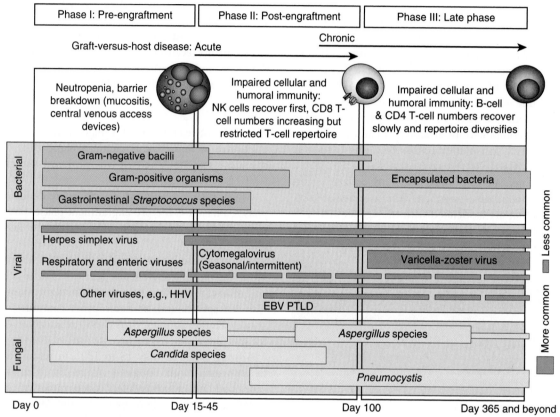

Three posttransplantation phases of infections and contributory factors. (From Tomblyn, M., Chiller, T., Einsele, H., et al.: (2009). Guidelines for preventing infectious complications among hematopoietic cell transplantation recipients: A global perspective. *Biology of Blood Marrow Transplantation 15*(10):1143-1238.)

Factors Affecting the Risk of Infection

Factor	Risk of Infection
Type of transplantation	Higher risk with allogeneic; lower risk with autologous or syngeneic, depending on graft manipulation and the clinical setting, including previous therapies
Time from transplantation	Lower risk with more time elapsed from transplantation
Pretransplantation factors	Higher risk with extensive pretransplantation immunosuppressive therapy (e.g., fludarabine, clofarabine), prolonged pretransplantation neutropenia or pretransplantation infection
Graft-versus-host disease (GVHD)	Higher risk with grades III and IV acute GVHD or extensive, chronic GVHD
Human leukocyte antigen (HLA) match	Higher risk with HLA-mismatched donors, particularly with haploidentical donors
Disease (e.g., leukemia)	Higher risk with more advanced disease at the time of transplantation (heavy pretreatment chemotherapy or radiotherapy)
Donor type	Higher risk with unrelated donor marrow or umbilical cord blood than with a fully matching sibling donor
Graft type	Highest risk with T-cell depletion and umbilical cord blood, intermediate risk with bone marrow, and lowest risk with colony-stimulating factor–mobilized blood stem cells; higher risk with T-cell–depleted grafts, depending on method used
Immunosuppression after transplantation	Higher risk with immunosuppressive drugs, particularly with corticosteroids, antithymocyte globulin, alemtuzumab, delayed immune recovery (umbilical cord blood, T-cell depletion), chronic GVHD
Conditioning intensity	Lower risk in the first 1 to 3 months after transplantation with reduced-intensity regimen; higher with total body irradiation regimens

Adapted from McAdams, F. W., & Burgunder, M. R. (2013). Transplant treatment course and acute complications. In S. Ezzone (Ed.). *Hematopoietic stem cell transplantation: A manual for nursing practice* (2nd ed., pp. 44-47). Pittsburgh, PA: Oncology Nursing Society; Tomblyn, M., Chiller, T., Einsele, H., Gress, R., Sepkowitz, K., Storek, J., Boeckh, M. J. (2009). Guidelines for preventing infectious complications among hematopoietic cell transplantation recipients: A global perspective. *Biology of Blood Marrow Transplantation, 15*(10), 1143-1238.

The Centers for Disease Control and Prevention (CDC) in its *Morbidity and Mortality Weekly Report* provides guidelines for preventing opportunistic infections in patients undergoing HSCT (CDC, 2000). Hospitals that perform HSCT should have appropriately designed facilities that have rooms with more than 12 air exchanges per hour and point-of-use high-efficiency particulate air (HEPA) filtration. HEPA filters should be able to remove particles at least as small as 0.3 µm in diameter. Rooms should have positive air pressure compared with the hallway unless housing a patient who has active disease with a pathogen that has airborne transmission (e.g., VZV); in such cases, a negative-pressure room is recommended.

Policies and procedures should be in the hospital infection-control manual to address issues of construction and renovation, cleaning, and isolation and barrier precautions. Hand washing should be strongly emphasized to prevent nosocomial transmission of infection. Most transplantation centers recommend that plants and dried or fresh flowers should not be allowed in HSCT patient rooms, although exposure has not been conclusively shown to cause fungal infections. Health care workers should follow a policy with regard to their immunizations and vaccinations. Health care workers with symptoms of viral illness should not care for HSCT patients (Chawala & Greenstein, 2013).

Strict adherence to visitor policies is required, particularly for children with potentially infectious conditions (e.g., varicella, community-acquired respiratory viruses). Oral and skin care should be stressed to patients throughout the bone marrow transplantation process. All patients undergoing HSCT should receive a dental evaluation before initiation of the preparative phase of transplantation. Patients with mucositis during conditioning or after transplantation should maintain a regimen of proper oral care (CDC, 2000).

Strategies for safe living after discharge from the hospital are important to discuss with HSCT recipients. Many centers provide controlled patient housing for HSCT recipients who are in the early posttransplantation phase. Patient education at discharge should include a discussion of how to avoid environmental infectious exposures, safe sex practices, pet safety, food and water safety, travel safety, and the need for posttransplantation vaccinations (CDC, 2000; Chawala & Greenstein, 2013).

Bacterial Infection Prophylaxis. The use of prophylactic antibiotic therapy in HSCT remains controversial (CDC, 2000; Chawala & Greenstein, 2013; Tomblyn et al., 2009). During the pre-engraftment phase, fluoroquinolones are often used in adult HSCT recipients to decrease the incidence of gram-negative bacteremia. β-lactam and macrolide prophylactic antibiotics have also been used prophylactically to reduce the incidence of gram-positive bacteremia (CDC, 2000; Chawala & Greenstein, 2013; Tomblyn et al., 2009). However, the use of prophylactic antibiotics may lead to the development of resistant organisms. Another concern is the increased risk of *Clostridium difficile* infection.

Mucosal injury, which results from the conditioning regimen, leads to translocation of bacteria, with approximately 40% of infections due to gram-negative organisms such as *Pseudomonas, Enterobacter, Escherichia coli,* and *Klebsiella*. Gram-positive bacteria, especially *Staphylococcus epidermidis, Streptococcus viridians,* and *Staphylococcus aureus*, colonize central venous catheters, leading to bacteremia that requires prompt initiation of appropriate antibiotics (Chalwala & Greenstein, 2013; Kedia et al., 2013). The treatment of bacterial infections before engraftment is usually empiric, with broad-spectrum antibiotic therapy started at the onset of any fever. Treatment is then tailored with the isolation of organisms but remains broad spectrum for continued coverage of all pathogens that are likely in HSCT patients who are profoundly neutropenic for a prolonged period. Treatment with empiric antibiotics usually continues until the engraftment of neutrophils.

Empiric coverage usually consists of one or more antipseudomonal agents alone or in combination with an antistaphylococcal antibiotic. Common choices include a carbapenem, such as imipenem or meropenem, and a cephalosporin, such as cefepime and ceftazidime, alone or in combination. Gram-positive coverage such as vancomycin or linezolid should also be considered for empiric antibiotic coverage due to the high risk of gram-positive bacteremia in these patients (Kedia et al., 2013). Local antimicrobial resistance patterns at the transplantation center should be considered when choosing the specific antimicrobial agents.

The use of hematopoietic colony-stimulating factors, such as G-CSF, can reduce the period of neutropenia, but the incidence of bacteremia and overall HSCT outcomes have not been influenced (CDC, 2000; Chawala & Greenstein, 2013; McAdams & Burgunder, 2013; Tomblyn et al., 2009). Granulocyte transfusion does not appear to be beneficial, even in the setting of profound neutropenia, but it may be used for the treatment of severe, documented, gram-negative bacterial and fungal infections in HSCT patients with anticipated prolonged neutropenia (Goldfinger & Lu, 2015).

In the late posttransplantation phase because of the increased risk of infection with encapsulated organisms, some centers suggest the use of penicillin prophylaxis and vaccination with the 23-valent polysaccharide *S. pneumoniae* vaccine (CDC, 2000). The role of the newer conjugate pneumococcal vaccines in younger children who have undergone HSCT is being investigated (Kedia et al., 2013; Tomblyn et al., 2009).

Fungal Infections. Factors that increase the HSCT patient's risk of invasive fungal infection include prolonged neutropenia, an indwelling central venous catheter, empiric antibiotic therapy, potent immunosuppressive agents, corticosteroids, GVHD, total parenteral nutrition, and severe mucositis (CDC, 2000; Chawala & Greenstein, 2013; Kedia et al., 2013; McAdams & Burgunder, 2013; Tomblyn et al., 2009). The risk of fungal infection is particularly increased after 5 to 7 days of continuous neutropenia, and most centers begin prophylactic therapy for fungi around this time. More than 80% of HSCT patients who develop fungal infection after transplantation are infected with *Candida* or *Aspergillus* species (Kedia et al., 2013; Nucci & Anaissie, 2009).

Fluconazole prophylaxis has been effective in reducing the number of infections with *C. albicans* and is most commonly used as prophylaxis in HSCT patients who are at lower risk of developing invasive *Aspergillus* infection (i.e., autologous and matched sibling donor transplants) because fluconazole possesses no significant activity against *Aspergillus*. With improved control of CMV infection, *Aspergillus* species have become the most common cause of infectious mortality after HSCT (Chawala & Greenstein, 2013; Kedia et al., 2013; Tomblyn et al., 2009).

For high-risk patients, such as those undergoing unrelated donor, haploidentical, or UCB HSCT, fungal prophylaxis is broadened to include prophylaxis against fungi and molds that are resistant to fluconazole. The newer antifungal agents (e.g., posaconazole, voriconazole, caspofungin) are the most common, effective prophylactic agents against most candidal species and are active against the more resistant fungi such as *Aspergillus* and *Fusarium* and the Mucormycetes class of organisms. In HSCT patients with documented fungal infection, a combination of these pharmacologic agents may be used due to the associated severity and high mortality rates.

Viral Infections

Herpes Simplex Virus. Reactivation of HSV infection can occur at any time after HSCT. The use of prophylactic acyclovir has been very effective in reducing the rate of HSV reactivation from 80% to less than 5% for HSV-seropositive recipients (Kedia et al., 2013; Tomblyn et al., 2009). Prophylactic acyclovir should be started during the conditioning regimen, and it should continue until the HSCT patient's immune system is reconstituted. Higher dose acyclovir is the treatment of choice when HSV infection does develop. When patients do not respond to acyclovir, foscarnet is used until the infection resolves. If foscarnet is unsuccessful, therapy with cidofovir should be attempted (CDC, 2000; Chawala & Greenstein, 2013; Kedia et al., 2013; Tomblyn et al., 2009).

Cytomegalovirus. Allogeneic HSCT recipients should be tested before transplantation for serum anti-CMV immunoglobulin G (IgG) antibodies before transplantation to determine the risk of primary CMV infection and reactivation after HSCT. Before the advent of early detection techniques and the use of ganciclovir prophylaxis in the mid-1990s, CMV was the leading cause of morbidity and mortality among HSCT recipients.

CMV infection can cause fatal pneumonia, enteritis, and retinitis. Up to 70% of allogeneic HSCT patients who are seropositive for CMV or who receive a graft from a seropositive donor will reactivate CMV after transplantation (Boeckh & Ljungman, 2009; Ljungman, 2008). Risk factors for CMV reactivation and disease include acute or chronic GVHD, steroid use, low CD4 counts ($<50/mm^3$), CMV-seronegative donors for CMV seropositive recipients, and unrelated, haploidentical, UCB, or TCD HSCTs. To minimize the risk of CMV primary infection, all blood products (except stem cell and granulocyte products) should be leukocyte filtered.

Two approaches are used when treating patients at risk for CMV disease. The older approach is to administer prophylaxis with ganciclovir to every patient at risk for CMV disease. The newer and more common approach is to perform active CMV surveillance to evaluate evidence of CMV in the body by pp65 cytomegalovirus (CMV) antigenemia assay or by viral polymerase chain reaction (PCR). Because of the potential harmful side effects of prophylactic ganciclovir and advances in viral testing for CMV on which to base early therapy, the preference at most transplantation centers is to use a preemptive approach (Boeckh & Ljungman, 2009; CDC, 2000; Chawala & Greenstein, 2013; Kedia et al., 2013; Tierny & Robinson, 2013; Tomblyn et al., 2009).

Preemptive therapy is based on at least weekly CMV surveillance of allogeneic HSCT patients who are CMV seropositive or who have a CMV seropositive donor. The trend in CMV diagnostics is to use the PCR-determined viral load instead of the antigenemia assay. PCR has better quantitation, less assay variability, and increased sensitivity. After CMV is detected, early preemptive therapy with intravenous ganciclovir is initiated for a minimum of 3 weeks after clearance of the virus (Boeckh & Ljungman, 2009). Oral ganciclovir (i.e., the prodrug valganciclovir) is then used for the maintenance phase of CMV therapy. Foscarnet and cidofovir are also used in patients with apparent or documented ganciclovir-resistant CMV disease. Both drugs have significant nephrotoxicity and must be used with caution in patients on other nephrotoxic medications.

Supplemental intravenous immune globulin (IVIG) is administered to assist in the prevention and treatment of CMV infection in allogeneic HSCT patients. IVIG is usually administered to allogeneic HSCT patients who are hypogammaglobulinemic (i.e., quantitative IgG level <400 mg/dL). IVIG is also used as prophylaxis against myriad other viral infections. CMV-specific immunoglobulin (CMVIG) has been used in addition to ganciclovir in HSCT patients who show signs of CMV; studies of CMVIG versus standard IVIG have had conflicting results (Alexander et al., 2010; Boeckh & Ljungman, 2009).

Treatment of CMV viremia with antivirals does not improve virus-specific immunity, and CMV reactivation and infection can often recur. Cellular immunotherapy for patients with deficient or absent CMV-specific immune system function can be an effective means to provide immediate and long-term protection from CMV. Several small, phase I/II studies have been published using adoptive transfer of donor CMV-specific CD4[+] and CD8[+] T cells, especially in patients developing repeated episodes of CMV disease. However, none of these adoptive T-cell transfer techniques is used in routine clinical practice.

Recipients of autologous HSCT can develop CMV viremia, but they are much less likely to develop CMV infection because they are less immunosuppressed. Patients undergoing autologous HSCT are not routinely screened or administered prophylactic ganciclovir therapy (CDC, 2000; Chawala & Greenstein, 2013; Kedia et al., 2013).

Varicella-Zoster Virus. Varicella-zoster infections can occur in the late posttransplantation phase. Although prophylaxis is not recommended during this period, prevention should be attempted after exposure to chickenpox or shingles.

Varicella-zoster immunoglobulin (VZIG) should be given to patients who are less than 24 months out from an allogeneic HSCT and to those more than 24 months out from allogeneic HSCT who are on immunosuppressive therapy or have chronic GVHD (CDC, 2000). For at-risk patients, VZIG is ideally administered within 48 to 96 hours after exposure to a person with chickenpox or shingles. Patients who have undergone HSCT who develop varicella should be treated for 7 to 10 days with intravenous acyclovir (Chawala & Greenstein, 2013; Kedia et al., 2013; Tierny & Robinson, 2013; Tomblyn et al., 2009).

Community-Acquired Respiratory Viruses and Adenoviruses. Treatment for respiratory viruses and adenoviruses in the patient who has undergone HSCT is not standardized. Adenoviral infections, including hemorrhagic cystitis, gastroenteritis, and pneumonitis, have been managed with some degree of success with cidofovir therapy and supplemental IVIG. Adenovirus is more common in pediatric patients and is often fatal after HSCT.

Many respiratory viruses (e.g., respiratory syncytial virus [RSV], influenza, parainfluenza, rhinovirus) do not have a standard treatment protocol. These community-acquired viral infections can be life-threatening after HSCT. Ribavirin treatment has been attempted using the intravenous or inhalation forms, but results have been inconclusive (Kedia et al., 2013). In some studies, the addition of RSV immune globulin (i.e., palivizumab) in conjunction with a traditional intravenous or inhalation form of ribavirin therapy has shown promise in preventing the progression of RSV upper respiratory infection to the lower respiratory tract and in the treatment of RSV pneumonia.

Autologous and allogeneic stem cell transplant recipients who are more than 6 months beyond transplantation should receive an annual influenza vaccine unless they are on corticosteroids for acute GVHD. Allogeneic HSCT patients more than 6 months but less than 1 year after transplantation should receive an influenza vaccine plus a booster vaccination. For individuals unlikely to receive benefit from influenza vaccine (i.e., less than 6 months after transplantation or on corticosteroids), all household contacts should consider immunization.

Oseltamivir is safe when given to HSCT patients and appears to play an important role in the prevention of the complications of influenza infection in those who test positive for influenza A and B viruses. Patients who test positive for influenza should receive treatment with this medication (Tierny & Robinson, 2013).

Human herpes virus 6 (HHV-6) infection in the HSCT patient is a consequence of viral reactivation. HHV-6 reactivation affects 40% to 60% of allogeneic HSCT patients and usually occurs 2 to 4 weeks after transplantation. Multiple risk factors are associated with HHV-6 reactivation, including mismatched transplants, UCB transplants, younger age, conditioning regimens, acute GVHD, and use of corticosteroids (Chawala & Greenstein, 2013; Kedia et al., 2013).

HHV-6 reactivation has been associated with graft failure, prolonged pancytopenia, and encephalitis after HSCT. HHV-6–associated meningoencephalitis has been treated with ganciclovir and with foscarnet with limited success. Ganciclovir has also been used as prophylaxis to prevent HHV-6 disease. There are no randomized, controlled trials to prove treatment or prophylaxis with ganciclovir is effective against HHV 6.

Epstein-Barr Virus and Posttransplantation Lymphoproliferative Disorder. Stem cell donors and candidates for transplantation should be tested for serum anti-EBV IgG antibodies before transplantation to determine risk for Epstein-Barr virus (EBV) DNA Anemia after HSCT. The recommendation is stronger for pediatric patients than adults. Although fever and mononucleosis can occur in primary EBV infection, the most significant clinical syndrome associated with EBV replication is posttransplantation lymphoproliferative disease (PTLD). It is the result of EBV-infected B cells, resulting in clonal abnormalities with resultant proliferation of lymphoid tissue (i.e., EBV-related lymphoma).

PTLD occurs principally in recipients who have profound T-lymphocyte cytopenia (e.g., after TCD, use of anti–T-cell antibodies, UCB transplants, haploidentical transplants). Early recognition in high-risk patients is important because PTLD tends to be rapidly progressive, and weekly surveillance with PCR may have a role in preventing progression. EBV DNA loads rise as early as 3 weeks before PTLD onset. Monitoring blood loads of EBV DNA allows preemptive reduction in immunosuppression as the first phase of managing PTLD.

Because of the variability of PCR techniques and the difference in risk for EBV-related PTLD (due to the degree of T-cell lymphopenia), no firm recommendation can be made about the threshold for initiation of preemptive therapy. If there is no response to a reduction in immunosuppression, preemptive treatment with immune-based therapies such as rituximab can prevent the progression to PTLD. Infusion of donor-derived, EBV-specific cytotoxic lymphocytes (CTLs) has demonstrated promise in the prophylaxis of EBV lymphoma. Expanded, donor-derived, EBV-specific T cells have also been used to control blood loads of EBV DNA in this setting, but the procedure remains experimental. Immunotherapies are offering promising results (Heslop, 2009).

Managing the Risk of Infection. HSCT is characterized by a variable period of early infectious complications caused largely by neutropenia and mucosal damage because of the preparative regimen. The complications are predictable based on clinical findings of mucositis and absolute neutrophil count. Allogeneic HSCT patients experience a prolonged period of immunosuppression characterized by profound defects in cell-mediated and humoral immunity. Unfortunately, there are no readily available markers with which to accurately measure the relative risk for individual patients. Patients must be monitored carefully and receive early intervention for signs or symptoms of an infectious disease. For most patients, immunocompetence improves progressively with increasing time after transplantation. However, many hematopoietic stem cell recipients remain immunocompromised far beyond 2 years after transplantation, especially those with chronic GVHD, for whom infection remains the most important cause of morbidity and mortality. Work is needed to augment immune reconstitution, for early pathogen detection, and to identify accurate surrogate markers of immunocompetence to guide the long-term treatment of this high-risk population.

Important nursing responsibilities include maintaining a protective environment, practicing consistent and thorough provider hand hygiene, delivering meticulous oral and skin care, monitoring vital signs frequently, and conducting a thorough review of systems and a physical examination to identify potential locations (e.g., alimentary tract, skin, lungs, sinuses, intravascular access device sites) of infection. Although there is limited evidence to support their effectiveness, most transplantation centers provide additional protective measures that may include low-microbial diets, protective isolation with masks and gloves, laminar air filtration, gowning, and gut and skin decontamination.

Sinusoidal Obstructive Syndrome of the Liver

Sinusoidal obstructive syndrome (SOS), also called hepatic veno-occlusive disease (VOD), is part of a spectrum of organ injury syndromes that occur after HSCT. SOS usually affects 10% to 30% of patients after allogeneic stem cell transplantation (Sousa, 2012). The box in the left column outlines risk factors for developing hepatic SOS. The incidence of SOS is lower after autologous HSCT and with RIC regimens.

SOS occurs as a result of tissue injury to sinusoidal endothelial cells and hepatocytes caused by TBI or high-dose alkylating chemotherapy agents. Endothelial injury to the liver activates cytokine and tumor necrosis factor, which stimulates coagulation and thrombosis in the hepatic sinusoids and eventually in the venules. The resulting impairment of blood flow leads to SOS (Anderson-Reitz & Clancy, 2013). The figure below shows the pathophysiology that leads to the development of SOS.

Clinical manifestations of SOS usually begin within the first 2 weeks after transplantation and include hyperbilirubinemia, rapid weight gain, ascites, right upper quadrant pain, hepatomegaly, splenomegaly, jaundice, coagulopathy, and increased platelet consumption. Progression of SOS can lead to fatal liver failure. Treatment usually is supportive and focuses on

---

Risk Factors for Hepatic Veno-occlusive Disease

- Pretransplantation preparative regimen with busulfan or total body irradiation
- Previous abdominal irradiation
- Pretransplantation hepatotoxic drug therapy (amphotericin)
- Abnormal liver function study results before transplantation
- HLA-mismatched or unrelated donor
- Active infection
- Metastatic liver disease
- Poor pretransplantation performance status
- Second transplantation
- Older recipient age
- Female gender
- Prior exposure to gemtuzumab

From Anderson-Reitz, L., & Clancy, C. (2013). Hepatorenal complication of hematopoietic stem cell transplantation. In S. Ezzone (Ed.). *Hematopoietic stem cell transplantation: A manual for nursing practice* (2nd ed., pp. 191-199). Pittsburgh, PA: Oncology Nursing Society; McDonald, G. B. (2010). Hepatobiliary complications of hematopoietic stem cell transplantation: 40 years on. *Hepatology, 51,* 1450-1460; Strasser, S. I., & McDonald, G. B. (2009). Gastrointestinal and hepatic complications. In F. R. Appelbaum, S. J., Forman, R. S. Negrin, & F. Blume (Eds.). *Thomas' hematopoietic cell transplantation: Stem cell transplantation* (4th ed., pp. 1393-1455). Hoboken, NJ: Wiley-Blackwell.

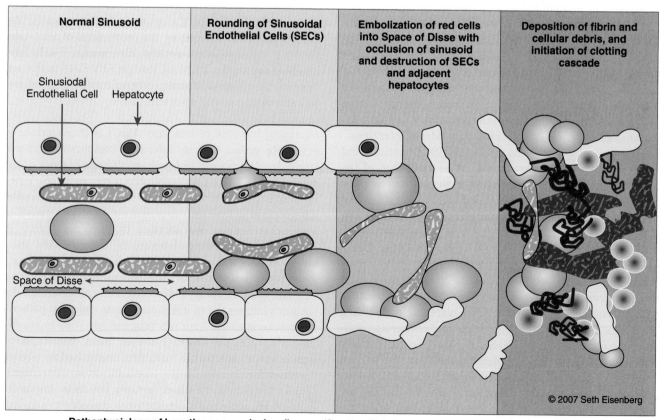

Pathophysiology of hepatic veno-occlusive disease. (Courtesy Seth Eisenberg, RN, OCN. Used with permission.)

maintaining intravascular volume and renal perfusion while minimizing fluid accumulation. Astute nursing care of these patients is critical. Nurses provide much of the supportive care essential to successful treatment of patients with SOS (see table below).

Nursing Management of Hepatic Veno-occlusive Disease or Sinusoidal Obstructive Syndrome

Management	Procedures
Laboratory monitoring	Perform liver function studies, coagulation studies (e.g., prothrombin time, partial thromboplastin time, international normalized ratio, fibrinogen D-dimer), frequent platelet counts, renal function tests, ammonia level assessment, complete blood count
Fluid management	Frequent weights, strict input and output measurements, daily abdominal girths, fluid restriction, concentrate medications in minimal fluid
Medication and transfusion administration	Administer colloid, blood productions (e.g., packed red blood cells, platelets, fresh frozen plasma), defibrotide, ursodiol; monitor for overuse of hepatotoxic medications
Renal function	Review medications for renal adjustments based on change in renal function, monitor during dialysis
Pain management	Frequent pain assessment, position patient to alleviate stress on liver capsule
Patient safety	Evaluate for mental status changes and provide a safe environment
Patient/family education	Educate regarding veno-occlusive disease or sinusoidal obstructive syndrome risks, signs, and symptoms
Identification of risk factors	Review patient's risk factors (e.g., busulfan- or TBI-containing regimen), posttransplantation infection, history of liver function abnormalities, second transplantation, unrelated or haploidentical donor

From Anderson-Reitz, L., and Clancy, C. (2013). Hepatorenal complication of hematopoietic stem cell transplantation. In S. Ezzone (Ed.), *Hematopoietic stem cell transplantation: A manual for nursing practice* (2nd ed., pp. 191-199). Pittsburgh, PA: Oncology Nursing Society; Sousa, E. C. (2012). Veno-occlusive disease in hematopoietic stem cell transplantation recipients. *Clinical Journal of Oncology Nursing, 16*(5), 507-513; Wikle Shapiro, T. J. (2015). Hematopoietic stem cell transplantation. In J. K. Itano, J. Brant, F. Conde, & M. Saria (Eds.). *Core curriculum for oncology nursing* (5th ed., pp. 212-225). Pittsburgh, PA: Oncology Nursing Society.

The most promising pharmacologic agent for treating SOS is defibrotide, with complete response rates of 30% to 60% (Anderson-Reitz & Clancy, 2013; McDonald, 2010; Cheuk, 2012). Defibrotide, a polydisperse oligonucleotide mixture of single-stranded oligonucleotides that has protective effects for vascular hepatic endothelium, is approved for patients with SOS in Europe; it is available in the United States only in clinical trials. Studies have demonstrated that defibrotide is also an effective agent for SOS prophylaxis after transplantation in patients at high risk for this complication (Cheuk, 2012; Sousa, 2012). The drug has antithrombotic, antiischemic, and antiinflammatory effects. Systemic anticoagulants or thrombolytics have been studied but are associated with excessive bleeding complications and have not improved survival.

The prognosis for SOS depends on the extent of hepatic injury, liver dysfunction, and existence of multiorgan

failure. Seventy percent of patients diagnosed with SOS spontaneously recover, but severe SOS is associated with an all-cause mortality rate of more than 90% by day 100 after HSCT (Anderson-Reitz & Clancy, 2013; McDonald, 2010; Cheuk, 2012). Until defibrotide is FDA-approved, standard therapy for SOS in North America continues to be supportive care.

Options for preventing SOS in patients who are at highest risk for the complications include anticoagulation with low-dose heparin, low-molecular-weight heparin, antithrombin III concentrates, prostaglandin E, and ursodeoxycholic acid. Despite many studies evaluating SOS prophylaxis, none has found a dramatic improvement in overall incidence and severity of SOS (Anderson-Reitz & Clancy, 2013; Strasser & McDonald, 2009; Wikle Shapiro, 2015).

Pulmonary Complications

Research suggests that pulmonary complications are the leading cause of posttransplantation morbidity and death in 25% to 50% of HSCT patients (Antin & Raley, 2009; Chi, Soubani, White, & Miller, 2013; Soubani & Pandya, 2010). The rate of significant pulmonary complications is lower for autologous transplant recipients than for allogeneic transplant recipients because of the absence of GVHD and posttransplantation immunosuppression. Few autologous HSCT preparative regimens include TBI, a significant factor for the development of pulmonary issues after transplantation. Posttransplantation pulmonary complications are classified as infectious or noninfectious and follow a predictable timeline after transplantation (see table on page 194).

Common pulmonary complications seen in the first 30 days after transplantation include pulmonary edema, bacterial or fungal pneumonia, pulmonary hemorrhage, diffuse alveolar hemorrhage, and acute respiratory distress syndrome (ARDS) associated with septic shock. Through day 100, patients remain at risk for these complications and for viral pneumonia, *Pneumocystis jiroveci* pneumonia, and idiopathic interstitial pneumonitis due to TBI.

Late pulmonary complications that can occur after day 100 include bronchiolitis obliterans syndrome as a result of chronic GVHD, idiopathic interstitial pneumonitis from TBI, PTLD involving the lung, infectious pneumonias due to encapsulated bacteria (e.g., pneumococcus), fungal disease due to *Aspergillus* or viral pneumonias caused by CMV, VZV, or community-acquired viruses (e.g., RSV, parainfluenza, human metapneumovirus, adenovirus).

Early detection and prompt investigation of pulmonary symptoms are essential for successful management of pulmonary complications. Early diagnosis and prompt intervention can reduce disease progression and premature death. Patients at risk can be screened weekly with viral PCRs for adenovirus, CMV, and EBV; a serum galactomannan immunoassay for early *Aspergillus* detection; and a comprehensive respiratory viral panel for a broad range of viruses before transplantation. Periodic chest radiographs, chest computed tomography (CT) for persistent fever, and intermittent evaluations of pulmonary function are obtained.

Timeline of Typical Onset of Pulmonary Complications After Hematopoietic Stem Cell Transplantation

Cause	Pulmonary Complications
Day 0 to 30	
Infectious and noninfectious causes related to the preparative regimen and neutropenia	Pulmonary edema Pleural effusion Transfusion-related lung injury IPS Engraftment syndrome Diffuse alveolar hemorrhage Aspergillosis Candidemia or candidal infection Respiratory viruses (community-acquired RSV, parainfluenza, or influenza) Bacterial pneumonia ARDS due to sepsis Chemotherapy-associated lung injury
Day 31 to 100	
Opportunistic infections due to impairment of cellular and humoral immunity and delayed lung injury from the preparative regimen	Diffuse alveolar hemorrhage Cytomegalovirus Adenovirus reactivation Aspergillosis *Pneumocystis jiroveci* pneumonia Respiratory viruses (community-acquired RSV, parainfluenza, or influenza) Toxoplasmosis ARDS due to many infections Idiopathic pneumonia syndrome Radiation-induced pneumonitis Busulfan-induced pneumonitis
Day 100+	
Infection from encapsulated bacteria and opportunistic infections due to delayed immune recovery, continued immunosuppressive therapy, and chronic GVHD	Aspergillosis Respiratory viruses (community acquired RSV, parainfluenza, or influenza) Varicella zoster Cytomegalovirus *Pneumocystis jiroveci* pneumonia Posttransplantation lymphoproliferative disorder ARDS Bronchiolitis obliterans due to chronic GVHD Bronchiolitis obliterans organizing pneumonia Busulfan-induced chronic lung injury Radiation-induced chronic lung injury

ARDS, Acute respiratory distress syndrome; *GVHD*, graft-versus-host disease; *IPS*, idiopathic pneumonia syndrome; *RSV*, respiratory syncytial virus.
From Antin, J. H., & Raley, D. Y. (Eds.). (2009). *Manual of stem cell and bone marrow transplantation.* New York: Cambridge Press; Polovich, M., Olsen, M., & LeFebvre, K. B. (2014). *Chemotherapy and biotherapy guidelines and recommendations for practice* (4th ed.). Pittsburgh, PA: Oncology Nursing Society; Wikle Shapiro, T. J. (2015). Hematopoietic stem cell transplantation. In J. K. Itano, J. Brant, F. Conde, & M. Saria (Eds.). *Core curriculum for oncology nursing* (5th ed., pp. 212–225). Pittsburgh, PA: Oncology Nursing Society.

HSCT patients should have frequent assessment for new rhinorrhea, cough, shortness of breath, fever, or a change in activity tolerance. Prophylactic measures include frequent incentive spirometry, encouraging activity, compliance with prophylactic antimicrobials, influenza vaccination, and avoidance of sick contacts.

Engraftment and Recovery

Complete engraftment after HSCT is usually defined as an absolute neutrophil count greater than $0.5 \times 10^9/L$ for 3 consecutive days and a platelet count greater than $20 \times 10^9/L$ achieved without transfusion support. The rate of engraftment depends on the source of the progenitor cells. For patients who receive marrow or PBSCs, neutrophil engraftment can occur as early as 10 days after transplantation, but it is more common between days 14 and 20. Patients who receive UCB cells typically take about 25 days after transplantation for engraftment, but it can take as long as 42 days (CIBMTR & NMDP, 2015).

The total number of progenitor cells transplanted, the use of colony-stimulating factors to prevent GVHD, and infection or other posttransplantation complications may affect the patient's time to engraftment (Gonçalves, Benvegnú, & Bonfanti, 2009; Mattson, Ringdén, & Storb, 2008).

Graft Failure

A significant obstacle to the success of allogeneic HSCT is graft failure, defined as a lack of initial engraftment of donor cells (i.e., primary graft failure) or loss of donor cells after initial engraftment (i.e., secondary graft failure). Graft failure caused by the immune cells of the recipient attacking the donor stem cells before they have the opportunity to engraft is called *graft rejection*. Factors associated with graft failure include HLA disparity between the donor and recipient, the patient's underlying disease, viral infections, type of conditioning regimen, and stem cell source (Locatelli, Lucarelli, & Merli, 2014).

The overall incidence of graft failure is less than 5%. It occurs most often in patients with aplastic anemia who are chemotherapy naïve or those receiving unrelated donor UCB transplants. The cause is multifactorial and may include insufficient dose intensity of the conditioning regimen, inadequate stem cell dose, insufficient posttransplantation immunosuppression, posttransplantation administration of medications with myelosuppressive side effects, viral infection, and folate or vitamin B_{12} deficiency (Satwani et al., 2013). Medications with myelosuppressive side effects (e.g., cotrimoxazole, ganciclovir) should be administered with caution after HSCT. Treatment of graft failure may include larger doses of hematopoietic growth factors and administration of additional donor-derived hematopoietic stem cells, also called a *stem cell boost*. If graft failure persists, a second transplantation with additional immunosuppressive drugs may be indicated.

Engraftment Syndrome

During neutrophil recovery after HSCT, a constellation of signs and symptoms, including fever, erythrodermatous rash, weight gain, and noncardiogenic pulmonary edema, often occur. These clinical findings are usually referred to as *engraftment syndrome* or *capillary leak syndrome*, which reflects the manifestations of increased capillary permeability. Although this syndrome was first described after autologous HSCT, a more severe manifestation has been observed after allogeneic HSCT.

Distinguishing engraftment syndrome from hyperacute GVHD in the allogeneic setting can be difficult. In some cases, engraftment syndrome may be a manifestation of graft rejection by the host. Experience with nonmyeloablative conditioning for stem cell transplantation revealed that engraftment syndrome may occur independent of GVHD. Although cellular and cytokine interactions are thought to be responsible for these clinical findings, a distinct effector cell population and cytokine profile have not been identified. Engraftment syndromes have been associated with increased TRM, mostly from pulmonary and associated multiorgan failure.

Corticosteroid therapy and supportive measures are often dramatically effective for engraftment syndrome, particularly for the treatment of pulmonary manifestations. A more uniform definition of engraftment syndrome is being developed to allow reproducible reporting of complications and evaluation of prophylactic and therapeutic strategies (Chang et al., 2014).

Graft-Versus-Host Disease

GVHD is a complication unique to allogeneic HSCT. GVHD results when the infused donor stem cells (i.e., graft) recognize the recipient (i.e., host) as foreign tissue. The attack of donor-derived T lymphocytes damages recipient (host) tissues.

GVHD is classified as acute or chronic. Classically, this determination has been made on the basis of the time at which GVHD occurs after transplantation. Clinical manifestations that occur before day 100 after transplantation are often designated as acute GVHD. Chronic GVHD is a set of clinical manifestations that occur 100 or more days after transplantation. Historically, a clear distinction was drawn between an early acute form of GVHD and a delayed chronic form of GVHD. However, recent observations of patients receiving UCB transplants, reduced-intensity conditioning regimens, and DLIs after transplantation confirmed that acute GVHD can occur several months after transplantation and that the classic characteristics of chronic GVHD can occur as early as 2 months after transplantation (Dhir, Slatter, & Skinner, 2014; Mitchell, 2013). There is growing recognition that acute and chronic GVHD are best differentiated by their features rather than the time at which they occur.

A new paradigm for identifying acute and chronic GVHD and for diagnosing and staging chronic GVHD (Dhir, Slatter, & Skinner, 2014; Mitchell, 2013) includes classic acute GVHD (i.e., maculopapular rash, nausea, vomiting or diarrhea, and elevated liver function test results); persistent, recurrent, or late acute GVHD (i.e., features of acute GVHD occurring beyond 100 days, often during withdrawal of immune suppression); classic chronic GVHD without features of acute GVHD; and an overlap syndrome that includes the diagnostic or distinctive features of chronic GVHD and acute GVHD.

The incidence of acute and chronic GVHD is 30% to 60% in cases involving histocompatible, sibling-matched allografts, with more GVHD occurring with greater HLA mismatches between the donor and recipient. The mortality rate directly or indirectly related to GVHD may reach 50% (Dhir, Slatter, & Skinner, 2014). Risk factors other than histoincompatibility include sex mismatching, donor parity, older age at the time of transplantation, posttransplantation infection (i.e., viral infections), the use of DLIs after transplantation, and the type of GVHD prophylaxis used.

Acute Graft-Versus-Host Disease

The reported incidence of acute GVHD varies from 20% to 80%, depending principally on the degree of HLA mismatch and donor type (i.e., matched or mismatched, sibling or unrelated donor), stem cell source (i.e., bone marrow, peripheral blood, or UCB), and to a lesser extent, donor age (i.e., older adult donors are associated with a higher risk of acute GVHD) and sex (i.e., multiparous female donor) (Martin et al., 2012).

In order of frequency, acute GVHD predominantly affects the skin, gastrointestinal tract, and liver. Skin involvement commonly starts as an erythematous maculopapular rash on the palms and soles but can involve any part of the skin, and when severe, it can lead to bullae formation. The figure on page 196 illustrates the typical findings of the various severities of acute GVHD skin manifestations. The differential diagnosis of cutaneous acute GVHD includes engraftment syndrome rash, infections (especially viral), and drug reactions, and it may require pathologic identification through a skin biopsy.

Gastrointestinal acute GVHD manifests with secretory diarrhea (i.e., copious and sometimes bloody in severe cases) and may cause abdominal pain, nausea, vomiting, and anorexia. The differential diagnosis includes treatment-related mucositis or enteritis and infection. Endoscopies of the upper and lower gastrointestinal tract with biopsies of multiple sites may be needed to differentiate infection from acute GVHD.

Hepatic acute GVHD usually manifests with cholestatic jaundice and raised levels of liver enzymes (typically γ-glutamyl transpeptidase). Differential diagnoses include SOS, viral infections, sepsis, and drug toxicity. Hepatic acute GVHD with prominent transaminitis is rare but well described. Transjugular liver biopsy may be necessary, but the risk of bleeding from this procedure must be considered (Dhir, Slatter, & Skinner, 2013).

The Glucksberg grading and staging of acute GVHD are shown in the table on page 196. They assess the degree of skin, liver, and gut involvement with the staging of each organ system, and the sum total provides the overall grade (Mitchell, 2013; Przepiorka et al., 1995; Wikle Shapiro, 2015).

With the significant improvements in post-HSCT supportive care in the past 2 decades, particularly the reduction of infection-related mortality, there is greater focus on preventing and managing GVHD. Guidelines for the diagnosis and management of acute GVHD were published in 2012 by the American Society of Blood and Marrow Transplantation (Martin et al., 2012) in an attempt to standardize the care of patients. The strategies used for prophylaxis of acute GVHD depend on the nature of the conditioning regimen, donor type, stem cell source, and degree of HLA mismatch. Acute GVHD prophylaxis for myeloablative full-intensity

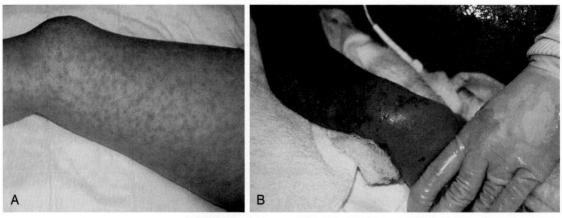

Acute graft-versus-host disease of the skin.

Glucksberg Staging and Grading System for Acute Graft-Versus-Host Disease

CLINICAL STAGING OF INDIVIDUAL ORGAN MANIFESTATIONS

Organ*	Stage	Description
Skin†	0	No evidence of graft-versus-host disease
	1	Maculopapular eruption over <25% of body area
	2	Maculopapular eruption over 25%-50% of body
	3	Generalized erythroderma
	4	Generalized erythroderma with bullous formation and often with desquamation
Liver	0	Bilirubin <2.0 mg/dL
	1	Bilirubin 2.0-3.0 mg/dL
	2	Bilirubin 3.1-6.0 mg/dL
	3	Bilirubin 6.1-15 mg/L
	4	Bilirubin >15 mg/dL
Gut	0	Diarrhea <500 mL/day
	1	Diarrhea 500-999 mL/day or persistent nausea with histologic evidence of graft-versus-host disease in the stomach or duodenum
	2	Diarrhea 1000-1499 mL/day
	3	Diarrhea ≥1500 mL/day
	4	Severe abdominal pain with or without ileus

OVERALL GRADE

Grade	Skin Stage‡	Liver Stage	Gut Stage
0	None	None	None
I	1 to 2	0	0
II	1 to 3	1 and/or Gut GVHD	1
III	2 to 3	2 to 3 and/or Gut GVHD	2 to 3
IV	2 to 4	2 to 4 and/or Gut GVHD	2 to 4

*Criteria for staging minimum degree of organ involvement required to confer that stage.
†Use rule of nines or burn chart to determine extent of rash.
‡If no skin disease is present, the overall grade is the highest isolated liver or gut stage.
From Przepiorka, D., Weisdorf, D., Martin, P., Klingemann, H. G., Beatty, P., Hows, J., & Thomas, E. D. (1995). 1994 Consensus conference on acute GVHD grading. *Bone Marrow Transplantation, 15*(6), 825-828; Mitchell, S. A. (2013). Graft versus host disease. In S. A. Ezzone (Ed.), *Peripheral blood stem cell transplant: Guidelines for oncology nursing practice* (pp. 103-157). Pittsburgh, PA: Oncology Nursing Society Press; Wikle Shapiro, T. J. (2015). Hematopoietic stem cell transplantation. In J. K. Itano, J. Brant, F. Conde, & M. Saria (Eds.). *Core curriculum for oncology nursing.* (5th ed., pp. 212-225). Pittsburgh, PA: Oncology Nursing Society.

HSCT usually includes cyclosporine for approximately 2 to 12 months (depending on the underlying disease) with or without a short course of intravenous methotrexate (usually three to four doses). Tacrolimus is preferred to cyclosporine in many transplantation centers, although published evidence comparing these two calcineurin inhibitors (CNIs) is lacking (Martin et al., 2012). Pre-HSCT anti–T-cell serotherapy with ATG or alemtuzumab is usually added for the use of unrelated donor transplants (i.e., PBSC, bone marrow, or UCB), and it provides additional prophylaxis against graft rejection (Deeg, 2011). Prophylaxis for reduced-intensity HSCTs usually includes cyclosporine and mycophenolate mofetil (MMF), although some centers prefer a corticosteroid to MMF. Serotherapy (i.e., ATG or alemtuzumab) is usually added when an unrelated donor or UCB donor is used. Despite these common regimens, there are wide variations in drug scheduling and dosing for acute GVHD prophylaxis (Dhir, Slatter, & Skinner, 2013; Martin et al., 2012; Mitchell, 2013).

For some patients, no suitably matched related or unrelated donor can be found. A haploidentical graft (i.e., using a parent or sibling) is feasible, and various TCD strategies have been used to minimize GVHD and maximize sustained engraftment and early immune reconstitution. TCD techniques are used by some centers regardless of donor matching.

Historical methods to remove viable T lymphocytes include in vitro alemtuzumab, antilymphocyte antibody, soy lectin, and sheep red cell rosetting. Newer TCD techniques using CD34+ stem cell selection devices (e.g., Miltenyi Biotech's CliniMACS system) are showing promise (Tonon et al., 2013). Other techniques that focus on preserving the GVT effect while removing the T cells responsible for acute GVHD are being explored.

The table on page 197 reviews prophylaxis and first-line, second-line, and third-line treatment options for acute GVHD. The modified Glucksberg clinical grades correlate with overall survival and are usually employed to stratify treatment for acute GVHD (Martin et al., 2012). The components of first-line management have changed little over the past 30 years. Grade I acute GVHD is managed by continuing the prophylactic CNI and applying topical steroids (and sometimes topical tacrolimus) to affected skin. Systemic immunosuppression with intravenous methylprednisolone (2 mg/kg/day) is added for grades II through IV, although an adult trial suggested that 1 mg/kg/day is sufficient for grade II acute GVHD (Mielcarek et al., 2009). Higher steroid doses

(>2 mg/kg/day) appear to offer no additional benefit and contribute to increased toxicity and the risk of fatal infection. In gastrointestinal acute GVHD, the addition of nonabsorbable steroids (i.e., budesonide and beclomethasone) may facilitate reduction of systemic steroid doses.

Management Options for Acute Graft-Versus-Host Disease

Options	Applications
Prophylaxis	Myeloablative HSCT: cyclosporine (or tacrolimus) ± short-course methotrexate
	Reduced-intensity HSCT: cyclosporine (or tacrolimus) + MMF or a corticosteroid
	Unrelated donor (or UCB) HSCT: serotherapy (ATG or alemtuzumab) + cyclosporin (or tacrolimus) + methotrexate
	Haploidentical donor HSCT: T-cell depletion or CD34+ selection ± cyclosporine
First-line treatment for acute GVHD	Continue cyclosporine (or tacrolimus) to optimize blood level
	Add corticosteroid (usually intravenous methylprednisolone, 1 to 2 mg/kg/day)
	Add topical corticosteroid ± topical tacrolimus for skin acute GVHD
	Consider enteral administration of nonabsorbable corticosteroids (e.g., budesonide) for gastrointestinal acute GVHD
Second-line treatment for steroid-refractory acute GVHD	Consider addition of one or more of anti-TNF-α antibodies (e.g., infliximab, etanercept), MMF, mTOR inhibitor (e.g., sirolimus), IL-2 receptor antibodies (e.g., daclizumab), or extracorporeal photopheresis
Third-line treatment: after failure of at least two second-line treatments	Consider alemtuzumab. methotrexate, pentostatin, and mesenchymal stem cells

ATG, Antithymocyte globulin; *GVHD*, graft-versus-host disease; *HSCT*, hematopoietic stem cell transplantation; *IL-2*, interleukin-2; *MMF*, mycophenolate mofetil; *mTOR*, mammalian target of rapamycin; *TNF*, tumor necrosis factor; *UCB*, umbilical cord blood.
From Dhir, S., Slatter, M., & Skinner, R. (2014). Recent advances in the management of graft versus host disease. *Archives of Diseases in Childhood, 99*(12), 1150-1157; Martin, P. J., Rizzo, J. D., Wingard, J. R., Ballen, K., Curtin, P. T., Cutler, C., Carpenter, P. A. (2012). First- and second-line systemic treatment of acute graft-versus-host disease: Recommendations of the American Society of Blood and Marrow Transplantation. *Biology of Blood and Marrow Transplantation, 18*(8), 1150-1163; Mitchell, S. A. (2013). Graft versus host disease. In S. A. Ezzone (Ed.). *Peripheral blood stem cell transplant: Guidelines for oncology nursing practice* (pp. 103-157). Pittsburgh, PA: Oncology Nursing Society Press.

Unfortunately, a complete response to steroid treatment is seen in only about 70% of cases of acute GVHD (Dhir, Slatter, & Skinner, 2013; Martin et al., 2012). However, newer treatments have been introduced for steroid-refractory acute GVHD, which is usually defined as failure to respond to 5 days of intravenous methylprednisolone and a CNI or deterioration after 3 days. Acute GVHD refractory to initial treatment is associated with a survival rate of less than 25% over 1 to 2 years due to the adverse consequences of GVHD itself (i.e., organ damage or subsequent development of chronic GVHD) and of its treatment (i.e., infectious complications due to severe immunosuppression) (Dhir, Slatter, & Skinner, 2013; Martin et al., 2012).

Chronic Graft-Versus-Host Disease
Chronic GVHD typically occurs 100 to 400 days after transplantation, although it can begin as early as 45 days after transplantation. It can be a debilitating, chronic condition that mimics autoimmune disease. Chronic GVHD usually occurs in patients who have had acute GVHD, although it can occur in the absence of acute GVHD. Among patients who survived 150 days after allogeneic HSCT, chronic GVHD was observed in 33% to 49% of HLA-identical related transplantations and in 64% of matched unrelated donor transplantations (Jacobsohn, 2010).

Risk factors for chronic GVHD include previous acute GVHD, older recipient age, and sex mismatching (i.e., female donor and male recipient). The incidence of chronic GVHD is also higher among recipients of PBSCs than recipients of bone marrow–derived stem cells.

Clinical manifestations of chronic GVHD are graded and may be mild, moderate, or severe. They are commonly observed in the skin, liver, eyes, oral cavity, lungs, gastrointestinal system, neuromuscular system, and other body systems. The table on page 198 outlines the first National Institutes of Health (NIH) consensus publication with proposed diagnostic criteria and an improved classification for chronic GVHD (Baird et al., 2013; Flowers & Martin, 2015). For assessing the severity of chronic GVHD, each organ or site is assigned a grade between 0 and 3 according to the clinical manifestations and resultant disability, and an overall grade of mild, moderate, or severe is assigned according to the extent of involvement of each organ. The grade has clinical relevance because moderate chronic GVHD implies at least one organ with clinically significant features but without major disability, whereas severe chronic GVHD (with a score of 3 in at least one organ) reflects major disability.

Sclerodermatous cutaneous and oral manifestations of chronic GVHD are seen in the figure on page 198. The table on page 199 summarizes the clinical features, screening, evaluation and recommended interventions for patients with chronic GVHD. Because other conditions can mimic chronic GVHD, a systematic, multidisciplinary evaluation of the patient with chronic GVHD is essential.

Chronic GVHD is usually treated with a combination of steroids, cyclosporine, tacrolimus, rapamycin, MMF, rituximab, pentostatin, hydroxychloroquine, methotrexate, and extracorporeal photopheresis (Dhir, Slatter, & Skinner, 2013; Flowers & Martin, 2015; Mitchell, 2013; Wikle Shapiro, 2015). Early recognition and treatment of chronic GVHD before disability ensues is critical. First-line therapy for mild chronic GVHD includes topical and oral steroids, cyclosporine or tacrolimus, and azathioprine. Patients refractory to first-line therapies or those with moderate to severe chronic GVHD may be placed on azathioprine alternating with cyclosporine, steroids, or thalidomide. Clofazimine, an antileprosy agent, has been effective in treating cutaneous and oral lesions of chronic GVHD and may be useful as a steroid-sparing agent.

MMF is the most commonly used agent to treat steroid-refractory chronic GVHD. Responses of 90% and 75% in first- and second-line settings are seen when MMF is added to standard tacrolimus, cyclosporine, and prednisone treatments (Flowers & Martin, 2015). MMF does not seem to increase the rate of infection or relapse.

Psoralen and ultraviolet A radiation (PUVA) therapy plays a role for patients with refractory cutaneous chronic GVHD. In one study, it resulted in a 78% response rate and improvement in a few extracutaneous sites. Extracorporeal photopheresis, a modification of PUVA treatment, has also shown benefit, with the best responses in the skin, liver, eye, and oral mucosa (Baird et al., 2013; Greinix & Antin, 2009).

The anti-CD20 monoclonal antibody rituximab has also been used effectively for musculoskeletal and cutaneous chronic GVHD, with durable responses 1 year after initiation, and it allowed a 75% reduction in steroid doses. Intravenous pentostatin given every 2 weeks for 6 months produced 50% response rates among patients with chronic GVHD who failed two prior immunosuppressive regimens (Pidala et al., 2010). Low-dose (100 cGy) total lymphoid irradiation to thoracoabdominal areas has also been attempted for patients with severe chronic GVHD. Patients with refractory GVHD with fibrotic features who have antibodies activating the platelet-derived growth factor receptor pathway have responded to imatinib (Flowers & Martin, 2015).

The immunosuppressive agents commonly used in patients undergoing HSCT and the associated nursing implications are presented in the table on page 200. Drug levels of cyclosporine or tacrolimus should be monitored at regular intervals and dosing adjusted to maintain levels within the therapeutic range. Because many drug-drug interactions are associated with cyclosporine and tacrolimus, it is important to regularly review the patient's medication profile to identify potentially deleterious interactions. Patients should be instructed to take their immunosuppressive medications exactly as instructed and to contact their transplant provider before starting new medications. Because sun exposure may activate or exacerbate GVHD of the skin, patients should be advised about appropriate methods for minimizing exposure.

Chronic GVHD is a cause of significant morbidity after allogeneic stem cell transplantation. Supportive care measures such as infection prophylaxis and nutritional management (Baird et al., 2013; Dhir, Slatter, & Skinner, 2013; Flowers & Martin, 2015; Jacobsohn, 2010; Mitchell, 2013) and coordinated multidisciplinary care are essential to improve the length and quality of life for patients with chronic GVHD. Antiviral prophylaxis against HSV, VZV, and CMV can prevent oropharyngeal infection and interstitial pneumonia in patients with refractory GVHD on long-term immunosuppression. Antifungal agents that cover mold species are also needed to prevent and treat fungal infections in patients with chronic GVHD on active treatment.

Grading of Chronic Graft-Versus-Host Disease Severity

Severity	Definition*
Mild	Involves one or two organs or sites (except the lung), with no clinically significant functional impairment (maximum score of 1 in all affected organs or sites)
Moderate	At least one organ or site with clinically significant impairment but no major disability (maximum score of 2 in any affected organ or site) *or* 3 or more organs or sites with no clinically significant functional impairment (maximum score of 1 in all affected organs or sites) *or* lung with a score of 1
Severe	Major disability caused by chronic graft-versus-host disease (score of 3 in any affected organ or site) *or* a lung score of ≥2

*Each organ is scored between 0 and 3 depending on physical manifestations and disabilities caused by graft-versus-host disease (0, no symptoms/signs; 1 to 3, increasingly severe symptoms, signs, or abnormal studies). These scores and the number of organs or sites involved are used to grade the overall severity.
From Dhir, S., Slatter, M., & Skinner, R. (2014). Recent advances in the management of graft versus host disease. *Archives of Diseases in Childhood, 99*(12), 1150-1157; Flowers, M. E. D., & Martin, P. (2015). How we treat chronic graft versus host disease. *Blood, 125*(4), 606-615; Jacobsohn, D. (2010). Optimal management of chronic graft-versus-host disease in children. *British Journal of Haematology, 150*:278-292.

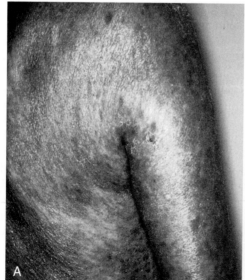
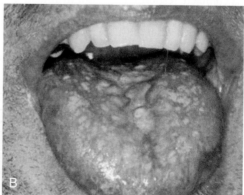

Chronic graft-versus-host disease of the skin.

Chronic Graft-Versus-Host Disease: Clinical Manifestations, Screening, and Interventions

Organ or System	Clinical Manifestations	Screening Studies or Evaluation	Interventions
Dermal	Dyspigmentation, xerosis (dryness), hyperkeratosis, pruritus, scleroderma, lichenification, onychodystrophy (nail ridging or nail loss), alopecia	Clinical examination Skin biopsy: 3-mm punch biopsy	Immunosuppressive therapy Psoralen and ultraviolet A radiation (PUVA) Topical with steroid creams, moisturizers or emollients, antibacterial ointments to prevent superinfection Avoid sunlight exposure, use sunblock lotion with a large hat that shades the face when outdoors
Oral	Lichen planus, xerostomia, ulceration	Oral biopsy	Steroid mouth rinses, PUVA, pilocarpine and anethole trithione for xerostomia, fluoride gels or rinses Careful attention to oral hygiene; regular dental evaluations
Ocular	Keratoconjunctivitis sicca syndrome	Schirmer test, ophthalmic evaluation Slit-lamp test	Regular ophthalmologic follow-up Preservative-free artificial tears and moisturizing lotions Temporary or permanent lacrimal duct occlusion; system-specific interventions, pancreatic enzyme supplementation
Hepatic	Jaundice, abdominal pain	Liver function tests	Actigall orally
Pulmonary	Shortness of breath, cough, dyspnea, wheezing, fatigue, hypoxia, pleural effusion	Pulmonary function studies, peak flow, arterial blood gas, high-resolution computed tomography of chest	Prevent and treat pulmonary infections Aggressively investigate changes in pulmonary function because they may represent graft-versus-host disease of lung or bronchiolitis obliterans
Gastrointestinal	Nausea, odynophagia, dysphagia, anorexia, early satiety, malabsorption, diarrhea, weight loss	Esophagogastroduodenoscopy, colonoscopy, nutritional assessment, fecal studies	Referral to gastroenterologist, nutrition support
Nutritional	Protein and calorie deficiency, malabsorption, dehydration, weight loss, muscle wasting	Weight, fat store measurement, prealbumin	Nutritional monitoring, supplementation, symptom-specific interventions
Genitourinary	Vaginal sicca; vaginal atrophy, stenosis, or inflammation	Pelvic examination	Efficacy of intravaginal steroid cream being evaluated
Immunologic	Hypogammaglobulinemia, autoimmune syndromes, recurrent infections, including cytomegalovirus, herpes simplex virus, varicella-zoster virus, fungi, *Pneumocystis jiroveci*, and encapsulated bacteria	Quantitative immunoglobulin levels, CD4/CD8 lymphocyte subsets	Intravenous immunoglobulins, prophylactic antimicrobials for prophylaxis against *P. jiroveci* pneumonia and encapsulated organisms, surveillance for cytomegalovirus reactivation
Musculoskeletal	Contractures, debility, muscle cramps	Performance status, formal quality of life evaluation, rehabilitation needs	Physical therapy

Data from Dhir, S., Slatter, M., & Skinner, R. (2014). Recent advances in the management of graft versus host disease. *Archives of Diseases in Childhood, 99*(12), 1150-1157; Mitchell, S. A. (2013). Graft versus host disease. In S. A. Ezzone (Ed.), *Peripheral blood stem cell transplant: Guidelines for oncology nursing practice* (pp. 103-157). Pittsburgh, PA: Oncology Nursing Society Press.

Pain control with analgesics for patients with mouth sores allows oral intake. Oral beclomethasone can improve oral intake, nausea, and diarrhea without causing systemic or local toxicity. Retinoic acid is used for ocular sicca syndrome, and pilocarpine (Salagen) is used for oral sicca manifestations. Clonazepam may be used to treat neuromuscular manifestations (e.g., muscular aches, cramping, carpal spasm). Patients receiving chronic corticosteroid therapy are at risk for osteoporosis and fractures. For patients on long-term steroids or female patients, estrogen replacement, calcium supplements, and antiosteoporosis agents (e.g., alendronate, calcitonin) should be considered. A skin care specialist may be needed for moderate to severe cutaneous chronic GVHD (Mandanas, 2014; Mitchell, 2013).

Specialists in dentistry or oral medicine, dermatology, endocrinology, gynecology, ophthalmology, pulmonology, nutrition, physical therapy, and occupational therapy are essential in caring for patients with acute or chronic GVHD.

Chronic GVHD is a primary factor in late transplantation-related morbidity, including abnormalities of growth and development in children, functional performance status, somatic symptoms; and decreased quality of life, psychological functioning, sexual satisfaction, and employment of adults. Support groups, individual and family psychotherapy, physical therapy, occupational therapy, and preventive and preemptive rehabilitation may help to prevent functional decline and emotional distress, thereby improving quality of life (Liu & Hockenberry, 2011; Mitchell, 2013). Complicating care is the fact that by the time chronic GVHD develops, many patients have returned to their local community and are at a distance from health care providers with expertise in the identification and management of the diverse manifestations of chronic GVHD.

Alternative approaches to the prevention, treatment, and control of GVHD are being developed and evaluated

Nursing Implications of Selected Immunosuppressants Used in Allogeneic Stem Cell Transplantation

Agent	Nursing Implications
Cyclosporine	• Bioavailability differs for the oral solution and capsule formulation. After a regimen is established, patients should be instructed not to change their formulation or brand. • Take with food. • Capsules have a foul odor: open to air before taking. • Instruct the patient to notify the health care team immediately if unable to take because of gastrointestinal side effects. • Monitor serum creatinine, blood urea nitrogen, potassium, magnesium, glucose, and triglyceride levels. • Monitor levels carefully in patients with renal or hepatic dysfunction. • Doses should be adjusted for renal dysfunction, as ordered. • Avoid potassium-sparing diuretics. • Replete electrolytes as indicated. • Avoid grapefruit juice or grapefruit-containing products due to interference with pharmacokinetics. • Drug-drug interactions can lead to subtherapeutic or toxic cyclosporine levels. Patients should advise their health care providers of changes made in concurrent medications. • Cyclosporine trough levels should be drawn before administration of morning dose. • Tacrolimus should be discontinued for at least 24 hours before cyclosporine is started.
Tacrolimus (Prograf)	• Take on an empty stomach. • Instruct patient to notify the health care team immediately if unable to take because of gastrointestinal side effects. • Monitor serum creatinine, blood urea nitrogen, potassium, magnesium, phosphorus, glucose, and triglyceride levels. • Monitor levels carefully in patients with renal or hepatic dysfunction. • Doses should be adjusted for renal dysfunction, as ordered. • Avoid potassium-sparing diuretics. • Replete electrolytes as indicated. • Avoid grapefruit juice or grapefruit-containing products due to interference with pharmacokinetics. • Drug-drug interactions can lead to subtherapeutic or toxic tacrolimus levels. Patients should advise their health care providers of changes made in concurrent medications. • Tacrolimus trough levels should be drawn before administration of morning dose. • Cyclosporine should be discontinued for at least 24 hours before tacrolimus is started.
Corticosteroids	• Consult physical therapy for proximal muscle-strengthening exercise program. • Monitor serum chemistries. • Instruct patient in strategies to prevent or treat hyperglycemia and in diabetic self-management. Consult with diabetes educator, as indicated. • Administer oral corticosteroids with food or milk to minimize gastrointestinal upset. • Administer H_2-blockers or proton pump inhibitors to decrease gastric acidity. • Consider need for antiviral, antibacterial, and antifungal prophylaxis. • May increase tacrolimus or cyclosporine levels. • Report complaints of visual changes and consult ophthalmology. • For patients on long-term steroids at risk for osteopenia, ensure regular dual-energy x-ray absorptiometric scans, calcium and vitamin D supplementation, and specific treatment for osteopenia with antiresorptive agents such as alendronate (Fosamax). • A tapering calendar specifying the dosage to be taken each day can help facilitate adherence by patients who are on tapering doses of steroids or an alternate-day steroid regimen.
Mycophenolate mofetil	• Take on an empty stomach. • Monitor complete blood cell count at regular intervals, and adjust dosage for pancytopenia, as ordered. • Monitor liver function tests (i.e., bilirubin and serum transaminases) at regular intervals, and adjust dosage for liver function abnormalities, as ordered. • Monitor plasma levels of mycophenolic acid (i.e., metabolite of mycophenolate mofetil) to guide treatment of patients with renal dysfunction. • There may be decreased absorption when coadministered with magnesium oxide, aluminum- or magnesium-containing antacids, or cholestyramine.
Azathioprine	• Dose reduction required when given with allopurinol. • May lead to anemia and leukopenia when given with angiotensin-converting enzyme inhibitors; synergistic with other bone marrow suppressants. • Use with caution in patients with hepatic or renal impairment. • Teratogenic; advise patient and partner about the need for contraception.
Methotrexate	• Dose and schedule for methotrexate prophylaxis for graft-versus-host disease varies by institution. • A common regimen is 5 to 15 mg/m^2 on days 1, 3, 6, and 11 after transplantation. • Dose may be adjusted or held for severe mucositis and renal or liver insufficiency. Dose may need to be adjusted for hypoalbuminemia. • Use with caution in patients with ascites or pleural or pericardial effusion due to risk of drug accumulation. • Consider the need to monitor methotrexate levels. • Wait until at least 24 hours after stem cell infusion to give day +1 dose.
Infliximab (Remicade)	• Monitor patient for development of infusion-related toxicities. • Consider premedication with acetaminophen and diphenhydramine. • Medications for treating hypersensitivity reactions (e.g., acetaminophen, antihistamines, corticosteroids, epinephrine) and supplemental oxygen should be available for immediate use in the event of a reaction. • Incompatible with polyvinyl chloride equipment or devices. Use glass infusion bottles and polyethylene-lined administration sets.

Continued

Nursing Implications of Selected Immunosuppressants Used in Allogeneic Stem Cell Transplantation—cont'd

Agent	Nursing Implications
Antithymocyte globulin (Atgam [equine], Thymoglobulin [rabbit])	• Monitor patient closely during and after infusion for signs of serum sickness and anaphylaxis. • Consider premedication with corticosteroids, acetaminophen, and H_1- and H_2-blockers. • Medications for treating hypersensitivity reactions (e.g., acetaminophen, antihistamines, corticosteroids, epinephrine) and supplemental oxygen should be available for immediate use in the event of a reaction. • Evaluate need for blood pressure support (e.g., fluid boluses, dopamine, dobutamine). • Because transient and sometimes severe thrombocytopenia may occur after antithymocyte globulin administration in patients with platelet counts less than 100,000/μL, the platelet count should be evaluated 1 hour after administration and as ordered and platelets transfused as indicated.
Alemtuzumab (Campath-1)	• Premedicate patient with acetaminophen and diphenhydramine. • Medications for treating hypersensitivity reactions (e.g., acetaminophen, antihistamines, corticosteroids, epinephrine) and supplemental oxygen should be available for immediate use in the event of a reaction. • Consider treatment with meperidine to control infusion-related rigors. • Administer fluid bolus as ordered to treat hypotension. • Produces rapid and prolonged lymphopenia; patients require broad antifungal, antibacterial, antiviral, and antiprotozoal prophylaxis for at least 4 months after treatment and continuing surveillance for cytomegalovirus infection.
Rapamycin (sirolimus)	• May suppress hematopoietic recovery if used in patients who have recently undergone high-dose therapy. • Oral bioavailability is variable and may be improved when administered with a high-fat meal. • Like tacrolimus and cyclosporine, it is metabolized through the cytochrome P450-3A system; anticipate drug-drug interactions.
Thalidomide	• Thalidomide is a potent teratogen and is contraindicated in patients who are or who are likely to become pregnant. A systematic counseling and education program, written informed consent, and participation in a confidential survey program at the start of treatment and throughout treatment are required for all patients receiving thalidomide. Men and women who are of childbearing potential must practice protected sex while on this drug. • Perform pregnancy test before initiating treatment and periodically throughout treatment course. • Obtain baseline electrocardiogram before treatment. • Thalidomide should not be started if the absolute neutrophil count is less than 750/mm³, and therapy should be reevaluated if the absolute neutrophil count drops below this level. • Administer doses in the evening to minimize impact of drowsiness on lifestyle and safety. • Teach patient to use caution when taking thalidomide with other drugs that can cause drowsiness or neuropathy. • Teach patient to rise slowly from a supine position to avoid lightheadedness. • Teach patient to report immediately signs or symptoms suggesting peripheral neuropathy, including numbness or tingling in the hands or feet or the development of rash or skin ulcerations. These may require immediate cessation of the drug until the patient can be evaluated. • Teach patient to use protective measures (e.g., sunscreens, protective clothing) against exposure to ultraviolet light or sunlight. • Prevent constipation with a stool softener or mild laxative.
Methoxsalen (Oxsoralen)	• Patients who have received cytotoxic chemotherapy or radiation therapy and who are taking methoxsalen are at increased risk for skin cancers. • Toxicity increases with concurrent use of phenothiazines, thiazides, and sulfanilamides. • Instruct patient to take methoxsalen with milk or food and to divide the dose into two portions, taken approximately 1/2 hour apart. • Severe burns may occur from sunlight or ultraviolet A exposure. • Pretreatment eye examinations are indicated to evaluate for cataracts. Repeat eye examinations should be performed every 6 months while patients are undergoing psoralen and ultraviolet A therapy.

From Baird, K., Steinberg, S. M., Grkovic, L., Pulanic, D., Cowen, E. W., Mitchell, S. A., Pavletic, S. Z. (2013). National Institutes of Health chronic graft-versus-host disease staging in severely affected patients: Organ and global scoring correlated with established indicators of disease severity and prognosis. *Biology of Blood and Marrow Transplantation, 19*(4), 632-639; Flowers, M. E. D., & Martin, P. (2015). How we treat chronic graft versus host disease. *Blood, 125*(4), 606-615; Mitchell, S. A. (2013). Graft versus host disease. In S. A. Ezzone (Ed.). *Peripheral blood stem cell transplant: Guidelines for oncology nursing practice* (pp. 103-157). Pittsburgh, PA: Oncology Nursing Society Press.

preclinically and clinically. They include the application of cytokine shields to decrease the inflammatory tissue responses thought to promote acute GVHD, identification of GVHD biomarkers, and more selective TCD and other graft engineering strategies. Gene transfer technologies are promising tools for manipulating donor T-cell immunity to enforce GVT or graft-versus-infection while preventing or controlling acute GVHD (Baird et al., 2013; Quian, Zhengcheng, & Shen, 2013).

Posttransplantation Relapse

Because HSCT is an intensive curative treatment for many high-risk malignancies, its failure to prevent relapse leaves few options for successful salvage treatment. Although the mortality rate due to relapse is high, some patients respond to transplantation and have sustained remissions, and some may have another chance of cure after a second HSCT.

The prognosis for relapsed hematologic malignancies after stem cell transplantation depends on four factors: the time elapsed between HSCT and relapse (i.e., relapses within 6 months have the worst prognosis); the disease type (i.e., chronic leukemias and some lymphomas have a possibility of cure with further treatment); the disease burden and site of relapse (i.e., improved success if disease is treated early); and the conditions of the first transplantation (i.e., superior outcomes for patients with an opportunity to increase the GVT effect or the intensity of conditioning in a second transplantation). These features guide further treatment toward modified second transplantations, chemotherapy, targeted antileukemia therapy, immunotherapy, or palliative care (Barrett & Bartiwalla, 2010; Shannon, 2013).

Treatment of relapsed disease continues to evolve. A classic approach is to rapidly withdraw immunosuppressive agents in an attempt to trigger a GVT effect. DLIs are also an option for patients without rapidly progressing relapse and whose donor is readily available to donate lymphocytes. Second myeloablative or reduced-intensity HSCT after allogeneic HSCT carries significant TRM, and few patients are candidates due to organ dysfunction, inability to achieve remission status, or poor performance status. More clinical trials are needed to determine which patients could benefit from a second transplantation.

Ongoing clinical trials are under way using cellular adoptive immunotherapy after allogeneic HSCT in an attempt to harness the powerful GVT effect of the donor's immune system against residual tumor cells. Some of these trials include ex vivo activated T cells (i.e., activated DLI), cytokine-induced killer cells, natural killer cells, and antigen-specific cytotoxic T cells (Laport & Negrin, 2009; Shannon, 2013).

Patients with certain subtypes (CD19 positive) of post-transplantation-relapsed acute lymphoblastic leukemia (ALL) remain difficult to treat, but the use of adoptive transfer of T cells engineered to express a chimeric antigen receptor (CAR) has emerged as a powerful targeted immunotherapy, showing striking responses in patients with highly refractory disease. Complete remission rates as high as 90% have been reported in children and adults with relapsed and refractory ALL treated with CAR-modified T cells targeting the B-cell–specific antigen CD19 (Maude, Teachey, Porter, & Grupp, 2015). Research that focuses on other antigens is ongoing.

Patients with relapse after HSCT who are not eligible for DLI or clinical trials may choose palliative supportive care. This can be a difficult decision. Information should be provided to patients and their families so that informed decisions regarding end-of-life care can be made. If patients desire to receive no further treatment, nurses can help facilitate their transition to palliative and hospice care (Shannon, 2013).

Long-Term Complications of Hematopoietic Stem Cell Transplantation: Assessment, Prevention, and Management

Long-term disease-free survival after HSCT has greatly improved, resulting in an expanding number of long-term survivors. The preparative regimen and GVHD are considered the main risk factors in allogeneic HSCT. Continuous changes in the transplantation practice and in the types of patients selected are responsible for the evolving pattern of late effects after HSCT over time. Relevant changes include the avoidance of TBI conditioning when possible, the higher age of patients receiving transplants, the increasing use of unrelated and haploidentical donors, and the introduction of RIC. The detection of an increasing number of late effects should not be considered a drawback in HSCT.

Although patients often are cured of their initial disease, several malignant and nonmalignant late effects can cause substantial morbidity with a considerable impact on the health status and quality of life of long-term HSCT survivors. Broad expertise and continued coordination by the transplantation team is mandatory to care for long-term survivors. Aftercare includes standardized screening, patient counseling, and prevention or treatment of late effects.

The potential for care fragmentation exists because health care providers include the transplantation team, the hematology-oncology team who referred the patient, the primary care provider, and many medical specialists, such as dentists, gynecologists, pulmonologists, cardiologists, endocrinologists, and ophthalmologists. Counseling should include self-examination for early cancer detection, compliance with routine testing or screening, and advice for healthy lifestyle behavior.

Beyond immediate survival, allogeneic HSCT is a lifelong commitment between long-term survivors and the transplantation team, involving the recipient's family and the general health care providers. Proper information about life after HSCT should be provided to the whole community, which plays a key role in the social reinsertion of long-term survivors.

Long-term and late complications result from the interplay of high-dose chemotherapy, total body irradiation, medication side effects, infections, acute and chronic GVHD, prolonged immunosuppression, and disease recurrence, along with the effects of prior treatment and preexisting medical conditions (Mohty & Mohty, 2011; Tierney & Robinson, 2013). In addition to chronic GVHD and infection, a wide range of complications may be experienced months or years after HSCT.

HSCT patients require lifelong surveillance and preventive care for some complications, including second malignancies, cardiovascular and pulmonary effects, and relapse. Most transplantation centers have protocol-specific requirements for continued follow-up care, and the frequency of clinic visits is determined by the nature of the patient's complications. The table on pages 203 to 204 summarizes guidelines for screening and evaluation of the potential late effects of HSCT. Guidelines for surveillance and follow-up are available to direct long-term supportive care, fertility preservation, and healthy nutrition and physical activity for HSCT patients (Mohty & Mohty, 2011; Tichell et al., 2012; Tierney & Robinson, 2013). Routine follow-up should include the promotion of a healthy lifestyle and risk reduction strategies, including nutrition, exercise, safe sexual practices, breast and colorectal screening, avoidance of sun exposure, and smoking cessation (Mohty & Mohty, 2011; Tierney and Robinson, 2013).

Evaluation and Screening of Late Effects of Hematopoietic Stem Cell Transplantation

System or Dimension	Possible Late Effects	Evaluation or Screening
Disease status	Relapse or recurrence	Determined on the basis of the site of original disease (complete blood cell count [CBC], periodic imaging) Evaluation for minimal residual disease as indicated
Engraftment	Graft failure or marrow dysfunction with cytopenias	CBC with differential count Bone marrow aspirate and biopsy Engraftment/chimerism studies Viral studies (cytomegalovirus, human herpesvirus 6, parvovirus polymerase chain reaction [PCR])
Immunologic function or recovery	Disorders of B- and T-lymphocyte quantity and function Hypogammaglobulinemia	CD4 and CD8 lymphocyte subsets Mitogen stimulation studies Quantitative immunoglobulin levels Vaccination titers
Cardiopulmonary	Interstitial pneumonitis Bronchiolitis obliterans Hypertension, cardiomyopathy, pericardial damage, peripheral vascular disease	Chest radiograph Pulmonary function tests with single-breath diffusing capacity Electrocardiogram Echocardiogram History and physical examination
Neurologic	Peripheral and autonomic neuropathies Cognitive changes (shortened attention span, difficulty with concentration) Leukoencephalopathy Ototoxicity	Health history Neurologic examination Neuropsychological testing Rehabilitation medicine Audiologic testing
Gastrointestinal	Liver dysfunction Chronic graft-versus-host disease Malabsorption syndromes	Liver function tests Hepatitis B serologies, hepatitis C PCR, qualitative Upper and lower gastrointestinal endoscopies Transjugular liver biopsy
Genitourinary	Renal dysfunction Radiation nephritis Hematuria, proteinuria Cancer of the bladder	Blood urea nitrogen, creatinine levels Urinalysis with microscopy 24-hour urine for creatinine clearance and total protein, if indicated
Thyroid function	Hypothyroidism	Thyroid-stimulating hormone, triiodothyronine, thyroxine, free thyroxine
Gonadal function	Decreased production of gonadal hormones	Luteinizing hormone, follicle-stimulating hormone, estradiol (women) Pelvic examination Luteinizing hormone, follicle-stimulating hormone, testosterone (men)
Hypothalamic-pituitary	Abnormal pituitary gland function	Prolactin, follicle-stimulating hormone, luteinizing hormone, thyroid-stimulating hormone, growth hormone levels (children)
Metabolic syndrome	Increased blood pressure Elevated glucose level Central obesity Abnormal cholesterol levels	Fasting glucose, lipid profile
Ophthalmic	Cataracts	Ophthalmologic examination that includes slit-lamp examination and Schirmer test
Dental or oral cavity	Sicca syndrome Caries Periodontal disease Xerostomia Oral malignancy	Regular dental evaluations Meticulous attention to oral hygiene Fluoride gels or rinses
Musculoskeletal	Osteoporosis Avascular necrosis Myopathy	Dual-energy x-ray absorptiometry (DEXA) scan Magnetic resonance imaging (MRI) if pain in a joint, limited range of motion, or a limp Neurologic examination Electromyelogram
Second malignancy	Nonmelanoma skin cancer Breast cancer (especially in patients with history of chest irradiation)	Complete physical examination with biopsy of suspicious lesions Skin photographs may help to monitor status Breast MRI, mammogram, self-examination

Continued

Evaluation and Screening of Late Effects of Hematopoietic Stem Cell Transplantation—cont'd		
System or Dimension	**Possible Late Effects**	**Evaluation or Screening**
	Thyroid cancer	History and physical examination Ultrasonography Iodine-131 scan
	Treatment-related acute leukemia	CBC with differential count Bone marrow aspirate and biopsy
	Myelodysplastic syndrome	Bone marrow aspirate and biopsy (if CBC abnormal), cytogenetics
	Posttransplantation lymphoproliferative disorder (PTLD)	Computed tomography if PTLD is suspected Epstein-Barr viral load by PCR weekly in first few months after allogeneic hematopoietic stem cell transplantation CD4 count >200 cells/mm^3
	Cancer of the uterine cervix	Gynecologic examination with Papanicolaou smear
	Cancer of the bladder	Urinalysis with microscopy to detect microhematuria, urine cytology, follow-up cystoscopy
Integumentary	Increased incidence of benign and malignant nevi	Complete physical examination Skin biopsy of suspicious lesions
Psychologic or rehabilitation quality of life	Changes in body image, roles, family relationships, lifestyle, occupation, discrimination, overcoming stigma, living with compromises, coping with symptoms	Assessment of individual adjustment, achievement of normal developmental tasks, marital stress, sexual function, body image, rehabilitation needs, symptom distress through systematic and structured evaluation

From Deeg, H. J. (2007). How I treat refractory acute graft versus host disease. *Blood, 109,* 4119-4126; Tierny, D. K., & Robinson, T. (2013). Long-term care of hematopoietic cell transplant survivors. In S. A Ezzone (Ed.). *Hematopoietic stem cell transplantation: A manual for nursing practice* (2nd ed., pp. 251-267). Pittsburgh, PA: Oncology Nursing Society; Roziakova, L., & Mladosievicova, B. (2010). Endocrine late effects after hematopoietic T stem cell transplantation. *Oncology Research, 18*(11-12):607-615.

References

Alexander, B. T., Hladnik, L. M., Casabar, E., McKinnon, P. S., Reichley, R. M., Richie, D. J., & Dubberke, E. R. (2010). Use of cytomegalovirus intravenous immune globulin for the adjunctive treatment of cytomegalovirus in hematopoietic stem cell transplant patients. *Pharmacotherapy, 30*(6), 554–561.

Alousi, A., & de Lima, M. (2008). Ablative preparative regimens for hematopoietic stem cell transplantation. In R. Soiffer (Ed.), *Hematopoietic stem cell transplantation* (2nd ed.) (pp. 321–347). New York: Humana Press.

Alpdogan, O., Grosso, D., & Flomenberg, N. (2013). Recent advances in haploidentical stem cell transplantation. *Discovery Medicine, 16*(88), 159–165.

Anderson-Reitz, L., & Clancy, C. (2013). Hepatorenal complication of hematopoietic stem cell transplantation. In S. Ezzone (Ed.), *Hematopoietic stem cell transplantation: A manual for nursing practice* (2nd ed.) (pp. 191–199). Pittsburgh, PA: Oncology Nursing Society.

Antin, J. H., & Raley, D. Y. (Eds.). (2009). *Manual of stem cell and bone marrow transplantation.* New York: Cambridge Press.

Appelbaum, F. (2012). Improved outcomes with allogeneic hematopoietic stem cell transplantation. *Best Practice Research in Clinical Hematology, 25*(4), 465–471.

Appelbaum, F., Forman, S. J., Negrin, R. S., & Blume, K. G. (Eds.). (2009). *Thomas' hematopoietic cell transplantation; stem cell transplantation.* Hoboken, NJ: Wiley-Blackwell.

Baird, K., Steinberg, S. M., Grkovic, L., Pulanic, D., Cowen, E. W., Mitchell, S. A., & Pavletic, S. Z. (2013). National Institutes of Health chronic graft-versus-host disease staging in severely affected patients: Organ and global scoring correlated with established indicators of disease severity and prognosis. *Biology of Blood and Marrow Transplantation, 19*(4), 632–639.

Ballen, K. K., Gluckman, E., & Broxmeyer, H. E. (2013). Umbilical cord blood transplantation: The first 25 years and beyond. *Blood, 122*(4), 490–498.

Barrett, A. J., & Battiwalla, M. (2010). Relapse after allogeneic stem cell transplantation. *Experts Reviews in Hematology, 3*(4), 429–441.

Boeckh, M., & Ljungman, P. (2009). How we treat cytomegalovirus in hematopoietic cell transplant recipients. *Blood, 113*(23), 5711–5719.

Center for International Blood and Marrow Transplant Research (CIBMTR) & National Marrow Donor Program (NMDP). (2015). Data. Available at www.CIMBTR.org (accessed February 18, 2016).

Centers for Disease Control and Prevention (CDC), Infectious Diseases Society of America, & American Society of Blood and Marrow Transplantation. (2000). Guidelines for preventing opportunistic infections among hematopoietic stem cell transplant recipients. *Morbidity and Mortality Weekly Report Recommendation Report, 49*(RR-10), 1–125.

Chang, L., Frame, D., Braun, T., Gatza, E., Hanauer, D. A., Zhao, S., & Choi, S. W. (2014). Engraftment syndrome after allogeneic hematopoietic cell transplantation predicts poor outcomes. *Biology of Blood and Marrow Transplantation, 20*(9), 1407–1417.

Chawala, R., & Greenstein, S. (2013). *Infections after bone marrow transplantation.* Available at http://emedicine.medscape.com/article/1013470-overview#aw2aab6b6 (accessed February 20, 2016).

Cheuk, D. K. L. (2012). Hepatic veno-occlusive disease after hematopoietic stem cell transplantation: Prophylaxis and treatment controversies. *World Journal of Transplantation, 2*(2), 27–34.

Chi, A. K., Soubani, A. O., White, A. C., & Miller, K. B. (2013). An update on pulmonary complications of hematopoietic stem cell transplantation. *Chest, 144*(6), 1913–1922.

Childs, R. W. (2011). Allogeneic stem cell transplantation. In T. S. Lawrence & S. A. Rosenberg (Eds.), *Cancer: Principles and practice of oncology* (9th ed.) (pp. 2244–2263). Philadelphia: Lippincott, Williams & Wilkins.

Deeg, H. J. (2011). GVHD free with Campath? *Blood, 118*(11), 2033–2036.

De la Morena, M. Y., & Gatti, R. A. (2010). A history of bone marrow transplantation. *Hematology Oncology Clinics of North America, 25*(1), 1–15.

de Lima, M., Alousi, A., & Giralt, S. (2015). Preparative regimens for hematopoietic cell transplantation. In R. Hoffman, B. Furie, E. J. Benz, Jr., P. McGlave, L. E. Silberstein, & S. J. Shattil (Eds.), *Hematology: Basic principles and practice.* Philadelphia: Elsevier.

Dhir, S., Slatter, M., & Skinner, R. (2014). Recent advances in the management of graft versus host disease. *Archives of Diseases in Childhood, 99*(12), 1150–1157.

Di Bartolomeo, P., Santarone, S., De Angelis, G., Picardi, A., Cudillo, L., Cerretti, R., & Arcese, W. (2013). Haploidentical, unmanipulated, G-CSF-primed bone marrow transplantation for patients with high-risk hematologic malignancies. *Blood, 121*(5), 849–857.

Flowers, M. E. D., & Martin, P. (2015). How we treat chronic graft versus host disease. *Blood, 125*(4), 606–615.

Forman, S. J., & Nakamura, R. (2011). Hematopoietic cell transplantation. In R. Pazdur, L. D. Wagman, K. A. Camphausen, & W. J. Hoskins (Eds.), *Cancer management: A multidisciplinary approach: Medical, surgical, and radiation oncology* (online edition). Available at http://www.cancernetwork.com/cancer-management/hematopoietic-cell-transplantation (accessed February 18, 2016).

Fürst, D., Müller, C., Vucinic, V., Bunjes, D., Herr, W., Gramatzki, M., & Mytilineos, J. (2013). High-resolution HLA matching in hematopoietic stem cell transplantation: A retrospective collaborative analysis. *Blood, 122*(18), 3220–3229.

Goldfinger, D., & Lu, Q. (2015). *Granulocyte transfusions.* Available at http://www.uptodate.com/contents/granulocyte-transfusions (accessed February 21, 2016).

Gonçalves, T. L., Benvegnú, D. M., & Bonfanti, G. (2009). Specific factors influence the success of autologous and allogeneic hematopoietic stem cell transplantation. *Oxidative Medicine and Cellular Longevity, 2*(2), 82–87.

Greinix, H. T., & Antin, J. A. (2009). Salvage therapy for chronic graft versus host disease. In G. B. Vogelsberg & S. Pavletic (Eds.), *Chronic graft versus host disease: Interdisciplinary management* (pp. 134–156). New York: Cambridge University Press.

Gyurkocza, B., & Sandmaier, B. M. (2014). Conditioning regimens for hematopoietic cell transplantation: One size does not fit all. *Blood, 124*(3), 344–353.

Harris, D. J. (2010). Transplantation. In J. Eggert (Ed.), *Cancer basics* (pp. 317–342). Pittsburgh, PA: Oncology Nursing Society.

Heslop, H. (2009). How I treat lymphoproliferation. *Blood, 114*(19), 4002–4008.

Jacobsohn, D. (2010). Optimal management of chronic graft-versus-host disease in children. *British Journal of Haematology, 150*, 278–292.

Kedia, S., Acharya, P. S., Mohammad, F., Nguyen, H., Deepak, A., Mehta, S., & Mobarakai, N. (2013). Infectious complications of hematopoietic stem cell transplantation. *Journal of Stem Cell Research and Therapy*, S3–002. Available at http://www.omicsonline.org/infectious-complications-of-hematopoietic-stem-cell-transplantation-2157-7633.S3-002.pdf (accessed February 2, 2016).

Laport, G. G., & Negrin, R. S. (2009). Management of relapse after hematopoietic stem cell transplantation. In F. R. Appelbaum, S. J. Forman, R. S. Negrin, & F. Blume (Eds.), *Thomas' hematopoietic cell transplantation: Stem cell transplantation* (4th ed.) (pp. 1059–1075). Hoboken, NJ: Wiley-Blackwell.

Liu, Y.-M., & Hockenberry, M. (2011). Review of chronic graft-versus-host disease in children after allogeneic stem cell transplantation: Nursing perspective. *Journal of Pediatric Oncology Nursing, 28*(1), 6–15.

Ljungman, J. (2008). CMV infections after hematopoietic stem cell transplantation. *Bone Marrow Transplantation, 42*(Suppl), S70–S72.

Locatelli, F., Lucarelli, B., & Merli, P. (2014). Current and future approaches to treat graft failure after allogeneic hematopoietic stem cell transplantation. *Expert Opinions in Pharmacotherapeutics, 15*(1), 23–36.

Koreth, J., Pidala, J., Oerex, W. S., Deeg, J. H., Garcia-Manero, G., Malcovati, L., & Cutler, C. (2013). Role of reduced-intensity conditioning allogeneic hematopoietic stem-cell transplantation in older patients with de novo myelodysplastic syndromes: An International Collaborative decision analysis. *Journal of Clinical Oncology, 10*(12), 1–10.

Mandanas, R. A. (2014). *Graft versus host disease treatment and management.* Available at http://emedicine.medscape.com/article/429037-treatment (accessed February 22. 2016).

Maude, S. L., Teachey, D. T., Porter, D., & Grupp, S. A. (2015). CD19-targeted chimeric antigen receptor T-cell therapy for acute lymphoblastic leukemia. *Blood, 125*(26), 4017–4024.

Mielcarek, M., Storer, B. E., Boeckh, M., Carpenter, P. A., McDonald, G. B., Deeg, H. J., & Martin, P. J. (2009). Initial therapy of acute graft-versus-host disease with low-dose prednisone does not compromise patient outcomes. *Blood, 113*(13), 2888–2894.

Martin, P. J., Rizzo, J. D., Wingard, J. R., Ballen, K., Curtin, P. T., Cutler, C., & Carpenter, P. A. (2012). First- and second-line systemic treatment of acute graft-versus-host disease: Recommendations of the American Society of Blood and Marrow Transplantation. *Biology of Blood and Marrow Transplantation, 18*(8), 1150–1163.

Mattson, J., Ringdén, O., & Storb, R. (2008). Graft failure after allogeneic hematopoietic cell transplantation. *Biology of Blood Marrow Transplantation, 14*(Suppl 1), 165–170.

McAdams, F. W., & Burgunder, M. R. (2013). Transplant treatment course and acute complications. In S. Ezzone (Ed.), *Hematopoietic stem cell transplantation: A manual for nursing practice* (2nd ed.) (pp. 44–47). Pittsburgh, PA: Oncology Nursing Society.

McDonald, G. B. (2010). Hepatobiliary complications of hematopoietic stem cell transplantation: 40 years on. *Hepatology, 51*, 1450–1460.

Mitchell, S. A. (2013). Graft versus host disease. In S. A. Ezzone (Ed.), *Peripheral blood stem cell transplant: Guidelines for oncology nursing practice* (pp. 103–157). Pittsburgh, PA: Oncology Nursing Society Press.

Mohty, B., & Mohty, B. (2011). Long-term complications and side effects after allogeneic hematopoietic stem cell transplantation: An update. *Blood Cancer Journal, 1*(16), 1–5.

National Cancer Institute (NCI). (2015). *A multi-center, phase III, randomized trial of reduced intensity (RIC) conditioning and transplantation of double unrelated umbilical cord blood (dUCB) versus HLA-haploidentical related bone marrow (haplo-BM) for patients with hematologic malignancies (BMT CTN 1101).* Available at https://clinicaltrials.gov/ct2/show/NCT01597778 (accessed February 18, 2016).

National Marrow Donor Program (NMDP). (2015). *Marrow donor program.* Available at https://network.bethematchclinical.org/ (accessed February 18, 2016).

Neiss, D. (2013). Basic concepts of transplantation. In S. A Ezzone (Ed.), *Hematopoietic stem cell transplantation: A manual for nursing practice* (2nd ed.) (pp. 13–21). Pittsburgh, PA: Oncology Nursing Society.

Nucci, M., & Anaissie, E. (2009). Fungal infections in hematopoietic stem cell transplantation and solid-organ transplantation—Focus on aspergillosis. *Clinical Chest Medicine, 30*(2), 295–306.

Ooi, J. (2009). Cord blood transplantation in adults. *Bone Marrow Transplantation, 44*, 661–666.

Perumbeti, A. (2014). *Hematopoietic stem cell transplantation: Indications.* Available at http://emedicine.medscape.com/article/208954-overview#a3 (accessed February 17, 2016).

Pidala, J., Roman-Diaz, J., Shapiro, J., Nishihori, T., Bookout, R., Anasetti, C., & Kharfan-Dabaja, M. A. (2010). Pentostatin as rescue therapy for glucocorticoid-refractory acute and chronic graft-versus-host-disease. *Annals of Transplantation, 15*(4), 21–29.

Przepiorka, D., Weisdorf, D., Martin, P., Klingemann, H. G., Beatty, P., Hows, J., & Thomas, E. D. (1995). 1994 Consensus conference on acute GVHD grading. *Bone Marrow Transplantation, 15*(6), 825–828.

Quian, L., Zhengcheng, W., & Shen, J. (2013). Advances in the treatment of acute graft versus host disease. *Journal of Cellular and Molecular Medicine, 17*(8), 966–975.

Satwani, P., Jin, Z., Duffy, D., Morris, E., Bhatia, M., Garvin, J. H., & Cairo, M. S. (2013). Transplantation-related mortality, graft failure, and survival after reduced-toxicity conditioning and allogeneic hematopoietic stem cell transplantation in 100 consecutive pediatric recipients. *Biology of Blood and Marrow Transplantation, 19*(4), 552–561.

Schmit-Pokorny, K. (2013). Stem cell collection. In S. A. Ezzone (Ed.), *Hematopoietic stem cell transplantation: A manual for nursing practice* (2nd ed.) (pp. 23–46). Pittsburgh, PA: Oncology Nursing Society.

Shannon, S. (2013). Relapse and secondary malignancy. In S. A. Ezzone (Ed.), *Hematopoietic stem cell transplantation: A manual for nursing practice* (2nd ed.) (pp. 245–249). Pittsburgh, PA: Oncology Nursing Society.

Shaughnessy, P., Uberti, J., Devine, S., Maziarz, R. T., Vose, J., Micallef, I., & McSweeney, P. (2013). Plerixafor and G-CSF for autologous stem cell mobilization in patients with NHL, Hodgkin's lymphoma and multiple myeloma: Results from the expanded access program. *Bone Marrow Transplantation, 48*(6), 777–781.

Sousa, E. C. (2012). Veno-occlusive disease in hematopoietic stem cell transplantation recipients. *Clinical Journal of Oncology Nursing, 16*(5), 507–513.

Soubani, A. O., & Pandya, C. M. (2010). The spectrum of noninfectious pulmonary complications following hematopoietic stem cell transplantation. *Hematology/Oncology and Stem Cell Therapy, 3*(3), 143–157.

Strasser, S. I., & McDonald, G. B. (2009). Gastrointestinal and hepatic complications. In F. R. Appelbaum, S. J. Forman, R. S. Negrin, & F. Blume (Eds.), *Thomas' hematopoietic cell transplantation: Stem cell transplantation* (4th ed.) (pp. 1393–1455). Hoboken, NJ: Wiley-Blackwell.

Tay, J., Allan, D., Tinmouth, A., Coyle, D., & Hébert, P. (2013). Donor selection for patients undergoing allogeneic hematopoietic SCT: Assessment of the priorities of Canadian hematopoietic SCT physicians. *Bone Marrow Transplantation, 48*, 314–316.

Tichell, A., Ravo, A., & Socie, G. (2012). Late effects after hematopoietic stem cell transplantation—Critical issues. *Current Issues in Dermatology, 43*, 132–149.

Tiercy, J. M. (2014). HLA-C incompatibilities in allogeneic unrelated hematopoietic stem cell transplantation. *Frontiers in Immunology, 5*(216), 1–5.

Tierny, D. K., & Robinson, T. (2013). Long-term care of hematopoietic cell transplant survivors. In S. A. Ezzone (Ed.), *Hematopoietic stem cell transplantation: A manual for nursing practice* (2nd ed.) (pp. 251–267). Pittsburgh, PA: Oncology Nursing Society.

Tomblyn, M., Chiller, T., Einsele, H., Gress, R., Sepkowitz, K., Storek, J., & Boeckh, M. J. (2009). Guidelines for preventing infectious complications among hematopoietic cell transplantation recipients: A global perspective. *Biology of Blood Marrow Transplantation, 15*(10), 1143–1238.

Tonon, J., Koehne, G., Collins, N. H., Malloy, M., Chen, X., Bleau, S., & Meagher, R. C. (2013). Final product composition after ex vivo T-cell reduction: Miltenyi CliniMACS versus Baxter Isolex 300I in a large cohort of allogeneic transplant patients. *Cytotherapy, 15*(4), S22–S23.

Wang, F. R., Wang, J. Z., Sun, Y. Q., & Huang, X. J. (2013). Long-term follow-up of haploidentical hematopoietic stem cell transplantation without in vitro T cell depletion for the treatment of leukemia: Nine years of experience at a single center. *Cancer, 119*(5), 978–985.

Wikle Shapiro, T. J. (2015). Hematopoietic stem cell transplantation. In J. K. Itano, J. Brant, F. Conde, & M. Saria (Eds.), *Core curriculum for oncology nursing* (5th ed.) (pp. 212–225). Pittsburgh, PA: Oncology Nursing Society.

Chemotherapy

Anna Christofanelli

This chapter provides basic concepts and principles related to chemotherapy and its primary mechanisms of action in the treatment goals of oncology patients. In addition, standards related to safe handling, administration, preadministration patient and family education, and special populations are reviewed.

Biologic and Pharmacologic Bases for Cancer Chemotherapy

Cancer is characterized as a growth of abnormal cells, mainly stemming from genetic alterations, that lead to unregulated cell growth, invasion into neighboring tissues, and metastasis to distant sites (Brown, 2014). Chemotherapy is used to prevent cancer cells from multiplying, invading, or metastasizing. Cancer spreads through the lymph nodes or the bloodstream or by direct extension, as in ovarian cancer. Chemotherapy is a systemic treatment that combats primary disease sites, areas of known metastasis, and possibly microscopic spread of disease.

The biologic basis of cancer chemotherapy is grounded in cell division or the cell cycle, which is reviewed in Section One: Cancer Pathophysiology of this book. Briefly, the cell cycle is the mechanism by which all cells divide and replicate, including both normal and neoplastic cells. See the figure below for phases of the cell cycle. In general, the cell is most vulnerable during active division. The cell cycle is the process by which the cell replicates and passes on all the information needed to make an identical replication of itself. Most chemotherapeutic agents are classified according to where they affect cell cycle activity and how they affect cellular function.

The goals of chemotherapy are cure, control, or palliation. Cure is the desired outcome for all patients, but its likelihood depends on several factors at the time of diagnosis and other factors throughout the planned treatment course. The extent of disease at diagnosis, the functional status of the patient, the physiologic presentation at diagnosis, and other socioeconomic influences determine the goal of cancer treatment for each patient. Cure may be further defined as a prolonged absence of disease. The term *remission*, which is the absence of detectable disease, may be used instead of cure because some cancers, such as adult leukemia and lymphoma, are likely to recur. Control is the goal of most chemotherapy when a cure is unrealistic. Control is also a cautious approach to treatment outcomes. Control focuses on maintaining or improving functional status in the presence of known disease without complete elimination of disease. Palliation is the goal of chemotherapy when neither cure nor control is possible because of the extent of disease. Quality of life, disease symptom management, and end-of-life issues or hospice are primary concerns when palliation is the goal.

Chemotherapy may be given as a primary, adjuvant, neoadjuvant, or chemopreventive treatment.

- Primary chemotherapy is used to treat a tumor when used primarily as the sole treatment—for example with leukemia and lymphomas.
- Adjuvant therapy is given after a primary treatment (e.g., surgery, radiation); the goal is to reduce the chance of

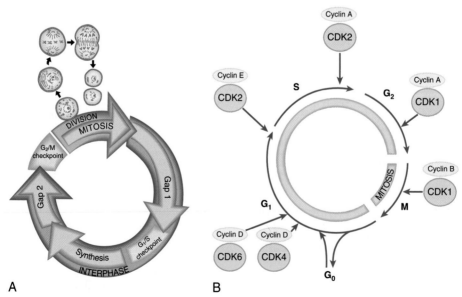

Phases of the cell cycle. (From Huether, S.E. & McCance, K.L. [2017]. *Understanding pathophysiology* [6th ed.]. St. Louis: Mosby.)

recurrence by targeting remaining disease after primary treatment for patients at high risk of recurrence.

- Neoadjuvant therapy is given before another treatment (e.g., surgery, radiation) to improve outcomes. Neoadjuvant therapy also helps to reduce morbidity and mortality from treatment and to treat micrometastasis (Polovich, Olsen, & LeFebvre, 2014).
- Chemoprevention is the use of natural, synthetic, or biologic agents to prevent cancer from occurring in high-risk individuals, such as those with inherited cancer syndromes, a family history of cancer, or a previous diagnosis of cancer.

It is very important that patients and family members be informed of treatment goals before the initiation of therapy so that they can set realistic goals in their personal lives. The information needs to be repeated throughout the course of planned treatments.

Chemotherapy is usually given as combination therapy—that is, two or more agents are used together in an effort to combat drug resistance and increase therapeutic effect. The different agents affect the cell at different points in the cell cycle, allowing for maximum cell kill while minimizing toxicities. Chemotherapeutic agents for combination therapy include those drugs that (1) are effective when used singly against the specific cancer, (2) do not pose the same toxicity or have similar dose-limiting toxicities, and (3) do not have the same time of onset of toxicity. Intermittent therapy may be more effective, less immunosuppressive, and less toxic than continuous therapy given in lower doses (Brown, 2014).

Tumor cells exposed to chemotherapy sometimes develop mechanisms to protect themselves against the drugs' effects; this is termed *drug resistance*. Resistance may result from drug exclusion, drug metabolism, or alteration of the target for the drug by mutation or overexpression. The most significant mechanism of drug resistance is the P-glycoprotein efflux pump, which is associated with overexpression of the multidrug resistance gene, *MDR1* (Tortorice, 2011). Drug resistance may involve many factors that affect response to therapy. Resistance may be inherent or acquired, single-agent or multidrug, temporary or permanent. Prevention of drug resistance is another justification for combination chemotherapy.

Cell Cycle Specificity and Chemotherapy

Chemotherapy uses knowledge of the cell cycle in the attempt to destroy or disrupt the abnormal growth of cancer cells. Most chemotherapeutic agents are classified according to where their effects are produced in the cell cycle. Cell cycle–specific agents exert effect when the cell is actively dividing (i.e., G_1, S, G_2, or M phases). Agents that are cell cycle specific tend to be schedule dependent, because the greatest tumor kill is obtained when the drug is given in frequent divided doses or in continuous infusions to capture the cell in a specific phase. Cell cycle–nonspecific agents are effective in all cell cycle phases, including the resting phase (G_0). Cell cycle–nonspecific agents also exhibit a steep dose-response curve, meaning

that the higher the dose, the greater the response. Dose dense chemotherapy relies on this premise.

Chemotherapy Classifications

Chemotherapeutic agents are classified by mechanism of action and specificity. See the figure in page 208 for a diagram of chemotherapeutic agent mechanisms of action. Each classification contains agents that have similar characteristics and side effect profiles. Although they agents are similar, each agent must be addressed on an individual basis or in combination during finalization of a treatment plan.

Alkylating Agents

Alkylating agents are cell cycle–nonspecific agents that bind with DNA and protein molecules, resulting in DNA strand breakage. Common toxicities include myelosuppression, hypersensitivity, renal impairment, gastrointestinal (GI) toxicities (e.g., nausea and vomiting, diarrhea), and cutaneous toxicities (e.g., alopecia, skin rashes). Side effects are dose dependent and may be cumulative. Alkylating agents are also strongly associated with secondary malignancies (usually different malignancies from the original disease), which can occur months to years after treatment for a primary cancer. Routes of administration include oral, intravenous (IV), intraperitoneal, and topical, depending on the agent and the treatment plan. Common alkylating agents include altretamine, bendamustine, busulfan, carboplatin, chlorambucil, cisplatin, cyclophosphamide, dacarbazine, ifosfamide, mechlorethamine, oxaliplatin, temozolomide, and thiotepa.

Nitrosoureas

Nitrosoureas are cell cycle–nonspecific agents that have a mechanism of action and toxicity profile similar to those of alkylating agents. They have a high lipid solubility, which enables them to pass freely across membranes; therefore, they rapidly penetrate the blood-brain barrier, whereas most other agents are unable to do so (Polovich, Olsen, & LeFebvre, 2014). Blood-brain barrier penetration allows nitrosoureas to be prominently used in the treatment of brain tumors and other central nervous system (CNS) diseases. Common nitrosourea agents include carmustine, lomustine, and streptozocin.

Antimetabolites

Antimetabolites are cell cycle–specific agents that work during the S phase of the cell cycle. Specifically, they interfere with DNA synthesis by imitating the chemical structure of essential enzymes needed for DNA replication or by becoming incorporated into the structure of the DNA molecule. These agents are most effective against cancers that have a high growth fraction or rapidly dividing cells. Common toxicities include myelosuppression, GI toxicities (e.g., nausea and vomiting, mucositis, diarrhea), and cutaneous toxicities (e.g., rash, alopecia, photosensitivity, hyperpigmentation). Routes of administration are based on agent and treatment plan and may include topical, oral, IV, intrathecal (IT), and intramuscular routes. Common antimetabolites include

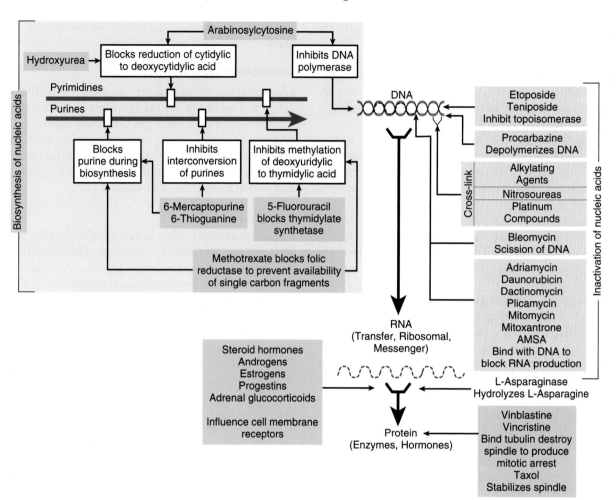

Mechanism of action of chemotherapeutic agents. (From Krakoff, I. [1991]. Cancer chemotherapeutic and biologic agents. *CA: A Cancer Journal for Clinicians, 41*, 264-278.)

capecitabine, cladribine, cytarabine, cytarabine liposomal, floxuridine, fludarabine, fluorouracil, gemcitabine, mercaptopurine, methotrexate, nelarabine, pentostatin, pemetrexate, praltrexate, and thioguanine.

Antitumor Antibiotics

Antitumor antibiotics are cell cycle–nonspecific agents that have different mechanisms of action depending on the agent used. Antitumor antibiotics are referred to as natural products because they occur naturally or are synthesized from microorganisms and have both antimicrobial and cytotoxic activity. Antitumor antibiotics have two primary mechanisms of cell kill: free radical formation and the inhibition of topoisomerase II enzyme, which results in DNA disruption and, eventually, cell death. Some antitumor antibiotics are also known as anthracyclines. Metabolism of anthracyclines can produce free radicals that form iron-containing complexes that are especially harmful to cardiac tissue (Volkova & Russell, 2011). Common toxicities include myelosuppression and GI, cutaneous, and primary organ (e.g., cardiac, pulmonary) toxicities. Routes of administration include IV, intraarterial, and intravesical (bladder instillation). Common antitumor antibiotics include bleomycin, dactinomycin, daunorubicin, daunorubicin citrate liposomal, doxorubicin, doxorubicin liposomal, epirubicin, idarubicin, mitomycin, mitoxantrone, and valrubicin.

Plant Alkaloids

Plant alkaloids are cell cycle–specific agents that act by binding to specific cell proteins that cause mitotic arrest, resulting in depletion of amino acids that are necessary for cell replication and apoptosis. Plant alkaloids are naturally occurring alkaloids isolated from plant material or synthetic and semisynthetic compounds originally extracted from plants. Common side effects include myelosuppression, GI toxicities (e.g., constipation, diarrhea), hypersensitivity reactions, cutaneous toxicities (alopecia), and autonomic and peripheral neurologic toxicities. Routes of administration are based on the agent and the treatment plan and include oral, IV, and IT. Plant alkaloids are divided into four categories:

1. Camptothecins (e.g., irinotecan, topotecan)
2. Epipodophyllotoxins (e.g., etoposide, teniposide)
3. Taxanes (e.g., cabazitaxel, paclitaxel, docetaxel)
4. Vinca alkaloids (e.g., vinblastine, vincristine, vinorelbine)

Microtubular Stabilizing Agents

A number of agents in clinical development target microtubules. Intact microtubules are needed for the formation of mitotic spindles in the process of cell division. This class of chemotherapy drugs is called *epothilones* (Chang, Bradley, & Budman, 2008). They were isolated from the mycobacterium, *Sporangium cellulosum*. The drugs work in the G_2/M phase of the cell cycle to initiate apoptosis. Although their mechanisms of action are similar to the taxanes, epothilones... resistance, because they seem to be less susceptible to p-glycoprotein overexpression, a mechanism of resistance in taxanes.

Epothilones have shown activity in several cancers, including breast, lymphoma, renal, prostate, and ovarian cancers. Side effects are similar to those of taxanes. Hypersensitivity reactions have been reported in cremophor-based epothilone agents. Other side effects to monitor for are neutropenia, peripheral neuropathy, fatigue, arthralgia, myalgia, nausea and vomiting, diarrhea, and stomatitis. Ixabepilone is currently in use, and several more epothilone agents are in clinical trials (Chang, Bradley, & Budman, 2008).

Miscellaneous Agents

Additional miscellaneous agents exist that are cell cycle nonspecific and have different mechanisms of action. They inhibit protein synthesis, block DNA replication, or trigger mechanisms that mediate cell death. Common side effects include myelosuppression, GI toxicity, and hepatotoxicity. Routes of administration include IV, subcutaneous (SC), intramuscular (IM), and oral. Commonly used miscellaneous agents include arsenic trioxide, asparaginase, bortezomib, mitotane, and pegaspargase.

See the table below for a list of chemotherapy agents, their classifications, mechanisms of action, and common uses.

Chemotherapy Drug Classes and Agents

Drug Class and Mechanism of Action	Drug Name	Oncologic Indications
Alkylating Agents		

Cell cycle nonspecific
Break DNA helix strand,
    thereby interfering with DNA replication
	Altretamine (Hexamethyl-
	    melamine, Hexalen)
		Ovarian cancer

	Bendamustine (Treanda)	Chronic lymphocytic leukemia (CLL) B-cell non-Hodgkin lymphoma
	Busulfan (Myleran, Busulfex)	Chronic myelogenous leukemia Blood disorders: polycythemia vera, myeloid metaplasia
	Carboplatin (Paraplatin)	Ovarian cancer Lung cancer Head and neck cancers Endometrial cancer Esophageal cancer Bladder cancer Breast cancer Cervical cancer CNS tumors Germ cell tumors Osteogenic sarcoma
	Chlorambucil (Leukeran)	Chronic lymphocytic leukemia (CLL) Non-Hodgkin lymphoma Hodgkin disease Breast cancer Ovarian cancer Testicular cancer Waldenström macroglobulinemia Thrombocythemia Choriocarcinoma
	Cisplatin (Platinol, PlatinolAQ, CDDP)	Testicular cancer Ovarian cancer Bladder cancer Head and neck cancer Small cell lung cancer Non–small cell lung cancer Esophageal cancer Breast cancer Cervical cancer Stomach cancer Prostate cancer Hodgkin lymphoma Non-Hodgkin lymphoma Neuroblastoma Sarcomas Multiple myeloma Melanoma Mesothelioma

Continued

Chemotherapy Drug Classes and Agents—cont'd

Drug Class and Mechanism of Action	Drug Name	Oncologic Indications
	Dacarbazine (DTIC-Dome, DTIC, DIC, Imidazole Carboxamide)	Metastatic malignant melanoma Hodgkin disease Soft tissue sarcomas Neuroblastoma Fibrosarcoma Rhabdomyosarcoma Islet cell carcinoma Medullary thyroid carcinoma
	Ifosfamide (Ifex)	Testicular cancer Soft tissue sarcoma Ewing sarcoma Osteogenic sarcoma Non-Hodgkin lymphoma Hodgkin disease Non–small cell lung cancer Small cell lung caner Bladder cancer Head and neck cancer Cervical cancer
	Mechlorethamine (Nitrogen Mustard, Mustargen, Mustine)	Hodgkin disease Non-Hodgkin lymphoma Lung cancer Breast cancer Cutaneous T-cell lymphoma
	Melphalan (Alkeran)	Multiple myeloma Ovarian cancer Neuroblastoma Rhabdomyosarcoma Breast cancer
	Oxaliplatin (Eloxatin)	Metastatic colorectal cancer
	Procarbazine (Matulane)	Hodgkin disease Non-Hodgkin lymphoma Brain tumor Melanoma Lung cancer Multiple myeloma
	Temozolomide (Temodar)	Anaplastic astrocytoma Glioblastoma multiforme
	Thiotepa (Thioplex, TESPA, TSPA)	Breast cancer Ovarian cancer Non-Hodgkin lymphoma Hodgkin lymphoma Bladder cancer
Antitumor Antibiotics Cell cycle nonspecific Varying mechanisms Antimicrobial and cytotoxic	Bleomycin (Blenoxane)	Squamous cell cancers Melanoma Sarcoma Testicular cancer Hodgkin's and non-Hodgkin lymphoma
	Dacarbazine (DTIC-Dome, DTIC, DIC, Imidazole Carboxamide)	Metastatic malignant melanoma Hodgkin disease Soft tissue sarcomas Neuroblastoma Fibrosarcoma Rhabdomyosarcoma Islet cell carcinoma Medullary thyroid carcinoma
	Daunorubicin (Cerubidine)	Acute myelogenous leukemia (AML) Acute lymphoblastic leukemia (ALL)

Chemotherapy Drug Classes and Agents—cont'd

Drug Class and Mechanism of Action	Drug Name	Oncologic Indications
	Daunorubicin Liposome (DaunoXome)	Advanced Kaposi sarcoma with HIV
	Doxorubicin HCl (Adriamycin, Rubex)	Bladder cancer Breast cancer Head and neck cancers Leukemia (some types) Liver cancer Lung cancer Lymphoma Mesothelioma Multiple myeloma Neuroblastoma Ovarian cancer Pancreatic cancer Prostate cancer Sarcomas Stomach cancer Germ cell tumors Thyroid cancer Uterine cancer
	Doxorubicin Liposome (Doxil)	Kaposi sarcoma in AIDS
	Epirubicin (Ellence)	Breast cancer
	Idarubicin (Idamycin PFS)	Acute myelogenous leukemia (AML) Acute lymphoblastic leukemia (ALL) Chronic myelogenous leukemia (CML) Myelodysplastic syndrome (MDS)
	Mitomycin (Mutamycin)	Adenocarcinoma of the stomach or pancreas Anal cancer Breast cancer Bladder cancer Cervical cancer Colorectal cancer Head and neck cancer Non–small cell lung cancer
	Mitoxantrone (Navantrone)	Prostate cancer Acute myelogenous leukemia (AML) Breast cancer Non-Hodgkin lymphoma
	Valrubicin (Valstar)	Bladder cancer
Plant Alkaloids: Camptothecins, Epipodophyllotoxins, Taxanes, and Vinca Alkaloids		
Cell cycle specific Bind to certain cell proteins to initiate mitotic arrest	Camptothecins: Irinotecan (Camptosar, CPT-11)	Metastatic colorectal cancer
	Topotecan HCl (Hycamptin)	Ovarian cancer Small cell lung cancer
	Epipodophyllotoxins: Etoposide (Toposar, Etopophos,VP-16, VePesid)	Testicular cancer Prostate cancer Bladder cancer Lung cancer Stomach cancer Uterine cancer Hodgkin lymphoma Non-Hodgkin lymphoma Mycosis fungoides Kaposi sarcoma Wilms tumor Rhabdomyosarcoma Ewing sarcoma Neuroblastoma Brain tumors
	Teniposide (Vumon)	Acute lymphoblastic leukemia
	Taxanes: Cabazitaxel (Jevtana)	Prostate cancer

Continued

Chemotherapy Drug Classes and Agents—cont'd

Drug Class and Mechanism of Action	Drug Name	Oncologic Indications
	Docetaxel (Taxotere)	Breast cancer Non–small cell lung cancer Advanced stomach cancer Head and neck cancer Metastatic prostate cancer
	Paclitaxel (Taxol, Onxal)	Breast cancer Ovarian cancer Lung cancer Bladder cancer Prostate cancer Melanoma Esophageal cancer
	Paclitaxel protein-bound particles (Abraxane)	Breast cancer Non–small cell lung cancer Pancreatic cancer
	Vinca Alkaloids: Vinblastine (Velban, Alkaban-AQ, VLB, vinblastine sulfate)	Hodgkin disease Non-Hodgkin lymphoma Testicular cancer Breast cancer Lung cancer Head and neck cancers Bladder cancer Kaposi sarcoma T-cell lymphoma Choriocarcinoma
	Vincristine (Oncovin, Vincasar Pfs, vincristine sulfate)	Acute leukemias Hodgkin lymphoma Non-Hodgkin lymphoma Neuroblastoma Rhabdomyosarcoma Ewing sarcoma Wilms tumor Multiple myeloma Chronic leukemias Thyroid cancer Brain tumors
	Vinorelbine (Navelbine)	Non–small cell lung cancer Breast cancer Ovarian cancer Hodgkin disease
Antimetabolites Cell cycle specific Act in S phase; interfere with DNA and RNA function	Azacitidine (Vidaza)	Chronic myelomonocytic leukemia (CMML) Myelodysplastic syndrome (MDS)
	Capecitabine (Xeoloda)	Metastatic breast cancer Metastatic colorectal cancer
	Cladribine (Leustatin, 2-CDA, 2-Chlorodeoxyadenosine)	Hairy cell leukemia Chronic lymphocytic leukemia (CLL) Non-Hodgkin lymphomas
	Clofarabine (Clolar)	Relapsed or refractory acute lymphoblastic leukemia (aged 1-21 years)
	Cytarabine (Arabinosylcytosine, ARA-C, Cytosar-U)	Acute myelogenous leukemia (AML) Chronic myelogenous leukemia (CML) Acute lymphoblastic leukemia (ALL) Lymphoma Meningeal leukemia and lymphoma
	Cytarabine liposomal (DepoCyt)	Meningeal lymphoma
	Decitabine (Dacogen)	Myelodysplastic syndrome (MDS)
	Floxuridine (FUDR)	Colon cancer Kidney cancer Stomach cancer
	Fludarabine (Fludara)	Chronic lymphocytic leukemia Non-Hodgkin lymphoma Acute leukemias
	5-Fluorouracil (5FU, Adrucil)	

Chemotherapy Drug Classes and Agents—cont'd

Drug Class and Mechanism of Action	Drug Name	Oncologic Indications
	Gemcitabine (Gemzar)	
	Hydroxyurea (Droxia, Hydrea, Mylocel)	Chronic myeloid leukemia Essential thrombocytosis Polycythemia vera Head and neck cancer Melanoma Ovarian cancer
	Mercaptopurine (6-MP, Purine-thol)	Acute lymphoblastic leukemia
	Methotrexate (Rheumatrex, Trexall)	Breast cancer Head and neck cancers Lung cancer Stomach cancer Esophagus cancer Acute lymphoblastic leukemia (ALL) Sarcomas Non-Hodgkin lymphoma Gastrointestinal trophoblastic cancer Cutaneous T-cell lymphoma
	Nelarabine (Arranon)	T-cell acute lymphoblastic leukemia T-cell lymphoblastic leukemia
	Pemetrexed (Alimta)	Malignant mesothelioma Non-squamous non–small cell lung cancer
	Pentostatin (Nipent)	Hairy cell leukemia Non-Hodgkin lymphoma
	Pralatrexate (Folotyn)	Peripheral T-cell lymphoma
	Thioguanine (Thioguanine Tabloid, 6-thioguanine, 6-TG)	Acute myelogenous leukemia Chronic myelogenous leukemia
Nitrosoureas Cell cycle nonspecific Bind with DNA protein molecules, cross the blood-brain-barrier	Carmustine (BCNU, BiCNU)	Brain tumors Multiple myeloma Hodgkin disease Non-Hodgkin lymphoma Melanoma Lung cancer Colon cancer
	Lomustine (CCNU, CeeNu)	Brain tumors Hodgkin disease Non-Hodgkin lymphoma Melanoma Lung cancer Colon cancer
	Streptozocin (Zanosar)	Islet cell carcinoma of the pancreas Carcinoid tumor and syndrome
Microtubule-Stabilizing Agents: Epothilones Cell cycle specific Act in G_2/M phase	Eribulin (Halaven)	Metastatic breast cancer
	Ixabepilone (Iaxempra)	Breast cancer
Miscellaneous Varying mechanisms	Amifostine (Ethyol, WR-2721)	Help relieve dry mouth from radiation for head and neck cancers Protect kidneys from harmful effects of repeated doses of cisplatin for advanced ovarian cancer
	Arsenic trioxide (Trisenox)	Acute promyelocytic leukemia (APL) Multiple myeloma (MM) Chronic myelogenous leukemia (CML) Acute myelogenous leukemia (AML)
	Bacillus Calmette-Guerin (TICE, TheraCys, BCG)	Bladder cancer Immunization against tuberculosis
	Bexarotene (Targretin)	Cutaneous T-cell lymphoma
	Dexrazoxane (Zinecard)	Avoid cardiotoxic side effects of doxorubicin for breast cancer
	Enzalutamide (Xtandi)	Metastatic castration resistant prostate cancer
	Estramustine (Emcyt)	Prostate cancer

Continued

Principles of Cancer Management 3

Chemotherapy Drug Classes and Agents—cont'd

Drug Class and Mechanism of Action	Drug Name	Oncologic Indications
	Isotretinoin (Accutane, 13-cis retinoic acid)	Severe acne Investigated in multiple cancers
	L-Asparaginase (Elspar, Kidrolase)	Acute lymphocytic leukemia (ALL)
	Leucovorin (Folinic Acid, Citrovo-rum Factor)	Colorectal cancer Head and neck cancers Gastrointestinal tract cancers Antidote to effects of certain chemotherapies such as methotrexate
	Mesna (Mesnex)	Prevention of ifosfamide-induced hemorrhagic cystitis Prevention of high-dose cyclophosphamide-induced hemorrhagic cystitis
	Octreotide (Sandostatin LAR)	Control symptoms of diarrhea and flushing for: Carcinoid tumors Pancreatic islet cell tumors Gastroma Vasoactive intestinal peptide-secreting tumors
	Pegaspargase (Oncaspar, PEG-L-asparaginase)	Acute lymphocytic leukemia (ALL) Non-Hodgkin lymphoma
	Thalidomide (Thalomid)	Investigational: Multiple myeloma Renal cell carcinoma Glioblastoma multiforme Waldenström macroglobulinemia Graft-versus-host disease after bone marrow transplant
	Tretinoin (Vesanoid)	Acute promyelocytic leukemia

From National Comprehensive Cancer Network Clinical Practice Guidelines in Oncology. Accessed May 10, 2016 at https://www.nccn.org/professionals/physician_gls/f_guidelines.asp; Gaddis, J. S., & Gullatte, M. M. (2014). Cellular mechanisms of chemotherapy. In M. M. Gullatte (Ed.). *Clinical guide to antineoplastic therapy: A chemotherapy handbook* (3rd ed., pp. 1-19). Philadelphia, PA: Oncology Nursing Society; and Polovich, M., Olsen, M., & LeFebvre, K. B. (Eds.). (2014). Chemotherapy and biotherapy guidelines and recommendation for practice (4th ed.). Pittsburg, PA: Oncology Nursing Society.

Patient and Family Assessment and Preparation

Nurses administering chemotherapy should conduct a pretreatment assessment of the patient, keeping in mind the individual characteristics of the patient and comorbidities that can affect the response to and toxicities of treatment. Past experiences can affect how patients perceive chemotherapy treatments and interactions with the health care team. Preconceived ideas of cancer, cultural and ethnic background, adult learning style, educational background, socioeconomic status, past coping mechanisms, and numerous other influences affect the needed preparation for chemotherapy. Inclusion of family, significant others, and existing support systems is critical in preparation for chemotherapy initiation (see box below).

Patient Education Regarding Chemotherapy

1. Review the treatment plan and protocol.
   - Names and actions of the drugs to be administered
   - Names and actions of the drugs to be taken by the patient at home
   - Schedule of drug administration
   - Length of the treatment plan
2. Review the purpose or goals (i.e., cure or palliation) of the chemotherapeutic treatment.
3. Review the potential side effects of chemotherapy and self-care activities to prevent or treat the side effects.
4. Review the schedule and rationale for diagnostic tests.
5. Provide the patient and family members with information on when and how to contact the nurse or the provider.

Data from Oncology Nursing Society. (2014). *Chemotherapy and biotherapy guidelines and recommendations for practice* (4th ed.). Pittsburg, PA: Oncology Nursing Society.

Safe Handling

One of the most prevailing issues for staff is the inherent potential for harm in the delivery of care to cancer patients. Chemotherapy agents are hazardous drugs and require caution in their administration. Hazardous drug handling guidelines have been available for almost 30 years. According to the American Society of Health-System Pharmacists (ASHP), any drug that requires special handling is referred to as a hazardous drug (ASHP, 2006). Recommendations for practice have been established by the Oncology Nursing Society (ONS), the Occupational Safety and Health Administration (OSHA), and the National Institute for Occupational Safety and Health (NIOSH) for safe handling of chemotherapy agents.

For an agent to be classified as a hazardous drug, one or more of the following criteria must be met: genotoxicity, carcinogenicity, teratogenicity or reproductive/fertility toxicity, and mimicking of existing drugs that have been determined to be hazardous by these standards (NIOSH, 2004). Drugs classified as hazardous include antineoplastic or cytotoxic agents, biological agents, antiviral agents, and immunosuppressive agents. Health care professionals involved in preparation, administration, and disposal of hazardous drugs and waste face potential work-related exposure (NIOSH, 2004). Each institution that uses hazardous drugs must have a hazardous drug safety and health plan.

Potential routes of exposure are limited to the following: absorption through skin or mucous membranes, injection, ingestion, and inhalation (Polovich & Martin, 2011). Recommended guidelines focus on eliminating or minimizing these routes of possible exposure. Safety guidelines must be used in storage and labeling, transportation, preparation, administration, and disposal of hazardous drugs. Environmental safety must also be a major portion of safety guidelines.

Environmental

The compounding and preparation of hazardous drugs should be performed in a controlled area with access limited to authorized personnel specially trained in handling requirements. The ASHP further recommends that the following considerations be addressed in the hazardous drug safety and health plan for drug preparation areas:

- Establishment of a designated hazardous drug handling area
- Use of containment devices such as biological safety cabinets (BSC)
- Procedures for safe removal of contaminated waste
- Decontamination procedures

Chemotherapy should be prepared sterilely in a BSC. The BSC also provides a means for safe preparation of chemotherapy agents, minimizing airborne exposure of the health care worker. Criteria for BSCs are given in the Biological Safety Cabinet Criteria box below. Additional guidelines for chemotherapy preparation and administration are presented in the Hazardous Drug Safety Guidelines box in the next column.

Biological Safety Cabinet (BSC) Criteria

1. Provide vertical laminar air flow.
2. Eliminate exhaust through a high-efficiency particulate air filter. Ideally a BSC should be vented to the outside (NIOSH, 2004).
3. Have a blower that operates continuously (ASHP, 2006).
4. Locate the BSC in a low-traffic area to reduce interference with air flow.
5. Individuals using the BSC should be trained to use techniques that reduce interference with air flow.
6. The BSC should be serviced according to the manufacturer's recommendation.
7. The BSC should be recertified every 6 months (ASHP, 2006).

Adapted from Oncology Nursing Society. (2014). *Chemotherapy and biotherapy guidelines and recommendations for practice* (4th ed.). Pittsburgh, PA: Oncology Nursing Society.

Other critical safety guidelines incorporate the use of appropriate personal protective equipment (PPE), including gloves, gowns, respirator, and face/eye protection. The clinical setting and potential risks of exposure should determine PPE selection whenever there is a risk of exposure or release into the environment. Latex-containing materials should be avoided because of possible sensitivity reactions. See the Appropriate Personal Protective Equipment with Hazardous Drugs box in the next column for specific PPE recommendations on the use of hazardous drugs.

Hazardous Drug Safety Guidelines

1. Use a plastic-backed absorbent pad on work and delivery surfaces.
2. Use closed-system drug transfer devices.
3. Use safe technique in the opening of ampule necks.
4. Avoid pressure buildup when reconstituting drugs packaged in vials if a closed system not available.
5. Use tubing and syringes with Luer-Lok fitting.
6. Avoid overfilling syringes.
7. Prime all tubing with fluids that do not contain the hazardous drug.
8. Place a label on each container with the words "Cytotoxic Drug" or a similar warning.
9. Wipe outside of container with moist gauze before placing it in a sealable bag for transport.
10. Dispose of all materials that have come in contact with the hazardous drug in waste containers designated for hazardous waste.
11. Remove and discard outer gloves and gown before removing inner gloves.
12. Wash hands before leaving work area.

Data from Oncology Nursing Society. (2014). *Chemotherapy and biotherapy guidelines and recommendations for practice* (4th ed.). Pittsburgh, PA: Oncology Nursing Society.

Appropriate Personal Protective Equipment with Hazardous Drugs

Gloves

- Meet testing standards set by the American Society for Testing and Materials for use with hazardous drugs (designated "chemotherapy gloves").
- Inspect for defects before donning.
- Powder free
- Disposable
- Double-glove.
- Nitrile or neoprene material (with latex sensitivity)
- Change after 30-60 min or immediately if there is visible contamination or damage.

Gowns

- Disposable
- Lint free
- Low-permeability fabric
- Solid front with back closure
- Long sleeves with tight cuffs
- Glove cuffs that extend over the gown cuffs
- Gown should not be reused.
- Discard if visibly contaminated, before leaving drug preparation areas, and after handling hazardous drugs.

Respirators

- NIOSH-approved respirator mask
- Used when cleaning a hazardous drug spill
- Surgical masks *do not* provide respiratory protection.

Eye and Face Protection

- Wear protection whenever there is a possibility of splash.
- Goggles or face shield should be available wherever hazardous drugs are prepared, mixed, or administered.

Data from Oncology Nursing Society. (2014). *Chemotherapy and biotherapy guidelines and recommendations for practice* (4th ed.). Pittsburgh, PA: Oncology Nursing Society.

Storage and Labeling

Careful attention must be paid to all potential exposures, including during storage and labeling of chemotherapeutic agents. Agents should be stored in a location that permits appropriate temperature and safety inspections and meets regulations.

Labeling should indicate the contents as a hazardous drug. Standardized instructions (e.g., Material Safety Data Sheet) on what to do in the event of accidental exposure should be readily available in all areas where hazardous drugs are stored, prepared, transported, administered, or disposed of. In the home setting, the same guidelines are to be followed, and the patient and family are provided with extensive education.

When chemotherapy is given in the home setting, standardized safety guidelines must be followed. The patient and family should be instructed about proper handling in the home. Education should include the following:

- Keep drugs out of the reach of children and pets.
- Protect drugs and packages from puncture or breakage.
- Do not remove labels.
- Store in an area that is free of moisture and temperature extremes.
- Have a spill kit in the home with detailed instructions on appropriate use.
- Maintain a list of emergency contact numbers.

Transportation

Hazardous drugs should be transported in a sealed leak-proof container. Always Luer-Lok the end of the syringe, and *never* transport with needles in place. The outermost container should have a "hazardous waste" label. Transporters should receive education on hazardous risk, safety precautions, and spill kit use in the event of a spill or contamination.

Spill Kit

A hazardous drug spill kit should be available wherever hazardous drugs are stored, transported, prepared, or administered. All staff members who work with hazardous drugs should be trained in spill cleanup. Spill kits may be purchased commercially or prepared by the individual institution as long as they meet approved guidelines. The following are guidelines to be followed in the event of a hazardous drug spill (Polovich & Martin, 2011):

- Post signs to warn others of the spill.
- Don two pairs of chemotherapy-safe gloves, a disposable gown, and a face shield.
- Wear a respirator.
- Contain the spill with plastic-backed absorbent pads.
- Pick up glass fragments using scoop or utility gloves worn over chemotherapy gloves. Place glass in a puncture-proof container.
- Place the puncture-proof container inside a bag and seal it. Double-bag all material, and label outermost bag as hazardous waste.
- Remove PPE as previously instructed, place it in disposable waste bag, and seal.
- Place all items in a puncture-proof container.

Documentation of a spill should include the name of the drug, the approximate volume spilled, how the spill occurred, and spill management procedures followed, as well as the names of personnel, patients, and others exposed and a list of personnel notified of the spill (see table in the next column).

Contents of Antineoplastic Spill Kit

Number	Item
2 pairs	Disposable chemical-protective gloves (optional pair of utility gloves)
1	Low-permeability, disposable protective garments (coveralls or gown and show covers)
1	Face shield
1	Respirator
1	Absorbent, plastic-backed sheets or spill pads
3-4	Disposable towels
2	Sealable thick plastic hazardous waste disposal bags with an appropriate warning label
1	Disposable scoop for collecting glass fragments
1	Puncture-resistant container for glass fragments

Data from American Society of Health-System Pharmacists. (2006). ASHP guidelines on handling hazardous drugs. *American Journal of Hospital Pharmacy, 63,* 1172-1193.

Waste and Disposal

Universal precautions are used when handling the blood, emesis, or excreta of a patient who has received chemotherapy within the past 48 hours. A protective barrier ointment should be applied to the skin of patients who are incontinent, and the skin should be cleaned with each diaper change. It is recommended that the toilet be flushed with the lid down. Although lowering the lid in the home setting is applicable, most institutions do not have lids, so efforts must again focus on protective barriers for employees. Flushing the toilet twice has been a long-standing practice and may still be helpful with low-volume flush toilets found in home settings. However, most institutions have high-volume flush toilets that may not require double-flushing (Polovich, 2011). All linen with exposure to chemotherapy should be laundered separately in hot water. The use of leak-proof disposable pads for incontinent episodes is helpful. Disposable items should be discarded in an appropriately labeled hazardous waste container (Polovich, Olsen, & LeFebvre, 2014).

Proper Care of Vesicants and Irritants

Although all chemotherapy agents require special handling to minimize exposure, special considerations must be incorporated for patients receiving agents identified as vesicants or irritants.

- Vesicants are agents that have the ability to cause blistering or tissue necrosis.
- Irritants are agents that have the ability to cause aching, tightness, and phlebitis with or without a local inflammatory reaction but do not cause tissue necrosis.
- Extravasation is the passage of chemotherapeutic agents into tissue. Necrosis or sloughing may occur.
  Risk factors for extravasation include the following:
- Small or fragile veins
- Poor vascular integrity
- Peripheral neuropathy
- Previous multiple venipunctures
- Limited vein selection
- Peripheral edema
- Unstable venous access because of the patient's condition

- Altered mental status that renders the patient unable to report discomfort at IV site
- Site of venous access (avoid veins in hand, wrist, and antecubital fossa whenever possible)

Extravasation can occur in peripherally inserted central catheters (PICC) and central access devices (CAD). Factors related to potential extravasation in a PICC line or CAD include catheter damage, displacement, and migration.

Prevention and early detection are of primary importance to avoid extravasation. Signs and symptoms of extravasation include the following:

- Severe swelling
- Stinging, burning, or intense pain
- Blotchy redness around the needle site (not always present at the time of extravasation)
- Inability to obtain blood return
- Ulceration that develops within 48 to 96 hours

Nurses must know which agents can cause this damage, be aware of the warning symptoms, and be familiar with agents that can cause extravasation. If extravasation does occur, nursing management is critical to patient outcome. Initial management includes the following measures:

- Stop infusion.
- Disconnect IV tubing from site or device. Do not remove device or catheter.
- Attempt to aspirate residual drug from device with a small (1-3 mL) syringe.
- Notify physician.
- Apply hot or cold compress as indicated.
- Initiate antidote, if applicable.

After extravasation, the following measures should be taken:

- Photograph the extravasation site and repeat weekly if appropriate.
- Instruct patient to rest and elevate extremity for 48 hours.
- Give written instructions regarding what symptoms to report immediately.
- Arrange for return appointment.
- Consult plastic surgeon, if applicable.

Extravasation is a serious matter that causes added pain, discomfort, wound healing issues, and treatment delays. By following administration guidelines, nurses can limit the possibility of an extravasation (Polovich & Martin, 2011) (see table below).

Vesicant Treatments and Antidotes

Vesicant	Warm versus Cool Therapy	Pharmacologic Antidote
Alkylating Agents	Cool	Sodium thiosulfate indicated for mechlorethamine only – local injection
Anthracyclines	Cool	Dexrazoxane – systemic
Antitumor Antibiotics	Cool	None indicated
Taxanes	Cool	None indicated
Vinca Alkaloids	Warm	Hyaluronidase – local injection

Routes of Administration

After obtaining knowledge of the characteristics of the chemotherapeutic agents to be given, the next decision is route of administration selection. Chemotherapeutic agents are administered by multiple routes to achieve systemic or regional delivery to the tumor.

The goal of systemic therapy is to attain a drug concentration that is sufficient to achieve a therapeutic toxic effect against the presumed or known disease without causing excessive toxicity to normal tissue. Regional chemotherapy is directed toward the goal of delivering the agent directly into the blood supply of the tumor or into the cavity or area in which the tumor is located. Regional administration of chemotherapy often allows for higher concentrations of the drug to be delivered to the area of the tumor with fewer systemic side effects.

The major routes used for systemic administration are the oral, IV, SC, and IM routes. Regional routes include IT, intra-arterial, and intracavity. Once the route of administration has been identified, appropriate patient/family and staff education must occur.

Education should include the identified route of administration, potential complications of the identified route, and the possible use of a vascular access device. With administration routes that may be used in the home setting (i.e., oral, SC, IM, and IV), special attention should be given to instructions on keeping agents out of the reach of small children and pets, proper storage without temperature extremes, and the use of spill kits.

Oral Route

The use of oral chemotherapeutic agents has escalated in the past few years. Advantages of oral chemotherapeutic agents include ease of use, portability, and patient independence. Several factors need to be evaluated before oral therapy is initiated:

1. Availability of the drug in an oral formulation
2. Functional status of the patient's gastrointestinal tract
3. Presence of nausea, vomiting, or dysphasia
4. Patient's level of consciousness
5. Patient's willingness and ability to adhere to the dosing schedule
6. Cost and reimbursement issues for oral preparations

Although it may seem deceptively simple to administer oral preparations, oral agents require special consideration and planning. Extensive patient/family and staff education should occur. Teaching should include the name, dose, and time at which agents should be taken, known or anticipated side effects, established prophylaxis for known side effects, appropriate physician or nurse notification, and safe handling issues. To ensure compliance with the administration schedule, the following factors should be assessed: presence of a caregiver in the home, living conditions (e.g., plumbing, electricity), access to emergency assistance, and whether the patient will need nursing follow-up in the home. Patients may also benefit from some form of organized delivery system (e.g., pill box) and a daily diary. A diary will allow consistent documentation of agent administration, side effect occurrence, and barriers to agent administration. It will also serve as an incentive to maintain scheduled dosing of the medications. The website of the American College for Preventive Medicines and other sites have tools that nurses can use to help educate patients regarding adherence to oral medication regimens (see box below).

Oral Medication Adherence Tool	
S	Simplify the regimen (e.g., adjust timing, dosage, and frequency of medication use)
I	Impart knowledge (e.g., written information)
M	Modify patient beliefs and behaviors (e.g., assess barriers and benefits)
P	Provide communication and trust (e.g., actively listen)
L	Leave the bias (e.g., tailor education to the patient's level of understanding)
E	Evaluate adherence (e.g., count pills)

Data from the American College of Preventive Medicine. (2011). Provider strategies to improving adherence. Available at www.acpm.org/?MedAdherTT_ClinRef (accessed February 4, 2016).

Subcutaneous and Intramuscular Routes

As with the oral agents, administration of chemotherapy by SC or IM routes allows a high degree of patient independence. Education of the patient and family regarding self-injection, disposal of sharps, site rotation, and monitoring should be incorporated into the teaching plan, along with safe handling in the preparation, administration, and disposal of waste in the home setting. Although the advantages are similar to those of oral preparations, the disadvantages vary greatly. Disadvantages include pain or discomfort at site of injection, possible infection at injection sites, and bleeding.

Topical Route

Although the topical route of chemotherapy is not frequently used, it remains an option. Careful guidelines should be adhered to when applying topical chemotherapy. Strict adherence to PPE is critical, as is environmental control during application and disposal of waste.

Intravenous Route

Chemotherapy is most commonly administered by the IV route in most patient care settings (Camp-Sorrell, 2011). Methods of administration include the following:

- Push—agent administered through syringe directly into vein
- Free-flow with a direct push—agent administered with syringe into the side port of a free-flowing IV
- Piggyback—use of a secondary bag or bottle and tubing connected to a primary infusion of IV fluids
- Continuous infusion—usually given over 12 hours for up to 5 to 7 days

The choice of IV administration site depends on the venous status of the patient, the vesicant/irritant potential of the agent, and patient preference. In peripheral sites, several factors must be incorporated. The patient's age and vein status, the drugs infused, and the expected period of infusion determine selection of the appropriate site and equipment. A flexible catheter should be used rather than a steel-winged due to prevent damage to the vessel with patient movement. See the table below for vein selection guidelines.

Peripheral Vein Selection	
Existing intravenous site	Do not use site >24 hr old.
	Assess site for inflammation and infiltration; if present, choose an alternate site.
	Assess for blood return and patency.
New intravenous site	Select a vein that is smooth and pliable.
	Avoid small, fragile, injured, or sclerosed veins.
	Avoid extremity with altered venous return or lymphedema.
	Avoid lower extremities.
	Avoid veins in the wrist, hand, or antecubital areas.
	Use nondominant arm whenever possible.

Adapted from Oncology Nursing Society. (2014). *Chemotherapy and biotherapy guidelines and recommendations for practice* (4th ed.). Pittsburgh, PA: Oncology Nursing Society.

Other options for IV administration include the use of central venous catheters or central venous access devices (VAD). Types of devices include percutaneous subclavian catheters (e.g., Hickman, Groshon, Broviac), PICC, and implanted devices and ports (e.g., chemoport, Passport, Infuse-a-Port). With all devices, proper placement must initially be verified radiographically. Thereafter, placement is verified by aspirating for a blood return before each use. Manufacturer or institutional guidelines should be closely followed for care, maintenance, and use of CAD. Infection prevention should be a primary focus of VAD use because these devices allow direct entry to the vascular system (Marschall et al., 2014). Prevention of extravasation should be carefully considered with intravenous administration. Risk factors for intravenous extravasation are included in the box below.

Risk Factors for Extravasation
- Small or fragile veins
- Obesity
- Multiple venipunctures
- Disseminated skin diseases in the area of placement (e.g. eczema)
- Patient movement
- Low pH drugs
- Caustic drugs
- Limited vein availability due to other conditions (e.g. lymphedema)
- Sensory deficits resulting in patient inability to sense IV problems (e.g. paralysis)
- Cognitive impairment or somnolence
- Use of rigid IV devices such as steel-winged or butterfly catheters
- Inadequately secured catheter
- Probing the skin during insertion of a vascular access device (VAD)
- Long dwell time of the VAD (e.g. greater than 6 months)

Data from Polovich, M., Olsen, M., & LeFebvre, K. B. (Eds.). (2014). Chemotherapy and biotherapy guidelines and recommendation for practice (4th ed.) Pittsburg, PA: Oncology Nursing Society and Schulmeister, L. (2010). Extravasation management: Clinical update. Seminars in Oncology Nursing, 27, 82-90.

Intrathecal Route

Intrathecal chemotherapy is the direct installation of chemotherapy into the CNS by lumbar puncture or through an implanted intraventricular device (e.g., Ommaya reservoir). This method allows the therapeutic agent to bypass the blood-brain barrier and enter directly into the CNS, resulting in a direct and consistent drug concentration in the cerebrospinal fluid. Delivery requires multiple invasive procedures (lumbar punctures) or surgery for device implantation. Therapy administration requires a physician, specially trained registered nurse, or nurse practitioner to access and administer chemotherapy by the IT route. Patients should be monitored for headache or other signs of increased intracranial pressure.

Intraarterial Route

Intraarterial chemotherapy involves cannulation of the artery that provides a tumor's blood supply or administration directly into an organ by way of an artery. The primary use of this route is for management of liver metastasis (Goodman, 2005) and for retinoblastoma (Shields et al., 2014). For consistent delivery of chemotherapy, the drug is delivered via an implanted pump after correct placement has been verified. Using a noncoring needle, the pump is accessed and filled with either the chemotherapy agent or heparinized sterile saline solution. Nursing considerations involve monitoring for drug side effects and potential pump complications, such as infections, occlusion, extravasation, and malfunction.

Intracavity Route

Intracavity administration is the direct instillation of a chemotherapy agent into a body cavity. Examples include intrapleural (lung), intraperitoneal (abdomen), and intravesicular (bladder) administration. This route allows direct exposure of a known area of disease to the chemotherapy drugs. Side effects of this route are directly related to the cavity receiving instillation. The intrapleural instillation is usually aimed at sclerosing the pleural lining to prevent reoccurrence of effusions and requires placement of a thoracotomy (chest) tube. The intraperitoneal route requires instillation into a peritoneal catheter or intraperitoneal port. The intravesicular route requires the placement of a Foley catheter. Each of these methods carries the risk of infection along with other site-specific complications. Special attention must be given to PPE (including face shield) with the use of this route (Polovich, Olsen, & LeFebvre, 2014).

Administration in Special Populations

Many special populations in the treatment of cancer in adult populations exist. Although cancer is a difficult prospect in the best of situations, special-needs populations require increased knowledge about the unique group. Cancer in pregnant women and in the elderly is reviewed here, and appropriate interventions are discussed.

Pregnancy Considerations

Cancer is the second leading cause of death during the reproductive years. The most common cancers associated with pregnancy are lymphoma, leukemia, malignant melanoma, and cancers of the breast, cervix, ovary, and colorectum. A diagnosis of cancer during pregnancy is a devastating time for expectant mothers and family members. They must consider the mother's health but also cannot ignore the health of the unborn fetus.

Chemotherapy has been administered before and during pregnancy. The decision to initiate chemotherapy during the first trimester usually results in a therapeutic abortion before the chemotherapy treatment. Chemotherapy may be given in the second or third trimester of pregnancy with careful monitoring of mother and fetus and careful selection of the agent used. The decision of when to proceed with chemotherapy is ultimately the mother's choice. The options are to delay treatment until the fetus is viable or near term or to proceed with therapy during pregnancy (Goodman, 2005). Nursing interventions include incorporation of standardized education and emotional support for the patient and family in a nonjudgmental, professional manner.

Considerations for Older Adults

Cancer is a disease associated with aging; people older than 65 years of age have an 11-fold increase in the incidence of cancer. By the year 2030, it is estimated that 20% of the population in the United States will be aged 65 years or older. Data have shown that older adults and younger adults derive similar benefits from chemotherapy (Hurria et al., 2011). Physiologic changes are a part of the normal aging process. These changes affect treatment decisions for some elderly patients but not all. Physiologic and functional status, not chronological age, should dictate treatment options. Myths and misconceptions held by both elderly patients and the public in general are obstacles to prevention, early detection, diagnosis, and treatment of cancer in this group. Some of these misconceptions include the notion that poor health is a natural part of aging, the question of dementia and self-care issues, and the idea that multiple comorbidities eliminate the possibility of chemotherapy. Issues that factually affect treatment options include an impaired immune system, inadequate nutritional status, obesity, polypharmacy, poor or limited support systems, and limited financial resources. Although consideration of these issues must be incorporated into the plan of care for an elderly patient, they do not eliminate the possibility of productive treatment for a cancer diagnosis. A risk stratification schema developed by Hurria and associates (2011) can help to establish the risk of chemotherapy in older adults.

Palliative Chemotherapy

Palliative care is patient- and family-centered care that focuses on the distressing symptoms of cancer, such as pain.

Palliative care incorporates psychosocial, spiritual, and cultural beliefs. The goal of palliative care is to improve the quality of life of the patient by anticipating, preventing, and reducing suffering. This care should begin at diagnosis and should be delivered alongside curative therapy, becoming the focus of care when disease-directed care is no longer effective or desired (NCCN, 2014).

Common symptoms treated during palliative care include the following (NCCN, 2014):

- Pain
- Dyspnea
- Anorexia/cachexia
- Nausea/vomiting
- Constipation
- Malignant bowel obstruction
- Fatigue/weakness/asthenia
- Insomnia/sedation
- Delirium

See the box below for the NCCN guidelines for palliative care, which should be considered when discussing treatment goals and the overall chemotherapy treatment plan.

National Comprehensive Cancer Network Standards of Palliative Care

- Institutions should develop processes for integrating palliative care into cancer care, both as part of usual oncology care and for patients with specialty palliative care needs.
- All cancer patients should be screened for palliative care needs at their initial visit, at appropriate intervals, and as clinically indicated.
- Patients and families should be informed that palliative care is an integral part of their comprehensive cancer care.
- Educational programs should be provided to all health care professionals and trainees so that they can develop effective palliative care knowledge, skills, and attitudes.
- Palliative care specialists and interdisciplinary palliative care teams, including board-certified palliative care physicians, advanced practice nurses, physician assistants, social workers, chaplains, and pharmacists, should be readily available to provide consultative or direct care to patients and families who request or require their expertise.
- Quality of palliative care should be monitored by institutional quality improvement programs.

Conclusion

Although cancer treatment has significantly evolved, chemotherapy remains a mainstay of therapy. The number of drugs continues to expand, along with new side effects and toxicities experienced by the patient. Nurses are on the front line and must stay knowledgeable about newly developed agents. They must continue to assess patients diligently and optimally manage treatment toxicities.

References

American Society of Health-System Pharmacists. (2006). ASHP guidelines on handling hazardous drugs. *American Journal of Hospital Pharmacy, 63,* 1172–1193.

Brown, D. L. (2014). Cellular mechanisms of chemotherapy. In M. M. Gullatte (Ed.), *Clinical guide to antineoplastic therapy: A chemotherapy handbook* (3rd ed.) (pp. 1–19). Philadelphia, PA: Oncology Nursing Society.

Camp-Sorrell, D. (Ed.). (2011). *Access device guidelines: Recommendations for nursing practice and education.* Pittsburgh, PA: Oncology Nursing Society.

Chang, K. L., Bradley, T., & Budman, D. (2008). Novel microtubule-targeting agents: The epothilones. *Biologics: Targets & Therapy, 2*(4), 789–811.

Gaddis, J. S., & Gullatte, M. M. (2014). Cellular mechanisms of chemotherapy. In M. M. Gullatte (Ed.), *Clinical guide to antineoplastic therapy: A chemotherapy handbook* (3rd ed.) (pp. 1–19). Philadelphia, PA: Oncology Nursing Society.

Hayden, D. K., & Goodman, M. (2005). Chemotherapy: Principles of administration. In C. H. Yarbro, M. H. Frogge, M. Goodman, et al. (Eds.), *Cancer nursing: Principles and practice* (6th ed.) (pp. 351–411). Sudbury, MA: Jones & Bartlett.

Hurria, A., Togawa, K., Mohile, S. G., Owusu, C., Klepin, H. D., Gross, C. P., & Tew, W. P. (2011). Predicting chemotherapy toxicity in older adults with cancer: A prospective multicenter study. *Journal of Clinical Oncology, 29*(25), 3457–3465.

Krakoff, I. (1991). Cancer chemotherapeutic and biologic agents. *CA: A Cancer Journal for Clinicians, 41,* 264–278.

Marschall, J., Mermel, L. A., Fakih, M., Hadaway, L., Kallen, A., O'Grady, N. P., & Yokoe, D. S. (2014). Strategies to prevent central line–associated bloodstream infections in acute care hospitals: 2014 Update. *Infection Control, 35,* 753–771.

National Comprehensive Cancer Network. (2014). *Palliative care guidelines, version 1.2014.* Available at http://www.nccn.org/professionals/physician _gls/pdf/palliative.pdf (accessed February 4, 2016).

National Institute for Occupational Safety and Health. (2004). Preventing occupational exposure to antineoplastic and other hazardous drugs in health care settings. *DHHS (NIOSH) publication no. 2004-165.* Available at http://www.cdc.gov/noish/docs/2004-165 (accessed February 4, 2016).

Polovich, M. (Ed.). (2011). *Safe handling of hazardous drugs* (2nd ed.) Pittsburg, PA: Oncology Nursing Society.

Polovich, M., & Martin, S. (2011). Nurses' use of hazardous drug-handling precautions and awareness of national safety guidelines. *Oncology Nursing Forum, 38*(6), 718–726.

Polovich, M., Olsen, M., & LeFebvre, K. B. (Eds.). (2014). *Chemotherapy and biotherapy guidelines and recommendation for practice* (4th ed.). Pittsburg, PA: Oncology Nursing Society.

Shields, C. L., Manjandavida, F., Lally, S. E., Peiretti, G., Arepalli, S. A., Caywood, E. H., & Shields, J. A. (2014). Intra-arterial chemotherapy for retinoblastoma in 70 eyes: Outcomes based on international classification of retinoblastoma. *Ophthalmology, 121*(7), 1453–1460.

Tortorice, P. V. (2011). Cytotoxic chemotherapy: Principles of therapy. In C. H. Yarbro, D. Wujcik, & B. H. Gobel (Eds.), *Cancer nursing: Principles and practice* (7th ed.) (pp. 166–198). Burlington, MA: Jones & Bartlett.

Volkova, M., & Russell, R. (2011). Anthracycline cardiotoxicity: Prevalence, pathogenesis and treatment. *Current Cardiology Reviews, 7*(4), 214–220.

Immunotherapy

Sandra Remer

Overview

Immunotherapy, also known as biotherapy, uses the body's immune system to fight cancer. Knowledge of the immune system provides the foundation for understanding the mechanisms of immunotherapy and provides the rationale for combining immunotherapy with other modalities (Drake 2012).

The body is protected from pathogens by natural anatomic barriers such as the skin and mucous membranes and by physiologic barriers such as temperature elevation that augments some immune responses and stomach acid that digests harmful microorganisms.

The immune system itself is composed of many cell types that collectively protect the body from infections and the growth of tumor cells. Its two main arms are the innate and adaptive systems. Cells of the innate system recognize and respond to pathogens in a generic way to provide immediate defense against infection, but they do not confer long-lasting immunity. Because innate immunity has no memory cells, it reacts the same way every time an antigen is encountered.

The adaptive system consists of specialized cells (e.g., lymphocytes) that eliminate or prevent pathogen growth and provide long-lasting protection of the host. Because adaptive immunity includes memory cells, subsequent immune responses are faster and stronger after an initial exposure to a foreign antigen. Like the innate system, the adaptive system includes two broad classes of responses: humoral (antibody) immunity and cell-mediated immunity (Badini, 2011; Kannan, Madden, & Andrews, 2014):

- Humoral immunity: The immune response is mediated by specialized proteins and antibodies (i.e., immunoglobulins). Antibodies are secreted by activated B lymphocytes that are found in bone marrow. Antibodies travel through the bloodstream and bind to specific foreign antigens Binding signals phagocytes or other immune cells to attack and inactivate the foreign antigen, preventing it from binding to the host.
- Cell-mediated immunity: The immune response is controlled by T cells and involves the activation of lymphocytes and release of cytokines in response to an antigen. T cells are made in the bone marrow, and most then develop in the thymus. T cells specifically bind to antigens recognized on foreign or nonself cells and can eliminate tumor cells before they have a chance to grow and spread.

As research provided a better understanding of immunology, the potential role was recognized for activation of the immune system in antitumor therapies. Stimulatory and inhibitory factors in the immune response to cancer are shown in the figure on page 224.

An early hypothesis about tumor immunity was formulated by Paul Ehrlich, who postulated that tumors might express different cell structures that could be recognized by antibodies, increasing the humoral immune response. Unfortunately, early work in the field of tumor immunity was thwarted by the realization that the antitumor activity demonstrated in mice was the result of an allogeneic rejection response to foreign (nonself) tissue rather than direct antitumor immunity. This problem was later overcome by the development of rodent models that allowed for implantation and culturing of tumor grafts without allogeneic rejection. These mouse and rat models are used as a staple in antitumor drug development and therapy research and as a first step in the preclinical approach to understanding a molecule's potential for further study (Rothaermel & Baum, 2009).

The nomenclature for immunotherapy is extensive (see box below and on pages 222 and 223).

Terms Used in Immunotherapy

Antibody: An immunoglobulin that is produced by B cells and that tightly binds to the surface antigen of a cell, tagging it for attack or directly neutralizing it.

Antigen: Any substance that induces an immune response, especially the production of antibodies.

Bacillus Calmette-Guérin (BCG): A weakened form of the bacterium *Mycobacterium bovis* (i.e., bacillus Calmette-Guérin) that does not cause disease. It is used in a solution to stimulate the immune system in the treatment of bladder cancer and as a vaccine to prevent tuberculosis.

B lymphocytes: White blood cells that produce antibodies specific to the antigen that stimulated their production.

Basophils: White blood cells that release histamine (i.e., substance involved in allergic reactions) and produce substances to attract other white blood cells (i.e., neutrophils and eosinophils) to an antigen.

Biologic response modifiers (BRMs): Substances made from living organisms to treat disease. They may occur naturally in the body, or they may be made in the laboratory. Some BRM therapies stimulate or suppress the immune system to help the body fight cancer, infection, and other diseases. Other BRM therapies attack specific cancer cells to prevent their growth or kill them.

BRCA1: A gene on chromosome 17 that normally helps to suppress tumor cell growth. Inherited mutations of *BRCA1* confer a higher risk of breast, ovarian, prostate, and other types of cancers.

Continued

Terms Used in Immunotherapy—cont'd

BRCA2: A gene on chromosome 13 that normally helps to suppress tumor cell growth. Inherited mutations of *BRCA2* confer a higher risk of breast, ovarian, prostate, and other types of cancers.

Cell: The smallest unit of a living organism, composed of a nucleus and cytoplasm surrounded by a plasma membrane.

Center for Biologics Evaluation and Research (CBER): Organization within the FDA that regulates biologic products for human use and provides information to promote their appropriate use.

Chemotaxis: Process of using a chemical substance to attract cells to a particular site.

Complement system: Group of proteins that are involved in a series of reactions (i.e., the complement cascade) that help kill bacteria and other foreign cells by making them easier for macrophages to identify and ingest and by attracting macrophages and neutrophils to a foreign or nonself antigen.

Cytokines: Cell-signaling proteins that are secreted by immune and other cells and act as messengers to help regulate immune responses.

Cytotoxic T cells: T lymphocytes that attach to and kill cancer cells or cells that are otherwise infected or damaged; also known as *CD8+ T cells* or *killer T cells*.

Dendritic cells: Specialized white blood cells that reside in tissues and help T cells to recognize foreign antigens.

Effector T cells (Teffs): Mature T cells released into the bloodstream that are considered to be immunologically naïve until they encounter antigens for which their receptors have a high affinity; recognition of antigen leads to extensive T-cell proliferation and differentiation into effector cells.

Endogenous: Produced inside an organism or cell; the opposite of external (exogenous) production.

Eosinophils: White blood cells containing granules readily stained by eosin that can kill bacteria and other foreign cells too big to ingest, help immobilize and kill parasites, participate in allergic reactions, and help destroy cancer cells.

Ex vivo: A process performed or taking place outside of a living organism, such as genetic modification performed by taking tissue from an organ, modifying it in a controlled environment, and returning it to the original organ for therapeutic purposes.

Fibroblast: Connective tissue cell that makes and secretes collagen proteins.

Glycopeptide: A short chain of amino acids (i.e., building blocks of proteins) that has sugar molecules attached to it. Some glycopeptides have been studied for their ability to stimulate the immune system.

Glycoprotein: A protein that has sugar molecules attached to it.

Granulocyte-macrophage colony-stimulating factor (GM-CSF): Cytokine that promotes the growth of white blood cells, especially granulocytes, macrophages, and megakaryocytes (i.e., cells that become platelets); also called colony-stimulating factor 2. The pharmaceutical analogs of naturally occurring GM-CSF are sargramostim and molgramostim.

Helper T cells: T lymphocytes that carry the CD4 glycoprotein receptor on their surface; when stimulated by foreign antigens, they release cytokines that promote the activation and function of B cells and killer T cells.

Histocompatibility: Molecular profile of tissue defined by human leukocyte antigens and used to determine whether a transplanted tissue or organ will be accepted by the recipient.

Human leukocyte antigens (HLAs): Genetically determined system of proteins on the surface of cells that is almost unique for each person and thereby enables the body to distinguish self from nonself; the human version of the major histocompatibility complex (MHC) system found in most vertebrates.

Human papillomavirus (HPV): DNA Virus with more than 100 HPV subtypes, some of which cause diseases in humans ranging from common warts to cervical cancer.

IDH1: A gene (isocitrate dehydrogenase 1) that is associated with a form of acute myeloid leukemia, chondrosarcomas, and brain tumors called gliomas. Recurrent point mutations affecting codon 132 of *IDH1*, located on chromosome locus 2q33, play a unique role in the pathogenesis of gliomas. Mutated *IDH1* is a strong prognostic factor in diffuse gliomas: Patients whose tumors harbored the wild-type gene had a median overall survival time of 1 year, compared with more than 2 years for those with tumors of the same grade and *IDH1* mutations.

Immune complex: Combination of an antibody and its corresponding antigen.

Immune modulators: Active agents of immunotherapy, such as natural or synthetic monoclonal antibodies and cytokines, or processes such as plasmapheresis, that are used to activate cell-mediated or humoral immunity.

Immune-related response criteria (irRC): Set of rules that define tumor responses during treatment with a drug being evaluated; based on new understanding of efficacy and the timing of response after initial treatment with an immunotherapeutic agent.

Immune response: The reaction of the immune system to an antigen.

Immunoglobulin: An antibody.

Immunosuppression: The immune system may be deliberately downregulated with drugs to prepare for bone marrow transplantation or to prevent rejection of donor tissue. It may also result from diseases such as acquired immunodeficiency syndrome and lymphoma or from the use of anticancer drugs.

Interleukins: Glycoproteins produced by white blood cells; a type of cytokine that regulates immune responses by communicating with and affecting other white blood cells.

Investigational new drug (IND) application: Federal law requires that a drug be the subject of an approved marketing application before it is transported or distributed across state lines. Before a laboratory or other sponsor ships the investigational drug to clinical investigators in other states, it must seek an exemption from the legal requirement by submitting an IND application to the U.S. Food and Drug Administration.

In vivo: A process performed or taking place inside a living organism, such as a genetic modification done within a cell.

Lentivector: *Lentivirus* is a genus in the Orthoretrovirinae subfamily of the Retroviridae family. Lentiviral vectors (LVs) include pathogens of bovine, equine, feline, ovine, and primate origin. Like other retroviruses, lentiviruses are enveloped particles that bud from an infected cell's plasma membrane. The particles bind to a target cell by an interaction between the cell's receptor and the viral glycoprotein.

Leukocytes: White blood cells, such as monocytes, neutrophils, eosinophils, basophils, B lymphocytes, and T lymphocytes.

Lymphocytes: White blood cells responsible for adaptive (acquired) immunity. B cells produce antibodies, T cells distinguish self from nonself, and cytotoxic T cells kill infected cells and cancer cells.

Macrophages: Large cells that develop from white blood cells called monocytes. They ingest bacteria and other foreign cells, help T cells to identify microorganisms and other foreign substances, and are normally present in the lungs, skin, liver, and other tissues.

Major histocompatibility complex (MHC): System of genes that encode cell-surface proteins responsible for regulation of the immune system in vertebrates; in humans, these proteins are called *human leukocyte antigens* (HLAs).

Mast cells: Cells (i.e., granulocytes) found in connective tissues that release histamine and other substances during inflammatory and allergic reactions.

Mesenchymal cells: Loosely organized, mainly mesodermal embryonic cells that develop into connective and skeletal tissue, blood vessels, and lymphatic tissue.

MGMT: Gene that encodes O^6-methylguanine-DNA methyltransferase, which is a DNA repair enzyme that confers resistance to the effects of

Terms Used in Immunotherapy—cont'd

chemotherapy with nitrosourea derivatives (e.g., BCNU) or temozolomide in some tumors such as glioblastomas and astrocytomas.

Moiety: One half or any significant portion of a molecule that may include a functional group.

Molecule: A group of electrochemically bonded atoms that represent the smallest fundamental unit of a chemical compound that can take part in a chemical reaction.

Monoclonal antibody: An antibody produced by cloning of a single cell line in the laboratory that binds to only one antigen. They are used to treat some types of cancers and can be designed to carry drugs, toxins, or radioactive substances directly to cancer cells.

Monocytes: Large, phagocytic white blood cells that are made in the bone marrow and travel through the bloodstream to other sites, where they can differentiate into macrophages and dendritic cells. Macrophages surround and kill microorganisms, ingest foreign material, remove dead cells, and boost immune responses.

Myeloid growth factor: Natural substances that stimulate the bone marrow to make blood cells and can be used prophylactically reduce the severity and duration of neutropenia.

Natural killer (NK) cells: White blood cells that recognize, bind to, and kill virus-infected cells and cancer cells without having to be stimulated by antigens.

Nanoparticles: A microscopic particle that behaves as a whole unit in terms of its transport and other properties and can be designed to carry a drug to tiny metastatic tumors. They are further classified as ultrafine particles (1 to 100 nm), fine particles (100 to 2500 nm), and coarse particles (2500 to 10,000 nm).

Neutrophils: White blood cells that form an essential part of the innate immune system and are among the first responders to acute inflammation. They ingest and kill bacteria and other foreign cells.

Pathogen-associated molecular patterns (PAMPs): Molecules associated with groups of pathogens that activate innate immune responses, protecting the host from infection by identifying some non-self molecules.

Peptide: A molecule that contains two or more amino acids, which join together to form proteins. Peptides that contain many amino acids are called polypeptides or proteins.

Peripheral blood stem cells (PBSCs): A small number of stem cells have escaped the bone marrow before maturation into red blood cells, white blood cells, or platelets and circulate in the bloodstream.

Phagocyte: A type of cell (e.g., neutrophil, macrophage) that is capable of engulfing and absorbing invading microorganisms, other small cells, and cell fragments.

Phagocytosis: The process of engulfing and ingesting invading microorganisms, other small cells, or cell fragments.

Pleiotropic cytokines: A cytokine that affects the activity of multiple cell types. Cytokines are small proteins that have specific effects on the interactions between cells and the behavior of cells.

Polypeptide: A substance that contains many amino acids, which join together to form proteins.

Receptors: Proteins embedded in surface membranes of cells and organelles to which complementary molecules, such as hormones, neurotransmitters, antigens, or antibodies, may become bound.

Regulatory T cells (Tregs): White blood cells that modulate the immune system, maintain tolerance to self-antigens, and abrogate autoimmune disease; formerly known as suppressor T cells.

Ribonucleic acid (RNA): Single-stranded molecule that is transcribed from DNA and assembled from long chains of nucleotides.

Each nucleotide contains a nitrogenous base, a ribose sugar, and a phosphate group. RNA has roles in regulation and expression of genes.

RNA interference (RNAi): A process by which RNA molecules inhibit gene expression, as when microRNA (miRNA) or small interfering RNA (siRNA) molecules bind to specific messenger RNA (mRNA) molecules and increase or decrease their activity.

Signal transduction: Process by which a signal, such as a hormone or a change in the concentration of an ion, is converted into a biochemical response by activation of a receptor on the surface or interior of a cell.

Signal transduction pathways: Groups of molecules in a cell that transmit molecular signals, in a cascading fashion, to control cell functions. Some pathway components serve as markers of tumor activity or provide therapeutic targets, such as the PI3K/AKT/mTOR pathway, which plays a central role in cell growth and proliferation.

T lymphocytes: White blood cells that are involved in adaptive immunity ($\alpha\beta$ T cells) and innate immunity ($\gamma\delta$ T cells). Subpopulations include helper, killer (cytotoxic), and regulatory T cells.

Toll-like receptors (TLRs): A class of proteins that play a key role in the innate immune system. They are single, membrane-spanning, noncatalytic receptors, usually expressed in sentinel cells (e.g., macrophages, dendritic cells), that recognize structurally conserved molecules expressed by microbial pathogens.

TP53: A tumor suppressor gene that normally inhibits the growth of tumors and is mutated in many types of cancers. It is called the guardian of the genome because of its role in conserving stability by preventing genomic mutations.

Transcription: In biology, the first step of gene expression, in which a segment of DNA (gene) is copied (transcribed) into RNA by the enzyme RNA polymerase.

Transfer RNA (tRNA): A small RNA molecule that participates in protein synthesis. Each tRNA molecule has two important areas: a trinucleotide region called the anticodon and a region for attaching a specific amino acid. During translation, each time an amino acid is added to the growing chain, a tRNA molecule forms base pairs with its complementary sequence on the messenger RNA (mRNA) molecule, ensuring that the appropriate amino acid is inserted into the protein.

Tumor microenvironment: The normal cells, molecules, and blood vessels that surround and feed a tumor cell. A tumor can change its microenvironment, and the microenvironment can affect how a tumor grows and spreads.

U.S. Food and Drug Administration (FDA): The federal agency in the Department of Health and Human Services that is responsible for protecting and promoting public health.

Vaccine: One or more substances that are prepared from the causative agent of a disease and treated to act as an antigen (i.e., stimulate the immune system) without inducing the disease. A vaccine helps the body recognize and destroy cancer cells or microorganisms.

Vaccine adjuvant: A substance that is added to a vaccine to improve the immune response so that less vaccine is needed.

Vaccine therapy: Treatment that uses one or more substances to stimulate the immune response against tumor cells or infectious microorganisms such as bacteria or viruses.

Vector: In molecular cloning, a vehicle (e.g., virus, plasmid) whose DNA is used to carry a desired foreign DNA sequence into a host cell (also called recombinant DNA). Depending on the purpose of the cloning procedure, the vector may assist in multiplying, isolating, or expressing the foreign DNA insert.

Data from National Cancer Institute (NCI). (2015). The Cancer Genome Atlas: The next stage. Available at http://www.cancergenome.nih.gov/ (accessed February 8, 2016); U.S. Food and Drug Administration (FDA). (2015). Cellular and gene therapy products. Available at http://www.fda.gov/BiologicsBloodVaccines/CellularGeneTherapyProducts/default.htm (accessed February 8, 2016); National Comprehensive Cancer Network (NCCN). (2015a). Myeloid growth factors, version 2.2044. Available at NCCN.org (accessed February 8, 2016); E. C. Lattime & S. L. Gerson (Eds.). Ex vivo gene therapy in gene therapy for cancer (3rd ed.). Amsterdam: Elsevier; National Center for Biotechnology Information (NCBI). (2015). Resources. Available at www.ncbi.nlm.nih.gov/ (accessed February 8, 2016); National Human Genome Research Institute. (2015). Understanding the human genome project. Available at http://www.genome.gov/25019879-educational resources (accessed February 8, 2016); National Institutes of Health (NIH). (2015a). Human genome project: Time line. Available at www.genome.gov (accessed February 8, 2016); U.S. National Library of Medicine. (2015). Terms. Available at http://www.nlm.nih.gov/medlineplus/ency (accessed February 8, 2016)

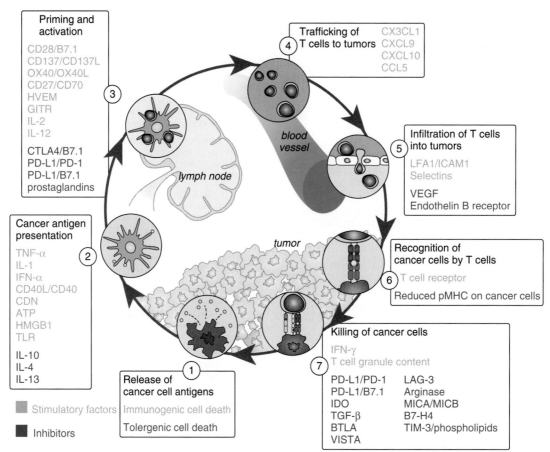

Stimulatory and Inhibitory Factors in the Cancer-Immunity Cycle Each step of the cancer-immunity cycle requires the coordination of numerous factors, both stimulatory and inhibitory in nature. Stimulatory factors shown in pink promote immunity, whereas inhibitors shown in red help keep the process in check and reduce immune activity and/or prevent autoimmunity. Immune checkpoint proteins, such as CTLA4, can inhibit the development of an active immune response by acting primarily at the level of T cell development and proliferation (step 3). We distinguish these from immune rheostat ("immunostat") factors, such as PD-L1, that can have an inhibitory function that primarily acts to modulate active immune responses in the tumor bed (step 7). Examples of such factors and the primary steps at which they can act are shown. *IL,* interleukin; *TNF,* tumor necrosis factor; *IFN,* interferon; *CDN,* cyclic dinucleotide; *ATP,* adenosine triphosphate; *HMGB1,* high-mobility group protein B1; *TLR,* Toll-like receptor; *HVEM,* herpes virus entry media-tor; *GITR,* glucocorticoid-induced TNFR family–related gene; *CTLA4,* cytotoxic T-lymphocyte antigen-4; *PD-L1,* programmed death-ligand 1; *CXCL/ CCL,* chemokine motif ligands; *LFA1,* lymphocyte function-associated antigen-1; *ICAM1,* intracellular adhesion molecule 1; *VEGF,* vascular endothe-lial growth factor; *IDO,* indoleamine 2,3-dioxygenase; *TGF,* transforming growth factor; *BTLA,* B- and T-lymphocyte attenuator; *VISTA,* V-domain Ig suppressor of T cell activation; *LAG-3,* lymphocyte-activation gene 3 protein; *MIC,* MHC class I polypeptide-related sequence protein; *TIM-3,* T-cell immunoglobulin domain and mucin domain-3. Although not illustrated, it is important to note that intratumoral T regulatory cells, macrophages, and myeloid-derived suppressor cells are key sources of many of these inhibitory factors. (From Chen, D. S., & Mellman, I. [2013]. Oncology meets im-munology: The cancer-immunity cycle. *Immunity, 39*[1], 1-10, 25.)

Biologic response modifiers (BRMs) are immunotherapy agents that are categorized as (1) cytokines and adjuvants, which enhance or stimulate the immune system without being antigen specific, and (2) vaccines and monoclonal antibod-ies, which provide antigen-specific immune responses and can have a direct effect on tumor cells (Dillman, 2011; Kuroki et al., 2012). This chapter focuses on BRMs, including their classes, approved indications, administration, side effects, and other pertinent information. These immunotherapy agents and their indications are shown in the table on page 225.

Cytokines

Cytokines are secreted by lymphocytes and monocytes, and they activate or deactivate downstream cellular function, activity, and division (Kuroki et al., 2012). They include the colony-stimulating factors, interferons, and interleukins.

Colony-Stimulating Factors

Colony-stimulating factors are a family of glycoproteins that help to regulate differentiation, proliferation, and activation of hematopoietic cell lineages. They act on different cells of the hematopoietic cascade at different times during the differen-tiation and proliferation phases.

Six colony-stimulating growth factors, also known as myeloid growth factors, are approved for use in the United States:

1. Granulocyte colony-stimulating factor (G-CSF)
2. Granulocyte-macrophage colony-stimulating factor (GM-CSF)
3. Erythropoietin (EPO)
4. Interleukin-11 (IL-11)
5. Keratinocyte growth factor
6. Thrombopoietin (TPO) receptor agonists

Approved Immunotherapy Agents

Agents	Drug Class	Oncologic Indications
Filgrastim Filgrastim-sndz Tbo-filgrastim Pegfilgrastim	Granulocyte colony-stimulating factor (G-CSF)	Tbo-filgrastim and pegfilgrastim are approved for use in patients with nonmyeloid malignancies receiving anticancer therapy. Filgrastim and filgrastim-sndz can be used in patients with acute myelogenous leukemia (AML), those undergoing peripheral blood progenitor cell collection, those undergoing bone marrow transplantation, and those with severe chronic neutropenia.
Sargramostim	Granulocyte-macrophage colony-stimulating factor (GM-CSF)	Used after induction therapy for AML and for stem cell transplantation
Epoetin alfa Erythropoietin	Erythropoiesis-stimulating agent (ESA)	Treatment of anemia in patients with nonmyeloid malignancies for anemia due to myelosuppressive chemotherapy and when there are at least 2 more months of planned chemotherapy
Oprelvekin	Thrombopoietic growth factor	Recombinant interleukin-11 prevents severe thrombocytopenia and reduces the need for platelet transfusions after myelosuppressive chemotherapy in adult patients with nonmyeloid malignancies.
Romiplostim Eltrombopag	Thrombopoietin (TPO) receptor agonists	Immune thrombocytopenia
Palifermin	Keratinocyte growth factor	Decreases incidence and duration of severe inflammation and ulceration of the lining of the mouth and throat (i.e., mucositis) in patients with bone marrow cancer who are receiving chemotherapy and radiotherapy to prepare the bone marrow for stem cell transplantation
Interferon alfa	Interferon	Chronic hepatitis B and C Kaposi sarcoma related to acquired immunodeficiency syndrome (AIDS) Condyloma acuminatum Malignant melanoma Follicular lymphoma Predominantly clear cell stage IV renal cell carcinoma
Human papillomavirus quadrivalent vaccine	Vaccine	Prevention of cervical, vulvar, vaginal, and anal cancer in women Prevention of anal and penile cancer in men
Interleukin-2	Interleukin	Renal carcinoma Melanoma
Ipilimumab	Monoclonal antibody and checkpoint inhibitor	Targets the CTLA4 receptor and stimulates the immune system Unresectable or metastatic melanoma
Nivolumab	Monoclonal antibody and immunomodulator	Targets the programmed cell death protein 1 (PD1) receptor on T cells Unresectable or metastatic melanoma Metastatic squamous non–small cell lung cancer

Granulocyte Colony-Stimulating Factor. G-CSF is a myeloid growth factor that regulates cell proliferation, maturation, and function of the neutrophil cell lineage of the myeloid cell line. Although G-CSF may have downstream effects on other cell lineages and their functions under certain circumstances, its primary role is to reduce the incidence of neutropenia and aid hematopoietic recovery from cytotoxic and radiotherapeutic treatments (Amgen, 2015d, 2015e; DeVita, Hellman, & Rosenberg, 2015; National Cancer Center Network [NCCN], 2015b; Rothaermel & Baum, 2009).

G-CSF can be secreted by a variety of cells in the body (DeVita, Hellman, & Rosenberg, 2015):

- Marrow stromal cells
- Epithelial cells
- Macrophages
- Endothelial cells
- Other immune cells such as natural killer cells

G-CSF can be readily detected in circulating serum at levels of 20 to 100 mg/dL. Circulating G-CSF levels and secretion are directly affected by inflammatory responses to toxins and tissue damage and are inversely affected by the total number of circulating neutrophils. In severely neutropenic subjects, detectable serum levels of G-CSF can be in excess of 2000 mg/dL (DeVita, Hellman, & Rosenberg, 2015; NCCN, 2015a).

Because of the ability of G-CSF to upregulate the function and proliferation of neutrophils, it is used in the treatment of neutropenia due to oncologic therapies. With this class of drugs, patients receiving marrow-toxic chemotherapeutic regimens have earlier neutrophil recovery and a decreased risk of opportunistic, potentially life-threatening infections.

Four G-CSFs are in use in the United States (see table above):

1. Filgrastim (Neupogen)
2. Pegfilgrastim (Neulasta)
3. Tbo-filgrastim (Granix)
4. Filgrastim-sndz (Zarxio)

Use of these agents has reduced the incidence of febrile neutropenia and decreased the length of hospital stays. Tbo-filgrastim and filgrastim-sndz are biosimilars and should not be used interchangeably with filgrastim or pegfilgrastim. Filgrastim is the parent molecule of this class of cytokines. Randomized clinical trials have demonstrated that the use of filgrastim results in the following (Amgen, 2015a; NCCN, 2015a):

- Reduction in occurrence of febrile neutropenia
- Significant decrease in hospital length of stay for infection
- Decrease in overall use of antibiotics
- Reduction in the absolute neutrophil count recovery time for patients with acute myeloid leukemia (AML) undergoing induction or consolidation therapy

- Reduction in the median number of days of severe neutropenia for patients receiving myeloablative chemotherapy for bone marrow transplantation (BMT)
- Significant elevation of colony-forming units of granulocytes and macrophages and CD34-positive progenitor cells in the setting of stem cell collection and mobilization

An increase in the number of these cells is a predictor of engraftment and time to platelet recovery after transplantation. The pegylated formulation of filgrastim, pegfilgrastim, is a covalent conjugate of filgrastim in which a glycol molecule has been bound to filgrastim, resulting in reduced renal clearance and prolonged persistence in vivo. This molecular change results in an average half-life of 15 to 80 hours for pegfilgrastim (compared with 3 to 4 hours for filgrastim), allowing single-dose administration after each course of chemotherapy associated with a significant risk of febrile neutropenia (Amgen, 2015b; NCCN, 2015a).

Pegfilgrastim produces equivalent reductions in days of severe neutropenia compared with filgrastim in patients receiving chemotherapy associated with a high risk of neutropenia. Because of its prolonged half-life, pegfilgrastim should not be used within the 14 days leading up to the administration of chemotherapy (Amgen, 2015b).

Granulocyte-Macrophage Colony-Stimulating Factor. GM-CSF is potent cytokine that directly affects hematopoiesis and has many implications for the care of patients with cancer (DeVita, Hellman, & Rosenberg, 2015; Rothaermel & Baum, 2009). GM-CSF is excreted by the following cell lines:

- Marrow stromal cells
- Fibroblasts
- Endothelial cells
- T lymphocytes

The most prolific production of GM-CSF is by activated T lymphocytes. GM-CSF affects a diverse population of cell lineages in the hematopoietic cascade, including all myeloid cell lines, and affects myeloid dendritic cell activation, proliferation, and differentiation. GM-CSF can increase circulating numbers of neutrophils, eosinophils, and macrophages (DeVita, Hellman, & Rosenberg, 2015; NCCN, 2015b).

Pharmacokinetic studies of GM-CSF have shown a significant increase in sustained circulating levels of GM-CSF in the serum when the recombinant cytokine is administered by subcutaneous injection compared with intravenous administration. Subcutaneous administration is therefore the preferred route (NCCN, 2015a).

The only form of GM-CSF approved by the U.S. Food and Drug Administration (FDA) is sargramostim. It is primarily used for myeloid reconstitution after autologous or allogeneic BMT. It is also used to treat neutropenia induced by chemotherapy for AML, after transplantation of autologous peripheral blood progenitor cells, and in the setting of BMT failure and engraftment delay (Berlex, 2015; NCCN, 2015b).

Additional clinical trials and studies are being conducted to better define the role of GM-CSF in the treatment of malignancies and treatment-related side effects. Investigations include the treatment of chemotherapy- and radiotherapy-induced mucositis, dendritic cell activation, and tumor vaccination (NCCN, 2015b).

Erythropoiesis-Stimulating Agents. Erythropoiesis-stimulating agents (ESAs), unlike other CSFs, act directly on pluripotent stem cells and in the later stages of hematopoietic development, targeting myeloid progenitor cells and erythrocytes. Erythropoietin (EPO) is also unique among cytokines in that it is almost exclusively secreted by the liver and kidneys rather than the bone marrow (NCCN, 2015a).

EPO production and secretion are inversely affected by the oxygen-carrying capacity of the circulating red blood cells (DeVita, Hellman, & Rosenberg, 2015). This negative feedback loop decreases EPO secretion when levels of oxygen-binding capacity are high and increases EPO secretion when levels are low, balancing the numbers of circulating red blood cells with the body's oxygen demands without overproduction of red blood cells. In some instances, EPO overproduction resulting in erythrocytosis is observed in patients with primary renal tumors that cause local renal hypoxic conditions or tumors that intrinsically oversecrete EPO (DeVita, Hellman, & Rosenberg, 2015).

In patients with cancer, ESAs are indicated for the effects of concomitant myelosuppressive but noncurative chemotherapy when at least 2 additional months of therapy are planned. Historically, ESAs have been widely used for the treatment of chemotherapy-associated anemia, but data have revealed that the agents may shorten overall survival time or increase the risk of tumor progression in some patients. When using ESAs, the lowest dose is recommended to avoid red blood cell transfusions, and the agent should be used only in patients with noncurative disease. Physicians must enroll in a specific monitoring program to prescribe ESAs for patients with cancer (Amgen, 2015e).

Interleukin-11. IL-11 (oprelvekin) is a thrombopoietic growth factor that directly stimulates the proliferation of hematopoietic stem cells and megakaryocyte progenitor cells and induces megakaryocyte maturation, resulting in increased platelet production (DeVita, Hellman, & Rosenberg, 2015; Wyeth-Pfizer Pharmaceuticals, 2015). IL-11 is approved for the prevention of severe thrombocytopenia after myelosuppressive, nonmyeloablative chemotherapy in patients with nonmyeloid malignancies (Rothaermel & Baum, 2009). In clinical studies, IL-11 has improved platelet nadirs, decreased the time to platelet recovery, and decreased the need for platelet transfusions in patients receiving chemotherapy (Wyeth-Pfizer Pharmaceuticals, 2015).

The use of IL-11 is absolutely contraindicated for patients receiving myeloablative chemotherapy because of the significantly increased risk of edema, conjunctival bleeding, hypotension, and tachycardia. Administration of IL-11 is also associated with a significant risk of allergic reaction, including anaphylaxis, and it should be discontinued immediately at the first sign of a drug-related allergic response (Wyeth-Pfizer Pharmaceuticals, 2015).

IL-11 therapy should begin 6 to 24 hours after chemotherapy completion. However, the safety and efficacy of IL-11 have not been determined in patients undergoing chemotherapy administration associated with prolonged or delayed myelosuppression, as is the case with mitomycin C and nitrosoureas (Wyeth-Pfizer Pharmaceuticals, 2015).

Keratinocyte Growth Factor. Keratinocyte growth factor (KGF), also known as *fibroblast growth factor 7*, is a cytokine originating from mesenchymal cells, fibroblasts, and microvascular endothelial cells. It activates epithelial cell repair and provides protection in response to inflammatory cytokines and steroidal hormones (Rothaermel & Baum, 2009; Sobi, 2015). Evidence suggests that the addition of KGF to chemotherapy for myeloid malignancies can prevent gastrointestinal graft-versus-host disease by acting as a cytokine protectant and by reducing the generation of proinflammatory cytokines. KGF can promote T-cell engraftment and reconstitution, indicating that KGF may play an important role in the prevention of epithelial toxicity in the treatment of myeloid malignancies (Sobi, 2015; Sonis, 2009).

Studies have also looked at the protective properties of KGF in the setting of chemotherapy- and radiotherapy-induced mucositis. For patients with hematologic malignancies, trials have demonstrated a direct correlation between KGF administration and a reduction in the severity and duration of oral mucositis due to intense chemotherapy regimens (Sonis, 2009). In vitro and in vivo studies have shown KGF to be an important cytoprotectant through its ability to positively affect epithelial cell differentiation, proliferation, and migration and because of having beneficial effects on epithelial cell survival, repair, and detoxification after exposure to cytotoxins. Results of a phase III trial of transplant recipients with hematologic malignancies receiving high-dose radiation therapy and chemotherapy before transplantation showed a significant reduction in the incidence and duration of severe oral mucositis ($P < 0.001$) in the KGF arm, which led to approval for use of palifermin (KGF) in this setting (Amgen, 2015c; Sonis, 2009).

Additional trials looking at the potential benefit of KGF in epithelial solid tumors are being conducted (Rothaermel & Baum, 2009). Studies are needed to determine further use of these growth factors.

The recommended dosage of palifermin is 60 mcg/kg/day, administered as an intravenous bolus for 3 consecutive days before and 3 consecutive days after myelotoxic therapy (total of 6 doses) for patients with hematologic malignancies planning to receive conditioning regimens in preparation for hematopoietic stem cell transplantation. It is not recommended if melphalan (200 mg/m^2) is used in the conditioning regimen (Sobi, 2015).

Thrombopoietin Agonists. Thrombopoietin (TPO) agonists are cytokines that increase platelet production through the regulation of thrombopoiesis. They are indicated for patients with chronic immune thrombocytopenia (ITP) and are activated by TPO receptors on the megakaryocyte cell surface. Two TPO receptor agonists, romiplostim and eltrombopag, are approved (Siegal, Crowther, & Cuker, 2013).

Gene Therapy

Gene therapy refers to any manipulation of the human genome with the intent of producing a therapeutic effect. This broad term can be used for any genomic manipulation, such as increasing immunization potential, adding cytotoxic agents directly to tumor cell lines, or increasing the immunologic effects of effector cells with the addition of tumor antigen genes (DeVita, Hellman, & Rosenberg, 2015).

Gene therapy is a technique that attempts to introduce engineered genetic material (DNA or RNA) into living cells to treat or prevent disease by compensating for abnormal genes or making a beneficial protein. Since its inception in the late 1980s, gene therapy has led a greater understanding of the potentials and limitations of manipulating the genes responsible for tumor growth and survival. For example, deletion or mutation of the *TP53* tumor supressor gene is associated with an increased risk of several malignancies (Adir et al., 2014). With the completion of the Human Genome Project in 2004 and the Cancer Genome Atlas project, the identification of many gene mutations opened the door for advanced treatment of many cancers. They include *BRCA1* and *BRCA2* mutations in breast cancer, *BRAF* mutations in melanoma, and *MGMT* and *IDH1* mutations in brain tumors (DeVita, Hellman, & Rosenberg, 2015; National Cancer Institute [NCI], 2015). The first human gene therapy trial was successfully conducted in 1990. Some human gene therapies have been approved in Europe, but none has been approved in the United States (FDA, 2015), although that could change as several therapies enter advanced trials.

Development of gene therapy is complex. Because genetic material cannot be inserted directly into cells, it is delivered using a carrier (i.e., vector). The vectors most commonly used in gene therapy are viruses because they can recognize certain cells and insert genetic material into them, as they do when they infect cells. To make them safer for humans, viruses are altered by inactivating genes that enable them to reproduce or cause disease, and they are altered to improve their ability to recognize and enter the target cell. A variety of liposomes (i.e., fatty particles) and nanoparticles are also being used as gene therapy vectors.

Technologic challenges to in vivo gene therapy have limited most studies in which immune cells or tumor cells are removed from a donor and then manipulated and cultured for later reintroduction to the host body (Baranyi, Slepuskin, & Dropulic, 2014; DeVita, Hellman, & Rosenberg, 2015). Several delivery systems are being evaluated in clinical trials:

- Nonviral vectors
- Nanoparticles
- Cationic liposomes
- Low-voltage electroporation
- Viral vectors
  - Retroviral vectors
  - Adenoviruses
  - Adeno-associated viruses

- Lentiviral vectors

In addition to the previous delivery systems for the transfer of foreign genes into host cells, many other methods are being studied to determine the most effective approach for various situations (DeVita, Hellman, & Rosenberg, 2015; Yuan, Pastoriza, Quinn, & Libutti, 2014).

RNA interference is another therapeutic modality used to treat various cancers by silencing the expression of cancer-related genes. Encouraging results warrant further research to employ the full capabilities of RNA interference as therapeutic cancer treatment (Baranyi, Slepushkin, & Dropulic 2014; Gujrati & Lu, 2014).

Oncolytic adenoviruses offer another therapeutic option. These agents can directly infect and kill tumor cells. Adenoviruses are double-stranded DNA viruses that normally cause mild respiratory, digestive, and ocular infections in humans. They have been used to deliver genes and are considered to be safe and easy to genetically manipulate. Advances have been seen in the use of oncolytic virotherapy in brain tumors and multiple myeloma (Balvers et al., 2014).

Direct modification of cells that cause the immune response continues to be an active area of research. Modifications may be accomplished by T-cell gene manipulation or by circumventing the tumor's ability to protect itself from or hide from immune cells. Tumor cells can be made more recognizable to immune cells by the induction of cytokine genes, noncytokine response genes, costimulatory signal expression genes, and genes that increase the number of T-cell receptor sites on the tumor surface. Increasing the immune system's response to tumor cells can be accomplished with the use of monoclonal antibodies and by amplifying the adaptive immune response with tumor-specific vaccines (discussed later) (Rothaermel & Baum, 2009).

Transduction of a cytokine gene into neoplastic cells elicits a strong inflammatory host reaction that impairs tumor growth. Cytokine gene therapy causes overexpression of the cytokines that upregulate and activate immune cells. One trial of interleukin-2 (IL-2) demonstrated an increase in $CD8^+$ T cells in tumors but not $CD4^+$ T cells, which may validate the lack of need for $CD4^+$ helper T cells with an increase in IL-2. Most trials, however, have failed to demonstrate clinical benefit in the setting of melanoma, breast cancer, renal cancer, and sarcoma.

IL-2 has also been studied for its role in enhancing the longevity of T cells. T cells transduced with the *IL2* gene can stimulate themselves in an autocrine fashion and thereby increase their life span and antigen specificity in an IL-2–independent state (DeVita, Hellman, & Rosenberg, 2015).

When gene therapy is planned as a treatment modality, it must first be determined how the transferred material will act in the long term. In certain circumstances, short-term gene expression is appropriate, in which case adenoviral transfer of genetic antigens is appropriate, whereas in the setting of permanent or long-term gene expression, retroviral transfer may be most suitable (DeVita, Hellman, & Rosenberg, 2015).

As gene therapy research continues to evolve, the clinical interpretation of anticancer gene transfer research raises ethical questions, which may not be addressed by the basic structure of research regulation. Current regulations underlined in pivotal documents emphasize the importance of research ethics. The Nuremberg Code, the Declaration of Helsinki, and the Belmont Report implicitly or explicitly refer to four important values underlying ethical conduct of research: scientific integrity, beneficence, respect for persons, and justice. Research regulations are evolving, and how they accommodate the ethical questions driven by translational gene transfer research will be shaped by people's philosophical interpretations of what core ethical values this type of research demands (Hyun & Kimmelman, 2014).

Interferons

Interferons (IFNs), named for their ability to interfere with viral replication, were first identified in 1957 by British researchers Isaacs and Lindemann at the National Institute for Medical Research in London (Gantz et al., 1995; Jonasch & Haluska, 2001). Interferons are part of a large family of immunoregulatory proteins that include type I IFNs called alpha (IFN-α), beta (IFN-β), delta (IFN-δ), epsilon (IFN-ε), kappa (IFN-κ), omega (IFN-ω), and tau (IFN-τ); a type II IFN called gamma (IFN-γ); and type III IFNs called lambda (IFN-λ), such as INF-λ or IL-29, INF-λ2, and IFN-λ3 or IL-28B (Borden & Sondel, 1990; Jonasch & Haluska, 2001; Kalliolias & Ivashkiv, 2010). These naturally occurring glycoproteins are secreted primarily by leukocytes, fibroblasts, macrophages, lymphocytes, and in some instances, epithelial cells.

Type I IFNs include at least 13 IFN-α members along with those of the IFN-β, IFN-ε, IFN-κ, and IFN-ω groups (Kalliolias & Ivashkiv, 2010). All type I IFNs bind to type I receptors on cell surfaces (i.e., IFNAR1 and IFNAR2), which then bind to the Janus-activated kinase (JAK) molecules TYK2 and JAK1, respectively. The IFN-γ receptors IFNGR1 and IFNGR2 are associated with JAK1 and JAK2, respectively. On binding, the receptor undergoes oligomerization, with transphosphorylation of JAKs followed by phosphorylation of the cytoplasmic tails of the receptor molecules. This provides a docking site for the signal transducers and activators of transcription (Jonasch & Haluska, 2001; Kalliolias & Ivashkiv, 2010; Rothaermel & Baum, 2009).

After binding, IFN exerts its effect by suppressing proliferation, inducing cell apoptosis, inhibiting angiogenesis, increasing the immunogenicity of tumor cells, and activating cytotoxicity against tumor cells. IFN plays an essential role in anticancer therapy through its immunomodulatory effects such as the upregulation of natural killer cells (key players in antibody-dependent cellular cytotoxicity), macrophages, dendritic cells, neutrophils, and T and B cells (Jonasch & Haluska, 2001; Rothaermel & Baum, 2009).

Interferon alfa-2b, an antiviral drug, first received FDA approval for the treatment of hairy cell leukemia (Dillman, 2011; Jonasch & Haluska, 2001). Over the next 8 years, it received approval for treating chronic hepatitis B and C, AIDS-related Kaposi sarcoma, condyloma acuminatum, malignant melanoma, follicular lymphoma, Philadelphia chromosome–positive chronic myelogenous leukemia (CML), and advanced renal cell carcinoma.

IFN-α remains the only approved interferon for the treatment of malignancies in the United States. IFN-β has received approval for use in multiple sclerosis, and IFN-γ is approved for use in chronic granulomatous disease. Approved interferons include the following (Dillman, 2011; Jonasch & Haluska, 2001; Rothaermel & Baum, 2009):

- Interferon alfa-2a (Roferon-A)
- Interferon alfa-2b (Intron-A)
- Interferon alfa-n3 (Alferon-N)
- Peginterferon alfa-2a (Pegasys)
- Peginterferon alfa-2b (PegIntron)
- Interferon beta-1a (Avonex)
- Interferon beta-1b (Betaseron)
- Interferon alfacon-1 (Infergen)
- Interferon gamma-1b (Actmmune)

Interferon is administered by subcutaneous injection, which results in a slow clearance of approximately 24 hours. Intravenous administration is not recommended due to the rapid clearance of the agent, nor is oral administration recommended because interferon is easily destroyed by digestive enzymes. Doses are determined by weight or body surface area and are commonly ordered with an induction (loading) dose followed by maintenance doses.

Interferons can cause constitutional, neuropsychiatric, hematologic, and hepatic side effects, which vary in severity and duration, and effective management requires different techniques. The severity of side effects appears to be related to the dose and duration of therapy.

Side effects are classified as acute or chronic. Acute toxicities include fever, chills, and rigors usually lasting between 3 and 6 hours after infusion. Patients may also experience flu-like symptoms, headache, myalgias, malaise, transaminitis, and neutropenia. Doses may be adjusted to control the latter. Transaminitis and neutropenia resolve after stopping therapy, but if transaminitis is not followed closely, it may result in fatal hepatotoxicity.

Fatigue is the most common symptom, which occurs in 70% to 100% of patients, and it is frequently the dose-limiting side effect. Chronic fatigue is multifaceted and must be investigated to ensure patient safety. Other chronic side effects include anorexia (40% to 70% of patients) and neurologic toxicities (up to 30%), which include somnolence, confusion, lethargy, dizziness, mental status changes, peripheral neuropathy (i.e., numbness and tingling), and extrapyramidal symptoms. Depression is common. Cognitive impairment can also occur, which can manifest as attention deficits, memory loss, reasoning problems, and impaired psychological adaptation and quality of life (Dillman, 2011; FDA, 2015; Jonasch & Haluska, 2001). Duration of therapy and dose appear to be highly correlated with the severity and duration of symptoms.

Additional toxicities include endocrine dysfunction such as hypothyroidism and significant stimulation of the hypothalamic-pituitary axis resulting in alterations of sex hormones. Dyspnea, pulmonary infiltrates, pneumonia, bronchiolitis obliterans, interstitial pneumonitis, pulmonary hypertension, and sarcoidosis are among the respiratory toxicities observed.

Interferon may cause drug interactions with the use of cytochrome P450 enzyme inducers (e.g., rifampin, phenobarbital, carbamazepine, phenytoin), and these agents should not be used with interferon due to a loss of efficacy. Obtaining a complete list of past medical problems and all drugs being taken by a patient, including over-the-counter and herbal medications, is essential to prevent and manage toxicities. Patients should receive adequate information about self-care and self-assessment of side effects. Nurses should encourage patients to report symptoms early. Education should include information about side effects and strategies to promote quality of life.

Interleukins

The class of cytokines referred to as interleukins (ILs) were named for their ability to interact with the leukocytes of the immune system. Interleukins are being studied in the treatment of malignancies. Many studies are investigating IL-2 and its ability to mediate antitumor responses by enhancing the proliferation and function of lymphokine-activated killer cells (Borden & Sondel, 1990; DeVita, Hellman, & Rosenberg, 2015; Dillman, 2011; Poust, Woolery, & Green, 2012).

Interleukins play a significant role in the maintenance of hematopoiesis and response to foreign body invasion. Interleukins are a key component in the inflammatory response and attraction of effector cells to the point of origin of infection. They play an important role in the stimulation and proliferation of effector and immune cell lines during the infection process. Of the 18 interleukins discovered, those with the greatest potential for anticancer use are IL-1, IL-2, IL-3, IL-6, IL-7, IL-11, IL-12, and IL-16.

IL-1 has a main role in inflammatory responses, is primarily produced by the macrophages in response to stimulation by toxins and other cytokines, and helps lymphocytes fight infection. It also helps leukocytes pass through blood vessel walls to sites of infection and causes fever by affecting areas of the brain that control body temperature. Two subtypes of IL-1 (IL-1α and IL-1β) share the same receptor site on cell surfaces, but each type affects cells in different ways. IL-1 locally affects cells by increasing production of adhesion molecules, prostaglandins, and chemokines (Wyeth-Pfizer Pharmaceuticals, 2015). A systemic response to invading toxins occurs through the production of fever and hypotension in the host.

The promise of IL-1 in cancer treatment has been limited by its significant side effect profile. However, potential utility may be seen in antiinflammatory diseases such rheumatoid arthritis and septic shock (DeVita, Hellman, & Rosenberg, 2015; NCI, 2015).

IL-3 is a group of related proteins that stimulates differentiation and proliferation of pluripotent stem cells into granulocytes, macrophages, and megakaryocytes. The primary clinical use of IL-3 made in the laboratory is to boost the immune system and help support cells ex vivo during cytotoxic therapy for reintroduction at a later time (DeVita, Hellman, & Rosenberg, 2015; NCI, 2015).

IL-6 is a group of related proteins that facilitates B lymphocytes to make more antibodies and causes fever by affecting areas of the brain that control body temperature. It has a direct effect on hematopoiesis and helps to increase immunoglobulin G formation by activating B cells. IL-6 is associated with cancer cachexia and acts as a growth factor for melanoma cell lines, which may outline its role in further clinical investigations. IL-6 made in the laboratory is used as a BRM to boost the immune system in cancer therapy (DeVita, Hellman, & Rosenberg, 2015; NCI, 2015).

IL-7 is an immunopotent regulatory cytokine that has been explored in clinical trials for many tumors. It is secreted by cells that cover and support organs, glands, and other structures in the body but not by normal lymphocytes. Because it is a hematopoietic growth factor, it is being investigated for use in the treatment of lymphoma and graft-versus-host disease and for prolongation of the lymphocyte life span (Zarogoulidis et al., 2014).

IL-11 is a cytokine that promotes hematopoiesis. IL-11 predominantly affects the proliferation, maturation, and function of megakaryocytes and thrombocytes (DeVita, Hellman, & Rosenberg, 2015; NCI 2015; Wyeth-Pfizer Pharmaceuticals, 2015).

IL-12 was identified as a natural killer–stimulating factor (NKSF) and a cytotoxic lymphocyte maturation factor (CLMF) (Mingli et al., 2010). IL-12, which consists of p40 and p35 subunits, stimulates proliferation of natural killer and T cells and the production of cytokines, especially IFN-γ. It enhances the generation and activity of cytotoxic T lymphocytes (CTLs). The most important role of IL-12 is stimulating the production of IFN by natural killer cells. Knockout mice models have demonstrated a direct relationship between IL-12 concentration and IFN production. In preclinical models, IL-12 administration demonstrated an antitumor effect. IL-12 is an essential cytokine for the differentiation of type 1 helper T cells, which is required for the generation of type 1 cell-mediated immunity to tumor cells and pathogenic organisms. The antitumor and antimetastatic activities of IL-12 have been extensively examined in a variety of murine tumor models, including melanoma, mammary carcinoma, colon carcinoma, renal cell carcinoma, and sarcoma. IL-12 is one of the most promising interleukins for cancer immunotherapy (Mingli et al., 2010; National Institutes of Health [NIH], 2015b).

IL-16 is a product of CD8[+] T cells that attracts and activates CD4[+] cells. It produces a chemotactic response by CD4[+] cells and promotes the G_0 to G_1 cell cycle transition in those cells. IL-16 may have a role in blast transformation in hematologic malignancies. Sources of IL-16 include epithelial cells, mast cells, lymphocytes, macrophages, synovial fibroblasts, and eosinophils. IL-16 may also be secreted by activated CD8[+] cells in response to histamine or serotonin. IL-16 expression has been linked to inflammation processes in asthma, rheumatoid arthritis, systemic lupus erythematosus, colitis, atopic dermatitis, and multiple sclerosis. The use of IL-16 or IL-16 antagonists may have therapeutic value in various pathologic immune responses.

In human immnodeficiency virus type 1 (HIV-1) infection, IL-16 may be used to promote reconstitution of CD4[+] T cells and repress HIV-1 replication. Treatment of severely immunodeficient HIV-infected individuals with the HIV protease inhibitor indinavir reduces plasma HIV RNA levels and results in significant increases in circulating levels of IL-16 (Cruikshank & Center, 2015).

Interleukin-2.   IL-2 has been the focus of clinical research in the treatment of malignancies and is the only interleukin to receive FDA approval for use in cancer. In 1992, the FDA approved its use in renal cell cancer, and it was approved for melanoma in 1997 because of its ability to upregulate proliferation and differentiation of natural killer cells and T lymphocytes. IL-2 also works with a cofactor to activate macrophages and B cells (DeVita, Hellman, & Rosenberg, 2015; Dillman, 2011).

Since its discovery in 1976 as a growth factor able to sustain T-cell proliferation for extended periods ex vivo, the effects of IL-2 have become better understood (Rothaermel & Baum, 2009). IL-2 is used as antitumor therapy because of its stimulation of T cells and the synthesis of secondary cytokines. IL-2 has no direct effect on tumor cells but instead provides sustained upregulation of the immune response, eliciting an antitumor response by immune cells and other cytokines (DeVita, Hellman, & Rosenberg, 2015).

During the mid-1980s, IL-2 was studied extensively in the setting of renal cell carcinoma and malignant melanoma. Trials in 1985 by Rosenberg using high-dose, intravenous IL-2 resulted in objective responses in 15% of the 255 patients participating. Outcomes included 17 complete responses, with a median survival time of 16 months, leading to FDA approval of IL-2 use for these diseases. Follow-up survival data from seven phase II studies demonstrated similar responses, with complete responses lasting more than 10 years (131+ months for the longest responders), suggesting a potential cure (DeVita, Hellman, & Rosenberg, 2015; Rothaermel & Baum, 2009).

A total of 270 patients with metastatic melanoma were enrolled in eight clinical trials at multiple centers using high-dose IL-2 (600,000 IU/kg or 720,000 IU/kg). Results included overall response rates of 15% to 17%, a partial response rate of 10%, and complete response rates of 6% to 8% for all tumor sites and regardless of tumor burden. Follow-up at 62 months revealed that 47% of responders were alive, with 15 surviving more than 5 years, and the longest duration was greater than 12 years. Demonstration of the potential for cure compelled the FDA to approve IL-2 for metastatic melanoma (DeVita, Hellman, & Rosenberg 2015; Dillman, 2011).

The greatest challenge with high-dose IL-2 therapy is the related morbidity and mortality. Adverse effects include severe flulike symptoms, fever, chills, nausea, vomiting, diarrhea, capillary leak syndrome, rash, anemia, thrombocytopenia, neutropenia, myalgias, arthralgias, exfoliative dermatitis, and confusion. Life-threatening side effects include the following:

- Hypotension
- Cardiac arrhythmia
- Pulmonary edema with dyspnea and severe respiratory distress

- Renal insufficiency with decreased renal perfusion causing acute oliguric and anuric renal failure
- Hepatic toxicity with hyperbilirubinemia or transaminitis
- Hemostatic changes in thromboplastin and prothrombin times
- Encephalopathy, primary delirium, depression, somnolence, and anxiety

Due to the significant impact of these adverse effects, IL-2 must be administered in carefully selected patients (i.e., Eastern Cooperative Oncology Group performance score of 0 or 1). It is infused in a closely controlled hospital setting according to NCCN guidelines (Dillman, 2011; NCCN, 2015b; Poust, Woolery, & Green, 2012). Appropriate monitoring, supportive care, and prophylactic medications are essential to prevent exacerbation of toxicities. Corticosteroids should not be used with IL-2 because they may blunt the immune response to IL-2, negating the therapeutic immunostimulatory effects against the cancer (Alwan et al., 2014; DeVita, Hellman, & Rosenberg, 2015; Poust, Woolery, & Green, 2012).

Clinical trials have used IL-2 in combination with cytotoxic chemotherapy such as cyclophosphamide, vinblastine, gemcitabine, and cisplatin or with biologics such as IFN, GM-CSF, thalidomide, bryostatin, and famotidine. Low-dose IL-2 has failed to demonstrate the same level of sustained response as high-dose regimens but is widely used in clinical practice because it produces similar clinical response rates without the additional cost and toxicity (Dillman, 2011; Rothaermel & Baum, 2009).

Cancer Vaccines

Prophylactic Cancer Vaccines

Although researchers once hoped for a general prophylactic approach against malignancy, the science has evolved to a more targeted approach for several reasons:

- Long-term, population-based immunizations can cause hereditary mutations and increased tolerance to the vaccine.
- Vaccination against self-directed antigens may have unwanted effects, resulting in an autoimmune response against healthy or nontargeted tissues.
- There is an inability to predict and compensate for the large number of genes that may be affected by a vaccine throughout the life span of the host.

The only feasible anticancer vaccine that may be used in the prophylactic setting in the future is vaccination against malignancies with a natural history directly related to infection of the host by a virus or toxin (Rothaermel & Baum, 2009). Two approved vaccines target viruses that can cause cancer. One that targets the hepatitis B virus, which can cause liver cancer, and another that targets several strains of HPV have been approved by the FDA (Guo et al., 2013).

Hepatitis B Vaccine

Liver cancer affects approximately 35,000 people each year in the United States, and about 25,000 die of the disease. The most common cause of liver cancer worldwide is chronic infection with the hepatitis B virus. Vaccinating against hepatitis B is a key strategy to prevent the disease (American Cancer Society [ACS], 2015). Hepatitis B vaccine has been available for several years and is recommended as part of childhood immunizations. Three doses are recommended for children from birth to 19 years. The first dose is recommended within the first 24 hours after birth, with second dose at 1 to 2 months and the third dose between 6 and 18 months. A two-dose regimen can be given to adolescents 11 through 15 years of age (Merck, 2015).

Human Papillomavirus Vaccine

Cervical cancer is the third leading cause of cancer deaths among women in the world, and more than 500,000 cases are diagnosed each year. In the United States, approximately 12,900 new cases of invasive cervical cancer are diagnosed annually, and approximately 4100 women die of the disease. Almost all cervical cancers can be attributed to the HPV infection (ACS 2015; Cancer Research UK, 2015).

Two HPV quadrivalent vaccines are approved to prevent HPV-related cancers, including cervical, vaginal, vulvar, and anal cancer in women and penile and anal cancer in men. The vaccines protect against HPV types 6, 11, 16, and 18, which account for 90% of infections. Vaccines are prepared from virus-like particles derived from the major capsid protein of HPV types 6, 11, 16, and 18 (Merck, 2015). Use of the vaccines has reduced the incidence of HPV infection and the development of genital warts by 90% to 100% in studies involving more than 20,000 participants (Rothaermel & Baum, 2009).

The recommended age for vaccination is between 9 and 26 years. The vaccine does not prevent the development of HPV-related neoplasms in those exposed before vaccination. Vaccination against HPV also does not take the place of regular Papanicolaou testing and physical examination (ACS, 2015).

Therapeutic Cancer Vaccines

Therapeutic cancer vaccines treat existing cancer. The goals are to eliminate the cancer by strengthening the patient's immune response while sparing normal cells and to inhibit further growth of advanced cancers or relapsed tumors that are refractory to conventional therapies such as surgery, radiation therapy, and chemotherapy (Guo et al., 2013; Drake, 2012).

Therapeutic vaccines work by upregulating specific T-cell responses and stimulating naïve T-cells by antigens offered by antigen-presenting cells (APCs). This is often accomplished through ex vivo culturing and growth of dendritic cells in a cytokine cocktail before reinfusion or reinjection into the host. The dendritic cells, which are the most potent APCs, can present tumor antigens to large numbers of naïve T cells, triggering an immune response against the malignant cells. Antigens for this process can be synthetically processed proteins specific to a malignant cell line or can be derived from an individual's tumor cells for a more specific antitumor vaccine.

Numerous therapeutic vaccines are being investigated. In April 2010, the FDA approved the first therapeutic cancer vaccine, sipuleucel-T (Provenge), for use in men with asymptomatic or minimally symptomatic metastatic, castration-resistant (i.e., hormone-refractory) prostate cancer. It is designed to stimulate an immune response to prostatic acid phosphatase (PAP), an antigen that is found on most prostate cancer cells. In the pivotal clinical trial, sipuleucel-T increased survival by about 4 months.

Sipuleucel-T is customized to each patient. The vaccine is created by isolating APCs from a patient's blood with a procedure called *leukapheresis*. The APCs are sent to a special facility, where they are cultured with a protein called *PAP-GM-CSF*. This protein consists of PAP linked to GM-CSF. GM-CSF stimulates the immune system and enhances antigen presentation.

APCs cultured with PAP-GM-CSF constitute the active component of sipuleucel-T. The cultured cells are reinfused into the patient. Patients receive three treatments, usually 2 weeks apart, with each round of treatment requiring the same manufacturing process. Although the precise mechanism of action of sipuleucel-T is unknown, it appears that the cultured APCs stimulate T cells of the immune system to kill tumor cells that express PAP (Kantoff et al., 2010).

Checkpoint Inhibitors

Advances in immunotherapy continue to occur with the discovery of novel anticancer mechanisms that stimulate or modulate the immune system, such as checkpoint inhibitors, which are also known as immunomodulators, coinhibitory molecules, or costimulatory molecules. These monoclonal antibodies exert their effects by blocking immune checkpoint molecules on T cells or associated ligands on APCs and tumor cells. This action restores and augments cytotoxic T cells. The mechanism of action can be described as releasing the brakes on the immune system to enhance the antitumor T-cell response (Ayumu, Kondo, Tada, & Kitano, 2015).

Anti-CTLA4 Antibody

Cytotoxic T-lymphocyte antigen 4 (CTLA4), a checkpoint inhibitor, is a member of the CD28 receptors. It is normally expressed at low levels on the surface of naïve effector cells (Teffs) and regulatory T cells (Tregs) and sequestered in vesicles in the cytosol. Although the mechanisms of Treg-mediated suppression are not completely understood, they are thought to involve the inhibitory surface molecules CTLA4 and programmed cell death protein 1 (PD1 or PDCD1); immunosuppressive soluble factors such as transforming growth factor-β (TGF-β), IL-10, and IL-35; and cytolytic molecules such as granzyme B and perforin (Zhou & Levitsky, 2012).

When a strong or long-lasting stimulus of the naïve T cell is supplied through the T-cell receptor (TCR), CTLA4 is recruited to the cell surface and is released in the immunologic synapse (i.e., interface between an APC or target cell and a lymphocyte). This happens several days after the initiation of the immune response. CTLA4 then competes with CD28 on the cell surface, preventing it from binding with CD80 (B7-1) and CD86 (B7-2) and effectively switching off TCR signaling and escalating an effective and sustained immunologic attack against tumors (Roman, 2011; Wolchok, Yang, & Weber, 2010; Zhou & Levitsky, 2012). The anti-CTLA4 monoclonal antibody (i.e., ipilimumab) does not reduce Treg cell numbers; it instead preferentially excludes Tregs from the tumor lesion, increasing the intratumoral Teff-to-Treg ratio and improving therapeutic efficacy (Zhou & Levitsky, 2012; Wolchok, 2012).

Ipilimumab is the first-in-class T-cell potentiator for metastatic melanoma and a fully human monoclonal antibody directed against CTLA4. It was approved by the FDA in March 2011 for the treatment of patients with unresectable or metastatic melanoma. The approved dosing schedule is 3 mg/kg, administered intravenously over 90 minutes every 3 weeks for a total of four doses (Bristol-Myers Squibb, 2015a).

Side Effects. Most side effects are related to the immune response and include fatigue, diarrhea, itching, and rash. Most are manageable with early detection, treatment (often with high-dose corticosteroids), and close monitoring. However, there is a black box warning for potentially severe and fatal immune-mediated adverse reactions due to T-cell activation and proliferation (Bristol-Myers Squibb, 2015b; Roman, 2011). The most common severe events include the following:

- Enterocolitis can cause intestinal perforation. Signs and symptoms include the following:
  - Diarrhea
  - Blood in stools or dark, tarry, sticky stools
  - Abdominal pain or tenderness
- Nonviral hepatitis can lead to liver failure. Signs and symptoms include the following:
  - Jaundice
  - Dark urine
  - Nausea or vomiting
  - Right-sided abdominal pain
  - Bleeding or bruising
- Dermatitis can lead to a severe skin reaction (i.e., toxic epidermal necrolysis). Signs and symptoms include the following:
  - Rash with or without itching
  - Oral mucositis
  - Dermatologic blistering or skin changes
- Neuropathy can lead to paralysis. Symptoms include the following:
  - Unusual weakness of legs, arms, or face
  - Numbness or tingling in hands or feet
- Endocrinopathy (especially of the pituitary, adrenal, and thyroid glands) may affect gland function. Signs and symptoms include the following:
  - Persistent or unusual headaches
  - Unusual sluggishness, feeling cold all the time, or weight gain
  - Changes in mood or behavior such as decreased sex drive, irritability, or forgetfulness
  - Dizziness or fainting
- Inflammation of the eyes. Symptoms include the following:
  - Blurry vision, diplopia, or other vision problems
  - Conjunctivitis

Patients should receive verbal and written materials on initiation of treatment about how to manage each side effect. Patients should have the medical oncology team contact information. Making sure patients understand the potential severity of problems encourages them to promptly report side effects.

Anti–Programmed Cell Death Protein 1 Antibodies

PD1 is similar to CTLA4 as a coinhibitor of the CD28 family molecule, but it instead works in the late phase of T-cell activation by inducing T-cell exhaustion. Antibodies that target the PD1 receptor and its ligand (PDL1) act primarily through inhibiting binding of PDL1 to PD1, freeing cancer antigen-specific CTLs to mediate killing of PDL1-expressing cancer cells.

Nivolumab (Opdivo) is a fully human IgG4 antibody that blocks the PD1 receptor. In 2014, nivolumab received accelerated FDA approval for treatment of patients with unresectable or metastatic melanoma and those with disease progression after ipilimumab therapy. For melanoma with the *BRAF* V600 mutation, a BRAF inhibitor is added. Another approval is indicated for the use of nivolumab metastatic squamous non–small cell lung cancer with progression on or after platinum-based chemotherapy. The most recent approval is for non–squamous cell lung cancer (Bristol-Myers Squibb, 2015b).

Phase III studies that led to the approval of nivolumab for patients with ipilimumab-refractory advanced melanoma demonstrated a 32% response rate, compared with 11% for the control group. In another trial of untreated patients with stage III or IV melanoma, the overall survival rate was 72.9%, compared with 42.1% in the other arm using treatment with dacarbazine (Sznol & Chen, 2013; Topalian, Sznol, McDermott, et al., 2014; Weber, Kudchadkar, Yu, et al., 2013). For non–small cell lung cancer, the overall response rate was 15%, with durable responses lasting more than 6 months for 59% of patients (Brahmer et al., 2015). The dosage is 3 mg/kg of nivolumab administered as an intravenous infusion over 60 minutes every 2 weeks.

Nivolumab has been well tolerated. Common side effects are pruritus, rash, diarrhea, fatigue, nausea, and decreased appetite. Gastrointestinal and hepatic effects are managed with interruption of treatment and steroids, and endocrine effects are managed with replacement therapy. Other PD1 inhibitors are being investigated.

Patterns of Response

Immunotherapeutic agents, including cytokines, vaccines, and immunomodulating antibodies, produce objective tumor responses similar to those from treatment with conventional chemotherapy. However, the timing of a response is quite different. In contrast to the immediate response of tumor shrinkage with chemotherapy, the immunotherapeutic agent response takes much longer to detect. It is often measured in months. Four main patterns of responses have been established:

- Response in baseline lesions, which is similar to chemotherapy-like responses
- Stable disease with a slow, steady decline in the total tumor burden
- Response after an initial increase in the total tumor burden (i.e., response with progressive disease)
- Response in the total tumor burden in the presence of new lesions (i.e., response with progressive disease)

The first two patterns of response are similar to conventional treatment responses under the irRC criteria. The criteria are based on a narrower definition of total disease burden, with progressive disease being established only after a 25% increase is established twice at least 4 weeks apart.

The latter two response patterns have been seen by health care professionals and are not completely understood. New lesions may not indicate progressive disease, and treatment should not be stopped. Responses occurring weeks to months after ipilimumab therapy likely reflect a combination of the indirect action of the ipilimumab, accumulation of sufficient antigens for immune recognition, and the chronic nature of the immune response. Radiographic imaging used to detect progressive disease may show a lymphocytic infiltrate or edema during an inflammatory response causing an increase in apparent volume that cannot be distinguished from tumor growth. These newly recognized response patterns mean that patients should not have treatment with ipilimumab stopped prematurely due to the appearance of early progressive disease because they may continue to receive benefit from the therapy (Pennock, Waterfield, & Wolchok, 2012; Roman, 2011; Wolchok, 2012). The irRC include the following four responses (Pennock, Waterfield, & Wolchok, 2012; Wolchok, 2012) (see the box below).

Immune-Related Response Criteria

- irCR: Decrease of 100% (complete disappearance)
- irPR: Decrease of 50% or more
- irPD: Increase of 25% or more
- irSD: Any response not covered by the previous criteria

irCR, Immune-related complete response; *irPD*, immune response with progressive disease; *irPR*, immune-related partial response; *irSD*, immune response with stable disease.

Programmed Cell Death Protein 1 Receptor and Ligand

The programmed cell death protein 1 (PD1) is a cell surface receptor and a member of the CD28 family. It functions as an immune checkpoint, downregulating the activation of T cells and preventing damage to normal tissue during the immune response. It also plays an important role in tumor immune escape.

PD1 is not detected on resting T cells, but it is expressed on active CD4+ and CD8+ T cells, natural killer cells, B cells, monocytes, and dendritic cells within 24 hours of activation (Chen, Irving, & Hodi, 2012; Sznol & Chen, 2013). The interaction of PD1 and its ligand PDL1 (B7-H1) inhibits T-cell proliferation, survival, and effector function; induces apoptosis of tumor-specific T cells; promotes the differentiation of CD4+ cells into immunosuppressive Tregs; and increases resistance of tumor cells to CTL attack.

Blockage of PD1 and PDL1 can revive exhausted T cells, augmenting their expansion, cytokine production, and cytolytic functions. Cancer as a chronic and often inflammatory disease can use this immunoprotective pathway during progression through upregulation of PD1 expression as a means to evade the host's immune response. PD1 is highly expressed in melanoma, non–small cell lung cancer, nasopharyngeal cancer, glioblastoma, hepatocellular carcinoma, multiple myeloma, and lymphomas and in several other cancers to some degree (Chen, Irving, & Hodi, 2012).

A challenge in developing immunotherapy is the highly aggressive, evolving nature of cancer, which limits the opportunity to generate an anticancer response. Advances in understanding signaling pathways, genetic markers, and tumor expression will expand the therapeutic options for patients with cancer. Combinations of various pathways for immunotherapy and targeted, and conventional regimens may be necessary to overcome resistance and produce better outcomes.

References

Adir, J. E., Johnson, S. K., Mrugala, M. M., Beard, B. C., Guyman, L. A., Baldock, A. L., Bridge, C. A., et al. (2014). Gene therapy enhances chemotherapy tolerance and efficacy in glioblastoma patients. *Journal of Clinical Investigation, 124*(9), P4082–4092. http://dx.doi.org/10.1172/JCI76739.

Alwan, L. M., Grossemann, K., Sageser, D., Van Atta, J., Agrwal, N., & Gilreath, J. A. (2014). Comparison of acute toxicities and mortality after two different dosing regimens of high-dose interleukin-2 for patients with metastatic melanoma. *Target Oncology*, 963–971.

American Cancer Society (ACS). (2015). Cancer immunotherapy. Available at http://www.cancer.org/treatment/treatmentsandsideeffects/treatmenttypes/immunotherapy/index (accessed February 8, 2016).

Amgen. (2015a). *Neupogen: Filgrastim full prescribing information.* Thousand Oaks, CA: Amgen.

Amgen. (2015b). *Neulasta: Pegfilgrastim full prescribing information.* Thousand Oaks, CA: Amgen.

Amgen. (2015c). *Kepivance: Palifermin, full prescribing information.* Thousand Oaks, CA: Amgen.

Amgen. (2015d). *Procrit epoetin alfa full prescribing information.* Raritan, NJ: Orthobiotech Products.

Amgen. (2015e). *Aranesp full prescribing information.* Thousand Oaks, CA: Amgen.

Badini, T. J. A. (2011). The role of innate immunity in spontaneous regression of cancer. *Indian Journal of Cancer, 48*(2), 246–251.

Balvers, R. K., Gomez-Manzano, C. G., Jiang, H., Piya, S., Klein, S. R., Lamfers, M. L. M., & Fueyo, J. (2014). Advances in oncolytic virotherapy for brain tumors. In E. C. Lattime & S. L. Gerson (Eds.), *Gene therapy for cancer* (3rd ed.) (pp. 137–151). Amsterdam: Elsevier.

Baranyi, L., Slepushkin, V., & Dropulic, B. (2014). Ex vivo gene therapy utilization of genetic vectors for the generation of genetically modified cell products for therapy. In E. C. Lattime & S. L. Gerson (Eds.), *Gene therapy for cancer* (3rd ed.) (pp. 3–18). Amsterdam: Elsevier.

Berlex. (2015). *Leukine: Sargramostim, full prescribing information.* Seattle, WA: Berlex.

Borden, E. C., & Sondel, P. M. (1990). Lymphokines and cytokines as cancer treatment: Immunotherapy realized. Presentation at the National Conference on Advances in Cancer Management, Los Angeles, CA, December 7–9, 1988. *Cancer, 65*, 800–814.

Brahmer, J., Reckamp, K. L., Baas, P., Crino, L., Eberhardt, W. E., Poddubskaya, E., & Spigel, D. R. (2015). Nivolumab versus docetaxel in advanced squamous-cell non-small-cell lung cancer. *New England Journal of Medicine, 373*(2), 123–135.

Bristol-Myers, Squibb (2015a). *Nivolumab package insert.* Available at http://packageinserts.bms.com/pi/pi_opdivo.pdf (accessed February 8, 2016).

Bristol-Myers, Squibb (2015b). Immuno-oncology. Available at www.immunooncology.bmsinformats.com (accessed February 8, 2016).

Cancer Research UK. (2015). @ http://www.cancerresearchuk.org/Gene therapy. Immunotherapy.

Cancer Research UK. (2015). @ http://www.cancerresearchuk.org/Gene therapy. Interferons and interleukins.

Chen, D. S., & Mellman, I. (2013). Oncology meets immunology: The cancer-immunity cycle. *Immunity, 39*(1), 1–10.

Chen, D. S., Irving, B. A., & Hodi, F. S. (2012). Molecular pathways: Next-generation immunotherapy—inhibiting programmed death ligand 1 and programmed death 1. *Clinical Cancer Research, 18*(24), 6580–6587.

Cruikshank, W. W., & Center, D. M. (2015). *Interleukin-16: Multiple roles in human pathology.* Boston University Pulmonary Center. Available at www.bu.edu/interleukin-16 (accessed February 8, 2016).

DeVita, V. T., Hellman, S., & Rosenberg, S. A. (2015). *Cancer principles and practice of oncology* (10th ed.). Philadelphia: Lippincott Williams & Wilkins.

Dillman, R. O. (2011). Cancer immunotherapy. *Cancer Biotherapy and Radiopharmaceuticals, 26*(1), 1–64.

Drake, C. G. (2012). Combination immunotherapy approaches. *Annals of Oncology, 23*(Suppl 8), viii41–viii46.

Gantz, S., Tomaszewski, J. G., DeLaPena, L., Molenda, J., Bernato, D. L., & Kryk, J. (1995). Programmed instruction: Biotherapy module III. Interferons. *Cancer Nursing, 18*(6), 479–494.

Gujrati, M., & Lu, Z. R. (2014). Targeted systemic delivery of therapeutic siRNA. In E. C. Lattime & S. I. Gerson (Eds.), *Gene therapy for cancer* (3rd ed.) (pp. 47–65). New York: Elsevier.

Guo, C., Manjili, M. H., Subjeck, J. R., Sarkar, D., Fisher, P. B., & Wang, X. Y. (2013). Therapeutic cancer vaccines: Past, present and future. *Advanced Cancer Research, 119*, 421–475.

Hyun, I., & Kimmelman, J. (2014). Ethics in translational gene transfer research. In E. C. Lattime & S. I. Gerson (Eds.), *Gene therapy for cancer* (3rd ed.) (pp. 517–525). New York: Elsevier.

Ito, A., Kondo, S., Tada, K., & Kitano, S. (2015). Clinical development of immune checkpoint inhibitors. *BioMed Research International, 2015*, 1–12. http://dx.doi.org/10.1155/2015/605478 ID 605478.

Jonasch, E., & Haluska, F. G. (2001). Inteferon in oncological practice: Review of interferon biology, clinical applications, and toxicities. *The Oncologist, 6*, 34–55.

Kalliolias, G. D., & Ivashkiv, L. B. (2010). Overview of the biology of type I interferons. *Arthritis Research & Therapy, 12*(Suppl 1), 51–58.

Kannan, R., Madden, K., & Andrews, S. (2014). Primer on immuno-oncology and immune responses. *Clinical Journal of Oncology Nursing, 18*(3).

Kantoff, P. W., Higano, C. S., Shore, N. D., Berger, E. R., Small, E. J., Penson, D. F., & IMPACT Study Investigators. (2010). Sipuleucel-T immunotherapy for castration-resistant prostate cancer. *New England Journal of Medicine, 363*, 411–422.

Kuroki, M., Miyamoto, S., Morisaki, T., Yotsumoto, F., Shirasu, N., & Soma, G. (2012). Biological response modifiers used in cancer biotherapy. *Anticancer Research, 32*, 2229–2234.

Merck. (2015). *Gardasil: Quadrivalent human papillomavirus (types 6, 11, 16, 18) recombinant vaccine, full prescribing information.* Whitehouse Station: Merck.

Mingli, X., Mizoguchi, I., Morishima, N., Chiba, Y., Mizuguchi, J., & Yoshimoto, T. (2010). Regulation of antitumor immune responses by the IL-12 family cytokines, IL-12, IL-23, and IL-27. *Clinical and Developmental Immunology, Vol. 2010*,ID832454 p1–9.doi:10.1155/2010/832454 et al., 2010.

National Cancer Institute (NCI). (2015). The Cancer Genome Atlas: The next stage. Available at http://www.cancergenome.nih.gov/ (accessed February 8, 2016).

National Center for Biotechnology Information (NCBI). (2015). Resources. Available at www.ncbi.nlm.nih.gov/ (accessed February 8, 2016).

National Comprehensive Cancer Network (NCCN). (2015a). *Myeloid growth factors, version 2.2014.* Available at NCCN.org (accessed February 8, 2016).

National Comprehensive Cancer Network (NCCN). (2015b). *Cancer and chemotherapy induced anemia, version 2.2015.* Available at NCCN.org (accessed February 8, 2016).

National Human Genome Research Institute. (2015). *Understanding the human genome project.* Available at http://www.genome.gov/25019879 (accessed February 8, 2016).

National Institutes of Health (NIH). (2015a). *Human genome project: Time line.* Available at www.genome.gov (accessed February 8, 2016).

National Institutes of Health (NIH). (2015b). Immune system. Available at www.niaid.nih.gov (accessed February 8, 2016).

Pennock, G. K., Waterfield, W., & Wolchok, J. D. (2012). Patient responses to ipilimumab, a novel immunopotentiator for metastatic melanoma—How different are these from conventional treatment responses? *American Journal of Clinical Oncology, 35*(6), 606611.

Poust, J. C., Woolery, J. E., & Green, M. R. (2012). Management of toxicities associated with high-dose interleukin-2 and biochemotherapy. *Anti-Cancer Drugs, 24*(1), 1–13.

Roman, R. A. (2011). Immunotherapy for advanced melanoma. *Clinical Journal of Oncology Nursing, 15*(5), E58–E65.

Rothaermel, J. M., & Baum, B. (2009) Biological response modifiers in Mosby's oncology nursing advisor: A comprehensive guide to clinical practice section 3, principles of Cancer Management, Newton, Hickey and Marrs (Ed) pp 161–182.

Siegal, D., Crowther, M., & Cuker, A. (2013). Thrombopoietin receptor agonists in primary ITP. *Seminars in Hematology, 50*(1), S18–S21.

Sobi. (2015). *Palifermin (Kepivance) keratinocyte growth factor by Swedish Orphan Biovitrum.* Stockholm, Sweden. Available at www.Kepivance.com (accessed February 8, 2016).

Sonis, S. (2009). Efficacy of palifermin (keratinocyte growth factor-1) in the amelioration of oral mucositis. *Core Evidence, 4,* 199–205.

Sznol, M., & Chen, L. (2013). Antagonist antibodies to PD-1 and B7-H1 (PD-L1) in the treatment of advanced human cancer. *Clinical Cancer Research, 19*(5), 1021–1034.

Topalian, S. L., Sznol, M., McDermott, D. F., Kluger, H. M., Carvajal, R. D., Sharfman, W. H., Brahmer, J. R., et al. (2014). survival, durable tumor remission, and long-term safety in patients with advanced melanoma receiving nivolumab. *Journal of Clinical Oncology, 32*(10), 1020–1030. http://dx.doi.org/10.1200/JCO.2013.53.0105.

U.S. Food and Drug Administration (FDA). (2015). Cellular and gene therapy products. Available at http://www.fda.gov/BiologicsBloodVaccines/CellularGeneTherapyProducts/default.htm (accessed February 8, 2016).

U.S. National Library of Medicine. (2015). *Terms.* Available at http://www.nlm.nih.gov/medlineplus/ency (accessed February 8, 2016).

Weber, S., Kudchadkar, R. R., Yu, B., Gallenstein, D., Horak, C. E., Inzunza, H. D., Zhao, X., Martinez, A. J., Wang, W., Gibney, G., Kroeger, J., Eysmans, C., Sarnaik, A. A., & Chen, Y. A. (2013). Safety, efficacy and biomarkers of nivolumab with vaccine in ipilimumab-refractory or naïve melanoma. *Journal of Clinical Oncology, 31*(34), 4311–4320. http://dx.doi.org/10.1200/JCO.2013.51.4802.

Wolchok, J. (2012). How recent advances in immunotherapy are changing the standard of care for patients with metastatic melanoma. *Annals of Oncology, 23*(Suppl 8), viii15–viii21.

Wolchok, J. D., Yang, A. S., & Weber, J. S. (2010). Immune regulator antibodies: Are they the next advance? *Cancer Journal, 16*(4), 311–317.

Wyeth-Pfizer Pharmaceuticals. (2015). *Neumega: Oprelvekin, full prescribing information.* Philadelphia: Wyeth Pharmaceuticals.

Yuan, Z., Pastoriza, J., Quinn, T., & Libutti, S. K. (2014). *Targeting tumor vasculature using adeno-associated virus phage vectors coding tumor necrosis factor-α in gene therapy of cancer* (3rd ed.). New York: Elsevier, 19–33. http://dx.doi.org/10.1016/B978-0-12-394295-1.00002-0.

Zarogoulidis, P., Lampaki, S., Yarmus, L., Kiroumis, J., Pitiou, G., Katsikogiannis, N., & Zarogoulidis, K. (2014). Interleukin-7 and interleukin-15 for cancer. *Journal of Cancer, 5*(9), 765–773.

Zhou, G., & Levitski, H. (2012). Towards curative cancer immunotherapy: Overcoming posttherapy tumor escape. *Clinical and Developmental Immunology, 2012,* 1–12. http://dx.doi.org/10.1155/2012/124187. Article ID 124187.

Targeted Therapy

Sandra Remer

Introduction

In the article, *Hallmarks of Cancer: The Next Generation*, Hanahan and Weinberg (2011) described the "six distinctive and complementary capabilities that enable tumor growth and metastatic spread, providing a solid foundation for understanding the biology of cancer." These capabilities include sustaining proliferative signaling, evading growth supressors, activating invasion and metastasis, enabling replicative immortality, inducing angiogenesis, and resisting cell death (Hanahan & Weinberg, 2000, 2011). This chapter considers how these concepts initiated the development of a new treatment modality for cancer, called *targeted therapy*.

Targeted anticancer therapy enables the precise destruction of cancer cells and therefore significantly improves the ability to treat cancer (Li et al., 2012). These therapies are designed to interfere with dysfunctional signaling of cells to stop cancer cell growth (Wujcik, 2014). Translational research applies discoveries generated during research in the laboratory and in preclinical studies to the development of trials and studies in humans and is aimed at enhancing the best practices in the community. Nurses should understand cancer treatment, from basic cell functioning to the processes involved in signaling pathways that control all cellular processes. Understanding these processes provides the oncology nurse with information needed to deliver appropriate patient care and effective education for patients and their families.

Signaling pathways work interdependently with one another. Cells contain many different receptors on their surfaces, and the surrounding microenvironment contains different ligands (i.e., proteins, enzymes) that are set into motion by various interactions that regulate the normal processes of cellular growth, differentiation, apoptosis, cell adhesion, and angiogenesis. A receptor remains dormant until a specific ligand binds with it, thereby initiating a cascade of intracellular signaling pathways. Examples are the binding of transforming growth factor-α (TGF-α) to the epidermal growth factor receptor (EGFR) and the binding of a monoclonal antibody (a protein designed in the laboratory) to a specific antigen located on the surface of a cancer cell. A list of terms specific to targeted therapy is presented in the box below and on page 237.

Targeted Therapy Terminology

Angiogenesis: Process by which new blood vessels form, sprouting from existing blood vessels.

Apoptosis: Programmed cell death. The normal process by which damaged cells are eliminated. Apoptosis is a tightly controlled process of normal cell function.

Cell-signaling cascades: Groups of factors that are linked and pass on messages from the cell surface to the inside of the cell.

Chromosomes: Thread-like structures inside the nucleus of cells. Each chromosome is made of protein and a single molecule of DNA. Passed from parents to offspring, DNA contains the specific instructions that make each type of living creature unique.

Comedone: A blackhead of discolored, dried sebum plugging an excretory duct of the skin.

Conjugated antibody: A tagged, loaded, or labeled antibody used as a honing device to direct treatment toward a specific cancer cell.

Cross-talk: Activation of a cell signaling pathway without growth factor binding; activation of a receptor by another activated receptor in the absence of ligand binding.

Cytokine: A small protein or biologic factor that is released by cells and has a specific effect on cell-cell interactions, communication, and behavior of other cells.

Cytoplasm: The intracellular portion of a cell where biochemical reactions take place.

Degradation: The breaking down of a substance.

Dimerization: Joining two molecular subunits through into a single dimer; results in little structural change

DNA: A molecule called deoxyribonucleic acid (DNA), which contains the biologic instructions that make each species unique. DNA, along with the instructions it contains, is passed from adult organisms to their offspring during reproduction.

Domain: Functional region or component of a protein.

Downstream regulation: Changes that take place below the site of a signaling inhibition.

Endothelial cells: Cells that line the vascular system. They act as a barrier between the bloodstream and target cells that hormones must pass through to reach their receptors and exert their biologic action.

Enzyme: A protein that speeds up chemical reactions in the body. Enzymes take part in many cell functions, including cell signaling, growth, and division.

Enzyme inhibitor: A substance that blocks the action of an enzyme. In cancer treatment, enzyme inhibitors may be used to block certain enzymes that cancer cells need to grow.

Epidermal growth factor (EGF): One of a family of ligands (growth factors) that bind to receptors, resulting in stimulation of cell growth.

Epidermal growth factor-like domain 7: A secreted angiogenic factor that is highly conserved in vertebrates; it is almost exclusively expressed by, and acts on, endothelial cells.

Epidermal growth factor receptor (EGFR): A member of a family of receptors, each composed of four similarly structured transmembrane receptor–tyrosine kinases; activation of these tyrosine kinases is usually dependent on ligand binding to the external portion of the receptor. ErbB1 is also called to as human EGF receptor 1 (HER1) and is commonly referred to as EGFR. Other members of this receptor

Targeted Therapy Terminology—cont'd

family are ErbB2 (HER2/neu), ErbB3 (HER3), and ErbB4 (HER4). These receptors are large proteins residing in the cell membrane.

Epidermal growth factor receptor–tyrosine kinase (EGFR-TK): The intracellular (cytoplasm) portion of the EGFR protein; essential for signaling transduction.

Expression: Production of proteins by messenger ribonucleic acids that result from transcription and translation of specific genes.

Extracellular matrix (ECM): The material that surrounds cells; important regulatory molecules in the ECM promote, inhibit, or guide growth of cells.

Genetic alteration: Changes in the instruction makeup of a cell that can cause a disruption in its signaling process so that the cell no longer grows and divides normally or dies when it should.

Genome: The complete set of DNA in a cell. DNA carries the instructions for building all of the proteins that make each living creature unique.

Growth factors: Function to regulate cell division and cell survival; produced by normal cells during embryonic development, tissue growth, and wound healing.

Hallmarks of cancer: Six distinctive and complementary capabilities that enable tumor growth and metastatic spread, providing a solid foundation for understanding the biology of cancer.

Heterodimerization: Pairing of two different (hetero) receptors.

Homodimerization: Pairing of two of the same (homo) receptors.

Integrins: Cell surface proteins that bind to components of the extracellular matrix.

Keratin: A protein that helps keep the skin hydrated by preventing water evaporation. It can also absorb water, further aiding hydration.

Keratinocytes: Cells of the hair, nails, and skin.

Kinase: An enzyme that catalyzes transfer of a phosphate molecule from adenosine triphosphate (ATP) to an acceptor molecule, resulting in a cascade of kinase-mediated activation reactions.

Ligand: A molecule that binds to another molecule and activates receptors on the cell surface.

Ligand binding: The process by which the ligand attaches itself to a specific receptor on the cell surface and activates the receptor, initiating the signaling pathway.

Lymphocytic perifolliculitis: Lymphocytic inflammation surrounding a hair follicle.

Malignant: Cancerous; a cell or mass that divides and grows without control and order.

Matrix metalloproteinases (MMP): Family of proteins that degrades the extracellular matrix ahead of sprouting vessels.

Monoclonal antibody: Genetically engineered protein designed to attach itself to a specific protein in order to recruit other parts of the immune system to destroy the cells containing the antigen.

Monomer: Single receptor in an inactivated state; also, a molecule of protein that can join with other identical monomers to form a polymer.

Naked monoclonal antibody: Antibody that works by itself, binding to antigens, free-floating proteins, or other noncancerous cells to boost the immune system response by targeting immune system checkpoints.

Oncogene: Mutated or overexpressed version of a normal gene that can release the cell from normal restraints on growth and promote or allow continuous growth and division, converting it into a tumor cell.

Papulopustular eruption: Small, circumscribed, superficial elevation of the skin containing pus; also, an elevation of the skin with an inflamed base or a pimple.

Paronychia: Acute or chronic infection of the folds of skin surrounding the nail.

Pericytes: Cells associated with the walls of small blood vessels that are neither smooth muscle cells nor endothelial cells.

P-glycoprotein: A protein that pumps substances out of cells. Cancer cells that have too much p-glycoprotein may not be killed by anticancer drugs.

Phosphorylation: Creation or generation of free phosphorus that results from binding of a molecule of ATP to the tyrosine receptor site on the intracellular portion of the receptor.

Proteases: Enzymes that aid in the breakdown of proteins in the body.

Protein: A molecule made up of amino acids; the basis of body structures, such as skin and hair, and of other substances such as enzymes, cytokines, and antibodies.

Receptor: A structure on the outside or inside of a cell (cell membrane protein) that selectively binds to a specific drug, hormone, or chemical mediators to alter cell function.

Signaling pathway: Series of interdependent proteins responsible for transmitting signals to the nucleus of the cell.

Small molecules: Targeted drugs that work inside the cell; generic names for most of these drugs end in -ib (e.g., imatinib, dasatinib)

Targeted therapy: Anticancer agent used to block a specific cellular cycle or pathway with the goal of preventing replication or invasion while preserving normal cellular function.

Transcription: Process by which DNA passes genetic information to RNA. Transcription is the first step in producing proteins.

Translational research: The process by which the results of research done in the laboratory are used to develop new ways to diagnose and treat disease.

Transmembrane: Refers crossing or passing through the cell membrane.

Tumorigenesis: The change of a normal cell into tumor cells.

Tumor suppressor gene: A normal gene that signals a cell to slow down growth and division.

Tyrosine kinase (TK): Enzyme that catalyzes the transfer of a phosphate molecule from adenosine triphosphate (ATP) to a tyrosine residue in proteins.

Tyrosine kinase receptor: Intracellular portion of the EGFR; activation of the TK receptor stimulates proliferation, invasion, angiogenesis, metastasis, and inhibition of apoptosis.

Upstream regulation: Changes that take place above the site of a signaling inhibition.

Vascular endothelial growth factor (VEGF): Growth factor essential to angiogenesis; binds to receptors on endothelial cells.

Data from National Cancer Institute. (2016). National Cancer Institute dictionary of cancer terms. Available at http//www.cancer.gov/dictionary/ (accessed February 5, 2016); American Cancer Society. (2015a). Cancer immunotherapy. Available at http://www.cancer.org/treatment/treatmentsandsideeffects/treatmenttypes/immunotherapy/index (accessed February 5, 2016); American Cancer Society. (2015b). Targeted therapy. Available at http://www.cancer.org/treatment/treatmentsandsideeffects/treatment types/targetedtherapy/index (accessed February 5, 2016).

Targeted Therapy Mechanism of Action

Targeted therapies work differently from chemotherapy agents in that they interfere with specific molecules involved in the processes of carcinogenesis, tumor growth, and metastasis. The specific molecule being targeted may be a "switch" that regulates growth and development of the tumor cell or one that allows the cancer cell to enter the process of apoptosis, or programed cell death (Hanahan & Weinberg, 2011; Wujcik, 2014). Targeted therapies may also involve the mounting of specifically designed proteins or antibodies that attach to antigens on the cell surface. These proteins are known as *monoclonal antibodies*.

Targeted therapies may also be directed at several other cellular changes specific to cancer cells, such as migration of cancer cells or the development of new blood vessels. Because targeted therapies focus on specific molecules or cellular changes, they may be more effective and less harmful to normal cells than other therapeutic modalities currently available. The benefit of targeted therapy may be a reduction in treatment-related side effects and improvement in quality of life. Targeted therapies are used alone or in combination with other chemotherapeutic or targeted agents and other treatment modalities. The combination of a molecular targeted therapy and radiation therapy is another promising therapeutic option. Overactivity of the EGFR pathway is associated with radiation resistance; therefore, combination therapy involving an agent that targets the EGFR pathway may increase the effectiveness of radiation therapy (Li, 2011).

Because each type of cancer involves a different set of genes and proteins involved in growth and spread, targeted therapies used to control each type of cancer are different. Once tumors have been more accurately classified by molecular and genetic mutations, treatments may be modified based on these mutations, DNA sequencing, and genomic data specific to the individual tumor type (Eggert, 2011). The most effective treatment may very well combine the older modalities of surgery, radiation, and chemotherapy with newer molecular targeted therapies.

The concept of targeted therapies has rapidly expanded within the past 2 to 5 years, and targeted therapies have become one of the most exciting treatment modalities entering the field of oncology. A list of approved targeted therapies may be found in the table below. Some of the categories of targeted agents are described more fully in later sections of this chapter.

Approved Targeted Therapies

Name of Agent	Drug Class	Oncologic Indications
Abiraterone acetate (Zytiga)	Adrenal inhibitor	Metastatic castration-resistant prostate cancer
Ado-trastuzumab emtansine (Kadcyla)	Monoclonal antibody	Metastatic breast cancer previously treated with trastuzumab
Afatinib (Gilotrif)	Tyrosine kinase inhibitor	Metastatic non–small cell lung cancer
Axitinib (Inlyta)	Angiogenesis inhibitor	Advanced renal cell carcinoma
Bacillus Calmette-Guerin (TICE, TheraCys, BCG)	Biologic response modifier	Bladder cancer Immunization against tuberculosis
Bevacizumab (Avastin)	Monoclonal antibody Angiogenesis inhibitor	Metastatic colorectal cancer Non-squamous, non–small cell lung cancer Glioblastoma (GBM) Metastatic renal cell carcinoma Cervical cancer Ovarian cancer
Blinatumomab (Blincyto)	Monoclonal antibody	Relapsed or refractory B-cell precursor acute lymphoblastic leukemia
Bosutinib (Bosuaftelif)	Tyrosine kinase inhibitor	Philadelphia chromosome–positive chronic myelogenous leukemia
Brentuximab vedotin (Adcetris)	Monoclonal antibody	Hodgkin lymphoma after failure of autologous stem cell transplantation Systemic anaplastic large cell lymphoma
Cabozantinib (Cometriq)	Tyrosine kinase inhibitor	Metastatic medullary thyroid cancer
Carfilzomib (Kyprolis)	Miscellaneous—Proteasome inhibitor	Multiple myeloma
Ceritinib (Zykadia)	Tyrosine kinase inhibitor	Non–small cell lung cancer—ALK positive
Cetuximab (Erbitux)	Monoclonal antibody	Metastatic colorectal cancer Squamous cell carcinoma of the head and neck
Crizotinib (Xalkori capsules)	Tyrosine kinase inhibitor	Non–small cell lung cancer—ALK positive
Dabrafenib (Tafinlar)	BRAF kinase inhibitor	Metastatic melanoma—BRAF positive
Dasatinib (Sprycel)	Tyrosine kinase inhibitor	Chronic myelogenous leukemia Philadelphia chromosome–positive acute lymphoblastic leukemia
Denosumab (Prolia, Xgeva)	Monoclonal antibody	Treatment of osteoporosis in postmenopausal women at high risk for fracture Treatment to increase bone mass in men at high risk for fracture receiving androgen deprivation therapy for nonmetastatic prostate cancer Treatment to increase bone mass in women at high risk for fracture receiving adjuvant aromatase inhibitor therapy for breast cancer Prevention of skeletal-related events (need for radiation, fracture due to cancer in the bone, surgery to the bone, or compression of the spinal cord) in patients with bone metastases from solid tumors Giant cell tumor of the bone
Eculizumab (Soliris)	Monoclonal antibody	Atypical hemolytic uremic syndrome Paroxysmal nocturnal hemoglobinuria
Erlotinib (Tarceva)	Tyrosine kinase inhibitor	Metastatic non–small cell lung cancer Metastatic pancreatic cancer
Everolimus (Afinitor)	mTOR inhibitor	Renal cell carcinoma Pancreatic neuroendocrine tumor Advanced breast cancer
Ibritumomab tiuxetan (Zevalin)	Monoclonal antibody-radiolabeled	Non-Hodgkin lymphoma
Ibrutinib (Imbruvica)	Tyrosine kinase inhibitor	Mantle cell lymphoma Chronic lymphocytic leukemia

Approved Targeted Therapies—cont'd

Name of Agent	Drug Class	Oncologic Indications
Idelalisib (Zydelig)	Phosphatidylinositol -3 kinase inhibitor	Chronic lymphocytic leukemia Follicular B-cell non-Hodgkin lymphoma Small lymphocytic lymphoma
Imatinib mesylate (Gleevac)	Tyrosine kinase inhibitor	Philadelphia chromosome–positive acute lymphocytic leukemia (ALL) Myelodysplastic syndrome Myeloproliferative disease Philadelphia chromosome–positive chronic myelogenous leukemia (CML)
Interferon alfa (Intron A, Roferon-A, IFN-alpha)	Biologic response modifier	Hairy cell leukemia AIDS-related Kaposi sarcoma Follicular non-Hodgkin lymphoma
Ipilimumab (Yervoy)	Monoclonal antibody	Metastatic melanoma
Lapatinib (Tykerb)	Tyrosine kinase inhibitor	Metastatic breast cancer that has been treated with Herceptin
Lenalidomide (Revlimid)	Antiangiogenic agent	Multiple myeloma Myelodysplastic syndrome Mantle cell lymphoma
Nilotinib (Tasigna)	Tyrosine kinase inhibitor	Philadelphia chromosome–positive chronic myelogenous leukemia (CML)
Nivolumab (Opdivo)	Monoclonal antibody	Metastatic melanoma
Obinutuzumab (Gayzva)	Monoclonal antibody	Chronic lymphocytic leukemia
Ofatumumab (Azerra)	Monoclonal antibody	Chronic lymphocytic leukemia
Omacetaxine mepesuccinate (Synribo)	Inhibitor of protein synthesis	Chronic myelogenous leukemia
Panitumumab (Victibix)	Monoclonal antibody	Metastatic colorectal cancer
Pazopanib (Votrient)	Tyrosine kinase inhibitor	Renal cell carcinoma
Pegaspargase (Oncaspar, PEG-L-asparaginase)	Miscellaneous—Enzyme	Acute lymphocytic leukemia (ALL) Non-Hodgkin lymphoma
Pembrolizumab (Keytruda)	Monoclonal antibody	Metastatic melanoma
Pertuzumab (Perjeta)	Monoclonal antibody	Breast cancer
Pomalidomide (Pomalyst)	Antiangiogenic agent	Multiple myeloma
Ponatinib (Iclusig)	Tyrosine kinase inhibitor	Chronic myelogenous leukemia Philadelphia chromosome–positive acute lymphoblastic leukemia
Ramucirumab (Cryamza)	Monoclonal antibody	Gastric cancer Gastroesophagael junction adenocarcinoma Metastatic non–small cell lung cancer
Regorafenib (Stivarga)	Tyrosine kinase inhibitor	Colorectal cancer GIST Tumor
Rituximab (Rituxan)	Monoclonal antibody	Non-Hodgkin lymphoma Chronic lymphocytic leukemia
Ruxolitinib (Jakafi)	Tyrosine kinase inhibitor	Myelofibrosis
Sorafenib (Nexavar)	Tyrosine kinase inhibitor	Renal cell carcinoma Hepatocellular carcinoma Thyroid cancer
Sunitinib (Sutent)	Tyrosine kinase inhibitor	Gastrointestinal stromal tumor Renal cell carcinoma Pancreatic neuroendocrine tumor
Temsirolimus (Torisel)	mTOR inhibitor	Renal cell carcinoma
Thalidomide (Thalomid)	Antiangiogenic agent	Multiple myeloma
Trametinib (Mekinist)	BRAF kinase inhibitor	Metastatic melanoma
Trastuzumab (Herceptin)	Monoclonal antibody	Breast cancer Gastric cancer
Vandetanib (Caprelsa)	Tyrosine kinase inhibitor	Medullary thyroid cancer
Vemurafenib (Zelboraf)	BRAF kinase inhibitor	Metastatic melanoma
Ziv-Aflibercept (Zaltrap)	Vascular endothelial growth factor inhibitor	Metastatic colorectal cancer

GIST, Gastrointestinal stromal tumor; mTOR, mechanistic target of rapamycin.
World Health Organization (2016). WHO Drug Information, Vol. 29, No. 4, 2015 Available at http://www.who.int/medicines/publications/druginformation/issues/PL_114.pdf (accessed 03/05/2016)
Food and Drug Administration (2016). Approved cancer drugs Available at http://www.accessdata.fda.gov/scripts/cder/drugsatfda/index.cfm?fuseaction=Search.Search_Drug_Name (accessed 05/15/15)

Antiangiogenesis

Angiogenesis is a process that occurs naturally throughout growth and development and at specific times in adult life. During embryonic development, vasculogenesis is the process that creates the primary network of vascular endothelial cells that become the major vessels (Ebos & Kerbel, 2011; National Cancer Institute [NCI], 2015; Wujcik, 2014). Angiogenesis continues throughout fetal development, transforming the new blood vessels and capillaries into a completed circulatory system. From this point and throughout adult life, the vascular system is generally associated with maintenance controlled by angiogenesis inhibitors and activators (see box on page 240). In the adult, new vessel formation is infrequent and is generally associated with repair of tissue during wound healing or cardiovascular injury (Hanahan & Weinberg, 2011). In women, angiogenesis is also active on a few days in each menstrual cycle in conjunction with the formation of new blood vessels in the lining of the uterus.

Angiogenesis Inhibitors and Activators

Inhibitors

- Angiostatin
- Endostatin
- Interferons
- Platelet factor 4
- Prolactin 16-kDa fragment
- Thrombospondin
- Tissue inhibitor of metalloproteinase-1 (TIMP-1)
- Tissue inhibitor of metalloproteinase-2 (TIMP-2)
- Tissue inhibitor of metalloproteinase-3 (TIMP-3)

Activators

- Acidic fibroblast growth factor
- Angiogenin
- Basic fibroblast growth factor (bFGF)
- Epidermal growth factor (EGF)
- Granulocyte colony-stimulating factor
- Hepatocyte growth factor
- Interleukin-8
- Placental growth factor (PGF)
- Platelet-derived endothelial growth factor (PDEGF)
- Scatter factor
- Transforming growth factor-α
- Tumor necrosis factor-α
- Vascular endothelial growth factor (VEGF)
- Adenosine
- 1-Butyryl glycerol
- Nicotinamide
- Prostaglandins E1 and E2

Data from National Cancer Institute. (2015). Angiogenesis. Available at http://www.cancer.gov/about-cancer/treatment/types/immunotherapy/angiogenesis-inhibitors-fact-sheet (accessed February 20, 2016); Rosen, L. S. (2005). VEGF-targeted therapy: Therapeutic potential and recent advances. *The Oncologist, 10,* 382-391; Ferrara, N. (2004). Vascular endothelial growth factor as a target for anticancer therapy. *The Oncologist, 9*(Suppl 1), 2-10. Hanahan, D., & Weinberg, R. A. (2011). Hallmarks of cancer: The next generation. *Cell,* 144(5), 646–674. Carmeliet, P., & Jain, R. K. (2011). Molecular mechanisms and clinical applications of angiogenesis. *Nature May*19, 473, 298–307. http://dx.doi. org/10.1038/nature10144. Albini, A., Tosetti, F., Li, V. W., Noonan, D. M., & Li, W. W. (2012). Cancer prevention by targeting angiogenesis. *National Review of Clinical Oncology,* 9(9), 498–509. Yoo, S. Y., & Kwon, S. M. (2013). Angiogenesis and Its Therapeutic Opportunities, Laboratory for Vascular Medicine and Stem Cell. *Mediators of Inflammation,* Volume 2013, 11. ID 127170 http://dx.doi.org/ 10.1155/2013/127170. Polverini, P.J. (2002) Angiogenesis in health and disease: Insights into basic mechanisms and therapeutic opportunities. *Journal of Dental Education*. 66(8), 962–975.

Angiogenesis is responsible for maintenance of the vascular system that controls delivery of oxygen and nutrients with corresponding elimination of metabolic wastes and carbon dioxide. Oxygen and nutrients are necessary for growth, maintenance, and survival of tissues supplied by the vasculature (see figure below).

The microenvironment surrounding the cell is highly specific for each type of tissue throughout the human body. Proteins located within the microenvironment perform important activities for the cell. Proteins are needed for the extracellular matrix to physically support the cell structure. Proteins can alter the behavior of the cell's matricellular proteins, growth factors, and proteases through interactions with membrane receptors (e.g., growth factor receptors, proteases) and adhesion proteins such as integrins (Goubran, Kotb, Stakiw, Emara, & Burnouf, 2014).

Other biologic functions, including extracellular matrix breakdown, proliferation, apoptosis, angiogenesis, and motility, are affected when signals from within the microenvironment influence ligand binding on the cell surface; this creates a signaling cascade inside the cell to the nucleus, leading to altered gene transcription and changed cell functions (Goubran et al., 2014; Hanahan & Weinberg, 2011).

The EGFR and vascular endothelial growth factor (VEGF) signaling pathways are two components that play major roles in the process of angiogenesis and the growth and spread of cancer cells. They therefore provide major targets for interfering with tumor growth (see figure on page 241).

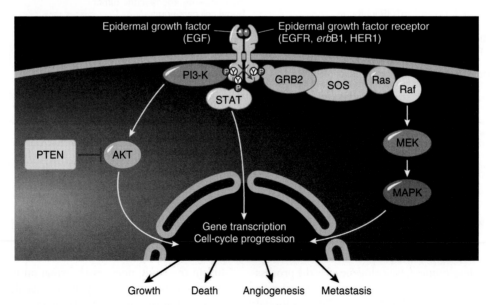

Cell signaling. Receptor activation is a multistep process. After ligand binding, receptors dimerize (form pairs). After which, the intracellular tyrosine kinase domains of the receptors are phosphorylated, activating the receptors and initiating downstream signaling cascades, such as the MAPK proliferation pathway. (Copyright © 2006 Oncology Nursing Society. Reprinted with permission.)

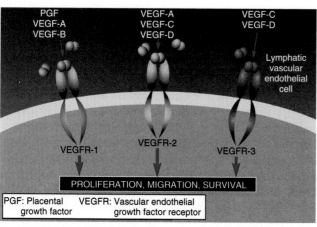

Targeting tumor vasculature. (Copyright © 2007 Oncology Nursing Society. Reprinted with permission.)

VEGF (a cytokine) is also known as VEGF-A. It stimulates vascular endothelial cell growth, survival, and proliferation and plays a significant role in the development of new blood vessels (angiogenesis). VEGF is a member of a family of six structurally related proteins that regulate the growth and differentiation of multiple components of the vascular system, especially blood and lymph vessels. It is known for its high permeability. The table below provides an overview of the VEGF family receptors and their functions.

Vascular Endothelial Growth Factor Family Receptors and Functions

VEGF Family	Receptors	Functions
VEGF (VEGF-A)	VEGFR-1, VEGFR-2, neuropilin-1	Angiogenesis, vascular maintenance
VEGF-B	VEGFR-1	Not established
VEGF-C	VGFR-2, VGFR-3	Lymphangiogenesis
VEGF-D	VGFR-2, VGFR-3	Lymphangiogenesis
VEGF-E (viral factor)	VGFR-2	Angiogenesis
PLGF (placental growth factor)	VGFR-1, neuropilin-1	Angiogenesis and inflammation

Data from Tejpar, S., Prenen, H., & Mazzone, M. (2012). Overcoming resistance to antiangiogenic therapies. *Oncologist*, 17(8), 1039–1050. http://dx.doi.org/10.1634/theoncologist.2012-0068. Shibuya, M. (2013). Vascular endothelial growth factor and its receptor system: physiological functions in angiogenesis and pathological roles in various diseases. *J Biochem*, 153(1), 13–19. http://dx.doi.org/10.1093/jb/mvs136 2013 Jan. Ferrara, N., Gerber, H. P., & LeCouter, J. (2003). The biology of VEGF and its receptors. *Nature Medicine*, 9, 669–676. Hicklin, D. J., & Ellis, L. M. (2005). Role of the vascular endothelial growth factor pathway in tumor growth and angiogenesis. *Journal of Clinical Oncology*, 23, 1011–1027. Ferrara, N. (2004). Vascular endothelial growth factor as a target for anticancer therapy. *The Oncologist*, 9(Supp. 1), 2–10.

Pathophysiology of Tumor Angiogenesis

Tumor angiogenesis involves the development of blood vessels that are structurally and functionally abnormal. Tumor vessels are irregular, distended capillaries with leaky walls and sluggish flow; they often demonstrate a lack of pericytes (Li et al., 2012). Both normal (physiologic) angiogenesis and tumor angiogenesis are regulated by a variety of growth factors and are targets for inhibitors and activators of angiogenesis (see box on page 240).

The growth of a tumor is dependent on its vascular supply. Absorption of oxygen and nutrients is possible only within 1 to 2 mm of the tumor borders (co-opting or appropriating vessels

from the surrounding tissue); further growth requires a process through which new vessels develop (NCI, 2015; Wujcik, 2011). Endothelial cells, the primary building blocks of vessels, are the cells that line the walls of blood vessels. The endothelial cell has the extraordinary ability to divide and migrate; however, most of the time, the endothelial cell remains dormant. The formation of new vessels involves recruitment of circulating endothelial cells.

Many factors activate angiogenesis; for example, hypoxia is an important stimulator of tumor angiogenesis (Carmeliet & Jain, 2011; Ebos & Kerbel, 2011). When a tumor can no longer obtain an adequate supply of oxygen and nutrients, its cellular environment secretes increased amounts of VEGF (upregulation) into the surrounding tissue and at the same time downregulates proteins that inhibit angiogenesis within the tumor and its microenvironment. This activation is referred to as the *angiogenic switch*. VEGF then binds to the appropriate receptor on the endothelial cell surface, activating the tyrosine kinase (TK) portion located inside the cell, which in turn initiates the signaling pathway. The signaling pathway transmits a series of molecules (proteins) to the nucleus, where gene transcription is altered, stimulating new endothelial cell growth. The extracellular matrix is degraded so that the endothelial cells are able to invade the matrix (i.e., migrate through the capillary basement membrane) and begin to divide and proliferate. As they divide, they produce a string of endothelial cells, which then forms a hollow tube. Eventually, a new network of blood vessels is created, making tissue growth and repair possible (Li et al 2012; Yoo & Kwon, 2013).

These new structures are tortuous, leaky, less organized, and less stable than normal blood vessels. As a result, the permeability of the vasculature is enhanced, and migration and proliferation of endothelial cells is increased, providing the pathway for metastasis (Carmeliet & Jain, 2011). It is also suggested that blocking VEGF and its receptor leads to apoptosis (programmed cell death) of the endothelial cells and a decrease in vessel diameter, density, and permeability. This decreases interstitial fluid pressure and, in some tumors, increases oxygen tension, improving the microenvironment of the tumor. This, in turn, allows not only for improved delivery of nutrients but also for increased delivery of therapeutic agents (Albini, Tosetti, Li, Noonan, & Li, 2012; Carmeliet & Jain, 2011; Mak et al., 2014, Yoo & Kwon, 2013).

Other triggers of VEGF expression include the following (Genentech, 2015; Wujcik, 2014):

- EGFR (HER1) activation associated with solid tumors such as breast, lung, colorectal, prostate, renal cell, and ovarian tumors
- HER2 overexpression associated with VEGF production in colon, pancreatic, gastric, breast, renal cell, non–small cell lung cancer, and glioblastoma multiforme tumors
- Insulin-like growth factor 1 receptor (IGF1R), which is also associated with increased VEGF production in breast, endometrial, pancreatic, and colorectal cancers
- Cyclooxygenase-2 (COX-2), which has been shown to mediate VEGF expression in numerous cell lines, although this effect is not evident in all tumors
- Platelet-derived growth factor (PDGF), which modulates angiogenesis by promoting endothelial cell survival and vascular maturation through the recruitment of pericytes and vascular smooth muscle cells.

Oncogenes and tumor suppressor genes are associated with increased production of VEGF. Examples include *SRC* (formerly *c-Src*), a proto-oncogene that regulates VEGF expression and promotes neovascularization in existing tumors; the *BCR-ABL* oncogene, which has a key role in the pathogenesis of leukemias; the *RAS* family of oncogenes, which are associated with increased VEGF production in pancreatic, colon, and non–small cell lung cancer and are part of the signaling cascade of growth factor–induced angiogenesis; and the *TP53* tumor suppressor gene, which is found in solid tumors such as colorectal, breast, and endometrial cancers and astrocytomas and functions as a regulator of the cell cycle, inducing apoptosis when DNA damage is beyond repair (Wujcik, 2014).

Other mechanisms for activation of VEGF expression include the link, in several solid tumors (including gastric, colon, prostate, breast, and pancreas tumors), between the prostaglandin COX-2 and PDGF in the regulation of host-derived VEGF for sustaining angiogenesis, as well as a recently emerged protein called *epidermal growth factor–like domain 7* (EGFL7), which is overexpressed in hepatocellular carcinoma, colorectal cancer, and glioma (Carmeliet & Jain, 2011; Ebos & Kerbel, 2011; Nichol & Stuhlmann, 2012).

The targeted therapy agents, which work by inhibiting angiogenesis within the tumor, include axitinib, pamalidomide, lenalidomide, and thalidomide (see table on pages 238 to 239). The monoclonal antibody bevacizumab also inhibits angiogenesis by binding to VEGF in the extracellular region and disrupting the angiogenic pathway.

Monoclonal Antibodies

An antibody is a protein that attaches itself to another specific protein called an *antigen*. Antibodies circulate in the body until they find and attach to their specific antigen and then recruit other parts of the immune system to destroy the cells containing that antigen. Monoclonal antibodies (mAbs or MoAbs) are genetically engineered (man-made) antibodies that are produced by identical immune cells cloned from a unique parent cell; as such, they have known affinity for a specific part of a particular antigenic protein.

History

Köhler and Milstein opened the door for discovery of tumor-associated antigens and production of immunoglobulins from a single clone of B cells (Dillman, 2011). Antibody-forming lymphocytes were harvested from immunized mice and fused with cancerous B cells from multiple myeloma. The process produced an immortal line of hybrid cells that recognized a known antigen. This hybridoma technology permitted production of large quantities of an antibody that seek out and bind with a specific antigen.

mAbs are used alone or in combination with chemotherapy. In addition, radioactive agents have been linked with mAbs (e.g., in ibritumomab tiuxetan) as a way to provide additional treatment options or diagnostic measures. In addition to oncology, mAbs have been developed for use in many other fields, such as immunohistochemistry, transplant rejection, and the management of autoimmune and inflammatory diseases (Castillo-Trivino, Braithwaite, Bacchetti, & Waubant, 2013; Duxbury, Combescure, & Chizzolini, 2013; Kuoki et al., 2012).

Originally, monoclonal antibodies were produced from mice (i.e., murine models). More than a decade later, techniques were developed that converted the murine constant (Fc) portion of the immunoglobulin molecule to a human subclass (chimerization). The chimeric model antibody is a combination of a mouse component in the variable region (about 30% mouse) and a human component in the constant region. Newer techniques allowed molecular conversion of all except the hypervariable region of the immunoglobulin (about 5%) to human amino acid sequences (humanization), and eventually 100% human mAbs were developed. Recombinant mAbs are engineered from viruses or yeast rather than mice and can be designed with desired specificities for stability, detectability, and therapeutic efficacy. These advances have resulted in antibodies that are far superior to the first generation of mouse mAbs and have fewer side effects (Dillman, 2011).

The nomenclature of mAbs identifies the type of antibody. Each antibody has an individual prefix, a substem that identifies the target—for example, *tu* is for tumor; a substem *b*, which is the prefix as shown below; and *mab* to indicate it is a monoclonal antibody. The common monoclonal antibody nomenclature for cancer agents is shown in the table below.

Monoclonal Antibody Nomenclature*

Prefix to Antibody	Type of Antibody	Example
o-	Murine (mouse)	Tositumomab
xi-	Chimeric	Rituximab
u-	Human	Efungumab
tu- substem a before antibody type	Tumor target	Panitumumab
ci- before antibody type	Circulatory target	Bevacizumab
li- before antibody type	Immunomodulating target	Ipilimumab
Xizu-	Chimeric/humanized	navicixizumab
Zu	Humanized	Trastuzumab
a	rat	
axo (pre-sub-stem)	Rat/mouse	
e	hamster	

All monoclonal antibodies contain the suffix -*mab* at the end of their name.
*Substem A indicates the target class, b- bacterial, f- fungal, k- interleukin, l- immunomodulating, n-neural,
s-bone, tox-toxin, v-viral.
The prefix should be random, e.g. the only requirement is to contribute to a euphonious and distinctive name.
From World Health Organization (2011). Available at Http://www.who.int/medicines/service/inn/bioRev.pdf

Mechanism of Action

mAbs target cells that are marked with a specific cell surface antigen. Two types of mAbs are used in cancer treatment: unconjugated and conjugated. Unconjugated mAbs are not fused to a toxin and therefore are called *naked* mAbs; they attach to a specific antigen on the cancer cell and prevent it from becoming active, then induce apoptosis and destroy the cell. Conjugated antibodies are attached to a radioisotope or chemotherapeutic agent. The mAb acts as a homing device, circulating in the body until it finds its targeted antigen, then delivering the toxic substance to the cancer cell. Conjugated antibodies are also called *labeled, loaded,* or *tagged* antibodies. Because they target cell surface markers instead of killing both tumor cells and normal, healthy cells, systemic side effects may be reduced. (American Cancer Society, 2015a; Behrend, 2015; Dillman, 2011; NCI, 2014).

Toxicities for Monoclonal Antibodies

The side effect profile for mAbs differs from that of chemotherapy. Early effects include infusion-related reactions. Chronic effects include fatigue and flu-like symptoms.

Most infusion reactions related to mAbs are caused by cytokine release. When the mAb binds to the antigen on the targeted cell, specific cytokines called *chemokines* recruit immune-effector cells (e.g., monocytes, macrophages, cytotoxic T cells, natural killer cells) and complement molecules. The immune-effector cells bind to the constant portion of the antibody (Fc region), targeting that cell for destruction. When they are destroyed, both target and immune-effector cells release cytokines into the circulation, further contributing to a group of symptoms. Immediate infusion-related events are common with the administration of mAbs (Vogel, 2010). The intensity of the event depends on the specific mAb administered and whether other treatment modalities are concomitantly used.

The following symptoms are described as an infusion reaction: chills, fevers, rigors, myalgias, arthralgias, urticaria, nausea, diarrhea, mucosal congestion, hypotension, fatigue, headache, tachycardia, and dyspnea (Bilotti, 2013; Edmonds et al., 2012; Grenon, 2011; Pilott et al., 2011).

Cytokine release syndrome typically occurs during the first infusion and may occur within the first 2 hours. Side effects may be mild to severe. To reduce the potential for cytokine release syndrome, pretreatment with acetaminophen and diphenhydramine 30 to 60 minutes before infusion is recommended. Should symptoms develop during the infusion despite premedication, the infusion should be interrupted and normal saline administered. Airway, breathing, and circulation should be assessed immediately, along with vital signs. Administration of meperidine and

additional histamine blockers may be warranted for rigors. Most reactions will subside on their own, and the infusion may then be reinitiated at a slower rate (Vogel, 2010). Severe reactions may require supplemental oxygen, steroids, bronchodilators, or emergency medications. Most patients who experience moderate infusion reactions may be considered for rechallenge because most reactions are likely caused by cytokine release and are not true anaphylaxic reactions. Nurses need to know basic immune actions, the mAb type, and the usual pattern of symptoms to provide expert care for those receiving mAb therapy.

Epidermal Growth Factor Inhibitors

EGFR (HER1) and its ligands, epidermal growth factor (EGF) and TGF-α, were first identified by Nobel Laureate Dr. Stanley Cohen in the 1960s (Seshacharyulu et al., 2012). Binding of this cell surface receptor to its ligand activates its intracellular tyrosine kinase domain, initiating multiple signaling pathways (Li et al., 2012; Wujcik, 2014).

The autocrine mechanism involving autostimulation of EGFRs on the surface of cancer cells by TGF-α, which cancer cells produce, was described in a landmark paper by Sporn and Todar (1980). In 1981, a subsequent article demonstrating that the EGFRs and the SRC oncogene product have the novel enzymatic activity of a TK (Alaoui-Jamali, Morand, & da Silva, 2015). Since these early discoveries, the number of known EGF-family ligands has increased from 2 to 11, with the autocrine mechanism being one of the major supports of tumor progression (Pines & Yarden, 2012). In addition to EGFR (HER1 or ErB1), other members of the EGFR family (also called the HER receptor family), a group of naturally occurring cell membrane–bound protein receptors, are HER2 (also called HER2/neu or ErbB2), which was discovered in 1985; HER3 (ErbB3); and HER4 (ErbB4) (see the figure below).

The two most studied and best understood members of the EGFR family are HER1 and HER2. These proteins are found on the surface or inside most normal cells and are overexpressed in many cancers (see table on page 244). The EGFR/

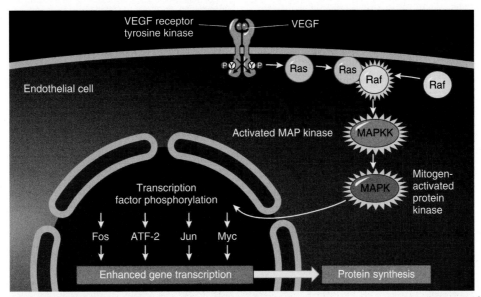

The HER family of receptors. HER family consists of 4 structurally related cellular receptors, which interact in many ways.[2] They include HER1 (EGFR), HER2, HER3, and HER4. HER1/EGFR, HER3, and HER4 are each associated with one or more specific ligands, whereas there are no known ligands that bind HER2. (Copyright © 2006 Oncology Nursing Society. Reprinted with permission.)

HER molecule is a membrane-bound protein that is structurally divided into three distinct regions. Region 1 is the extracellular ligand-binding region located on the outside of the cell; region 2 is the transmembrane lipophilic section that spans the cell membrane and holds the receptor to the cell; and region 3 is the intracellular (cytoplasmic) region, which has TK activity and regulatory function (see figure below). Each region plays an important role in cell function, growth, and interaction for the development and metastasis of malignant tumors.

In normal cells, EGFR signaling is very tightly controlled; however, oncogenic activation of this pathway occurs as a result of EGFR mutation, overexpression, structural rearrangements of genes, or release of normal autoinhibitory and regulatory constraints.

Epidermal Growth Factor—Tyrosine Kinase

As established earlier, EGFR is a member of the ErbB family with TK activity that is commonly altered in epithelial tumors. Kinases (serine, threonine, and tyrosine) were discovered in the 1980s and play a significant role in a variety of cellular processes such as growth and differentiation. Kinases are proteins that perform phosphorylation (i.e., carry phosphate molecules from one area in the signaling pathway to another). EGFR-TK is overexpressed or abnormally activated in most common solid tumors (see table below). Overexpression allows continuous activation of signaling pathways. These mutated proteins then transfer signaling messages independently to promote growth, interfere with the signals that should be telling them to stop growing, or increase invasiveness or metastatic potential.

Epidermal Growth Factor Receptor Overexpression in Solid Tumors

Tumor Type	Frequency of Overexpression (%)
Hereditary small cell lung cancer	80-100
Non–small cell lung cancer	40-80
Prostate	40-70
Glioma	40-63
Gastric	25-77
Breast	14-91
Colorectal	25-77
Pancreatic	30-50
Ovarian	35-70
Renal cell carcinoma	50-90
Bladder	31-48

Data from Ciardiello, F., & Tortota, G. (2008). EGFR Antagonists in Cancer Treatment. *N England Journal of Medicine*, 358, 1160–1174. http://dx.doi.org/10.1056/NEJMra0707704. Martinelli, E., De Palma, R., De Vita, F., & Ciardiello, F. (2009). Anti-epidermal growth factor receptor monoclonal antibodies in cancer therapy. *Clin Exp Immunol*, 158(1), 1–9. http://dx.doi.org/10.1111/j.1365– 2249.2009.03992.x Oct. Salomon, D. S., Brandt, R., Ciardielo, F., et al. (1995). Epidermal growth factor-related peptides and their receptors in human malignancies. Critical Reviews in Oncology/Hematology, 19, 183–232. Hanahan, D., & Weinberg, R. A. (2011). Hallmarks of cancer: The next generation. *Cell*, 144(5), 646–674. Rukazenkov, Y., Speake, G., Marshall, G., Anderton, J., Davies, BR., Wilkinson, RW.,et al. (2009) Epidermal growth factor receptor tyrosine kinase inhibitors: similar but different? Anti-Cancer Drugs 2009, Vol 20 No 10 pp856-866 doi: 10.1097/CAD.0b013e32833034e1. Readon, Da., and Wen, PY. (2006) Therapeutic Advances in the Treatment of Glioblastoma: Rational and Potential Role of Targeted Agents. The Oncologist, 11, pp 152-164. Soulieres, D., Senzer, NN., Vokes, EE. Et al. (2004) Multicenter phase II study of erlotonob, an oral epidermal growth factor receptor tyrosine kinase inhibitor, in patient with recurrent or metastatic squamous cell cancer of the head and neck. Journal of Clinical Oncology, 22, pp 77-85.

Epidermal Growth Factor Receptor–Tyrosine Kinase Overexpression in Human Solid Tumors

Tumor	% of Overexpression
Non–small cell lung cancer	40-80
Prostate	40
Head and neck (squamous cell cancer)	80-100
Colorectal	25-77
Breast	14-91
Ovarian	35-70
Pancreatic	30-50
Gastric	33
Glioblastoma	60

Data from Hanahan, D., & Weinberg, R. A. (2011). Hallmarks of cancer: The next generation. Cell, 144(5), 646–674. Rukazenkov, Y., Speake, G., Marshall, G., Anderton, J., Davies, BR., Wilkinson, RW.,et al. (2009) Epidermal growth factor receptor tyrosine kinase inhibitors: similar but different? Anti-Cancer Drugs 2009, Vol 20 No 10 pp856-866 doi: 10.1097/CAD.0b013e32833034e1. Readon, Da., and Wen, PY. (2006) Therapeutic Advances in the Treatment of Glioblastoma: Rational and Potential Role of Targeted Agents. The Oncologist, 11, pp 152-164. Soulieres, D., Senzer, NN., Vokes, EE. Et al. (2004) Multicenter phase II study of erlotonob, an oral epidermal growth factor receptor tyrosine kinase inhibitor, in patient with recurrent or metastatic squamous cell cancer of the head and neck. Journal of Clinical Oncology, 22, pp 77-85.

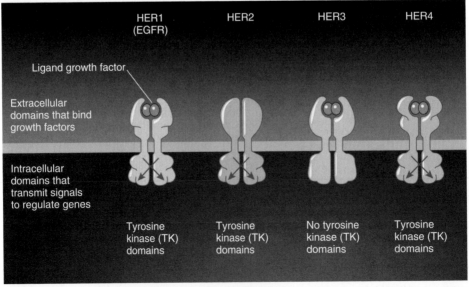

HER1/EGFR and angiogenesis. (Copyright © 2006 Oncology Nursing Society. Reprinted with permission.)

EGFR-TK activity in the normal cell is strictly controlled, allowing only limited cell growth for the processes of maintenance and repair. In tumor activity, EGFR-TK activation contributes to tumor development and progression by means of proliferation, differentiation, invasion, metastases, and inhibition of apoptosis. It also influences tumor angiogenesis by upstream regulation of VEGF and interleukin-8. Additionally, cross-talk with other signaling molecules, such as G protein–coupled receptors and integrins, increases the range of impact of EGFR-TK (Goetsch, 2011; van Leeuwen, van Gelder, Mathijssen, & Jansman, 2014).

More than 500 TKs have been identified in the human genome; 58 are the transmembrane receptor type and 32 the cytoplasmic nonreceptor type (Li et al., 2012; Vlahovic & Crawford, 2003). The nonreceptor type of TK is found in the cytoplasm of the cell, lacks the transmembrane domain segment, and functions downstream of the receptor TKs. The BCR-ABL fusion protein and SRC are examples of nonreceptor TKs. BCR-ABL is created by the chromosomal translocation that generates the Philadelphia chromosome found in some forms of leukemia, and SRC is a TK implicated in the control of cell division, production of autocrine growth factors, cell survival response, and cell motility. Upstream signaling occurs near the cell membrane, and downstream regulation occurs closer to the nucleus. *KRAS* is one of the genes involved in the EGFR pathway (Goetsch, 2011; van Leeuwen et al., 2014).

Activation of the receptor occurs when a ligand (EGF or TGF-α) binds to the extracellular domain on the cell surface, resulting in dimerization with either another EGFR protein or another ErbB receptor; HER2 is the preferred partner (Janmaat & Giaccone, 2003). This dimerization triggers autophosphorylation of TK at the intracellular domain segment, activating appropriate downstream signaling molecules. EGFR-activated pathways include Akt and signal transducer and activator of transcription cascades, which are important for cell survival, and the mitogen-activated protein pathway, which induces proliferation. EGFR can also be activated by stimuli that do not directly bind to the receptor, such as hormones, lymphokines, and stress factors (Vlahovic & Crawford, 2003).

High expression levels or mutations, as well as other potential mechanisms, can provoke abnormal EGFR-TK activity, including ligand overexpression, heterodimerization with other ErbB members (especially HER2), and transactivation by heterologous signaling networks. This, combined with the ability of EGFR-TK to affect tumor growth, including cell proliferation, angiogenesis, invasion, metastases, and survival, provides a rationale for inhibition of EGFR-TK as an anticancer therapy (Goetsch, 2011).

Toxicities

Targeted therapies have more promising safety profiles and fewer nonspecific toxicities than standard chemotherapy and generally do not exert an effect on the hematopoietic system, making them effective for primary treatment or in combination therapy with other treatment modalities. Some of the common side effects are rash, nail and hair changes, xerosis, diarrhea, ophthalmologic and otic toxicity, interstitial lung disease, infusion reactions, and drug interactions.

Rash

Papulopustular eruptions are one of the most common side effects of the EGFR inhibitors, affecting approximately two thirds of patients. The rash, which develops primarily on the face, neck, shoulders, and upper torso and is characterized by interfollicular and intrafollicular papulopustules, usually occurs within the first 2 weeks of treatment. The rash is usually mild to moderate, although some reports of severe rashes exist. It is generally considered dose dependent and usually resolves after discontinuation of treatment or with treatment interruptions (often within 1 to 2 weeks). However, the rash may spontaneously clear despite therapy continuation.

The EGFR-inhibitor rash is classified according to Common Toxicity Criteria from the National Cancer Institute (i.e., whether symptoms are present, how much of the body is affected by the rash, and whether there is a need for management) (National Cancer Institute, 2010). Rashes may be localized (<50% of the body) or spread (>50% of the body). One of the main problems with this type of classification system is that the grading scale does not accurately depict the true nature of the rash.

The EGFR-related rash has been called an acneiforme-like skin reaction, acneiforme follicular rash, maculopapular skin rash, and monomorphic pustular lesion (Boucher, Olson, & Piperdi, 2011; Lacouture et al., 2010, 2011). The distinguishing feature separating the EGFR-inhibitor rash from acne vulgaris is the lack of comedones (blackheads or whiteheads); therefore, these descriptive names should not be used.

Pathophysiology of Rash. The etiology of EGFR-related rash is not completely understood. It is well known, however, that EGFR/HER1 is expressed in epidermal and follicular keratinocytes, sebaceous epithelium, and various other epithelial and connective tissue cells. The rash is characterized by lymphocytic perifolliculitis or suppurative superficial folliculitis without an infectious etiology, but the rash occurs as a result of follicular rupture. Histologic inspection reveals that sebaceous (oil) glands are not affected, and there is no presence of microcomedones or comedones. Sterile neutrophils are observed within the follicle, along with a strong inflammatory element. As more targeted therapies are developed and used, more accurate descriptions and classification of these rashes will lead to a better understanding of the etiology and provide a comprehensive pathway to specific treatment. Management of this rash is crucial to the quality of life for patients because it is one of the leading toxicities to affect psychosocial well-being. Should the rash not be properly managed, quality of life may cause premature discontinuation of treatment (Lacouture et al., 2010, 2011). Interestingly, the degree of the rash has been correlated with disease response.

Management of Rash. The Multinational Association for Supportive Care in Cancer (MASCC) has developed guidelines for prevention and treatment of EGFR-associated skin toxicities. The guidelines recommend that EGFR rashes be treated symptomatically for symptoms such as erythema, dry skin, itching, and burning sensation (Lacouture et al., 2010, 2011). Complications such as herpes zoster and secondary infections may also occur. Patients should be referred to a dermatologist for atypical rash, symptoms of infection, necrosis, blistering, and petechiae.

Patients should also be instructed that the rash is not an allergic reaction but that they should notify the health care team as soon as a rash develops so that it can be evaluated. Because the EGFR rash is unlike acne, the use of makeup to hide the rash will not make it worse. A dermatologist-approved brand of makeup may be used; however, most water-based foundations are acceptable. Makeup should be removed with a gentle hypoallergenic cleanser. Recommendations for skin rash care are presented in the box in the next column. Products that contain alcohol or benzoyl peroxide should be avoided because they will dry the skin and worsen the condition. Patients should be encouraged to use emollients to alleviate skin dryness, applying them after showering. Tepid water will increase absorption of the emollients. Mild, nonperfumed skin cleansers such as Basis soap, Ivory, Dove, or Neutrogena should be used during showering. Patients should avoid direct sunlight. Use of a sun block, sun hats, and protective clothing is recommended when outdoors. Sun blocks should be reapplied frequently.

Painful rashes may be treated with standard analgesics. Patients should be encouraged to discuss the pain with their clinician. For itching, antihistamines such as diphenhydramine or hydroxyzine hydrochloride may be used. Topical agents such as menthol 0.5%, pramoxine 1%, or topical steroids including triamcinolone acetonide 0.025%, desonide 0.05%, or fluticasone proprionate 0.05% may be helpful (Lacouture et al., 2010, 2011).

Prophylactic use of intranasal mupirocin daily may prevent secondary infections (Lacouture et al., 2010, 2011). If a secondary infection develops, antibiotics are prescribed based on the bacterial strain. A short course of oral antibiotics, such as minocycline 100 mg daily or doxycycline 100 mg twice a day, is indicated (Lacouture et al., 2010, 2011). These antibiotics are used for their anti-inflammatory property and coverage of *Staphylococcus aureus*, one of the most common skin infections. Signs of an *S. aureus* infection are a yellowish-brown crust overlying the inflammatory lesions with significant fluid oozing from the lesion. Topical clindamycin, pimecrolimus (Elidel), or tacrolimus (Protopic) may also be applied.

Nail Changes

Paronychia, or inflammation of the lateral nail folds, can occur between 4 weeks and 6 months after treatment is initiated (average, 2 months). The incidence is 6% to 50% of patients being treated with EGFR inhibitors. Patients present with painful, erythematous, and edematous lateral nail folds, ingrown nails, and proliferation of granulation tissue. Fungal cultures are routinely negative; however, bacterial cultures may show the presence of *S. aureus*. Treatment with antibiotic therapy is necessary to prevent further complications. Paronychial inflammation may interfere with activities of daily living. Patients should be advised to avoid tight-fitting

---

Product Recommendations for EGFR-Inhibitor Skin Rash

Mild Soaps and Cleansers
Basis
Neutrogena
Cetaphil
Dove
Ivory Skin Cleansing Liquid-Gel
Aveeno Shower Gel

Makeup
Dermablend makeup
Hypoallergenic brands of makeup (e.g., Almay, Clinique)

Sunscreen
AntiHelios Sunscreen

Emollients for Dry Skin
Eucerin Cream
Eucerin Dry Skin Therapy
Cetaphil cream
Aquaphor healing ointment
Bag Balm
Udderly Smooth Udder Cream
Zim's Crack Cream products
Neutrogena Norwegian Formula Cream (hand/body)
Vaseline Intensive Care Advanced Healing Lotion

Pruritus
Gold Bond powder
Aveeno baths
Sween cream
Benadryl (diphenhydramine) lotion or oral tablets (25 mg) every 6 hr

Cracks and Fissures
Band-Aid Brand Liquid Bandage applied into cracks or fissures to relieve pain and promote healing
Bag Balm for soothing fissures on palms of hands and soles of feet
Zim's Crack Cream products
Aquaphor healing ointment

Data from Lacouture, M. E., Anadkat, M. J., Bensadoun, R. J., Bryce, J., Chan, A., Epstein, et al. (2011). Clinical practice guidelines for the prevention and treatment of EGFR inhibitor-associated dermatologic toxicities. *Supportive Care in Cancer*, 19(8), 1079–1095. Boucher, J., Olson, L., & Piperdi, B. (2011). Preemptive management of dermatologic toxicities associated with epidermal growth factor receptor inhibitors. Clinical Journal of Oncology Nursing, 15(5), 501–508.Culkin, A. (2006). Nursing management: Questions and answers. In Current Topics in Lung Cancer: Targeting EGFR (p. 4). North Miami, Florida: Institutes for Medical Education & Research. Accessed on 10/01/2007 at http://www.imeronline.com/109_lung_cancer/Lung_cancer_4.html. Dick, A. E., & Crawford, G. H. (2005). Managing cutaneous side effects of epidermal growth factor receptor (HER1/EGFR) inhibitors. *Community Oncology*, 2, 492–496. Perez-Soler, R., Delord, J. P., Halpern, A., Kelly, K., Krueger, J., Sureda, B. M., et al. (2005). HER1/EGFR inhibitor-associated rash: future directions for management and investigation outcomes from the HER1/EGFR inhibitor rash management forum. The Oncologist, 10, 345–356. Lacouture, M. E., Maitland, M. L., Segaert, S., Setser, A., Baran, R., Fox, L. P., & Trotti, A. (2010). A proposed EGFR inhibitor dermatologic adverse event-specific grading scale from the MASCC Skin Toxicity Study Group. Supportive Care in Cancer, 18(4), 509–522.

shoes, pushing back the cuticles around the nail beds, clipping nails too short, and biting nails. If nail lesions are severe, application of silver nitrate, antiseptic soaks, and cushioning may also be recommended.

Hair Alterations

Alterations in the hair are less common than rash and usually are not seen until 2 to 3 months after the start of therapy. The common complaint is that of brittle, finer, and curly hair, with frontal alopecia gradually developing. Progressive growth of facial hair and eyelashes may be particularly noticeable in some patients.

Unwanted facial hair may be cosmetically treated with wax depilation or electrolysis. Minoxidil has been found to be effective for some patients.

Xerosis

Dry skin (xerosis) is a common side effect of EGFR inhibitors. The mechanism for xerosis is similar to that of dry skin associated with the use of retinoids. It is the result of an unwoven epidermal layer that can no longer preserve moisture. Dry skin on the fingertips may result in painful fissures. Treatment with emollients containing 5% to 10% urea or 10% salicylic acid is recommended. Patients should be advised to avoid alcohol-containing lotions and gels as well as hot baths and showers, which tend to cause drying. Measures should be taken to avoid the development of folliculitis.

Acral erythema has also been seen 2 to 4 weeks after treatment with EGFR inhibitors; it appears to be dose dependent and disappears after therapy is stopped. Acral erythema manifests as painful, symmetric, erythematous, and edematous areas on the palms and soles, similar to the "hand-foot syndrome" observed with some chemotherapy agents. Paresthesias may be present, which can be aggravated by warmth. Although the palms and soles are the most common sites, other areas of the body may be affected. The use of mild soaps and shower gel and skin care products that promote and maintain hydration is indicated.

Ocular Toxicities

Ocular symptoms include blepharitis, epiphora, conjunctivitis, and trichomegaly. Blepharitis is inflammation of the eyelids; the most common form is the posterior type, which occurs in the inner eye around the meibomian glands. These glands secrete a substance that helps tears spread over the eye, keeping them from evaporating. Posterior blepharitis is accompanied by dry eye syndrome, conjunctivitis, and keratitis. Epiphora is watery eyes; it occurs with an overproduction of tears or when tears do not drain correctly. Treatment with bevacizumab and imatinib may lead to epiphora. Trichomegaly, or excess eyelash growth, is caused by agents such as erlotinib, gefitinib, and cetuximab. The receptors for the normal development of hair follicles are blocked, which leads to increased hair follicle maturation. Although trichomegaly may be irritating, corneal ulcerations are uncommon. Lashes need to be trimmed with scissors if too long. Otic symptoms are vertigo and tinnitus, which may be the result of damage to the cochlea, the vestibular system, or both. These symptoms may occur gradually or rapidly and are related to the dose of the drugs and their frequency of use (Boucher, Habin, & Underhill, 2014; O'Leary, 2014).

Conclusion

Nursing knowledge of these novel targeted therapies can affect patient outcomes. Thorough nursing care involves adequate teaching about targeted therapy, prompt recognition of side effects, and evidence-based practice treatment recommendations. Being well informed helps nurses promote quality of life for patients undergoing treatment with targeted therapy.

References

Alaoui-Jamali, M. A., Morand, G. B., & da Silva, S. D. (2015). ErbB polymorphisms: Insights and implications for response to targeted cancer therapeutics. *Frontiers of Genetics, 6*, 17.

Albini, A., Tosetti, F., Li, V. W., Noonan, D. M., & Li, W. W. (2012). Cancer prevention by targeting angiogenesis. *National Review of Clinical Oncology, 9*(9), 498–509.

American Cancer Society. (2015a). *Cancer immunotherapy.* Available at http://www.cancer.org/treatment/treatmentsandsideeffects/treatmenttypes/immunotherapy/index (accessed February 5, 2016).

Behrend, S. W. (2015). Update on…radiation oncology. *Oncology Nursing Forum, 42*(1), 103–104.

Bilotti, E. (2013). Carfilzomib: A Next-Generation Proteasome Inhibitor for Multiple Myeloma Treatment. *Clinical Journal of Oncology Nursing, 17*(2). http://dx.doi.org/10.1188/B.CJON.E35-E-44 E35-E-44.

Boucher, J., Habin, K., & Underhill, M. (2014). Cancer genetics and genomics: Essentials for oncology nurses. *Clinical Journal of Oncology Nursing, 18*(3), 355–359.

Boucher, J., Olson, L., & Piperdi, B. (2011). Preemptive management of dermatologic toxicities associated with epidermal growth factor receptor inhibitors. *Clinical Journal of Oncology Nursing, 15*(5), 501–508.

Carmeliet, P., & Jain, R. K. (2011). Molecular mechanisms and clinical applications of angiogenesis. *Nature May19, 473*, 298–307. http://dx.doi.org/10.1038/nature10144.

Castillo-Trivino, T., Braithwaite, D., Bacchetti, P., & Waubant, E. (2013). Rituximab in relapsing and progressive forms of multiple sclerosis: A systematic review. *PLoS One, 8*(7), e66308.

Dillman, R. O. (2011). Cancer immunotherapy. *Cancer Biotherapy and Radiopharmacy, 26*(1), 1–64.

Duxbury, B., Combescure, C., & Chizzolini, C. (2013). Rituximab in systemic lupus erythematosus: An updated systematic review and meta-analysis. *Lupus, 22*(14), 1489–1503.

Ebos, J. M., & Kerbel, R. S. (2011). Antiangiogenic therapy: Impact on invasion, disease progression, and metastasis. *National Review of Clinical Oncology, 8*(4), 210–221.

Edmonds, K., Hall, D., Spencer-Shaw, A., Koldenhof, T., Chrysou, M., Boers-Doets, C., & Molassiotis, A. (2012). Strategies for assessing and managing the adverse events of sorafenib and other targeted therapies in the treatment of renal cell and hepatocellular carcinoma: Recommendations from the European Nursing Task Group. *European Journal of Oncology Nursing, 16*, 172–184. http://dx.doi.org/10.1016/J.ejon.2011.05001.

Eggert, J. (2011). The biology of cancer: What do oncology nurses really need to know? *Seminars in Oncology Nursing, 27*(1), 3–12.

Ferrara, N. (2004). Vascular endothelial growth factor as a target for anticancer therapy. *The Oncologist, 9*(Suppl. 1), 2–10.

Ferrara, N., Gerber, H. P., & LeCouter, J. (2003). The biology of VEGF and its receptors. *Nature Medicine, 9*, 669–676.

Genentech, Inc. (2015). *Avastin (package insert).* Available at http://www.gene.com/download/pdf/avastin_prescribing.pdf (accessed February 5, 2016).

Goetsch, C. (2011). Genetic tumor profiling and genetic targeted cancer therapy. *Seminars in Oncology Nursing, 27*(1), 31–44.

Goubran, H. A., Kotb, R. R., Stakiw, J., Emara, M. E., & Burnouf, T. (2014). Regulation of tumor growth and metastasis: The role of tumor microenvironment. *Cancer Growth and Metastasis, 7*, 9–18.

Grenon, N. N. (2011). Managing toxicities associated with antiangiogenic biologic agents in combination with chemotherapy for metastatic colorectal cancer. *Clinical Journal of Oncology Nursing, 17*(4), 425–433 Doi:10.1188.13CJON.425-433.

Hanahan, D., & Weinberg, R. A. (2011). Hallmarks of cancer: The next generation. *Cell, 144*(5), 646–674.

Hicklin, D. J., & Ellis, L. M. (2005). Role of the vascular endothelial growth factor pathway in tumor growth and angiogenesis. *Journal of Clinical Oncology, 23*, 1011–1027.

Janmaat, M. L., & Giaccone, G. (2003). Small-molecular epidermal growth factor receptor tyrosine kinase inhibitors. *The Oncologist, 8*, 576–586.

Kuoki, M., Miyamoto, S., Morisaki, T., Yotsumoto, F., Shirasu, N., Taniguchi, Y., & Soma, G.-I. (2012). Biological response modifiers used in cancer biotherapy. *Anticancer Research, 32*, 2229–2234.

Lacouture, M. E., Anadkat, M. J., Bensadoun, R. J., Bryce, J., Chan, A., Epstein, et al. (2011). Clinical practice guidelines for the prevention and treatment of EGFR inhibitor-associated dermatologic toxicities. *Supportive Care in Cancer, 19*(8), 1079–1095.

Lacouture, M. E., Maitland, M. L., Segaert, S., Setser, A., Baran, R., Fox, L. P., & Trotti, A. (2010). A proposed EGFR inhibitor dermatologic adverse event-specific grading scale from the MASCC Skin Toxicity Study Group. *Supportive Care in Cancer*, 18(4), 509–522.

Li, M., Wang, I. X., Li, Y., Bruzel, A., Richards, A. L., Toung, J. M., & Cheung, V. G. (2011). Widespread RNA and DNA sequence differences in human transcriptome. *Science. 2011 Jul 1*, 333(6038), 53–58. http://dx.doi.org/10.1126/science.1207018. Epub 2011 May 19.

Li, J., Chen, F., Cona, M. M., Feng, Y., Himmelreich, U., Oyen, R., & Ni, Y. (2012). A review on various targeted anticancer therapies. *Target Oncology*, 7, 69–85.

Mak, A. B., Schnegg, C., Lai, C.-Y., Ghosh, S., Yang, M. H., Moffst, J., & Hsu, M.-Y. (2014). CD133-targeted niche-dependent therapy in cancer: A multipronged approach. *The American Journal of Pathology*, 184(5), 1256–1262.

National Cancer Institute. (2014). *Advances in targeted therapies tutorial*. Available at http://herenciageneticayenfermedad.blogspot.com/2014/07/advances-in-targeted-therapies-tutorial.html (English -language copy on this Spanish-language blog). / (accessed 03/05/2016).

National Cancer Institute. (2015). *Understanding angiogenesis*. Available at http://www.thyroidfnaqa.cancer.gov/images/understandingcancer/PDFs/ANGIOGEN.PDF (accessed February 4, 2016). (accessed February 5, 2016).

Nichol, D., & Stuhlmann, H. (2012). EGFL7: A unique angiogenic signaling factor in vascular development and disease. *Blood*, 119(6), 1345–1352.

O'Leary, C. (2014). Optic and otic side effects of molecular targeted therapies. *Seminars in Oncology Nursing*, 3(3), 169–174.

Pines, G., & Yarden, Y. (2012). The ERBB network: At last, cancer therapy meets systems biology. *Nature Reviews Cancer*, 12(8), 553.

Pilotte, A. P., Hohos, M. B., Polson, K. M., Huflalen, T. M., & Treister, N. (2011). Managing stomatitis in patients treated with Mammalian target of rapamycin inhibitors. *Clinical Journal of Oncology Nursing*, 15, E83–E89. http://dx.doi.org/10.1188/11.cjon.E83-E89.

Readon, Da., & Wen, P. Y. (2006). Therapeutic advances in the treatment of glioblastoma: Rational and potential role of targeted agents. *The Oncologist*, 11, 152–164.

Salomon, D. S., Brandt, R., Ciardielo, F., et al. (1995). Epidermal growth factor-related peptides and their receptors in human malignancies. *Critical Reviews in Oncology/Hematology*, 19, 183–232.

Seshacharyulu, P., Ponnusamy, M. O., Haridas, D., Jain, M., Ganti, A., & Batra, S. K. (2012). Targeting the EGFR signaling pathway in cancer therapy. *Expert Opinion Therapeutic Targets*, 16(1), 15–31. http://dx.doi.org/10.1517/14728222.2011.648617.

Sporn, M. B., & Todaro, G. J. (1980). Autocrine secretion and malignant transformation of cells. *New England Journal of Medicine*, 303(15), 878–880.

Tejpar, S., Prenen, H., & Mazzone, M. (2012). Overcoming resistance to antiangiogenic therapies. *Oncologist*, 17(8), 1039–1050. http://dx.doi.org/10.1634/theoncologist.2012-0068.

van Leeuwen, R. W., van Gelder, T., Mathijssen, R. H., & Jansman, F. G. (2014). Drug interactions between tyrosine-kinase inhibitors and acid suppressive agents: More than meets the eye. Authors' reply. *Lancet Oncology*, 15(11), e470–e471.

Vlahovic, G., & Crawford, J. (2003). Activation of tyrosine kinases in cancer. *The Oncologist*, 8, 531–538.

Vogel, W. H. (2010). Infusion reactions: Diagnosis, assessment and management. *Clinical Journal of Oncology Nursing*, 14(2), E10–E21.

Wujcik, D. (2011). Targeted therapy. In C. H. Yarbro, D. Wujcik, & B. H. Gobel (Eds.), *Cancer nursing: Principles and practice* (7th ed.) (pp. 561–583). Sudbury, MA: Jones and Bartlett.

Wujcik, D. (2014). Science and mechanism of action of targeted therapies in cancer treatment. *Seminars in Oncology Nursing*, 30(3), 139–146.

Yoo, S. Y., & Kwon, S. M. (2013). Angiogenesis and its therapeutic opportunities, laboratory for vascular medicine and stem cell. *Mediators of Inflammation*, Volume 2013, 11. ID 127170 http://dx.doi.org/10.1155/2013/127170.

Hormonal Therapy

Debbie Winkeljohn

Introduction

The importance of hormonal suppression in the treatment of breast cancer was recognized as early as the 19th century. In 1896, George Beatson observed an association between surgical removal of the ovaries and a reduction in some breast tumors (Beatson, 1896). Since that time, estrogen suppression has been attempted through many different mechanisms. Because hormonal therapies are highly specific in their ability to block specific receptors and various feedback loops, they were the first form of targeted therapy. Although hormone therapy was first used in the treatment of breast cancer, it was quickly added to the treatment regimens for prostate, endometrial, and ovarian cancers. Tumor growth that is stimulated by testosterone or estrogen can be suppressed by blocking these hormones, inhibiting cancer cell communication and growth.

Adrenocorticoids

Adrenocorticoids are primarily responsible for the control of glucose metabolism, gluconeogenesis, and immune system regulation. The major forms of adrenocorticoids are glucocorticoids (e.g., cortisol, corticosterone), mineralocorticoids (e.g., aldosterone), and androgens. Adrenocorticoids are synthesized in the adrenal cortex and regulated through the action of adrenocorticotropic hormone (ACTH), which is produced in the anterior pituitary. The regulation of ACTH depends on a precise and sensitive balance between serum levels and stimulation from the central nervous system.

The most commonly used corticosteroids in clinical practice are cortisone acetate, hydrocortisone, prednisolone, methylprednisolone, and dexamethasone. Because lymphoid cells are sensitive to glucocorticoids, which inhibit lymphocyte proliferation by encouraging apoptosis, adrenocorticoids are used commonly in treating lymphocyte-rich cancers such as acute lymphoblastic leukemia, chronic lymphocytic leukemia, Hodgkin disease, non-Hodgkin lymphoma, and multiple myeloma. The hormones also may be used as adjuvant treatment with routine antiemetics, with pain medications, and to reduce cerebral edema due to central nervous system metastasis.

The most common side effects from this class of drugs are hypersensitivity and the appearance of Cushing syndrome, hypertension, osteoporosis, diabetes mellitus, and profound immune system suppression. Additional side effects include euphoria, peptic ulcer disease, muscle weakness, and steroid psychosis.

Androgens

Androgens are the major sex steroids in males. The primary functions of the androgens are male development,

spermatogenesis, inhibition of fat deposition, increased muscle mass, and brain development. The best known adrenal androgen is testosterone, which is produced by the testes. Other androgens include the following:
- *Dehydroepiandrosterone* is a steroid produced from cholesterol in the adrenal cortex. This is the primary precursor of natural androgens and estrogens.
- *Androstenedione* is produced by the testes, adrenal cortex, and ovaries. Androstenediones are metabolically converted to androgens, including testosterone. In females, this androgenic steroid forms the parent structure of estrone. Supplementation with this steroid for athletic or body-building purposes is banned by many sporting organizations.
- *Androstanediol* is a steroid metabolite that acts as the main regulator of gonadotropin secretion.
- *Androsterone* is a chemical byproduct created during the breakdown of androgens or progesterone. It also exerts minor masculinizing effects. It is found in equal amounts in the urine and the plasma in males and females.
- *Dihydrotestosterone* is a metabolite of testosterone. It is an extremely potent androgen and binds strongly to androgen receptors.

Antiandrogens

Antiandrogens comprise a group of hormonal therapies used in men with castration-resistant prostate cancer (CRPC) for androgen-deprivation therapy (ADT). These medications block binding of dihydrotestosterone to the androgen receptor, inhibiting tumor growth that depends on the hormones (Dawson, 2014). ADT options include bilateral orchiectomy or luteinizing hormone–releasing hormone, also known as gonadotropin-releasing hormone (GnRH) agonist, or a combination of GnRH with antiandrogen. These regimens can be rotated in different combinations in men with CRPC (Basch et al., 2014).

Antiandrogen agents include bicalutamide, nilutamide, and flutamide (see table on page 250). Newer agents such as enzalutamide and abiraterone are available for CRPC, but their role and timing are still under investigation. Side effects of antiandrogens can include hot flashes, loss of libido, impotence, and gynecomastia (Dawson, 2014).

Antiestrogens

More than a century ago, estrogen was found to play an important role in the pathophysiologic mechanisms of breast cancer. In the early 1900s, approximately one third of premenopausal women with advanced breast cancer were found to respond to an oophorectomy (Singh, 2012). In the same way, some

Hormonal Therapy for Prostate Cancer*

Drug	Dose	Side Effects
GnRH agonist: leuprolide (Lupron)	7.5 mg for 1 mo, 22.5 mg for 3 mo, 30 mg for 4 mo, and 45 mg for 6 mo	Hot flashes, pain, testicular atrophy, flu-like syndrome, injection site pain
Antiandrogen: bicalutamide	50 mg by mouth daily	Hot flashes, decreased libido, impotence, nausea, and diarrhea
Antiandrogen: nilutamide	300 mg by mouth daily for 30 days, then 150 mg by mouth daily	Delayed adaptation to darkness, nausea, increased LFTs, interstitial lung disease
Antiandrogen: flutamide (not commonly used)	250 mg by mouth every 8 hr	Diarrhea, nausea and vomiting, fatal hepatotoxicity
Androgen receptor inhibitor: enzalutamide	160 mg by mouth daily	Seizure, fatigue, asthenia, back pain, decreased appetite, hot flashes, edema, hypertension
CYP17 inhibitor: abiraterone	1000 mg by mouth daily 1 hr before or 2 hr after meals With prednisone 5 mg by mouth twice daily	Hepatotoxicity, fatigue, edema, hot flashes, diarrhea, hypertension

*GnRH therapy is continued with all of the drugs listed.

CYP17, Cytochrome P450 17α-hydroxylase/17,20-lyase; *GnRH*, gonadotropin-releasing hormone; *LFTs*, liver function test results.
Data from National Comprehensive Cancer Network. (2015b). Prostate cancer. Available at http://nccn.org/professionals/physician_gls/pdf/prostate.pdf (accessed February 8, 2016); Dawson, N. A. (2014). Secondary endocrine therapies for castration-resistant prostate cancer. Available at http://www.uptodate.com/contents/secondary-endocrine-therapies-for-castration-resistant-prostate-cancer (accessed February 8, 2016); Astellas Pharma. (2012). Xtandi (enzalutamide) [package insert]. Northbrook, IL: Author.

postmenopausal women responded to adrenalectomy or hypophysectomy. With the discovery of the estrogen receptor, the mechanism of action for estrogen on the various target tissues became better understood.

Current knowledge reveals two major routes for estrogen production: ovarian production and peripheral aromatization. In premenopausal women, both routes are active. In postmenopausal women, only the peripheral aromatization pathway is active. This difference has significant implications for the use of hormonal therapy in women with breast cancer, depending on their premenopausal or postmenopausal status. In most postmenopausal women, androstenedione is released from the adrenal glands. This adrenal steroid goes through several metabolic steps before interacting with the aromatase enzyme and being converted to estrogen. This process is known as aromatization. The enzymatic conversion occurs in sites such as breast tissue, liver, muscles, and fat cells and is catalyzed by the aromatase enzyme complex. Blocking or inhibiting the aromatase enzyme makes the conversion to estrogen impossible.

The two most common drug classes used for their antiestrogen-like effects are selective estrogen receptor modulators (SERMs) and aromatase inhibitors (AIs).

Selective Estrogen Receptor Modulators

SERMs work by occupying the estrogen receptors inside cells to block the action of estrogen in breast and other estrogen-sensitive tissues. SERMs do not block all estrogen receptors. As the name suggests, they selectively inhibit certain estrogen receptors, such as those in breast tissue, while allowing stimulation of estrogen receptors in other organs, such as bone and uterus in postmenopausal women (although this is not the case for premenopausal women). Tamoxifen (Nolvadex) is the most commonly used SERM. Toremifene (Fareston) is another option, but it is not widely used in the United States.

Tamoxifen is the treatment of choice for hormone receptor–positive breast cancer in premenopausal women. It can

be used in postmenopausal women depending on a review of risk factors and the side effect profile (see table on page 251), but an AI should be used during some part of treatment in postmenopausal women. Tamoxifen can be used in adjuvant treatment of breast cancer and in the treatment of metastatic breast cancer (Pritchard, 2014).

Aromatase Inhibitors

Aminoglutethimide was the first drug used to block the aromatase enzyme in women with metastatic breast cancer. Since that time, several other agents have become available. Two major classes of AIs currently exist: nonsteroidal aromatase inhibitors and steroidal aromatase inhibitors.

Nonsteroidal aromatase inhibitors, also known as competitive aromatase inhibitors, bind reversibly to the receptor site on the enzyme and prevent the formation of estrogen for as long they occupy the site. These medications include anastrazole and letrozole (see table on page 251).

Steroidal aromatase inhibitors, also called noncompetitive aromatase inhibitors, are derivatives of androstenedione. This class of AIs retain the androgenic properties. Because these agents bind irreversibly to the aromatase enzyme, they are also called *suicide inhibitors.* New enzymes must be synthesized to overcome this inhibitor even after the drug has been cleared from the body. Hypothetically, these agents should have improved efficacy compared with the reversible inhibitors, although this has not been demonstrated in studies. Exemestane is the steroidal aromatase inhibitor currently used (see table on page 251).

Metastatic Therapy with Antiestrogens

SERMs and AIs are also given to women with metastatic breast cancer. Treatment for metastatic breast cancer needs to be individualized. If a woman does not present with acute visceral crisis, end-organ damage, or aggressive, immediately life-threatening disease, she can be treated with endocrine therapy (Ellis, Naughton, & Ma, 2014). For premenopausal women, options include ovarian suppression

Hormonal Therapy for Breast Cancer

Drug	Dose	Side Effects	Length of Use	Use
SERMs: tamoxifen (toremifene and raloxifene are rarely used)	20 mg PO daily	Hot flashes, stroke, thromboembolic risk, uterine cancer, vaginal discharge, menstrual irregularities	Premenopausal: 5 yr, and consider an additional 5 yr Postmenopausal: up to 5 yr	Premenopausal and post-menopausal DCIS Adjuvant and metastatic therapy Can be used with GnRH ovarian suppression
AIs: (1) Anastrozole (2) Letrozole (3) Exemestane (Aromasin)	(1) 1 mg PO daily (2) 2.5 mg PO daily (3) 25 mg PO daily	Osteoporosis, hot flashes, increased cholesterol, arthralgias, decreased sexual interest, decreased vaginal lubrication	Postmenopausal: up to 5 yr	Postmenopausal Premenopausal with ovarian suppression or ablation Adjuvant and metastatic therapy
GnRH agonists: (1) Lupron (2) Goserelin	Varies: every 1, 3, or 6 mo (subcut or IM)	Hot flashes, mood changes, weight gain, injection reaction	As indicated	Premenopausal Can be used with tamoxifen or an AI Metastatic breast cancer
Estrogen receptor down-regulator (antagonist): fulvestrant	500 mg IM on day 1, 15, and 29 and then monthly	Hot flashes, increased LFTs, arthralgias	As indicated	Metastatic breast cancer Adjuvant treatment May be beneficial in nonadherent patients because of IM injection
Kinase inhibitor: lapatinib	Varies: 1250 daily with capecitabine days 1-21; 1500 mg PO daily with letrozole	Nausea, diarrhea, fatigue, rash	As indicated	Metastatic breast cancer that is HER2 positive
Progestin: megestrol acetate	40 mg PO qid	Increased appetite, weight gain, diarrhea, rash	As indicated	Metastatic breast cancer

AI, Aromatase inhibitor; *DCIS,* ductal carcinoma in situ; *GnRH,* gonadotropin-releasing hormone; *HER2,* human epidermal growth factor receptor 2; *IM,* intramuscular; *LFTs,* liver function test results; *PO,* oral; *qid,* four times daily; *SERM,* selective estrogen receptor modulators; *subQ,* subcutaneous.
Data from National Comprehensive Cancer Network. (2015a). Breast cancer. Available at http://nccn.org/professionals/physician_gls/pdf/breast.pdf (accessed February 8, 2016); Pritchard, K. (2014). Adjuvant endocrine therapy for non-metastatic, hormone receptor-positive breast cancer. Available at http://www.uptodate.com/contents/adjuvant-endocrine-therapy-for-non-metastatic-hormone-receptor-positive-breast-cancer (accessed February 8, 2016); Ellis, M., Naughton, M. J., & Ma, C. X. (2014). Treatment approach to metastatic hormone receptor-positive breast cancer: Endocrine therapy. Available at http://www.uptodate.com/contents/treatment-approach-to-metastatic-hormone-receptor-positive-breast-cancer-endocrine-therapy (accessed February 8, 2016).

or oblation, SERM, or a combination of ovarian suppression and tamoxifen. Options for postmenopausal women include an AI, SERM, or fulvestrant (see table above). After the disease has progressed while on first-line endocrine therapy, second-line endocrine therapy options should be evaluated and offered. This may include newer agents such as the AI Aromasin (see table above). Women with HER2-positive tumors may be given endocrine therapy along with lapatinib (Ellis et al., 2014) (see table above). Current studies are evaluating newer endocrine agents such as entinostat (Ellis et al., 2014).

Gonadotropin-Releasing Hormone Agonists

Ovarian ablation has been recognized as an effective means for treating breast cancer for more than a century, in the same way that orchiectomy has been used to treat prostate cancer. Historically, surgical removal or irradiation of the ovaries or testes has been used to ablate hormonal stimulation, which can cause proliferation to sensitive tissues.

The development of GnRH agonists has allowed chemical ovarian or testicular ablation rather than surgical ablation. The use of a GnRH agonist may minimize morbidity, providing a preferable alternative to other, more invasive procedures. The GnRH agonist mimics the naturally occurring substance in the body and produces the same physiologic effects. By mimicking the normal GnRH, the agonists fill the receptor in the pituitary; they also occupy the receptors for a longer period of time compared with endogenous GnRH.

GnRH agonists suppress ovarian production of estrogen by binding to the GnRH pituitary receptors. This results in downregulation of the receptors. With continued administration, estrogen and progesterone production are greatly reduced, although estrogen initially surges because of the primary stimulating effects on the receptors. After 2 to 4 weeks of treatment, the negative feedback mechanism is activated, and the desired inhibition of luteinizing hormone (LH) and follicle-stimulating hormone (FSH) can be achieved. Estrogen and progesterone levels then begin to fall. This exact process happens the same way in males, resulting in decreased LH and FSH stimulation on the testicles and ultimately in a decrease in testosterone production. Lupron is an example of a GnRH agonist used in the treatment of prostate cancer (see on page 250).

Gonadotropin-Releasing Hormone Antagonists

GnRH antagonists are a class of peptide analogs with important oncologic and gynecologic applications. The antagonists act on the same receptor site as GnRH, causing immediate inhibition of the release of gonadotropins and sex steroids. The *flare response* is prevented because the antagonists induce immediate suppression. Just as with GnRH agonists, the ovaries are no longer stimulated to produce estrogen, and the testes are not stimulated to release testosterone. Degarelix is an example of this group of medications.

Progestins

In normal physiologic functioning, progesterone is involved in the differentiation of a broad spectrum of tissues. The specific effect of progesterone appears to depend on the type of tissue (Dunn, Wickerham, & Ford, 2005). For example, progesterone is required for the maintenance of pregnancy and produces changes in the uterus and breast tissue during the menstrual cycle.

Synthetic progestins exert their action on the hypothalamic-pituitary axis. This results in inhibition of GnRH and indirectly affects tissue growth. Progestins also appear to have a direct effect on cellular proliferation. This can result in growth or inhibition of cellular processes. The cellular effects are mediated through the progesterone receptor located in the cell nucleus.

Before the development of third-generation AIs, progestins were used as second-line hormonal therapy for estrogen receptor– or progesterone receptor–positive breast cancer in postmenopausal women. With the development the new AIs, progestins have become third- or fourth-line treatments for breast cancer and are commonly used in women with metastatic breast cancer.

Conclusion

The past century has brought many changes and advances in hormonal therapy for the treatment of cancer. One type of treatment that remains consistent is hormonal manipulation and hormonal blockade. Tumors that are stimulated to grow by hormones attached to specific receptor sites frequently respond to treatment that interrupts the communication between the hormone and receptor. Hormonal treatment has been used successfully since the 19th century and will continue to be used and improved in the future.

References

Basch, E., Loblaw, D. A., Oliver, T. K., Carducci, M., Chen, R., Frame, J., & Dusetzina, S. (2014). Systemic therapy in men with metastatic castrate resistant prostate cancer: American Society of Clinical Oncology and Cancer Care Ontario Clinical Practice Guideline. *Journal of Clinical Oncology, 32*(30), 3436–3448.

Beatson, G. T. (1896). On the treatment of inoperable cases of carcinoma of the mamma: Suggestions for a new method of treatment, with illustrative cases. *Lancet, 2,* 104–107.

Dawson, N. A. (2014). *Secondary endocrine therapies for castration-resistant prostate cancer.* Available at http://www.uptodate.com/contents/secondary-endocrine-therapies-for-castration-resistant-prostate-cancer (accessed February 8, 2016).

Dunn, B. K., Wickerham, D. L., & Ford, L. G. (2005). Prevention of hormone-related cancers: Breast cancer. *Journal of Clinical Oncology, 23*(2), 357–367. http://dx.doi.org/10.1200/jco.2005.08.028.

Ellis, M., Naughton, M. J., & Ma, C. X. (2014). *Treatment approach to metastatic hormone receptor positive breast cancer: Endocrine therapy.* Available at http://www.uptodate.com/contents/treatment-approach-to-metastatic-hormone-receptor-positive-breast-cancer-endocrine-therapy (accessed February 8, 2016).

Pritchard, K. (2014). *Adjuvant endocrine therapy for non-metastatic, hormone receptor-positive breast cancer.* Available at http://www.uptodate.com/contents/adjuvant-endocrine-therapy-for-non-metastatic-hormone-receptor-positive-breast-cancer (accessed February 8, 2016).

Singh, G. (2012). Oophorectomy in breast cancer: Controversies and current status. *Indian Journal of Surgery, 74*(3), 210–212.

Adherence and Persistence with Oral Therapies

Jody Pelusi

Introduction

With one third of all new oncologic agents being oral formulations, oncology practices and institutions are challenged to provide safe, efficient, and consistent quality care to all patients receiving oral cancer therapies. Initiating, managing, and supporting patients who are taking oral agents can have a substantial effect on the patient's experience with medication adherence and persistence, degree of toxicities, and overall potential outcome of therapy. The American Society of Clinical Oncology/Oncology Nursing Society (ASCO/ONS) Chemotherapy Administration Safety Standards and the Quality Oncology Practice Index (QOPI) provide recommendations for safe administration of chemotherapy- and hematology-based therapy. This chapter focuses on the role of the nurse in supporting patients to achieve the highest level of adherence with their oral therapy. Common terminology can be found in the box below.

Definition of Terms

Adherence rate: The percentage of time over a specified interval (e.g., per cycle, per month) during which the patient is able to be adherent to the medication plan.

Motivational interviewing: Encouraging the patient to adhere to his or her medication by using collaborative approaches and strategies between the patient and the team.

Oral adherence: The patient's ability to take the medication exactly as prescribed (e.g., daily, three times daily) and appropriately as related to food and other medications including over-the-counter (OTC) medications, herbs, and vitamins.

Persistence: The length of time from initiation of treatment to discontinuation. Persistence can be preset (e.g., 5 years of adjuvant therapy with an aromatase inhibitor), or it can last as long as the therapy continues to control the disease (e.g., tyrosine kinase inhibitors for chronic myelogenous leukemia).

Side effects (also known as adverse events or reactions): A myriad of symptoms a patient could experience while taking a medication.

Toxicity grading scale: A way in which medication symptoms are assessed. The one most commonly used is the National Cancer Institute (NCI) toxicity grading scale (Common Terminology Criteria for Adverse Events [CTCAE], version 4.03), and its use is encouraged to provide consistency in the evaluation process (National Cancer Institute, 2010). When medications are in development, the most current version of the CTCAE is used, and recommendations for dose holds or interruptions or dose reductions are based on these criteria. Over time, the grading toxicity scale has been updated, so nurses and nurse practitioners must be aware of the specific recommendations for each agent.

The Current Landscape of Oral Oncology-Hematology Therapies

Oral cancer therapies are on the rise; 9 out of 10 patients prefer an oral drug over intravenous (IV) therapy as long as the result is equal or better. Nurses are challenged to develop new skills to meet the needs of the growing number of patients on oral cancer therapies.

Oral cancer therapies have several advantages in that they allow patients to take a more active role in their care, feel more in control of their therapy, and experience greater independence and mobility (including less chemotherapy "chair" time). Therefore, oncology practices should evaluate how they are currently managing patients on oral therapies and determine strategies to enhance efficiency, consistency, and effectiveness in providing this service.

Oral regimens require patients to take responsibility for their care. Before the surge in oral chemotherapy, community oncology practices focused on an IV chemotherapy delivery model; minimal attention and resources were designated for patients receiving oral cancer therapy regimens. Creating a new oral therapy delivery model that can be used in tandem with the current IV delivery model is now a necessity, and nursing expertise is critical in this redesign. Nurses are often called on to assess and educate the patient, provide symptom management, determine treatment adherence, and coordinate the process of care—all of which promote optimal adherence to oral therapy.

Optimal patient adherence involves taking medications exactly as prescribed and appropriately as related to food and other medications. Early identification and management of side effects is based on the relationship between patients and caregivers and the oncology team's ability to provide consistent ongoing education, monitoring, and support. A more collaborative interaction among the patient, caregivers, and oncology team members enhances the likelihood that the patient will take the medications correctly, identify side effects early, use appropriate interventions to manage them, and thus be able to stay on the medication longer with less toxicity. If a patient is responding to an oral therapy, persistence can greatly be influenced by many factors, such as proactive symptom management and a supportive environment that enhances adherence.

Dose intensity applies to oral therapy just as it does to IV therapy. Ensuring that the right dose is delivered during treatment can have a significant impact on overall treatment outcomes. Ongoing assessment of the level of adherence is important; if the patient is not adherent, a plan to assist the patient in meeting this goal needs to be developed.

Patient Assessment: Initial and Ongoing

Evaluating patients to determine whether they are candidates for an oral drug is crucial for ensuring overall adherence. Assessment should answer the following questions:

- How many medications is the patient currently taking?
- What is the complexity of the cancer or hematology drug regimen?
- Is the patient adherent with his or her current medications?
- Are there any potential drug interactions with the patient's current medications, diet, or lifestyle activities?
- Is the patient able to physically take the medication?
- Can the patient or caregiver physically open the vial, bottle, or blister pack the medication comes in?
- Is the patient able to read the instructions and patient education material?
- Is the patient able to identify his or her medications and what they are for?
- Is the patient able to understand the treatment plan?
- Is the patient a good historian regarding his or her experience at home with medications and side effects?
- Is the patient able to identify side effects or symptoms?
- Is the patient able to articulate these symptoms to health care staff?
- Is the patient able to self-manage his or her own symptoms?
- Are there any safety issues to consider with the specific oral oncolytic agent?
- Is the patient able to come in for laboratory and imaging testing as needed for monitoring while taking the specific oral medication?
- Is the patient able to come in for routine follow-up and educational visits?
- Is the patient able to afford copays for the medication?
- Can the patient afford supportive care medications as well as imaging, laboratory testing, office visits, and so on?
- Does the patient have a physical address where he or she can receive the medication from specialty pharmacies if needed?
- Is an up-to-date baseline physical and/or mental assessment needed before starting the therapy (to be used for comparison throughout treatment)?
- Has pretreatment testing been conducted, if needed, to ensure accurate dosing?
- Is there a backup caregiver or care provider (depending on the home setting)?
- What is the level of support with family, friends, workplace, or care facility to assist the patient if needed?

These questions should be asked initially and throughout the course of treatment. Institutions should develop appropriate tools that address the following: a distress inventory that evaluates the patient's ability to be adherent, a cultural assessment that influences the education and symptom management approach, and a quality-of-life questionnaire that can identify issues that may influence adherence or possible symptoms from the medication. Each clinic should identify who will formally evaluate and document the outcomes of patients taking oral oncolytics. Although many patients are not able to meet all the criteria listed above, knowing the areas in which they need assistance can guide the nurse to help the patient and caregiver so that medication adherence and safety can be ensured. Often, unless a formal evaluation is conducted, patients and staff may not know what to prepare for; having such an evaluation at the beginning of treatment is helpful for avoiding pitfalls with oral therapy.

Treatment Plan

A treatment plan is critical to guide the patient and the care team in their treatment journey. The plan includes the goal of therapy; timing and dosing; monitoring plans (e.g., frequency of office visits, laboratory testing, imaging procedures); what specific foods, drugs, or lifestyle activities to avoid (e.g., smoking, alcohol); symptom management strategies; and the follow-up plan. A specific and consistent care team can provide guidance for the patient. The treatment plan serves as a guide and reminder for the patient and caregivers, which encourages patient autonomy.

Informed Consent Process

Informed consent should occur before the medication is dispensed. Several days may have passed since the treatment was decided, giving the patient and caregiver time to prepare questions about the treatment. This reflection allows the patient to make an informed decision about the treatment.

Providing informed consent and reviewing the goal of therapy, timing and dosing, potential side effects, and management of side effects as well as the patient's role in the overall process is paramount. Providing the patient with a copy of the consent form is encouraged so he or she will have it as a reference. During the informed consent visit, the nurse practitioner or physician should perform a head-to-toe physical examination and ask specific questions, contributing to the baseline assessment before the medication is started. Because grading of toxicities is based on what is "normal" for the patient, it is imperative that the baseline assessment be retrievable and referred to at every visit. Explaining what is assessed also helps educate the patient about potential side effects. This ultimately assists with adherence because the patient is able to identify and manage side effects early, resulting in fewer dose interruptions.

The informed consent visit provides an opportunity to discuss possible dose holds or interruptions and possible dose reductions. Patients should understand the importance of reporting side effects early so that a symptom management strategy can be initiated or the dose of the medication can be reduced. Many times patients are reluctant to report for fear of having the dose withheld or reduced; they worry that a reduced dose might not be as effective as a higher dose. Patients may also fear that if they miss doses the cancer may be advancing. It is important to explain at the beginning that side effects occur commonly with oral medications and that the sooner symptoms are addressed, the less likely the need for dose interruptions and reductions. Consistent laboratory testing and imaging also ensure that changes are detected early. Diligently managing symptoms and enhancing quality of life assist with patient adherence.

Patient Education

Patient education is the cornerstone to help the patient be successful with the oral therapy regimen. This is not a one-time occurrence but rather an ongoing process. Most oncology practices are set up for an IV therapy approach, which lends itself to education each time the nurse interacts with the patient, but currently less structure exists for patients receiving oral therapy. A system should be established that ensures continued patient support and education. Nurses have provided IV chemotherapy patient education for decades, but with oral agents, additional focus must be placed on the roles of adherence, medication safety, storage, administration, potential drug-drug interactions, refill policies, what to do with leftover medication, interacting with specialty pharmacies, and constant reinforcement regarding side effect identification and symptom management.

Because most oral therapies come from a specialty pharmacy and each pharmacy is different, the nurse needs to confirm what services are offered. The range of services include, but is not limited to, managing the delivery of the medication to the patient, obtaining authorization for the medication, monitoring for drug-drug interactions, providing educational materials, providing patient education and follow-up calls, working with pharmaceutical companies to provide the drug for free until the authorization process is complete, and monitoring adherence. Depending on which services the pharmacy provides, the nurse must be collaborative to ensure a seamless process that will not overwhelm the patient or duplicate services. Documentation of each step is critical in the overall management to optimize oral therapy adherence.

Having an individualized education plan for each patient can ensure that agent- and patient-specific elements are discussed and reinforced over time. Knowing who will provide that information, over what time frame, and the points to be discussed will guide the team so that the message remains consistent and comprehensive regardless of who sees or calls the patient. With adult learners, providing small sessions of information over time is more successful than one long educational session. The nurse first assesses the learning needs of the patient and caregivers and then determines which approaches will be best for them.

Motivational interviewing has been suggested as a technique to improve adherence with oral therapies. Although it has been used in behavioral settings, research is lacking in oncology settings. Key principles of motivational interviewing include a focus on the patient's right to determine his or her own care approach so as to successfully reach the outcome of therapy. It emphasizes the partnership and collaboration between the health care team and the patient to mutually share information. It also facilitates informed decision making, uses reflective listening and open-ended questions, affirms efforts, and encourages self-evaluation. It assumes that the health care professional is nonjudgmental

and has gained the respect of the patient. Many of these principles are inherent in the practice of nursing. Studies have demonstrated that patients who have more interactions and support during oral therapy have increased rates of adherence and increased persistence.

Measurement of Adherence

As the patient remains on the medication, it is important to understand the degree of adherence to the oral therapy to guide the treatment plan. It is important to know if the patient is overadherent or underadherent so that necessary adjustments can be made to assist the patient in having the best possible treatment outcome.

Many ways to assess adherence exist. First, it is recommended that adherence rate is documented in the patient's chart at each visit; based on those data, a plan should be proposed to assist the patient in improving adherence. Depending on the drug and treatment plan, adherence may be reported as a percentage based on a specific time (e.g., per cycle, over a certain number of months). Indirect or direct techniques may be used to monitor adherence.

Indirect Methods

Providing education for patient adherence takes time. Staff should be allocated time within their roles to measure adherence by one of the following methods.

Patient Self-Report. Patient self-report is the most common and easiest method to conduct in the clinical setting. If it is done in a nonjudgmental manner with a trusting relationship between the nurse or nurse practitioner and the patient, a fairly accurate report should be obtained. However, this technique is susceptible to human error.

Patient Questionnaires. Patient questionnaires work well in the research setting and can be simple and inexpensive to administer if the patient or caregiver is willing to consistently complete them. They are susceptible to human error and many times are completed just before a visit and not on a daily basis. Questionnaires also require someone to review them in depth. Because oral medications can be continued for months or years, many clinics have elected to use daily questionnaires when treatment is initiated and change to quarterly or semi-annual questionnaires once the patient seems to be adherent.

Patient Diaries. Patient diaries work well in the research setting and assist with recall ability, but they require patients to enter information daily and staff to read it. Diaries can be altered or updated by the patient and caregiver before the visit.

Calendar Check Sheets. Calendars can be used for daily tracking of doses taken and can be helpful for the patient to remember whether a scheduled dose was taken. They can be especially helpful if the regimen is complex. A small pocket calendar is most useful for the patient who travels or who is in and out of the home often to ensure that updates and tracking data are accurate.

Prescription Refill Count. Specialty pharmacies can provide information about whether a prescription is being filled on time. This is an objective count and does not reflect any dose interruption or whether the patient actually took the medication.

Medication Count. A medication count is used predominantely in the research setting as an objective measure, but it is subject to alteration. In the clinical setting, the patient brings in the medication bottles and has clinic staff count the pills. This is an objective count and does not reflect any dose interruption or the actual adherence.

Office Call Programs. An office call program can be very helpful to the patient to assess adherence along with symptoms. The call can also be a time for continued education and for patients to ask questions that might be forgotten by their scheduled visit. This interaction requires medical record documentation for each encounter.

Nurse Call Centers, Case Managers, and Pharmacy Call Programs. Calls may be made by nurse call centers supported by pharmaceutical companies, insurance companies, or specialty pharmacies. Interaction with patients and caregivers can be positive for reminders about adherence and education and for the evaluation of side effects. Each call center differs in terms of what the patient is asked. It is important for the health care team to know who is calling the patient, when, why, and what is done with that information. Collaboration and documentation are critical and sometimes limited. Patients may also have some confusion as to whom they should report information.

Electronic Medication Monitors. Electronic monitors provide a precise measurement with reminders to take the medication or a record of when the prescription bottle is opened. This technology is often considered initially until the patient becomes adherent. Such devices can track patterns of behavior and record trends over time, but they can be expensive, and the data must be downloaded and reviewed.

Clinical Response Rates. Many assume that if patients are having a clinical response, they must be taking their medication. This is a simple method to assess adherence, but other outside factors could influence the response. Some patients could be achieving a response at a lower dose level than recommended.

Direct Methods

Measurements of Physiologic Markers. It is easy to measure physiologic markers along with other laboratory testing, but the measurements may be limited based on disease state

and may be absent due to poor metabolism or lack of response to the oral agent.

Measurement of the Level of Medicine or Metabolite in the Blood. Blood analysis can be used to detect levels of the drugs taken or of their metabolites. This method is very objective, but the results vary with the degree of adherence, the method is expensive and drug specific, and very few drugs can be tested in this way.

Direct Observation. The most accurate technique is direct observation—watching the patient take each dose of medication and ensuring that it is swallowed. However, this method is impractical.

Conclusion

Each patient is unique in terms of what approaches will work best to assist their efforts toward adherence with oral therapy over time. Adherence begins at the initial assessment of the patient, reinforcing what is needed to be successful and establishing the trust relationship with the health care team. Building the right environment for the patient in terms of support, education, and monitoring is paramount for success with oral drug therapy. The nurse plays a key role in every step of an oral therapy regimen. Oral therapies are here to stay, and it is critical for nurses to embrace the challenges and develop skills to ensure quality care for patients receiving oral therapy.

Bibliography

American Society of Clinical Oncology. (2015). Quality oncology practice initiative (QOPI) certification standards. Available at http://www.instituteforquality.org/qopi/qopi-certification-standards (accessed February 10, 2016).

Barefoot, J., Blecher, C., & Emery, R. (2009, May/June). Keeping pace with oral chemotherapy. *Oncology Issues*, 36–39. Available at https://accc-cancer.org/oncology_issues/articles/MJ09/MJ09-Keeping-Pace-with-Oral-Chemotherapy.pdf (accessed February 10, 2016).

Given, B. A., Spoelstra, S. L., & Grant, M. (2011). The challenges of oral agents as antineoplastic treatments. *Seminars in Oncology Nursing, 27*(2), 93–103.

Moseley, W., & Nystrom, S. (2009). Dispensing oral medications: Why now and how? *Community Oncology, 8*(6), 358–361.

National Cancer Institute. (2010, March 1, 2010). Common Toxicity Criteria for Adverse Events. Retrieved from http://ctep.cancer.gov (accessed February 29, 2016).

Neuss, M. N., Polovich, M., McNiff, K., Esper, P., Gilmore, T. R., LeFebvre, K. B., & Jacobson, J. O. (2013). 2013 updated American Society of Clinical Oncology/Oncology Nursing Society chemotherapy administration safety standards including standards for the safe administration and management of oral chemotherapy. *Oncology Nursing Forum, 40*(3), 225–233.

Oncology Nursing Society. (2015). Oral therapies for cancer. Available at https://www.ons.org/content/oral-therapies-cancer (accessed February 10, 2016).

Oncology Nursing Society. (2015). ONS toolkit helps patients adhere to oral therapies for cancer. Available at https://www.ons.org/practice-resources/clinical-practice/ons-toolkit-helps-patients-adhere-oral-therapies-cancer (accessed February 10, 2016).

Pelusi, J. (2014). Managing oral oncology-hematology treatments in your practice. http://www.communityoncology.org/pdfs/Sat%20CL%202%20%20930%202013%20Pelusi%20Managing%20Oral%20Agents.pdf (accessed February 10, 2016).

Weingart, S. N., Brown, E., Bach, P. B., Eng, K., Johnson, S. A., Kuzel, T. M., & Walters, R. S. (2008). NCCN task force report: Oral chemotherapy. *Journal of the National Comprehensive Cancer Network, 6*(Suppl 3), S1–S14.

Complementary and Alternative Therapies

Georgia Decker

Introduction

Definitions

- Professionals in clinical practice, education, and research contribute to the practice of complementary and alternative medicine (CAM). National surveys confirm a continued interest in the use of CAM therapies in the United States and Europe (Eisenberg, 1993; Nahin, Barnes, Stussman, & Bloom, 2009).
- Approaches known as *conventional* or *traditional* are those associated with Western medicine.
- *Complementary* means "in addition to," and the term refers to therapies used *along with* conventional medical treatment.
- *Alternative* means "instead of," and this term is accurate when a therapy is used *instead of* conventional approaches.
- The more contemporary term, *integrative* (or *integrated*), refers to the combining of evidence-based CAM therapies with evidence-based conventional therapies.
- A therapy can be both complementary and alternative; it is the *intent* with which a therapy is used that defines it.

Background

- Before the 19th century, unconventional methods of treatment were considered folk medicine or quackery (Whorton, 1999).
- The Biologics Control Act of 1902 and the Food and Drug Act of 1906 formed the foundation of the present-day U.S. Food and Drug Administration (FDA) (FDA, 1906; Whorton, 1999).
- The Food, Drug, and Cosmetic Act, passed in 1938, required that new drugs provide evidence of safety before being placed on the market (Meadows, 2006).
- In 1994, because of increasing interest in CAM therapies, the Dietary Supplement Health and Education Act was passed. This act defined dietary supplements as food, established regulations under the FDA, and created the Office of Dietary Supplements within the National Institutes of Health (NIH) to promote, conduct, and compile research and maintain a database on supplements and individual nutrients (Office of Dietary Supplements, 1994).
- In 1998, the Office of Alternative Medicine (OAM), which had been established 6 years earlier, became the National Center for Complementary and Alternative Medicine (NCCAM). In December 2014, its name was changed to the National Center for Complementary and Integrative Health (NCCIH) (NCCIH, 2014, 2015a; NIH, 2015).
- Also in 1998, the National Cancer Institute (NCI) instituted an Office of Cancer Complementary and Alternative Medicine (OCCAM) to increase high-quality cancer research and information about CAM use (NCI, 2012).
- In 2000, the White House Commission on Complementary and Alternative Medicine Policy (WHCCAMP) was established to address issues of access to and delivery of CAM, priorities for research, and the need to educate consumers and health care professionals about these therapies; their final report was published 2 years later (WHCCAMP, 2002).
- In 2003 and 2004, the Institute of Medicine (IOM) of the National Academies sponsored meetings to explore scientific, policy, and practice questions related to increasing use of CAM by the American public; the committee's final report was released in 2005 (IOM, 2005).

Use of Complementary and Alternative Medicine

Studies conducted during the 1970s and 1980s revealed that users of CAM were most likely to be female, well educated, of higher socioeconomic class, and using more than one CAM therapy. That profile remains accurate in current surveys as well. Early surveys did not assess specific population or diagnostic information. By the late 1990s, more was known about CAM use among cancer patients in rural populations and among elderly patients (Basch & Ulbricht, 2004; Davis, Oh, Butow, Mullen, & Clarke, 2012; Mao, Palmer, Healy, Desai, & Amsterdam, 2011; Nahin et al., 2009; Vallerand, Fouladbakhsh, & Templin, 2003).

Cancer patients are among the top consumers of CAM, with researchers reporting that 28% to 91% of cancer patients use some form of CAM. Of concern is the fact that 40% to 70% of cancer patients using CAM are not reporting their use to their health care practitioners (Blaes, Kreitzer, Torkelson, & Haddad, 2011; Davis et al., 2012; Deng & Cassileth, 2005; Rausch et al., 2011; van Tonder, Herselman, & Visser, 2009). The reasons given for nondisclosure include fear of disapproval or being dismissed by the provider or practice. Health care professionals report that they do not always ask about CAM use because they believe they lack the knowledge to appropriately counsel patients regarding efficacy and safety. It is essential that nurses become informed and are prepared to initiate and participate in these conversations with patients (Bauer-Wu & Decker, 2012).

Cancer patients report that they use CAM therapies for a variety of reasons, often to manage symptoms such as fatigue, pain, or nausea that are related to their disease or its treatment. Those with recurrent or refractory disease are seeking ways to "boost" their immune system to help fight their disease. Others report a preference for "natural" or nontoxic therapies to provide a sense of hope and control (Blaes et al., 2011; Deng & Cassileth, 2005; Rausch et al., 2011; van Tonder et al., 2009).

Contributing to the appeal of CAM therapies is displeasure with decreased personal attention from conventional medical practitioners and feelings of depersonalization with increased technology in conventional medicine. Embedded in this is patients' belief that if a product is proclaimed to be *natural* it must be *safe*. Dr. David Eisenberg coined the phrase, *safety trumps efficacy*, meaning that even if a particular product or treatment is effective for the reason it is sought, it may not be safe for patients to use under their particular set of circumstances (Painter, 2001). For example, an important safety consideration is the potential for product contamination.

Complementary and Alternative Medicine Approaches

Two main approaches to categorizing and describing CAM therapies exist. The NCCAM described five main categories: natural products, mind-body medicine, manipulative and body-based practices, whole medical systems, and other CAM approaches (see table below).

The OCCAM extended these categories to include movement therapy and complex natural products (as a subcategory of pharmacologic and biologic treatments). There can be an overlap of categories, and some therapies may be represented in more than one category (see first table on page 259).

Levels of Evidence

Sorting through scientific evidence is intimidating to the clinician as well as the patient and family. The "gold standard" for clinical research is evidence from double-blind, randomized controlled trials (RCTs). However, some researchers contend that this is not the best approach to study some CAM therapies (e.g., mind-body interventions) because of the complexity of the therapy. They hold that qualitative research provides opportunities to reach a greater understanding of the patient's

well-being and to gather information that can be helpful for future CAM research (Centre for Evidence-Based Medicine [CEBM], 2009; Fonteyn & Bauer-Wu, 2005).

Although there remains much to be learned about CAM therapies, we now know far more than when the earliest surveys were conducted in the early 1990s. However, even the experts do not always agree on how to determine the level of evidence. Clinical trials determine the safety and efficacy of a particular product or intervention and provide the foundation of evidence-based medicine and the accepted evidence of efficacy. Effectiveness, as opposed to efficacy, incorporates the evaluation of a clinically meaningful effect and whether the risks outweigh the benefits (Barton & Pachman, 2012).

Levels of evidence are used by researchers and clinicians to assess the degree to which interventions meet preestablished criteria (CEBM, 2009; National Library of Medicine, 2015; OCEBM Levels of Evidence Working Group, 2011). A frequent outcome of level-of-evidence data is clinical practice guidelines that can be used as a basis for recommendations for the care of patients with specific conditions. The Society for Integrative Oncology published the first edition of its *Integrative Oncology Practice Guidelines* in 2007. The 2009 edition updated and expanded on the previous version and provided practical recommendations for the use of complementary therapies in the supportive care of cancer patients (Deng et al., 2009). The table on page 259 provides examples of descriptions of levels of evidence. Large amounts of CAM information are available online, in the media, and in lay literature.

The Internet

The Internet is increasingly used by patients and families to gain knowledge about specific diagnoses, treatment choices, and CAM and supportive care. Distinguishing high-quality from poor-quality information is essential. According to the NCI, websites that volunteer medical resources should openly discuss who visits the site, who pays for the site, the purpose of

National Institutes of Health NCCAM Categories

Category	Description	Examples
Natural products	The most popular form of CAM among both adults and children	Herbal medicines (botanicals), vitamins, minerals, and other natural products; some are sold as dietary supplements, including probiotics
Mind-body interventions	Mind and body practices focus on the interactions among brain, mind, body, and behavior, with the intent to use the mind to affect physical functioning and promote health	Meditation techniques, various types of yoga, acupuncture, deep-breathing exercises, guided imagery, hypnotherapy, progressive relaxation, and tai chi
Manipulative and body-based methods	Focuses on the structures and systems of the body: bones, joints, soft tissues, and circulatory and lymphatic systems	Spinal manipulation, massage
Whole medical systems	Distinct systems of theory and practice that have evolved over time in different cultures	Chinese (or Oriental) medicine, Ayurvedic medicine, homeopathy, naturopathy
Other CAM practices	Movement therapies	Feldenkrais method, Alexander technique, Pilates, Rolfing structural integration, and Trager psychophysical integration
	Practices of traditional healers	Native American healer/medicine man
	Energy field manipulation to affect health	Magnet and light therapies, qi gong, Reiki, healing touch, therapeutic touch

NCCAM, National Center for Complementary and Alternative Medicine.
From Bauer-Wu, S., & Decker, G. M. (2012). Integrative oncology imperative for nurses. *Seminars in Oncology Nursing, 28*(1), 2-9.

National Cancer Institute OCCAM Domains of CAM

Domain	Description	Examples
Alternative medical systems	Systems built upon completed systems of theory and practice	Traditional Chinese medicine, Ayurvedic medicine, homeopathy, naturopathy, acupuncture
Manipulative and body-based methods	Methods based on manipulation and/or movement of parts of the body	Chiropractic, therapeutic massage, osteopathy, reflexology
Energy therapies	Therapies involving the use of energy fields: biofield therapies and bioelectromagnetic-based therapies	Reiki, therapeutic touch, pulsed fields, magnet therapy
Mind-body interventions	Techniques designed to enhance the mind's capacity to affect body function and symptoms	Meditation, hypnosis, art therapy, biofeedback, mental healing, imagery, relaxation therapy, support groups, music therapy, cognitive-behavioral therapy, prayer, dance therapy, aromatherapy, animal-assisted therapy
Movement therapy	Modalities used to improve patterns of body movement	Tai chi, Feldenkrais, hatha yoga, Alexander technique, dance therapy, qi gong, Rolfing, Trager method
Nutritional therapeutics	The use of nutrients and nonnutrient, bioactive food components as chemopreventive agents and the use of specific foods or diets as cancer prevention or treatment strategies	Dietary regimens such as macrobiotics, vegetarian, Gerson therapy, Kelley/Gonzalez regimen, vitamins, dietary macronutrients, supplements, antioxidants, melatonin, selenium, coenzyme Q10, ephedrine, orthomolecular medicine
Pharmacologic and biologic therapies	Includes drugs, vaccines, off-label use of prescription drugs, and other biologic interventions not yet accepted in mainstream medicine	Vaccines, off-label use of drugs, antineoplastons, products from honeybees, 714-X, low-dose naltrexone, metencephalin, immunoaugmentative therapy, laetrile, hydrazine sulfate, Newcastle virus, melatonin, ozone therapy, thymus therapy, enzyme therapy, high-dose vitamin C
Complex natural products	Subcategory of pharmacologic and biologic treatments consisting of an assortment of plant samples (botanicals), extracts of crude natural substances, and unfractionated extracts from marine organisms used for healing and treatment of disease	Herbs and herbal extracts, mixtures of tea polyphenols, shark cartilage, essiac tea, Sun's Soup, MGN-3

From Bauer-Wu, S., & Decker, G. M. (2012). Integrative oncology imperative for nurses. *Seminars in Oncology Nursing, 28*(1), 2-9.

Levels of Evidence in Cancer CAM

Data Source	Strength of Study Design	Strength of End Points Measured	Level of Evidence Score
Centre for Evidence-Based Medicine Database, 2009	1a SR of RCTs 1b Individual RCT with narrow confidence interval 1c All or none 2a SR of cohort studies 2b Individual cohort study (including low-quality RCT) 2c Outcomes research, ecological studies 3a SR of case-controlled studies 3b Individual case-control study 4 Case-series (and poor-quality cohort and case-control studies 5 Expert opinion without explicit critical appraisal or based on physiology, bench research, or "first principles"	A Consistent level 1 studies B Consistent level 2 or 3 studies or extrapolation from level 1 studies C Level 4 or extrapolation from level 2 or 3 studies D Level 5 evidence or troublingly inconsistent or inconclusive studies of any level	1 A, B, C 2 A, B, C 3 A, B 4 5
Physician Data Query, National Library of Medicine, 2015	1 RCT (DB/NB) 2 Non-RCT 3 Case series 4 Best case series	A Total mortality B Cause-specific mortality C Quality of life D Indirect surrogates	1-4 (study design score) joined with A-D (strength of endpoints measured)
Natural Medicines, 2016	A Strong scientific evidence B Good scientific evidence C Unclear or conflicting scientific evidence D Fair negative scientific evidence F Strong negative scientific evidence Lack of evidence; unable to evaluate efficacy due to lack of adequate human data	Quality of study 0-2 Poor 3-4 Good 5 Excellent	A B C D F Lack of evidence
Oncology Nursing Society, 2014	Nursing experts summarize and synthesize the evidence	*Green level:* Recommended for practice/likely to be effective *Yellow level:* Effectiveness not established *Red level:* Effectiveness unlikely/not recommended for practice	

DB, Double blind; *NB,* not blinded; *NCI,* National Cancer Institute; *RCT,* randomized controlled trial; *SR,* systematic review.

the site, the source of information, how information is selected for inclusion, how recent the information is, how links to other sites are selected, and what information the site collects about visitors (NCI, 2015e).

Investigators examined websites to determine how CAM is represented. Among the 41 NCI-designated comprehensive cancer centers, 19 provided a link to NCCAM on their website; 12 did not have functional websites with CAM information. On the sites that did have CAM information, the most often mentioned therapies were acupuncture (59%); meditation, nutrition, spiritual support, or yoga (56%); massage therapy (54%); and music therapy (51%) (Brauer, El Sehamy, Metz, & Mao, 2010). The table below provides examples of reliable resources.

Alternative Medical Systems

Alternative medical systems are built on complete systems of theory and practice that typically developed before the conventional medical approaches used in the United States. Examples include traditional Chinese medicine, acupuncture, and homeopathy.

Traditional Chinese Medicine

- Traditional Chinese medicine has been used for thousands of years, primarily in Eastern countries.
- Clinical diagnosis and treatment are typically based on the *yin-yang* and *five elements* theories. These theories apply the occurrence and laws of nature to the study of the physiologic activities and pathologic changes of the human body and their interrelationships.
- Health is considered to be a balance of yin and yang (opposite forces present in everyone).
- Disease or any medical condition is a result of imbalance, usually a blockage or deficiency of energy.
- Typical Chinese medicine therapies include acupuncture, herbal medicine, and qi gong exercises.
- These therapies share the same underlying set of assumptions and insights on the nature of the human body and its place in the universe.

Acupuncture

- Acupuncture has been used to treat a variety of health conditions, including pain and other disorders of the musculoskeletal system, headaches, stress, ear-nose-throat conditions (e.g., sinusitis, tinnitus, vertigo), allergies, dental pain, addictions, and immune system support.
- Acupuncture usually involves the insertion of needles into the skin in specific sites (acupoints) for therapeutic purposes.
- Acupoint stimulation may also be achieved via electrical current, laser, moxibustion, pressure, ultrasound, or vibration.
- There are three types of acupuncture: Japanese, Korean, and Chinese.
- The underlying principle is that *qi* (pronounced "chee" and translated as meaning *energy*) is present at birth and maintained throughout life. *Qi* flows throughout the body via 12 major paths or meridians.
- There are approximately 350 acupoints along the 12 meridians, and additional acupoints lie outside the meridian pathways.
- Acupuncture theory holds that stimulation of the appropriate acupoints aids the body in correcting any imbalance in the flow of energy, thus restoring balance. Moreover, it is believed that changes in the balance of energy and flow of *qi* may be identified before disease has developed and therefore that acupuncture has a role in the prevention of illness and maintenance of health (Natural Medicines, 2016).

Level of Evidence

- More than 400 RCT results are reported in Medline.
- There is no scientific evidence of the physical existence of *qi* or meridians.
- The effects of acupuncture are reportedly better than those of placebo in most trials.
- Opioid peptides, serotonin, and other neurotransmitters are released by acupuncture.

Complementary and Alternative Medicine Resources

Organization	Website
American Cancer Society	http://www.cancer.org/treatment/treatmentsandsideeffects/complementaryand alternativemedicine/complementary-and-alternative-medicine-landing
Food and Drug Administration	http://www.fda.gov/OHRMS/DOCKETS/98FR/06D-0480-GLD0001.PDF
Medline Plus	https://www.nlm.nih.gov/medlineplus/druginfo/herb_All.html
National Cancer Institute (NCI) Office of Cancer Complementary and Alternative Medicine (OCCAM)	http://cam.cancer.gov/
National Center for Complementary and Integrative Health (NCCIH)	https://nccih.nih.gov/
	https://nccih.nih.gov/research/clinicaltrials/alltrials.htm
National Institutes of Health (NIH) National Center for Complementary and Alternative Medicine	https://nccih.nih.gov/health/supplements
NIH Office of Dietary Supplements	https://ods.od.nih.gov/
National Library of Medicine	https://www.nlm.nih.gov/medlineplus/complementaryandintegrativemedicine .html
	https://www.nlm.nih.gov/tsd/acquisitions/cdm/subjects24.html
Natural Medicine Comprehensive Database	http://naturaldatabase.therapeuticresearch.com/home.aspx?cs=CEPDA&s= ND&AspxAutoDetectCookieSupport=1
Physician's Data Query	http://www.cancer.gov/publications/pdq/information-summaries/cam

- Efficacy is considered inconclusive by some authors; whereas others suggest that the evidence is equivocal and/or promising for some indications, including addiction, stroke rehabilitation, postoperative and chemotherapy-related nausea and vomiting, tennis elbow, carpal tunnel syndrome, and asthma (Natural Medicines, 2016).
- The impact of acupuncture on chemotherapy-induced nausea and vomiting has been studied for 2 decades, and the results have been mostly favorable (Bao, 2009; Ma, 2009).

Contraindications

- The "needling" technique is contraindicated in those patients who have severe bleeding disorders or are at increased risk for infection (e.g., neutropenia).
- Acupuncture is contraindicated during the first trimester of pregnancy, with the exception of treatment for nausea.
- Patients with cardiac pacemakers should not be treated with electrical stimulation.
- Caution is advised for the first acupuncture treatment because some patients may become drowsy. Care should be taken if driving or operating machinery after treatment. Needles should not be reused, and strict asepsis should be mandatory. Potential side effects include bleeding, bruising, pain with needling, and worsening of symptoms. Reported adverse events are rare but include pneumothorax and death (Natural Medicines, 2016).

Practitioners

- Certification as an acupuncturist can be achieved in two ways: completion of a formal, full-time educational program that includes both classroom and clinical hours, or participation in an apprenticeship program. Practitioners must also complete a "Clean Needle Technique" approved course. Medical doctors with training in acupuncture may also become board certified.
- Some states require licensure. The National Certification Commission for Acupuncture and Oriental Medicine has established standards for certification that are accepted by some states for licensure (www.nccaom.org). Medical doctors must possess a valid medical license and be certified through the American Academy of Medical Acupuncture (www.medicalacupuncture.org).
- Some states require medical referral, whereas others allow nonmedical practitioners to see patients without referral (www.nccaom.org).
- A comparison of licensed versus certified acupuncturists is available on the Web site of the Acupuncture Society of New York (www.asny.org).

Homeopathy

- Homeopathic remedies have been used orally and topically for a range of conditions including the common cold, flu (influenza), allergic rhinitis, asthma, diarrhea, dermatitis, fibromyalgia, chronic fatigue syndrome, anxiety, depression, fatigue, migraine headache, osteoarthritis, muscle pain, motion sickness, otitis media, and many others.

- Homeopathy was started by the German physician Samuel Hahnemann in 1796 when he presented the paper, *A New Principle of Healing*. This new principle was *homeopathy*.
- The word *homeopathy* means "similar disease" (Greek origin).
- Hahnemann believed that *like cures like*. For example, if a substance in large amounts causes a certain disease, then that same substance in small amounts could cure the disease. This is known as the *Law of Similars*.
- In order to find homeopathic treatments, *provings* were conducted, in which substances such as herbs or minerals were tested in healthy people to see what kind of reaction occurred. These reactions were then documented in detail. For example, if a substance caused fever, then that substance was identified as a treatment for conditions involving fever.
- Homeopathic treatment consists of small doses of the *proved* substance, based on the *Law of Infinitesimals*. It is believed that the more dilute the substance, the more potent its effect; this is known as *potentiation through dilution*.
- Commonly used homeopathic remedies include arnica, belladonna, chamomile, nux vomica, and poison ivy (Natural Medicines, 2016).

Level of Evidence

- Homeopathic theories and principles are considered to be inconsistent with the current understanding of pharmacology, chemistry, and physics.
- There is insufficient reliable evidence to rate the safety of these preparations (Natural Medicines, 2016), but it is unlikely that they have any pharmacologic effect because they are so dilute that they have little or no active ingredient.
- Many clinical trials have found no benefit for homeopathic preparations compared with placebo; other research has found statistically significant benefits.
- The results of metaanalyses and systematic reviews are also inconsistent.
- When all evidence is pooled, regardless of study quality, findings often suggest that homeopathic preparations might offer some benefit.
- Homeopathic remedies are likely safe when used orally or topically and appropriately. Most preparations contain little or no active ingredient. Therefore, it is unlikely that they have any beneficial or harmful effects (Natural Medicines, 2016).

Contraindications

- Homeopathic treatments are contraindicated in pregnant or lactating women.
- There are no known interactions with drugs, herbs, foods, laboratory tests, diseases, or conditions (Natural Medicines, 2016).

Practitioners

- A Certificate of Classical Homeopathy is awarded by the Council for Homeopathic Certification (CHC). Information can be found on their website (http://www.homeopathicdirectory.com/).

- This practitioner certificate program is open to anyone who is interested in studying professional-level homeopathy. This program is appropriate for physicians or health care practitioners.

Manipulative and Body-Based Methods

Several methods based on manipulation and/or movement of body parts exist. Examples include chiropractic, therapeutic massage, osteopathy, and reflexology.

Therapeutic Massage

- Therapeutic massage includes various forms of therapeutic manipulation of soft tissue.
- Swedish massage is the most common form in the West and provides the core of most massage training curricula.
- An important concern regarding massage in cancer care is whether massage could contribute to metastasis (based on the concept that increased blood and lymph circulation might encourage the spread of cancer). Emphasis on evidence-based practices has led to critical examination of this issue, and the speed of circulation is no longer thought to influence cancer spread.

Levels of Evidence

- Studies consistently demonstrate the potential of massage to improve mood and quality of life. An early Cochrane review concluded that the short-term benefits of massage include improved psychological well-being and, in some cases, reduced severity of physical symptoms (Fellowes, Barnes, & Wilkinson, 2004).
- A systematic review of RCTs of Swedish methods for cancer patients identified 14 trials, and the evidence suggested that massage can alleviate a wide range of symptoms, including pain, nausea, anxiety, depression, anger, stress, and fatigue (Ernst, 2009b).

Contraindications

- Contraindications are based on the most common element of massage, pressure, which needs to be modified in patients with cancer (Collinge, MacDonald, & Walton, 2012; MacDonald, 2011).
- Examples include the following (Walton, 2011):
  - Solid tumors
    - Avoid pressure on a solid tumor in any area that is accessible to the hands. It is OK to touch, hold, or stroke using soft hands. Use moderate pressure elsewhere.
    - For patients with palmar plantar erythrodysesthesia (PPE), use soft touch only.
  - Known or suspected bone metastasis, including the spine
    - Avoid pressure on the area or jostling or moving the joints. It is OK to use moderate pressure elsewhere.
  - Tendency toward bruising or bleeding
    - Avoid pressure or aggressive kneading or gliding. It is OK to use gentle kneading or light stroking with just enough pressure to apply lotion, "holding" the body with soft hands.

- Removal or irradiation of lymph nodes in the armpit, groin, neck, or jaw
  - Avoid pressure on the limb and the area drained by those lymph nodes. Touch or hold the area with soft hands (no pressure). It is OK to use moderate pressure elsewhere in the body.

Practitioners. Consensus exists that licensed or certified massage therapists should have additional knowledge, skill, and experience in oncology massage to provide safe and effective therapy for cancer patients. (Myers, et al, 2008; Myers, Walton, & Small, 2008; Corbin, 2005; Walton, 2011). More information is available on the website of the Society for Oncology Massage (http://www.s4om.org/).

Reflexology

Reflexology is the application of pressure to the feet and hands with specific thumb, finger, and hand techniques in specific zones or reflex areas, without the use of oil or lotion, to cause a physical change in the corresponding area or the body.

Level of Evidence. Systematic reviews of RCTs concluded that the evidence to date does not demonstrate that reflexology is an effective treatment for any medical condition (Ernst, 2009a; Ernst, Posadzki, & Lee, 2011).

Contraindications. No contraindications have been reported.

Practitioners

- In the United Kingdom, reflexology is coordinated on a voluntary basis by the Complementary and Natural Healthcare Council (CNHC). Registrants are required to meet standards of proficiency outlined by profession-specific boards. CNHC registration is voluntary; therefore, anyone can describe him- or herself as a reflexologist.
- In Canada, reflexology is not regulated in any province, and the expenses incurred are not eligible as medical claims for income taxes. The Reflexology Association of Canada has reflexology therapists in all provinces, and British Columbia, Ontario, and Quebec have other associations (Natural Medicines, 2016).

Energy Therapies

Energy therapies involve the use of energy fields. There are two types of energy therapies. *Biofield therapies* are intended to affect energy fields that purportedly surround and penetrate the human body. The existence of such fields has not yet been scientifically proven. Examples of biofield therapies include qi gong, Reiki, and therapeutic touch. *Electromagnetic-based therapies* involve nontraditional use of electromagnetic fields, such as pulsed fields, magnetic fields, and alternating current or direct current fields. Examples include pulsed electromagnetic fields and magnet therapy.

Reiki

- Reiki an ancient form of healing that in Japanese means "universal life energy." The practitioner acts as a conduit for the movement of energy. It is the energy, not the healer, that influences healing. In this way, Reiki differs from other healing systems: Energy travels *through* the healer, not *from* the healer.

- Reiki is said to alleviate physical, emotional, and spiritual blockages. The practitioner gently places his or her hands on or over the client in a particular series of positions. About 5 minutes are spent on each of 12 positions although this may vary based on the needs of the client. The client is fully clothed at all times, and there is no direct pressure, massage, or manipulation applied to the client. The environment is kept quiet and soothing.

- The five premises of Reiki are as follows:
  - There is an energy of unique properties applicable to physical and psychological conditions.
  - The energy has a source.
  - This source can be tapped.
  - A person can be taught to use this energy.
  - The effects of this energy are palpable and subjective.

Level of Evidence
- More than 20 RCTs are reported in Medline for Reiki showing that it may be helpful in the treatment of pain, mood change, and fatigue. One study tested a standardized procedure for placebo Reiki in an effort to provide a foundation for subsequent randomized and placebo-controlled Reiki efficacy studies. An example of a clinical trial is the Reiki/Energy Healing in Prostate Cancer trial (NCT00065208) (ClinicalTrials.gov, 2012).

Contraindications. Contraindications for Reiki therapy are inability to let go of one's fear and need for control.

Practitioners. Typically, Reiki is taught in three parts:
- Reiki I includes history of Reiki, Reiki hand positions, Reiki symbols and their names, and meditation manifestation.
- Reiki II involves intense training focusing on advanced techniques and includes a review of Reiki I. The training for Reiki II brings knowledge of long-distance healing, scanning techniques, and the long-distance Reiki symbols and their names. Two Usui-REIKI-Tibetan attunements, named after the Japanese Buddhist Mikao Usui, are performed at intervals throughout the course. These are powerful spiritual

experiences during which the attunement energies are channeled into the student through the Reiki Master.
- Reiki III (Master) includes a review of previous training and practice and brings to the student knowledge for long-distance healing, scanning techniques, more meditation techniques, and an additional Reiki symbol. There is a Reiki attunement at the end of the course. There is no national curriculum or certifying body, although the Usui approach is the most prevalent. There are no states that license Reiki practitioners (Natural Medicines, 2016; NCCIH, 2015b).

Mind-Body Interventions

Mind-body interventions involve techniques designed to enhance the mind's capacity to affect body functions and symptoms. Examples include meditation, hypnosis, biofeedback, guided imagery, support groups, music therapy, cognitive-behavioral therapy, and aromatherapy

Mindfulness Meditation
- Mindfulness meditation, when it is practiced in Mindfulness-Based Stress Reduction (MBSR), is a self-regulatory approach to stress reduction and management of emotions. Mindfulness is a state in which an individual is highly aware and focused on the reality of the present moment, including acceptance and acknowledgment. Growing interest in the use of MBSR in cancer care reflects a desire for a more holistic approach to cancer treatment and acknowledges the links between social, psychological, and physiologic health determinants.
- MBSR programs are usually 6-8 weeks in length, involving daily individual activities and group activities up to several days per week. It is anticipated that individuals will continue to practice the activities for an extended period after completion of the structured program to receive the full benefit of the intervention.

Level of Evidence. Anxiety and emotional control improved in the treatment group as compared to the control group in an RCT assessing the effectiveness of an MBSR program in patients with heart disease. In two RCTs involving patients with cancer, MBSR was effective in decreasing mood disturbance and stress symptoms in both male and female patients (Branstrom, Kvillemo, Brandberg, & Moskowitz, 2010). Examples of clinical trials are listed in the table below.

Clinical Trials in Mindfulness-Based Stress Reduction

Branstrom et al. (2010) Phase II, N = 71	MC, wait-list control	Perceived stress and psychological well-being	Positive for stress, positive state of mind, avoidance (3 of 7 outcomes)
Foley et al. (2010) Phase II, N = 115	MC, wait-list control	Mindfulness, depression, anxiety, distress, QOL	Positive for depression, anxiety, distress, mindfulness (4 of 5 outcomes)
Lengacher et al. (2009) Phase II, N = 84	Breast cancer, wait-list control	Psychological status and psychological and physical subscales of QOL (23 outcomes)	Positive for 5 of 7 psychological measures, 3 of 10 QOL
Monti et al. (2006) Phase II, N = 111	MC, wait-list control	Distress, anxiety and depression, health-related QOL	Positive for psychological measures

MC, Multiple cancers; *QOL*, quality of life.
From Barton, D., & Pachman, D. R. (2012). Clinical trials in integrative therapies. *Seminars in Oncology Nursing, 28*(1), 19.

Contraindications. No contraindications have been reported.

Practitioners. Trained individuals may administer MBSR interventions either separately or in a group situation. It has been recommended that this therapy is best practiced by those licensed in counseling psychology or social work (Foley et al., 2010; Lengacher et al., 2009; Monti et al., 2006).

Aromatherapy

- Aromatherapy is the controlled use of plant essences for therapeutic purposes.
- *Essential oil* is the aromatic essence of a plant in the form of an oil or resin derived from the plant's leaf, stalk, bark, root, flower, fruit, or seed. The diluent, as the *carrier*, is used with a concentrated essential oil for application.
- Currently, there are about 150 recognized essential oils.
- The term *neat* refers to direct application of the essential oil compound (essential oil plus carrier) to the skin.
- The term *note* refers to the unique aromatic variable of an essential oil, which is important when blending combinations of essential oil compounds.
- Essential oils can be applied directly to the skin through a compressor massage, inhaled via a diffuser or steaming water, or added directly to bath water. The mechanism of action in the use of essential oils begins after the smell is sensed. The limbic system is activated in retrieving learned memories. Essential oils are also absorbed via the skin and subcutaneous fat into the bloodstream. Entry via the oral route into the digestive system is not recommended.
- Aromatherapy can be practiced with massage. Aromatherapy massage is used in palliative care settings to improve quality of life for patients with cancer.

Level of Evidence. Published data on dosing, comparative methods of administration, and therapeutic outcomes in the use of essential oils in aromatherapy are limited. Almost 40 RCTs were reported on Medline between 1998 and 2014 for the use of aromatherapy in various clinical settings, of which 4 involved patients with cancer. Six of these trials suggested that aromatherapy massage had a relaxing effect. One study measured the responses of 17 patients with cancer to humidified essential lavender oil, with a positive change noted in blood pressure, pulse, pain, anxiety, depression, and sense of well-being after both the humidified water treatment and lavender treatment. Another study compared drop size of six different essential oils; the bottles differed in their method of delivery, and the researchers recommended a universal standardization of measure to ensure equity and safety in administration.

Massage and aromatherapy massage seem to offer short-term benefits for psychological well-being, but there is limited evidence supporting the effect on anxiety. Mixed evidence exists as to whether aromatherapy enhances the effects of massage. Replication, longer follow-up, and larger trials are needed to accrue the necessary evidence (Fellowes, Barnes, & Wilkinson, 2004).

Contraindications

- Contraindications include allergy, pregnancy, contagious disease, epilepsy, venous thrombosis, varicose veins, open wounds on skin sites, and recent surgery of any type.
- Aromatherapy should not be administered orally and should not be applied to the skin before dilution.
- Possible adverse events associated with the use of essential oils include photosensitivity, allergic reactions, nausea, and headache. Many essential oils have the potential to either enhance or reduce the effects of prescribed medications, including antibiotics, tranquilizers, antihistamines, anticonvulsants, barbiturates, morphine, and quinidine. Cases of potentially serious reactions involving the use of essential oils have been reported in two individuals who were without known allergies or sensitivities before exposure (Fellowes, 2004; NCI, 2014).
- Special considerations
  - Check resources for safety precautions for each oil before use:
    - Oils should be diluted with a carrier oil such as grapeseed or apricot.
    - Check the FDA's Generally Regarded as Safe (GRAS) list.
    - Check for skin sensitivities and for oils that can increase skin sensitivity to sun exposure.
    - Check for oils that can be hepatotoxic and/or nephrotoxic with prolonged use.
    - Check for estrogenic effects that would make the oil contraindicated in patients with estrogen-sensitive tumors.
  - Some essential oils, such as oil of clove, may compete for receptor sites with chemotherapy drugs, so keep the oil dose low (1-2 drops/ounce of carrier oil) and do not use oils for 9 to 10 days before or after chemotherapy (Fellowes, 2004; NCI, 2014).

Practitioners

- Certification is available through the National Association for Holistic Aromatherapy (www.naha.org). Schools must provide practice in the fields of aromatherapy, essential oil studies, anatomy, and physiology. Holistic nursing certification is available through the American Holistic Nurses' Certification Corporation (www.ahncc.org). Requirements include a Bachelor of Science in Nursing (BSN) degree, continuing education, 1 year of practice, and a passing score on a written examination.
- Certification in aromatherapy or holistic nursing does not qualify a nurse to work independently, nor does it necessarily meet institutional requirements for practice.

Movement Therapies

Movement therapies are used to improve patterns of body movement. Examples include tai chi, hatha yoga, dance therapy, qi gong, Rolfing, and the Feldenkrais method. A few of the more common movement therapies are addressed here.

Qi Gong (Chi Kung)

- Qi gong means "energy cultivation" in Chinese, and the term refers to movements that are believed to improve health, longevity, and harmony within oneself and the world. Thousands of such movements exist, and qi gong may include any of these movements done with the intention of enhancing energy.
- Qi gong is a component of traditional Chinese medicine.
- It is based on four common principles, sometimes referred to as the "secrets" of qi gong:
  - Mind (the presence of intention)
  - Eyes (the focus of intention)
  - Movement (the action of intention)
  - Breath (the flow of intention)
- There are numerous styles of qi gong, which may include meditation, exercise, and self-massage.
- Mastery of qi gong is the achievement of a harmonious existence and action in all situations. Mastery does not exhibit as knowing everything but rather as a willingness to continue learning no matter what the level of achievement.
- Numerous books and teachers profess to teach the secrets of qi gong and the power of its applications, but authors agree that it is actually defined by a person's willingness to practice and experience it.

Level of Evidence

- Approximately 100 RCTs are reported in Medline of qi gong treatment for various conditions. Two trials involved patients with cancer and were aimed at training of inspiratory muscles and relief of breathlessness.

Contraindications. Psychosis has been reported, but it is not known whether there was a latent or undiagnosed psychiatric condition (Natural Medicines, 2016).

Practitioners. Because it is considered a form of Chinese medicine, patients should seek an acupuncturist and those appropriately credentialed in acupuncture and/or Oriental medicine (Natural Medicines, 2016).

Yoga

- Yoga is a mind and body practice with origins in ancient Indian philosophy.
- The various styles of yoga typically combine physical postures, breathing techniques, and meditation or relaxation. Hatha yoga is the most commonly practiced method in the United States and Europe. Other types of yoga include Iyengar, Ashtanga, Vini, Kundalini, and Bikram yoga.
- The 2007 National Health Interview Survey found that yoga is among the top 10 complementary and integrative health approaches used by U.S. adults. It has been used in the treatment of numerous medical conditions.

Levels of Evidence

- Studies suggest that yoga may be beneficial for a number of conditions, including pain and fatigue. Recent studies in people with chronic low-back pain suggest that a carefully adapted set of yoga poses can help reduce pain and improve function.
- Other studies suggest that practicing yoga may have other health benefits, such as reducing heart rate and blood pressure, and may also help relieve anxiety and depression.
- Iyengar yoga may help improve fatigue and vigor in breast cancer survivors, according to an NCCAM-funded study in 2011.

Contraindications

- Serious adverse events affecting the musculoskeletal, neurologic, and ocular systems have occurred in people using the "pranayam" or "Kapalabhati pranayama" technique.
- Yoga is contraindicated after abdominal surgery if the Valsalva maneuver is included.
- Research suggests that yoga is not helpful for asthma.
- Aggressive forms of yoga may raise blood pressure.
- Studies looking at yoga and arthritis have had mixed results.
- Those patients with hypertension, glaucoma, or sciatica and women who are pregnant should modify or avoid certain yoga poses (Natural Medicines, 2016).

Practitioners

- Certification is available through the Yoga Alliance (www.yogaalliance.org). There is no formal licensure process.
- Choice of instructor is important. The instructor must be able to adapt poses to individual needs (Natural Medicines, 2016).

Nutritional Therapeutics

Nutritional therapies include a variety of nutrients and non-nutrient bioactive food components used as chemopreventive agents, as well as specific foods or diets used as cancer prevention or treatment strategies. Examples include the macrobiotic diet, vegetarianism, Gerson therapy, the Gonzalez regimen, vitamins, soy phytoestrogens, antioxidants, selenium, and coenzyme Q10. Some of the most notable types are highlighted here.

Gonzalez Regimen

- This regimen was developed by Dr. Nicholas Gonzalez and is based on the theory that pancreatic enzymes help the body get rid of toxins that lead to cancer.
- It involves taking nutritional supplements and pancreatic enzymes thought to have anticancer activity, following prescribed diets, and taking coffee enemas.
- The Gonzalez regimen is purported to facilitate the body's getting rid of cancer-causing toxins from the environment and processed foods, balancing the part of the nervous system that controls automatic body functions, and maintaining a healthy immune system.
- Key components of the program include the following:
  - A special diet of mainly organic foods
  - Freeze-dried pancreatic enzyme capsules made from pigs and considered to be the main cancer fighter in the regimen

- Large numbers of nutritional supplements (130-160 per day) including magnesium citrate, papaya, vitamins, and other minerals
  - Coffee enemas twice daily
- The diets used in the Gonzalez regimen are planned for each patient's metabolic type. Metabolic typing is based on a theory that people fall into one of three groups based on the main type of food (protein, carbohydrate, or mixed) that their bodies need to maintain health.
- Side effects reported include gas, bloating and digestion problems, flu-like symptoms, low-grade fever, muscle aches, and skin rashes.
- No information is available regarding side effects of the coffee enemas.

Level of Evidence

- Animal studies of the Gonzalez regimen have examined the effect of pancreatic enzymes in cancer treatment but have not studied the regimen as a whole. Preclinical testing was conducted on the effects of pancreatic enzymes in several cancers. In 1999, an animal study tested the effect of various doses of pancreatic enzymes taken by mouth on the growth and metastasis of breast cancer in rats. Some of the rats received magnesium citrate in addition to the enzymes. Rats receiving the enzymes were compared with rats that did not receive the enzymes. Results showed that the enzyme did not affect the growth of the primary tumor; the rats that received the highest dose of enzymes had the greatest number of metastases; and the cancer spread to the fewest places in those rats that received the lowest dose of enzymes plus magnesium citrate.
- Another animal study looked at the effects of pancreatic enzymes on survival rates and tumor growth in rats with pancreatic cancer. Rats receiving the enzyme treatment were more active, lived longer, and had smaller tumors and fewer signs of disease than the control group rats that did not receive the enzyme.
- Nicholas Gonzalez first studied his regimen in 11 patients who had advanced pancreatic cancer. In 1993, he reported results of the study to the NCI: Patients treated with the Gonzalez regimen lived a median of 17 months, which is longer than usual for patients with this disease. Because of the small number of patients in the study, the NCI and NCCAM sponsored a second study with a much larger number of patients. This was a 7-year clinical study that included patients who had stage II, stage III, or stage IV nonoperable pancreatic cancer. One group of patients followed the Gonzalez regimen, while another group was given standard chemotherapy treatment. Patients treated with standard chemotherapy survived a median of 14 months, and patients treated with the Gonzalez regimen survived a median of 4.3 months. Patients treated with chemotherapy reported a better quality of life than those treated with the Gonzalez regimen. Dr. Gonzalez published comments on his website to express concerns about how the trial was conducted. One concern was how well patients in the Gonzalez

regimen group actually followed the regimen. The FDA has not approved the Gonzalez regimen or any of its components (NCI, 2015b).

Antioxidants

Antioxidant vitamins—vitamin C, vitamin E, and beta carotene—are believed to have health-promoting properties. Coenzyme Q 10 ubiquinone (CoQ10) is found in all living cells; it is involved in the production of energy within cells and is believed to have powerful antioxidant effects. It is estimated that 30% of Americans are taking some form of antioxidant supplement. Patients with cancer take antioxidants, typically at doses higher than the recommended daily allowances (RDAs). Antioxidants act by scavenging free radicals. The debate that surrounds antioxidants has focused on cancer therapies such as alkylating agents, antimetabolites, taxanes, and radiation therapy because of their purposeful creation of free radicals through cytotoxic mechanisms.

Level of Evidence

- The belief that antioxidants may interfere with the efficacy of cancer therapy is not new. Limited research supports the belief that chemotherapy diminishes total antioxidant status, but inconsistencies based on cancer site, cancer therapy, research methodologies, patient populations, variability in doses, duration of supplementation, and timing of interventions have prevented the formulation of conclusions or consensus (Harvie, 2014; Ladas, Jacobson, & Kennedy, 2004).
- More than 2000 RCTs involving antioxidants have been reported. The association between beta-carotene and increased risk of lung cancer in smokers is well known (Branstrom et al., 2010; Medline Plus, 2016). However, selective inhibition of tumor cell growth is an action of antioxidants, and it is suggested that antioxidants may promote cellular differentiation with enhanced cytotoxic effects. Researchers have been concerned that although antioxidants may decrease some kinds of toxicity associated with cancer chemotherapy, the therapeutic benefit of the cancer therapy may be compromised (Harvie, 2014).
- Antioxidants may have a role in primary and secondary cancer prevention. Early studies suggest that high vitamin C intake prior to a diagnosis of breast cancer may positively affect survival (Dixon, 2012; Greenlee, 2012; Harris, Orsini, & Wolk, 2014).
- Another study found that supplementation with vitamin E and vitamin B complex may provide protection against breast cancer among women with a low dietary intake of these vitamins (Dorjgochoo et al., 2008). A metaanalysis assessing the role of vitamin C among women with breast cancer suggested that supplementation with vitamin C after diagnosis may be associated with a lower risk of mortality (Harris et al., 2014).
- Selenium and vitamin E supplements were thought to reduce the risk of prostate cancer. Results of the Selenium and Vitamin E Clinical Trial (SELECT) in 2008 showed that selenium and vitamin E, taken alone or together for

an average of 5½ years, did not prevent prostate cancer, and trial participants were directed to discontinue trial supplements due to lack of benefit. In 2011, the data were updated and revealed that men taking vitamin E had a 17% increased risk for prostate cancer, compared with men taking placebo. A further analysis published in 2014 indicated that men who began the trial with high levels of selenium doubled their risk for developing high-grade prostate cancer by taking selenium supplements, and men who had low levels of selenium at the start of the trial doubled their risk of high-grade prostate cancer by taking vitamin E. Variability in doses, duration of supplementation, and timing of interventions have prevented the formulation of conclusions and specific recommendations except in clinical trials (NCI, 2015d).

Contraindications
- Contraindications do exist for specific antioxidants:
  - *Beta carotene* increases the risks of lung cancer and stomach cancer (Albanes et al., 1995; Medline Plus, 2016).
  - *Vitamin E* increases the risks of prostate cancer and colorectal adenoma (NCI, 2015d).
- Potential interactions (Harvie, 2014; Hendler & Rorvik, 2008; FDA, 2016):
  - *Vitamin C*: aluminum antacids, cyclosporine, statins, calcium channel blockers, protease inhibitors, iron, vitamin E
  - *Vitamin E*: cholestyramine, colestipol, mineral oil, anticonvulsants, anticoagulants, verapamil
  - *Beta carotene*: cholestyramine, colestipol, mineral oil, orlistat

Practitioners
- Registered dieticians have a minimum of a bachelor's degree in dietetics.
- Certified nutritional consultants have education and training in clinical nutrition and may be nurses or other health care professionals.
- Caution should be used when choosing a nutrition practitioner to be certain that he or she has expertise in cancer care as well as in supplements and nutrition (Dixon, 2012).

Pharmacologic and Biologic Therapies

The pharmacologic and biologic group of therapies includes drugs, vaccines, off-label use of prescription drugs, and other biologic interventions not yet accepted in conventional medicine. Some of the most common types are highlighted here.

Laetril
- Laetril is also known as amygdalin, apricot almonds, apricot kernel oil, apricot seed, laetrile, prunus kernel, vitamin B_{17}, and other names.
- It is taken orally or intravenously as a treatment for cancer.

Level of Evidence
- Laetril is considered to be unsafe when taken either orally or intravenously.

- Apricot kernel is a source of cyanide. Orally, apricot kernel can cause acute poisoning, with symptoms including dizziness, headache, nausea, vomiting, drowsiness, dyspnea, palpitations, marked hypotension, convulsions, paralysis, coma, and death within 15 minutes. The lethal dose is 50 to 60 kernels, but the amount may vary. It can also cause chronic poisoning, with symptoms of increased blood thiocyanate, goiter, thyroid cancer, optic nerve lesions, blindness, ataxia, hypertonia, cretinism, and mental retardation.
- Demyelinating lesions and neuromyopathies reportedly have occurred secondary to chronic exposure, including long-term therapy.

Practitioners. In 2000, the FDA sought permanent injunctions against three corporations for unlawfully promoting and marketing laetril and apricot seeds or kernels for treatment of cancer on their Internet websites: Without Cancer, Inc., located in Florida; Health World International, Inc., located in Florida; and Health Genesis Corporation, located in Arizona (NCI, 2015c).

714-X
- The main ingredient of 714-X is camphor, which is derived from the wood and bark of the camphor tree. Nitrogen, water, and salts are added to the camphor. It is believed that 714-X helps the immune system fight cancer. No study of 714-X has been published in a peer-reviewed scientific journal that demonstrates safe and/or effectiveness in treating cancer.
- 714-X was developed in the 1960s in Canada, where it is still being manufactured. The development of 714-X was based on the theory that there are tiny living things in the blood called *somatids*. Some types of somatids are found only in the blood of people who have cancer or other serious diseases. These types of somatids are said to make growth hormones that initiate uncontrolled cell growth. The makers of 714-X state that by looking at the numbers and types of somatids in the blood, doctors can see if cancer is starting to form or can diagnose cancer and predict where it will spread. The theory states that cancer cells trap nitrogen needed by normal cells and make a toxic substance that weakens the immune system.
- 714-X is reported to help the body fight cancer by preventing cancer cells from taking nitrogen from the body's normal cells. It is also said to help the immune system by increasing the flow of lymphatic fluid through the body carrying white blood cells that help fight infection and disease.
- 714-X is usually given by injection near the lymph nodes in the groin but can be sprayed into the nose using a nebulizer in specific cases.
- 714-X should not be injected into a vein (intravenously) or taken by mouth.
- 714-X can be used along with conventional treatments.
- Vitamin B_{12} supplements, vitamin E supplements, shark cartilage, and alcohol should not be used during treatment with 714-X.

Practitioners

- Patients in Canada can get 714-X only from a doctor, for compassionate use.
- It is used in Mexico and some western European countries.
- The FDA has not approved 714-X for use in the United States (NCI, 2015a).

Complex Natural Products

Complex natural products are a subcategory of pharmacologic and biologic therapies and include many botanicals and extracts of natural substances including marine organisms. The table below provides information on a number of herbs and herbal extracts in this category.

- Herbal products are rated by the American Herbal Products Association in their *Botanical Safety Handbook* (AHPA, 2013).
  - Class 1 herbs can be consumed safely when used appropriately.

- Class 2 herbs have some restrictions, unless otherwise directed by a qualified expert:
  - Class 2a herbs are for external use only.
  - Class 2b herbs are not to be used during pregnancy.
  - Class 2c herbs are not to be used by lactating women.
  - Class 2d herbs may have other restrictions.
- Class 3 herbs are those for which significant data exist to recommend the following labeling: "to be used only under the supervision of an expert qualified in the appropriate use of this substance." Labeling must include the following:
  - Dosage
  - Contraindications
  - Potential adverse events and drug interactions
  - Any other relevant information related to the safe use of the substance
- Class 4 herbs are those for which insufficient data are available for classification.

Examples of Commonly Used Herbs

Herb and AHPA Class*	Purported Properties/Actions	Availability	Potential Side Effects	Precautions/Contraindications
Aloe (*Aloe vera*) Class 2b	Antiseptic Laxative Antiinflammatory Antiviral Wound healing	Capsules, extract, powder, cream, gel, shampoo, conditioner	May increase risk of hypoglycemia if given concurrently with diabetic agents Risk of hypokalemia if taken concurrently with licorice *May alter serum potassium (laxative properties) May decrease serum glucose level*	Inflammatory bowel disease, fecal impaction, appendicitis, abdominal pain of unknown origin Any spasmodic gastrointestinal compliant, arrhythmia, neuropathy, edema Bone deterioration with long-term use Concurrent use with digoxin can cause digoxin toxicity
Bilberry (*Vaccinium myrtillus*) Class 4	Astringent Tonic Antioxidant Antiseptic Wound healing Antiulcer Vasoprotective	Capsules, fluid extract, fresh berries, dried berries, liquid, tincture, dried root, dried leaves	May cause bleeding, heartburn, hypoglycemia, hypertension *May decrease serum glucose level*	Increased risk of bleeding in individuals who are taking anticoagulants, antiplatelet agents, thrombolytic agents, or low-molecular-weight heparins
Chamomile (*Matricaria recutita*) Class 1	Anxiolytic Mild hypnotic Hypoglycemic effect Estrogen-dependent and estrogen-independent effects Antispasmodic Antimicrobial	Capsules, cream, fluid extract, lotion, shampoo, conditioner, tea, tincture, cosmetic	Topical use: burning of the face, eyes, and mucous membranes Systemic use: hypersensitivity and contact dermatitis, bruising, confusion, drowsiness, anaphylaxis	Increased risk of bleeding with concurrent use of aspirin, antiplatelet agents, heparin, NSAIDs, warfarin, thrombin inhibitors, thrombolytics, darunavir Caution when used concurrently with acetaminophen combination products Increased risk of sedation with benzodiazepines, dextromethorphan and pseudoephedrine combination products, cannabinoids, ethanol, gotu cola, kava, muscle relaxants, all SSRIs, all sedatives, and all hypnotics Increased risk of bleeding and sedation with concurrent use of capsaicin, dong quai, primrose oil, fenugreek, feverfew, fish oil, garlic, ginger, ginkgo, ginseng, feverfew, horse chestnut, licorice, SJW
Cinnamon (*Cinnamomum cassia*) Class 2b	Antifungal Analgesic Antiseptic Antidiarrheal Antiviral Antidiabetic (insulin potentiator) Also used for hypertension, loss of appetite, and bronchitis	Dried bark, essential oil, leaves, fluid extract, powder, tincture	Flushing, tachycardia, stomatitis, glossitis, gingivitis Increased gastrointestinal mobility, anorexia, Allergic dermatitis Shortness of breath Hypersensitivity	Avoid prolonged use in patients with intestinal or gastric ulcers

Examples of Commonly Used Herbs—cont'd

Herb and AHPA Class*	Purported Properties/Actions	Availability	Potential Side Effects	Precautions/Contraindications
Dong Quai or Chinese Angelica (*Angelica sinensis*) Class 2b	Menstrual irregularities and menopausal symptoms Headache Neuralgia Herpes infections Malaria	Capsules, fluid extract, powder, tablets, tea, tincture Primarily a combination product	Nausea, vomiting, diarrhea, anorexia Increased menstrual flow Hypersensitivity reactions Photosensitivity Fever, sweating Bleeding *May alter APTT, PT, INR*	Increases effects of anticoagulants, antiplatelets, estrogens, hormonal contraceptives Increases risk of bleeding when taken concurrently with chamomile, dandelion, horse chestnut, red clover, SJW Photosensitivity when taken concurrently with SJW Alters PT and INR Increases CNS depression and muscle relaxation with concurrent use of benzodiazepines Hypoglycemia with concurrent use of tolbutamide
Garlic (*Allium sativum*) Class 2b	Antimicrobial Antilipidemic Antitriglyceride Antiplatelet Antioxidant	Capsules, extract, fresh garlic, oil, powder, syrup, tablets, tea	Halitosis Alters coagulation Alters serum glucose Kyolic garlic has less impact on serum glucose Enteric-coated product lessens halitosis May decrease LDL, triglycerides, serum lipid profile *May increase PT, INR, and serum IgE*	Avoid with dacarbazine (CYP 2E1 inhibition) Avoid before and after surgery (alters coagulation) Caution with other chemotherapy (data inconclusive)
Ginkgo (*Ginkgo biloba*) Class 1	Cognitive enhancement Peripheral vascular insufficiency Antioxidant Enhances circulation throughout the body Antiarthritic and analgesic	Capsules, fluid extract, tablets, tinctures	Allergic reactions Alters coagulation Anxiety/restlessness Bleeding Gastrointestinal disturbances Insomnia Skin reactions Transient headache *May increase C-peptide concentrations, plasma insulin levels*	Caution with camptothecin, cyclophosphamide, EGFR-TK inhibitors, epiphodophyllotoxins, taxanes, vinca alkaloids (CYP 3A4 and CYP 2C19 inhibition) Discourage use with alkalating agents, antitumor antibiotics, and platinum analogs (free radical scavenging) *Subarachnoid hemorrhage without trauma has been associated with ginkgo* *One case was reported of acute CNS depression in a woman taking trazadone*
Grapeseed Extract (pycnogel) Class 4	Antioxidant Enhances circulation throughout the body Decreases visual stress	Capsules, tablets, drops, liquid concentrate, cream	Dizziness Nausea, anorexia Rash *Theoretically: hepatotoxicity*	Potential interactions with anticoagulant and antiplatelets (increases risk of bleeding) Caution with camptothecin, cyclophosphamide, EGFR-TK inhibitors, epiphodophyllotoxins, vinca alkaloids (CYP 3A4 inhibition) Discourage use with alkylating agents, antitumor antibiotics, and platinum analogs (free radical scavenging)
Kava (*Piper methysticum*) Class 2b, 2c, 2d	Antiinflammatory	Capsules, beverage, extract, tablets, tincture	Hyperreflexivity Drowsiness Blurred vision Nausea, vomiting, anorexia, weight loss Potential decrease in platelets, lymphocytes, bilirubin, protein, and albumin Increase in red blood cell volume Hypersensitivity reactions Shortness of breath (pulmonary hypertension) *Potential hepatotoxicity* *May increase hepatic function tests: AST, ALT, LDH* *Chronic use is associated with decreased lymphocyte count, decreases platelet size, hematuria* *May decrease albumin, bilirubin, total protein*	Avoid with antiparkinson drugs (increases the symptoms of Parkinson disease) Avoid with antipsychotic medications (may cause neuroleptic movement disorders) Avoid with barbiturates (increases sedation) Avoid with benzodiazepines (increases risk of sedation and/or coma) Avoid with CNS depressants (increased sedation) Avoid with CYP 1A2, 2C9, 2C19, 2D6, 3A4 substrates (significantly decreases these substrates) Oncology-specific guidelines: avoid in all patients with existing liver disease, evidence of hepatic damage, or herb-induced hepatotoxicity and in combination with hepatotoxic chemotherapy

Continued

Examples of Commonly Used Herbs—cont'd

Herb and AHPA Class*	Purported Properties/Actions	Availability	Potential Side Effects	Precautions/Contraindications
Milk Thistle (*Silybum marianum*) Class 1	Hallucinogenic Hepatoprotective Cirrhosis of the liver caused by alcohol or virus Antiinflammatory Antioxidant Nephroprotective	Tincture, capsules	Headache Nausea, vomiting, diarrhea, anorexia, abdominal bloating, and abdominal pain Menstrual changes Hypersensitivity reactions Erectile dysfunction Pruritus Joint pain *May decrease AST, ALT, alkaline phosphatase, and serum glucose levels*	Avoid with warfarin Avoid with combination products involving acetaminophen, dextromethorphan, pseudoephedrine, or estrogen/progestin May decrease levels of irinotecan, lorazepam, lovastatin, morphine, meprobamate
Purple Coneflower (*Echinacea purpura*) Class 1	Antiviral Immunostimulant Vulvovaginal candidiasis Psoriasis Allergic rhinitis	Capsules, fluid extract, juice, dried powered extract, sublingual tablets, tea, tincture	Hepatotoxicity Acute asthma attack Anaphylaxis, angioedema *May increase ALT, AST, lymphocyte counts, serum IgE, ESR*	Do not use in children <2 yr of age Avoid use in CYP 3A4 substrates such as immune-modulators (cyclosporine, protease inhibitors, corticosteroids, methotrexate) Alters ALT, AST, lymphocytes, IgG, sedimentation rates, and ESR
Valerian (*Valeriana officinalis*) Class 1	Antianxiety Anti-insomnia	Capsules, brewed herb, extract, tablets, tea, tincture, and in combination products with other herbs	Insomnia Headaches Restlessness Nausea, vomiting, anorexia Hepatotoxicity Hypersensitivity reactions Vision changes Palpitations *May increase ALT, AST, GGT, total bilirubin, alkaline phosphatase, urine bilirubin*	Increases CNS depression (alcohol, barbiturates, benzodiazepines, opiate, sedatives/hypnotics) Negates therapeutic effects of MAOs, phenytoin, warfarin Avoid in patients with preexisting liver disease Caution with tamoxifen (CYP 2C9 inhibition) Caution with cyclophosphamide, teniposide (CYP 2C19)

*Classification is for the general population; not cancer specific.

From Decker, G., & Lee, C. O. (2010). *Handbook of integrative oncology nursing: Evidence-based practice* (pp. 52-58). Pittsburgh, PA: Oncology Nursing Society Press.
AHPA, American Herbal Products Association; *ALT*, alanine aminotransferase; *APTT*, activated partial thromboplastin time; *AST*, aspartate transaminase; *CNS*, central nervous system; *CYP*, cytochrome P450 isoenzyme; *EGFR-TK*, epidermal growth factor receptor tyrosine kinase; *ESR*, erythrocyte sedimentation rate; *GGT*, gamma-glutamyl transpeptidase; *IgE*, immunoglobulin E; *IgG*, immunoglobulin G; *INR*, International Normalized Ratio; *LDH*, lactate dehydrogenase; *LDL*, low-density lipoprotein; *MAOs*, monoamine oxidase inhibitors; *NSAIDs*, nonsteroidal antiinflammatory drugs; *PT*, prothrobin time; *SJW*, St. John's wort; *SSRIs*, selective serotonin reuptake inhibitors.

Conclusion

CAM therapies are now commonplace in oncology practice. Nurses should understand the basic foundations of CAM therapies in order to provide patient education and safely incorporate these therapies into daily practice.

References

Albanes, D., Heinonen, O. P., Huttunen, J. K., Taylor, P. R., Virtamo, J., Edwards, B. K., & National Cancer Institute. (1995). Effects of alpha-tocopherol and beta-carotene supplements on cancer incidence in the Alpha-Tocopherol Beta-Carotene Cancer Prevention Study. *American Journal of Clinical Nutrition, 62*(6 Suppl), 1427S–1430S.

American Herbal Products Association. (2013). *Botanical safety handbook* (2nd ed.). Available at http://abc.herbalgram.org/site/DocServer/AHPABotanicalSafety_FMexcerpt.pdf?docID=4601 (accessed February 12, 2016).

Bao, T. (2009). Use of acupuncture in the control of chemotherapy induced nausea and vomiting. *Journal of the National Comprehensive Cancer Network, 7*(5), 606–612. Available at http://www.jnccn.org/content/7/5/606.abstract (accessed February 12, 2016).

Barton, D. L., & Pachman, D. R. (2012). Clinical trials in integrative therapies. *Seminars in Oncology Nursing, 28*(1), 10–28.

Basch, E., & Ulbricht, C. (2004). Prevalence of CAM use among U.S. cancer patients: An update. *Cancer Integrative Medicine, 2*, 13–14.

Bauer-Wu, S., & Decker, G. M. (2012). Integrative oncology imperative for nurses. *Seminars in Oncology Nursing, 28*(1), 2–9.

Blaes, A. H., Kreitzer, M. J., Torkelson, C., & Haddad, T. (2011). Nonpharmacologic complementary therapies in symptom management for breast cancer survivors. *Seminars in Oncology, 4*, 274–286.

Branstrom, R., Kvillemo, P., Brandberg, Y., & Moskowitz, J. T. (2010). Self-report mindfulness as a mediator of psychological well-being in a stress reduction intervention for cancer patients: A randomized study. *Annals of Behavioral Medicine, 39*(2), 151–161.

Brauer, J. A., El Sehamy, A., Metz, J. M., & Mao, J. J. (2010). Complementary and alternative medicine and supportive care at leading cancer centers: A systematic analysis of websites. *Journal of Alternative and Complementary Medicine, 16*(2), 183–186.

Centre for Evidence-Based Medicine, University of Oxford. (2009). *Levels of evidence*. Available at http://www.cebm.net/oxford-centre-evidence-based-medicine-levels-evidence-march-2009/ (accessed February 12, 2016).

ClinicalTrials.gov. (2012). *Reiki/energy healing in prostate cancer*. Available at https://www.clinicaltrials.gov/ct2/show/NCT00065208 (accessed February 12, 2016).

Collinge, W., MacDonald, G., & Walton, T. (2012). Massage in supportive cancer care. *Seminars in Oncology Nursing, 28*(1), 45–54.

Corbin, L. (2005). Safety and efficacy of massage therapy for patients with cancer. *Cancer Control, 12*, 158–164.

Davis, E. L., Oh, B., Butow, P. N., Mullen, B. A., & Clarke, S. (2012). Cancer patient disclosure and patient-doctor communication of complementary alternative medicine use: A systematic review. *The Oncologist, 17*, 1475–1481.

Deng, G., & Cassileth, B. R. (2005). Integrative oncology: Complementary therapies for pain, anxiety and mood disturbances. *CA: A Cancer Journal for Clinicians, 55*, 109–116.

Deng, G. E., Frenkel, M., Cohen, L., Cassileth, B. R., Abrams, D. I., Capodice, J. L., & Sagar, S. (2009). Evidence-based clinical practice guidelines for integrative oncology: Complementary therapies and botanicals. *Journal of the Society for Integrative Oncology*, 7(3), 85–120.

Dixon, S. (2012). Nutrition in complementary and alternative medicine. *Seminars in Oncology Nursing*, 28(1), 75–84.

Dorjgochoo, T., Shrubsole, M. J., Shu, X. O., Lu, W., Ruan, Z., Zheng, Y., & Zheng, W. (2008). Vitamin supplement use and risk for breast cancer: the Shanghai Breast Cancer Study. *Breast Cancer Res Treat*, 111(2), 269–278. http://dx.doi.org/10.1007/s10549-007-9772-8.

Eisenberg, D. M., Kessler, R. C., Foster, C., Norlock, F. E., Calkins, D. R., & Delbanco, T. L. (1993). Unconventional medicine in the United States: Prevalence, costs, and patterns of use. *New England Journal of Medicine*, 328(4), 246–252.

Ernst, E. (2009a). Is reflexology an effective intervention? A systematic review of randomized controlled trials. *Medical Journal of Australia*, 191(5), 263–266.

Ernst, E. (2009b). Massage therapy for cancer palliation and supportive care: A systematic review of randomized clinical trials. *Supportive Care in Cancer*, 17(4), 333–337.

Ernst, E., Posadzki, P., & Lee, M. S. (2011). Reflexology: An update of a systematic review of randomised clinical trials. *Maturitas*, 68(2), 116–120.

Fellowes, D., Barnes, K., & Wilkinson, S. (2004). Aromatherapy and massage for symptom relief in patients with cancer. *Cochrane Database of Systematic Reviews* (2), CD002287.

Foley, E., Baillie, A., Huxter, M., Price, M., & Sinclair, E. (2010). Mindfulness-based cognitive therapy for individuals whose lives have been affected by cancer: A randomized controlled trial. *Journal of Consulting and Clinical Psychology*, 78(1), 72–79.

Fonteyn, M., & Bauer-Wu, S. (2005). Using qualitative evaluation in a feasibility study to improve and refine a complementary therapy intervention prior to subsequent research. *Complementary Therapies in Clinical Practice*, 11, 247–252.

Food and Drug Administration. (1906). *Federal Food and Drugs Act of 1906.* Available at http://prescriptiondrugs.procon.org/sourcefiles/FEDERAL_FOOD_AND_DRUGS_ACT_1906.pdf (accessed February 12, 2016).

Food and Drug Administration. (2016). *Dietary supplements.* Available at http://www.fda.gov/Food/DietarySupplements/ (accessed February 12, 2016).

Greenlee, H. (2012). Natural products for cancer prevention. *Seminars in Oncology Nursing*, 28(1), 29–44.

Harris, H. R., Orsini, N., & Wolk, A. (2014). Vitamin C and survival among women with breast cancer: A meta-analysis. *European Journal of Cancer*, 50(7), 1223–1231.

Harvie, M. (2014). Nutritional supplements and cancer: Potential benefits and proven harms. *American Society of Clinical Oncology Educational Book*, 2014, e478–3486.

Hendler, S. S., & Rorvik, D. M. (2008). *PDR for nutritional supplements* (2nd ed.). Montvale, NJ: Thomson Reuters.

Institute of Medicine (U.S.) & Committee on the Use of Complementary and Alternative Medicine by the American Public. (2005). *Complementary and alternative medicine in the United States.* Washington, DC: National Academies Press.

Ladas, E. J., Jacobson, J. S., & Kennedy, D. D. (2004). Antioxidants and cancer therapy. *Journal of Clinical Oncology*, 22, 517–528.

Lengacher, C. A., Johnson-Mallard, V., Post-White, J., Moscoso, M. S., Jacobsen, P. B., Klein, T. W., & Kip, K. E. (2009). Randomized controlled trial of mindfulness-based stress reduction (MBSR) for survivors of breast cancer. *Psycho-oncology*, 18(12), 1261–1272.

Ma, L. (2009). Acupuncture as a complementary therapy in chemotherapy-induced nausea and vomiting. *Baylor University Medical Center Proceedings (BUMC Proceedings)*, 22(2), 138–141. Available at http://www.baylorhealth.edu/Documents/BUMC%20Proceedings/2009%20Vol%2022/No.%202/22_2_ma.pdf (accessed February 12, 2016).

MacDonald, G. (2011). The progression of oncology massage: Difficult lessons learned. *Massage and Bodywork*, 26, 32–39.

Mao, J. J., Palmer, C. S., Healy, K. E., Desai, K., & Amsterdam, J. (2011). Complementary and alternative medicine use among cancer survivors: A population-based study. *Journal of Cancer Survivorship*, 5(1), 8–17.

Meadows, M. (2006). *Promoting safe and effective drugs for 100 years.* Available at http://www.fda.gov/AboutFDA/WhatWeDo/History/CentennialofFDA/CentennialEditionofFDAConsumer/ucm093787.htm (accessed February 12, 2016).

Medline Plus. (2016). *Beta-carotene.* Available at https://www.nlm.nih.gov/medlineplus/druginfo/natural/999.html (accessed February 12, 2016).

Monti, D. A., Peterson, C., Kunkel, E. J., Hauck, W. W., Pequignot, E., Rhodes, L., & Brainard, G. C. (2006). A randomized, controlled trial of mindfulness-based art therapy (MBAT) for women with cancer. *Psycho-oncology*, 15(5), 363–373.

Myers, C., Walton, T., Bratsman, L., et al. (2008). Massage modalities and symptoms reported by cancer patients: narrative review. *J Soc Integr Oncol*, 6, 19–28.

Myers, C., Walton, T., & Small, B. (2008). The value of massage therapy in cancer care. *Hematol Oncol Clin North Am*, 22: 649–660.

Nahin, R. L., Barnes, P. M., Stussman, B. J., & Bloom, B. (2009). *Costs of complementary and alternative medicine (CAM) and frequency of visits to CAM practitioners: United States, 2007. National Health Statistics Reports no. 18.* Available at http://www.cdc.gov/NCHS/data/nhsr/nhsr018.pdf (accessed February 12, 2016).

National Cancer Institute. (2012). *About CAM.* Available at http://cam.cancer.gov/health_aboutcam.html (accessed February 12, 2016).

National Cancer Institute. (2014). *Aromatherapy and essential oils (PDQ).* Available at http://www.cancer.gov/about-cancer/treatment/cam/patient/aromatherapy-pdq (accessed February 12, 2016).

National Cancer Institute. (2015a). *714-X (PDQ) overview.* Available at http://www.cancer.gov/about-cancer/treatment/cam/patient/714-x-pdq (accessed February 12, 2016).

National Cancer Institute. (2015b). *Gonzalez regimen (PDQ) overview.* Available at http://www.cancer.gov/about-cancer/treatment/cam/patient/gonzalez-pdq (accessed February 12, 2016).

National Cancer Institute. (2015c). *Laetrile/Amygdalin (PDQ).* Available at http://www.cancer.gov/about-cancer/treatment/cam/patient/laetrile-pdq (accessed February 12, 2016).

National Cancer Institute. (2015d). *Selenium and Vitamin E Cancer Prevention Trial (SELECT): Questions and Answers.* Available at http://www.cancer.gov/types/prostate/research/select-trial-results-qa (accessed February 12, 2016).

National Cancer Institute. (2015e). *Using trusted resources.* Available at http://www.cancer.gov/about-cancer/managing-care/using-trusted-resources (accessed February 12, 2016).

National Center for Complementary and Integrative Health. (2014). *NIH complementary and integrative health agency gets new name.* Available at https://nccih.nih.gov/news/press/12172014 (accessed February 12, 2016).

National Center for Complementary and Integrative Health. (2015). *Complementary, alternative or integrative health: What's in a name?* Available at https://nccih.nih.gov/health/whatiscam (accessed February 12, 2016).

National Center for Complementary and Integrative Health. (2015b). *Reiki information.* Available at https://nccih.nih.gov/health/reiki (accessed February 12, 2016).

National Institutes of Health. (2015). *The NIH almanac: National Center for Complementary and Integrative Health (NCCIH).* Available at http://www.nih.gov/about-nih/what-we-do/nih-almanac/national-center-complementary-integrative-health-nccih (accessed February 12, 2016).

National Library of Medicine. (2015). *Levels of evidence for human studies of cancer complementary and alternative medicine (PDQ).* Available at http://www.ncbi.nlm.nih.gov/pubmedhealth/PMH0032708/ (accessed February 12, 2016).

Natural Medicines. (2016). Available at https://naturalmedicines.therapeuticresearch.com/search.aspx?q=levels+of+evidence&go.x=0&go.y=0 (accessed February 12, 2016).

OCEBM Levels of Evidence Working Group. (2011). *The Oxford Centre for Evidence-Based Medicine (OCEBM) levels of evidence 2.* Available at http://www.cebm.net/ocebm-levels-of-evidence/ (accessed February 12, 2016).

Office of Dietary Supplements. (1994). *Dietary Supplement Health and Education Act of 1994.* Available at https://ods.od.nih.gov/About/DSHEA_Wording.aspx#sec4 (accessed February 12, 2016).

Oncology Nursing Society. (2014). *Putting Evidence into Practice (PEP) rating system overview.* Available at https://www.ons.org/practice-resources/pep (accessed February 12, 2016).

Painter, F. M. (2001). *David Eisenberg, M.D., speaks to WHCCAMP on May 15, 2001.* Available at http://www.chiro.org/alt_med_abstracts/CAM/Eisenberg.shtml (accessed February 12, 2016).

Rausch, S. M., Winegardner, F., Kuruk, K. M., Phatak, V., Wahner-Roedler, D. L., Bauer, B., & Vincent, A. (2011). Complementary and alternative medicine: Use and disclosure in radiation oncology community practice. *Supportive Care in Cancer*, 19, 521–529.

Vallerand, A. H., Fouladbakhsh, J. M., & Templin, T. (2003). The use of complementary/alternative medicine for pain among residents of urban, suburban and rural communities. *American Journal of Public Health*, 93, 923–925.

van Tonder, E., Herselman, M. G., & Visser, J. (2009). The prevalence of dietary-related complementary and alternative therapies and their perceived usefulness among cancer patients. *Journal of Human Nutrition and Dietetics, 22*, 528–535.

Walton, T. (2011). *Medical conditions and massage therapy: A decision tree approach.* Philadelphia, PA: Lippincott Williams & Wilkins.

Weiger, W. A., Smith, M., Boon, H., Richardson, M. A., Kaptchuk, T. J., & Eisenberg, D. M. (2002). Advising patients who seek complementary and alternative medical therapies for cancer. *Annals of Internal Medicine, 137*(11), 889–903.

White House Commission on Complementary and Alternative Medicine Policy. (2002). *Final report.* Available at http://www.whccamp.hhs.gov/ (accessed February 12, 2016).

Whorton, J. C. (1999). The history of complementary and alternative medicine. In W. B. Jonas & J. S. Levin (Eds.), *Essentials of complementary and alternative medicine* (pp. 16–30). Philadelphia, PA: Lippincott Williams & Wilkins.

Clinical Trials

Marlon Garzo Saria

Introduction

"Today's standard cancer treatments were yesterday's clinical trials" (National Cancer Institute [NCI], 2002). Cancer research has significantly expanded understanding of the biologic mechanisms that contribute to cancer development, progression, and metastasis. Although success at the bench in preclinical studies does not always translate to success at the bedside, lessons learned from previous translational experiments provide insight for designing better translational studies that yield clinically relevant data (Lieu, Tan, Leong, Diamond, & Eckhardt, 2013). Clinical trials make up the significant final steps in an arduous research process that translates basic research findings into clinical interventions for cancer risk reduction, detection, and treatment, allowing many individuals to survive diseases that in the past were almost universally fatal.

The contribution of clinical trials to modern medicine can readily be seen in the advances made in the treatment of pediatric cancers. Only 3% of adults with cancer participate in clinical trials; in contrast, more than 60% of children with cancer participate in clinical trials. The higher rate of participation has resulted in improved outcomes, with a 15% increase in the 5-year survival rate for children with cancer—70%, compared with only 55% four decades ago (NCI, 2002).

Drug Development Process

It takes about 10 to 15 years at a cost of $800 million to $1 billion to develop a new drug. Development begins with the discovery of a potentially effective agent and includes a series of steps that takes 3 to 6 years.
- Prediscovery: understanding the disease
- Target identification: choosing a molecule to target with a drug
- Target validation: testing the target and confirming its role in the disease
- Drug discovery: finding a promising molecule that could become a drug
- Early safety tests: performing initial tests on promising compounds
- Lead optimization: altering the molecule to improve drug properties
- Preclinical testing: laboratory and animal testing to determine whether the drug is safe enough for human testing

Candidate drugs are extensively studied in humans before they are approved by the U.S. Food and Drug Administration (FDA). This process involves a series of steps designed with specific goals and requirements, taking an average of 6 to 7 years to complete.

Types of Clinical Trials

Several types of cancer clinical trials exist; each is designed to answer different research questions (NCI, 2002, 2012).
- *Prevention trials:* Involve otherwise healthy individuals who may have higher risk characteristics for developing cancer. This type of trial evaluates the safety and efficacy of various risk reduction strategies that may include "action" interventions (e.g., being more active, quitting smoking, eating more fruits and vegetables) or "agent" interventions (e.g., taking certain medications, vitamins, and supplements). Agent trials are also referred to as chemoprevention trials.
- *Screening trials:* Evaluate the effectiveness of new techniques for early detection of cancer in the general population. Screening effectiveness is measured by the reduction in the number of deaths from the cancer being screened.
- *Diagnostic trials:* Examine tests or procedures that can better identify cancer in symptomatic individuals; they can provide clinicians with improved tools to classify types and phases of cancer and evaluate techniques designed to measure and monitor treatment response more accurately or less invasively.
- *Quality-of-life or supportive care trials:* Evaluate interventions designed to improve the comfort and quality of life of individuals diagnosed with cancer and their families. Supportive care trials explore pharmacologic or nonpharmacologic therapies suggested to minimize cancer-related and cancer treatment–related toxicities.
- *Treatment (therapeutic) trials:* Evaluate the safety and efficacy of new drugs, vaccines, biologic agents, approaches to surgery or radiation therapy, treatment combinations, or other interventions in people diagnosed with cancer.

Phases of Clinical Trials

Cancer therapeutic trials evaluate the safety and efficacy of new pharmaceutical agents, biologic therapies, procedures, or other interventions in people with cancer. Cancer clinical trials include a series of steps, called phases (NCI, 2002; National Library of Medicine, 2008; Pharmaceutical Research and Manufacturers of America, 2007). Each phase is designed to answer a distinct research question (see figure on page 274).

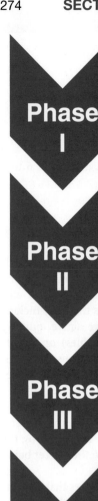

Phase I
- Sample: Patients with advanced disease that is resistant to standard therapy
- Sample size: 15-30 patients
- Objective: Determine a dose that will be appropriate for use in phase II studies
- End Point: Safety
- Specific End Points: Toxicities, dose-limiting toxicity, pharmacokinetics, metabolism, maximum tolerated dose, schedule, pharmacodynamics/biomarkers, early evidence of effectiveness
- Time to complete: 1-6 months

Phase II
- Sample: Patients with maximum performance status and minimum exposure to prior chemotherapy
- Sample size: <100 patients
- Objectives: Determine antitumor activity against specific tumor type; determine short-term side effects and risks
- End Point: Efficacy
- Specific End Point: Tumor response, toxicity
- Time to complete: 6 months to 2 years

Phase III
- Sample: Patients with specific types of cancer
- Sample size: 100s to 1000s, multiple sites
- Objectives: Determine whether new therapy is more effective or has better toxicity profile than standard treatment
- End Point: Efficacy
- Specific End Point: Survival time, symptom control, quality of life, long-tern side effects and risks, progression-free survival, disease-free survival, cost-benefit analysis
- Time to complete: 1-10 years

Phase IV
- Objectives: Monitor ongoing safety of marketed drugs and identify additional potential uses of the drug
- End Point: Safety and efficacy
- Specific End Point: Long-term side effects
- Time to complete: 6 months to 5 years

Phases of cancer clinical trials. (From U.S. Food and Drug Administration. [2007]. *Guidance for industry: Clinical trial endpoints for the approval of cancer drugs and biologic.* Rockville, MD: Author; Jayson, G., & Harris, J. [2006]. How participants in cancer trials are chosen: Ethics and conflicting interests. *National Review of Cancer, 6*[4], 330-336; National Cancer Institute. [2002]. Cancer clinical trials: The in-depth program. Bethesda, MD: National Institutes of Health.)

Phase I: Initial testing in a small group of volunteers
- *Goal:* Evaluate safety, determine a safe dosage range, and identify side effects of a new drug or treatment in a small group of people.
- *Benefits:* If the new drug or treatment under study demonstrates anticancer activity, participants will be among the first to benefit; the intervention may benefit future patients.
- *Risks:* Unpredictable side effects can occur because phase I trials are often the first study of the drug or treatment that involves human subjects.

Phase II: Testing in a small group of patients
- *Goal:* Evaluate the efficacy and further determine the safety of a drug or treatment in a larger group of people.

- *Benefits:* Participants may be among the first to benefit from the treatment.
- *Risks:* Unpredictable side effects may occur.

Phase III: Testing in a large group of patients to show safety and efficacy
- *Goal:* Evaluate the effectiveness, monitor side effects, and compare the drug or treatment with other, commonly used treatments (also known as standard of care).
- *Benefits:* Regardless of randomization, participants will receive the best widely accepted standard treatment.
- *Risks:* New drugs or treatments are not always better than, or even as good as, standard treatment; new treatments may have toxicities that are worse than those of the standard treatment; despite phase I and II testing, unexpected

side effects may still occur; participants who are randomized to standard treatment may not benefit as much as those receiving the experimental drug or treatment.

Phase IV: Ongoing studies, sometimes called postmarketing surveillance studies
- *Goal:* Evaluate the drug's effect in various populations and any side effects associated with long-term use after the treatment has been marketed.

Components of a Clinical Trial

Clinical trials adhere to strict scientific and ethical guidelines to protect participants. Multiple regulatory groups and independent review and advisory boards oversee participation of human subjects in research, monitor progress of clinical trials, and guarantee that the studies are conducted, recorded, and reported according to the protocol, standard operating procedures, good clinical practices, and regulatory requirements.

Clinical Research Team

The design and implementation of a clinical trial requires the talents and expertise of a multidisciplinary research team. The team may include clinical research associates, research nurses, data managers, and study coordinators who have varying responsibilities, including screening for potential study candidates, determining eligibility, coordinating the patient calendar, preparing documents for submission to institutional review boards (IRBs), filing amendments, submitting safety data, conducting patient education, obtaining informed consent, and assessing potential adverse events (Baer, Zon, Devine, & Lyss, 2011):
- *Principal investigator (PI) or clinical investigator:* Conducts research that contributes to generalizable knowledge; ultimately responsible for the equitable and fair conduct of research and the protection of human participants (Baer, Devine, Beardmore, & Catalano, 2011).
- *Clinical research associate (CRA):* Also known as a clinical or trial monitor; monitors all aspects of a clinical trial.

Responsibilities include protection of the rights and well-being of human subjects; accurate, complete, and verifiable reporting of trial data; and compliance with currently approved protocols and amendments, good clinical practices, and applicable regulatory requirements (Ajay & Bhatt, 2010). CRAs are often required to have a degree in life sciences and to have knowledge of good clinical practice and local regulations. Certification is available as a Certified Clinical Research Associate (CCRA).
- *Research nurse:* Coordinates and manages the collection of data throughout the clinical trial; responsible for education of staff, patients, and referring health care providers about the trial; assists the PI with toxicity and response monitoring, quality assurance, audits, data management, and analysis (NCI, 2002).
- *Data manager:* Supervises clinical trial data, including electronic data entry; provides data to monitoring agencies; prepares summaries for data analysis (NCI, 2002).
- *Staff physicians and nurses:* Administer treatments to participants as dictated by the protocol; assess and document toxicities, drug tolerance, and adverse events; collaborate with the PI and research nurse in monitoring clinical trends; provide direct care and patient and family education (NCI, 2002).

Clinical Trial Protocol

A clinical trial protocol is a clear, detailed, and transparent action plan that guides the conduct of a clinical trial. Protocols provide investigators with a written plan to carry out the clinical trial; provide trial participants with a precise description of the methodology; provide ethics committees and IRBs with information on the safety plan and assurances to protect participants' welfare and rights; provide funding agencies with a mechanism to evaluate proposed methodologies; and provide systematic reviewers with a description of *a priori* methods to address potential biases. The table below outlines the sections to be included in a clinical trial protocol as reported by an expert consensus panel (Tetzlaff et al., 2012; Tetzlaff, Moher, & Chan, 2012).

Minimum Clinical Trial Protocol Content

Section and Topic	Brief Description
General Information	
Title	Descriptive title identifying study design
Trial identifier	Unique number/name and registration information
Protocol version	Version or amendment number and date
Protocol summary	Short summary of proposed research
Names and addresses	Contact information for primary investigators and sponsor
Table of contents	List of contents and page numbers
Introduction	
Rationale	Outlines topic and provides justification for the study
Background of the study	Summary of all previous studies
Preliminary data	Describe preliminary studies
Objectives	Specific objectives and hypotheses for the study
Study locations	Description of intended site or sites
Methods: Participants	
Population	Target and study population and source of the latter
Eligibility criteria	Description of inclusion and exclusion criteria
Sample size	Estimated number; calculations and assumptions
Recruitment	Process of recruitment and enrollment (e.g., advertisements)

Continued

Minimum Clinical Trial Protocol Content—cont'd

Section and Topic	Brief Description
Methods: Design	
Type of study	Description of type/design and trial framework
Study timeline	Diagram of procedures/visits through trial stages
Sequence generation	Random sequence method; details of any restriction
Allocation concealment	Random sequence implementation and whether concealed
Random implementation	How participants will be assigned to groups
Blinding	Who (e.g., participants, investigators, outcome assessors)
Methods: Interventions	
Interventions A	Precise details; how administered (e.g., dosage, form)
Interventions B	Justification of control
Schedule of interventions	Number and duration of treatment periods (run-in, washout)
Concomitant interventions	Treatments permitted or not before or during trial
Risks or harms	Known or potential risks for each intervention
Methods: Data Collection and Management	
Outcomes	Describes and defines primary and secondary outcomes
Data collection	Instruments and timing of data collection and recording
Biologic specimens	Laboratory evaluation, specimen collection and handling
Validation of instruments	Instrument reliability/validity or plans to validate
Follow-up	Description and schedule of visits and logistics
Data management	Plans for data entry, editing, coding, and storage
Quality control	Quality of outcome assessment and data records
Compliance	Monitoring of participant compliance
Methods: Statistical Methods	
Statistical methods	Methods for primary/secondary outcomes and additional analyses
Withdrawals A	Criteria to withdraw or exclude participants from the intervention
Withdrawals B	Data collected and follow-up, withdrawn participants
Missing data	Methods to account for missing or erroneous data
Interim trial monitoring	Process and timing of any planned interim analyses
Stopping guidelines A	Predefined statistical stopping boundaries
Stopping guidelines B	Nonstatistical criteria for the early trial termination
Methods: Safety and Monitoring	
Safety evaluations	Monitoring of safety plans including methods, timing
Data and Safety Monitoring Board (DSMB)	If relevant, composition and role of DSMB
Adverse event reporting	Recording and reporting events; methods to handle
Emergency code breaking	Establishment and storage of code; when and by whom it can be broken
Trial monitoring	Plans and frequency, whether independent
Trial Organization and Administration	
Monetary and material support	Sources of financial and material support
Data ownership	Who has ownership; contractual limits for principal investigators
Ethical Considerations	
Potential benefits and risks	Potential benefits and risks to participants, society
Agreement and consent	Materials for potential participants
Surrogate consent/assent	Method of obtaining surrogate consent or assent
Confidentiality/Anonymity	Provisions for protecting personal data and privacy
Ethics approval	Whether obtained, names of committees
Role of sponsor	Role of sponsor in design, data collection, analysis, dissemination
Conflict of interest	Real or perceived conflicts of interest
Posttrial care	Posttrial follow-up, access to treatment, duration; who is responsible
Reporting and Dissemination	
Protocol amendments	Methods of communicating to investigators and institutional review boards, documentation
Dissemination	How results will be disseminated to participants, practitioners, public
Publication policy	Publication rights, restrictions, authorship guidelines
Reporting of early stopping	Dissemination of results if trial is stopped early
Other	
Limitations	Limitations of study, including risk of bias
References	List of references cited in protocol
Data collection forms	Summary table of data collection forms and times

From Tetzlaff, J. M., Moher, D., & Chan, A. W. (2012). Developing a guideline for clinical trial protocol content: Delphi consensus survey. *Trials, 13,* 176.

Eligibility Criteria (National Cancer Institute, 2002; The Clearity Foundation, 2015)

Eligibility criteria include demographic characteristics and specific disease- and treatment-related characteristics; they may vary with the specific phase of the clinical trial (NCI, 2002; The Clearity Foundation, 2015). Phase I and II trials often seek participants who may better tolerate the treatment or have fewer risk factors for potential toxicities. Phase II and III trials often add criteria that include disease type, stage, and exposure to prior treatments.

Common Inclusion Criteria

- *Cancer status:* Most inclusion criteria relate to cancer status, such as participants who are in remission or have progressive disease, whose cancer responded to a particular drug class, or who did not respond to treatment.
- *Health and performance status:* Blood counts, blood chemistry tests, and performance status must be within well-defined parameters.
- *Measurable disease:* Disease must be measurable by imaging procedures such as computed tomography (CT) or positron-emission tomography (PET)/CT scans; response to drug treatment often is monitored by tumor size.
- *Tumor biopsy for biomarker evaluation:* This criterion applies to trials measuring biomarkers that correlate with drug response or studies identifying new biomarkers predictive of response.

Common Exclusion Criterion

- *Prior treatment:* Patients may be excluded if they have received numerous prior treatments or have been exposed to a drug that is being given in combination with the experimental drug.

End Points

End points are measurable outcomes that indicate an intervention's effectiveness. Early-phase trials evaluate safety and identify evidence of biologic drug activity (e.g., tumor response). Later, efficacy studies commonly evaluate the clinical benefit of a drug, such as increased survival or reduced toxicities (see table below) (U.S. FDA, 2007). End points should show clinically meaningful benefit for the participant (Wilson et al., 2015).

Comparison of Important Cancer Approval End Points

End Point	Regulatory Evidence	Study Design	Advantages	Disadvantages
Overall survival	Clinical benefit for regular approval	Randomized studies essential Blinding not essential	Universally accepted direct measure of benefit Easily measured Precisely measured	May involve larger studies May be affected by crossover therapy and sequential therapy Includes noncancer deaths
Symptom end points (patient-reported outcomes)	Clinical benefit for regular approval	Randomized blinded studies	Patient perspective of direct clinical benefit	Blinding is often difficult Data frequently missing or incomplete Clinical significance of small changes unknown Multiple analyses Lack of validated instruments
Disease-free survival	Surrogate for accelerated approval or regular approval*	Randomized studies essential Blinding preferred Blinded review recommended	Smaller sample size and shorter follow-up necessary compared with survival studies	Not validated as surrogate for survival in all settings Not precisely measured; subject to assessment bias, particularly in open-label studies Definitions vary
Objective response rate	Surrogate for accelerated approval or regular approval*	Single-arm or randomized studies may be used Blinding preferred in comparative studies Blinded review recommended	Can be assessed in single-arm studies Assessed earlier and in smaller studies compared with survival studies Effect attributable to drug, not natural history	Not a direct measure of benefit Not a comprehensive measure of drug activity Only a subset of patients benefit
Complete response	Surrogate for accelerated approval or regular approval*	Single-arm or randomized studies may be used Blinding preferred in comparative studies Blinded review recommended	Can be assessed in single-arm studies Durable complete responses can represent clinical benefit Assessed earlier and in smaller studies compared with survival studies	Not a direct measure of benefit in all cases Not a comprehensive measure of drug activity Small subset of patients with benefit
Progression-free survival	Surrogate for accelerated approval or regular approval*	Randomized studies essential Blinding preferred Blinded review recommended	Smaller sample size and shorter follow-up necessary compared with survival studies Measurement of stable disease included Not affected by crossover or subsequent therapies Generally based on objective and quantitative assessment	Not validated as surrogate for survival in all settings Not precisely measured; subject to assessment bias particularly in open-label studies Definitions vary Frequent radiologic or other assessments Involves balanced timing of assessments of treatment arms

From Wilson, M. K., Karakasis, K., & Oza, A. M. (2015). Outcomes and endpoints in trials of cancer treatment: The past, present, and future. *Lancet Oncology, 16*(1), e32-e42.

*Adequacy as a surrogate end point for accelerated approval or regular approval is highly dependent on other factors such as effect size, effect duration, and benefits of other available therapies.

Oncology Clinical Trials Nurse Competencies

Functional Area	Competency
Protocol compliance	Facilitate compliance with requirements of the research protocol and good clinical research practice while remaining cognizant of the needs of diverse patient populations.
Communication	Utilize multiple communication methods to facilitate the effective conduct of clinical trials.
Informed consent process	Demonstrate leadership in ensuring patient comprehension and safety during initial and ongoing clinical trial informed consent discussions.
Management of clinical trial patients	Use a variety of resources and strategies to manage the care of patients participating in clinical trials, ensuring compliance with protocol procedures, assessments, and reporting requirements as well as management of symptoms.
Documentation	Provide leadership to the research team in ensuring collection of source data and completion of documentation that validates the integrity of the conduct of the clinical trial.
Patient recruitment	Utilize a variety of strategies to enhance recruitment while being mindful of the needs of diverse patient populations.
Ethical issues	Demonstrate leadership in ensuring adherence to ethical practices during the conduct of clinical trials in order to protect the rights and well-being of patients and the collection of quality data.
Financial implications	Identify the financial variables that affect research and support good financial stewardship in clinical trials.
Professional development	Take responsibility for identifying one's ongoing professional development needs and seek resources and opportunities to meet those needs, such as through membership in nursing, oncology, or research organizations.

Data from Oncology Nursing Society. (2010). *Oncology clinical trials nurse competencies*. Pittsburgh, PA: Author.

Randomization

In phase III trials (and some phase II trials), participants are randomly assigned to either the experimental or the control group with the use of a computer program or table of random numbers. This allows an equal chance of being assigned to either group. Randomization reduces selection biases that may influence trial results (NCI, 2002).

Stratified Randomization

Stratified randomization is a two-step process by which participants are grouped into categories according to clinical features that may influence outcomes. Participants are randomly assigned to an experimental or a control group (Kernan, Viscoli, Makuch, Brass, & Horwitz, 1999).

Blinding

Blinding usually refers to keeping study participants, the clinical research team, and the disease management team unaware of the assigned treatment. In clinical research, there is a risk that access to information and study expectations could introduce bias, especially when there is subjectivity in the measurement of outcomes (e.g., alleviation of pain, increased quality of life). Blinding aims to minimize such bias (Day & Altman, 2000).

Considerations for Nursing Care (Oncology Nursing Society, 2010)

The Oncology Clinical Trials Nurse (OCTN) requires specialized preparation and qualifications for providing direct care to participants in a cancer clinical trial (see table in the left column). The OCTN coordinates the trial, identifies eligible participants for studies, and often recognizes those who may not be able to complete the study for reasons not evident in the protocol. This nurse also identifies significant trends in toxicities and collaborates with the PI to develop and evaluate management strategies and effectively communicate with participants, caregivers, the research team, the disease management team, and sponsors (Oncology Nursing Society, 2010).

References

Ajay, S., & Bhatt, A. (2010). Training needs of clinical research associates. *Perspectives on Clinical Research, 1*(4), 134–138.

Baer, A. R., Devine, S., Beardmore, C. D., & Catalano, R. (2011). Clinical investigator responsibilities. *Journal of Oncology Practice, 7*(2), 124–128.

Baer, A. R., Zon, R., Devine, S., & Lyss, A. P. (2011). The clinical research team. *Journal of Oncology Practice, 7*(3), 188–192.

Day, S. J., & Altman, D. G. (2000). Statistics notes: Blinding in clinical trials and other studies. *British Medical Journal, 321*(7259), 504.

Jayson, G., & Harris, J. (2006). How participants in cancer trials are chosen: Ethics and conflicting interests. *National Review of Cancer, 6*(4), 330–336.

Kernan, W. N., Viscoli, C. M., Makuch, R. W., Brass, L. M., & Horwitz, R. I. (1999). Stratified randomization for clinical trials. *Journal of Clinical Epidemiology, 52*(1), 19–26.

Lieu, C. H., Tan, A. C., Leong, S., Diamond, J. R., & Eckhardt, S. G. (2013). From bench to bedside: Lessons learned in translating preclinical studies in cancer drug development. *Journal of the National Cancer Institute, 105*(19), 1441–1456.

National Cancer Institute. (2002). *Cancer clinical trials: The in-depth program*. Bethesda, MD: National Institutes of Health.

National Cancer Institute. (2012). *Types of clinical trials*. Available at http://www.cancer.gov/clinicaltrials/learningabout/what-are-clinical-trials/types (accessed February 10, 2016).

National Library of Medicine. (2008). *FAQ: Clinical trial phases*. Available at http://www.nlm.nih.gov/services/ctphases.html (accessed February 10, 2016).

Oncology Nursing Society. (2010). *Oncology clinical trials nurse competencies*. Pittsburgh, PA: Author.

Pharmaceutical Research and Manufacturers of America. (2007). *Drug discovery and development*. Washington, DC: Author.

Tetzlaff, J. M., Chan, A. W., Kitchen, J., Sampson, M., Tricco, A. C., & Moher, D. (2012). Guidelines for randomized clinical trial protocol content: A systematic review. *Systematic Review, 1*, 43.

Tetzlaff, J. M., Moher, D., & Chan, A. W. (2012). Developing a guideline for clinical trial protocol content: Delphi consensus survey. *Trials, 13*, 176.

The Clearity Foundation. (2015). *Clinical trial eligibility criteria*. Available at http://www.clearityfoundation.org/clinical-trials/ (accessed February 29, 2016).

U.S. Food and Drug Administration. (2007). *Guidance for industry: Clinical trial endpoints for the approval of cancer drugs and biologic*. Rockville, MD: Author.

Wilson, M. K., Collyar, D., Chingos, D. T., Friedlander, M., Ho, T. W., Karakasis, K., & Oza, A. M. (2015). Outcomes and endpoints in cancer trials: Bridging the divide. *Lancet Oncology, 16*(1), e43–e52.

Wilson, M. K., Karakasis, K., & Oza, A. M. (2015). Outcomes and endpoints in trials of cancer treatment: The past, present, and future. *Lancet Oncology, 16*(1), e32–e42.

Oncology Symptoms

Alopecia

Wendy H. Vogel

Definition

- Alopecia is the absence or loss of hair.
- It can result from genetic factors, aging, or local or systemic disease, or it can be therapy induced.
- Loss of less than 25% of the hair is considered minimal, 25% to 50% is considered moderate hair loss, and more than 50% is severe hair loss.
- At least 50% of hair must be lost for it to be noticeable.
- In oncology settings, toxic alopecia typically occurs because of chemotherapeutic agents or radiation therapy; the estimated incidence is 65% (see table below). Some targeted therapies, such as kinase inhibitors, may cause varying degrees of alopecia.
- Toxic alopecia is usually temporary and can include body hair as well as the hair of the head.
- The average daily hair loss (under normal conditions) is approximately 100 hairs.
- Because hair follicles are mitotically active structures, they are at risk for damage from radiation therapy and chemotherapy.
- The scalp is the area most sensitive to hair damage, followed by the male beard, the eyebrows, axillary hair, pubic hair, and fine hair.
- The degree of alopecia depends on the treatment given, the dose, the schedule, and the route of administration.
- Bolus-dosing schedules of chemotherapy cause more alopecia than cumulative doses given over an extended period.
- Radiation doses of 2500 to 3000 cGy fractionated over 2 or 3 weeks will cause hair loss. A single dose as small as 500 cGy may cause hair loss.
- Radiation doses greater than 4500 cGy can cause permanent alopecia.
- Radiation doses greater than 6000 cGy may cause sebaceous and sweat glands to stop functioning.

Oncology Agents That Cause Hair Loss (Listed in Order of Toxicity)

Class	Drug Examples	Incidence of Hair Loss (%)*
Antimicrotubule agents	Docetaxel, paclitaxel, vincristine	>80
Topoisomerase	Doxorubicin, epirubicin, etoposide	60-100
Alkylators	Bendamustine, cisplatin, cyclophosphamide	>60
Antimetabolites	5-Fluorouracil, capecitabine, pemetrexed	10-50

*Incidence and severity vary by selected agent and dose density. The combination of agents may increase toxicity.

Pathophysiology and Contributing Factors

- When cells in the hair bulb absorb the chemotherapeutic agent or are damaged by radiation therapy, cellular division and protein synthesis may be suppressed or halted.
- Cells can enter the telogen phase early, enabling the hair to be shed, either in clumps or gradually, depending on the mitotic activity of the hair follicle at the time of the exposure.
- Hair loss usually occurs within 2 to 3 weeks after the first exposure to the toxin.
- Continued loss can occur over the next 3 to 4 weeks, although this varies according to the chemotherapeutic agent.
- In general, hair loss begins on the crown and on the sides of the head above the ear.
- Regrowth occurs within 3 to 5 months. New hair growth may be of a different texture, color, or consistency.
- Regrowth may occur before the end of therapy because of the tricyclic nature of hair growth phases.
- Permanent alopecia is rare after cancer treatment, although it has been reported after bone marrow transplantation and it is associated with chronic graft-versus-host reaction, previous exposure to radiation, and advanced age.

Signs and Symptoms

- Loss of hair usually begins 2 to 3 weeks after exposure. The scalp may become sensitive before hair is lost.

Assessment Tools

- Thorough history
  - Comorbid diseases
  - Nutrition
  - Drug history
  - Psychiatric history
- Physical examination
  - Inspection for a pattern of hair loss
  - Density of remaining hair
  - Color (dull or bright)
  - Condition of scalp
  - Length and texture of hair
- A hair pull test involves gentle traction on about 50 hairs. If two to three or more hairs are dislodged, then accelerated hair loss is likely.
- Common Terminology Criteria for Adverse Events (version 4.03)
  - Grade 1 indicates thinning or patchy hair.
  - Grade 2 is complete hair loss.
- Eastern Cooperative Oncology Group grading scale
- World Health Organization toxicity grading criteria

Laboratory and Diagnostic Tests

- None

Differential Diagnoses

- Malnutrition
- Hypothyroidism
- Noncytotoxic drugs such as allopurinol, amphetamines, anticoagulants, antithyroid drugs, heavy metals, hypocholesterolemic drugs, levodopa, oral contraceptives, propranolol, and retinoids
- Chronic stress
- Postpartum state
- Lupus erythematosus
- Alopecia of other causes, such as congenital alopecia, alopecia areata, androgenetic alopecia, alopecia associated with trauma, tinea capitis, folliculitis decalvans, and alopecia neoplastica

Interventions

- Prevention has been a subject of debate since the 1960s.
- Various preventive methods have been used, including scalp tourniquets and scalp hypothermia. Discomfort and the risk of creating a "drug-free area" that could be a site for recurrence (e.g., skin metastases) have discouraged these practices.

Pharmacologic Interventions

- None is used as the standard of care.
- Several agents for prevention and treatment of alopecia have been studied with varying results, although none has been approved by the U.S. Food and Drug Administration (FDA):
  - Tocopherol (vitamin E)
  - ImuVert, a biological response modifier
  - Minoxidil (topical) may shorten duration or severity but does not prevent hair loss

Nonpharmacologic Interventions

- Alopecia can cause the skin to be sensitive or tender. Warmth, lotions, massage, or other symptomatic treatments may be used, although there are no guidelines in the medical literature to advise these.
- Scalp cooling is generally contraindicated for hematologic malignancies and is controversial for those undergoing curative treatment. Side effects of scalp cooling include headaches and feelings of cold throughout the body.
- Patients should be reassured that hair regrowth will occur.
- Psychosocial adjustment should be continually assessed throughout the treatment period until regrowth occurs.

Patient Teaching

- Instruct the patient as to when hair loss will occur.
- Advise the patient to obtain a wig or head covering, if desired, before hair loss occurs, while a good color and style match can be made.

- Encourage use of sunscreen and sun hats.
- Care should be taken to avoid cuts or nicks to the scalp if the head is shaved.

Follow-up

- Hair should begin to regrow within 3 to 5 months after therapy ends. The rate of growth depends on the individual's growth rate. If hair has not begun to regrow within 6 months, alopecia may be permanent.

Resources

- American Academy of Dermatology: www.aad.org/default.htm
- Cancer Care.org: www.cancercare.org
- Oncolink: www.oncolink.com

Bibliography

Callaghan, M., & Cooper, A. (2014). Alopecia. In C. Yarbro, D. Wujcik, & B. Gobel (Eds.), *Cancer symptom management* (4th ed.) (pp. 495–503). Burlington, MA: Jones & Bartlett.

Camp-Sorrell, D. (2011). Chemotherapy toxicities and management. In C. Yarbro, D. Wujcik, & B. Gobel (Eds.), *Cancer nursing principles and practice* (7th ed.) (pp. 458–503). Sudbury, MA: Jones & Bartlett.

Eaby-Sandy, B., Grande, C., & Viale, P. (2012). *Journal for the Advanced Practitioner in Oncology, 3*(3), 138–150.

Haas, M. (2011). Radiation therapy: Toxicities and management. In C. Yarbro, D. Wujcik, & B. Gobel (Eds.), *Cancer nursing principles and practice* (7th ed.) (pp. 312–351). Sudbury, MA: Jones & Bartlett.

Nail, L., & Lee-Lin, F. (2015). Alopecia. In C. Brown (Ed.), *Guide to oncology symptom management* (pp. 17–25). Pittsburg, PA: Oncology Nursing Society.

National Cancer Institute, National Institutes of Health. (2010). *Common terminology criteria for adverse events, version 4.03*. Available at http://evs.nci.nih.gov/ftp1/CTCAE/CTCAE_4.03_2010-06-14_QuickReference_8.5x11.pdf (accessed February 10, 2016).

Paus, R., Haslam, I., & Botchkarev, V. (2013). Pathobiology of chemotherapy-induced hair loss. *Lancet Oncology, 14*(2), e50–e59.

Polovich, M., Olsen, M., & LeFebvre, K. (2014). *Chemotherapy and biotherapy guidelines and recommendations for practice* (4th ed.). Pittsburgh, PA: Oncology Nursing Society.

Trueb, R. (2010). Chemotherapy-induced hair loss. *Skin Therapy Letter, 15*(7), 5–7.

Anorexia

Kristin A. Cawley

Definition

- Anorexia is the involuntary loss of appetite.
- It is characterized by loss of greater than 10% of body weight within a 6-month period.

- It occurs in as many as 40% of cancer patients at diagnosis and up to 80% in patients in advanced stages.
- The highest incidences are in patients with gastrointestinal cancers.
- Anorexia is often associated with cachexia (lean tissue wasting).
- Weight loss is a major cause of morbidity and mortality in patients with advanced cancer.
- Anorexia is associated with a lower quality of life, poor response to chemotherapy, reduced performance status, and shorter survival times.

Pathophysiology and Contributing Factors
- End result of altered central and peripheral neurohormonal signals that govern appetite
- Involuntary systemic effect of underlying disease
- Predisposed by disease progression
- Direct result of supportive treatment modalities, including surgery, radiation therapy, and chemotherapy
- Secondary effect of
  - Taste alterations
  - Pain
  - Nausea
  - Lowered immune competence
- Humoral and inflammatory responses
  - Production of inflammatory cytokines
- Local effects of tumor
  - Dysphagia
  - Gastric obstruction
- Psychological factors, including depression
- Metabolic disturbances

Signs and Symptoms
- Lack of appetite
- Weight loss
- Muscle wasting
- Early satiety
- Fatigue
- Nausea
- Vomiting
- Weakness
- Sleep disturbances

Assessment Tools
- Patient history and physical examination
- The Functional Assessment of Anorexia/Cachexia Therapy Questionnaire
- Simplified Nutrition Assessment Questionnaire (SNAQ)
- Rotterdam Symptom Checklist

Laboratory and Diagnostic Tests
- Complete blood cell count
- Creatinine clearance
- Albumin, prealbumin, transferrin, and retinol-binding protein levels

Differential Diagnoses
- Dysphagia
- Malnutrition
- Cachexia
- Nausea and vomiting
- Dehydration
- Fatigue
- Depression
- Hypercalcemia

Interventions
- Treat underlying causes.
- Provide nutritional counseling.

Pharmacologic Interventions
- Progestational agents
  - Megestrol acetate (Megace)
  - Medroxyprogesterone
- Corticosteroids
  - Dexamethasone
  - Prednisone
- Cannabinoids
  - Dronabinol
- Dietary supplements
- Treatment of hypercalcemia, if present

Nonpharmacologic Interventions
- Increased food intake
- Screening at diagnosis and at regular intervals
  - Weight change
  - Dietary intake
  - Physical examination findings
  - Laboratory findings
- Management of underlying causes
  - Nausea
  - Constipation
  - Mucositis
- Nutritional counseling
- Enteral or parenteral nutrition
- Minimizing factors that decrease food intake

Patient Teaching
- Eat small, frequent meals.
- Decrease energy expenditure.
- Minimize factors that decrease food intake.
- Avoid offensive odors.
- Eat energy-dense foods.
- Limit fat intake.
- Avoid extremes in taste and smell of food.
- Enhance presentation of food.

Follow-up
- Consultation with nutritionist or dietician as needed
- Reassessment of patient status
- Assessment of new-onset or continued weight loss

Resources

- Oncology Nursing Society: https://www.ons.org/practice-resources/pep/anorexia
- FAACT Version 4: obtained from FACIT.org

Bibliography

Aapro, M., Arends, J., Bozzetti, F., Fearon, K., Grunberg, S. M., & European School of Medical Oncology. (2014). Early recognition of malnutrition and cachexia in the cancer patient: A position paper of a European School of Oncology Task Force. *Annals of Oncology, 25*(8), 1492–1499.

Baldwin, C., Spiro, A., Ahern, R., & Emery, P. W. (2012). Oral nutritional interventions in malnourished patients with cancer: A systematic review and meta-analysis. *Journal of the National Cancer Institute, 104*(5), 371–385.

Dy, S. M., Lorenz, K. A., Naeim, A., Sanati, H., Walling, A., & Asch, S. M. (2008). Evidence-based recommendations for cancer fatigue, anorexia, depression, and dyspnea. *Journal of Clinical Oncology, 26*(23), 3886–3895.

Esper, P., & Heidrich, D. (2005). Symptom clusters in advanced illness. *Seminars in Oncology Nursing, 21*, 20–28.

Molfino, A., Muscaritoli, M., & Rossi-Fanelli, F. (2015). Anorexia assessment in patients with cancer: A crucial issue to improve the outcome. *Journal of Clinical Oncology, 33*(13), 1513.

Ravasco, P., Monteiro-Grillo, I., Vidal, P. M., & Camilo, M. E. (2005). Dietary counseling improves patient outcomes: A prospective, randomized, controlled trial in colorectal cancer patients undergoing radiotherapy. *Journal of Clinical Oncology, 23*(7), 1431–1438.

Yavuzen, T., Davis, M. P., Walsh, D., LeGrand, S., & Lagman, R. (2005). Systematic review of the treatment of cancer-associated anorexia and weight loss. *Journal of Clinical Oncology, 23*, 8500–8511.

Anxiety

Denice Economou

Definition

- Anxiety is a subjective feeling of distress, apprehension, tension, insecurity, or uneasiness, usually without a known stimulus or cause, and a fear of real or perceived threat to oneself.
- It is most often rated as mild, moderate, or severe.
- Anxiety related to cancer is considered a normal reaction to a potentially life-threatening illness.

Pathophysiology and Contributing Factors

- Anxiety is thought to result from an inappropriate activation of the sympathetic nervous system.
- Increased levels of norepinephrine and decreased levels of serotonin and γ-aminobutyric acid are present.
- Hormonal inputs, such as from the hypothalamus, pituitary, and adrenal glands, interfere with normal processes, leading to feelings of panic or a sense of dread.
- Cardiovascular abnormalities contribute to anxiety as a result of altered regulation of the autonomic nervous system.

- Anxiety can be medication induced (see list under "Assessment Tools").
- It can be caused by withdrawal from alcohol or nicotine.
- It can be related to disease stage: Anxiety increases as disease advances or physical status declines.
- It can be related to difficulty with treatment regimens or lifestyle changes and financial concerns.
- It can be related to dealing with family issues or conflicts and facing death.
- Family and staff anxiety can contribute to the patient's level of anxiety, and vice versa.

Signs and Symptoms

- Restlessness, panic, tachycardia, difficulty concentrating, palpitations, sweating, dizziness, urinary frequency, abdominal discomfort, sleep disturbances
- Chest pain, irritability, headache, apprehension, and anorexia
- Repetitive behaviors to prevent discomfort (e.g., pacing, rubbing hands)
- Changes in vital signs: elevated heart rate, blood pressure, or respiratory rate and temperature
- Endocrine-associated changes to the skin that contribute to anxiety (e.g., dry skin in thyroid disorder, Addison disease symptoms), facial puffiness, and increased skin pigmentation
  - Skin turgor may predict poor appetite, dehydration, or hypernatremia.

Assessment Tools

- Depression and anxiety screening tools to help evaluate subjective feelings of anxiety and the level of anxiety the patient is experiencing. Anxiety can be rated on a visual analog scale or on a verbal rating scale from 1 to 10 (similar to pain ratings).
  - Screening tools include the GAD-7 scale, which is used to measure the level of anxiety.
  - Ask questions such as, "Do you feel nervous?" and "Do you worry about your diagnosis or treatment?" The goal is to understand what may be contributing to the anxiety.
- The history should include any history of psychosocial disorders, adjustment disorders, or panic attacks.
- Any history of generalized anxiety disorders or phobias or a history of agitated depression.
- What are the presenting symptoms, including precipitating factors, onset, and duration?
- What makes the symptoms better or worse?
- How does the patient cope with anxiety? What methods does the patient use to manage anxiety?
- Medication history, including over-the-counter medications. Medications associated with anxiety include stimulants, thyroid replacement medications, corticosteroids, bronchodilators and decongestants, epinephrine, antihypertensives, antihistamines, anticholinergics, anesthetics, and analgesics.
- Uncontrolled pain, hypoxia, sepsis, adverse drug effects, and withdrawal effects
- Cardiac examination to identify irregular heart rate or abnormal heart sounds
- Pulmonary examination to rule out hypoxia related to pneumonia, pleural effusions, or embolus

- Neurologic examination to identify cranial nerve palsies and neuropathies

Laboratory and Diagnostic Tests

- Complete blood cell count to identify infections
- Thyroid-stimulating hormone to detect thyroid abnormalities
- Oxygen saturation measurement to identify respiratory conditions
- Electrocardiography to evaluate cardiac functioning
- Chest radiography to rule out pneumonia, pleural effusion, and embolus

Differential Diagnoses

- Phobic disorders
- Panic attack
- Obsessive-compulsive disorder
- Posttraumatic stress disorder
- Delirium (may be misdiagnosed as anxiety or depression)
- Medications that contribute to anxiety
  - Stimulants: caffeine, amphetamines, cocaine
  - Psychotropics: antipsychotics, buspirone
  - Central nervous system depressant withdrawal: barbiturates, benzodiazepines
  - Antihistamines
  - Anticholinergics
  - Other medications: steroids, theophylline, thyroid replacement hormones, cannabis

Interventions

- Treatment of anxiety is related to the patient's subjective level of distress.
- Moderate to severe anxiety can interfere significantly with a patient's ability to comply with treatments.
- The goal of treatment is to diagnose the presence and level of anxiety and to modify potential contributing factors.

Pharmacologic Interventions

- Benzodiazepines: diazepam, alprazolam, temazepam
- Azapirones: buspirone
- Antidepressants: amitriptyline, imipramine, nortriptyline, doxepin, fluoxetine, sertraline, paroxetine, venlafaxine
- Other medications used for anxiety: propranolol, haloperidol
- Atypical neuroleptics: olanzapine, risperidone

Nonpharmacologic Interventions

- Cognitive-behavioral interventions provide the greatest evidenced-based benefit.
- Initiate a discussion of concerns that may be contributing to the feeling of anxiety, such as pain, fear, or dependence issues. Use open-ended questions and clarification remarks.
- Help the patient identify what has helped him or her get through times like this before. How we can help you use those strategies now?
- Encourage the patient to identify people who can support him or her through this anxiety.

- Recognize that as patients move from mild to severe anxiety, the cause may be lost as the anxiety takes over. Preventive strategies can be useful to minimize anxiety or stabilize the escalation.
- Increase opportunities for control.
- Evaluate dietary intake to reduce caffeine and alcohol intake to promote sleep.
- Relieve pain.

Patient Teaching

- Provide patient and family education to support reduction of fear and anticipatory reactions. Give instructions on medications and management of side effects. The goal of education is to reduce stress and anxiety.
- Increase patient and family participation in activities.
- Encourage hope.
- Use a family member or friend as the support person to stay present and help the patient.
- Provide accurate information to help restructure unrealistic fearful beliefs.
- Teach anxiety-reducing interventions such as relaxation, visualization, deep breathing, massage, touch, and physical exercise.
- Stress management may include music and art therapy, yoga, and meditation.

Follow-up

- Refer patients to supportive psychiatric care when necessary.
- Multidisciplinary management can be the most effective way to achieve relief of anxiety. Social workers and chaplains should be part of the team to help support patients experiencing anxiety.

Resources

- National Cancer Institute: Adjustment to cancer: Anxiety and distress. www.cancer.gov/cancertopics/pdq/SupportiveCare/Adjustment//Patient/page1
- Cancer.Net: Coping with cancer: Anxiety. http://www.cancer.net/coping-and-emotions/managing-emotions/anxiety
- MentalHelp.Net: www.mentalhelp.net

Bibliography

Andersen, B. L., DeRubeis, R. J., Berman, B. S., Gruman, J., Champion, V. L., Massie, M. J., & Rowland, J. H. (2014). Screening, assessment, and care of anxiety and depressive symptoms in adults with cancer: An American Society of Clinical Oncology guideline adaptation. *Journal of Clinical Oncology, 32*(15), 1605–1620.

Breitbart, W., Chochinov, H. M., & Passik, S. (2010). Psychiatric symptoms in palliative medicine. In G. Hanks, N. Cherny, N. Christakis, M. Fallon, S. Kassa, & R. K. Portenoy (Eds.), *Oxford textbook of palliative medicine* (4th ed.) (pp. 1453–1482). New York: Oxford University Press.

Dahlin, C. (2006). Anxiety. In D. Camp-Sorrell & R. A. Hawkins (Eds.), *Clinical manual for the oncology advanced practice nurse* (pp. 1105–1111). Pittsburgh: Oncology Nursing Society.

Jacobsen, P., & Jim, H. (2008). Psychosocial interventions for anxiety and depression in adult cancer patients: Achievements and challenges. *CA: A Cancer Journal for Clinicians, 58*, 214–230.

Pasacreta, J., Minarik, P. A., Nield-Anderson, L., & Paice, J. (2015). Anxiety and depression. In B. Ferrell, N. Coyle, & J. Paice (Eds.), *Textbook of palliative nursing* (4th ed.) (pp. 366–384). New York: Oxford University Press.

Rucker, Y., & Gobel, B. C. (2014). Anxiety. In C. Yarbro, D. Wujcik, & B. H. Gobel (Eds.), *Cancer symptom management* (4th ed.) (pp. 619–635). Burlington, MA: Jones & Bartlett Learning.

Spitzer, R., Kroenke, K., William, J., & Lowe, B. (2006). A brief measure for assessing generalized anxiety distress: The GAD-7. *Archives of Internal Medicine, 166*, 1092–1097.

Zigmond, A. S., & Snaith, R. P. (1983). The hospital anxiety and depression scale. *Acta Psychiatrica Scandinavica, 67*(6), 361–370.

Arthralgias and Myalgias

Carol S. Blecher

Definition

- Arthralgias are pains in the joints.
- Myalgias are diffuse generalized muscle pains.
- Both symptoms may be accompanied by a general feeling of malaise.

Pathophysiology and Contributing Factors

- The pathophysiology of arthralgias and myalgias in the oncology context is unclear.
- Proposed theories include the following:
  - They occur in response to a noxious stimulus or trauma that damages the muscle tissue, leading to release of bradykinin and stimulation of muscle nociceptors.
  - They may be related to the taxanes and vinca alkaloids and possibly to microtubule stabilization or an inflammatory reaction to the drug.
- Risk factors include the following:
  - History of peripheral neuropathy
  - History of diabetes
  - Alcohol use
  - Chemotherapy agents including 13-*cis*-retinoic acid, alemtuzumab, altretamine, aromatase inhibitors as a class, azacytidine, bacille Calmette-Guérin (BCG), bevacizumab, bleomycin, cetuximab, cladribine, cytarabine, dacarbazine, docetaxel, etoposide, filgrastim, fludarabine, 5-fluorouracil, gemcitabine, interferon, interleukin-2, isotretinoin, L-asparaginase, olaparib, paclitaxel (especially in combination with cisplatin), procarbazine, rituximab, sargramostim, topotecan, trastuzumab, trimetrexate, vincristine, vinblastine, and vinorelbine
  - Age
  - Prior neurotoxic chemotherapy
  - History of arthritis
  - History of neuromuscular disease

Signs and Symptoms

Myalgias

- Generalized or localized muscle aches
- Edema
- Induration
- Fever
- Warm, flushed skin
- Tachycardia
- Shortness of breath
- Headache
- Thirst

Arthralgias

- Painful joints
- Swelling and redness of joints
- Fever and chills
- Fatigue
- Depression

Assessment Tools

Assessment of the patient with arthralgias or myalgias should include the following:

- History, including diagnosis and cancer treatment, current medications, presenting symptoms, precipitating factors, location, and duration
- Vital signs
  - Elevated temperature
  - Tachycardia
  - Tachypnea
- Musculoskeletal system
  - Edema
  - Spasm
  - Erythema
  - Warmth and tenderness
  - Strength and range of motion
- Complete pain assessment
  - Character of the pain
  - Location
  - Quality
  - Onset
  - Factors that cause pain to worsen
  - Factors that alleviate pain
    - Current medication
    - Severity of the pain—current pain score, worst pain score, best pain score, and pain goal
    - Effects of pain on activities of daily living (ADLs) and quality of life
- National Cancer Institute (NCI), Common Terminology Criteria for Adverse Events (CTCAE)
  - Grade 1: Mild pain not interfering with function
  - Grade 2: Moderate pain, limiting instrumental ADLs
  - Grade 3: Severe pain, limiting self-care ADLs
  - Grade 4: Disabling pain

Laboratory and Diagnostic Tests

- Complete blood cell count (CBC) with differential to evaluate neutropenia and rule out infection
- Chemistry studies to rule out hypokalemia, hyperkalemia, hypomagnesemia, hypocalcemia, hyponatremia, hypernatremia, and hypophosphatemia
- Creatine phosphokinase levels to rule out muscle inflammation or damage
- Urinalysis focusing on red blood cells
- Thyroid-stimulating hormone (TSH) level

- Blood cultures if neutropenia is suspected
- Electromyelography (EMG) to differentiate myelopathy from neuropathy
- Muscle biopsy to identify specific myopathies

Differential Diagnoses

- Cancer or metastatic disease
- Hematoma
- Ruptured tendon
- Thrombophlebitis
- Pyomyositis
  - Bacterial infection of the skeletal muscles that results in a pus-filled abscess
  - Most often caused by *Staphylococcus aureus*
- Fasciitis
- Sarcoidosis
- Ischemia or infarction
- Alcoholic myopathy
- Exertional muscle damage
- Fibromyalgia
- Inflammation
- Infections such as toxoplasmosis, trichinosis, influenza, herpes
- Electrolyte imbalance such as hypokalemia, hyperkalemia, hypomagnesemia, hypocalcemia, hyponatremia, hypernatremia, or hypophosphatemia
- Hypothyroidism
- Drugs: steroid withdrawal, paclitaxel (especially in combination with cisplatin), docetaxel, vincristine, vinblastine, vinorelbine, rituximab, etoposide, BCG, filgrastim, sargramostim, interferon, interleukin-2, dacarbazine, altretamine, topotecan, gemcitabine, procarbazine, fludarabine, letrozole (aromatase inhibitors as a class), azacytidine, cladribine, L-asparaginase, olaparib
- Amyloidosis
- Osteomalacia
  - The adult equivalent of the disease rickets
  - Defective mineralization of newly formed bone matrix
- Guillain-Barré syndrome
- Polymyalgia rheumatica
- Fabry disease
  - An X-linked recessive inherited lysosomal storage disease
- Parkinson disease

Interventions

- Treatment of the underlying disease
- Frequent rests interspersed with activity
- Maintain adequate nutrition and hydration

Pharmacologic Interventions

- Add medications as needed using the World Health Organization analgesic ladder as a reference
  - Acetaminophen (Tylenol), 650 mg orally every 4 hr as needed not to exceed 4 g/day
  - Ibuprofen (Motrin, Advil, Nuprin), 200-400 mg every 6 hr

- Indomethacin (Indocin), 25-50 mg orally twice or three times a day, not to exceed 200 mg/day
- Prednisone, 10 mg orally twice a day for 5 days after chemotherapy
- Amitriptyline, 25 mg orally at night
- Terfenadine (Seldane), 60 mg twice daily
- Glutamine, 10 g orally three times daily

Nonpharmacologic Interventions

- Heating pad or hot water bottle on the painful area
- Ice pack on the painful area
- Warm baths
- Complementary therapies such as massage, relaxation techniques, whirlpool, magnets

Patient Teaching

- Keep a diary of your pain
- If you are having pain for any reason, your health care provider will ask certain questions to determine the cause of your pain. Things to include are:
  - Onset: when did the pain start? What was I doing when I had pain?
  - Quality: What does the pain feel like? Is it knifelike and stabbing or dull and constant?
  - Location: Where is the pain? Can I point to it with my finger, or is it spread all over?
  - Intensity: How bad is your pain all the time? How bad is it with certain activities that cause you to feel pain, on a 1-10 scale, with the number "10" being the worst pain imaginable?
  - Duration: How long did the pain last?
  - Character: Does the pain come and go whenever I perform a certain activity, or is it unpredictable?
  - Relieving factors: What can I do to make the pain go away? Does anything help? What have I used in the past that has worked, and does this work now?
  - Your mood: Are you depressed or anxious? Does this make the pain worse?

Follow-up

- Pain service referral
- Physical therapy
- Occupational therapy
- Instruct patients to call the health care provider if they experience
  - New and increasingly severe back pain
  - A new symptom of numbness and tingling down the legs
  - Weakness or decreased sensation in the lower extremities
  - Loss of bowel function or bladder control

Resources

- Arthritis Foundation: Arthritis pain management. Available at http://www.arthritis.org/living-with-arthritis/pain-management/ (accessed February 10, 2016).

Principles of Symptom Management

- Chemocare: Muscle pain (myalgias). Available at http://chemocare.com/chemotherapy/side-effects/muscle-pain-myalgias.aspx (accessed February 10, 2016).

Bibliography

Brant, J. M. (2014). Bone pain. In D. Camp-Sorrell & R. A. Hawkins (Eds.), *Clinical manual for the oncology advanced practice nurse* (3rd ed.) (pp. 843–847). Pittsburgh: Oncology Nursing Press.

Chemocare: Pain & chemotherapy. Available at http://chemocare.com/chemotherapy/side-effects/pain-and-chemotherapy.aspx (accessed February 10, 2016).

Garrison, J. A., Mccune, J. S., Livingston, R. B., Linden, H. M., Gralow, J. R., Ellis, G. K., & West, H. L. (2003). *Myalgias and arthralgias associated with paclitaxel.* Available at http://www.cancernetwork.com/review-article/myalgias-and-arthralgias-associated-paclitaxel (accessed February 10, 2016).

Jones, C., Gilmore, J., Saleh, M., & Simmons, S. (2012). Therapeutic optimization of aromatase inhibitor–associated arthralgia: Etiology, onset, resolution, and symptom management in early breast cancer. *Community Oncology, 9,* 94–101.

Martin, V. R. (2014). Arthralgias and myalgias. In C. H. Yarbro, M. H. Frogge, & M. Goodman (Eds.), *Cancer symptom management.* Sudbury, MA: Jones & Bartlett.

MedlinePlus Medical Encyclopedia. (2016). *Joint pain.* Available at http://www.nlm.nih.gov/medlineplus/ency/article/003261.htm (accessed February 10, 2016).

MedlinePlus Medical Encyclopedia. (2016). *Muscle aches.* Available at http://www.nlm.nih.gov/medlineplus/ency/article/003178.htm (accessed February 10, 2016).

National Cancer Institute. (2010). *Common terminology criteria for adverse events, version 4.03.* Available at http://evs.nci.nih.gov/ftp1/CTCAE/CTCAE_4.03_2010-06-14_QuickReference_5x7.pdf (accessed February 10, 2016).

Niravath, P. (2013). Aromatase inhibitor-induced arthralgia: A review. *Annals of Oncology, 24,* 1443–1449.

Noonan, K. A. (2014). Arthralgia. In D. Camp-Sorrell & R. A. Hawkins (Eds.), *Clinical manual for the oncology advanced practice nurse* (3rd ed.) (pp. 849–857). Pittsburgh: Oncology Nursing Press.

Noonan, K. A. (2014). Myalgia. In D. Camp-Sorrell & R. A. Hawkins (Eds.), *Clinical manual for the oncology advanced practice nurse* (3rd ed.) (pp. 865–870). Pittsburgh: Oncology Nursing Press.

World Health Organization. website: http://www.who.int/cancer/palliative/painladder/en/ (accessed March 10, 2016).

Confusion

Carol S. Blecher

Definition

- Confusion, or cognitive failure, is a symptom or a description of a person's mental state.
- It has variable subjective symptoms and objective behaviors.
- It may be operationally defined as behaviors that fall into the following four categories:
  - Disorientation to time, place, or person
  - Inappropriate communication
  - Inappropriate behavior
  - Illusions, misinterpretation of real stimuli, or hallucinations, which are subjective sensory perceptions without real stimuli

- End-of-life confusion refers to cognitive failure caused by metastatic cancer and multiorgan system failure.

Pathophysiology and Contributing Factors

- The pathogenesis is not well understood.
- Contributing factors may include:
  - Reduced cerebral oxygen metabolism
  - Damaged neuronal enzyme synthesis
  - Neurotransmitter imbalance
  - Neuronal loss
  - Metabolic abnormality

Signs and Symptoms

- Hypoactive behavior, such as mental slowness, a generalized slowing down, or somnolence
- Hyperactive behavior, such as restlessness, pacing, searching, or picking
- Delusions
- Paranoia
- Poor memory or forgetfulness
- Inability to concentrate
- Changes in personality
- Changes in habits or ability to care for self

Assessment Tools

- Brief Cognitive Assessment/Mini Mental Status Examination including
  - Orientation to time and place
  - Memory test through repetition of the names of three unrelated objects
  - Attention and calculation with serial numbers testing
  - Language testing through identification of two items and repetition of a sentence
  - Following a multistep command, writing a sentence, and then copying a sentence
  - Confusion assessment measurement: 10-item scale administered by the clinician to assess nine domains of cognitive function
- Common terminology criteria for adverse events (CTCAE): grading for confusion and its associated symptoms, cognitive disturbances, and concentration impairments
  - Confusion
    - Grade 1: Mild disorientation
    - Grade 2: Moderate disorientation, limiting instrumental activities of daily living (ADLs)
    - Grade 3: Severe disorientation, limiting self-care ADLs
    - Grade 4: Life-threatening consequences, urgent intervention indicated
    - Grade 5: Death
  - Cognitive disturbance
    - Grade 1: Mild cognitive disability not interfering with work/school/life performance; specialized educational services or devices not indicated
    - Grade 2: Moderate cognitive disability interfering with work/school/life performance but capable of independent living; specialized resources on a part-time basis indicated

- Grade 3: Severe cognitive disability; significant impairment of work/school/life performance
- Concentration impairment
  - Grade 1: Mild inattention or decreased level of concentration
  - Grade 2: Moderate impairment in attention or decreased level of concentration, limiting instrumental ADLs
  - Grade 3: Severe impairment in attention or decreased level of concentration, limiting self-care ADLs
- Physical examination to rule out neurologic problems
- Cardiovascular examination to rule out cardiac abnormalities
- Pulmonary examination to rule out adventitious breath sounds

Laboratory and Diagnostic Tests

- Chemistry panel to evaluate for metabolic abnormalities:
  - Hypernatremia
  - Hyponatremia
  - Hypercalcemia
  - Hypomagnesemia
  - Hyperglycemia
  - Hypoglycemia
  - Liver function
- Complete blood cell count (CBC) to evaluate for
  - Leukocytosis
  - Anemia
- Serum therapeutic drug levels of
  - Digoxin
  - Lithium
  - Alcohol
  - Phenytoin
  - Gabapentin
- Ammonia level
- Magnetic resonance imaging (MRI) of the head to rule out brain metastases or hemorrhage
- Pulse oximetry or arterial blood gas (ABG) analysis to rule out hypoxia
- Lumbar puncture to assess for carcinomatous meningitis
- Electroencephalography (EEG)

Differential Diagnoses

- Electrolyte abnormalities
- Dehydration
- Renal failure
- Cirrhosis
- Sepsis
- Hypothermia
- Hyperthermia
- Meningitis
- Airway obstruction
- Syndrome of inappropriate antidiuretic hormone (SIADH) secretion
- Tumor lysis syndrome
- Constipation

- Drug-induced confusion related to
  - Cardiac drugs such as procainamide, propranolol, quinidine, lidocaine, clonidine, methyldopa, reserpine, digitalis
  - Gastrointestinal drugs such as atropine, belladonna, phenothiazine, scopolamine, cimetidine, ranitidine, metoclopramide
  - Musculoskeletal drugs such as corticosteroids, indomethacin, salicylate, diazepam
  - Neurologic/psychiatric drugs such as barbiturates, phenytoin, levodopa, amantadine, chloral hydrate, glutethimide, benzodiazepines, lithium salts, antidepressants
  - Respiratory/allergy drugs such as chlorpheniramine, cyproheptadine, diphenhydramine, theophylline
  - Analgesics such as opioids
  - Antidiabetic drugs such as insulin, oral hypoglycemics
  - Antineoplastic agents such as methotrexate, mitomycin, procarbazine, ifosfamide, interferon, L-asparaginase, cytarabine

Interventions

Pharmacologic Interventions

- Haloperidol (Haldol)
  - Mild confusion: 0.5-1.0 mg orally (PO), intramuscularly (IM), or intravenously (IV) twice a day
  - Agitated confusion: 1-2 mg every 30-60 min; after agitation is controlled, assess the 24-hr dose and adjust to a twice-daily dose
  - Terminal confusion: treat per protocol for mild confusion
- Lorazepam (Ativan) for use in confusion associated with alcohol withdrawal and hepatic encephalopathy; dose is 0.5-2.0 mg every 1-4 hr PO, IM, or IV
- Phenothiazine (Thorazine) for severe symptoms when sedation is required. Usual dose is 12.5-50 mg every 12 hr PO, IM, or IV.
- Diazepam (Valium) may be used but with caution because the active metabolites can cause prolonged sedation; dose is 2-10 mg PO or IV two to four times a day
- Midazolam (Versed), used only if all other methods fail to control symptoms; short half-life, so titration is easy; dose is 1-4 mg continuous IV or subcutaneous infusion.

Nonpharmacologic Interventions

- Correct or manage causative factors.
- Orient patient frequently with calendars, clocks, and reorientation to place.
- Ensure safety:
  - Keep bed in low position; if patient is hospitalized, keep call bell within reach.
  - Assist with toileting, ambulation, and positioning.
  - Check often for thirst, dry mouth, indigestion, hunger, pain, and hypothermia or hyperthermia.
  - Have support people stay with the patient, and avoid restraints.
  - Encourage the patient to use hearing aids and glasses if necessary.

- Patient is not to drive.
- Reassure patient frequently.

Patient Teaching

- If the patient has early-stage confusion, aim patient teaching toward offering reassurance, frequent orientation, and encouraging the safety mechanisms listed above while correcting or managing the causative factors.
- If the patient has late-stage confusion, direct education efforts toward the caregiver or family, offering reassurance and teaching them how to assist the patient according to the nonpharmacologic interventions listed above.

Follow-up

- Short term:
  - Monitor the effectiveness of the drug regimen over the first 24-48 hr.
  - Correct the underlying cause of confusion, and monitor for clearing of confusion.
  - Continue safety measures to reduce the risk for falls or self-injury.
  - In terminal-stage confusion, balance sedation with wakefulness to facilitate patient/caregiver/family communication.
- Long term:
  - Follow at-risk patients closely (e.g., elopement, self-injury)
  - Refer patient to psychiatrist or psychologist.
  - Refer patient for home care.
  - Refer patient to hospice if appropriate.

Resources

- Common terminology criteria for adverse events: http://evs.nci.nih.gov/ftp1/CTCAE/CTCAE_4.03_2010-06-14_QuickReference_5x7.pdf MedlinePlus Medical Encyclopedia. Confusion: http://www.nlm.nih.gov/medlineplus/ency/article/003205.htm
- National Comprehensive Cancer Network palliative care guidelines addressing distress: http://www.nccn.org/professionals/physician_gls/pdf/distress.pdf

Bibliography

Dahlin, C. (2014). Confusion/delirium. In D. Camp-Sorrell & R. A. Hawkins (Eds.), *Clinical manual for the oncology advanced practice nurse* (3rd ed.) (pp. 1099–1107). Pittsburgh, PA: Oncology Nursing Society.
National Institutes of Health, U.S. Library of Medicine. (2014). *Confusion.* Available at http://www.nlm.nih.gov/medlineplus/ency/article/003205.htm (accessed February 10, 2016).

Constipation

Carolyn Grande

Definition

- Passage of hard, dry stools with difficulty or discomfort
- Decrease in frequency of defecation
- Obstipation
  - A more severe form of constipation

- Absence of bowel movement despite large volumes of stool in the bowel
- Occurs in approximately 50% of cancer patients and in as many as 75% of terminally ill patients
- More common in women and the elderly

Pathophysiology and Contributing Factors

- Bowel function is determined by the state of intestinal motility and management of fluid in terms of absorption and secretion.
- Primary causes are related to extrinsic and lifestyle factors, including the following:
  - Age
  - Low-fiber diet
  - Dehydration
  - Decreased activity
  - Weakness/poor muscle tone
  - Extreme fatigue
- Secondary causes are related to medical conditions or disease processes that may cause hypomotility or obstruction.
- Iatrogenic causes result from medical interventions or from pharmacologic agents including the following drug classes:
  - Opioids
  - Anticonvulsants
  - Anesthetics
  - Anticholinergics
  - Tricyclic antidepressants
  - Diuretics
  - Iron supplements
  - Serotonin antagonists
  - Vinca alkaloids
- Surgical anastomosis may lead to narrowing of the colon lumen from scar tissue.

Signs and Symptoms

- Abdominal fullness
- Bloating
- Nausea
- Vomiting
- Excessive gas
- Cramping
- Change in bowel elimination pattern (size and consistency of stools)

Assessment Tools

- Comprehensive history:
  - Extent of cancer, past and current treatments
  - Dietary habits including fluid intake
  - Alcohol use
  - Medication list of prescribed and over-the-counter drugs with doses and frequency
  - Previous laxative or enema use and its effect
- Baseline frequency pattern of bowel elimination
- Description of last bowel movement:
  - When
  - Amount

- Consistency and color of stool
- Presence of blood
- Distinct odor change
- Comprehensive physical examination:
  - Abdominal examination, including auscultation for bowel sounds, percussion of all four quadrants, palpation for masses or hepatomegaly
  - Examination of anus for fissures, external hemorrhoids, inflammation
  - Rectal or stoma examination for masses, fecal impaction, stricture
  - Examination of stool for occult blood
- Accurate assessment tools are lacking in making the diagnosis of constipation. Given the subjective nature of constipation, the Rome criteria were developed to assist in diagnosing this symptom. Criteria to establish a diagnosis of constipation require that a patient has experienced the following within the past 3 months:
  - Straining with defecation
  - Hard stools
  - Incomplete evacuation
  - Anorectal blockage
  - Disimpaction
  - Fewer than three bowel movements in a week
  - The patient should not have loose stools or symptoms of irritable bowel syndrome.
- The National Cancer Institute has outlined the common terminology criteria for adverse events (CTCAE) grading system to assist in categorizing the severity of the event. Grading for constipation is as follows:
  - Grade 1: occasional or intermittent symptoms; occasional use of stool softeners, laxatives, dietary modification, or enema
  - Grade 2: persistent symptoms with regular use of laxatives or enemas indicated
  - Grade 3: symptoms interfering with activities of daily living, obstipation with manual evacuation indicated
  - Grade 4: life-threatening consequences (e.g., obstruction, toxic megacolon)
  - Grade 5: death

Laboratory and Diagnostic Tests

- Complete blood cell count, electrolyte panel including calcium and potassium, renal and liver function tests, thyroid function tests
- Supine and upright radiographic films to differentiate between mechanical obstruction and ileus
- Computed tomography of abdomen and pelvis if an extraluminal site is suspected
- Barium enema
- Sigmoidoscopy or colonoscopy

Differential Diagnosis

- Cancer
  - Mass obstruction
  - Spinal cord tumor compression at T8-L3
- Metabolic causes
  - Hypercalcemia
  - Hypokalemia
  - Uremia
  - Hypothyroidism
- Diseases and other conditions
  - Anorectal abscess
  - Anal fissure
  - Cirrhosis
  - Depression
  - Diabetes
  - Diverticulosis
  - Hepatic porphyria
  - Intestinal obstruction
  - Irritable bowel syndrome
  - Mesenteric artery ischemia
- Other
  - Dehydration
  - Nutritional compromise
  - Extreme fatigue/weakness
  - Poor muscle tone

Interventions

Pharmacologic Interventions

- Laxatives and cathartics are divided into categories on the basis of the mechanism of action.
- Bulk formers: onset of effect in 12 hours to 3 days
  - Psyllium (Metamucil)
  - Methylcellulose (Cologel, Citrucel)
- Bowel stimulants: onset of effect in 6-10 hours, rectally in 15-60 minutes
  - Phenolphthalein (Ex-lax, Feen-a-mint, Correctol)
  - Bisacodyl (Dulcolax), 5 mg tablet one to three times a day; suppository 10 mg as needed
  - Senna (Senokot), 187 mg tablet, maximum eight per day
  - Cascara sagrada, 5 mL or 1 tablet as needed at bedtime
  - Casanthranol, 30 mg usually in combination with docusate
- Osmotic laxatives
  - MiraLax: onset of effect in 2 to 4 days; 1 tablespoon (17 g) in 4-8 ounces of water, juice, soda, coffee, or tea daily
  - Lactulose: onset of effect in 24-48 hours
    - Cephulac, 30-45 mL three or four times daily, or hourly to induce rapid effect
    - Chronulac, 15-30 mL/day, maximum 60 mL/day
    - Sorbitol, 3-150 mL/day
  - Polyethylene glycol electrolyte solution: onset of effect within 1 hour
    - GoLYTELY, 8 ounces orally every 15 minutes as tolerated over 3-4 hours until 1 L has been taken or diarrhea results
  - Glycerin suppositories: onset of effect within 30 minutes; one or two per day as needed or 5-15 mL as enema
- Lubricants: onset of effect within 8 hours
  - Mineral oil, 15-40 mL/day, once or in divided doses; as a retention enema, 60-150 mL/day

- Detergent laxatives: onset of effect in 24-72 hours
  - Docusate, 50-500 mg/day, once or in divided doses
    - Docusate sodium (Colace)
    - Docusate calcium (Surfak)
- Saline laxatives
  - Magnesium salts:
    - Magnesium citrate, $^1/_2$ to 1 full bottle orally as needed, onset of effect in 30 minutes to 6 hours depending on dose
    - Magnesium hydroxide (milk of magnesia), 30-60 mL/day orally in single or divided doses, onset of effect in 4-8 hours
  - Sodium salts:
    - Sodium phosphate (Fleet Phospho-soda), 20-30 mL as a single dose, onset of effect in 3-6 hours
    - Fleet enema, onset of effect in 3-5 minutes
- Use of these agents can be initiated with a four-step approach. Advancement to the next step is indicated if the prior step at maximal doses was ineffective. Allow at least 48 hours to evaluate effectiveness of an intervention:
  - Step 1: bulk laxatives or milk of magnesia
  - Step 2: docusate sodium, senna, or milk of magnesia
  - Step 3: sorbitol or lactulose
  - Step 4: magnesium citrate or GoLYTELY
- Drug and dosage should be determined by patient condition, response, and tolerance of side effects. For patients receiving opioids for chronic pain or who have vinca alkaloid–containing chemotherapy regimens, prophylaxis for constipation with a stool softener and a stimulant laxative should be used.

Nonpharmacologic Interventions

- Increase daily intake of dietary fiber, gradually titrate 3-4 g/day to total of 10-20 g/day. For patients with structural blockage, this method should be avoided because it may increase the obstruction. Sources of fiber include the following:
  - Wheat bran
  - Whole grain breads
  - Peanuts
  - Peanut butter
  - Peas
  - Unpeeled pears
  - Dried apricots
  - Beans
- Increase fluid intake to six to eight 8-ounce glasses of water daily; avoid coffee, tea, and grapefruit juice because they can have a diuretic effect.
- Establish a toileting routine after breakfast, when contractions within the intestines are strongest.
- Increase exercise to improve gastrointestinal motility.

Patient Teaching

- Prevention of constipation is the goal.
- Recommend that patients consistently carry a water bottle to sip on throughout the day.
- Develop a routine for toileting, at the same time each day.
- Establish an exercise routine of at least 30 minutes/day.

- Incorporate at least 10 g of dietary fiber/day into the meal plan.
- Initiate bowel regimen as specified by physician or nurse concurrently with chronic opioid use for pain management.
- Initiate prophylactic bowel regimen as specified by physician or nurse with chemotherapy regimens containing vincristine or vinblastine.

Follow-up

- Contact the nurse or physician for persistent constipation or if pain or bleeding ensues.

Resources

- Chemocare: Constipation and chemotherapy. Available at http://chemocare.com/chemotherapy/side-effects/constipation-and-chemotherapy.aspx (accessed January 6, 2016).

Bibliography

http://www.cancercare.org/publications/218-coping_with_constipation (accessed March 19, 2016).

Clark, K., Urban, K., & Currow, D. C. (2010). Current approaches to diagnosing and managing constipation in advanced cancer and palliative care. *Journal of Palliative Medicine, 13*(4), 473–476.

Gibson, R. J., & Keefe, D. M. K. (2006). Cancer chemotherapy-induced diarrhea and constipation: Mechanisms of damage and prevention strategies. *Support Care Cancer, 14*, 890–900.

Lagman, R. L. (2006). Constipation: Not a mundane symptom. *The Journal of Supportive Oncology, 4*, 223–224.

Sykes, N. P. (2006). The pathogenesis of constipation. *The Journal of Supportive Oncology, 4*, 213–218.

Thomas, J. (2006). Strategies to manage constipation. *The Journal of Supportive Oncology, 4*, 220–223.

National Cancer Institute, National Institutes of Health. (2010). *Common terminology criteria for adverse events (CTCAE)*, version 4.03. Available at http://ctep.cancer.gov/protocolDevelopment/electronic_applications/ctc.htm (accessed February 18, 2016).

Woolery, M., Bisanz, A., Lyons, H., Gaido, L., Yenulevich, M., Fulton, S., & McMillan, S. C. (2008). Putting evidence into practice: Evidence-based interventions for the prevention and management of constipation in patients with cancer. *Clinical Journal of Oncology Nursing, 12*, 317–337.

Cough

Ruth Canty Gholz

Definition

- A pulmonary protective reflex
- An explosive expiration for clearing the tracheobronchial tree
- Categorized as acute or chronic
- May become excessive and nonproductive, possibly harming the airway mucosa

Pathophysiology and Contributing Factors

- Common causes include asthma, gastroesophageal reflux disease, and upper airway cough syndrome (formerly called postnasal drip syndrome).
- It can result from aspiration, inhalation of matter, pathogens, inflammation, or inflammatory mediators.
- It may be voluntary or involuntary.
- It starts with an inspiratory gasp to the closing of the glottis, followed by a Valsalva maneuver, and ending with an expiratory release.
- Vagal afferent nerves initiate the cough reflex. They are plentiful in the airway mucosa and airway wall.
- The "cough center" in the medulla generates an efferent signal.
- During cough, intrathoracic pressures rise and expiratory pressures may near 500 mph.
- Excessive cough interferes with breathing and sleep and may cause headache, pain, nausea, vomiting, syncope, and urinary incontinence.

Signs and Symptoms

- Patients present with cough interfering with quality of life.
- Cough is persistent.
- There is frequent throat clearing
- Cough may be accompanied by wheezing or dyspnea.
- Cough becomes worse with exposure to fragrances, cold dry air, or pollutants.
- Cough may be productive or nonproductive of sputum.
- Air flow obstruction may be present.

Assessment Tools

- Patient history
- Medication review, being alert to use of angiotensin-converting enzyme (ACE) inhibitors
- Character and timing of cough
- Precipitating factors
- Smoking history or exposure to environmental or occupational irritants
- Physical assessment
  - Oropharynx examination: assess for mucus or erythema
  - Pulmonary examination: assess respiratory muscles, lung sounds
  - Cardiovascular examination: jugular venous distention, wet lung sounds

Laboratory and Diagnostic Tests

- Sputum cytology, sputum culture, arterial blood gas analysis
- Chest radiographic film
- Computed tomography of chest, bronchoscopy, and pulmonary function tests if indicated
  - Methacholine challenge
  - Monitoring of esophageal pH

Differential Diagnoses

- Asthma, chronic obstructive pulmonary disease (COPD), pulmonary fibrosis, interstitial lung disease
- Infection, aspiration, superior vena cava syndrome
- Obstruction, pericardial or pleural effusion, endobronchial tumor
- Lymphangitis, paraneoplastic syndrome
- Gastroesophageal syndromes
- Esophagorespiratory fistula
- Radiation pneumonitis

Interventions

- Must treat the underlying disease process as well as the cough

Pharmacologic Interventions

- Centrally acting antitussives: codeine, hydrocodone, dextromethorphan
- Peripherally acting antitussives: benzonatate levodropropizine, moguisteine
- Antihistamine/decongestant combination
- Expectorants
- Anticholinergics
- Morphine
- Over-the-counter lozenges
- Nasal spray, ipratropium bromide
- Inhaled bronchodilators or inhaled corticosteroids or oral steroids
- Antibiotic if infection is present
- Palliative chemotherapy and/or radiation therapy
- If no improvement: inhaled cromolyn sodium or lidocaine, nebulized morphine, paroxetine, benzodiazepines

Nonpharmacologic Interventions

- Warm humidified air
- Deep breathing exercises
- Sleeping or resting lying on side
- Splinting with pillow to reduce strain

Patient Teaching

- Take medications as prescribed.
- Reduce exposure to irritants.
- Stop smoking, and maintain a smoke-free environment.
- Perform coughing and deep breathing exercises including splinting with pillow to reduce strain.
- Sleep in a semi-upright position.
- Add warm humidified air to room.
- Keep a journal to document the course of the cough.

Follow-up

- Report change in sputum production: change in color, odor, blood tinged.
- Report fevers or chills.
- Report sudden onset of chest pain or shortness of breath.

Resources

- National Institute of health: www.nih.gov
- Lungcancer.org: www.lungcancer.org
- Oncology Nursing Society: www.ons.org
- Coughjournal.com

- Chemocare: Cough and chemotherapy. Available at http://chemocare.com/chemotherapy/side-effects/cough-and-chemotherapy.aspx (accessed January 6, 2016).

Bibliography

Harle, A. S., Blackhall, F. H., Smith, J. A., & Molassiotis, A. (2012). Understanding cough and its management in lung cancer. *Current Opinion in Supportive and Palliative Care, 6*(2), 153–162.

Lechtzin, N. (2014). *Cough in adults.* Available at http://www.merckmanuals.com/professional/pulmonary_disorders/symptoms_of_pulmonary_disorders/cough_in_adults.html (accessed February 18, 2016).

Molassiotis, A., Bailey, C., Caress, A., Brunton, L., & Smith, J. (2010). Interventions for cough in cancer. *Cochrane Database of Systematic Reviews* (9), CD007881.

Pratter, M., Brightling, C., Boulet, L., & Irwin, R. S. (2006). An empiric integrative approach to the management of cough: ACCP evidence-based clinical practice guidelines. *Chest, 129*(1 Suppl), 222S–231S.

Silvestri, R., & Weinberger, S. (2014). *Evaluation of subacute and chronic cough in adults.* Available at http://www.uptodate.com/contents/evaluation-of-subacute-and-chronic-cough-in-adults?source=see_link (accessed February 18, 2016).

Von Gunten, C., & Bucholz, G. (2014). *Palliative care: Overview of cough, stridor, and hemoptysis.* Available at http://www.uptodate.com/contents/palliative-care-overview-of-cough-stridor-and-hemoptysis?source=search_result&search=cough+stridor+hemoptysis&selectedTitle=1%7E150 (accessed February 18, 2016).

Depressed Mood

Denice Economou

Definition

- Major depressive disorder is diagnosed according to the *Diagnostic and Statistical Manual of Mental Disorders, Fourth Edition* (DSM-IV).
- Patients report a depressed mood or state that they have experienced a loss of interest or pleasure, lasting most of the day, in almost all of their activities for at least 2 weeks.
- Four of the following additional conditions must exist:
  - Decreased energy
  - Feelings of guilt or lack of worth
  - Difficulty concentrating or making decisions
  - Recurrent thoughts of death or suicidal thoughts or plans
  - Changes in appetite or weight
  - Changes in sleep patterns
- Many of the physical symptoms that relate to appetite, concentration, and lack of energy also can result from a cancer patient's treatment regimen. For this reason, depression in oncology patients is often missed or undertreated.
- Depression affects treatment adherence due to lack of motivation, withdrawal, and isolation.

Pathophysiology and Contributing Factors

- Both biologic and psychosocial factors influence mood disturbances in patients.
- Genetic factors may make some patients more susceptible to the development of depression.
- Physiologic stressors including medications, endocrine or nutritional disturbances, and infections can induce biochemical changes that precipitate depression.
- Developmental events or multiple losses may sensitize a patient, causing the patient to lose the ability to cope with their illness.
- These factors contribute to changes in neurotransmission, affecting mood, motivation, and psychomotor function. Norepinephrine and serotonin are the neurotransmitters most often associated with depression. Medications used to manage depression are related to regulation of these transmitters.
- Medication classes associated with depressive side effects include analgesics, anticonvulsants, antihypertensives, antiinflammatory agents, antimicrobials, antineoplastics, cytotoxics, hormones, immunosuppressive agents, sedatives, steroids, stimulants, tranquilizers, and benzodiazepines.
- Cancer diagnosis causes fear of pain, dependence, and altered body image; distress; and fear of death.
- Psychological factors contribute to feelings of depression (i.e., coping ability, emotional maturity, disruption of life's plans).
- Social factors associated with depressed mood include financial stability, emotional support from family or friends, and occupational successes or failures.
- The mood state of depression includes feelings of gloom, despair, numbness, emptiness, lack of worth, hopelessness, and helplessness.

Signs and Symptoms

- Mood that seems depressed for at least 2 weeks
- Unable to find pleasure in activities that used to be enjoyable
- Feelings of worthlessness
- Difficulty concentrating
- Difficulty sleeping or sleeping too much
- Fatigue
- Verbalizes thoughts of dying or committing suicide

Assessment Tools

- All patients should be screened for depression at their initial visit and as appropriate thereafter.
- One of the most accurate screening measurements is a single question: "Are you depressed most of the day nearly every day?" A positive response necessitates further evaluation. A study of 197 patients with advanced cancer found that this question showed 100% sensitivity and 100% specificity for depression.
- The Beck Depression Inventory (BDI) is a 21-item questionnaire that takes about 2-5 minutes to complete and has an average specificity of 90%.
- Hospital Anxiety and Depression Scale (HADS)
- National Comprehensive Cancer Network (NCCN) Distress Thermometer Scale
- Two items from the nine-item Personal Health Questionnaire (PHQ-9), based on American Society of Clinical Oncology (ASCO) guideline for screening and assessment of depression in adults with cancer, to guide further assessment:
  - Little interest or pleasure in doing things
  - Feeling down, depressed or helpless (depressed mood)

- Assessment should include the following:
  - Report of depression
  - Signs and symptoms (four or more of those listed in the "Definition" section)
  - History of depression or substance abuse (drugs or alcohol)
  - Medications associated with depression
  - Patient with head and neck, gastrointestinal, or lung cancer (higher risk for suicide)
  - Unrelieved pain
- Social worker assessment can be beneficial to assist with evaluation and management of appropriate problems.
- Predictors of risk include a history of poor coping or psychological adjustment skills. Patients with a history of clinically significant anxiety or depression or major psychiatric syndromes should be monitored closely throughout treatment.
- Social support: Patients who are able to maintain close connections with family and friends cope more effectively with their illness and their outlook for the future.
- Cultural considerations: What is the language used to describe feelings of depression? Latin and Mediterranean cultures may complain of nerves or headaches. Asian or Chinese cultures may use words related to weakness, tiredness, or imbalance. Middle Eastern cultures may refer to problems of the heart or feeling heartbroken.

Laboratory and Diagnostic Tests

- There are no laboratory or diagnostic tests to screen for depressed mood (refer to "Assessment Tools").

Differential Diagnoses

- Fatigue
- Hypothyroidism
- Bipolar disorder
- Anxiety

Interventions

Pharmacologic Interventions

- Antidepressant medications used in the cancer setting include selective serotonin reuptake inhibitors (SSRIs) and serotonin-norepinephrine reuptake inhibitors (SNRIs) aimed at symptomatic benefit. Antidepressants are especially effective when used in conjunction with behavioral interventions and follow-up.
  - SSRIs: fluoxetine, mirtazapine, paroxetine, sertraline (helpful for sleep aid, appetite stimulant, less gastrointestinal effects, few P450 interactions)
  - SNRIs: duloxetine, venlafaxine (helpful for hot flashes and neuropathic pain; least interaction with tamoxifen)
  - Atypical antidepressants: trazodone (helpful as a sleep aid)
  - Psychostimulants: buproprion (may be helpful for low energy or concentration issues)
  - When prescribing, consider the short- and long-term side effects, possible interactions with other medications and other illnesses, and prior response to antidepressants.
  - Monitor patients who are taking psychotropic medications for dosing accuracy, especially when therapies change or invasive procedures (e.g., surgery, chemotherapy) or disease progression occurs.
- Common side effects of antidepressants include sedation, anticholinergic effects, orthostatic hypotension, and weight gain.

Nonpharmacologic Interventions

- If a patient verbalizes thoughts or plans for committing suicide, immediate evaluation is necessary. If a patient verbalizes thoughts of jumping out a window, shooting himself or herself, or self-harm in other ways, the nurse must assess whether the patient has access to complete these threats and must remove the patient from harm. The patient's psychiatrist should be called at this time.
  - Statements such as "I should just kill myself" or "I have no reason to go on living" require further evaluation. Always ask "Do you have a plan?" "Can you tell me what it is?"
  - Statements of feeling hopeless or helpless must be evaluated because these patients are at high risk for suicide.
- Help patients identify and build adaptive coping mechanisms.
- Help patients regain a sense of control over their lives; provide options when possible.
- Be available to your patient. Help to normalize the patient's feelings and maintain realistic hope.
- Any reference to suicide must be referred for further evaluation beyond the nurse who is taking care of the patient.
- Counseling

Patient Teaching

- Patients with depressed mood are at higher risk for noncompliance with their treatments. Monitor and encourage adherence.
- Reinforce hope and educate family and caregivers on the patient's needs as appropriate.
- If suicidal thoughts have been identified, caregivers must be aware of these feelings and take preventive actions in the home to remove items that may be used to complete these threats (e.g., guns, knives, ropes). A suicide hotline phone number should be accessible.
- Discuss plans with the patient so that suicide is not thought of as an automatic solution to problems. Interventions should be provided to relieve extreme symptoms and improve quality of life.
- Feelings of hopelessness, helplessness, and worthlessness need to be discussed, and the patient's ability to mobilize personal support systems needs to be established.
- Caregiver support is essential.

Follow-up

- If the patient screens positively for depression, notify the physician for referral to a psychiatric professional for further assessment.
- If the patient reports a desire to commit suicide, discuss the plan with the patient and notify the physician immediately. Take necessary steps to protect the patient from self-harm, and arrange for immediate psychiatric follow-up.

- Ask specific questions regarding mood. Be aware of statements that refer to feelings of hopelessness, being a burden to one's family, financial concerns, or unrelieved symptoms.
- Assess distress levels related to fatigue, pain, mood, or family and financial concerns.
- Continue to provide hope and support.

Resources

- http://www.cancer.net/coping-and-emotions/managing-emotions/depression

Bibliography

Andersen, B. L., DeRubeis, R. J., Berman, B. S., Gruman, J., Champion, V. L., Massie, M. J., & Rowland, J. H. (2014). Screening, assessment, and care of anxiety and depressive symptoms in adults with cancer: An American Society of Clinical Oncology guideline adaptation. *Journal of Clinical Oncology, 32*(15), 1605–1620.

Albright, A. V., & Valente, S. (2006). Depression and suicide. In R. M. Carroll-Johnson, L. M. Gorman, & N. J. Bush (Eds.), *Psychosocial nursing care along the cancer continuum* (pp. 241–274). Pittsburgh, PA: Oncology Nursing Press.

Fulcher, C. (2014). Depression. In C. Yarbro, D. Wujcik, & B. H. Gobel (Eds.), *Cancer symptom management* (4th ed.) (pp. 655–671). Burlington, MA: Jones & Bartlett Learning.

Jacobsen, P., & Jim, H. (2008). Psychosocial interventions for anxiety and depression in adult cancer patients: Achievements and challenges. *CA A Cancer Journal for Clinicians, 58*, 214–230.

Pasacreta, J., Minarik, P. A., Nield-Anderson, L., & Paice, J. (2015). Anxiety and depression. In B. Ferrell, N. Coyle, & J. Paice (Eds.), *Textbook of palliative nursing* (4th ed.) (pp. 366–384). New York: Oxford University Press.

Trill, M. D. (2012). Psychological aspects of depression in cancer patients: An update. *Annals of Oncology, 23*(10 Suppl.), 302–305.

Diarrhea

Carolyn Grande

Definition

- Increase in frequency, volume, and consistency of stool
- Passage of ≥200 g of stool/day
- Can be acute or chronic
- Experienced by 10% of advanced cancer patients and 43% of bone marrow transplantation patients
- Diarrhea classifications:
  - *Osmotic diarrhea* is related to mechanical disturbances resulting from ingestion of hyperosmolar substances such as sorbitol or enteral feeding solutions (J-tubes, G-tubes). The diarrhea is watery and voluminous, resolving when the causative agent is withdrawn.
  - *Secretory diarrhea* is related to biochemical disturbances causing a mechanical response. The origins of these disturbances are enterotoxin-producing pathogens such as *Clostridium difficile* and *Escherichia coli* or endocrine tumors. The diarrhea is watery and voluminous.
  - *Exudative diarrhea* is often the toxic effect of radiation therapy to the bowel mucosa. This diarrhea is characterized by high frequency (>6 stools/day) with variable volume, although less than 1000 mL/day. Stools are characterized by mucus and blood.
  - *Malabsorptive diarrhea* is related to both mechanical and biochemical disturbances. These disturbances can result from enzyme deficiencies. Stools are voluminous, foul smelling, and steatorrhea type.
  - *Dysmotility-associated diarrhea* is related to a mechanical disturbance or peristaltic dysfunction that results in rapid transit time of stool through the small and large intestine. Stools are small, semisolid to liquid in consistency, with variable volume and frequency.
  - *Chemotherapy-induced diarrhea* results from mechanical and biochemical disturbances caused by the effects of chemotherapy on the bowel mucosa. Stools are watery or semisolid.

Pathophysiology and Contributing Factors

- Gastrointestinal (GI) motility involves processes that promote the absorption of nutrients. Movement through the GI tract requires coordination of intraluminal pressures and smooth muscle contractions controlled by the enteric nervous system and peptide hormonal release. Diarrhea is caused by an imbalance in the physiologic mechanisms of the GI tract. It is the result of impaired absorption and excessive secretion.
- Decreased absorption of fluid and electrolyte can result from
  - Presence of osmotically active substances in the lumen
  - Increased intestinal motility
- Increased secretion of fluid and electrolytes can result from
  - Endogenous secretions
  - Exogenous toxins
- With radiation therapy that involves the abdomen or pelvis and in chemotherapy-induced diarrhea, acute damage to the epithelial crypt cells results in necrosis, inflammation, and ulceration of the intestinal mucosa. Atrophy and fibrosis of the lining can occur over time, resulting in decreased absorption of water and electrolytes and producing diarrhea.
- Risk factors for diarrhea:
  - Chemotherapy
    - Diarrhea from previous chemotherapy cycles
    - Types of chemotherapeutic agents, including fluoropyrimidines, topoisomerase I inhibitors (irinotecan, topotecan), antitumor antibiotic (actinomycin D), and toxoid (paclitaxel)
  - Other factors, such as the presence of primary tumor
  - Radiation therapy (RT)—diarrhea is dependent on
    - Total RT dose
    - Size of the RT field
    - Site being irradiated
    - Dose per fraction

Signs and Symptoms

- Increased number of stools/day
- Nocturnal stool
- Incontinence
- Cramping
- Patient may have other symptoms:
  - Nausea/vomiting
  - Hypotension

- Dizziness
- Decreased skin turgor
- Dry mouth
- Perianal irritation

Assessment Tools

- Comprehensive history:
  - Cancer diagnosis, past and current treatments
  - Sites of metastasis
  - Complete medication list:
    - Laxatives
    - Opioids or recent opioid withdrawal
    - Recent antibiotic therapy
    - Regular and as-needed prescription medications
    - Over-the-counter medications
    - Herbal and vitamin supplements
    - Chemotherapy/biotherapy agents
- The hallmark assessment tool is the patient report.
  - Description of baseline bowel movements and current bowel movement history:
    - When
    - Amount
    - Consistency and color of stool
    - Incontinence
    - Presence of blood
    - Distinct odor change
- Assess for signs and symptoms of dehydration:
  - Orthostatic hypotension
  - Dry mouth
  - Excessive thirst
  - Dizziness
  - Feelings of weakness
  - Decreased urination
  - Weight loss
- Comprehensive physical examination
  - Abdomen
    - Palpate for tenderness, distention
    - Percuss—dullness may indicate obstruction, fecal impaction
    - Auscultate for bowel sounds
- The National Cancer Institute has outlined the common terminology criteria for adverse events (CTCAE) grading system to assist in categorizing the severity of the event (see table below).
- Diarrhea can originate in the small bowel or in the colon, or it can occur in an ostomy.

Laboratory and Diagnostic Tests

- Complete blood cell count
- Stool test for occult blood
- Metabolic panel to assess electrolyte levels, blood urea nitrogen (BUN)/creatinine, albumin
- Stool cultures for enteric pathogens, *Clostridium difficile*, and ova and parasites
- Radiography: flat plate of the abdomen or obstruction series (as indicated by history and physical examination)

Differential Diagnoses

- Carcinoid syndrome
- Chemotherapy-induced or targeted therapy–induced diarrhea
- Radiation therapy–induced diarrhea
- *C. difficile* infection
- Enzyme deficiency
- Crohn disease
- Acute viral, bacterial, or protozoal infections
- Intestinal obstruction
  - Tumor
  - Stool
  - Scar tissue
- Irritable bowel disease
- Ischemic bowel disease
- Lactose intolerance
- Pseudomembranous enterocolitis
- Rotavirus gastroenteritis
- Thyrotoxicosis
- Ulcerative colitis
- Laxative overuse
- Opioid withdrawal

Interventions

Pharmacologic Interventions

The intervention selected should be correlated with the root cause of the diarrhea. Maximizing the use of a particular intervention, while monitoring patient adherence to the prescribed regimen, is critical in determining efficacy. Antidiarrheal agents are divided into categories based on the mechanism of action:

- Opioids
  - Lomotil: 2.5 mg diphenoxylate with 0.025 mg atropine sulfate/tablet. May give a loading dose with 2 tablets, then 1 to 2 tablets four times daily, not to exceed 8 tablets/day
  - Codeine: 15-60 mg orally every 4-6 hours as needed

Common Terminology Criteria for Adverse Events (CTCAE) Reporting: Diarrhea*

Adverse Event	Grade 1	Grade 2	Grade 3	Grade 4	Grade 5
Diarrhea	Increase of <4 stools/day over baseline; mild increase in ostomy output compared with baseline	Increase of 4-6 stools/day over baseline; moderate ostomy output compared with baseline	Increase of ≥7 stools/day; incontinence; hospitalization indicated; severe increase in ostomy output compared with baseline; limiting self-care activities of daily living (ADLs)	Life-threatening consequence; urgent intervention needed	Death

*A semicolon indicates "or" in the grade description.
From National Cancer Institute, National Institutes of Health. (2010). Common terminology criteria for adverse events (CTCAE), version 4.03. Available at http://ctep.cancer.gov/protocolDevelopment/electronic_applications/ctc.htm (accessed February 18, 2016).

- Opium tincture: 10% opium liquid (10 mg morphine/mL with 19% alcohol); 0.3-1 mL orally every 2-6 hours until controlled, not to exceed 6 mL/24 hours.
- Paregoric: 0.4 mg morphine/mL orally one to four times daily or 4 mL every 4 hours
- Nonopioids
  - Imodium (loperamide): 2-mg capsules or liquid 1 mg/mL or 1 mg/5 mL; may give a loading dose of 4 mg orally, then 2 mg after each loose stool, not to exceed 16 mg/day
- Absorbents
  - Bismuth subsalicylate (Pepto-Bismol): chewable tablets 262 mg or suspensions 262 mg/15 mL or 524 mg/15 mL. Dosing is 524 mg every 30 minutes, not to exceed 5 g/day
  - Kaopectate (5.85 gm kaolin and 130 mg pectin/30 mL): 2-6 g every 4 hours as needed
- Somatostatin analog
  - Octreotide acetate: 50-200 mcg subcutaneously three times daily
  - Sandostatin LAR 20-30 mg intramuscular injection every 28 days

Nonpharmacologic Interventions

- Diet modifications, including
  - Foods that build stool consistency (i.e., low in fiber, pectin containing)
  - Foods high in potassium
  - Foods at room temperature to minimize peristalsis
  - Lactose-free diet if indicated
  - Fluid intake at least 3 L/day

Patient Teaching

- Encourage foods that are low in fiber and that contain pectin (* = high in potassium):
  - Beets
  - Applesauce (without spice)
  - Peeled apple
  - White rice
  - Banana*
  - Baked potato without skin
  - White bread
  - Plain pasta
  - Avocados*
  - Asparagus tips*
- Encourage foods high in potassium:
  - Peach and apricot nectar
  - Boiled or mashed potatoes without skin
  - Lactose-free milk
  - Fish
  - Bananas
- Avoid high-fiber, high-fat, greasy, or spicy foods or caffeine-containing foods:
  - Whole grain breads or cereals
  - Raw vegetables
  - Nuts
  - Seeds
  - Popcorn
  - Relishes or pickles

- High-fat spreads or dressings
- Chocolate
- Coffee/tea
- Increase fluids to at least 3 L/day:
  - Bouillon
  - Fruitades
  - Gatorade, Propel, or other sports drinks
  - Pedialyte or Pedialyte ice pops
  - Ice pops
  - Gelatin
- Avoid alcohol and carbonated beverages.
- Maintain a lactose-free diet when indicated.
  - Avoid milk and dairy products
  - May use lactose-free dairy products or soy milk products
- Maintain skin integrity.
  - Cleanse rectal area after each bowel movement with soft wipes; pat rather than rub perianal area when cleansing.
  - Apply a topical skin barrier ointment such as Desitin or A&D ointment.
  - Take sitz baths as needed.
- Take antidiarrheal medication as prescribed.

Follow-up

- Have patient or caregiver record number and consistency of stools.
- Call physician or nurse if diarrhea persists in frequency and volume >24 hours after following outlined plan of care.

Resources

- Chemocare: Diarrhea and chemotherapy. Available at http://chemocare.com/chemotherapy/side-effects/diarrhea-and-chemotherapy.aspx (accessed January 6, 2016).

Bibliography

Benson, A. B., III, Ajani, J. A., Catalano, R. B., Engelking, C., Kornblau, S. M., Martenson, J. A., Jr., & Wadler, S. (2004). Recommended guidelines for the treatment of cancer treatment-induced diarrhea. *Journal of Clinical Oncology, 22,* 2918–2926.

Gibson, R. J., & Keefe, D. M. K. (2006). Cancer chemotherapy-induced diarrhea and constipation: Mechanisms of damage and prevention strategies. *Supportive Care in Cancer, 14,* 890–900.

Muehlbauer, P. M., Thorpe, D., Davis, A., Drabot, R., Rawlings, B. L., & Kiker, E. (2009). Putting evidence into practice: Evidence-based interventions to prevent, manage and treat chemotherapy and radiotherapy-induced diarrhea. *Clinical Journal of Oncology Nursing, 13,* 336–341.

O'Brien, B. E., Kaklamani, V. G., & Benson, A. B. (2005). The assessment and management of cancer treatment related diarrhea. *Clinical Colorectal Cancer, 4*(6), 375–381.

Richardson, G., & Dobish, R. (2007). Chemotherapy induced diarrhea. *Journal of Oncology Pharmacy Practice, 13,* 181–198.

National Cancer Institute, National Institutes of Health. (2010). *Common terminology criteria for adverse events (CTCAE), version 4.03.* Available at http://ctep.cancer.gov/protocolDevelopment/electronic_applications/ctc.htm (accessed February 18, 2016).

Dizziness and Vertigo

Ruth Canty Gholz

Definition

- Described in terms of sensations
- Lightheadedness, fainting, spinning, confusion, blurred vision, tingling
- Nonspecific symptoms
- Clustered with vertigo, dizziness, disequilibrium, and presyncope (prodromal symptom for fainting or near fainting)
- Unsteadiness
- Must fit patient into category of dizziness, vertigo, or presyncope
- May include nausea and/or vomiting

Pathophysiology and Contributing Factors

- Vertigo (a symptom of dizziness) is caused by a disturbance in the vestibular system: sensory, visual, or somatosensory. The vestibular system includes apparatus in inner ear, the vestibular nerve and nucleus in the medulla, and connections from the cerebellum.
- Contributing factors may be specific or nonspecific.
- Symptoms are never continuous.
- It may be made worse by movement of the head or cervical spine.
- There is a disruption between vestibular apparatus and the brain.
- A prior psychological disorder may be a factor.

Signs and Symptoms

- Lightheadedness
- Feeling of spinning (similar to coming off a roller coaster or when spun multiple times)
- Imbalance, tipping to one side
- Nausea and vomiting with the spinning
- Visual changes
- Auditory changes
- May be episodic or regular, in short or long duration
- Out-of-body feeling
- Additional paresthesias of face or limbs possible

Assessment Tools

- Patient history, including head injury, comorbid conditions
- Identify what dizziness means to patient, full sensations, duration, and aggravating, triggering, and alleviating factors
- Neurologic examination
- Orthostatic assessment
- Ear, nose, and throat (ENT) examination (dizziness with vertigo involves the peripheral vestibular system)
- Medication review
- Assessment for nystagmus, hearing loss, ataxic gait, nausea, vomiting, visual changes, numbness, incoordination
- Social history, including any history of substance abuse
- Psychological assessment

Laboratory and Diagnostic Tests

- Complete blood count (CBC), blood glucose level, thyroid-stimulating hormone (TSH) level
- Range of motion with emphasis on cervical spine
- Cervical spine radiographic film
- Vestibular function tests
- Stimulate to hyperventilate
- Magnetic resonance imaging (MRI) if focal neurologic symptoms are present

Differential Diagnoses

- Meniere disease
- Diseases of the central nervous system (CNS)
- Cerebrovascular disease
- Orthostasis
- Neurologic deficit
- Dehydration
- Hyperventilation
- Parkinson disease
- Medication side effect
- Labyrinthitis
- Malignancy
- Cervical spine disorders

Interventions

Pharmacologic Interventions

- Antihistamines: meclizine
- Anticholinergics: scopolamine
- Benzodiazepines
- Antiemetics as needed

Nonpharmacologic Interventions

- Hydration
- Repositioning
- Vestibular rehabilitation
- Bed rest if needed
- Treat the cause
- Physical and occupational therapy
- Sodium-restricted diet

Patient Teaching

- Avoid sudden changes in position.
- Chief concern is patient safety.
- Sit or lie down if feeling dizzy.
- Increase fluids; drink 3 L/day.
- Ensure good lighting to prevent falls.
- Use assistive devices as needed for support.
- Do not drive or use machinery if dizzy.
- Do not use alcohol, tobacco, or caffeine if symptomatic.
- Use energy conservation techniques.

Follow-up

- Seek immediate medical assistance if there is a change in level of consciousness, respiratory difficulty, or sudden loss of vision or hearing.
- Alert health care provider if there is sudden, severe ear pain or a temperature greater than 100.5° F or 38.3° C.

- Report all ear infections, sinus congestion, and respiratory complaints.
- Ensure that the patient's environment remains safe.

Resources

- Mayo Clinic (Mayo Foundation for Medical Education and Research): www.mayoclinic.com
- WebMD: www.webmd.com
- Chemo Care (Cleveland Clinic): http://www.chemocare.com/

Bibliography

ADAM Medical Encyclopedia [Internet]. (2015). *Light-headedness, dizzy, loss of balance, vertigo.* Available at https://www.nlm.nih.gov/medlineplus/ency/article/003093.htm (accessed February 18, 2016).

Branch, W., & Barton, J. (2015). *Approach to the patient with dizziness.* Available at http://www.uptodate.com/contents/approach-to-the-patient-with-dizziness?source=search_result&search=dizziness&selectedTitle=1%7E150 (accessed February 18, 2016).

Tucci, D. L. (2013). *Dizziness and vertigo.* Available at http://www.merckmanuals.com/professional/ear,-nose,-and-throat-disorders/approach-to-the-patient-with-ear-problems/dizziness-and-vertigo (accessed February 18, 2016).

Dysphagia

Kristin A. Cawley

Definition

- Dysphagia is difficulty swallowing.
- It is a ommon sequela of head and neck cancer and its treatment, occurring in 96% of those patients.
- It is described as food getting "stuck" and as choking.
- Classifications:
  - Oropharyngeal dysphagia—difficulty initiating the swallowing process and propelling food through esophagus
  - Esophageal dysphagia—ability to swallow food, yet having the sensation that food is not able to pass from esophagus into the stomach (often associated with pain)
- Chemotherapy and radiation therapy often reduce symptoms of dysphagia, thus prolonging life.
- Dysphagia is strongly associated with lower quality of life for patients.

Pathophysiology and Contributing Factors

- Narrowing (stricture) of the lower part of the esophagus
- Inflammatory changes in the esophagus
- Results from any condition that weakens or damages the muscles and nerves involved in swallowing:
  - Obstructive lesions
  - Tumors
  - Inflammatory masses
  - Trauma/surgical resection
  - Zenker diverticulum
  - Esophageal webs
  - Extrinsic structural lesions
  - Anterior mediastinal masses
  - Esophageal spasms
  - Mucositis
  - Xerostomia
  - Postirradiation sequelae
  - Laryngeal penetration
  - Age-related factors

Signs and Symptoms

- Difficulty swallowing
- Pain with swallowing
- Weight loss
- Dehydration
- Taste alterations
- Atrophy of neck muscles
- Aspiration
- Infection

Assessment Tools

- History and physical examination, including history of gastroesophogeal reflux disease (GERD), hiatal hernia, aspiration, or pneumonia
- Character and quality of pain
- Precipitating factors

Laboratory and Diagnostic Tests

- Comprehensive metabolic panel (creatinine)
- Albumin, prealbumin, transferrin, and retinol-binding protein
- Clinical swallowing evaluation (CSE)
- Water swallow test (WST)
- Barium study (esophagram)/barium swallow
- Videofluoroscopy (VFSS)
- Fiberoptic endoscopic examination of swallowing (FEES)
- Nasopharyngoscopy
- Endoscopy
- Manometry—measures pressure within the esophagus
- Chest radiographic film

Differential Diagnoses

- Xerostomia
- Anorexia
- Aspiration
- Malnutrition
- Dehydration
- Pain
- Cough
- Mucositis
- Gastroesophageal reflux
- Tissue fibrosis
- Aspiration pneumonia
- Anxiety
- Infection
- Depression
- Isolation (may avoid social gatherings where food is involved)

Interventions

Treat the underlying causes.

Pharmacologic Interventions

- Histamine-2 receptor antagonists (blockers)
- Proton pump inhibitors

- Prokinetic agents
- Antacids
- Hydration
- Pain management

Nonpharmacologic Interventions

- Positioning exercises:
  - Chin tuck for improved airway closure
  - Head rotation to modify pharyngeal pressure
- Parenteral nutrition
- Esophageal dilation
- Pharyngeal electrical stimulation

Patient Teaching

- Eat sitting upright at a 90-degree angle.
- Avoid lying down after meals for 30 minutes.
- Keep head of bed elevated while sleeping.
- Avoid solid, abrasive foods; incorporate a pureed, liquid diet.
- Maintain adherence with medications.

Follow-up

- Nutritional counseling
- Speech pathologist consultation
- Surgery consultation
- Call health care provider if experiencing the following:
  - Difficulty or pain when swallowing continues
  - Pain is unrelieved.
  - Continued weight loss

Resources

- Dysphagia Resource Center: www.dysphagiaonline.com
- Cancer.net—Difficulty swallowing or dysphagia: http://www.cancer.net/navigating-cancer-care/side-effects/difficulty-swallowing-or-dysphagia
- The Oral Cancer Foundation—Dysphagia: http://oralcancer foundation.org/complications/dysphagia.php
- Oncology Nursing Society: www.ons.org

Bibliography

Balusik, B. (2014). Management of dysphagia in patients with head and neck cancer. *Clinical Journal of Oncology Nursing, 18*(2), 149–150.

Dawson, C. J., Hickey, M. M., & Newton, S. (2011). Dysphagia. In C. J. Dawson, M. M. Hickey, & S. Newton (Eds.), *Telephone triage for otorhinolaryngology and head-neck nurses.* Pittsburg, PA: Oncology Nursing Society.

Massey, S. (2011). Esophageal cancer and palliation of dysphagia. *Clinical Journal of Oncology Nursing, 15*(3), 327–329.

Nguyen, N. P., Moltz, C. C., & Frank, C. (2004). Dysphagia following chemo-radiation for locally advanced head and neck cancer. *Annals of Oncology, 15*(3), 383–388.

Patterson, J., & Wilson, J. (2011). The clinical value of dysphagia preassessment in the management of head and neck cancer patients. *Current Opinion in Otolaryngology and Head and Neck Surgery, 19*(3), 177–181.

Peyrade, F., Cupissol, D., Geoffrois, L., et al. (2013). Systemic treatment and medical management of metastatic squamous cell carcinoma of the head and neck: Review of the literature and proposal for management changes. *Oral Oncology, 49*(6), 482–491.

Starmer, H. M. (2014). Dysphagia in head and neck cancer: Prevention and treatment. *Current Opinion in Otolaryngology and Head & Neck Surgery, 22*(3), 195–200.

Dyspnea

Ruth Canty Gholz

Definition

- An uncomfortable sensation or awareness of breathing
- May have a feeling of doom
- A subjective experience of breathing discomfort that consists of qualitative distinct sensations that vary in intensity; derived from interactions among multiple physiologic, psychological, social, and environmental factors and may induce secondary physiologic and behavioral responses
- Shortness of breath
- Subjective sensation of breathlessness
- Inability to get air
- Feeling of suffocation
- Severity may be related to the perception of dyspnea.
- Heavy or hard breathing
- Described as "air hunger"
- Occurs in up to 70% of persons with advanced cancer
- Most common symptom in lung cancer

Pathophysiology and Contributing Factors

- Dyspnea is not completely understood.
- Dyspnea is multifactorial.
- Although the respiratory center controls breathing, dyspnea results from cortical stimulation.
- The cortex overrides the respiratory center, stimulating chemoreceptors in the lung and respiratory muscles and mechanoreceptors.
- Respiratory effort increases.
- There is increased use of respiratory muscles.
- Amplification of ventilatory requirements occurs.
- Dyspnea may be divided into respiratory system dyspnea and cardiovascular dyspnea.
- It can be acute or chronic and may occur with exertion or at rest.
- Contributing factors include the following:
  - Hypoxia
  - Hypercapnia
  - Interstitial lung disease
  - Pleural or cardiac effusion
  - Malignancy: direct tumor effects, indirect tumor effects, or treatment-related causes
  - Chronic obstructive pulmonary disease (COPD)
  - Neuromuscular weakness
  - Bronchoconstriction or spasm
  - Air flow obstruction
  - Myocardial dysfunction
  - Anemia
  - Pain
  - Deconditioning
  - Thyroid disorders
  - Cardiovascular disease
  - Aspiration
  - Pneumonia
  - Anxiety
  - Radiation pneumonitis

Signs and Symptoms

- Air hunger
- Feeling of suffocation
- Cyanosis, pallor
- Anxiety
- Tachypnea
- Tachycardia
- Use of accessory muscles when breathing

Assessment Tools

- Visual or verbal analog scale for dyspnea
- Subjective descriptors/self-report
- Functional assessment tools: shuttle walking test, reading aloud of numbers
- Medical, social, smoking, and exposure history
- Physical examination and review of systems with emphasis on cardiopulmonary
- Respiratory rate and quality, use of accessory muscles
- Onset and aggravating or alleviating factors

Laboratory and Diagnostic Tests

- Pulse oximetry (may be within normal limits despite dyspnea)
- Complete blood count, blood chemistry, plasma brain natriuretic peptide (BNP) level
- Pulmonary function tests
- Maximal inspiratory pressure (MIP)
- Arterial blood gas measurement
- Chest radiographic films
- Echocardiogram

Differential Diagnoses

- Lung cancer
- COPD
- Pulmonary embolism
- Myocardial infarction
- Congestive heart failure
- Cardiomyopathy
- Anxiety/panic attack
- Pain
- Asthma
- Obesity

Interventions

Pharmacologic Interventions

- Treat the underlying cause.
- Opioids
- Anxiolytics
- Glucocorticoids for spasm or inflammation
- Bronchodilators
- Diuretics
- No strong evidence to support nebulized opioids for dyspnea

Nonpharmacologic Interventions

- Oxygen for hypoxia only
- Cool air blowing on the face
- Breathing exercises
- Pulmonary rehabilitation

Patient Teaching

- Take medications as directed.
- Keep a dyspnea diary.
- Report changes in sputum production.
- Cool air from a fan may be effective.
- Monitor temperature and report if greater than 100.5° F (38° C).
- Pursed-lip breathing
- Relaxation techniques
- Diaphragmatic breathing
- Inspiratory muscle training
- Positioning for comfort; keep head tilted
- Exercise
- Nutrition
- Energy conservation and pacing
- Get rid of smoking and pet dander in the home.

Follow-up

- Reinforce need for prompt communication with health care providers if future episodes of dyspea occur or if interventions are not effective.

Resources

- Oncology Nursing Society: www.ons.org
- Chemo Care (Cleveland Clinic): www.chemocare.com

Bibliography

DiSalvo, W., Joyce, M., Tyson, L., Culkin, A., & Mackey, K. (2008). Putting evidence into practice: Evidence-based interventions for cancer-related dyspnea. *Clinical Journal of Oncology Nursing, 12*(2), 341–352.

Dudgeon, D., & Shadd, J. (2016). *Assessment and management of dyspnea in palliative care.* Available at http://www.uptodate.com/contents/assessment-and-management-of-dyspnea-in-palliative-care (accessed February 22, 2016).

National Cancer Institute. (2015). *Cardiopulmonary syndromes: Dyspnea in patients with advanced cancer (PDQ).* Available at http://www.cancer.gov/about-cancer/treatment/side-effects/cardiopulmonary-hp-pdq (accessed February 22, 2016).

Oncology Nursing Society. (2016). *Dyspnea.* Available at https://www.ons.org/practice-resources/pep/dyspnea (accessed February 22, 2016).

Parshall, M., Schwartzstein, R., Adams, L., Banzett, R., Manning, H., Bourbeau, J., & ATS Committee on Dyspnea. (2012). An official American Thoracic Society statement: Update on the mechanisms, assessment, and management of dyspnea. *American Journal of Respiratory Critical Care Medicine, 185*(4), 435–457.

Schwartzstein, R. (2015). *Approach to the patient with dyspnea.* Available at http://www.uptodate.com/contents/approach-to-the-patient-with-dyspnea (accessed February 22, 2016).

Epistaxis

Joshua Carter

Definition

- Epistaxis is defined as nasal bleeding.
- Severity can range from minor to intractable.
- Approximately 10% of epistaxis cases require medical treatment; 1-2% require surgery.
- Epistaxis can be spontaneous with hematologic disorders, malignancies, or thrombocytopenia.

Pathophysiology and Contributing Factors

- Epistaxis is described as either anterior or posterior, depending on origin site.
- Epistaxis from the anterior region accounts for 80% of cases.
- Local causes of epistaxis include trauma to the nasal cavity, facial injury, and a foreign body in the nasal cavity.
- Systemic causes of epistaxis include environmental factors (e.g., temperature, humidity, being at a high altitude) and other systemic causes (e.g., inflammation, neoplastic conditions, organ failure).
- Antiplatelet or anticoagulant therapy is a common cause of epistaxis. In these cases, epistaxis usually is caused by nasal dryness, trauma, and the effects of therapy.
- For nasopharyngeal carcinoma patients treated with radiation therapy, epistaxis can be a treatment-related toxicity.
- Immune thrombocytopenia can cause a sudden onset of epistaxis.

Signs and Symptoms

- Bleeding from the nose
- Blood running into throat from nose
- Difficulty breathing
- Fatigue
- Disorientation (from uncontrolled epistaxis)

Assessment Tools

- History, including all past medical history; medications and supplements that the patient is currently taking
- Nasal examination by primary care physician; ear, nose, and throat (ENT) doctor; and/or head and neck surgeon
- From patient's report, suspected cause for epistaxis (if from trauma or other preceding known cause)
- To establish the cause of uncontrolled epistaxis, the head and neck surgeon may evaluate the patient under anesthesia, examining the patient's nose and nasopharynx; biopsy procedures may be warranted.
- Establish whether the patient has any hematologic disorders or malignancies.

Laboratory and Diagnostic Tests

- Complete blood count
- Platelet studies
- Coagulation studies
- Angiography
- Computed tomography, magnetic resonance imaging

Differential Diagnoses

- Trauma
- Head and neck malignancy
- Medication-related
- Treatment-related
- Environment-related
- Immune-related thrombocytopenia
- Hematologic disorders and malignancies

Interventions

Invasive Interventions

- Cauterization of the bleeding site
- Angiography with embolization
- Surgical biopsy if the lesion is in the nasal passage
- Transnasal endoscopic sphenopalatine artery ligation

Noninvasive Interventions

- Patient sits upright with head tilted forward and applies direct external pressure to the nares with index finger and thumb.
- Anterior nasal packing
- Posterior nasal packing

Patient Teaching

- Avoid nonsteroidal antiinflammatory drugs (NSAIDs), alcoholic beverages, and smoking.
- Do not blow, pick, or clean the inside of the nose.
- Inform patient that there may be a dark red or brown discharge from the nose.
- Use a cool-mist room humidifier.
- Use strategies to prevent constipation and straining.
- Avoid forceful blowing of the nose.
- If packing is in place, moisturize lips and nostrils with water-soluble ointment.
- For 24 hours after epistaxis episode, avoid bending over.
- Before starting any supplements, discuss with physician.
- If epistaxis remains uncontrolled, present to emergency department for a full workup and evaluation.

Follow-up

- Reinforce need for prompt communication with health care providers when future epistaxis episodes occur.

Resources

- Chemo Care (The Cleveland Clinic Foundation): www.chemocare.com
- Uptodate.com: Patient Information, beyond the basics: www.uptodate.com; http://www.uptodate.com/contents/search?search=epistaxis&x=0&y=0

Bibliography

Bansal, D., Rajendran, A., & Singhi, S. (2014). Newly diagnosed immune thrombocytopenia: Update on diagnosis and management. *Indian Journal of Pediatrics, 81*(10), 1033–1041.

Dawson, C. J., Hickey, M. M., & Newton, S. (2010). Epistaxis. In C. J. Dawson, M. M. Hickey, & S. Newton (Eds.), *Telephone triage for otorhinolaryngology and head-neck nurses.* Pittsburg, PA: Oncology Nursing Society.

Gilyoma, J., & Chalya, P. (2011). Etiological profile and treatment outcome of epistaxis at a tertiary care hospital in Northwestern Tanzania: A prospective review of 104 cases. *BMC Ear, Nose and Throat Disorders, 11*(8). http://dx.doi.org/10.1186/1472-6815-11-8.

He, C., Si, F., Xie, Y., & Yu, L. (2013). Management of intractable epistaxis in patients who received radiation therapy for nasopharyngeal carcinoma. *European Archives of Oto-Rhino-Laryngology, 270*(10), 2763–2767.

Kristensen, V., Nielsen, A., Gaihede, M., Boll, B., & Delmar, C. (2011). Mobilisation of epistaxis patients: A prospective, randomised study documenting a safe patient care regime. *Journal of Clinical Nursing, 20*(11/12), 1598–1605.

Minni, A., Dragonetti, A., Gera, R., Barbaro, M., Magliulo, G., & Filipo, R. (2010). Endoscopic management of recurrent epistaxis: The experience of two metropolitan hospitals in Italy. *Acta Oto-Laryngologica, 130*(9), 1048–1052.

4

Rudmik, L., & Leung, R. (2014). Cost-effectiveness analysis of endoscopic sphenopalatine artery ligation vs arterial embolization for intractable epistaxis. *JAMA Otolaryngology Head and Neck Surgery, 140*(9), 802–808.

Rushing, J. (2009). Managing epistaxis. *Nursing 2009, 39*(6), 12.

Strand, M., Meyers, J., & Boyer, H. (2014). Epistaxis in a patient on antiplatelet therapy: Not always benign. *American Journal of Otolaryngology Head and Neck Medicine and Surgery, 35*(3), 411–413.

Esophagitis

Kristin A. Cawley

Definition

- An inflammatory process that causes erythematous and ulcerative lesions to develop in the lining of the esophagus
- A common complication associated with patients receiving radiation therapy with concurrent chemotherapy
- May cause significant pain; may affect nutritional status and quality of life
- Affects the course of treatment, causing delays or dose reductions in therapy
- Usually begins to occur in the first 2-3 weeks after starting radiation therapy.
- If left untreated, can become very uncomfortable, causing problems with swallowing, ulcers, and scarring of the esophagus. In rare instances, a condition known as Barrett esophagus may develop, which is a risk factor for cancer of the esophagus.

Pathophysiology and Contributing Factors

- Breakdown of rapidly dividing epithelial cells caused by chemotherapy and radiation treatment, primarily in the gastrointestinal (GI) tract
- History of esophagitis or mucositis
- Age
- Poor oral hygiene, prior dental disease
- Alcohol and tobacco use are risk factors
- Treatment regimen, dose and frequency

Signs and Symptoms

- Difficult swallowing (dysphagia) or painful swallowing (odynophagia)
- Heartburn or acid reflux
- Mouth sores
- Bleeding
- Infection
- A feeling of something of being stuck in the throat
- Nausea
- Vomiting

Assessment Tools

- History, physical examination, and oral examination
- Radiation Therapy Oncology Group (RTOG) scoring
- Common Terminology Criteria for Adverse Events (CTCAE), version 4.0
- Nutritional status
- Symptomatic functional assessment based on ability to swallow
- Pain, using scale of 0 to 10 or a categorical scale (none, mild, moderate, or severe)

Laboratory and Diagnostic Tests

- Complete blood cell count (CBC)
- Blood, urine, and sputum culture
- Upper endoscopy
- Biopsy of esophageal tissue sample
- Upper GI series (or barium swallow)

Differential Diagnoses

- Gastroesophageal reflux disease (GERD)
- Esophageal stricture
- Dysphagia
- Pain
- Dehydration
- Anorexia
- Infection

Interventions

- Managed symptomatically

Pharmacologic Interventions

- Topical anesthetics: viscous lidocaine, analgesics
- Antacid therapy (proton pump inhibitor)
- Promotility agents (metoclopramide)
- Amifostine
- Antibiotics, antifungals, or antivirals to treat an infection
- Pain medications that can be gargled or swallowed
- Corticosteroid medication to reduce inflammation
- Enteral/Parenteral nutrition to allow the esophagus to heal and to reduce the likelihood of malnourishment or dehydration

Nonpharmacologic Interventions

- Nutritional support with intravenous hydration, feeding tube, or parenteral nutrition
- Sodium bicarbonate rinses

Patient Teaching

- Dental evaluation before treatment is initiated
- Dental cleaning:
  - Brush with soft toothbrush.
  - Continue despite thrombocytopenia or neutropenia unless uncontrolled bleeding develops.
  - Use fluoride toothpaste.
- Rinsing:
  - Normal saline solution (NS), sodium bicarbonate ($NaHCO_3$), NS/$NaHCO_3$, water
  - Nonalcoholic unsweetened mouthwash
- Dental appliances:
  - Should be left out as much as possible once mucous membranes become irritated
- Report any pain that is unrelieved with pain medication.

- Dietary modifications:
  - Follow a low-acid and bland diet.
  - Avoid coffee, hot beverages, spicy foods, citrus fruits and juices, alcohol, and tobacco.
- Report any fever of 100.5° F (38° C) or greater.

Follow-up

- Assess for increased risk of esophagitis with continuing treatments.
- Assess for pain unrelieved with pain medication.
- Monitor nutritional status closely.
- Reinforce the importance of communication with the physician and nurse.

Resources

- Kornmehl, C. (2005). Esophagitis: A common radiation side effect. *Cure.* Available at http://www.curetoday.com/publications/cure/2005/spring2005/esophagitis--a-common-radiation-side-effect (accessed February 22, 2016).
- National Cancer Institute. (2016). Oral complications of chemotherapy and head/neck radiation: For health professionals (PDQ). Available at http://www.cancer.gov/cancertopics/pdq/supportivecare/oralcomplications/healthprofessional (accessed February 22, 2016).
- Metz, J. (2014). Esophagitis. *Oncolink.* Available at http://www.oncolink.org/treatment/article.cfm?c=157&id=554 (accessed February 22, 2016).
- Oncology Nursing Society. (2014). Mucositis. *Putting evidence into practice.* Available at https://www.ons.org/practice-resources/pep/mucositis (accessed February 22, 2016).

Bibliography

Harris, D. J., Eilers, J., Harriman, A., Cashavelly, B. J., & Maxwell, C. (2015). Putting evidence into practice: Evidence-based interventions for the management of oral mucositis. *Clinical Journal of Oncology Nursing, 12*(1), 141–152.

Lalla, R. V., Bowen, J., Barasch, A., Elting, L., Epstein, J., Keefe, D. M., & Mucositis Guidelines Leadership Group of the Multinational Association of Supportive Care in Cancer and International Society of Oral Oncology (MASCC/ISOO). (2014). MASCC/ISOO clinical practice guidelines for the management of mucositis secondary to cancer therapy. *Cancer, 120,* 1453–1461.

Lalla, R. V., Sonis, S. T., & Peterson, D. E. (2008). Management of oral mucositis in patients with cancer. *Dental Clinics of North America, 52*(1), 61–77.

Sauer, A. C., & Coble Voss, A. (2012). *Improving outcomes with nutrition in patients with cancer. ONS Edge White Paper.* Pittsburgh, PA: Oncology Nursing Society.

Fatigue

Susie Newton

Definition

- Fatigue is a distressing, persistent, and subjective sense of physical, emotional, and/or cognitive tiredness or exhaustion that is not proportional to activity and interferes with usual function.
- Cancer-related fatigue is a subjective feeling of weariness or tiredness that is different from any other fatigue that the person has experienced.
- It is typically not relieved by sleep or rest.
- It has a serious detrimental effect on the cancer patient's quality of life.
- It affects as many as 80-100% of cancer patients.

Pathophysiology and Contributing Factors

- Exact pathophysiologic mechanism unknown
- Many contributing factors:
  - Underlying disease
  - Treatment-related toxicity:
    - Chemotherapy
    - Radiation therapy
    - Surgery
    - Biotherapy
  - Cytokines
  - Performance status
  - Pain
  - Depression
  - Anemia
  - Dyspnea
  - Infection
  - Anorexia
  - Metabolic disturbances
  - Sleep disorders

Signs and Symptoms

- Fatigue is reported as the most distressing symptom associated with cancer and its treatment.
- It is rated as more distressing than pain, nausea, and vomiting, which can frequently be treated with medications.
- Patients report whole-body tiredness and inability to perform basic tasks.
- Other reported physical symptoms include the following:
  - Dyspnea
  - Heart palpitations
  - Depressed mood
  - General lack of energy
- Fatigue often manifests with other symptoms:
  - Pain
  - Insomnia
  - Depression or anxiety

Assessment Tools

- The key assessment finding is the patient's self-report.
  - Fatigue is whatever the patient says it is.
  - Neither clinicians, family members, nor anyone else cannot judge fatigue level.
- Other assessment information includes the following:
  - Physical examination
  - Related laboratory data
  - Caregiver information
- Methods and tools for measuring fatigue include the following:
  - FACT-G (general)
  - FACT-F (fatigue)
  - FACT-An (anemia)
  - Brief Fatigue Inventory (BFI)
  - Linear Analog Scale Assessment (LASA)

- Visual Analog Scale (VAS)
- Multidimensional Fatigue Symptom Inventory—Short Form (MFSI-SF)

Laboratory and Diagnostic Tests

- Laboratory tests to assess for the cause of fatigue include the following:
  - Complete blood cell count (CBC)
  - Serum iron testing, including transferrin, total iron-binding capacity, ferritin, and iron levels
  - Folic acid and vitamin B_{12}
  - Thyroid function, including thyroxine (T_4) total, triiodothyronine (T_3) uptake, thyroid-stimulating hormone (TSH)
- There are no diagnostic tests to screen for fatigue.

Differential Diagnoses

- Anemia
- Depression
- Infection
- Sleep disturbances
- Anorexia
- Hypothyroidism
- Dehydration
- Medications that cause fatigue

Interventions

Pharmacologic Interventions

- Ginseng
  - There are two types of ginseng: Asian and American. Ginseng is reported to have many effects, including boosting of the immune system, antidepressive properties, and increased energy, concentration, and libido.
- Erythropoiesis stimulating factors (ESFs), if fatigue is related to anemia
  - ESAs such as erythropoietin, darbepoetin, and erythropoietin alfa are agents that control red blood cell production.
  - The effects of erythropoietin on fatigue and cognitive impairment have been studied in patients with chemotherapy-related anemia. The U.S. Food and Drug Administration has issued several warnings related to the use of ESAs. Related concerns include risk of increased tumor growth, decreased survival time, and cardiovascular side effects.
- Antidepressants, if depression is suspected
  - The prevalence and incidence of depression in patients with cancer vary widely depending on the diagnostic criteria and the instruments used; however, a significant number of patients with cancer have depression.
  - Patients who are at greatest risk of depression are those with advanced disease, those who have uncontrolled physical symptoms, and those who have had previous psychiatric disorders.
  - Oncology professionals should seek the expertise of mental health providers if they have questions regarding the prescribing of antidepressants or for referral to cognitive/psychological counseling.

- Corticosteroids such as methylprednisolone (prednisone) have been shown to reduce the significance of fatigue in some patient populations (e.g., those with chronic fatigue syndrome). However, because of the side effects associated with long-term use of these drugs (e.g., alterations in bone metabolism, adrenal suppression), they are not good options for the cancer population.

Nonpharmacologic Interventions

- Exercise, such as walking on a regular basis
  - Exercise is the one intervention recommended in the "Putting Evidence into Practice" (PEP) resource guide published by the Oncology Nursing Society.
- Yoga
- Delegating tasks
- Energy conservation principles
- Frequent rest periods that do not interfere with nighttime sleep
- Stress reduction techniques, such as progressive muscle relaxation or relaxation breathing

Patient Teaching

- Instruct patient regarding factors that contribute to fatigue:
  - Cancer itself
  - Cancer treatments
  - Anemia
  - Nutritional problems
  - Sleep problems
- Teach patient to recognize the signs of fatigue:
  - Feeling weary or exhausted (may be physical, emotional, or mental exhaustion)
  - A feeling of heaviness in the body, especially arms and legs
  - Less desire to do normal activities such as eating or shopping
  - Difficulty concentrating or thinking clearly
- Instruct patient regarding ways to manage fatigue:
  - Take time to rest, but be aware that too much rest can decrease energy levels.
  - Stay as active as possible; take part in enjoyable physical activities at least three times a week.
  - Practice yoga.
  - Eat nutritious foods and drink plenty of liquids.
  - Conserve energy when possible.
  - Perform stress-relieving activities.

Follow-up

Fatigue is one of the most common side effects experienced by patients with cancer. Patients will need education before beginning therapy for their cancer, as well as continuing evaluation and support to help them through the effects of this symptom.

After consulting with a health care provider, patients may begin an exercise program with activities such as walking, stretching, or riding a bicycle. Begin slowly with exercise for 5-10 minutes twice a day. Increase the exercise by 1 minute per day. Strive for consistency in the exercise without overdoing it.

Resources

- Abramson Cancer Center of the University of Pennsylvania: www.oncolink.com
- American Society of Clinical Oncology (ASCO): Cancer.net
- CancerCare, Inc.: www.cancercare.org
- Oncology Nursing Society: www.ons.org

Bibliography

Andersen, C., Rørth, M., Ejlertsen, B., Stage, M., Møller, T., Midtgaard, J., & Adamsen, L. (2013). The effects of a six-week supervised multimodal exercise intervention during chemotherapy on cancer-related fatigue. *European Journal of Oncology Nursing, 17*, 331–339.

Barton, D. L., Liu, H., Dakhil, S. R., Linquist, B., Sloan, J. A., Nichols, C. R., & Loprinzi, C. L. (2013). Wisconsin ginseng (*Panax quinquefolius*) to improve cancer-related fatigue: A randomized, double-blind trial, N07C2. *Journal of the National Cancer Institute, 105*, 1230–1238.

Chandwani, K. D., Perkins, G., Nagendra, H. R., Raghuram, N. V., Spelman, A., Nagarathna, R., & Cohen, L. (2014). Randomized, controlled trial of yoga in women with breast cancer undergoing radiotherapy. *Journal of Clinical Oncology, 32*, 1058–1065.

Cramp, F., & Byron-Daniel, J. (2012). Exercise for the management of cancer-related fatigue in adults. *Cochrane Database of Systematic Reviews* (11), CD006145.

Eton, D. T., & Cella, D. (2011). Do erythropoietic-stimulating agents relieve fatigue? A review of reviews. *Cancer Treatment and Research, 157*, 181–194.

Mitchell, S. A., Hoffman, A. J., Clark, J. C., DeGennaro, R. M., Poirier, P., Robinson, C. B., & Weisbrod, B. L. (2014). An update of evidence based interventions for cancer related fatigue during and following treatment. *Clinical Journal of Oncology Nursing, 18*(6), 38–58.

Berger, A. M., Mooney, K., Alvariz-Perez, A., Brietbart, W. S., Carpenter, K. M., Cella, D., & Smith, C. (2015). NCCN clinical practice guidelines in oncology: Cancer-related fatigue, version 2.2015. *Journal of the National Comprehensive Cancer Network, 13*, 1012–1039.

Oncology Nursing Society. (2016). *Putting evidence into practice: Fatigue.* Available at https://www.ons.org/practice-resources/pep/fatigue (accessed February 22, 2016).

Wenzel, J. A., Griffith, K. A., Shang, J., Thompson, C. B., Hedlin, H., Stewart, K. J., DeWeese, T., & Mock, V. (2013). Impact of a home-based walking intervention on outcomes of sleep quality, emotional distress, and fatigue in patients undergoing treatment for solid tumors. *The Oncologist, 18*, 476–484.

Fever

Ruth Canty Gholz

Definition

- Fever is elevation of core body temperature.
- The mean oral temperature is 98.6 ± 7° F or 37 ± 0.4° C

- A single temperature of 101° F (or 38.3° C) is significant.
- Fever is an emergency in a person who has neutropenia or is on immunosuppressive therapy

Pathophysiology and Contributing Factors

- The hypothalamus regulates and controls body temperature in the thermoregulatory center.
- The thermoregulatory center balances heat production with heat dissipation.
- When the balance is disrupted (i.e., elevation of the hypothalamic set point), vasoconstriction and heat production occur.
- Fever can be induced by disease or pyrogens.
- Exogenous pyrogens originate from outside the body; they are primarily infectious agents and toxins. Endogenous pyrogens originate from inside the body; normal flora are altered by neutropenia, toxins, and tumors.
- Pyrogenic cytokines cause fever when activated; they include interleukins, interferons, and tumor necrosis factor.
- Fever has three phases: chill, fever, and flush.
- Elderly persons are more susceptible to temperature change; they may present apyrexic or manifest a lower fever than others.
- Persons with cancer may mount a febrile response to infection, drugs, tumor, thrombosis, graft-versus-host disease, or a blood transfusion.

Signs and Symptoms

- Vasoconstriction of hands and feet
- Shivering, followed by need for warmth
- Chills, rigors
- Flush
- Dry skin
- Diaphoresis

Assessment Tools

- Determine whether the patient is at high or low risk for febrile neutropenia if he or she is undergoing chemotherapy or has marrow disease.
- High-risk assessment of fever:
  - Inpatient
  - Comorbidities
  - Neutropenia
  - Elevated serum creatinine level
  - Elevated liver function tests
- Low-risk assessment of fever:
  - Outpatient
  - No comorbidities
  - Short duration of neutropenia
  - Good performance status
- Risk assessment tools:
  - Multinational Association for Supportive Care in Cancer (MASCC) risk score
  - Talcott Risk Assessment
  - History and physical examination

- Areas to examine:
  - Skin assessment for areas of pressure, ulcerations, or wounds
  - Vascular access devices as sources of infection
  - Lungs and sinuses
  - Alimentary canal: mouth, pharynx, esophagus, rectum, bowel
  - Perineal, vaginal, perirectal areas
  - Lymph nodes
- Assessment for nausea, vomiting, diarrhea
- Review of the medical history
- Medications, previous or current use of antibiotics
- Review of potential exposures: family, friends, pets, travel, recent blood transfusion, exposure to tuberculosis
- Time from last treatment and agents received
- Neurologic assessment (confusion and cognitive impairment can occur with high fevers)
- Vital signs: evaluate for any signs of sepsis; check temperature frequently
- In persons with cancer, consider infection as the cause of fever unless proven otherwise\
- Foreign bodies (e.g., prosthetic joint)

Laboratory and Diagnostic Tests

- Complete blood cell count (CBC) with differential, sedimentation rate
- Renal panel, liver function tests
- Chest radiographic film
- Cultures: urine, sputum, blood, stool, central and peripheral devices

Differential Diagnoses

- Tumor/paraneoplastic fever
- Transfusion-associated fever
- Drug-associated fever
- Infection: neutropenic fever (bacterial, viral, fungal, or opportunistic)
- Fever of unknown origin (FUO)
- Deep vein thrombosis

Interventions

- Determined by cause of fever
- Treat the cause of fever

Pharmacologic Interventions

- Antipyretics to reduce temperature, myalgias, rigors
- Empirical broad-spectrum antibiotics based on institutional isolates
- Anaerobic therapy as needed
- Specific therapy for documented infection sites or pathogens
- Prophylaxis as required

Nonpharmacologic Interventions

- Hydration
- Nutritional support
- Comfort care, oral care, keep mucous membranes moist, sponge bathing with cool or cold cloths, changing bed linen and clothes, use of a fan for cooling

Patient Teaching

- Prevention includes good hand washing and hygiene.
- Report fevers (>38.3° C or 100.5° F) or chills to health care provider as soon as possible.
- Take the complete course of antibiotics or other medications as prescribed
- Monitor temperature at least two times daily at home throughout duration of chemotherapy.
- Future treatments may include a colony-stimulating factor.
- Teach when to contact a health care provider (e.g., presenting with unusual symptoms, signs of infection or bleeding).
- A neutropenic person will not experience the usual signs of infection (i.e., redness, swelling, pus); fever may be the first sign of infection.
- Instruct the patient and family to not take any rectal medications or treatments.
- Educate the patient and family to avoid contact with anyone who is ill.
- Instruct patient to avoid dental work unless approved by the health care provider.
- Oral care hygiene should be performed at least 4 times a day.

Follow-up

- Daily follow-up when hospitalized
- Outpatient daily follow-up for the first 72 hours at home or in the clinic and then as needed for signs and symptoms of persistent or recurrent fever

Resources

- Centers for Disease Control and Prevention: www.cdc.gov
- National Comprehensive Cancer Network: www.NCCN.org
- Oncology Nursing Society: www.ons.org
- National Cancer Institute: www.cancer.gov
- American Cancer Society: www.cancer.org

Bibliography

Bor, D. (2015). *Approach to the adult with fever of unknown origin.* Available at http://www.uptodate.com/contents/approach-to-the-adult-with-fever-of-unknown-origin (accessed February 22, 2016).

Marinella, M. Fever in patients with cancer. Available at http://www.antimicrobe.org/new/e13.asp (accessed February 22, 2016).

National Comprehensive Cancer Network. (2014). *Prevention and treatment of cancer-related infections.* Available at http://www.nccn.org/professionals/physician_gls/PDF/infections.pdf (accessed February 22, 2016).

Flu-like Symptoms

Ruth Canty Gholz

Definition

- Cluster of constitutional symptoms similar to those of influenza; may occur in various combinations
- Not influenza
- Characterized by fever, chills, rigors, myalgias/arthralgias, malaise, headache, cough, and nasal congestion
- Occurs after specific oncologic therapies

- Symptoms resolve within a specific time frame and lessen with each exposure to the specific agent

Pathophysiology and Contributing Factors

- Flu-like symptoms occur as a result of pyrogens causing an increase in the thermoregulatory set point.
- Pyrogens may be exogenous (virus, bacteria, neoplastic cells, or drugs) or endogenous (cytokines).
- Chill is a muscle contraction that occurs in response to the rise in temperature.
- Flu-like symptoms occur with the following agents (a representative but not inclusive list):
  - Interferons
  - Interleukins
  - Granulocyte colony-stimulating factor (G-CSF)
  - Granulocyte-macrophage colony-stimulating factor (GM-CSF)
  - Monoclonal antibodies
  - Tumor necrosis factor
  - Bacille Calmette-Guérin (BCG)
  - Bleomycin
  - Cladribine
  - Cytarabine
  - Dacarbazine
  - Fluorouracil
  - L-Asparaginase
  - Paclitaxel
  - Pamidronate disodium
  - Procarbazine
  - Trimetrexate
  - Zoledronic acid

Signs and Symptoms

- Chills or rigors that occur 3-6 hours after therapy
- Fever that occurs, on average, 30-90 minutes after a chill
- Myalgia or arthralgia
- Headache
- Malaise
- Fatigue
- Nausea or vomiting
- Anorexia
- Diarrhea
- Nasal congestion (runny nose, clear)

Assessment Tools

- Physical examination with review of systems: cardiopulmonary, abdomen, lymph nodes, musculoskeletal, and skin
- Vital signs: blood pressure, temperature, pulse, respirations, and pulse oximetry
- Neurologic assessment

Laboratory and Diagnostic Tests

- Complete blood cell count (CBC) to determine whether the symptoms are related to neutropenia
- If patient is neutropenic, need to pan culture and rule out infection
- Chest x-ray film if neutropenic

Differential Diagnosis

- Infection
- Toxic shock syndrome
- Influenza
- Cold
- Drug-induced symptoms

Interventions

Pharmacologic Interventions

- Antipyretics such as nonsteroidal antiinflammatory drugs (NSAIDs, if patient is not thrombocytopenic) or acetaminophen
- Antihistamines
- Opiates to relieve rigors (e.g., meperidine, morphine, hydromorphone)
- Monitor temperature patterns; if there is no response to antipyretics, an infectious process may be present.
- Analgesics for headache, myalgias, arthralgias
- Premedicate before administration of causative agent to potentially block flu-like syndrome.

Nonpharmacologic Interventions

- Provide warm blankets, heating pads, warm bath.
- Provide a quiet, dark room for patients with headache.
- Increase fluids.
- Encourage relaxation techniques.
- Provide emotional support and reassurance.
- Provide for rest.

Patient Teaching

- Teach patient that this is a possible side effect of therapy.
- Use antipyretics for fever.
- Use warm blankets to relieve chills.
- Use an NSAID (if no thrombocytopenia) or acetaminophen for myalgias or arthralgias.
- Instruct patient that this side effect is short lived and usually reduces with future drug administration.

Follow-up

- Report fevers or chills not controlled with above interventions.
- Obtain emergency care if vomiting, seizures, mental status change, or uncontrolled fever occurs.
- Patients have 24-hour emergency numbers for access to providers.

Resources

- Oncology Nursing Society: www.ons.org/patientEd
- Chemocare.com

Bibliography

Polovich, M., White, J., & Kelleher, L. (2005). *Chemotherapy and biotherapy guidelines and recommendations for practice* (pp. 156–158). Pittsburgh, PA: Oncology Nursing Society.

Shelton, R. (2001). Flu-like syndrome. In P. Reiger (Ed.), *Biotherapy: A comprehensive review* (pp. 519–543). Boston: Jones & Bartlett.

Tovey, M. G., & Lallemand, C. (2011). Immunogenicity and other problems associated with the use of biopharmaceuticals. *Therapeutic Advances in Drug Safety, 2*(3), 113–128. http://dx.doi.org/10.1177/2042098611406318 (accessed June 2011).

Hand-Foot Syndrome

Laura S. Wood

Definition

- Dermatologic reaction associated with certain anti-cancer therapies
- Presentation varies depending on agent, dose, and patient characteristics
- Involvement of hands and feet is most common but can involve other skin surfaces.
- Hand-foot syndrome (HFS) is also known as
  - Palmar-plantar erythrodysesthesia (PPE)
  - Acral erythema
  - Hyperkeratosis
  - Hand-foot skin reaction

Pathophysiology and Contributing Factors

- HFS is a cutaneous eruption of the integument of the hands and feet.
- Chemotherapy drugs with sustained serum levels (e.g., liposomal doxorubicin, capecitabine) are most likely to cause HFS.
- Multikinase inhibitors, including sorafenib, sunitinib, pazopanib, and axitinib, are associated with HFS.
- HFS results from prolonged drug exposure via superficial capillaries.
- It is dependent on both peak drug concentration and total cumulative dose.
- It may occur earlier and more severely with bolus or short-term dose-intensive therapy.
- It may result from friction and pressure (weight bearing) on hands, feet, or other areas.
- Patients with diabetes or peripheral vascular disorders are at increased risk.
- Cytochrome P450 subsystem inhibitors must be considered as potential contributing factors.

Signs and Symptoms

- Often characterized by initial paresthesias (tingling sensations, numbness, or sensitivity to warmth) followed by erythema
- May occur concurrently with dry skin
- May include hyperkeratosis and callus formation
- May include blisters, bullae, or fissures
- Acral erythema consists of painful symmetric erythematous and edematous areas.
- Dry or moist desquamation may occur.

- May include swelling or edema
- May become painful and/or interfere with both function and activities of daily living (ADLs)
- May have a negative impact on quality of life

Assessment Tools

- Patient history
- Medication review during each interaction
- Physical examination of hands and feet before initiation of therapy and at every clinic visit
- Common Toxicity Criteria (CTC, version 4.0) grading scale:
  - Grade 1 (mild): minimal skin changes or dermatitis (e.g., erythema, edema, hyperkeratosis without pain)
  - Grade 2 (moderate): skin changes (e.g., peeling, blisters, bleeding, edema, hyperkeratosis) with pain; limiting instrumental ADLs
  - Grade 3 (severe): severe skin changes (e.g., peeling, blisters, bleeding, edema, hyperkeratosis) with pain; limiting self-care ADLs

Laboratory and Diagnostic Tests

- There are no specific laboratory tests.
- Physical examination and patient-reported symptoms facilitate accurate diagnosis.
- Patients with diabetes, peripheral vascular disease, or peripheral neuropathy should have more frequent examinations of the hands and feet.

Differential Diagnoses

- Cellulitis
- Rash
- Contact dermatitis
- Allergic reaction

Interventions

Pharmacologic Interventions

- Topical high-potency steroids twice daily for erythema and burning sensation associated with HFS
- Dexamethasone for severe HFS not responsive to other interventions
- Pain control: nonsteroidal antiinflammatory agents (NSAIDs, as long as thrombocytopenia is not present), γ-aminobutyric acid (GABA) agonist
- Celecoxib 200 mg/m^2 twice daily plus topical high-potency steroid twice daily for capecitabine-induced HFS
- Treatment interruption and/or dose reduction for severe HFS

Nonpharmacologic Interventions

- Prevention is not possible. Patient education regarding frequent self-assessment and compliance with skin care regimen is critical to minimize risk of severe or treatment-limiting HFS.
- Initiation of skin care regimen with first dose of therapy:
  - Frequent application of moisturizing lotion (e.g., Bag Balm, Udderly Smooth cream, Eucerin cream, Aquaphor)

- Urea 10% cream
- Avoidance of activities resulting in excessive friction or pressure to hands or feet
- Minimize duration of exposure to heat (i.e., bathing, dishwashing)
- Well-fitting, cushioned, comfortable shoes
- Gel insole liners
- Early notification of provider for development of symptoms associated with HFS
- Exfoliating agents for hyperkeratotic areas
- Referral to podiatrist for evaluation and management

Patient Teaching

- Emphasize compliance with skin care regimen.
- Emphasize early notification for development of symptoms associated with HFS.
- If skin blisters are noted, soak the area with cool water for 10 minutes, and then apply petroleum jelly to the wet skin to trap the moisture.

Follow-up

- If the patient reports any changes to the palms or soles, a physical assessment with diagnosis and a treatment plan must occur.

Resources

- http://ctep.cancer.gov/protocolDevelopment/electronic_applications/docs/ctcaev3.pdf http://www.chemocare.com
- http://www.mascc.org
- http://www.nccn.org
- http://evs.nci.nih.gov/ftp1/CTCAE/CTCAE_4.03_2010-06-14_QuickReference_5x7.pdf

Bibliography

Anderson, R., Jatoi, A., Robert, C., Wood, L. S., Keating, K. N., & Lacouture, M. E. (2009). Search for evidence-based approaches for the prevention and palliation of hand-foot skin reaction (HFSR) caused by multikinase inhibitors (MKIs). *The Oncologist, 14*, 291–302.

Balagula, Y., Wu, S., Xiao, S., Feldman, D. R., & Lacouture, M. E. (2012). The risk of hand foot skin reaction to pazopanib, a novel multikinase inhibitor: A systematic review of literature and meta-analysis. *Investigational New Drugs, 30*, 1773–1781.

Bardia, A., Loprinzi, C. L., & Goetz, M. P. (2006). Hand-foot syndrome after dose-dense adjuvant chemotherapy for breast cancer: A case series. *Journal of Clinical Oncology, 24*(13), 18–19.

Bhojani, N., Jeldres, C., Patard, J. J., Perrotte, P., Suardi, N., Hutterer, G., & Karakiewicz, P. I. (2008). Toxicities associated with the administration of sorafenib, sunitinib, and temsirolimus and their management in patients with metastatic renal cell carcinoma. *European Urology, 53*, 917–930.

Lacouture, M. E., Wu, S., Robert, C., Atkins, M. B., Kong, H. H., Guitart, J., & Durcher, J. P. (2008). Evolving strategies for the management of hand-foot skin reaction associated with multitargeted kinase inhibitors sorafenib and sunitinib. *The Oncologist, 12*, 1001–1011.

Manchen, E., Robert, C., & Porta, C. (2011). Management of tyrosine kinase inhibitor-induced hand-foot skin reaction: Viewpoints from the medical oncologist, dermatologist, and oncology nurse. *Journal of Supportive Oncology, 9*(1), 13–23.

National Cancer Institute. (2010). *Common Terminology Criteria for Adverse Events (CTCAE)*, version 4.03. Available at http://evs.nci.nih.gov/ftp1/CTCAE/CTCAE_4.03_2010-06-14_QuickReference_5x7.pdf (accessed April 5, 2016).

Robert, C., Soria, J. C., Spatz, A., Le Cesne, A., Malka, D., Pautier, P., & Le Chevalier, T. (2005). Cutaneous side effects of kinase inhibitors and blocking antibodies. *Lancet Oncology, 6*(7), 491–500.

Rosen, A., Amitay-Laish, J., & Lacouture, M. E. (2014). Management algorithms for dermatologic adverse events. In M. E. Lacouture (Ed.), *Dermatologic principles and practice in oncology: Conditions of the skin* (pp. 367–383). Hoboken, NJ: Wiley-Blackwell.

Von Moos, R., Thuerlimann, B. J., Aapro, M., Rayson, D., Harrols, K., Sehouli, J., & Hauschild, A. (2008). Pegylated liposomal doxorubicin hand-foot syndrome. *European Journal of Cancer, 44*(6), 781–790.

Wilkes, G. M., & Doyle, D. (2005). Palmar-plantar erythrodysesthesia. *Clinical Journal of Oncology Nursing, 9*(1), 103–106.

Wood, L. S., Gornell, S., & Rini, B. I. (2012). Maximizing clinical outcomes with axitinib therapy in advanced renal cell carcinoma through proactive side effect management. *Community Oncology, 9*, 46–55.

Wood, L. S., Lemont, H., Jatoi, A., Lacouture, M. E., Robert, C., Keating, K., & Anderson, R. (2010). Practical considerations in the management of hand-foot skin reaction caused by multikinase inhibitors. *Community Oncology, 7*(1), 23–29.

Wyatt, A. J., Leonard, G. D., & Sachs, D. L. (2006). Cutaneous reactions to chemotherapy and their management. *American Journal of Clinical Dermatology, 7*(1), 45–63.

Yang, C. H., Lin, W. C., Chuang, C. K., Chang, Y. C., Pang, S. T., Lin, Y. C., & Chang, J. W. (2008). Hand-foot skin reaction in patients treated with sorafenib: A clinicopathological study of cutaneous manifestations due to multitargeted kinase inhibitor therapy. *British Journal of Dermatology, 158*, 592–596.

Zhang, R. X., Wu, X. J., Wan, D. S., Lu, Z. H., Kong, L. H., Pan, Z. Z., & Chen, G. (2012). Celecoxib can prevent capecitabine-related hand-foot syndrome in stage II and III colorectal cancer patients: Result of a single-center, prospective randomized phase III trial. *Annals of Oncology, 23*, 1348–1353.

Headache

Carol S. Blecher

Definition

Headache is defined as pain that is referred to the surface of the head from deep structures.

Pathophysiology and Contributing Factors

- Headache can be caused by some other physical disorder, or it can be an independent disorder.
- When there is damage to the venous sinuses or to the membranes that cover the brain, intense pain may occur, although the brain itself is almost completely insensitive to pain.
- There are three major types of headaches:
  - Tension (or stress) headache: caused by the tightening of muscles in the head and neck
  - Migraine headache: caused by vasodilation of the blood vessels in the brain
  - Cluster headache: a form of chronic, recurrent headaches characterized by sudden onset with no specific cause, although it appears to be related to a sudden release of histamine or serotonin
- Contributing factors vary with the type of headache; in cancer patients, headaches are most frequently related to
  - Primary brain tumors or brain metastases
  - An increase in intracranial pressure from mass effect or edema
  - Radiation therapy treatments that initially increase edema and cause headaches

- Intrathecal chemotherapy causing headaches and the procedure of administering chemotherapy by Ommaya reservoir or lumbar puncture
- Chemotherapy and biotherapy agents including but not limited to the following:
  - Antithymocyte globulin (ATG)
  - Erythropoietin
  - Granulocyte colony-stimulating factor (G-CSF)
  - Granulocyte-macrophage colony-stimulating factor (GM-CSF)
  - Oprelvekin (Neumega)
  - Immunoglobulin G (IgG)
  - Interferon
  - Interleukin
  - Levamisole
  - All-*trans* retinoic acid (ATRA)
  - Monoclonal antibodies in general
  - Tumor necrosis factor
  - Dacarbazine
  - Gemcitabine
  - Paclitaxel
  - Targretin
  - Temozolomide

Signs and Symptoms

- Patients with brain tumors may have headaches that are worse in the morning.
- Initially these headaches ease during the day, but ultimately they become persistent.
- Pain is usually described as dull, but if it occurs during sleep, it awakens the patient.
- The pain may be associated with morning nausea and vomiting, papilledema, and seizures.

Assessment Tools

- History, including diagnosis and cancer treatment, current medications, presenting symptoms, precipitating factors, location, and duration (assess for any associated symptoms)
- Neurologic examination, evaluating for confusion, decrease in attention span, memory loss, drowsiness, weakness, or ataxia
- Vital signs: Changes in vital signs may indicate an increase in intracranial pressure (ICP). Blood pressure should be monitored for a widening pulse pressure and for hypertension. Heart rate should be monitored for bradycardia and for irregular or thready pulse.
- Examine the head for signs of trauma, skull tenderness (subdural hematoma), poor dentition or grinding of the teeth, bogginess of the sinuses, papilledema, otitis media, and mastoiditis.
- Examine the neck for nuchal rigidity, tenderness of the shoulders or neck, and decreased range of motion.
- National Cancer Institute (NCI) common terminology criteria adverse events (CTCAE) grading system:
  - Grade 1: mild pain not interfering with function
  - Grade 2: moderate pain; pain or analgesics interfering with function but not interfering with activities of daily living (ADLs)

- Grade 3: severe pain; pain or analgesics severely interfering with ADLs
- Grade 4: disabling pain

Laboratory and Diagnostic Tests

- Complete blood cell count (CBC) with differential to rule out infection or anemia
- Chemistry studies to rule out renal failure and other underlying systemic diseases
- Platelet count, prothrombin time (PT), international normalized ratio (INR)/partial thromboplastin time (PTT) to identify a risk for intracranial bleeding
- Arterial blood gas analysis (ABGs) to assess for hypoxia
- Drug screening for cocaine and amphetamines
- Computed tomography (CT) scan of the head to identify a tumor, metastases, or edema
- Magnetic resonance imaging (MRI) of the head to identify a tumor, metastases, or edema
- Lumbar puncture to assess infection (meningitis or encephalitis) or meningeal carcinomatosis

Differential Diagnoses

- Acute glaucoma
- Anemia
- Arteriovenous malformation
- Brain metastases
- Dental abscess
- Hypertension
- Meningeal carcinoma
- Meningitis
- Migraine
- Primary brain tumor
- Sinusitis
- Stroke
- Subarachnoid hemorrhage
- Subdural hematoma
- Systemic lupus erythematosus
- Trigeminal neuralgia
- Drug-related headaches from chemotherapy and biotherapy agents including but not limited to the following:
  - ATRA
  - Dacarbazine
  - Erythropoietin
  - 5-Fluorouracil (5FU)
  - G-CSF
  - GM-CSF
  - Gemcitabine
  - Oprelvekin (Neumega)
  - IgG
  - Interferon
  - Interleukin
  - Intrathecal chemotherapy
  - Levamisole
  - Monoclonal antibodies in general
  - Paclitaxel
  - Procarbazine
  - Tumor necrosis factor

- Drug-related headaches from analgesics including but not limited to the following:
  - Acetaminophen (Tylenol)
  - Caffeine
  - Ergot preparations
  - Opioids
  - Tranquilizers/muscle relaxers
- Drug-related headaches from other agents including but not limited to the following:
  - Amphotericin B
  - Azathioprine
  - Aztreonam
  - Cyclosporine
  - Foscarnet
  - Ganciclovir
  - Pamidronate
  - Rifampicin
  - Voriconazole

Interventions

Treatment of the Underlying Disease

- Surgery for primary brain tumor, radiation therapy, chemotherapy, targeted therapy
- Radiation therapy for metastatic disease
- Steroids for cerebral edema due to increased intracranial pressure

Pharmacologic Interventions

- Acetaminophen (Tylenol)
- Aspirin
- Aspirin or acetaminophen/caffeine
- Beta-blockers: propranolol (Inderal), nadolol (Corgard), metoprolol (Lopressor)
- Calcium channel blockers: verapamil (Calan) for prevention of migraines
- Ergotamine tartrate/caffeine (Cafergot, Wigraine, Ergomar)
- Naproxen (Naprosyn, Anaprox, Aleve)
- Ibuprofen (Motrin, Advil, Nuprin)
- Indomethacin (Indocin)
- Ketorolac (Toradol)
- Sumatriptan (Imitrex)
- Tricyclic antidepressants: amitriptyline (Elavil, Endep), nortriptyline (Pamelor)

Nonpharmacologic Interventions

- Complementary therapies such as biofeedback, acupuncture, acupressure, massage, relaxation, transcutaneous electrical nerve stimulation (TENS)
- Dietary modifications: avoid dairy products, caffeinated drinks, chocolate, salted or preserved meats, and foods containing monosodium glutamate (MSG)
- Herbal and nutrient therapies suggested for relief of headaches include skullcap, rosemary, thyme, chamomile, feverfew, valerian, white willow, vitamin B complex, vitamin E, calcium, and magnesium

Patient Teaching

- Treatment for headache is determined on the basis of the following:
  - Age, health status, and medical history
  - Severity of symptoms
  - Individual tolerance of specific medications, procedures, or therapies
  - Expectations for the course of the condition
  - Personal opinions and preferences
- Treatment may include the following:
  - Biofeedback training
  - Complementary medicine
  - Dietary evaluation to eliminate foods that might contribute to headaches
  - Drug therapy (medication)
  - Regular exercise, such as swimming or vigorous walking
  - Stress reduction
  - Use of cold packs

Follow-up

- Call health care provider if any of the following occurs:
  - This is the first time the person has had a headache.
  - The headache occurs rapidly or is persistent.
  - The headache is associated with fever, stiff neck, or projectile or uncontrollable vomiting.
  - The headache is associated with confusion, seizures, or loss of consciousness.
  - There is numbness, weakness, or vision loss with the headache.
  - The headache interferes with the ability to function normally.
  - Medication for the headache is taken on more than 2 days per week.
- Also consider the following:
  - Pain service referral
  - Headache center referral
  - Physical therapy
  - Occupational therapy

Resources

- American Council for Headache Education: www.achenet.org
- National Headache Foundation: www.headaches.org

Bibliography

Association of Migraine Disorders. (2015). *Prescription medications for migraines.* Available at http://www.migrainedisorders.org/treatments/prescription-medications-migraines/ (accessed February 29, 2016).

Cancer.Net. (2014). *Headaches.* Available at http://www.cancer.net/navigating-cancer-care/side-effects/headaches (accessed February 29, 2016).

National Cancer Institute. (2010). *Common terminology criteria for adverse events,* version 4.03. Available at http://evs.nci.nih.gov/ftp1/CTCAE/About.html (accessed February 29, 2016).

MedlinePlus Medical Encyclopedia. (2013). *Headache.* Available at http://www.nlm.nih.gov/medlineplus/ency/article/003024.htm (accessed February 29, 2016).

Rice, L. (2014). Headache. In D. Camp-Sorrell & R. A. Hawkins (Eds.), *Clinical manual for the oncology advanced practice nurse* (pp. 1179–1187). Pittsburgh, PA: Oncology Nursing Press.

Hiccups

Denice Economou

Definition

- Sudden, involuntary diaphragmatic spasm causing a sudden inhalation and interrupted by a spasmodic closure of the glottis resulting in the "hic" sound
- Three types of hiccups:
  - Benign: lasting as long as 48 hours
  - Persistent or chronic: lasting longer than 48 hours but less than 1 month
  - Intractable: lasting longer than 1 month

Pathophysiology and Contributing Factors

- A reflex arc in the cervical spine (C3-C5) travels afferent pathways over fibers of the phrenic and vagus nerves and thoracic segments T6-T12.
- Hiccups are a response to vagus and phrenic nerve irritation.
- Causes of hiccups are organized into four conditions:
  - Structural
  - Metabolic
  - Inflammatory
  - Infectious
- Hiccups can contribute to fatigue and exhaustion, especially if sleep and eating are interrupted.
- Unrelieved hiccups can also lead to feeling of depression, anxiety, and frustration over the long term.
- Common causes of hiccups in terminal illness include stroke, brain tumor, sepsis, and nerve irritation such as gastric distention, gastritis, gastroesophageal reflux disease (GERD), pancreatitis, *Helicobacter pylori* infection, hepatitis, and myocardial infarction.
- Excessive drinking or smoking can be a factor.
- Medications that may contribute to hiccups include the following:
  - Steroids
  - Chemotherapy agents
  - Nicotine
  - Opioids
  - Muscle relaxants

Signs and Symptoms

- Brief, irritable spasms of the diaphragm

Assessment Tools

- Obtain a history of presenting symptoms.
- Identify precipitating factors or triggers (e.g., eating, drinking, positioning).
- Obtain medical history regarding abdominal, thoracic, or neurologic surgery and social history of alcohol use.
- Determine the level of distress hiccups are causing.
- Determine interference with activities of daily living (ADLs), including eating and sleeping.
- Observe patient for other causes of hiccups.
- Evaluate for other causes such as temporal artery tenderness and hair or foreign body in the ear.
- Perform an oral examination to identify any swelling or obstruction that may be contributing to hiccups.
- Evaluate for infection or a septic process.
- Assess for pneumonia, pericarditis, abdominal distention, or ascites.
- Identify peritumor edema in the abdominal area.

Laboratory and Diagnostic Tests

- Complete blood cell count (CBC) and electrolytes to rule out infection or renal failure
- Chest radiographic film to rule out pulmonary processes
- Fluoroscopy to determine whether one hemidiaphragm is dominant
- The extent of the workup is proportional to the duration of hiccups and the impact on the patient's quality of life.

Differential Diagnoses

- Diaphragmatic or phrenic nerve irritation
- Gastric dilation
- Hiatal hernia
- Pancreatitis
- Alcohol abuse
- Central nervous system (CNS) dysfunction
- Psychogenic cause

Interventions

Pharmacologic Interventions

- Attempt to decrease gastric distention with medications such as simethicone and metoclopramide. A nasogastric (NG) tube or fasting may be necessary to help relieve this symptom.
- Anecdotal results have been seen with baclofen, chlorpromazine (Thorazine), haloperidol.
- Additional medications may include muscle relaxants, anticonvulsants, antidepressants, and dopamine agonists.

Nonpharmacologic Interventions

- Respiratory measures may help. Consider having the patient perform breath-holds. Try rebreathing in a paper bag or causing sneeze or cough with spices. Try an ice-cold wet cotton tip applied between the hard and soft palates for 1 minute.
- Drinking large gulps of water, swallowing sugar, or sucking on a lemon wedge may interfere with hiccups.
- Psychological interventions include distraction techniques and breathing exercises.
- Intractable hiccups may require anesthetic block of the phrenic and cervical nerves, acupressure, or acupuncture.
- Peppermint water helps to relax the lower esophagus.

Patient Teaching

- Provide education and information regarding different classes of medications used for relief along with nonpharmacologic management approaches.

Follow-up

- Gastrointestinal (GI) consultation if the cause is GI related
- Anesthesia consultation if nerve block is necessary

- Provide support to the patient and continual assessment of interventions until hiccups are relieved.

Resources

- Mayo Clinic http://www.mayoclinic.com/health/hiccups/DS00975

Bibliography

Calsina-Berna, A., Garcia-Gomez, G., Gonzalez-Barboteo, J., & Porta-Sales, J. (2012). Treatment of chronic hiccups in cancer patients: A systematic review. *Journal of Palliative Medicine, 15*(10), 1142–1150.

Camp-Sorrell, D. (2006). Hiccups. In D. Camp-Sorrell & R. A. Hawkins (Eds.), *Clinical manual for the oncology advanced practice nurse* (pp. 13–17). Pittsburgh, PA: Oncology Nursing Society.

Dahlin, C., & Cohen, A. (2015). Dysphagia, xerostomia, and hiccups. In B. R. Ferrell, N. Coyle, & J. Paice (Eds.), *Textbook of palliative nursing* (4th ed.) (pp. 191–216). New York: Oxford University Press.

Moretto, E., Wee, B., Wiffen, P., & Murchison, A. (2013). Interventions for treating persistent and intractable hiccups in adults. [Review]. *Cochrane Database of Systematic Reviews* (1), CD008768.

Hyperglycemia

Deborah Kirk Walker

Definition

- Increased amount of glucose in the blood
- Type 1: destruction of pancreatic beta cells due to a cellular-mediated autoimmune response
  - Rate of destruction is variable
- Type 2: combination of insulin resistance and insulin deficiency
  - Usually develops gradually

Pathophysiology and Contributing Factors

Prolonged elevated insulin levels may stimulate cancer cell proliferation in certain cancers. Diabetes increases risk for pancreatic, liver, breast, colorectal, urinary tract, gastric, and female reproductive cancers. Diabetes increases mortality rates in the cancer population. Glucose control is important for survivors to protect the health of their organs (e.g., eyes, heart, kidneys). Cancer survivors are often at increased risk for comorbidities such as diabetes, with variations seen based on risk factors and type of treatment.

- Type 1: Insulin deficiency is usually related to beta cell destruction.
  - Family history: A first-degree relative with diabetes greatly increase a person's risk.
  - The presence of certain genes may increase risk.
  - There is an increased risk for those farthest away from the equator.
  - Age: There are two peak periods, between 4 and 7 years, and between 10 and 14 years.
- Type 2: Defective insulin secretion with insulin resistance (typically obese)
  - Women with polycystic ovary syndrome or who delivered a baby weighing more than 9 pounds or who had a diagnosis of gestational diabetes mellitus
  - Physical inactivity

- Age 45 years or older
- Overweight and obesity
- Dietary factors:
  - High-fat foods
  - Processed foods
  - Red meats
  - Excessive alcohol intake
- Hypertension
- Hyperlipidemia
  - Fasting triglyceride level 250 mg/dL or greater
  - High-density lipoprotein cholesterol level 35 mg/dL or lower
- Smoking
- Family history: First-degree relative with diabetes greatly increases risk
- Race/ethnicity:
  - African American
  - Latino
  - Native American
  - Asian American
  - Pacific Islander
- History of cardiovascular disease
- Infections
- Kidney and liver disease
- Glycated hemoglobin (A_{1C}) 5.7% or higher, impaired glucose tolerance (IGT), or impaired fasting glucose (IFG) on previous testing
- Drugs (may alter glucose homeostasis)
  - Mechanistic target of rapamycin (mTor): hyperglycemia
  - Tyrosine kinase inhibitor (TKI): hyperglycemia or hypoglycemia
  - Corticosteroids
  - Octreotide
  - L-Asparaginase
  - Thiazides
  - Thyroid hormone
  - Atypical antipsychotics

Signs and Symptoms

- Symptoms vary from none to severe and life-threatening (e.g., diabetic ketoacidosis [DKA])
  - DKA: frequent urination, extreme thirst, nausea, vomiting, abdominal pain, confusion, breath that smells fruity, a flushed face, fatigue, weakness, increased ketones in urine
- Type 1 diabetics are more likely to present with elevated glucose levels and to have acute symptoms.
- Elevated glucose
- Frequent infections
- Slow wound healing
- Weight loss that is not intentional
- Visual changes
- Polyuria, polydipsia, polyphagia
- Tremors
- Tingling in hands and feet (early)
- Neuropathy in hands and feet (late)
- Fatigue
- Mood changes

Assessment Tools

- A complete past medical history, social history, and family history
- Vital signs, including body mass index (BMI)
- Physical examination
  - Eye examination to evaluate for retinopathy
  - Skin evaluation to evaluate for integrity and any infections
  - Cardiac examination for look for any evidence of cardiac disease caused by elevated blood sugar levels
  - Peripheral vascular examination (pulses may be decreased with vascular disease)
  - Abdominal examination for hepatomegaly and assessment of injection sites if injecting insulin
  - Neurologic examination including reflexes and evaluation of proprioception
  - Foot examination that includes evaluation for any fungal infection or breaks in skin
  - Psychiatric examination

Laboratory and Diagnostic Tests

- Consider testing overweight adults (BMI ≥ 25 kg/m^2, or 23 kg/m^2 in Asian Americans)
- Hemoglobin A_{1C}
  - Fasting is not required.
  - Stress and illness do not affect results as much as they do for random glucose levels.
  - Hemoglobinopathies and anemia may alter results.
  - Levels of hemoglobin A_{1C}: normal, >5.7; prediabetes, 5.7-6.4%; diabetes, 6.5% or higher
- Plasma glucose levels
  - Fasting plasma glucose (FPG): 100-125 mg/dL
  - 2-Hour plasma glucose (on the 75-g oral glucose tolerance test [OGTT]): 140-199 mg/dL
- Other
  - Fasting lipid profile
  - Liver function studies
  - Serum creatinine and calculated glomerular filtration rate (GFR)
  - Thyroid-stimulating hormone level in type 1
  - Screen for increased urinary albumin excretion yearly
  - Serum creatinine level yearly

Differential Diagnoses

- Secondary diabetes mellitus
  - Drugs
  - Chemicals
- Pancreatitis
- Infection
- Paraneoplastic syndrome
- Cushing disease
- Diabetes insipidus

Interventions

- Individualized: weight loss through healthy diet and exercise if obese

- Prevention
- Treatment of disease
- Prevention and treatment of secondary effects and complications

Pharmacologic Interventions

- Type 1
  - Insulin
- Type 2
  - Metformin initially
  - May add a second oral agent (or basal insulin) if monotherapy is ineffective:
    - Orlistat
    - Thiazolidinediones
    - Gamma-glucosidase inhibitors
- For those with hypertension, the goal is <140/90 mm Hg
  - Angiotensin-converting enzyme inhibitor (ACEI), angiotensin receptor blocker (ARB), thiazide diuretics
- Cholesterol management and control
  - Statin therapy should be initiated for those with cardiovascular disease

Nonpharmacologic Interventions

- Psychosocial assessment for depression, distress, anxiety, eating disorders, cognitive impairment
- Lifestyle modifications
  - Weight loss
  - Moderate-intensity physical activity 150 minutes per week
  - Nutrition

Patient Teaching

- Emphasis on self-management, helping the patient understand the following:
  - Diabetes as a disease
  - Healthy eating
  - Physical activity
  - Medications
  - Blood glucose monitoring
  - Blood pressure monitoring
  - Increased needs during illness
  - Long-term complications of diabetes
  - Health promotion
  - Behavior change
- Lifestyle
  - Nutrition
    - Healthy eating patterns that are personalized and culturally appropriate
    - Carbohydrate management with portion control and healthy food choices
    - Weight loss
    - Limited alcohol
    - Individualized sodium reduction
    - Limited calories from fat
    - Low-fat protein sources
    - Encouragement to record food intake

- Importance of a healthy breakfast
- Small portions when eating out
- Self-weighing once per week
- Choosing water to drink
- Avoiding television watching while eating
- Exercise
  - 150 Minutes per week of moderate-intensity aerobic physical activity
  - No more than 2 days in a row without exercise
  - Resistance training twice a week
  - Exercise record keeping
  - Setting goals
- Home blood pressure monitoring and blood pressure control (<140/90 mm Hg)
- Routine cholesterol screening and control
- Smoking cessation
  - Because of the increased risk of cardiovascular disease in those with diabetes, smoking cessation is recommended.
  - Refer to counseling if needed.
- Self-monitoring of blood glucose
  - Frequency is individualized based on severity of hyperglycemia and agents used for treatment.
- Foot care
- Risk of diabetic kidney disease
  - Importance of blood pressure control

Follow-up

A multidisciplinary, comprehensive approach is needed and is individualized based on severity of symptoms. Follow-up and referrals should be made for the following:

- Eye care: annual eye examination for evaluation of retinal disease
- Foot examination at least annual, including pulse check
- Dietitian or diabetes educator
- Diabetes self-management support
- Dentist
- Mental health
- Immunizations (influenza, pneumococcus, hepatitis A)
- Hemoglobin A_{1C} measured at least twice a year, more often with changes in management or if not well controlled
- Endocrinology referral
- Cardiovascular workup including blood pressure control and monitoring
- Nephrologist if renal disease is apparent
- Neurologist for neuropathy

Resources

- List of interferences with A_{1C} measurement: www.ngsp.org/interf.asp
- Evidence-based lifestyle change programs: www.cdc.gov/diabetes/prevention/index.html
- Small steps. Big rewards. Your GAME PLAN to Prevent Type 2 diabetes: Information for patients: http://go.usa.gov/8n7F
- DASH Eating Plan: http://go.usa.gov/GUZV
- ChooseMyPlate: http://go.usa.gov/8Qax
- 2008 Physical Activity Guidelines for Americans: http://go.usa.gov/8QC4
- Resource for smoking cessation:
  - www.smokefree.gov
  - 1-877-44U-QUIT
- American Association of Diabetes Educators
- American Diabetes Association

Bibliography

American Diabetes Association (ADA). (2015). Standards of medical care in diabetes—2015. *Diabetes Care, 38*(Suppl. 1), S1–S94.

Brady, V. J., Grimes, D., Armstrong, T., & LoBiondo-Wood, G. (2014). Management of steroid-induced hyperglycemia in hospitalized patients with cancer: A review. *Oncology Nursing Forum, 41*(6), E355–E365.

Dieli-Conwright, C. M., Mortimer, J. E., Schroeder, E. T., Courneya, K., Demark-Wahnefried, W., Buchanan, T. A., & Bernstein, L. (2014). Randomized controlled trial to evaluate the effects of combined progressive exercise on metabolic syndrome in breast cancer survivors: rationale, design, and methods. *BMC Cancer, 14,* 238.

Kurtin, S. (2014). Diabetes mellitus, types 1 and 2. In D. Camp-Sorrell & R. A. Hawkins (Eds.), *Clinical manual for the oncology advanced practice nurse* (pp. 1257–1274). Pittsburgh, PA: Oncology Nursing Society.

National Diabetes Education Program. (2014). *Guiding principles for the care of people with or at risk for diabetes.* Available at http://ndep.nih.gov/media/Guiding_Principles_508.pdf (accessed February 29, 2016).

Verges, B., Walter, T., & Cariou, B. (2014). Endocrine side effects of anti-cancer drugs: Effects of anti-cancer targeted therapies on lipid and glucose metabolism. *European Journal of Endocrinology, 170,* R43–R55.

Xu, C. X., Zhu, H. H., & Zhu, Y. M. (2014). Diabetes and cancer: Associations, mechanisms, and implications for medical practice. *World Journal of Diabetes, 5*(3), 372–380.

Hypersensitivity Reactions

Colleen O'Leary

Definition

- Terms such as *drug reaction*, *drug allergy*, and *drug hypersensitivity* are often used interchangeably.
- Drug reaction includes all adverse events from a drug regardless of cause.
- Drug allergies are specifically mediated by the immune system.
- Drug hypersensitivity is an immune-mediated response to a drug in a patient who has been sensitized to the drug.
- Hypersensitivity reactions (HSR) to chemotherapy and/or biotherapy are unexpected reactions with symptoms that are different from the normal side effects of the agent.
- Severity ranges from mild to anaphylaxis.
- Four categories have been identified:
  - Type I: immediate immunoglobulin E (IgE) mediated (most common type with chemotherapy)
  - Type II: antibody mediated
  - Type III: immune complex mediated
  - Type IV: delayed or cell mediated

Pathophysiology and Contributing Factors

- Type I reactions
  - They occur after exposure to a foreign substance or antigen.

- Exposure causes immunoglobulin E (IgE) antibodies to form; they bind to receptors on mast cells in tissues or basophils in the peripheral blood.
- With subsequent exposure to the antigen, the antigen attaches to the IgE antibody, causing mast cells to degranulate and release chemical mediators of this type of reaction into the peripheral blood.
- Histamines, leukotrienes, prostaglandins, and chemotactins are the chemical mediators.
- Some drugs such as paclitaxel and docetaxel require mixture with synthetic solvents such as cremaphor so they can be given parenterally. These solvents have been connected with severe to life-threatening reactions.
- Nanoparticle albumin-bound paclitaxel (nabP) is solvent free, and there are few to no reactions associated with its administration.
- Type II reactions
  - They are caused by immunoglobulin G (IgG) or immunoglobulin M (IgM).
  - The immunoglobulin is released and forms an antibody-antigen complex, resulting in the signs and symptoms of this reaction type.
- Type III reactions
  - Antibody-antigen interactions cause immune complexes to be formed in the circulation and deposited in various tissues.
- Type IV reactions
  - These are cell-mediated or delayed-type reactions that involve the interaction of sensitized T lymphocytes with the antigen.
- Factors that influence the development and severity of reactions include the amount of antigen introduced, the route of entry (i.e., PO, IV), and the rate of absorption (length of infusion).
- Cytokine release syndrome
  - It is a drug reaction common to biologic agents.
  - It is associated with drugs that are directed to specific immune system targets, such as anti-CD19 and anti-CD20 antibodies.
  - The drug reacts with the antibody and releases cytokines such as tumor necrosis factor- α (TNF-α), interleukin-6 (IL-6), and interferons.
- Risk factors for HSR include type of drug administered, high doses, female gender, and history of prior allergic reactions.
  - Chemotherapy drugs with the highest potential for HSR include L-asparaginase, taxanes, platinum compounds, epidophyllotoxins, and procarbazine.
  - Chemotherapy drugs that occasionally cause HSR include anthracyclines, dacarbazine, and 6-mercaptopurine.
  - Biotherapy drugs associated with HSR and cytokine release syndrome include interferons, interleukins, and monoclonal antibodies.
  - Patients with a history of prior allergic reactions to food, insulin, opiates, penicillins, bee stings, blood products, or contrast media are at a higher risk for HSR.

Signs and Symptoms

- Type I HSR: fever, rash, nausea, vomiting, flushing, urticaria, bronchospasm, hypotension, angioedema, feeling of impending doom, respiratory and cardiovascular collapse
- Type II HSR: hemolysis
- Type III HSR: tissue injury including vasculitis, nephritis, and arthritis
- Type IV HSR: contact dermatitis, graft rejection, formation of granulomas

Assessment Tools

- Baseline vital signs and assessment; frequent measurement of vital signs and assessment of symptoms throughout administration

Laboratory and Diagnostic Tests

- There are no specific laboratory or diagnostic tests for HSR; diagnosis is based on symptom assessment.

Differential Diagnosis

- Drug allergy
- Drug reaction

Interventions

Pharmacologic Interventions

- Prevention is the mainstay of interventions. Premedication with corticosteroids such as dexamethasone; histamine receptor 1 (H$_1$) antagonists such as diphenhydramine; histamine receptor 2 (H$_2$) antagonists such as cimetidine, famotidine, and ranitidine; and antipyretics such as acetaminophen are commonly used.
- Desensitization protocols have been used, but none has proved highly effective.
- Medications for severe HSR include adrenaline, crystalloid solutions, and oxygen.
- Rechallenge with premedications is often accomplished.

Nonpharmacologic Interventions

- At the first suspicion of HSR, administration of the drug should be stopped.
- Place patient in supine position to promote organ profusion.
- Maintain airway, breathing, and circulation as indicated.
- Vital signs should be taken every 2 to 5 minutes until stable, and then every 15 minutes.

Patient Teaching

- Patients should be taught to tell the nurse of any changes experienced during their treatment, including itching, hives, shortness of breath, and cough.
- Often patients cannot verbalize exactly what is wrong, but they know they just don't feel right. This is often the first indication of HSR and should be taken seriously.

Follow-up

- As needed to assess resolution of symptoms.

Resources

- American Cancer Society: www.cancer.org
- Chemocare.com: www.chemocare.com
- Canadian Cancer Society: www.cancer.ca
- National Cancer Institute: www.cancer.gov
- Oncology Nursing Society: www.ons.org

Bibliography

Boulanger, J., Boursiquot, J. N., Cournoyer, G., Lemieux, J., Masse, M. S., Almanric, K., & Comité de l'évolution des pratiques en oncologie. (2014). Management of hypersensitivity to platinum- and taxane-based chemotherapy: CEPO review and clinical recommendations. *Current Oncology, 21*, e630–e641.

Castells Guitart, M. C. (2014). Rapid drug desensitization for hypersensitivity reactions to chemotherapy and monoclonal antibodies in the 21st century. *Journal of Investigative Allergology and Clinical Immunology, 24*, 72–79.

Lee, C., Gianos, M., & Klaustermeyer, W. B. (2009). Diagnosis and management of hypersensitivity reactions related to common cancer chemotherapy agents. *Annals of Allergy, Asthma and Immunology, 102*, 179–187.

Mezzano, V., Giavina-Bianchi, P., Picard, M., Caiado, J., & Castells, M. (2014). Drug desensitization in the management of hypersensitivity reactions to monoclonal antibodies and chemotherapy. *BioDrugs, 28*, 133–144.

Ruggiero, A., Triarico, S., Trombatore, G., Battista, A., Dell'acqua, F., Rizzari, C., & Riccardi, R. (2013). Incidence, clinical features and management of hypersensitivity reactions to chemotherapeutic drugs in children with cancer. *European Journal of Clinical Pharmacology, 69*, 1739–1746.

Syrigou, E., Triantafyllou, O., Makrilia, N., Kaklamanos, I., Kotanidou, A., Manolopoulos, L., & Syrigos, K. (2010). Acute hypersensitivity reactions to chemotherapy agents: an overview. *Inflammation and Allergy Drug Targets, 9*, 206–213.

VanGerpen, R. (2009). Chemotherapy and biotherapy-induced hypersensitivity reactions. *Journal of Infusion Nursing, 32*, 157–165.

Zetka, E. S. (2012). The essentials of chemotherapy-induced infusion reactions. *Clinical Journal of Oncology Nursing, 16*, 527–529.

Hypertension

Deborah Kirk Walker

Definition

- Blood pressure is the force of blood on arterial walls.
  - Systolic blood pressure is the pressure measured when the heart beats.
  - Diastolic blood pressure is the pressure measured when the heart is at rest.
- Blood pressure goals have been established for different age groups (see table below).
- Diagnosis is made after three consecutive elevated readings.

Blood Pressure Goals

Classification	Systolic (mm Hg)	Diastolic (mm Hg)
Patients >60 years of age with no comorbidities	<150	<90
Patients 18-59 years of age with no comorbidities	<140	<90
Patients ≥60 years of age with diabetes, chronic kidney disease, or both	<140	<90

- In primary (essential) hypertension, the cause is unknown; it develops gradually over years.
- Secondary hypertension is caused by an underlying condition or stimulus; it is often sudden in onset.

Pathophysiology and Contributing Factors

- Increased vascular stiffness, systemic resistance, and responsiveness contribute to hypertension.
- Contributing factors:
  - Age: men, >55 years; women, >65 years
  - Gender: men > women
  - Race: African Americans are at greatest risk and can develop hypertension early in life.
  - Heredity
  - Diabetes
  - Diets high in sodium (often found in processed foods) or table salt
  - Diets low in potassium
  - Physical inactivity causing weight gain
  - Overweight or obesity
  - Alcohol in excess (women, >1 drink per day; men, >2 drinks per day)
  - Smoking
  - Stressful situations
  - Pain
  - Drugs: vascular endothelial growth factor (VEGF) inhibitors, angiogenesis inhibitors, oral contraceptives, over-the-counter cold medications, illegal drugs
  - Kidney problems
  - Adrenal gland problems

Signs and Symptoms

- Some patients experience no signs or symptoms.
- Some patients have headaches, dizziness, nosebleeds, or flushing.
- Peripheral edema, blurred vision, and dyspnea may be seen with uncontrolled blood pressure.

Assessment Tools

- Medical and family history for evaluation of any conditions that may contribute to development of high blood pressure
- Review of current medications
- Social history including alcohol, tobacco, and illegal drugs, diet history, and job-related stress
- Physical examination:
  - Vital signs including several blood pressure readings at different times and in different positions
  - Height and weight
  - Eye examination, noting any narrowing of blood vessels, retinopathy, papilledema, or exudate
  - Neck examination, evaluating carotid arteries, jugular veins, and thyroid
  - Cardiovascular examination
  - Pulmonary examination, noting any adventitious breath sounds
  - Abdominal evaluation for enlarged kidneys, aneurysms, hepatomegaly

- Peripheral vascular system, evaluating pulses, edema, muscle weakness or atrophy
- Neurologic evaluation including reflexes

Laboratory and Diagnostic Tests

- Chest radiograph for evaluation of heart size, lung disease, or other heart abnormalities
- Electrocardiograph to evaluate for any damage to the heart
- Complete blood cell count (CBC) looking for anemia or polycythemia
- Urine analysis to evaluate for proteinuria
- Complete metabolic panel
  - Evaluation of electrolytes before any treatment with diuretics is started
  - Blood sugar level for diabetes
  - Creatinine and blood urea nitrogen (BUN) for kidney disease

Differential Diagnoses

- Renal artery stenosis
- Kidney disease
- Cushing syndrome
- Tumors of the pituitary
- Tumors of the adrenal glands
- Blood vessel diseases
- Thyroid disorders
- Alcoholism
- Arteriosclerosis
- Drug-induced hypertension
  - Steroids, erythropoietin, certain chemotherapy agents (i.e., antiangiogenesis agents)
  - Over-the-counter cold preparations

Interventions

- Individualized treatment plans to help lower blood pressure
- Patients 60 years of age or older without comorbid conditions should have a blood pressure goal of <150/90 mm Hg.
- Patients 18 to 59 years of age without major comorbid conditions and those 60 years or older with diabetes and/or chronic kidney disease should have a blood pressure goal of <140/90 mm Hg.
- Considerations should be made for those with chronic kidney disease and/or diabetes, with a blood pressure goal of <140/90 mm Hg.

Pharmacologic Interventions

First-line treatment should consist of a thiazide-type diuretic, calcium channel blocker, angiotensin-converting enzyme inhibitor (ACEI), or angiotensin receptor blocker (ARB), as follows:

- For blacks: initial treatment with a thiazide-type diuretic or calcium channel blocker or both
- For races other than black: initial treatment with a thiazide-type diuretic, an ACEI, an ARB, or a calcium channel blocker
- For patients with chronic kidney disease: initial treatment with an ACEI or ARB or both

- Thiazide diuretics are the preferred agents; monitor electrolytes and blood sugar
- ACEIs are less effective in African Americans; monitor electrolytes and creatinine; may cause a cough
- Alternative classes of drugs to consider as additional therapy in late management of hypertension or include the following:
  - Beta-blockers
  - Alpha-blockers (give at bedtime)
  - Alpha/beta-blockers (more effective in African Americans)
  - Vasodilators (use in combination with other agents)
  - Peripherally acting adrenergic antagonists
  - Loop diuretics
  - Aldosterone antagonists
  - Central alpha$_2$-adrenergic agonists

Nonpharmacologic Interventions

- Lifestyle changes
  - Low-sodium, low-fat diet
  - Weight loss
  - Regular exercise
  - Smoking cessation
  - Reduced alcohol consumption
  - Stress management

Patient Teaching

- Monitor blood pressure at home.
- Control of high blood pressure is important to avoid complications such as damage to heart or other organs.
- Maintain regular medication administration to control blood pressure.
- Avoid or eliminate known modifiable risk factors.
- Reduce salt and fat in the diet.
- Lose or control weight.
- Exercise regularly.
- Cease smoking.
- Limit alcohol consumption.

Follow-up

- One month after initiation of treatment to monitor progress
- Monthly until desired blood pressure is met
- Every 3 to 6 months for maintenance follow-up
- If goal is not met, medication dose should be increased or a second agent added.
- Consider referral to cardiology, if needed.

Resources

- http://www.nlm.nih.gov/medlineplus/highbloodpressure.html
- http://www.heart.org/HEARTORG/Conditions/HighBloodPressure/High-Blood-Pressure_UCM_002020_SubHomePage.jsp
- http://www.nhlbi.nih.gov/health/health-topics/topics/hbp/
- http://www.fda.gov/Drugs/ResourcesForYou/SpecialFeatures/ucm358442.htm
- http://www.cdc.gov/bloodpressure/docs/novella_spanish.pdf
- http://www.cdc.gov/bloodpressure/hypertension_iom.htm

- http://smokefree.gov/
- http://www.cdc.gov/dhdsp/data_statistics/fact_sheets/fs_bloodpressure.htm
- http://millionhearts.hhs.gov/Docs/MH_SMBP.pdf
- http://www.cdc.gov/bloodpressure/

Bibliography

American Heart Association (AHA). (2014). What are the symptoms of high blood pressure? Available at http://www.heart.org/HEARTORG/Conditions/HighBloodPressure/SymptomsDiagnosisMonitoring ofHighBloodPressure/What-are-the-Symptoms-of-High-Blood-Pressure_UCM_301871_Article.jsp (accessed February 29, 2016).

Curigliano, G., Cardinale, D., Suter, T., Plataniotis, G., de Azambuja, E., Sandri, M. T., & Roila, F. (2012). Cardiovascular toxicity induced by chemotherapy, targeted agents and radiotherapy: ESMO Clinical Practice Guidelines. *Annals of Oncology, 23*(Suppl. 7), vii155–vii166.

GroupHealth. (2014). *Hypertension diagnosis and treatment guideline.* Available at https://www.ghc.org/all-sites/guidelines/hypertension.pdf (accessed February 29, 2016).

James, P. A., Oparil, S., Carter, B. L., Cushman, W. C., Dennison-Himmelfarb, C., Handler, J., & Ortiz, E. (2014). 2014 Evidence-based guideline for the management of high blood pressure in adults: Report from the panel members appointed to the Eighth Joint National Committee (JNC8). *Journal of the American Medical Association, 311*(5), 507–520.

Sharp, K. (2014). Hypertension. In D. Camp-Sorrell & R. A Hawkins (Eds.), *Clinical manual for the oncology advanced practice nurse* (pp. 403–417). Pittsburgh, PA: Oncology Nursing Society.

Lymphedema

Wendy H. Vogel

Definition

- Lymphedema is swelling from abnormal production of lymph fluid or because of an obstruction in the lymph circulation, usually in the upper or lower extremities.
- It occurs in approximately 20% of patients after a radical mastectomy and in 6% to 7% after modified radical mastectomy (worldwide statistics report incidences of up to 40%).
- Lower extremity lymphedema after pelvic or inguinal lymphadenectomy occurs in about 20% of patients.

Pathophysiology and Contributing Factors

- Primary lymphedema is rare, most often occurring as a birth defect.
- Secondary lymphedema usually develops as the result of obstruction or disruption of the lymphatic system by a tumor or trauma such as infection, surgery, or radiation therapy.
  - It may occur acutely or chronically, years after treatment.
  - Acute lymphedema subsides within a few weeks after surgery, when collateral circulation has developed.
  - The most common sites of lymph obstruction are the axillary, pelvic, and inguinal nodes.
- After surgery, if lymph fluid does not get rerouted or collateral circulation does not develop, the lymph system may not be able to accommodate the demand for drainage, and fluid may accumulate in the interstitial spaces, resulting in edema.
- If edema persists, the high protein concentration causes fibrosis of the subcutaneous tissue, leading to irreversible damage to the lymph system. Chronic lymphedema increases the risk of cellulitis, infections, and lymphangitis and decreases the quality of life.
- Lymphedema is more common in women who have undergone axillary dissection and radiation therapy with a dose greater than 46 Gy.
- Most patients develop lymphedema within 3 years after cancer treatment.
- Chronic lymphedema is lymphedema that persists for longer than 3 months.
- Risk factors include the following:
  - Lymph node dissection (usually, the greater the number of lymph nodes removed, the greater the risk of lymphedema)
  - Radiation therapy
  - Infection
  - Obesity
  - Trauma
  - Age
  - Breast cancer, ovarian cancer, lymphoma, or prostate cancer
  - Comorbidities such as congestive heart failure and neurologic, kidney, or liver disease
- Lymphedema is considered incurable; treatment is palliative, to prevent disease progression and alleviate symptoms.

Signs and Symptoms

- Swollen limb
- Swollen axilla or groin area
- May extend to face, neck, or genitalia
- Signs of infection or inflammation may be present.
- Patients may report edema, heaviness, tightness, firmness, pain, aching, numbness, tingling, stiffness, limb fatigue, or impaired limb mobility even in early stages before lymphedema is visually noticeable.

Assessment Tools

- Obtain a thorough history:
  - Possible sources, signs, and symptoms of infection
  - Any unusual or heavy lifting or activity
  - Repetitive-type movements
  - Time frame with regard to surgery or trauma
  - Activity level
  - Nutrition
  - Comorbid conditions
- Evaluate psychosocial factors:
  - Assess impact on body image, sexuality, social activities, work.
  - Assess for anger, social avoidance, sexual dysfunction, poor adjustment.
- Assess for pain.
- Perform a physical examination:
  - Measure the affected limb, using anatomic landmarks for accuracy in follow-up assessments. Compare with unaffected limb. Serial measurements allow assessment of changes over time.
  - Assess for signs and symptoms of infection.
  - Measure pulses and range of motion.
  - Assess the strength of the affected limb.

Principles of Symptom Management 4

- Check affected areas for presence of suspicious masses or tumor recurrence.
- Grade the severity (International Society of Lymphology):
  - *Stage 0:* Subclinical lymphedema—no visible edema, but symptoms of heaviness (may be present for months or years before progressing)
  - *Stage I:* Mild—2- to 3-cm difference between limbs; feelings of heaviness, throbbing or soreness. May subside with elevation.
  - *Stage II:* Moderate—3- to 5-cm difference between limbs, visibly noticeable; skin may be stretched and shiny; pitting edema may be present; tissue is soft. Elevation rarely reduces edema.
  - *Stage III:* Severe—>5-cm difference between limbs; skin stretched and discolored to purple or brown; skin tough, brawny, with peau d'orange appearance; tissue may be firm, nonpitting.

Laboratory and Diagnostic Tests

- Rule out venous swelling (e.g., venous obstruction or thrombus) with color flow Doppler ultrasonography or venography.
- Perform computed tomography (CT) or magnetic resonance imaging (MRI) of the axilla or groin to rule out tumor recurrence
- Bioelectric impedance analysis measures impedance and resistance of extracellular fluid.
- Perform lymphoscintigraphy as indicated.
- Perform blood urea nitrogen (BUN), creatinine, liver function tests, albumin, urinalysis, and liver function tests to rule out possible systemic causes.

Differential Diagnoses

- Thrombus
- Infection
- Cirrhosis
- Nephrosis
- Congestive heart failure
- Myxedema (severe hypothyroidism)
- Hypoalbuminemia
- Chronic venous stasis
- Obstruction from pelvic or abdominal malignancy

Interventions

- Gold standard: complete decongestive physiotherapy (CDP) after recurrent malignancy is ruled out:
  - Phase I: Therapist administers manual lymphatic massage, compression bandaging, exercises, and skin care.
  - Phase II: Patient self-care activities, including use of compression garments, night wrappings, skin care, self-massage (manual lymph drainage), and continued exercises
  - Maintenance activities are time-consuming and are required lifelong; cost may be problematic for some patients. Adherence can be difficult but is necessary to prevent progression.
- Intermittent pneumatic gradient sequential pump therapy

- Compression garments that are properly fitted
- Elevation of edematous extremity
- Referral to physical therapy or surgery as indicated; specific exercises and surgical interventions may improve mobility but must be balanced with potential harms
- Pain management
- Referral to support group or support resources as appropriate
- Diuretics, used only temporarily if at all; effects are generally minimal. Little evidence exists for pharmacologic therapy of cancer-related lymphedema.
- Prevention is key:
  - Encourage exercise, particularly strengthening exercises and aerobic activities
  - Perform no heavy, dependent lifting of more than 15 lb.
  - Avoid breaks in the skin (e.g., wear gloves when gardening)
  - Prevent infection or treat promptly if it occurs.
  - Encourage good hygiene and precautions against trauma.
  - Encourage a well-balanced, low-sodium, high-fiber diet.
  - Maintain ideal body weight.
  - Consider wearing a well-fitted compression garment on long flights (National Lymphedema Network, Position Statement on Air Travel, May 2011. Available at http://www.lymphnet.org/pdfDocs/nlnairtravel.pdf (accessed March 1, 2016).

Patient Teaching

- Prevention education is the best risk reduction tool.
- Avoid trauma and breaks in the skin in the affected extremity.
- Practice good hygiene to avoid introduction of bacteria to potential open areas of the affected extremity.
- Avoid heavy, dependent lifting or vigorous repetitive motions against resistance.
- Avoid venipuncture, chemotherapy, blood product administration, injection, and assessment of blood pressure in the affected extremity unless need outweighs the potential consequences.
- Be aware of and report signs and symptoms of infection.
- Avoid having the limb in a dependent position for long periods, as with travel.
- Refer to patient teaching sheet in Section Seven.

Follow-up

- Periodically assess for intervention success with visual inspection and serial measurements of anatomic landmarks.
- Provide referrals as appropriate, especially for CDP if necessary.

Resources

- American Cancer Society: www.cancer.org
- Breast cancer.org: www.breastcancer.org
- Lymphedema Resources, Inc.: http://www.lymphedemaresources.org
- National Cancer Institute: www.cancer.gov

- National Comprehensive Cancer Network: http://www.nccn.org/patients/resources/life_with_cancer/managing_symptoms/lymphedema.aspx
- The National Lymphedema Network: www.lymphnet.org

Bibliography

Brayton, K., Hirsch, A., O Brien, P., Cheville, A., Karaca-Mandic, P., & Rockson, S. (2014). Lymphedema prevalence and treatment benefits in cancer: Impact of a therapeutic intervention on health outcomes and costs. *PLoS One, 9*(12), e114597.

Chang, C., & Cormier, J. (2013). Lymphedema interventions: Exercise, surgery, and compression devices. *Seminars in Oncology Nursing, 29*(1), 28–40.

Fu, M. (2014). Breast cancer-related lymphedema: Symptoms, diagnosis, risk reduction, and management. *World Journal of Clinical Oncology, 5*(3), 241–247.

Fu, M., Deng, J., & Armer, J. (2014). Putting evidence into practice: Cancer-related lymphedema. *Clinical Journal of Oncology Nursing, 18*(6), 68–79.

Fu, M., & Kang, Y. (2013). Psychosocial impact of living with cancer-related lymphedema. *Seminars in Oncology Nursing, 29*(1), 50–60.

International Society of Lymphology. (2013). The diagnosis and treatment of peripheral lymphedema: 2013 Consensus Document of the International Society of Lymphology. *Lymphology, 46*, 1–11. Available at http://www.u.arizona.edu/~witte/2013consensus.pdf (accessed March 1, 2016).

Marrs, J. (2015). Lymphedema. In C. Brown (Ed.), *Guide to oncology symptom management* (pp. 315–332). Pittsburg, PA: Oncology Nursing Society.

Ridner, S. (2014). Lymphedema. In C. Yarbro, D. Wujcik, & B. Gobel (Eds.), *Cancer symptom management* (4th ed.) (pp. 555–564). Burlington, MA: Jones & Bartlett.

Ridner, S. (2013). Pathophysiology of lymphedema. *Seminars in Oncology Nursing, 29*(1), 4–11.

Ryan, J., Cleland, C., & Fu, M. (2012). Predictors of practice patterns for lymphedema care among oncology advanced practice nurses. *Journal for the Advanced Practitioner in Oncology, 3*(5), 307–318.

Wanchai, A., Armer, J., & Stewart, B. (2013). Complementary and alternative medicine and lymphedema. *Seminars in Oncology Nursing, 29*(1), 41–49.

Menopausal Symptoms

Wendy H. Vogel

Definition

- Menopause is a hormonal change that occurs when estrogen and progesterone levels begin to drop.
- It usually occurs between the ages of 45 and 55 years; however, it can also be surgically or chemically induced.
- The average age at menopause in the United States is 51 years.
- There are increasing numbers of women who have menopausal symptoms after treatment for cancer.
- Early menopause can have long-lasting effects on a woman's quality of life.

Pathophysiology and Contributing Factors

- Physiologic menopause is caused by exhaustion of the ovarian follicles, which contain the germ cells that produce the steroid hormones estrogen and progesterone.
- Premature ovarian failure is cessation of ovarian function before the age of 40 years.
- Ovarian failure may be induced by radiation therapy, chemotherapy, surgery, or infection.
- When a decreased level of hormone is detected by the hypothalamus, the pituitary gland secretes follicle-stimulating hormone (FSH) and luteinizing hormone (LH). In menopause, the ovaries are unable to respond to the FSH and LH; therefore, estrogen deficiency occurs, ovulation does not occur, and the woman becomes amenorrheic.
- Vasomotor instability (a hot flash) is caused by dysfunction of the thermoregulatory center in the hypothalamus.
  - There is a sharp rise in epinephrine, which stimulates heart function, a rise in blood pressure, and an intense feeling of warmth throughout the upper body with flushing and perspiration that may last as little as a few seconds or as long as 20 minutes.
  - Estrogen influences the firing rate of the thermosensitive neurons in the preoptic area of the hypothalamus and affects how responsive vascular smooth muscle is to vasoactive substances such as epinephrine and norepinephrine.
  - Symptoms may resolve spontaneously over time without treatment.
- Cancer survivors, especially those who have had breast cancer (65-80% of breast cancer survivors), may experience more vasomotor symptoms and at an earlier age.
- A few years after estrogen deprivation, women begin to experience genitourinary symptoms, primarily as a result of decreased arterial blood flow to vagina and vulva. This occurs in an estimated 50% to 75% of breast cancer survivors. The following symptoms may increase over time and may persist indefinitely:
  - Atrophy of the vaginal wall
  - Vaginal dryness, infections, bleeding, and burning sensations
  - Dyspareunia
  - Urinary symptoms occurring as a result of urogenital atrophy
  - Decreased libido, which may occur because loss of ovarian function also decreases serum androgen levels.
- Psychological changes:
  - Estrogen increases the degradation rate of monoamine oxidase, the enzyme that catabolizes serotonin.
  - Serotonin deficiency is believed to contribute to depression.
  - Decreased bone density occurs because of the imbalance of bone resorption and formation. Early estrogen deprivation can lead to osteoporosis and potential fractures.
  - The risk for heart disease is increased because risk is relative to the age at which estrogen deprivation occurs.

Signs and Symptoms

- Can be mild or severe
- Change in or cessation of menses
- Vasomotor symptoms such as hot flashes and night sweats
- Vaginal atrophy, thinning of the vaginal wall, dryness, dyspareunia, postcoital bleeding
- Urinary symptoms such as urgency, stress incontinence, and frequent urinary tract infections
- Emotional lability, mood changes, irritability
- Cognitive changes such as forgetfulness or decreased ability to concentrate or make decisions; depression
- Weight gain in hips and thighs
- Sleep disturbances
- Decreased skin elasticity

Assessment Tools

- Thorough history and physical examination to determine the cause of menopausal symptoms.
- Pelvic examination, observing for vaginal atrophy and associated difficulties
- Assessment of the characteristics, frequency, and severity of symptoms

Laboratory and Diagnostic Tests

- FSH
- LH
- Serum estradiol
- Mean estrone level
- Urinalysis, presence of urinary tract symptoms
- Bone density testing
- Lipid panel

Differential Diagnoses

- Ovarian abnormalities
- Polycystic ovarian syndrome
- Pregnancy
- Hypothalamic dysfunction
- Hypothyroidism
- Pituitary tumors
- Adrenal abnormalities
- Ovarian neoplasm
- Tuberculosis
- Bone loss
- Lipid profile elevations

Interventions

Pharmacologic Interventions

- Hormone replacement therapy (HRT) is a controversial subject in postmenopausal women because of various health risks, including breast cancer. However, it is not always contraindicated.
  - HRT options involve different doses of estrogen or combinations of estrogen and progesterone or testosterone and different levels of systemic absorption depending on the route of administration.
  - HRT is contraindicated in patients who have experienced a stroke or thromboembolic event, recent myocardial infarction, acute liver or pancreatic disease, or undiagnosed vaginal bleeding.
  - For menopausal symptoms, HRT may be considered but should be given for the shortest period possible (ideally, <5 yr).
  - HRT should be chosen to match the specific menopausal complaints and to provide maximum safety.
  - HRT options include oral estrogens, vaginal estrogens, and transdermal estrogens, each of which can involve various hormone combinations. A full discussion of benefits and risks of HRT should ensue between the patient and the health care provider.
  - In the oncology patient, careful consideration should be given to hormone-related cancer, and the risks of cancer stimulation should be evaluated.
  - The lowest possible dose of estrogen should be chosen. Oral doses and vaginal doses as low 0.3 mg may provide relief from hot flashes and vaginal discomfort, although the lower doses may have a somewhat delayed response. Consider adding a progestin if a patient remains symptomatic.
  - Local estrogen products may be used for vaginal and urinary complaints and have less systemic absorption.
  - Minimizing progestin exposure decreases the rate of endometrial hyperplasia. Progestins may be given less frequently, such as quarterly or biannually, to women taking lower dose estrogens.
  - Topical estrogens may be useful for vaginal and urinary symptoms, but the potential risks should be reviewed with the patient.
- Zoledronic acid is in clinical trials for the prevention of bone loss in postmenopausal women with breast cancer who are taking an aromatase inhibitor.
- Nonhormonal pharmacologic options for vasomotor symptoms include the following:
  - Clonidine, oral or transdermal

Venlafaxine, fluoxetine, citalopram, or paroxetine (caution is advised because of possible interactions between selective serotonin reuptake inhibitors or serotonin-norepinephrine reuptake inhibitors and tamoxifen)

  - Bellergal or Bellergal-S (ergotamine, belladonna, and phenobarbital)
  - Propranolol
  - Lofexidine
  - Vitamin E 400 IU twice daily; also vitamins B and C
  - Ginseng
  - Megace acetate and medroxyprogesterone have been used; however, their safety in patients with a hormonally sensitive tumor is not fully known. Progestins can stimulate proliferation of the endometrium when given alone. Potential risks and benefits of treatment must be considered carefully and discussed with the patient.
  - Phytoestrogens and black cohosh have been used, but the safety of these interventions is not known, and the results in many studies show effects similar to those of placebo.

- Gabapentin is being evaluated in clinical trials for the treatment of hot flashes, but side effects may limit its use.

Nonpharmacologic Interventions

- For hot flashes (effectiveness not established):
  - Acupuncture
  - Paced respirations
  - Trained relaxation techniques
  - Avoidance of hot flash triggers such as alcohol, hot drinks, or spicy foods
- Follow a low-fat diet, cease smoking, allow low to moderate alcohol intake, maintain a healthy weight, and avoid a sedentary lifestyle.
- Weight reduction and moderate exercise of 30 minutes or more on most days of the week should be recommended.
- Vaginal lubricants, such as Replens (Auspharm, Australia), may be helpful for vaginal dryness (refer to Sexuality Alterations, page 347).
- Insomnia may be treated both pharmacologically and nonpharmacologically (refer to Sleep Disturbances, page 350).
- Osteoporosis prevention and treatment:
  - Bisphosphonates may be prescribed for patients with osteopenia or osteoporosis.
  - Raloxifene, a selective receptor modulator, is also approved for the prevention and treatment of osteoporosis. It should not be given with an aromatase inhibitor or with tamoxifen. Raloxifene may increase hot flashes.
  - Patients should be advised to take calcium and vitamin D, to perform weight-bearing exercise, and to avoid smoking and excessive alcohol intake.

Patient Teaching

- Patients should understand the fertility risks and the potential for early menopause before undergoing cancer treatment.
- If HRT is considered, the risks and benefits must be fully explored with the patient.
- Prevention and screening for osteoporosis and maintenance of bone health are important.

Follow-up

- Follow up as needed to assess symptom management
- Sleep hygiene or bladder training as appropriate

Resources

- American Cancer Society: www.cancer.org
- Breastcancer.org: www.breastcancer.org
- Chemocare.org: www.chemocare.org
- National Cancer Institute: www.cancer.gov

Bibliography

Desmarais, J., & Looper, K. (2010). Managing menopausal symptoms and depression in tamoxifen users: Implications of drug and medicinal interactions. *Maturitas, 67*(4), 296–308.

Engstrom, C. (2010). Hot flashes. In C. Brown (Ed.), *Guide to oncology symptom management* (pp. 299–314). Pittsburg, PA: Oncology Nursing Society.

Erickson, J., & Berger, A. (2010). Sleep-wake disturbances. In C. Brown (Ed.), *Guide to oncology symptom management* (pp. 473–496). Pittsburg, PA: Oncology Nursing Society.

Frazier, S., & Egger, M. (2014). Menopausal symptoms. In C. Yarbro, D. Wujcik, & B. Gobel (Eds.), *Cancer symptom management* (4th ed.) (pp. 45–61). Burlington, MA: Jones & Bartlett.

Hickey, M., Saunders, C., Partridge, A., Santoro, N., Joffe, H., & Stearns, V. (2008). Practical guidelines for assessing and managing menopausal symptoms after breast cancer. *Annals of Oncology, 19*, 1669–1680.

Kaplan, M., & Mahon, S. (2014). Hot flash management: Update of the evidence for patients with cancer. *Clinical Journal of Oncology Nursing, 18*(6), S59–S67.

Michaelson-Cohen, R., & Beller, U. (2009). Managing menopausal symptoms after gynecological cancer. *Current Opinions in Oncology, 21*(5), 407–411.

Misiewicz, H. (2014). *Acupuncture for the management of hot flashes in breast cancer survivors.* Abstract 210 at JADPRO Live10/30/2014-11/2/ 2014, Orlando, FL.

Trinkaus, M., Shin, S., Wolfman, W., Simmons, C., & Clemons, M. (2008). Should urogenital atrophy in breast cancer survivors be treated with topical estrogens? *The Oncologist, 13*, 222–231.

Mucositis

Kristin A. Cawley

Definition

- Mucositis is an inflammatory process that affects the mucous membranes of the oral cavity and gastrointestinal tract.
- It is commonly associated with chemotherapy, radiation therapy, and bone marrow transplantation.
- It can occur anywhere along the digestive tract from the mouth to the anus; in the mouth or oropharynx, it is referred to as oral mucositis.
- It occurs in 40% of patients treated with chemotherapy.
- Almost 100% of patients receiving chemotherapy and radiation therapy for head and neck cancer and as many as 80% of patients undergoing hematopoietic stem cell transplantation (HSCT) experience mucositis.
- It is the most significant adverse symptom of cancer treatment reported by patients.

Pathophysiology and Contributing Factors

- Breakdown of rapidly dividing epithelial cells caused by chemotherapy and radiation treatment, primarily in the gastrointestinal tract
- Previous history of mucositis
- Poor oral hygiene, prior dental disease
- Treatment and dose regimen
- History of kidney disease, diabetes, or HIV infection
- Ill-fitting dentures
- Age younger than 20 years or older than 50 years
- History of alcohol use and smoking

Signs and Symptoms

- Dry, cracked lips
- Pain and difficulty swallowing

- Soreness or pain in the mouth or throat; usually begins as asymptomatic erythema of the oral mucosa that may feel like burning or tingling in the mouth
- Red, shiny, or swollen mouth and gums
- Ulcers or sores in the mouth, on gums, and on the tongue; the sores may be reddish and may have white centers
- Mucosal bleeding
- Sensitivity to hot and cold foods
- Feeling of dryness (xerostomia), mild burning, or pain
- Infection
- Weight loss
- Dehydration

Assessment Tools

- Oral Assessment Guide (OAG)
- Oral Mucositis Index (OMI)
- Oral Mucositis Assessment Scale (OMAS)
- Common toxicity criteria common terminology criteria for adverse events, v4.0 (CTCAE)
- World Health Organization (WHO) scale for oral mucositis
- Eastern Cooperative Oncology Group (EGOG) common toxicity criteria
- History and physical examination; clinical examination based on inspection of oral cavity
- Risk for mucositis
- Current oral hygiene and dental care
- Nutritional status
- Symptomatic functional assessment based on ability to swallow
- Pain, using a scale of 0 to 10 or a categorical scale (none, mild, moderate, or severe)

Laboratory and Diagnostic Tests

- Complete blood cell count (CBC)
- Blood, urine, sputum cultures

Differential Diagnoses

- Pain
- Malnutrition
- Infection
- Dysphagia
- Bleeding
- Anorexia
- Xerostomia
- Dehydration

Interventions

- Treat the underlying cause.

Pharmacologic Interventions

- Palifermin (Kepivance)
- Viscous lidocaine
- Opioid narcotics
- Total parenteral nutrition (TPN), if mucositis is severe

Nonpharmacologic Interventions

- Monitor nutritional intake and weight; consult a dietician

- Cryotherapy
- Low-level laser therapy (LLLT) for patients undergoing HSCT
- Saline and sodium bicarbonate rinses

Patient Teaching

- Dental evaluation before initiation of treatment and throughout
- Cleaning:
  - Brush with a soft toothbrush.
  - Continue despite thrombocytopenia or neutropenia unless uncontrolled bleeding develops.
  - Use fluoride toothpaste.
- Floss daily
  - Patients who floss regularly should continue unless there is uncontrolled bleeding, the platelet level falls to less than 20,000 per microliter, or the absolute neutrophil count (ANC) is less than 1 per microliter.
- Rinsing:
  - Normal saline solution (NS), sodium bicarbonate ($NaHCO_3$), NS/$NaHCO_3$, water
  - Nonalcoholic, nonmedicated, unsweetened mouthwash
  - Before meals, increasing to every 2 hours as needed for comfort (swish/gargle for 15-30 seconds).
- Dental appliances should be left out as much as possible once mucous membranes become irritated.
- Maintain adequate hydration.
- Avoid tobacco, alcohol, and foods that are spicy, acidic, hot, or rough.
- Report any fever of 100.5° F (38° C) or greater.
- Report any pain that is unrelieved with pain medication.
- Dietary modifications:
  - Encourage a soft diet or a liquid diet supplement, which may be more tolerable.

Follow-up

- Assess for increased risk of mucositis with continuing treatments.
- Assess for pain that is unrelieved with pain medication.
- Reinforce the importance of communication with physician and nurse.

Resources

- American Cancer Society. Caring for the Patient with Cancer at Home: Mouth sores. http://www.cancer.org/treatment/treatmentsandsideeffects/physicalsideeffects/dealingwithsymptomsathome/caring-for-the-patient-with-cancer-at-home-mouth-sores
- National Cancer Institute. Oral complications of chemotherapy and head/neck radiation (PDQ): http://www.cancer.gov/about-cancer/treatment/side-effects/mouth-throat/oral-complications-pdq
- National Institute of Dental and Craniofacial Research. Oral complications of cancer treatment: What the oncology team can do: http://www.nidcr.nih.gov/oralhealth/Topics/CancerTreatment/OralComplicationsCancerOncology.htm

- Oncolink: Cancer resources for patients and health care professionals. Mucositis: The basics: http://www.oncolink.org/coping/article.cfm?id=965
- Oncology Nursing Society. Putting Evidence into Practice: Mucositis: https://www.ons.org/practice-resources/pep/mucositis

Bibliography

Bensinger, W., Schubert, M., Ang, K. K., Brizel, D., Brown, E., Eilers, J. G., & Trotti, A. M., 3rd. (2008). NCCN Task Force Report: Prevention and management of mucositis in cancer care. *Journal of the National Comprehensive Cancer Network*, 6(Suppl. 1), S1–S21; quiz S22–S24.

Bhatt, V., Vendrell, N., Nau, K., Crumb, D., & Roy, V. (2010). Implementation of a standardized protocol for prevention and management of oral mucositis in patients undergoing hematopoietic cell transplantation. *Journal of Oncology Pharmacy Practice*, 16(3), 195–204.

Brown, C. G., Beck, S. L., Peterson, D. E., McGuire, D. B., Dudley, W. N., & Mooney, K. H. (2009). Patterns of sore mouth in outpatients with cancer receiving chemotherapy. *Supportive Care in Cancer*, 17(4), 413–428.

Dawson, C. J., Hickey, M. M., & Newton, S. (2011). Mucositis. In C. J. Dawson, M. M. Hickey, & S. Newton (Eds.), *Telephone triage for otorhinolaryngology and head-neck nurses*. Pittsburg, PA: Oncology Nursing Society.

Eilers, J. E., Harris, D., Henry, K., & Johnson, L. A. (2014). Evidence-based interventions for cancer treatment-related mucositis: Putting evidence into practice. *Clinical Journal of Oncology Nursing*, 18(Suppl.), 80–96.

Epstein, J. B., & Schubert, M. M. (2003). Oropharyngeal mucositis in cancer therapy: Review of pathogenesis, diagnosis, and management. *Oncology*, 17, 1767–1779.

Harris, D. J., Eilers, J., Harriman, A., Cashavelly, B. J., & Maxwell, C. (2015). Putting evidence into practice: Evidenced-based interventions for the management of oral mucositis. *Clinical Journal of Oncology Nursing*, 12(1), 141–152.

Keefe, D. M., Schubert, M. M., Elting, L. S., Sonis, S. T., Epstein, J. B., Raber-Durlacher, J. E., & Mucositis Study Section of the Multinational Association of Supportive Care in Cancer and the International Society for Oral Oncology. (2007). Updated clinical practice guidelines for the prevention and treatment of mucositis. *Cancer*, 109, 820–831.

Lalla, R. V., Sonis, S. T., & Peterson, D. E. (2008). Management of oral mucositis in patients with cancer. *Dental Clinics of North America*, 52(1), 61–77.

Lalla, R. V., Bowen, J., Barasch, A., Elting, L., Epstein, J., Keefe, D. M., & The Mucositis Guidelines Leadership Group of the Multinational Association of Supportive Care in Cancer and International Society of Oral Oncology (MASCC/ISOO). (2014). MASCC/ISOO clinical practice guidelines for the management of mucositis secondary to cancer therapy. *Cancer*, 120, 14531461.

McGuire, D. B., Fulton, J. S., Park, J., Brown, C. G., Correa, M. E., Eilers, J., & Lalla, R. V. (2013). Systematic review of basic oral care for the of oral mucositis in cancer patients. On behalf of the Mucositis Study Group of the Multinational Association of Supportive Care in Cancer/International Society of Oral Oncology (MASCC/ISOO). *Supportive Care in Cancer*, 21(11), 3165–3177.

Rubenstein, E. B., Peterson, D. E., Schubert, M., Keefe, D., McGuire, D., Epstein, J., & International Society for Oral Oncology. (2004). Clinical practice guidelines for the prevention and treatment of cancer therapy-induced oral and gastrointestinal mucositis. *Cancer*, 100(9 Suppl.), 2026–2046.

Sonis, S. T., Elting, L. S., Keefe, D., Peterson, D. E., Schubert, M., & Hauer-Jensen, M. (2004). Perspectives on cancer therapy-induced mucosal injury: Pathogenesis, measurement, epidemiology, and consequences for patients. *Cancer*, 100(9 Suppl.), 1995–2025.

Stricker, C. T., & Sullivan, J. (2003). Evidence-based oncology oral care clinical practice guidelines: Development, implementation, and evaluation. *Clinical Journal of Oncology Nursing*, 7, 222–227.

Worthington, H. V., Clarkson, J. E., & Eden, O. B. (2004). Interventions for treating oral mucositis for patients with cancer receiving treatment. *Cochrane Database of Systematic Reviews* (2), CD001973.

Yamagata, K., Arai, C., & Sasaki, H. (2012). The effect of oral management on the severity of oral mucositis during hematopoietic stem cell transplant. *Bone Marrow Transplant*, 47(5), 725–730.

Nail Changes

Colleen O'Leary

Definition

- The types and severity of nail changes depend on the drug, dose, duration, and frequency of treatment.
- Nail changes include the following:
  - Changes in nail color
  - Growth reduction
  - Beau's lines—deep horizontal grooves across the nails
  - Mees' lines—horizontal lines of white/opaque discoloration across nails reflecting damage to the distal nail matrix and moving distally with nail growth
  - Onycholysis—lifting of the nail from nail bed
  - Paronychia—inflammation of skin folds around nail
  - Onychomycosis—fungal nail infection
  - Ingrown toenails
  - Pincer nails—type of ingrown nail in which an overcurvature causes the nail to penetrate into the soft tissue
- Nail changes occur frequently, especially with the use of taxanes, epidermal growth factor receptor (EGFR) inhibitors, and mammalian target of rapamycin (mTOR) inhibitors.
- Nail changes seen with chronic graft-versus-host disease (GVHD) can range from mild nail dystrophy to anoychia and include the following:
  - Longitudinal ridging
  - Splitting or brittle nails
  - Onycholysis
  - Pterygium—abnormal adherence of the nail plate to the proximal nail fold
- It is important to distinguish between GVHD nail changes and infectious processes.
- The most common nail infections are paronychial infections and onychomycosis.

Pathophysiology and Contributing Factors

- There are multiple mechanisms of adverse nail changes, including changes to the nail bed and surrounding tissue and sensitivity to environmental factors such as exposure to chemicals, polishes, or harsh detergents and prolonged water or ultraviolet exposure.
- Often more than one process is involved.
- Changes to the nail bed and nail can be caused by defective nail matrix production, resulting from effects of cancer treatments (chemotherapy and molecularly targeted agents) on maturation of cells, and by direct toxicity to structures surrounding the nail.

- Nail color changes result from toxins related to chemotherapy that alter melanocytes in the epithelium of the nail matrix.
- Toxins from the chemotherapy can cause damage to the nail bed and edema under the nail bed, resulting in onycholysis.
- Toxin-related damage to soft tissue surrounding the nail toxins can lead to paronychia and possible secondary infection.
- Changes such as splinter hemorrhage and subungual hemorrhage may result when patients are thrombocytopenic.
- Frequency and duration of treatment contribute to nail changes; patients receiving taxanes for longer than 6 weeks are predisposed to nail changes.
- More adverse nail changes are seen with patients receiving treatments every week rather than every 3 weeks.
- Some research indicates that chemotherapy makes nails more sensitive to ultraviolet light, which can cause further damage.
- Certain types of chemotherapies, such as taxanes, EGFR inhibitors, and mTOR inhibitors, confer a greater risk for nail changes.

Signs and Symptoms

- The National Cancer Institute's common terminology criteria for adverse effects (CTCAE) are used to grade nail changes based on symptoms.
  - Grade 1 includes nail discoloration, asymptomatic nail loss, nail ridging, localized nail infection, and paronychia without pain.
  - Grade 2 includes symptomatic nail loss limiting activities of daily living (ADLs), nail infection requiring oral antibiotics, paronychia with pain interfering with ADLs, and nail plate separation.
  - Grade 3 includes nail infections requiring intravenous, radiologic, or operative treatment and paronychia limiting self-care with intravenous treatment indicated.
- Painful paronychias are most common and can involve multiple nails, especially the thumbs and great toes.
- Paronychial lesions may bleed easily.

Assessment Tools

- Observation of nails and surrounding skin is the most effective means of assessing for nail changes.

Laboratory and Diagnostic Tests

- There are no specific tests for nail changes other than observation. However, if infection is suspected, consideration should be given to obtaining cultures to tailor treatment.

Differential Diagnoses

- Infection
- Trauma

Interventions

Pharmacologic Interventions

- Oral or intravenous antibiotics for culture-proven paronychia.
- Empiric antibiotics initiated in immunocompromised patients.
- Soaks with Burrows solution (4% thymol in alcohol with aluminum acetate).
- Silver nitrate and ferric subsulfate to act as chemical cautery
- Topical corticosteroids to reduce inflammation

Nonpharmacologic Interventions

- Soaking nails in warm water two or three times a day can help reduce swelling and pain.
- Soaks with white vinegar (1:10) or bleach (0.25 cup bleach to 3 gallons water) for 10 minutes a day can provide relief from pain, decrease the microbe count, and prevent superinfections.

Patient Teaching

- Keep nails trimmed and clean.
- Wear gloves when gardening or house cleaning.
- Paint nails to hide blemishes and increase nail strength.
- Remove nail polish with nonacetone remover only.
- Do not bite or tear nails.
- Do not pick at cuticles.
- Use cuticle removal cream or gel.
- Massage cuticle cream into nail area daily to avoid dryness and hangnails.
- Limit the time your hands are in water.
- Avoid professional manicures unless you bring all of your own equipment.
- Do not use artificial nails.
- If ingrown nails occur, soak in warm water and apply antibiotic cream. If area is painful, is swollen, or has discharge, contact your health care provider.
- Tell your health care provider about any signs of inflammation or infection.
- If you need to bandage an area, use paper tape.
- Soak nails in vegetable or olive oil daily and gently massage.
- Wear comfortable shoes that do not rub.
- If an infectious organism is identified, discard or wash in hot soapy water with bleach any slippers, socks, or gloves that might have become contaminated.

Follow-up

- As needed to assess signs and symptoms.
- Refer patient to podiatry and/or dermatology specialists for assistance in management of nail disorders.
- Consult with an infectious disease specialist if infection is suspected.

Resources

- American Cancer Society: www.cancer.org
- Patient Resource: www.patientresource.com
- Breastcancer.org: www.breastcancer.org
- Chemocare.org: www.chemocare.org
- American Podiatric Medical Association: www.apma.org
- American Academy of Dermatology: www.aad.org
- Podiatry Today: http://www.podiatrytoday.com/diagnosing-and-treating-chemotherapy-induced-nail-changes
- National Cancer Institute: http://evs.nci.nih.gov/ftp1/CTCAE/CTCAE_4.03_2010-06-14_QuickReference_5x7.pdf

Bibliography

Balagula, Y., Garbe, C., Mysowski, P., Hauschild, A., Rapoport, B., Boers-Doets, C. B., & Lacouture, M. E. (2011). Clinical presentation and management of dermatologic toxicities of epidermal growth factor inhibitors. *International Journal of Dermatology, 50,* 129–146.

Boussemart, L., Routier, E., Mateus, C., Opletalova, K., Sebille, G., Kamsu-Kom, N., & Robert, C. (2013). Prospective study of cutaneous side-effects associated with the BRAF inhibitor vemurafenib: A study of 42 patients. *Annals of Oncology, 24,* 1691–1697.

Bryce, J., & Boers-Doets, C. B. (2014). Non-rash dermatologic adverse events related to targeted therapies. *Seminars in Oncology Nursing, 30*(3), 155–168.

Eames, T., Grabein, B., Kroth, J., & Wolleberg, A. (2010). Microbiological analysis of epidermal growth factor receptor inhibitor therapy-associated paronychia. *Journal of the European Academy of Dermatology and Venereology, 24,* 958–960.

Hoffman, K. (2014). Diagnosing and treating chemotherapy-induced nail changes. *Podiatry Today, 27*(2), 42–50.

McLellan, B., & Kerr, H. (2011). Cutaneous toxicities of the multikinase inhibitors sorafenib and sunitanib. *Dermatologic Therapy, 24*(4), 396–400.

Miller, K. K., Gorcey, L., & McLellan, B. N. (2014). Chemotherapy-induced hand-foot syndrome and nail changes: A review of clinical presentation, etiology, pathogenesis, and management. *Journal of the American Academy of Dermatology, 71,* 787–794.

National Cancer Institute. (2009). *Common terminology criteria for adverse events, v4.0.* National Cancer Institute, National Institutes of Health, Department of Health and Human Services. Available at http://evs.nci.nih.gov/ftp1/CTCAE/CTCAE_4.03_2010-06-14_QuickReference_5x7.pdf (accessed March 1, 2016).

National Institutes of Health. (2014). *Medline Plus Medical Encyclopedia: paronychia.* U.S. Library of Medicine. Available at http://www.nlm.nih.gov/medlineplus/ency/article/001444.htm (accessed March 1, 2016).

Peuvrel, L., Bachmeyer, C., Reguiai, Z., Bachet, J. B., André, T., Bensadoun, R. J., & Dréno, B. (2012). Semiology of skin toxicity associated with epidermal growth factor receptor (EGFR) inhibitors. *Supportive Care in Cancer, 20,* 909–921.

Sinha, R., Edmonds, K., Newton-Bishop, J. A., Gore, M. E., Larkin, J., & Fearfield, L. (2012). Cutaneous adverse events associated with vemurafenib in patients with metastatic melanoma: Practical advice on diagnosis, prevention and management of the main treatment-related skin toxicities. *British Journal of Dermatology, 167,* 987–994.

Tosti, A., & Piraccini, B. A. (2012). Nail disorders. In J. L. Bolognia, J. L. Jorizzo, & J. V. Schaffer (Eds.), *Dermatology* (3rd ed.). Philadelphia, PA: Saunders.

Wu, P. A., Balagula, Y., Lacouture, M. E., & Anadkat, M. J. (2011). Prophylaxis and treatment of dermatologic adverse events from epidermal growth factor receptor inhibitors. *Current Opinions in Oncology, 23,* 343–351.

Nausea and Vomiting

Carolyn Grande

Definition

Nausea

- Nausea is s sensation of profound revulsion to food or of impending vomiting, a feeling of being sick at one's stomach.
- It can be classified as anticipatory, acute, delayed, breakthrough, or refractory.
- Severity can lead to poor compliance with treatment regimen and decreased quality of life.

Vomiting

- Vomiting is forceful expulsion of gastric contents from the stomach through the mouth.
- Matter is ejected from the stomach through the mouth.

Patterns of Nausea and Vomiting

- *Anticipatory*: a conditioned response that occurs before chemotherapy. It typically occurs after a negative experience with chemotherapy.
- *Acute*: onset within a few minutes to several hours after drug administration; usually resolves within 24 hours
- *Delayed*: onset more than 24 hours after chemotherapy; achieves maximum intensity 48 to 72 hours after chemotherapy and can last up to 7 days
- *Breakthrough*: occurs if preventive regimen fails
- *Refractory*: occurs in subsequent chemotherapy cycles when prior antiemetic prophylactic or rescue therapies have failed

Pathophysiology and Contributing Factors

- Mechanisms include activation of afferent impulses to the vomiting center (medulla) in the brain from the chemotherapy trigger zone (CTZ); peripheral mechanisms in the gastrointestinal (GI) tract; vestibular mechanisms; cortical mechanisms; and alterations of taste and smell.
- Efferent impulses sent from the medulla (vomiting center) initiate a series of events leading to vomiting. Several neuroreceptors are involved in emesis, most notably serotonin (5-hydroxytryptamine [5-HT3]) and neurokinin-1 (NK-1). Anticipatory nausea and vomiting involves a psychological mechanism because the experience is not related to the administration of chemotherapy or radiation therapy.
- The exact mechanism of radiation-induced vomiting is not clear; however, it is believed that a peripheral mechanism in the GI tract or central mechanisms in the CTZ may contribute.
- Contributing factors include the following:
  - Underlying tumor
  - Treatment-related toxicity:
    - Surgery
    - Chemotherapy
    - Radiation therapy
    - Blood and marrow transplantation
- Patient-specific factors:
  - Sex—women more susceptible
  - Age—younger patients more susceptible
  - Alcohol history—higher consumption correlates with lower incidence
  - Performance status—lower performance status correlates with higher incidence
  - History of morning sickness or motion sickness—positive history increases susceptibility
  - Level of chemotherapy emetogenicity: low, moderate, or high (see table on page 328)
  - Tumor burden—greater susceptibility as tumor burden increases
  - Combined-modality therapy—greater susceptibility compared with monotherapy
  - Dehydration—increases incidence.
  - Comorbid conditions: anxiety, GI malignancies, intestinal obstruction, impaired liver or renal function, hypercalcemia, hepatitis, pancreatitis, peritonitis, cerebellar metastasis

Signs and Symptoms

- Ill feeling of the stomach
- Hypersalivation
- Diaphoresis
- Tachycardia
- Tachypnea

Emetic Risk Classifications for Chemotherapy-Induced Nausea and Vomiting

Risk	Emesis Risk Without Use of Antiemetics (%)
High	>90
Moderate	30-90
Low	10-30
Minimal	<10

Modified from Grunberg, S., & Hawkins, R. (2009). Chemotherapy-induced nausea and vomiting: Challenges and opportunities for improved patient outcomes. *Clinical Journal of Oncology Nursing, 13*(1), 54-64; Multinational Association of Supportive Care in Cancer (MASCC). (2014). MASCC/ESMO antiemetic guideline 2013. Available at http://www.mascc.org/assets/Guidelines-Tools/mascc_antiemetic_english_2014.pdf (accessed March 1, 2016); National Comprehensive Cancer Network. (2015). NCCN clinical practice guidelines in oncology (NCCN guidelines): Antiemesis, v1.2015. Available at http://www.nccn.org/professionals/physician_gls/pdf/antiemesis.pdf (accessed March 1, 2016).

Assessment Tools

- The hallmark assessment tool is patient report.
- Other assessment information:
  - Physical examination including vital signs and weight
  - Laboratory data
  - Caregiver report

The common terminology criteria for adverse events (CTCAE) provides a grading system ranked from 1 to 5 for assessing severity of side effects associated with cancer therapy. Grade 1 represents the mildest and 5 the most severe effects (see table below).

Laboratory and Diagnostic Tests

- Laboratory tests to assess for a primary cause or secondary complications from persistent nausea and vomiting.
- Diagnostic tests to rule out differential diagnoses. There are no diagnostic tests for nausea/vomiting.

Common Terminology Criteria for Adverse Events (CTCAE) for Nausea and Vomiting

CTCAE Grade	Nausea	Vomiting
1	Loss of appetite without alteration in eating habits	1-2 episodes (separated by 5 min) in 24 hr
2	Oral intake decreased without significant weight loss, dehydration, or malnutrition	3-5 episodes (separated by 5 min) in 24 hr
3	Inadequate oral caloric or fluid intake; tube feeding, total parenteral nutrition, or hospitalization indicated	≥6 episodes (separated by 5 min) in 24 hr; tube feeding, total parenteral nutrition, or hospitalization indicated
4	—	Life-threatening consequences; urgent intervention indicated
5	—	Death

Adapted from National Cancer Institute. (2010). Common terminology criteria for adverse events (CTCAE), version 4.03. Available at http://ctep.cancer.gov/protocolDevelopment/electronic_applications/ctc.htm (accessed March 1, 2016).

- Complete blood cell count (CBC), electrolyte panel including sodium, potassium, and chloride; carbon dioxide level; blood urea nitrogen (BUN) and creatinine; liver function tests
- Radiography: flat plate of the abdomen, obstruction series

Differential Diagnoses

- Chemotherapy–induced nausea/vomiting
- Radiation therapy–induced nausea/vomiting
- Underlying disease
- Intestinal obstruction
- Cholecystitis
- Cirrhosis
- Diverticulitis
- Gastritis
- Hepatitis
- Migraine headache
- Pancreatitis
- Medication–induced nausea

Interventions

- Prevention of nausea and vomiting is the goal.

Pharmacologic Interventions
Anticipatory Nausea or Vomiting

- Benzodiazepines (select one)
  - Alprazolam (Xanax) 0.5-1 mg orally three times a day, starting the night before treatment, then repeated the next day 1-2 hours before chemotherapy OR
  - Lorazepam (Ativan) 0.5-2 mg orally the night before treatment and on the morning of treatment, then repeated the next day 1-2 hours before chemotherapy

Acute and Delayed Nausea/Vomiting: Highly Emetogenic Chemotherapy

- NK-1 receptor antagonist–containing regimen (select one)
  - Aprepitant (Emend) 125 mg orally on day 1, 80 mg orally daily on days 2 and 3 OR
  - Fosaprepitant (Emend Injectable) 150 mg IV on day 1 only AND
- Corticosteroid (select one)
  - Dexamethasone (Decadron) 12 mg orally or IV on day 1, 8 mg orally or IV on days 2-4 (with aprepitant 125 mg on day 1) OR
  - Dexamethasone 12 mg orally or IV on day 1, 8 mg orally on day 2, then 8 mg orally twice daily on days 3 and 4 (with fosaprepitant 150 mg IV on day 1) AND
- 5-HT3 receptor antagonist (select one)
  - Dolasetron (Anzemet) 100 mg orally on day 1
  - Granisetron (Kytril) either 2 mg orally, 1 mg orally twice a day, or 0.01 mg/kg IV on day 1, or transdermal patch (Sancuso), 3.1 mg/24-hour patch, applied 24-48 hours before chemotherapy administration, to remain in place no longer than 7 days
  - Ondansetron (Zofran) 16-24 mg orally or 8-16 mg IV on day 1
  - Palonosetron (Aloxi) 0.25 mg IV on day 1 OR

- Olanzapine (Zyprexa)-containing regimen
  - Olanzapine 10 mg orally on days 1-4 AND
  - Palonosetron 0.25 mg IV on day 1 AND
  - Dexamethasone 20 mg IV on day 1

Acute and Delayed Nausea/Vomiting: Moderately Emetogenic Chemotherapy
- 5-HT3 receptor antagonist (select one)
  - Dolasetron 100 mg orally on days 1-3
  - Granisetron either 2 mg orally, 1 mg orally twice a day, or 0.01 mg/kg IV on days 1-3
  - Transdermal patch (Sancuso), 3.1 mg/24-hour patch, applied 24-48 hours before chemotherapy administration to remain in place no longer than 7 days
  - Ondansetron 16-24 mg orally or 8-16 mg IV on day 1; then 8 mg orally twice a day or 16 mg orally daily or 8-16 mg IV daily on days 2 and 3
  - Palonosetron 0.25 mg IV on day 1
- Corticosteroid
  - Dexamethasone 12 mg orally or IV once day 1 and 8 mg orally or IV on days 2 and 3, WITH OR WITHOUT
- NK-1 antagonist (select one)
  - Aprepitant (Emend) 125 mg orally on day 1, 80 mg orally daily on days 2 and 3
  - Fosaprepitant (Emend Injectable) 150 mg IV on day 1 only AND
- Netupitant-containing regimen
  - Netupitant 300 mg/palonosetron 0.5 g (Akynzeo) orally, AND
- Olanzapine (Zyprexa)-containing regimen
  - Olanzapine 10 mg orally on days 1-4 AND
  - Palonosetron 0.25 mg IV on day 1 AND
  - Dexamethasone 20 mg IV on day 1

Acute and Delayed Nausea/Vomiting: Low Emetogenic Chemotherapy.
Start before chemotherapy and repeat daily for multiday doses:
- Dexamethasone 12 mg orally or IV on day of treatment, OR
- Prochlorperazine (Compazine) 10 mg orally or IV every 6 hr as needed or 15-mg spansule every 8-12 hr as needed, OR
- Metoclopramide (Reglan) 10-40 mg orally or IV every 4-6 hr as needed OR
- 5-HT3 antagonist (select one)
  - Dolasetron 100 mg orally daily
  - Granisetron 2 mg orally daily or 1 mg twice daily
  - Ondansetron 8-16 mg orally daily

Breakthrough Nausea or Vomiting.
The general rule is to consider administering an additional agent from a different class not previously given:
- Corticosteroid: Dexamethasone 12 mg orally or IV daily, OR
- 5-HT3 receptor antagonist (select one)
  - Dolasetron 100 mg orally
  - Granisetron either 1-2 mg orally daily, 1 mg orally twice daily, or 0.01 mg/kg (maximum 1 mg) IV
  - Ondansetron 16 mg orally or IV daily, OR
- Phenothiazine

- Prochlorperazine either 25 mg suppository every 12 hr, 10 mg orally, or IV every 6 hr, or 15 mg
- Promethazine 25 mg suppository per rectum every 6 hr or 12.5-25 mg orally or IV (central line only) every 4-6 hr
- Substituted benzamide: metoclopramide 10-40 mg orally every 4-6 hr
- Butyrophenone: haloperidol (Haldol) 0.5-2 mg orally every 4-6 hr
- Benzodiazepine: lorazepam 0.5-2 mg orally, sublingual, or IV every 4-6 hr
- Cannabinoid (select one)
  - Dronabinol (Marinol) 5-10 mg orally every 3-6 hr
  - Nabilone (Cesamet) 1-2 mg orally twice a day
- Atypical antipsychotic: olanzapine 10 mg orally daily for 3 days
- Anticholinergic belladonna alkaloid: scopalamine transdermal patch, 1 patch every 72 hr

Nonpharmacologic Interventions
- Behavioral management
- Acupuncture, acupressure
- Guided imagery, progressive muscle relaxation
- Music therapy

Patient Teaching
- Take antinausea medication on a timed schedule before nausea begins.
- Eat small, frequent meals. Nausea is more likely to occur on an empty stomach.
- Avoid spicy, greasy, or fatty foods and overly sweet foods.
- Cold foods, salty foods, dry crackers, and dry toast may be more tolerable.
- Consider diversionary activities (i.e., music therapy, relaxation techniques).
- Reduce food aromas and other strong odors.

Follow-up
- If vomiting is severe, restrict diet to clear liquids and notify doctor or nurse.
- If emesis is red or brown (coffee-ground appearance), recall foods eaten and notify doctor or nurse.

Resources
- Chemocare: http://chemocare.com/chemotherapy/side-effects/nausea-vomiting-chemotherapy.aspx (accessed January 6, 2016).
- CancerCare.org: http://www.cancercare.org/publications/212-chemotherapy-induced_nausea_and_vomiting_cinv. (accessed January 6, 2016).

Bibliography

Basch, E., Prestrud, A. A., Hesketh, P. J., Kris, M. G., Feyer, P. C., Somerfield, M. R., & American Society of Clinical Oncology. (2011). Antiemetics: American Society of Clinical Oncology clinical practice guidelines update. *Journal of Clinical Oncology, 29*(31), 4189–4198.

Grunberg, S., & Hawkins, R. (2009). Chemotherapy-induced nausea and vomiting: Challenges and opportunities for improved patient outcomes. *Clinical Journal of Oncology Nursing, 13*(1), 54–64.

Multinational Association of Supportive Care in Cancer (MASCC). http://www.mascc.org/assets/Guidelines-Tools/mascc_antiemetic_guidelines_english_2016_v.1.1.pdf (accessed April 3, 2016).

National Cancer Institute. (2010). *Common terminology criteria for adverse events (CTCAE), version 4.03.* Available at http://ctep.cancer.gov/protocolDevelopment/electronic_applications/ctc.htm (accessed March 1, 2016).

National Cancer Institute. (2015). *Nausea and vomiting—For health professionals (PDQ).* Available at http://www.cancer.gov/about-cancer/treatment/side-effects/nausea/nausea-hp-pdq (accessed March 1, 2016).

National Comprehensive Cancer Network. (2015). *NCCN clinical practice guidelines in oncology (NCCN guidelines): Antiemesis.* v. 1.2015. Available at http://www.nccn.org/professionals/physician_gls/pdf/antiemesis.pdf (accessed March 1, 2016).

Navari, R. M. (2009). Pharmacological management of chemotherapy-induced nausea and vomiting. *Drugs, 69*(5), 515–533.

Roila, F., Herrstedt, J., Aapro, M., Gralla, R. J., Einhorn, L. H., Ballatori, E., & ESMO/MASCC Guidelines Working Group. (2010). Guideline update for MASCC and ESMO in the prevention of chemotherapy- and radiotherapy-induced nausea and vomiting: Results of the Perugia consensus conference. *Annals of Oncology, 21*(Suppl. 5), v232–v243.

Tipton, J., McDaniel, R., Barbour, L., Johnston, M. P., Kayne, M., LeRoy, P., & Ripple, M. L. (2007). Putting evidence into practice: Evidence-based interventions to prevent, manage and treat chemotherapy-induced nausea and vomiting. *Clinical Journal of Oncology Nursing, 11*(1), 69–78.

Ocular and Visual Changes

Colleen O'Leary

Definitions

- Blepharitis
  - Inflammation of the eyelids that may include reddened eyelids with drainage and crusting around the eyelashes
  - Often accompanied by eye redness
- Epiphora
  - Watery eyes or excessive tearing
  - Excessive painless tearing, not related to crying
- Dry eye syndrome (ocular sicca)
  - It occurs when the eyes do not produce enough tears.
  - Although the eyes may produce excessive tearing, dry eye syndrome may cause a lack of the chemicals needed to form tears in order to lubricate eyes, which makes them feel dry.
- Conjunctivitis (see figure below)
  - Commonly called "pink eye"
  - Redness and inflammation around the conjunctiva

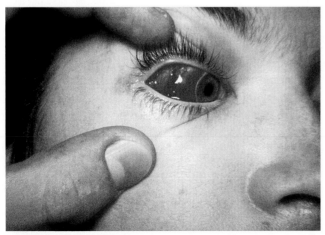

Conjunctivitis. (From Dr. Thomas F. Sellers, Emory University, Centers for Disease Control and Prevention.)

- Can be caused by allergies, bacteria, or viruses
- Conjunctival injection, commonly referred to as red or bloodshot eyes
- Chemosis: the conjunctiva may have the appearance of a blister or appear filled with fluid.
- Trichomegaly
  - Excessive growth of eyelashes as a result of cancer treatment
- Cataracts (see figure below)
  - A cloudy area in the lens of the eye that prevents light from passing through
  - Painless but lead to progressive loss of vision over time
  - Most often develops symmetrically in both eyes

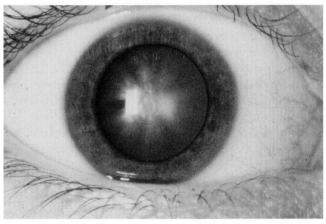

Cataracts. (From National Eye Institute, National Institutes of Health, retrieved from https://www.flickr.com/photos/nationaleyeinstitute/7544344214.)

- Glaucoma
  - Glaucoma occurs when the optic nerve is damaged, most commonly from an increase in intraocular pressure (IOP) greater than 22 mm Hg.
  - Increased IOP results from a buildup of the aqueous humor fluid, which normally flows through the eye and is subsequently drained.
  - There are several types, with the most common being open angle glaucoma, which occurs over time.
  - Closed angle glaucoma occurs suddenly.
  - Because the only symptom is loss of peripheral vision, regular ophthalmic evaluations are critical to early detection.
- Photophobia
  - Photophobia is the avoidance of light due to eye pain.
  - It is a common result of injury to the cornea.
  - Swelling of any eye structure may cause pain when the pupil is constricting.
  - Pain may be noticed when changing from dark to brightly lit environments or when going outside into the bright light.

Pathophysiology and Contributing Factors

- Blepharitis
  - Anterior blepharitis is less common and is found mainly around eyelashes and follicles.

- Posterior blepharitis involves inflammation of the inner portion of the eye around the meibomian gland.
- Meibomian glands secrete an oily layer of tear film to help prevent tears from evaporating.
- Posterior blepharitis often occurs with dry eye syndrome, conjunctivitis, and keratitis.
- Between 25% and 50% of patients receiving 5-fluorouracil (5-FU) develop blepharitis.
- Eighty percent of patients receiving cetuximab develop blepharitis, and 15% experience severe blepharitis.
- Patients with chronic graft-versus-host disease (cGVHD) are at greater risk for ocular GVHD, which can affect the lids, meibomian glands, and cornea.
- Epiphora
  - Epiphora is divided into four categories: lid-globe growth abnormalities, obstructive lacrimal drainage disorders, ocular surface disorders, and neurogenic lacrimal hypersecretory disorders.
  - Epiphora resulting from cancer treatment is most often caused by ocular surface disorders.
  - Blepharitis, foreign bodies, ptosis, or allergies can contribute to epiphora.
  - Agents known to be associated with epiphora include 5-FU, high-dose cytarabine, doxorubicin, bevacizumab, and imatinib.
  - Epiphora is a typical symptom of ocular GVHD.
- Dry eye syndrome (ocular sicca)
  - In dry eye syndrome, the eyes fail to produce a sufficient amount of tears.
  - Tears provide moisture, oxygen, and nutrients for the eye.
  - A decrease in tear production results in irritation.
  - The decrease in tear formation is usually caused by lacrimal aqueous insufficiency.
  - Ocular sicca is commonly seen with the use of 5-FU and retinoids as well as antihistamines, antidepressants, and antipsychotic medications.
  - The retinoid isotretinoin, used in the treatment of acute promyelocytic leukemia, is often associated with dry eye syndrome.
  - Ocular sicca is commonly seen with ocular GVHD.
- Conjunctivitis
  - Conjunctivitis is usually caused by viral infections, but noninfectious conjunctivitis is seen with the use of certain chemotherapeutic agents, including doxorubicin, 5-FU, capecitabine, carmustine, methotrexate, erlotinib, and epirubicin.
  - The conjunctiva, the transparent mucous membrane that lines the inner surface of the eyelid and covers the front part of the orbit, becomes inflamed, causing cellular infiltration, vascular engorgement, and diffuse exudation accompanied by itching and irritation.
  - Conjuctival injection and chemosis are common manifestations.
- Trichomegaly
  - The epidermal growth factor receptor (EGFR) pathway is important to normal development of hair follicles.
  - The biotherapy agents cetuximab, gefitinib, and erlotinib block the EGFR signaling pathway.
  - The cyclin-dependent kinase inhibitor 1C (P57) pathway is important in the regulation of hair follicle growth. EGFR inhibitors upregulate P57, causing an increase in maturation of hair follicles and leading to trichomegaly.
- Cataracts
  - The lens of the eye, which is normally clear, allows light to pass through the iris to the retina, where it is converted into nerve signals that are sent to the brain.
  - The lens is made mostly of water and crystalline proteins that are arranged in a particular pattern to allow light to pass through the lens.
  - When the crystalline proteins change over time, most often due to aging, they begin to clump together, resulting in the clouding seen with cataracts.
  - Cataracts can occur secondary to treatment with specific anticancer therapies or supportive care medications commonly used in cancer treatment (e.g., corticosteroids).
  - Patients with leukemia or lymphoma who are receiving long-term prednisone or dexamethasone therapy can experience cataracts.
  - Tamoxifen has been associated with the development of cataracts.
  - Patients who receive total body irradiation with bone marrow transplantation are at a greater risk for development of cataracts.
  - Patients with diabetes are at a greater risk for cataract formation.
- Glaucoma
  - The aqueous humor flows through the posterior and anterior chambers of the eye and eventually drains out of the eye through outflow mechanisms.
  - The flow of aqueous humor helps to preserve the integrity and functioning of ocular structures.
  - When the outflow mechanisms do not function correctly, the fluid builds up, causing increased IOP.
  - Increased IOP can cause damage to the optic nerve, resulting in loss of vision.
  - Glaucoma associated with chemotherapy is related to capillary protein leakage.
  - Administration of paclitaxel or docetaxel is associated with increased risk of glaucoma.
  - Corticosteroids, especially in eye drops, increase the risk for glaucoma.
  - Other medications that can increase the risk for development of glaucoma include sulfamethoxazole and trimethoprim, topiramate, ranitidine, epinephrine, and venlafaxine.
- Photophobia
  - When the rapidly dividing cells of the corneal epithelium are exposed to chemotherapeutic agents, small (pinpoint) areas on the outer layer of the epithelium are destroyed, resulting in oversensitivity to light.
  - Agents associated with photophobia include procarbazine, vincristine, vinblastine, and 5-FU.

Signs and Symptoms

- Blepharitis
  - Conjunctival injection
  - Foreign body or gritty sensation

- Burning sensation
- Excessive tearing
- Itchy eyelids
- Red, swollen eyelids
- Crusting or matting of eyelashes
- Flaking or scaling of the eyelid
- Light sensitivity
- Blurred vision
- Epiphora
  - Watery eyes
  - Excessive tearing when not crying
  - Painless
- Dry eye syndrome
  - Dry or gritty feeling in the eye
  - Sensation of foreign body in eye
  - Excessive watering of eyes
- Conjunctivitis
  - Redness or swelling of eyelids
  - Chemosis, scleral injection, and conjunctival erythema
  - Scratchy, watery, itchy eyes
  - Purulent discharge from the eye
  - Sensitivity to light
- Trichomegaly
  - Long, wiry eyelashes or eyebrows
- Cataracts
  - Cloudy or blurry vision
  - Difficulty seeing in the dark or at night
  - Difficulty driving at night
  - Lights appearing bright or with a halo around them
  - Frequent changes in eyeglasses prescription
  - Diplopia (double vision) that worsens over time
- Glaucoma
  - Loss of side vision over time
- Photophobia
  - Pain in the eye when changing from dark to light areas, especially when going outside in bright light

Assessment Tools

- A comprehensive history and assessment are important to help determine the etiology of the ocular signs and symptoms.
  - Symptom initiation, duration, and exacerbation
  - Smoking history
  - Allergies
  - History of light sensitivity
  - History of eye pain
- Physical examination
  - Thorough eye examination:
    - Visual acuity
    - Visual field testing
    - Examination of eye structures for erythema, edema, and crusting of eyelashes or eyelids
    - Examination of eyelashes for
      - Misdirected eyelashes
      - Loss of lashes
      - Loss of pigmentation
      - Abnormal growth

- If glaucoma is suspected, a complete ophthalmoscopic examination, including examination of the optic disc, should be performed and intraocular pressures should be measured.

Laboratory and Diagnostic Tests

- There are no laboratory or diagnostic tests to confirm most ocular toxicities.
- Tear cultures can be used with epiphora.
- Schirmer's test is used with ocular sicca to evaluate millimeters of wetting.
  - Filter paper is placed inside the lower eyelid pouch to measure tear production.

Differential Diagnoses

- Allergy
- Injury to eye
- Foreign body in eye
- Viral, bacterial, or fungal infection

Interventions

Pharmacologic Interventions

- Blepharitis
  - Erythromycin or bacitracin ointment
  - Topical azithromycin ophthalmic solution
  - Doxycycline or tetracycline for prolonged cases
- Epiphora
  - Antibiotic eye drops with bacterial infections
- Dry eye syndrome
  - Preservative-free single-use artificial tears or ointment
  - Topical cyclosporine
  - Topical steroids
  - Punctal plugs or punctal cautery
  - Scleral lenses
- Conjunctivitis
  - Antihistamine (tablets or drops)
  - Antibiotic eye drops for bacterial infections
- Glaucoma
  - Prostaglandin drops
  - β-Blocker drops
  - α_2-Adrenergic agonist drops
  - Carbonic anhydrase inhibitor drops
  - Parasympathomimetic drops
  - Epinephrine drops
  - Hyperosmotic drops
  - Combination drops

Nonpharmacologic Interventions

- Blepharitis
  - Warm compresses placed over eyes for 5-10 minutes two to four times a day
  - Lid massage after warm compresses, massaging the edge of the eyelid toward the eye with circular motions
  - Lid washing using warm water or warm water and baby shampoo
- Epiphora
  - Warm compresses applied to eyes to help them drain if there is an infection

- Use of an air cleaner to help eliminate other eye irritants such as dust
- Wearing dark or colored glasses to help protect eyes from light
- Dry eye syndrome
  - Preservative-free, single-use artificial tears should be used routinely.
  - Panoptx eyewear for use in windy conditions
- Conjunctivitis
  - Wash hands often, and avoid people with compromised immune systems.
  - Gently wash eyelids with a warm, clean, moist towel to remove drainage.
- Trichomegaly
  - Carefully trim eyelashes with small scissors.
  - Electrolysis, laser or phototherapy, and/or waxing can be used to remove eyelashes in severe cases.
- Cataracts
  - Intraocular lens implant to improve vision
- Photophobia
  - Wear dark glasses to decrease the amount of light that reaches the eyes

Patient Teaching

- Patients should be taught how to cleanse around eyes and how to instill eye drops.
- Protecting eyes from light with dark glasses and/or the use of Panoptx eyewear in windy conditions should be encouraged to limit environmental sources of irritation.
- Use of a bright light when reading can be helpful to patients with cataracts.
- Patients with conjunctivitis should be taught to avoid sharing cosmetics, towels, sheets, contacts lenses, and lens cleaning products and to use a separate washcloth for each eye when cleansing.
- Teach patients to call their health care provider in the following situations:
  - Sudden severe eye pain
  - Eyelashes that are growing in toward the eye
  - Sudden loss of vision, floaters
  - Eyes becoming sensitive to light
  - Seeing halos around lights
  - Worsening symptoms or no improvement in symptoms

Follow-up

- Follow-up with any new or worsening symptoms
- Follow-up as needed to assess prior symptoms

Resources

- American Cancer Society: www.cancer.org
- Chemocare.org: www.chemocare.org
- National Cancer Institute: Chemotherapy and you: www.cancer.gov
- American Academy of Ophthalmology: www.aao.org
- Eye Health: www.myeyes.com
- National Eye Institute: https://nei.nih.gov/health

Bibliography

Agustoni, R., Platania, M., Vitali, M., Zilembo, N., Haspinger, E., Sinno, V., & Garassino, M. C. (2014). Emerging toxicities in the treatment of non-small cell lung cancer: Ocular disorders. *Cancer Treatment Reviews*, 40, 197–203.

American Academy of Ophthalmology. (2013). *Blepharitis: Preferred practice pattern.* Available at http://www.aao.org/preferred-practice-pattern/blepharitis-ppp–2013 (accessed March 1, 2016).

Blomquist, P. H. (2011). Ocular complications of systemic medications. *American Journal of Medical Science*, 342(1), 62–69.

Criado, P. R. (2010). Blepharitis and trichomegaly induced by cetuximab. *Anais Brasileiros de Dermatologia*, 85(6), 919–920.

Foroozan, R. (2010). *North American Neuro-ophthalmology (NANO) annual meeting: Neuro-ophthalmic complications of chemotherapy.* Available at http://www.nanosweb.org/files/Neuro-Ophthalmology.of.Cancer.pdf (accessed March 1, 2016).

Huillard, O., Bakalian, S., Levy, C., Desjardins, L., Lumbroso-Le Rouic, L., Pop, S., & Le Tourneau, C. (2014). Ocular adverse events of molecularly targeted agents approved in solid tumours: A systematic review. *European Journal of Cancer*, 50, 638–648.

LaCouture, M. E., Anadkat, M. J., Bensadoun, R. J., Bryce, J., Chan, A., Epstein, J. B., & MASCC Skin Toxicity Study Group. (2011). Clinical practice guidelines for the prevention and treatment of EGFR inhibitor-associated dermatologic toxicities. *Supportive Care in Cancer*, 19, 1079–1095.

Lindsey, K., Matsumura, S., Hatef, E., & Akpek, E. K. (2012). Interventions for chronic blepharitis. *Cochrane Database of Systematic Reviews* (5), CD005556.

Lowery, R. S. (2015). *Adult blepharitis.* Available at http://emedicine.medscape.com/article/1211763-overview (accessed March 1, 2016).

O'Leary, C. (2014). Ocular and otic complications. In C. H. Yarbro, D. Wujcik, & B. H. Gobel (Eds.), *Cancer symptom management* (4th ed.) (pp. 569–586). Burlington, MA: Jones & Bartlett.

O'Leary, C. (2014). Optic and otic side effects of molecular targeted therapies. *Seminars in Oncology Nursing*, 30(3), 169–174.

Renouf, D. J., Velazquez-Martin, J. P., Simpson, R., Siu, L. L., & Bedard, P. L. (2012). Ocular toxicity of target therapies. *Journal of Clinical Oncology*, 30, 3277–3286.

Singh, P., & Singh, A. (2012). Ocular adverse effects of anti-cancer chemotherapy and targeted therapy. *Journal of Cancer Research and Therapy*, 1(1), 5–12.

Pain

Denice Economou

Definition

- Pain is an unpleasant sensory and emotional experience associated with actual or potential tissue damage.
- One third of patients actively receiving treatment for cancer and two thirds of patients with end-stage cancer have pain.
- Pain is whatever the person says it is, experienced whenever the person says it is.

Pathophysiology and Contributing Factors

- The basic causes of cancer pain are associated with the cancer or its treatment or with unrelated iatrogenic causes.
- Somatosensory primary afferent fibers carry sensory information to the spinal cord; these can be grouped on the basis of transduction properties of the individual nerve fibers.
- Noxious stimuli activate nociceptor A-delta and C-fibers in the peripheral nerve.
- Nociceptors are polymodal and respond to mechanical, thermal, and chemical stimuli; the resulting action potentials are conducted by the axon to the dorsal horn of the spinal cord and the brainstem.

- Transmission of acute pain involves the activation of sensory receptors on peripheral C-fibers (nociceptors).
- Once tissue damage and inflammation occur, prostaglandins, bradykinin, histamine, adenosine triphosphate (ATP), and acetylcholine act on excitatory receptors on the sensory ending and play a major role in sensitization and activation.
- Impaired nerve fibers, either at the site of nerve injury or in the cell body of impaired fibers in the dorsal root ganglia, have ectopic discharges that are characterized as neuropathic pain.
- Multiple factors come together to determine a patient's perception of pain and his or her ability to get relief from the pain. Gender, culture, and social and societal inputs affect a patient's pain response.
- Major barriers to pain management continue to be related to the patient's belief in myths associated with the management of pain, including fear of tolerance, addiction, and dependence.
  - *Tolerance*: the physiologic adaptation of receptors that are continually exposed to opioids in circulation such that the dose of medication needs to be increased to achieve the same level of pain relief. Tolerance is not an issue in cancer patients because studies have shown that the primary reason for oncology patients to need an increase in dose is related to a change in the source of their pain (e.g., metastasis, bone fractures, impingement of nerves from growing tumors). Oncology patients on stable doses of opioids over time can reduce the dose of their medications and achieve the same level of pain relief.
  - *Addiction*: a neurobehavioral syndrome with genetic and environmental influences that results in psychological dependence on the use of a substance for its psychic effects. Addiction is characterized by compulsive use despite harm. Use of opioids to relieve pain cannot by itself lead to addiction to the medications.
  - *Physiologic dependence*: symptoms of withdrawal are experienced when opioids are discontinued immediately, without tapering of the medication. The experience of dependence does not signify addiction; acute symptoms occur with abrupt withdrawal because the receptors are used to being bathed in the medication. Other drugs that may cause withdrawal symptoms if stopped abruptly include sedative-hypnotics, β-blockers, corticosteroids, and antidepressants.

Signs and Symptoms

- There is no truly objective test to establish a patient's experience of pain.
- Verbal report of pain is the single most accurate tool in identifying pain.
- Subjective signs may include the following:
  - Facial grimacing
  - Furrowed brow
  - Contracted muscles
  - Moaning
  - Guarding or decreased movement
  - Agitation or restlessness
- Cognitive responses include withdrawn behaviors, inability to concentrate, and irritability.
- Associated symptoms may include lack of appetite, depressed mood, and sleep disorders.

Assessment Tools

- A visual analog scale (VAS) may be used with anchor words or numbers (e.g., a scale of 0 to 10).
- Verbal scale
- Faces (Wong-Baker scale or Revised Faces Scale [RFS])
- Nonverbal pain scale (Odhner et al., 2003)
- Pain assessment is the most important intervention for the successful management of pain.

Pain Assessment

- Pain history: Past experience with pain or pain medications. Include the family or caregiver when assessing pain; the patient may be stoic and may underreport the pain, or the family may overrate their loved one's pain. What do they call the pain (e.g., discomfort, hurt)? Is this pain acute (i.e., lasting less than 1-3 months) or chronic (i.e., lasting longer than 1-3 months)?
- Location: Where does the patient report pain? There may be more than one site of pain. If the patient complains of pain all over, assess the emotional state of the patient for depression, anxiety, fear, or hopelessness.
- Intensity: How does the patient rate the level of pain? The most common tool is the numerical rating scale that asks the patient to rate the pain on a scale of 0 to 10. The VAS is a 10-cm line on which the patient marks (starting at the left end of the line) how intense the pain is, after which the distance to the mark is measured in centimeters, indicating the pain rating. Children older than 3 years of age and adults who have difficulty using the 0-to-10 scale may use one of the faces scales.
- Description: What words does the patient use to describe the pain: sharp, shooting, dull, aching? These are indicators of the potential source of pain. General types of pain include the following:
  - *Somatic*: Pain in skin, muscle, tendon, joints, fasciae, and bones. Usually the patient can point to a specific area of pain. This type of pain responds to heat or cold, massage, transcutaneous electrical nerve stimulation (TENS), and nonopioids such as acetaminophen or nonsteroidal antiinflammatory drugs (NSAIDs). Bone pain related to cancer may respond to radiation therapy, steroids, calcitonin, or bisphosphonates in addition to opioids and nonopioid therapy.
  - *Visceral*: Pain related to the stretching of viscera and surrounding organs, including the gastrointestinal tract, lungs, gallbladder, kidneys, and bladder. Visceral pain is characteristically vague in distribution and quality. It can be described as deep, dull, aching, or squeezing and can be associated with nausea, vomiting, and diaphoresis. It is called referred pain when the area that hurts

is not the specific site of origin but appears to "travel" because of the related nerve distribution. Opioids and adding additional nonopioid and nonpharmacologic approaches may be beneficial.

- *Neuropathic:* Injury to some element of the peripheral or central nervous system. Chemotherapy drugs that can cause nerve injury include bortezomib, platinum, taxanes, thalidomide, and vinca alkaloids.
- Dysesthesia: burning, tingling, numbing, or shooting pain
- Hyperalgesia: increased response to a normally painful stimulus
- Allodynia: response to a stimulus that is not normally painful (e.g., light touch). Treatments include antidepressants, antiseizure medications such as gabapentin, Lyrica, and membrane stabilizers.
- Other risk factors: diabetes, alcohol abuse, autoimmune disease, kidney disease or failure, and HIV/AIDS
- Aggravating and relieving factors: What makes the pain better or worse?
- Effect on physical or social functioning: Does the pain affect the patient's ability to complete activities of daily living (ADLs) or cause the patient to withdraw from normal activities?
- Medication history: What opioids has the patient tolerated in the past? This information aids in treatment planning. If the patient has had pain relief with an opioid previously, relief will likely happen again.
- Physical examination
  - Examine the site of pain and any patterns of referred pain.
  - Perform a neurologic examination as appropriate to the site of pain.
    - Head and neck pain: cranial nerve and funduscopic evaluation
    - Back and neck pain: examine patient for motor and sensory function in limbs, gross motor weakness, or sensory deficit. Report deficits to physician immediately.
    - Bowel and bladder control: assess urinary and rectal sphincter control. Report deficits to physician immediately.
- Diagnostic evaluation: Evaluate disease status as appropriate to cancer diagnosis and treatment, including tumor markers and radiologic examinations (e.g., computed tomographic [CT] scan, bone scan, magnetic resonance imaging [MRI] scan).
- Reassess pain frequently. Patient comfort is the primary indicator of successful pain management.

Pain in the Geriatric Population

- Patients 65 years of age and older are at increased risk for inadequate pain assessment.
- Additional assessment in the geriatric patient should include the following: cognitive impairment, review of ADLs, gait and balance, sensory deprivation, and visual and auditory function.
- Accurate assessment is important for effectiveness of treatment

- Use of morphine, hydromorphone, oxymorphone, and tapentadol in older adults may lower the potential for drug-drug interactions. Use caution with metabolite-forming drugs such as morphine in older adults with renal insufficiency.

Pain Assessment in Cognitively Impaired Patients (Hierarchy of Pain Assessment)

- Do not assume that patients who cannot self-report their pain are not experiencing pain.
- Identify procedures or pathologic conditions that may cause pain.
- Observe for behavior associated with painful conditions. Use a behavioral assessment tool.
- Gather information from family members or caregivers familiar with the patient.
- If pain is expected, medicate for pain and observe for changes in pain-related behaviors.

Laboratory and Diagnostic Tests

- No blood test can identify the existence of pain. Laboratory testing (such as carcinoembryonic antigen [CEA] or cancer antigen [CA] 125 levels) would be important for documentation of possible disease recurrence or metastasis.
- Diagnostic testing is related to the location of the pain or to known disease locations or both and may include CT scans, positron emission tomographic (PET) scans, and radiology examinations.

Differential Diagnoses

- Rule out a history of nonmalignant chronic pain.
- Arthritis
- Neuralgia
- Chronic abdominal pain
- Fibromyalgia
- Headaches
- Low back pain
- Peripheral neuropathy related to diabetes
- AIDS
- Phantom limb pain
- Reflex sympathetic dystrophy
- Sickle cell disease

Interventions

- The World Health Organization offers a three-step analgesic ladder to help guide medication management of patients with newly diagnosed pain. Based on the level of pain a patient describes, the appropriate medication class combination can be initiated (on the basis of a VAS).
  - 0-3 = mild pain, nonopioid/adjuvants
  - 4-7 = moderate pain, opioid/nonopioid/adjuvants
  - 8-10 = severe pain, opioid/nonopioid/adjuvants/etc.

  If patient's pain is rated as severe (8-10 on a 0-10 scale), the route of choice should be subcutaneous or intravenous to allow for rapid effect from the medication in a shorter amount of time.

Pharmacologic Interventions

- Combined opioid/nonopioid medications: acetaminophen with codeine (Tylenol 3), hydrocodone with acetaminophen (Vicodin), hydrocodone with acetaminophen (Norco, Lortab), oxycodone with acetaminophen (Percocet, Tylox), and hydrocodone with ibuprofen (Vicoprofen) (see box below)
- Compounded opioids are dose limited by the amount (milligrams) of acetaminophen and NSAIDs. The maximum recommend total dose of acetaminophen has been changed to 2.6 g/24 hours (i.e., 8 regular-strength tablets maximum per day).
- Pain medication must be titrated for effectiveness. Increasing or decreasing the dose for comfort is essential to achieve effective management of a patient's pain.
- If patients are not receiving effective management of their pain and are experiencing multiple side effects related to their medication, opioid rotation may be necessary. Another opioid may provide more effective pain management with fewer side effects.
- If a patient becomes overly sedated from the medication and is experiencing respiratory distress, reversal of the opioid dose may be necessary. Dilute naloxone in 10 mL of normal saline solution and titrate until alertness and respirations are improved.
- Consult with an anesthetist for management with appropriate pain blocks.
- Radiopharmaceuticals may be used for bone pain if appropriate.
- Spinal infusion of medications (epidural/intrathecal) may be necessary if large doses of opioids, orally or peripherally, are required to achieve pain relief.

Types of Pharmacologic Interventions

Opioids
- Morphine
- Hydromorphine
- Oxycodone
- Hydrocodone
- Methadone
- Fentanyl (transdermal and transmucosal)
- Tramadol

Nonopioids
- Aspirin
- Acetaminophen
- Nonsteroidal antiinflammatory drugs (NSAIDs)

Adjuvants
- Steroids
- Antidepressants
- Anticonvulsants
- Bisphosphonates
- Benzodiazepines

Nonpharmacologic Interventions

- Radiation therapy for pain related to bone metastases
- Heat or cold compresses for musculoskeletal pain (somatic)
- Surgical interventions to relieve compression
- Physical activity to maintain mobility and prevent secondary pain sources
- Cutaneous stimulation (TENS), massage, pressure, or vibration for pain associated with muscle tension or muscle spasm
- Relaxation or visualization techniques for distraction
- Acupuncture
- Community resources such as pastoral care and psychosocial care based on patient assessment
- The table below describes pain interventions related to quality of life domains.

Treatments for Pain Related to Quality-of-Life Domains

Domain	Category and Type of Treatment
Physical	Pharmacologic
	Interventional
Psychological	Cognitive-behavioral
	Relaxation, guided imagery, stress management
	Psychoeducational
Social	Supportive/Complementary
	Acupuncture, massage, movement therapy
	Rehabilitative—occupational therapy
Spiritual	Existential—spiritual support
	Chaplaincy
	Religious resources as requested

Modified from Ferrell, B.R., Dow, K. H., & Grant, M. (1995). Measurement of the quality of life in cancer survivors. *Quality of Life Research*, 4(6), 523-531.

Patient Teaching

- Help patients understand how to rate their pain, and document the tool and words they use to describe their pain.
- The right dose is the one that relieves a patient's pain with minimal side effects.
- Anticonstipation medications should be started as soon as pain medication is started.
- Anticonstipation medications must include both a laxative and a softener for relief of opioid-related constipation.

Follow-up

- Reassess the patient's pain ratings daily (or every shift if inpatient and no pain is reported).
- Reassess the patient's comfort level 30 minutes after an intravenous or subcutaneous injection and 1 hour after oral medications. If pain is not improved, the physician or advanced practice nurse must be notified to increase or change the pain management plan as necessary.
- Documentation is the most important follow-up intervention. Communicating the patients' medication regimen and response can prevent needless suffering.

Resources

- Pain Medicine and Palliative Care at Beth Israel NY: www.stoppain.org
- Pain Resource Center at City of Hope: http://prc.coh.org
- National Comprehensive Cancer Network (NCCN): Cancer pain guidelines: https://www.nccn.org/store/login/login.aspx?ReturnURL=http://www.nccn.org/professionals/physician_gls/pdf/pain.pdf

Bibliography

American Pain Society. (2008). *Principles of analgesic use in the treatment of acute pain and cancer pain* (6th ed.). Glenview, IL: American Pain Society Press.

Brant, J. (2014). Pain. In C. Yarbro, D. Wujcik, & B. Gobel (Eds.), *Cancer symptom management* (4th ed.) (pp. 69–92). Burlington, MA: Jones & Bartlett Learning.

Fink, R., Gates, R., & Montgomery, R. (2015). Pain assessment. In B. Ferrell, N. Coyle, & J. Paice (Eds.), *Oxford textbook of palliative nursing care* (4th ed.) (pp. 113–153). New York: Oxford University Press.

Merskey, H., & Bogduk, N. (1994). Classification of chronic pain. In *International Association for the Study of Pain, Task Force on Taxonomy* (2nd ed.) (pp. 209–214). Washington, DC: IASP Press.

National Comprehensive Cancer Network (NCCN). (2015). *Practice guidelines: Adult cancer pain*. version 1.2015. Available at http://www.nccn.org/professionals/physician_gls/pdf/pain.pdf (accessed March 1, 2016).

Odhner, M., Wegman, D., Freeland, N., Steinmetz, A., & Ingersoll, G. L. (2003). Assessing pain control in nonverbal critically ill adults. *Dimensions of Critical Care Nursing, 22*(6), 260–267.

Pasero, C., & McCaffery, M. (2011). *Pain assessment and pharmacologic management*. St. Louis: Mosby Elsevier.

Portenoy, R. K., & Ahmed, E. (2014). Principles of opioid use in cancer pain. *Journal of Clinical Oncology, 32*(16), 1662–1670.

Redinbaugh, E. M., Baum, A., DeMoss, C., Fello, M., & Arnold, R. (2002). Factors associated with the accuracy of family caregiver estimates of patient pain. *Journal of Pain and Symptom Management, 23*, 31–38.

Reisner, L. (2011). Pharmacological management of persistent pain in older persons. *Journal of Pain, 12*(3 Suppl.), S21–S29.

Schaible, H. G., & Richter, F. (2004). Pathophysiology of pain. *Langenbecks Archiv für Chirurgie, 389*, 237–243.

Simmon, C., MacLeod, N., & Laird, B. (2012). Clinical management of pain in advanced lung cancer. *Clinical Medicine Insights: Oncology, 6*, 331–346.

Peripheral Neuropathy

Carol S. Blecher

Definition

- A functional or structural disorder of the motor, sensory, and autonomic neurons that lead from the skin, joints, and muscles of the face, arms, legs, and torso to the central nervous system
- Causes a lack of communication between the brain and the periphery
- Characterized by symptoms of pain and numbness

Pathophysiology and Contributing Factors

- Direct damage to the neurons
- Chemotherapy-induced peripheral neuropathy: damage to the nerve fibers caused by demyelination of the large-fiber sensory nerves (cisplatinum), microtubule inhibition resulting in axonal degeneration (vinca alkaloids), or axonal degeneration and demyelination (taxanes)
- Tumor pressing on the nerves
- Many contributing factors, including the following:
  - Alcohol abuse
  - Arthrosclerosis/ischemic disease
  - Concurrent neuropathic medication (isoniazid, gentamicin, ciprofloxacin hydrochloride, phenytoin)
  - Infections: human immunodeficiency virus (HIV) infection, syphilis, Epstein-Barr virus, shingles, sarcoidosis
  - Metabolic disorders: diabetes mellitus, hypothyroidism, acromegaly
  - Nutritional imbalance: vitamin B_{12} deficiency
  - Treatment-related toxicity
    - Radiation
    - Phantom limb pain
    - Postherpetic neuralgia

Signs and Symptoms

- A perception of wearing a sock or glove when there is none
- Extreme sensitivity to touch
- Muscle weakness, tremor, cramps or spasms, loss of dexterity or coordination
- Numbness or tingling and loss of feeling
- Pain, which may be described as burning, pins-and-needles, sharp, stabbing, or an electric or shooting type of pain

Assessment Tools

- Clinical evaluation of sensory, motor, autonomic, and cranial nerve functions
- History, including risk factors for the development of neuropathy (e.g., diabetes, alcoholism)
- Any concomitant medications that cause neuropathy
- Symptom assessment: onset, intensity, location, quality, intermittent or constant, alleviating and aggravating factors, accompanying symptoms, and impact on ability to perform activities of daily living (ADLs) and quality of life
- Physical examination: monitoring for orthostatic hypotension, cranial nerve examination, assessment of motor function, reflexes, and sensory function
- Common terminology criteria for adverse events (CTCAE):
  - Neuropathy, motor
    - Grade 1—asymptomatic; clinical or diagnostic observations only; intervention not indicated
    - Grade 2—moderate symptoms; limiting instrumental ADLs
    - Grade 3—severe symptoms; limiting self-care ADLs; assistive device indicated
    - Grade 4—life-threatening consequences; urgent intervention indicated
    - Grade 5—death
  - Neuropathy, sensory
    - Grade 1—asymptomatic; loss of deep tendon reflexes or paresthesia
    - Grade 2—moderate symptoms; limiting instrumental ADLs
    - Grade 3—severe symptoms; limiting self-care ADLs
    - Grade 4—life-threatening consequences; urgent intervention indicated
    - Grade 5—death
  - Neuropathy, cranial
- Toxicity grading scales
  - World Health Organization (WHO) toxicity criteria
  - Eastern Cooperative Oncology Group (ECOG)

Principles of Symptom Management

④

- National Cancer Institute of Canada (NCIC) common toxicity criteria:
  - Sensory neuropathy
  - Motor neuropathy
- Ajani Motor Neuropathy tool for assessing chemotherapy-induced neuropathy in patients with cancer
  - Sensory neuropathy
  - Motor neuropathy
- Total neuropathy scale
  - Sensory symptoms
  - Motor symptoms
  - Pin sensibility
  - Vibration sensibility
  - Reflex
  - Autonomic symptoms
  - Vibration sensation
  - Sural amplitude: The sural nerve is the nerve leading from the tibial nerve that enervates the gastrocnemius and lateral portion of the leg. The conduction amplitude may be decreased in chemotherapy-induced peripheral neuropathies.
  - Peroneal amplitude: The peroneal nerve is the nerve leading from the sciatic nerve to the biceps femoris and gastrocnemius muscles. The conduction amplitude may be decreased in chemotherapy-induced peripheral neuropathies.
- Functional Assessment of Cancer Therapy/Gynecologic Oncology Group—Neurotoxicity (FACT/GOG-Ntx)
- Functional Assessment of Cancer Therapy—Taxane
- Peripheral Neuropathy Scale

Laboratory and Diagnostic Tests

- Audiometry to assess hearing
- Electromyelography (EMG) to evaluate axonal neuropathy and muscle atrophy related to the neuropathy
- Nerve biopsy to assess for abnormalities
- Nerve conduction studies to identify the severity and location of the peripheral neuropathy
- Blood screening for
  - Anemia
  - Diabetes
  - Electrolyte imbalance
  - Hepatitis
  - Homocysteine/methylmalonic acid levels
  - Lupus erythematosus
  - Lyme disease
  - Thyroid-stimulating hormone (TSH) deficiency
  - Vitamin deficiency

Differential Diagnoses

- Alcoholism/Malnutrition
- Diabetes mellitus
- Motor neuron disease
- Disorders of the neuromuscular junction
- Myopathy
- Myelopathy

- Syringomyelia
- Dorsal column disorders
  - Tabes dorsalis
- Hysterical disorders

Interventions

Pharmacologic Interventions

- Anticonvulsants
  - Phenytoin
  - Carbamazepine
  - Gabapentin
  - Pregabalin (Lyrica)
- Lidocaine patches
- Opioid analgesics
- Over-the-counter pain relievers
  - Acetaminophen
  - Nonsteroidal antiinflammatory drugs (NSAIDs)
- Tricyclic antidepressants
  - Amitriptyline (Elavil)
  - Nortriptyline (Pamelor)
  - Desipramine (Norpramin)
  - Imipramine (Tofranil)
- Vitamin B_{12} supplements

Nonpharmacologic Interventions

- Treatment of the underlying disease
- Physical therapy
- Massage
- Exercise
- Occupational therapy
- Transcutaneous electrical nerve stimulation (TENS)
- Biofeedback
- Acupuncture
- Hypnosis
- Relaxation techniques
- Support groups
- Safety measures
  - Orthotics
  - Ergonomic chairs
  - Braces
  - Splints
  - Positioning
  - Adequate lighting
  - Rails or other appliances to promote safety
  - Removal of obstacles such as loose rugs
  - Bed frames to keep sheets off tender body parts

Patient Teaching

- Help patients to describe their symptoms
  - Pain
  - Numbness or tingling and loss of feeling
  - Feeling as if one is wearing a sock or glove
  - Muscle weakness, loss of dexterity or coordination
  - Burning pain
  - Sharp stabbing or electric type of pain
  - Extreme sensitivity to touch

- Prevention
  - Avoid alcohol.
  - Increase intake of B vitamins.
  - Avoid repetitive activities that may place stress on a nerve (e.g., golf, tennis, playing a musical instrument, typing at a computer keyboard).
- Management
  - Controlling diabetes
  - Correction of vitamin deficiency
  - Relieving nerve pressure by eliminating the source of the pressure, if possible, or through surgical repair of the problem
  - Medications: pain relief medication following the WHO ladder, antiseizure medication, lidocaine patches, tricyclic antidepressants
  - Therapies: TENS, biofeedback, acupuncture, hypnosis, relaxation techniques
- Safety
  - Orthotics
  - Ergonomic chairs
  - Braces
  - Splints
  - Positioning
  - Adequate lighting
  - Rails or other appliances to promote safety
  - Removal of obstacles such as loose rugs
  - Bed frames to keep sheets off tender body parts
- Coping skills
  - Setting priorities
  - Getting out of the house
  - Seeking and accepting support
- Mayo Clinic Patient Education Tool

Follow-up

- Physician
- Physical therapy
- Occupational therapy
- Laboratory data for underlying disease state
- Have the patient call the health care team immediately for tingling or weakness in hands or feet or for pain that is new.

Resources

- Center for Peripheral Neuropathy: http://peripheralneurop athycenter.uchicago.edu
- National Institute of Neurological Disorders and Stroke (NINDS): Peripheral Neuropathy Information: www.ninds .nih.gov/disorders/peripheralneuropathy/peripheralneurop athy.htm
- Pain Medicine and Palliative Care at Mount Sinai Beth Israel NY: www.stoppain.org
- American Society of Clinical Oncology: Cancer.Net http://www.cancer.net/navigating-cancer-care/side-effects/peripheral-neuropathy
- National Cancer Institute: Common terminology criteria for adverse events, version 4.03: http://www.oncology.tv/ SymptomManagement/NationalCancerInstituteUpdates CTCAEtov403.aspx

Bibliography

Center for Peripheral Neuropathy. (2010). *About peripheral neuropathy.* Available at http://peripheralneuropathycenter.uchicago.edu/learnaboutpn/ aboutpn/whatispn/ (accessed March 1, 2016).

Grisdale, K. A., & Armstrong, T. S. (2014). Peripheral neuropathy. In D. Camp-Sorrell & R. A. Hawkins (Eds.), *Clinical manual for the oncology advanced practice nurse* (3rd ed.) (pp. 1137–1149). Pittsburgh, PA: Oncology Nursing Press.

Medline Plus Medical Encyclopedia. (2014). *Peripheral neuropathy.* Available at http://www.nlm.nih.gov/medlineplus/ency/article/000593.htm (accessed March 1, 2016).

Oncology Nursing Society. (2011). *PEP topic: Peripheral neuropathy.* Available at https://www.ons.org/practice-resources/pep/peripheral-neuropathy (accessed March 1, 2016).

Postma, T. J., & Heimans, J. J. (2000). Grading of chemotherapy-induced peripheral neuropathy. *Annals of Oncology, 11,* 509–513.

Wilkes, G. M. (2014). Peripheral neuropathy. In C. H. Yarbro, M. H. Frogge, & M. Goodman (Eds.), *Cancer symptom management* (4th ed.) (pp. 333–358). Sudbury, MA: Jones & Bartlett.

Pleural Effusion

Pamela Garnier

Definition

- Accumulation of excess fluid in the pleural space
- Classified as *transudative* (from a systemic problem such as heart failure) or *exudative* (from a localized inflammatory or malignant dysfunction)
- Prevalence: Approximately 45% of all pleural effusions are malignant.
- Associated most commonly with lung, breast, or ovarian cancer; lymphoma; and cancer of unknown primary

Pathophysiology and Contributing Factors

- Normally there is only 10 to 20 mL of pleural fluid, spread thinly over the visceral and parietal pleurae, which facilitates chest wall movement.
- Excess fluid is formed in, or fluid is removed from, the pleural space, resulting in imbalance between the osmotic and hydrostatic pressures controlling the secretion and reabsorption of pleural fluid.
- May be benign or malignant
- May result from direct tumor involvement or from indirect sequelae of disease progression due to pleural involvement or mediastinal cancer with blockage of lymphatics
- Superior vena cava syndrome (SVC)
- Pericardial constriction
- Obstruction of mediastinal lymphatics by tumor
- Obstruction of pulmonary vessels by tumor or a pulmonary infarction
- Shedding of malignant cells into the pleural space
- Intraabdominal cancer draining through the right diaphragm

Signs and Symptoms

- Dependent on the amount and rate of fluid accumulation and comorbid illnesses (e.g., chronic obstructive pulmonary disease [COPD], heart failure)
- Malignant pleural effusions usually develop slowly.

- Presenting symptoms:
  - Resting or exertional dyspnea
  - Cough
  - Pleuritic pain and chest discomfort
  - Weight loss from advancing cancer
  - Malaise

Assessment Tools

- Patient history (both medical and oncologic). The temporal pattern of symptoms is important when assessing the cluster of symptoms experienced with the effusion.
- Physical examination
  - Vital signs: evaluate for pulsus paradoxus with superior vena cava (SVC), respiratory rate, pulse rate
  - Jugular venous pressure: increased, changes with respiration
  - Distended chest veins and elevated jugular pulse with SVC
  - Lung auscultation and percussion
    - Dullness to percussion measured on both sides of the chest, decreased breath sounds, egophony above the effusion
    - Absence of fremitus on affected side
    - Cardiac sounds: distant, gallop and murmur
- Common toxicity criteria (CTC version 4.0):
  - Grade 1 (mild)
  - Grade 2 (moderate)
  - Grade 3 (severe)
  - Grade 4 (life threatening)

Laboratory and Diagnostic Tests

- Resting and ambulatory pulse oximetry
- Chest radiographic film
- Chest ultrasonography
  - Can detect small volumes (5 mL) of fluid
  - Useful in guiding thoracentesis as well as chest tube insertion
  - No radiation exposure
  - Can be repeated frequently at the bedside
- Chest computed tomographic (CT) scan with contrast: high-resolution scanning for pulmonary embolism depending on history
- Thoracentesis procedure with cytologic analysis of pleural fluid and assessment for symptom relief
- Video-assisted thoracoscopic surgery (VATS)
  - Used when thoracoscopy fails to confirm malignancy or tissue type remains in question

Differential Diagnoses

- Congestive heart failure
- Nephrotic syndrome
- Cirrhosis
- Infection
- Malignancy
- Hemothorax
- Pulmonary embolism
- Pancreatitis

Interventions

- Oxygen therapy if clinically appropriate
- Thoracentesis
- Chest tube placement for drainage
- Indwelling pleural catheter
- Talc or chemical pleurodesis procedure for large or recurrent pleural effusions
- External beam radiation therapy
- Pleuroperitoneal shunt
- Treatment of underlying malignancy in breast cancer or lymphoma
- PleurX catheter

Patient Teaching

- The patient and family should be educated that a malignant pleural effusion is a sign of advanced disease.
- The treatment plan should be based on patient goals, performance status, and general prognosis.
- If the patient is asymptomatic, observation alone is reasonable until symptoms occur.
- Provide information about specific procedures.

Follow-up

- Provide routine follow-up to assess the effects of treatment.
- Plan for early diagnosis and intervention for recurrent pleural effusions.
- Assess patient goals to ensure that treatments are in keeping with the patient's wishes.
- An interdisciplinary approach should be used to provide continued education and support to the patient and family.
- Educate the patient or family when to contact the provider (e.g., if the patient becomes symptomatic or experiences a sudden change in respiratory status).

Resources

- Chemo Care (The Cleveland Clinic Foundation): www.chemocare.com
- National Cancer Institute: Common terminology criteria for adverse events, version 4.03: http://www.oncology.tv/SymptomManagement/NationalCancerInstituteUpdatesCTCAEtov403.aspx

Bibliography

Balmanoukkian, A., & Brahmer, J. R. (2011). Pleural and pericardial effusions. In M. Davis, P. Feyer, P. Ortner, & C. Zimmerman (Eds.), *Supportive oncology* (pp. 354–357). Philadelphia, PA: Elsevier.

Davies, H., & Lee, Y. C. (2013). Management of malignant pleural effusions: Questions that need answers. *Current Opinion in Pulmonary Medicine, 19,* 374–379.

Demmy, T. L., Gu, L., Burkhalter, J. E., Toloza, E. M., D'Amico, T. A., Sutherland, S., & Kohman, L. (2012). Optimal management of malignant pleural effusions (results of CALGB 30102). *Journal of the National Comprehensive Cancer Network, 10,* 975–982.

Fabian, T., & Bakhos, C. (2014). Evaluation and management of pleural conditions. In H. S. Smith & J. G. Pilitsis (Eds.), *The art of palliative medicine* (pp. 542–548). Sheung Wan, Hong Kong: AME Publishing Company.

Hass, A. R., & Sterman, D. H. (2014). Advances in pleural disease management, including updated procedural coding. *Chest, 146,* 508–513.

Heffner, J. E., & Klein, J. S. (2008). Recent advances in the diagnosis and management of malignant pleural effusions. *Mayo Clinic Proceedings, 83,* 235–250.

Heffner, J. E. (2016). Management of malignant pleural effusions. In E. K. King, & J. R. Jett (Eds.), *UpToDate.* Available at http://www.uptodate.com/contents/management-of-malignant-pleural-effusions (accessed March 1, 2016).

Pruritus and Xerosis

Denice Economou

Definition

- Pruritus refers to the pathologic condition that is a stimulus for the sensory discomfort, and itching is a symptom related to localized and systemic diseases.
- Itching can affect patients on many different levels.
- Pruritus is a systemic issue with multiple causes.
- Itching is subjective and affects patients' quality of life in all domains.
- Words used to describe itching include stinging, pins and needles, tickle, crawling sensation, and pain.

Pathophysiology and Contributing Factors

- Pruritus begins in the free nerve endings in the epidermis and dermis and is transmitted through C-fibers to the dorsal horn of the spinal cord and to the cerebral cortex by the spinothalamic tract.
- A spinal reflex response, scratching, is as innate as a deep tendon reflex.
- Itching most commonly occurs in skin and is exacerbated by skin inflammation, dry or hot weather conditions, sunburn, skin vasodilation, and psychological stressors.
- Chemical causes include caustic substances, perfumes, and cleaning products.
- Repeated scratching itself can promote itching.

Signs and Symptoms

- Pruritus occurs when the nerves in the skin react to the release of chemicals such as histamine. The signals from these nerves are processed in the brain and perceived as itching.
- What makes it better or worse? Applying heat may make it worse, whereas ice or cool cloths may provide some relief. Hodgkin disease and myeloid metaplasia are two diseases in which heat or hot showers worsen the itch. This may be the symptom that leads the patient to the physician for diagnosis.

Assessment Tools

- Assessment is aimed at identifying the cause.
- Assessment should include dermatologic causes (local chemical reactions; skin disorders such as eczema, psoriasis, or infestation), systemic causes (opioid-induced pruritus, organ failure, endocrine dysfunction, connective tissue disorder), neuropathic causes, and psychological causes (psychiatric disorder).
- The intensity of the discomfort or distress can be identified by using a 0-10 rating system.
- Check the area for signs of secondary infection.
- Check the family history for allergies, exposure to known infectious agents or insect bites, and other family members who may also be experiencing itching symptoms.
- Evaluate the patient's medication profile for potential causes, including chemotherapy and biologic medications.

- Physical examination
  - Follow a systematic approach, as in pain assessment.
  - Location of the itch: general site, specific site, or pattern. This information may reveal, for example, whether the symptoms are related to a fungal infection in skin creases or a scabies mite infestation. Also assess whether the pattern of itch is following a dermatomal distribution, which may relate to a past herpes zoster infection.
  - Is there a rash related to the itch? A rash is usually not related to a systemic cause. Evaluate whether the "rash" is really skin irritation related to physical scratching of the site. Focal rash may indicate a contact sensitivity or infection.
  - Quality of the itch: Is the itch relieved even briefly by scratching? Is it described as a tickling sensation (usually associated with contact dermatitis) or as burning or painful sensation (usually associated with herpes zoster)?
  - Chemotherapy drugs associated with itching or rash include asparaginase, cisplatin, carboplatin, cytarabine, etoposide, interferon alfa-2a and interferon alfa-2b, doxorubicin, melphalan, and daunorubicin. Gemcitabine is associated with perianal pruritus.
  - Obtain a thorough history of any new products being used, any recent travel, exposure to outdoor plants (e.g., poison oak, poison ivy), or pets in the home. Assess any new medications or use of over-the-counter herbal preparations or vitamins.

Laboratory and Diagnostic Tests

- Complete blood cell count (CBC), including a differential leukocyte count
- Liver function tests (alkaline phosphatase, serum bilirubin)
- Renal function tests (blood urea nitrogen [BUN], creatinine)
- Thyroid panel (free thyroxine [FT_4], thyroid-stimulating hormone [TSH])
- Serum iron and ferritin
- Stool examination for occult blood, ova, and parasites
- Human immunodeficiency virus (HIV) testing
- Skin biopsy (assess whether pruritus is related to chemotherapy—biopsy may not be necessary)

Differential Diagnoses

- Dry skin
- Hives
- Rash
- Eczema
- Psoriasis
- Chickenpox
- Insect bite
- Medications (opioid induced)
- Hormonal changes
- Infestations of the skin with a parasite, such as scabies or head lice
- Allergic reactions
- Shingles

- Blood disorders, such as anemia, polycythemia, multiple myeloma
- Kidney failure
- Liver disease, including hepatitis C and cirrhosis
- Thyroid disease
- Diabetes
- Acquired immunodeficiency syndrome (AIDS)

Interventions

Management of pruritus requires multiple approaches to reduce the symptoms. Depending on the severity and cause, use of topical, systemic, and behavioral interventions may be necessary.

- Preventive treatment when possible: Prevent dry skin or skin breakdown.
- Topical treatments related to source of pruritus:
  - Xerosis (dry skin): Hydrate the skin by soaking in a warm/tepid bath and then patting dry and applying an occlusive moisturizer to trap in the moisture.
  - Lotions should be alcohol and fragrance free; examples include Aquaphor, Vanicream, Moisturel, and Eucerin or Cetaphil. If cost is an issue, cooking shortening (e.g., Crisco) can be used.
- Soothing oatmeal baths and the use of cold packs can be helpful.
- Alcohol and spicy foods may worsen the itch.

Pharmacologic Interventions

- Systemic interventions to improve pruritus include the following:
  - Opioid antagonists (Narcan) may be used for systemic or intraspinal opioid-associated itching.
  - Systemic corticosteroids can be helpful when the itch is generalized and related to inflammatory conditions; however, long-term use is contraindicated and may increase preexisting pruritus
  - Antihistamines are useful for itching associated with histamine-mediated causes such as hives. However, the side effect of sedation may make its use less attractive. Use of this approach at bedtime is most helpful.
  - Local anesthetics such as mexiletine have provided relief to patients with intractable itching.
  - Antidepressants have provided some relief for itching related to neuropathic pain. (Doxepin may be most effective because it is most "antihistaminic.") The selective serotonin reuptake inhibitor (SSRI) and antidepressant paroxetine has been shown to reduce itching in patients with advanced cancer or opioid-induced itch.
- Topical lotions containing calamine and Benadryl as an antihistamine or a menthol-containing ointment may have a local anesthetic or cooling response that relieves the itch. Capsaicin cream applied four to five times per day can also be helpful. It reduces substance P, decreasing both pain and itching sensations.
- Antidepressant-compounded creams may decrease pain and itching by local inhibition of H_1 and H_2 receptors and antiserotonergic effects (e.g., doxepin, Zonalon).

- Topically applied corticosteroids can reduce the sensation of itch, but long-term use can cause secondary problems such as skin infections, acne, and thinning of the skin.
- Use the higher percentage ointment or cream initially, and decrease the strength as itching improves. The choice of ointment depends on the area to be covered and the percentage potency needed. Examples of these preparations include Diprolene 0.05% and Topicort 0.25% (high potency), Kenalog 0.1% and Valisone 0.1% (mid-range), and hydrocortisone ointment 1% (low potency).
- Applying topical steroids to skin that has been hydrated improves local absorption.
- Itching is commonly caused by a fungal infection, such as *Candida albicans*, which is especially present in skin folds. Topical antifungal medications such as nystatin, ketoconazole, and the newest group, allylamine/benzalamine drugs, can cure the infection and relieve the itch.
- Fungal infections not responding to topical antifungal agents may require systemic treatments.
- Tar products can be used to reduce inflammation and itching. These products reduce the need for topical steroids in patients with chronic pruritus, but the smell and associated staining with these products make them less preferred than other products.

Nonpharmacologic Interventions

- Acupuncture or a transcutaneous electrical nerve stimulation (TENS) unit can be helpful in reducing pruritus.
- Behavioral techniques (e.g., distraction, relaxation techniques) may reduce the sensation of itching and break the cycle of itching and scratching.

Patient Teaching

- Moisturize the skin with lubricants frequently, especially after bathing.
- Avoid known irritants such as pet hair and cleaning products.
- Wear loose-fitting cotton clothing.
- Drink plenty of fluids.
- Keep a humid and cool environment.
- Keep fingernails cut short to limit damage from scratching, and wear soft mittens and socks at bedtime.
- Skin cleansing is important if skin breakdown has occurred related to scratching or open lesions. Skin cleansers must have a neutral pH. Dove, Oil of Olay, and Aveeno are some products that can be used.

Follow-up

- Have the patient call the health care team if pruritis is not relieved.
- Ascertain what the cause of the pruritis is and treat the underlying cause.
- Refer patient to dermatology specialists for assistance in management

Resources

- Mayo Clinic: http://www.mayoclinic.org/diseases-conditions/itchy-skin/basics/definition/CON-20028460?p=1

Bibliography

Larkin, P. (2015). Pruritus, fever, and sweats. In B. Ferrell, N. Coyle, & J. Paice (Eds.), *The Oxford textbook of palliative nursing* (4th ed.) (pp. 341–348). New York: Oxford University Press.

Polovich, M., Olsen, M., & LeFebre, K. (2014). *Side effects of cancer therapy*. In *Chemotherapy and biotherapy guidelines and recommendations for practice* (4th ed.). Pittsburgh, PA: Oncology Nursing Press.

Roebuck, H. L. (2006). For pruritus, combination therapy works best. *The Nurse Practitioner, 31*, 12–13.

Yarbro, C. H., & Seiz, A. M. (2014). Pruritus. In C. H. Yarbro, M. H. Frogge, & M. Goodman (Eds.), *Cancer symptom management* (4th ed.). Boston: Jones & Bartlett.

Rash

Laura S. Wood

Definition

- A rash is a dermatologic reaction that can be treatment related or associated with a malignancy.
- Rashes are more commonly associated with targeted therapies but also occur with chemotherapy and other cancer therapies.
- With targeted therapies, the precise etiology of most rashes remains unclear but is thought to be related to pathway inhibition.
- Rashes may be associated with xerosis, pruritus, and/or pain.
- The incidence and severity of rash associated with epidermal growth factor receptor (EGFR) inhibitor therapies may correlate with outcome.
- Rashes should be described by using phenotypic terms for appearance and location (see box below).

Phenotypic Terms Used to Describe Rashes
• Acneiform
• Acral erythema
• Bullous dermatitis
• Desquamation
• Erythema
• Erythema multiforme
• Erythroderma
• Folliculitis
• Macule
• Mobilliform
• Nodule
• Papule
• Papulopustular
• Plaque
• Pustule
• Urticaria

From Balagula, Y., Rosen, A., Tan, B., Busam, K. J., Pulitzer, M. P., Motzer, R. J., et al. (2012). Clinical and histopathologic characteristics of rash in cancer patients treated with mammalian target of rapamycin inhibitors. *Cancer, 118*, 5078-5083; Chen, A. P., Setser, A., Anadkat, M. J., Cotliar, J., Olsen, E. A., Garden, B. C., & Lacouture, M. E. (2012). Grading dermatologic adverse events of cancer treatments: The common terminology criteria for adverse events, version 4.0. *Journal of the American Academy of Dermatology, 67*, 1025-1039; Esper, P., Gale, D., & Muehlbauer, P. (2007). What kind of rash is it? Deciphering the dermatologic toxicities of biologic and targeted therapies. *Clinical Journal of Oncology Nursing, 11*(5), 659-666.

Pathophysiology and Contributing Factors

- EGFR is expressed in the epidermal and follicular keratinocytes, sebaceous epithelium, and hair follicles.
- Inhibition of EGFR may result in follicular occlusion due to lack of differentiation in the epithelium; this may cause sebaceous glands to produce a rosacea-like reaction that results in increased production of inflammatory mediators.

Signs and Symptoms

- Rash associated with targeted therapies typically occurs within the first few weeks of treatment.
- Erythema, dry skin, pruritus, and pain may accompany the rash at any point in time.
- Areas of involvement, severity, and duration vary greatly.
- Eruptions associated with EGFR inhibitors commonly involve the seborrheic areas, the face, neck, retroauricular area, shoulders, upper trunk, and scalp.
- Erythematous papules associated with EGFR inhibitors may evolve into pustules with pus that dry out with the formation of yellow crusts.

Assessment Tools

- Patient history (both medical and oncologic)
  - Review of prior dermatologic reactions
  - Review of allergies and sensitivities to medications and environmental factors
- Physical examination including assessment of
  - Area of involvement
  - Appearance of the dermatologic reaction
  - Date of onset
    - Any change in type, extent, or severity of rash since onset
  - Associated symptoms
    - Erythema, swelling, pruritus, blisters, desquamation
    - Determination of which side effects are affecting the patient. Treatment for mild or moderate side effects should be initiated before they become dose limiting.
- Common toxicity criteria for adverse events (CTCAE, version 4.0) (see table on page 344)

Considerations for Diagnosing Cancer Therapy-Associated Rash

- Rash presentation: Appearance, area of involvement
- Associated symptoms: Pruritus, pain or burning, paresthesias
- Characteristics of secondary infection: Fluid or drainage from lesions, crusting, fever or chills.
- Refer to dermatologist when:
  - Abrupt change in appearance of rash or associated symptoms
  - Worsening of rash or associated symptoms in spite of several OTC or prescription topical interventions
  - Atypical dermatologic manifestations unrelated to the rash

Laboratory and Diagnostic Tests

- Swab culture (to evaluate possible secondary infection)
- Biopsy (typically a punch biopsy)

Differential Diagnosis

- Folliculitis, often referred to as an acneiform eruption or acne-like rash, consists of inflammatory follicular papules and pustules.
- Bacterial culture may be appropriate but is often negative.

Dermatologic Terminology Criteria (CTCAE, Version 4.0)

	Grade 1	Grade 2	Grade 3	Grade 4
Dry skin	Covering <10% BSA and no associated erythema or pruritus	Covering 10-30% BSA and associated with erythema or pruritus; limiting instrumental ADLs	Covering >30% BSA and associated with pruritus; limiting ADLs	—
Palmar-plantar erythrodysesthesia syndrome	Minimal skin changes or dermatitis (e.g., erythema, edema, hyperkeratosis) without pain	Skin changes (e.g., peeling, blisters, bleeding, edema, hyperkeratosis) with pain; limiting instrumental ADLs	Severe skin changes (e.g., peeling, blisters, bleeding, edema, hyperkeratosis) with pain; limiting self-care ADL	—
Rash: acneiform	Papules and/or pustules covering <10% BSA, which may or may not be associated with symptoms of pruritus or tenderness	Papules and/or pustules covering 10-30% BSA, which may or may not be associated with symptoms of pruritus or tenderness; associated with psychosocial impact; limiting instrumental ADLs	Papules and/or pustules covering >30% BSA, which may or may not be associated with symptoms of pruritus or tenderness; limiting self-care ADLs; associated with local superinfection with oral antibiotics indicated	Papules and/or pustules covering any % BSA, which may or may not be associated with symptoms of pruritus or tenderness; associated with extensive superinfection with IV antibiotics indicated; life-threatening consequences
Rash: maculopapular	Macules/papules covering <10% BSA, with or without symptoms (e.g., pruritus, burning, tightness)	Macules/papules covering 1-30% BSA, with or without symptoms (e.g., pruritus, burning, tightness); limiting instrumental ADLs	Macules/papules covering >30% BSA, with or without associated symptoms; limiting self-care ADLs	—

ADLs, Activities of daily living; *BSA,* body surface area; *IV,* intravenous.
Adapted from National Cancer Institute. (2010). Common terminology criteria for adverse events (CTCAE), version 4.03. Available at http://www.oncology.tv/SymptomManagement/NationalCancerInstituteUpdatesCTCAEtov403.aspx (accessed March 1, 2016).

Interventions

- Treatment is based on the clinical phenotype and associated symptoms and focuses on maintaining quality of life while maximizing clinical outcomes.
- Evidence-based recommendations continue to evolve.
- Prophylactic strategies continue to evolve, and evolving data should be incorporated into clinical practice.

Pharmacologic Interventions

- Prophylactic approaches may decrease severity of the rash and improve quality of life
- Use of topical or systemic steroids or antibiotics may be indicated (see table below)

Nonpharmacologic Interventions

- Initiation of cleansing and moisturizing skin care regimen with initiation of treatment
- Non-deodorant, non–fragrance-containing soaps
- Frequent applications of lotion
- Use of lotions with higher dimethicone content to provide a higher degree of moisture barrier

- Water-based makeup (may also be used to camouflage rashes involving the face)
- Gentle makeup remover
- Avoidance of sun exposure and use of sunscreen with a strong sun protection factor (SPF) rating

Patient Teaching

- Educate patient and family on adherence to the recommended skin care regimen.
- Emphasize prevention, early intervention, and ongoing management to maximize clinical benefit of therapy and quality of life.
- Follow good hygiene practices to avoid introduction of bacteria to potential open areas.
- Treatment interruptions and dose reduction may be needed for intolerable symptoms.
- Educate patient and family on early and ongoing communication with the health care team regarding interventions and management of rash.

Follow-up

- Periodically assess for intervention success.
- Make referrals as appropriate, especially to a dermatologist and for psychosocial support if necessary.

Resources

- National Cancer Institute: Common terminology criteria for adverse events, version 4.03: http://www.oncology.tv/SymptomManagement/NationalCancerInstituteUpdatesCTCAEtov403.aspx
- Chemo Care (Cleveland Clinic): http://www.chemocare.com

Pharmacologic Interventions

Topical Products	Systemic Steroids	Systemic Antibiotics
Diphenhydramine lotion Lachydrin lotion Clindamycin lotion or gel Metrogel (topical Flagyl) Temovate (clobetasol propionate)	Dexamethasone Methylprednisolone (Medrol dose-pack)	Clindamycin Doxycycline Minocycline hydrochloride Trimethoprim/ sulfamethoxazole

- Multinational Association of Supportive Care in Cancer (MASCC). http://www.mascc.org
- National Comprehensive Cancer Network: http://www.nccn.org

Bibliography

Balagula, Y., Rosen, A., Tan, B., Busam, K. J., Pulitzer, M. P., Motzer, R. J., & Lacouture, M. E. (2012). Clinical and histopathologic characteristics of rash in cancer patients treated with mammalian target of rapamycin inhibitors. *Cancer, 118,* 5078–5083.

Burtness, B., Anadkat, M., Basti, S., Hughes, M., Lacouture, M. E., McClure, J. S., & Spencer, S. (2009). NCCN Task force report: Management of dermatologic and other toxicities associated with EGFR inhibition in patients with cancer. *Journal of the National Comprehensive Cancer Network, 7*(Suppl. 1), 5–21.

Chen, A. P., Setser, A., Anadkat, M. J., Cotliar, J., Olsen, E. A., Garden, B. C., & Lacouture, M. E. (2012). Grading dermatologic adverse events of cancer treatments: The common terminology criteria for adverse events, version 4.0. *Journal of the American Academy of Dermatology, 67,* 1025–1039.

Eaby, B., Culkin, A., & Lacouture, M. E. (2008). An interdisciplinary consensus on managing skin reactions associated with human epidermal growth factor receptor inhibitors. *Clinical Journal of Oncology Nursing, 12*(2), 283–290.

Esper, P., Gale, D., & Muehlbauer, P. (2007). What kind of rash is it? Deciphering the dermatologic toxicities of biologic and targeted therapies. *Clinical Journal of Oncology Nursing, 11*(5), 659–666.

Gomez-Fernandez, C., Garden, B. C., Wu, S., Feldman, D. R., & Lacouture, M. E. (2012). The risk of skin rash and stomatitis with the mammalian target of rapamycin inhibitor temsirolimus: A systemic review of the literature and meta analysis. *European Journal of Cancer, 48,* 340–346.

Lacouture, M. E., Anadkat, M. J., Bensadoun, R. J., Bryce, J., Chan, A., Epstein, J. B., & MASCC Skin Toxicity Study Group. (2010). Clinical practice guidelines for the prevention and treatment of EGFR inhibitor-associated dermatologic toxicities. *Supportive Care in Cancer, 19,* 1079–1095.

Lacouture, M. E., Maitland, M. L., Segaert, S., Setser, A., Baran, R., Fox, L. P., & Trotti, A. (2010). A proposed EGFR inhibitor dermatologic adverse event-specific grading scale from the MASCC skin toxicity group. *Supportive Care in Cancer, 18,* 509–522.

Lacouture, M. E., Mitchell, E. P., Piperdi, B., Pillai, M. V., Shearer, H., Iannotti, N., & Yassine, M. (2010). Skin toxicity evaluation protocol with panitumumab (STEPP), a Phase II, open-label, randomized trial evaluating the impact of a pre-emptive skin treatment regimen on skin toxicities and quality of life in patients with metastatic colorectal cancer. *Journal of Clinical Oncology, 28,* 1351–1357.

National Cancer Institute. (2010). *Common terminology criteria for adverse events (CTCAE),* version 4.03. Available at http://www.oncology.tv/SymptomManagement/NationalCancerInstituteUpdatesCTCAEtov403.aspx (accessed March 1, 2016).

Oishi, K. (2008). Clinical approaches to minimize rash associated with EGFR inhibitors. *Oncology Nursing Forum, 35,* 103–111.

Perez-Soler, R., DeLord, J. P., Halpern, A., Kelly, K., Krueger, J., Sureda, B. M., & Leyden, J. (2005). HER1/EGFR inhibitor-associated rash: Future directions for management and investigation outcomes from the HER1/EGFR inhibitor rash management forum. *The Oncologist, 10,* 345–356.

Rhee, J., Oishi, K., Garey, J., & Kim, E. (2005). Management of rash and other toxicities in patients treated with epidermal growth factor receptor-targeted agents. *Clinical Colorectal Cancer, 5*(Suppl. 2), S101–S106.

Robert, C., Soria, J. C., Spatz, A., Le Cesne, A., Malka, D., Pautier, P., & Le Chevalier, T. (2005). Cutaneous side effects of kinase inhibitors and blocking antibodies. *The Lancet Oncology, 6,* 491–500.

Segaert, S. (2008). Management of skin toxicity of epidermal growth factor receptor inhibitors. *Targeted Oncology, 3,* 245–251.

Segaert, S., & Cutsem, E. V. (2005). Clinical signs, pathophysiology and management of skin toxicity during therapy with epidermal growth factor receptor inhibitors. *Annals of Oncology, 16,* 1425–1433.

Thatcher, N., Nicolson, M., Groves, R. W., Steele, J., Eaby, B., Dunlop, J., & U.K. Erlotinib Skin Toxicity Management Consensus Group. (2009). Expert consensus on the management of erlotinib-associated cutaneous toxicity in the U.K. *The Oncologist, 14,* 840–847.

Wacker, B., Nagrani, T., Weinberg, J., Witt, K., Clark, G., & Cagnoni, P. J. (2007). Correlation between development of rash and efficacy in patients treated with the epidermal growth factor receptor tyrosine kinase inhibitor erlotinib in two large phase III studies. *Clinical Cancer Research, 13,* 3913–3921.

Wright, L. G. (2006). Maculopapular skin rashes associated with high-dose chemotherapy: Prevalence and risk factors. *Oncology Nursing Forum, 33,* 1095–1103.

Seizures

Carol S. Blecher

Definition

- A seizure may be defined as a sudden overactivation of cerebral neurons that may cause changes in sensory and motor function. There may also be changes in autonomic function, behavior, and level of consciousness.

Pathophysiology and Contributing Factors

- Seizures are a symptom of irritation of the central nervous system (CNS) that results in an abnormal discharge of neurons.
- Cerebral function is disturbed by electrical discharges that are synchronous, abnormal, and excessive.
- This abnormal discharge of neurons can cause an alteration of consciousness or any other cerebral cortical function.
- Classification is either focal or generalized, but all seizures are characterized by sudden involuntary contraction of groups of muscles.
- Causes
  - Neuronal loss or scarring from surgery or head trauma
  - Primary brain cancer or metastatic brain tumors
  - Acquired immunodeficiency syndrome (AIDS) or a history of seizures
  - Metabolic disturbances such as syndrome of inappropriate antidiuretic hormone secretion (SIADH), hypoglycemia, hyponatremia, hypercalcemia (a late sign), hypocalcemia, hypomagnesemia, renal or hepatic failure, alcohol or drug withdrawal
  - Chemotherapeutic agents including bevacizumab, busulfan, carmustine, cisplatin, cyclosporine, cytarabine, cyclophosphamide, etoposide, gemcitabine, ifosfamide, interferon-alfa, intrathecal methotrexate, oxaliplatin, rituximab, vincristine
- Types
  - Primary generalized seizures
    - *Absence:* Brief loss of consciousness
    - *Myoclonic:* Sporadic (isolated), jerking movements
    - *Atonic:* Loss of muscle tone
    - *Tonic:* Muscle stiffness, rigidity

- *Clonic*: Repetitive, jerking movements
- *Tonic-clonic*: Unconsciousness, convulsions, muscle rigidity
- Partial seizures: preceded by an aura
  - *Simple partial*: Characterized by focal activity with no loss of consciousness
  - *Complex partial*: Characterized by loss of consciousness
  - *Secondarily generalized*
- Absence (petit mal): brief, characterized by no obvious motor symptoms
- Unclassified epileptic seizures characterized by abrupt onset, unconsciousness, involuntary motor activity, involuntary sensory activity, and incontinence. There is also a postictal state after the seizure that is characterized by somnolence or headache.

Signs and Symptoms

- Change in level of consciousness
- Aura before the event: an unusual feeling, smell, or sensation
- Change in muscle tone and movement
- Activity that is involuntary and uncontrolled
- A postictal state after the seizure is characterized by somnolence or headache
- No memory regarding the event

Assessment Tools

- History, including diagnosis and cancer treatment, current medications, presenting symptoms, changes in activities of daily living (ADLs), social history, family history, and history of recent infections
- Signs and symptoms, including clinical symptoms regarding the episode. This information may need to be obtained from an individual who observed the event because the patient may have no memory of the seizure.
- Neurologic examination evaluating for automatism (repetitive movements), hyperreflexia, positive Babinski sign, localized neurologic deficits
- Vital signs: orthostatic changes
- Skin examination for signs of intravenous (IV) drug abuse or trauma, including lacerations, bruises, and oral trauma
- Precipitating factors such as stress, exercise, alcohol, barbiturates, recreational drugs, fatigue, heat, flashing lights, focusing on a computer screen, driving, antihistamines, nonadherence to therapy
- National Cancer Institute (NCI) common toxicity criteria
  - Grade 1: brief partial seizure; no loss of consciousness
  - Grade 2: brief generalized seizure
  - Grade 3: multiple seizures despite medical intervention
  - Grade 4: life-threatening; prolonged repetitive seizures
  - Grade 5: death

Physical Examination

- Neurologic examination
- Cranial nerve examination
- Motor examination
- Reflex examination
- Sensory examination
- Coordination examination

Laboratory and Diagnostic Tests

- Complete blood cell count (CBC) to rule out thrombocytopenia, which can cause intracerebral bleeding
- Chemistry studies to assess for SIADH, hypoglycemia, hyponatremia, hypercalcemia, hypocalcemia, hypomagnesemia, renal or hepatic failure
- Pregnancy test for women of childbearing age; because anticonvulsives are pregnancy category D, they can cause harmful effects to the fetus.
- Drug screening for cocaine, crack cocaine, and heroin because these medications or their withdrawal can cause seizures
- Drug levels of current anticonvulsive medications
- Alcohol blood level
- Computed tomographic (CT) scan of the head to identify tumor, metastases, or head trauma
- Electroencephalogram (EEG) to differentiate seizure activity from psychogenic symptoms and motor activity caused by neuromuscular conditions
- Lumbar puncture to assess for infection (meningitis, abscess, toxoplasmosis) or meningeal carcinomatosis

Differential Diagnoses

- Alcohol withdrawal
- Cerebrovascular event
- Drug toxicity: busulfan, carmustine, cisplatin, cyclosporine, high-dose 5-fluorouracil (5-FU), ifosfamide, intrathecal methotrexate, cocaine, crack cocaine, and heroin
- Infectious meningitis, abscess, toxoplasmosis
- Metabolic imbalance
- Migraine headache
- Psychiatric disorders
- Tumor: primary brain tumor or metastatic disease
- Trauma

Interventions

Pharmacologic Interventions

- Carbamazepine (Tegretol) 600-1200 mg PO
- Diazepam (Valium) 2-10 mg PO bid to qid
- Gabapentin (Neurontin) 900-3600 mg PO
- Lamotrigine (Lamictal) 50-200 mg PO bid
- Levetiracetam (Keppra) 1000-3000 mg PO
- Lorazepam (Ativan) 1-8 mg PO
- Phenytoin (Dilantin) 300-400 mg PO
- Phenobarbital 60-200 mg PO at night
- Valproic acid (Depakote) 250-750 mg PO

Nonpharmacologic Interventions

- During an active seizure
  - Secure airway
  - Obtain IV access
  - Protect from injury

- Provide oxygen supplementation
- Obtain blood work: blood glucose level for hypoglycemia
- If patient has a history of seizures and is taking antiseizure medications, monitor serum levels of anticonvulsants.
- If the seizure is caused by underlying metabolic disturbances, these should be corrected and any medications contributing to the conditions should be discontinued.
- If appropriate, transfer patient to the nearest emergency department.

Patient Teaching

- Instructions should include the following:
  - Follow seizure precautions.
  - Do not drive or operate dangerous machinery.
  - Report blurred vision, ataxia, or drowsiness caused by anticonvulsive medications to health care provider immediately.
  - Avoid alcohol while taking anticonvulsants.
  - Contact health care provider if
    - This is a first-time seizure.
    - A seizure lasts more than 2-5 minutes.
    - The person does not awaken or have normal behavior after a seizure.
    - Another seizure starts soon after a seizure ends.
    - The person had a seizure in water.
    - The person is pregnant, injured, or has diabetes.
    - The person does not have a medical ID bracelet (instructions explaining what to do).
    - There is anything different about this seizure compared with the person's usual seizures.

Follow-up

- Monitor the patient's clinical state, seizure frequency, and serum anticonvulsant levels.
- CBC, chemistries, liver enzymes; monitor renal and hepatic function
- Patients who have a 2-year seizure-free period and no risk factors may be taken off the antiseizure medications. Anticonvulsive medication must be tapered slowly. Patients with risk factors should be maintained on medication for 5 years.
- If the patient's disease is terminal, the seizure activity should be controlled with lorazepam or a barbiturate.
- Referrals should be made to a neurologist, a radiation oncologist, and an epilepsy center.

Resources

- Common terminology criteria for adverse events, version 4.03 (2010). http://evs.nci.nih.gov/ftp1/CTCAE/About.html
- Epilepsy Foundation of America: http://www.epilepsy.com/
- MedlinePlus Patient Education Tools http://www.nlm.nih.gov/medlineplus/ency/patientinstructions/000128.htm
- Ohio State University Patient Education Tool https://patienteducation.osumc.edu/pages/patienteducation/atoztopicdetail.aspx?t=Seizures

Bibliography

Common terminology criteria for adverse events, version 4.03 (2010). Available at http://evs.nci.nih.gov/ftp1/CTCAE/About.html (accessed March 1, 2016).

Epilepsy Foundation of America (Homepage). Available at http://www.epilepsy.com/ (accessed March 1, 2016).

Medline Plus. Seizures. Available at http://www.nlm.nih.gov/medlineplus/ency/article/003200.htm (accessed March 1, 2016).

Medline Plus. Epilepsy or seizures—Discharge. Available at http://www.nlm.nih.gov/medlineplus/ency/patientinstructions/000128.htm (accessed March 1, 2016).

Ohio State University. Wexner Medical Center: Health Topics—Seizures. Available at https://patienteducation.osumc.edu/pages/patienteducation/atoztopicdetail.aspx?t=Seizures (accessed March 1, 2016).

Schwartz, M. A. (2015). Neurological disturbances. In B. R. Ferrell & N. Coyle (Eds.), Textbook of palliative nursing (4th ed.) (pp. 349–365). New York: Oxford University Press.

Walker, J. G., & Le, E. M. (2014). Seizures. In D. Camp-Sorrell & R. A. Hawkins (Eds.), Clinical manual for the oncology advanced practice nurse (pp. 1217–1230). Pittsburgh, PA: Oncology Nursing Press.

Wilkes, G. M. (2014). Increased intracranial pressure. In C. H. Yarbro, M. H. Frogge, & M. Goodman (Eds.), Cancer symptom management (4th ed.). Sudbury, MA: Jones & Bartlett.

Zielke, K. A. (2008). Seizures. In K. K. Kuebler & P. Esper (Eds.), Palliative practices A-Z (2nd ed.) (pp. 211–213). Pittsburgh, PA: Oncology Nursing Society.

Sexuality Alterations

Wendy H. Vogel

Definition

- Sexuality is a multidimensional concept that encompasses sexual self-concept, sexual function, sexual roles, sexual relationships, and sexual orientation. It includes intimacy and is not limited to just sexual function, intercourse, and reproduction. Sexuality is ultimately defined by each person.
- Sexual health is a component of overall health.
- Sexual dysfunction is a group of disorders, both physiologic and psychological, that adversely affect sexuality. This can include (but is not limited to) dyspareunia, loss of libido, impotence, infertility, anorgasmia, and delayed ejaculation.
- Estimates of prevalence of alterations in sexuality range from 40% to 100%. Long-term dysfunction may occur (50% of breast cancer survivors).
- Alterations in sexuality are underdiagnosed often because of health care professionals' discomfort, lack of knowledge, or embarrassment of the subject.

Pathophysiology and Contributing Factors

- Gonadal function is regulated by the anterior pituitary and the hypothalamus.
  - Hypothalamic hormones induce glandular secretions that control the hypothalamus and pituitary
    - Luteinizing hormone-releasing hormone (LHRH) or gonadotropin-releasing hormone (GnRH), secreted by the hypothalamus, stimulates the pituitary to produce luteinizing hormone (LH) and follicle-stimulating hormone (FSH)

- LH and FSH stimulate the testis to produce testosterone or the ovary to produce estrogen and progesterone, hormones that control sexual function.
- Disruption of the neurovasculature of the genitalia or changes in hormonal status can occur secondary to cancer or cancer treatments.
- Chemotherapy, radiation therapy, or surgery may cause direct injury to gonads.
- Ovarian failure may be induced by radiation therapy, chemotherapy, hormonal therapy, surgery, or infection.
  - Estrogen deficiency, resulting in amenorrhea and vaginal and urogenital atrophy
  - Depletion of primordial follicles and oocytes, resulting in loss of fertility
  - Disruption of the hypothalamic-pituitary-gonadal axis
- Testicular aplasia, azoospermia, and erectile dysfunction in males may occur because of direct organ damage from surgery or radiation therapy or because of changes in hormonal status secondary to systemic cancer treatment (chemotherapy or hormonal therapy).
  - Disruption of the hypothalamic-pituitary-gonadal axis
  - Loss of or damage to germ cells and developing sperm
  - Leydig cell dysfunction resulting in decreased testosterone
  - Mechanical dysfunction resulting from surgery
- Other causes of sexual dysfunction include the following:
  - Medications (e.g., antihypertensives, anticonvulsants, antiemetics, psychotropic agents, narcotics, hormonal agents, histamine H_2 receptor blockers)
  - Alcohol, nicotine, cocaine, and other illegal drugs
  - Depression, stress, relationship difficulties
  - Body image (e.g., related to colostomy, head and neck surgery, amputation, cachexia, radiation skin changes, surgery)

Signs and Symptoms

- Women: Vaginal atrophy, thinning of the vaginal wall, dryness, dyspareunia, postcoital bleeding, premature menopause, decreased libido, impaired fertility, hot flashes, emotional lability, mood changes, irritability, body image changes, sexual identity issues (see Menopausal Symptoms on page 321)
- Men: decreased testosterone, decreased libido, decreased to no production of semen, erectile dysfunction, ejaculatory difficulties, impotence, impaired fertility, gynecomastia, body image changes, sexual identity issues

Assessment Tools

- PLISSIT model (Permission, Limited Information, Specific Suggestions, Intensive Therapy)
- Men
  - International Index of Erectile Function
  - Brief Male Sexual Function Inventory
  - Sexual Health Inventory for Men

- Women
  - Brief Index of Sexual Functioning for Women
  - Changes in Sexual Functioning Questionnaire
  - Female Sexual Function Index
- Risk factors for sexual dysfunction
  - Increasing age
  - Certain medications
  - Psychological issues such as alterations in body image, depression, low self-esteem, decreased sense of femininity/masculinity, poor coping mechanisms, poor communication skills
  - Comorbidities such as arthritis, chronic obstructive pulmonary disease (COPD), diabetes, myocardial infarction, spinal cord injury
- Review medication list for medications that could be affecting sexual function.
- Assess relationship status, reasons and incentives to be sexually active.
- Assess sexual functioning before cancer diagnosis and current sexual functioning.

Laboratory and Diagnostic Tests

- Females: FSH, LH, serum estradiol, mean estrone, human chorionic gonadotropin (hCG); genital, pelvic, and breast examination
- Males: testosterone, Rigiscan, penile ultrasound studies, genital examination
- Both sexes as indicated: urinalysis if urinary tract symptoms are present, prolactin levels, rectal examination; testing for sexually transmitted diseases; fertility studies
- Computed tomography (CT), magnetic resonance imaging (MRI), or ultrasound of the abdomen/pelvis if vascular or neurologic damage is suspected

Differential Diagnoses

- Females: ovarian abnormalities, polycystic ovarian syndrome, ovarian neoplasia
- Hypothyroidism
- Pituitary tumors
- Adrenal abnormalities

Interventions

Pharmacologic Interventions

- Hormone replacement therapy (HRT) in postmenopausal women is a controversial subject because of various health risks, including breast cancer (see Menopausal Symptoms on page 321).
- Testosterone replacement in men or women
  - Contraindicated in prostate cancer
  - In female patients, the route is not established nor is safety in hormonally related cancers.
- In the oncology patient, careful consideration should be given to hormone-related cancer, and the risks of cancer stimulation should be evaluated.
- Treatment of comorbidities affecting sexuality

- In females, menopausal symptoms should be treated as noted in Menopausal Symptoms on page 321
- Medications for erectile dysfunction: sildenafil, vardenafil, tadalafil (contraindicated with concurrent use of nitrates or the α-blockers terazosin and doxazosin)

Nonpharmacologic Interventions

- Refer patients to a fertility preservation specialist before cancer treatment, as appropriate.
- Refer patients to a surgeon, urologist, or reconstructive surgeon as appropriate.
- Proactively approach patients about sexual dysfunction, giving them permission to ask questions or express concerns. Discuss common issues related to the type of treatment and some ways to work through it.
- Fatigue issues must be addressed.
- Advise smoking cessation, low to moderate alcohol intake, maintenance of a healthy weight, and exercise as tolerated.
- For dyspareunia (painful intercourse), recommend vaginal moisturizers or lubricants, position changes for comfort, relaxation exercises, stress reduction techniques, topical lidocaine, regular sexual activity, adequate foreplay, vaginal dilation; provide instruction in Kegel exercises, EROS clitoral therapy device.
- Vaginal lubricants, such as Replens (Auspharm, Australia), may be helpful for vaginal dryness (see Menopausal Symptoms on page 321).
- For erectile dysfunction, penile suppositories, vacuum devices, penile injections, and penile implants may be used.
- For sexual issues related to colostomies or iliostomies
  - Refer to national organization resources.
  - Limit food intake before anticipated sexual activities.
  - Plan times for intimacy when bowel movement is less likely.
  - Empty pouch when intimacy is anticipated.
  - Roll up or tape down empty, flat ostomy bag.
  - Use decorative covers.
  - Review selection of ostomy products.
- Refer patients to a sex therapist or couples counseling as needed.
- Do not assume because a patient is elderly, terminally ill, or without a partner that sexual concerns are not an issue.
- Nurses must assume a nonjudgmental, open, caring attitude with all patients regardless of sexual orientation.

Patient Teaching

- Patients should understand the fertility risks and the potential for sexual dysfunction before undergoing cancer treatment.
- If hormonal therapy is considered, the risks and benefits must be fully explored with the patient.
- Reassure patients and significant others that there are many ways to express love and intimacy and that communication is key.
- Information regarding safe sex must be discussed with each oncology patient as part of chemotherapy teaching.
- Contraception discussion is needed for female patients of child-bearing age.
- Avoid sexual relations at times of low blood counts.
- Explore other means of sexual expression besides intercourse.

Follow-up

- Provide follow-up as needed to assess symptom management.

Resources

- American Cancer Society: www.cancer.org
- Chemocare.org: www.chemocare.org
- National Cancer Institute: www.cancer.gov
- Oncology Nursing Society: www.ons.org
- American Association of Sex Educators: www.aasect.org

Bibliography

Anderson, J. (2013). Acknowledging female sexual dysfunction in women with cancer. *Clinical Journal of Oncology Nursing, 17*(3), 233–235.

Brennan, A., Barnsteiner, J., Siantz, M., Cotter, V., & Everett, J. (2012). Lesbian, gay, bisexual, transgendered, or intersexed content for nursing curricula. *Journal of Professional Nursing, 28*(2), 96–104.

De Vocht, H., Hordern, A., Notter, J., & van de Wiel, H. (2011). Stepped skills: A team approach towards communication about sexuality and intimacy in cancer and palliative care. *Australasian Medical Journal, 4*(11), 610–619.

Hickey, M., Saunders, C., Partridge, A., Santoro, N., Joffe, H., & Stearns, V. (2008). Practical guidelines for assessing and managing menopausal symptoms after breast cancer. *Annals of Oncology, 19*, 1669–1680.

Johnson, R., & Kroon, L. (2013). Optimizing fertility preservation practices for adolescent and young adult cancer patients. *Journal of the National Comprehensive Cancer Network, 11*(1), 71–77.

Krebs, L. (2014). Altered body image and sexual health. In C. Yarbro, D. Wujcik, & B. Gobel (Eds.), *Cancer symptom management* (4th ed.) (pp. 507–540). Burlington, MA: Jones & Bartlett.

Krebs, L. (2011). Sexual and reproductive dysfunction. In C. Yarbro, D. Wujcik, & B. Gobel (Eds.), *Cancer nursing principles and practice* (7th ed.) (pp. 879–912). Sudbury, MA: Jones & Bartlett.

McCallum, M., Jolicoeur, L., Lefebvre, M., Babchishin, L., Robert-Chauret, S., Le, T., & Lebel, S. (2014). Supportive care needs after gynecologic cancer: Where does sexual health fit in? *Oncology Nursing Forum, 41*(3), 297–306.

Misiewicz, H. (2012). Fertility issues of breast cancer survivors. *Journal for the Advanced Practitioner in Oncology, 3*, 289–298.

Moore, A., Higgins, A., & Sharek, D. (2013). Barriers and facilitators for oncology nurses discussing sexual issues with men diagnosed with testicular cancer. *European Journal of Oncology Nursing, 17*, 416–422.

National Cancer Institute. (2016). *Sexuality and reproductive issues (PDQ).* Available at https://www.oncolink.org/resources/nci.cfm?id=CDR0000062862 (accessed March 1, 2016).

Nishimoto, P., & Mark, D. (2014). Altered sexuality patterns. In C. Brown (Ed.), *Guide to oncology symptom management* (pp. 423–456). Pittsburgh, PA: Oncology Nursing Society.

Trinkaus, M., Shin, S., Wolfman, W., Simmons, C., & Clemons, M. (2008). Should urogenital atrophy in breast cancer survivors be treated with topical estrogens? *The Oncologist, 13*, 222–231.

Principles of Symptom Management

④

Polovich, M., Olsen, M., & LeFebvre, K. (2014). *Chemotherapy and biotherapy guidelines and recommendations for practice* (4th ed.) (pp. 383–391). Pittsburg, PA: Oncology Nursing Society.

Williams, A., Reckamp, K., Freeman, B., Sidhu, R., & Grant, M. (2013). Sexuality, lung cancer, and the older adult: An unlikely trio? *Journal for the Advanced Practitioner in Oncology, 4*(5), 331–340.

World Health Organization (WHO). (2014). *Sexual health.* Available at http://www.who.int/topics/sexual_health/en/ (accessed March 1, 2016).

Sleep Disturbances

Wendy H. Vogel

Definition

- Sleep disturbances include insomnia and hypersomnia.
  - Insomnia is the inability to sleep when needed; it may include difficulty falling asleep, difficulty maintaining sleep, or early-morning awakenings with difficulty resuming sleep.
  - Hypersomnia is the inability to maintain wakefulness when needed.
- Sleep disturbances are a common problem in oncology patients; they can be transient, chronic, or recurring and can affect quality of life.

Pathophysiology and Contributing Factors

- Sleep disturbances are common in oncology patients.
- Sleep impairment risk increases with age.
- The most common cause of insomnia is uncontrolled pain.
- Insomnia or hypersomnia can also occur because of use of certain medications, withdrawal from certain medications, anxiety, depression, hypoxia, sleep apnea, urinary frequency, pruritus, endocrine disorders, hot flashes, restless legs, sleeping during the day, caffeine intake, change in environment, or psychological stress.
- Insomnia could also be an independent disorder with no known etiology (primary insomnia).
- Cancer patients often complain of daytime sleepiness and nighttime insomnia.
- Sleep deprivation is linked to changes in mentation, such as a decline in cognitive function and behavioral changes.
- Studies have shown a decrease in certain immune functions associated with insomnia.
- Pathophysiology of sleep: an interrelated process involving the balance between being asleep and being awake, the circadian rhythm, and the cycles (stages) of sleep.
- There are two stages of sleep, non–rapid eye movement (NREM) sleep and rapid eye movement (REM) or dreaming sleep. Circadian factors control the wake and sleep patterns over a 24-hour period. NREM sleep, REM sleep, and circadian rhythms may be disrupted in oncology patients.
- The normal amount of sleep needed to maintain healthy functioning varies from 6 to 10 hours per night.
- Types
  - Transient: lasting less than 2 weeks
  - Short-term: lasting between 2 and 4 weeks
  - Chronic: lasting longer than 4 weeks

- Incidence
  - The incidence of sleep disturbances range from 25% to 95% in oncology patients.
  - About 50% of these sleep disturbances are insomnias (in the general population, insomnia occurs in 30-35% of people).
  - Sleep disturbances are more likely during the initial diagnosis, during cancer treatments, and at the end of life.
  - Up to 44% of patients continue to report insomnia several years after diagnosis and treatment.

Signs and Symptoms

- Inability to fall asleep or sleeping too much
- Awakenings in the night, early-morning awakening and inability to return to sleep, difficulty staying asleep
- Daytime sleepiness, daytime napping, fatigue, irritability, depression, anxiety, decreased concentration, irregular sleep schedules

Assessment Tools

- Routinely assess for sleep disturbances, including sleep quality, daytime sleepiness, and symptoms of insomnia. Include assessments of frequency, severity, and duration of symptoms.
- Knowing the patient's normal sleep habits enables the health care provider to establish a baseline normal pattern.
- Assess the amount and timing of daily physical exercise.
- Determine the bed partner or family member's perceptions of sleep disturbance.
- Bedtime/wake times
- Diet, caffeine, and alcohol intake
- Environmental conditions (e.g., lighting, noise, ventilation, bedding, temperature, positioning)
- Medication review
- Patient's belief about the cause of sleep disturbance
- Presence of daytime napping
- Presleep routines (e.g., food and fluid intake, hygiene, stimulation)
- Total hours slept during a 24-hour period
- Assess for risk factors
  - Active chemotherapy treatment
  - Chronic medical illness (e.g., asthma, gastroesophageal reflux, and chronic obstructive pulmonary disease)
  - Depression/anxiety
  - Distress of symptoms such as pain, nausea, or diarrhea
  - Fatigue
  - Female sex
  - Lower educational level
  - Lower socioeconomic status
  - Menstruation
  - Older age
  - Perimenopause
  - Personal or family history of insomnia
  - Recent life stressors
  - Specific cancer type (e.g., breast, colorectal, prostate, ovarian, lung, hematologic, and malignant melanoma)

- Unpleasant environment
- Use of alcohol
- Shift work
- Polypharmacy
- Assess for medications known to cause insomnia
  - Amphetamines
  - Anticonvulsants
  - Biologicals (e.g., interferons, interleukins, tumor necrosis factor)
  - Bronchodilators
  - Caffeine
  - Chemotherapy
  - Corticosteroids
  - Decongestants
  - Dieting agents
  - Hormonal agents
  - Illicit drugs
  - Long-term use of analgesic medications
  - Monoamine oxidase inhibitors (MAOIs)
  - Selective serotonin reuptake inhibitors (SSRIs)
  - Theophyllines
- Physical examination
  - Neurologic assessment
  - Oropharyngeal examination, observing for anatomic obstruction

Laboratory and Diagnostic Tests

- No standard quantitative criteria exist to diagnose insomnia.
- A sleep study (polysomnography) may be useful in a primary sleep disorder such as narcolepsy, parasomnias, or sleep apnea (not indicated for evaluation of transient or chronic insomnia or insomnia associated with psychiatric disorders).
- It is useful to determine cause factors for sleep disturbances such as obstructive sleep apnea and periodic leg movements.

- A sleep journal (1- to 2-week log) may be helpful in obtaining the specific information related to the assessments described.
- Underlying physical and emotional causes should be ruled out and treated as necessary. This could include obtaining a urinalysis and a complete blood cell count.

Differential Diagnoses

- It is important to differentiate between a primary cause of sleep disturbance (e.g., narcolepsy, parasomnia) and secondary causes of sleep disturbance.
- Cancer-related fatigue

Interventions

- Rule out any physical or emotional causes of sleep disturbances. Management of these causes (e.g., uncontrolled pain, depression) may correct the sleep disturbance.

Pharmacologic Interventions

- For insomnia, benzodiazepines, benzodiazepine-receptor agonists, melatonin-receptor agonists, or sedative-hypnotics may be used.
- Medications should be closely monitored.
- Tolerance to short-acting benzodiazepines could occur in as little as 2 weeks, and these medications should be used intermittently and for as short a period as possible (ideally, no longer than 3-4 weeks).
- Tapering and then discontinuing the medication once a therapeutic point is reached should be considered.
- Pharmacotherapy is not recommended for chronic insomnia except for a short-term period and only as an adjunct to other treatment, such as cognitive behavioral treatment (see table below).
- Alternative treatments for insomnia (efficacy and safety not established):
  - Melatonin
  - Valerian root extract

Pharmacologic Treatment for Short-Term Insomnia

Class	Drugs	Benefits	Complications
Benzodiazepines	Clonazepam Lorazepam Oxazepam	Class of choice for short-term treatment Useful in insomnia caused by anxiety or restless legs Useful in insomnia that is refractory to other treatments	Long-acting agents may cause daytime drowsiness, dizziness, cognitive impairment. Short-acting agents may have tolerance and dependence issues, rebound insomnia, daytime anxiety.
Nonbenzodiazepines	Eszopiclone Zaleplon Zolpidem	More receptor selectivity Fewer residual side effects the next day Do not lead to tolerance and have less potential for abuse Quick onset of action	May cause amnesias, paresthesias, arthralgias, flu-like symptoms
Tricyclic antidepressants with sedative effects	Amitriptyline Doxepin Nortriptyline	Useful in depressed patients or insomnia from neuropathic pain High sedative effects	May cause dry mouth, somnolence, dizziness, constipation, palpitations
Second-generation antidepressants with sedative effects	Trazodone (low dose) Nefazodone Mirtazapine	Useful in depressed patients Mirtazapine can stimulate appetite and decrease nausea	May cause dry mouth, somnolence, dizziness, constipation
Antihistamines	Diphenhydramine Hydroxyzine	Useful for sedation, reducing nausea and vomiting	May cause daytime sedation and delirium, especially in elderly May cause constipation, urinary retention, and confusion
Melatonin-receptor agonists	Ramelteon	Useful with difficulty falling asleep; little to no hangover effect	Caution in mild-moderate hepatic impairment

- Treatment for daytime hypersomnia
  - Psychostimulants such as methylphenidate or a cholinesterase inhibitor such as donepezil
  - Modafinil, a nonamphetamine stimulant, may be considered. Use in small doses, and give early in the day; this may help prevent daytime napping, thus improving insomnia

Nonpharmacologic Interventions

- Review medications; adjust timing so that patient does not have to awaken to take medications. Ensure that medications such as diuretics are taken no later than 3 PM.
- Instruct in good sleep hygiene. Sleep hygiene includes therapies for stimulus control, sleep restriction, and relaxation.
- Cognitive control techniques such as counting, refocusing, meditation, or guided imagery may assist in controlling racing thoughts or worries.
- Thought stopping is performed by repeating the word "the" or "stop" every 3 seconds.
- Relaxation training includes progressive muscle relaxation, biofeedback, yoga, hypnosis.

Patient Teaching

- Educate the patient on sleep hygiene (specific behaviors that promote good sleep).
  - Stay in the bed only during the hours intended for sleep.
  - Establish a routine wake time and bedtime.
  - Avoid stimulants such as caffeine.
  - Refrain from exercising at least 6 hours before bedtime.
  - Decrease or eliminate nighttime use of tobacco products.
  - Determine the best sleep environment.
  - Do not nap during the day, or limit naps to 20 minutes, and avoid all naps after 3 PM.
  - Create a bedtime routine.
  - If not asleep within 15 to 20 minutes, get out of bed and do a nonstimulating activity until sleepy, then return to bed.
  - Avoid heavy foods at bedtime.
  - Keep a sleep log.
  - Remove bedroom clock.

Follow-up

- Follow-up as indicated to assess pharmacologic success and as needed for cognitive-behavioral training.

Resources

- American Cancer Society: www.cancer.org
- American Academy of Sleep Medicine: http://www.aasmnet.org
- National Cancer Institute: http://www.cancer.gov/cancertopics/pdq/supportivecare/sleepdisorders/HealthProfessional/page1/AllPages
- National Institutes of Health, National Center on Sleep Disorder Research: http://www.nhlbi.nih.gov/about/org/ncsdr/
- OncoLink: http://www.oncolink.org/coping/coping.cfm?c=486

Bibliography

Enderlin, C., Coleman, E., Cole, C., Richards, K., Hutchins, L., & Sherman, A. (2010). Sleep across chemotherapy treatment: A growing concern for women older than 50 with breast cancer. *Oncology Nursing Forum, 37*(4), 461–468.

Erickson, J., & Berger, A. (2014). Sleep-wake disturbances. In C. Brown (Ed.), *Guide to oncology symptom management* (pp. 473–496). Pittsburg, PA: Oncology Nursing Society.

Lamberti, M. (2014). Improving sleep-wake disturbances in patients with cancer. *Clinical Journal of Oncology Nursing, 18*(5), 509–511.

Matthews, E., & Berger, A. (2014). Sleep disturbances. In C. Yarbro, D. Wujcik, & B. Gobel (Eds.), *Cancer symptom management* (4th ed.) (pp. 93–109). Burlington, MA: Jones & Bartlett.

National Cancer Institute. (2014). *Sleep disorders (PDQ).* Available at http://www.cancer.gov/cancertopics/pdq/supportivecare/sleepdisorders/Health Professional/page1/AllPages (accessed March 1, 2016).

Page, M., Berger, A., & Johnson, L. (2006). Putting evidence into practice: Evidence-based interventions for sleep-wake disturbances. *Clinical Journal of Oncology Nursing, 10*(6), 753–767.

Woodward, S. (2011). Cognitive-behavioral therapy for insomnia in patients with cancer. *Clinical Journal of Oncology Nursing, 15*(4), 42–52.

Yamamoto, D. (2010). Identifying and treating insomnia in the adult cancer patient. *Journal for the Advanced Practitioner in Oncology, 1*, 107–115.

Xerostomia

Kristin A. Cawley

Definition

- Changes in the quantity and composition of saliva due to a lack of salivary secretion, referred to as dry mouth
- May be acute or chronic
- The most common acute and late side effect of radiation treatment for head and neck cancer, if the major salivary glands are affected by treatment
- Often chronic, affecting taste perception, chewing, swallowing, speech, and overall quality of life (QOL)
- Has a profound impact on a patient's QOL

Pathophysiology and Contributing Factors

- Radiation therapy to the head and neck causes direct injury to salivary glands by damaging blood vessels. Damage depends on the total dose and volume of tissue irradiated.
- Major and minor salivary glands become atrophic and fibrotic.
- Saliva consistency changes from thin and watery to thick, ropy, tenacious secretions.
- Surgical excision of head and neck tumors involving salivary glands may be causal.
- Chemotherapy is a contributing factor.
- Pharmacologic causes include anticholinergics, antidepressants, antihistamines, antihypertensives, diuretics, opiates, phenothiazines, and sedatives.
- Gastroesophageal reflux may contribute.

Signs and Symptoms

- Dry mouth
- Dysphagia
- Gagging sensation

- Anorexia
- Gingival bleeding
- Halitosis
- Ulcerations in the oral cavity
- Sore throat
- Hoarseness and difficulty speaking
- Tenacious secretions
- Weight loss and malnutrition
- Dental caries
- Painful tongue (glossodynia)
- Oral candidiasis
- Pain, mild to burning
- Difficulty wearing dentures
- Taste alterations
- Infection
- Dehydration

Assessment Tools

- Common terminology criteria for adverse Events (CTCAE), version 4.0
- History and physical examination, clinical examination based on inspection of oral cavity. Ask the patient to describe the saliva (e.g., thin, watery, scant, thick, ropy).
- Review of all prescription and over-the-counter medications
- Current oral hygiene and dental care
- Nutritional status
- Symptomatic functional assessment based on ability to swallow
- Rule out differential diagnoses.
- Pain, using a rating scale from 0 to 10 or a categorical scale (none, mild, moderate, and severe)

Laboratory and Diagnostic Tests

- Blood, urine, sputum culture
- Sialometry—measurement of the rate of saliva production
- Biopsy taken from salivary glands in the lip, if ruling out Sjögren syndrome

Differential Diagnoses

- Sjögren syndrome
- Pain
- Malnutrition
- Infection
- Dysphagia
- Anorexia
- Mucositis
- Dehydration

Interventions

- Treat the underlying cause to restore moisture and lubrication to the oral cavity.

Pharmacologic Interventions

- Pilocarpine (Salagen)
- Cevimeline (Evoxac)
- Amifostine (Ethyol)
- Viscous lidocaine

Nonpharmacologic Interventions

- Dental care using soft toothbrushes and fluoride toothpaste
- Fluoride gels and rinses
- Nutritional status monitoring
- Saliva substitutes
- Sugar-free candy and sugar-free gum
- Increased fluid intake during and between meals (e.g., water, nonacidic juices)
- Avoidance of dry foods
- Avoidance of irritants such as tobacco, alcohol, carbonated beverages, caffeine, and spicy or acidic foods

Patient Teaching

- Rinse mouth frequently throughout the day.
- Have a comprehensive dental evaluation before treatment is initiated.
- Report any pain, tenderness, or burning sensations in the oral cavity.
- Practice oral care daily using fluoride treatments during radiation therapy; wait 30 minutes afterward before rinsing, eating, or drinking.
- Brush teeth three to four times daily, using a soft toothbrush.
- Floss daily with unwaxed dental floss.
- Rinse with nonalcoholic mouthwashes.
- After completion of therapy, patients require dental follow-up every 3 to 4 months to monitor for oral complications because they can deteriorate rapidly in irradiated patients with head and neck cancer.
- Report fever of 100.5° F (38° C) or greater.
- Report unrelieved pain.
- Follow dietary modifications.

Follow-up

- Assess the patient's current oral intake and ability to maintain adequate hydration and nutrition.
- Assess for pain unrelieved by pain medication.
- Reinforce the importance of communication with physician and nurse.

Resources

- National Cancer Institute: Oral complications of chemotherapy and head/neck radiation (PDQ): http://www.cancer.gov/cancertopics/pdq/supportivecare/oralcomplications/HealthProfessional/page16#_592_toc
- Oncology Nursing Society: Mucositis: https://www.ons.org/practice-resources/pep/mucositis

Bibliography

Bardet, E., Martin, L., Calais, G., Alfonsi, M., Feham, N. E., Tuchais, C., & Bourhis, J. (2011). Subcutaneous compared with intravenous administration of amifostine in patients with head and neck cancer receiving radiotherapy: Final results of the GORTEC2000-02 Phase III randomized trial. *Journal of Clinical Oncology, 29*, 127–133.

Bomeli, S. R., Desai, S. C., Johnson, J. T., & Walvekar, R. R. (2008). Management of salivary flow in head and neck cancer patients: A systematic review. *Oral Oncology, 44*, 1000–1008.

Brennan, M. T., Elting, L. S., & Spijkervet, F. K. (2010). Systematic reviews of oral complications from cancer therapies: Methodology and quality of the literature. Oral Care Study Group, MASCC/ISOO. *Supportive Care in Cancer, 18,* 979–984.

Dawson, C. J., Hickey, M. M., & Newton, S. (2011). Xerostomia. In C. J. Dawson, M. M. Hickey, & S. Newton (Eds.), *Telephone triage for otorhinolaryngology and head-neck nurses.* Pittsburg, PA: Oncology Nursing Society.

Dirix, P., Nuyts, S., & Van den Bogaert, W. (2006). Radiation-induced xerostomia in patients with head and neck cancer: A literature review. *Cancer, 107,* 2525–2534.

European Society for Radiotherapy and Oncology (ESTRO). (2013). New radiotherapy approach reduces dry mouth symptoms in patients with head and neck cancer. *British Journal of Hospital Medicine, 74,* 248.

Structural Emergencies

Jennifer S. Webster

Bowel Obstruction

Definition

- Bowel obstruction is interference with or cessation of the normal passage of intestinal contents through the gastrointestinal (GI) tract.
- The obstruction may be partial or complete.
- It may involve the small or large bowel.
- Paralytic ileus is a failure of normal motility in the absence of mechanical obstruction.
- Obstipation refers to intractable constipation refractory to normal interventions.

Epidemiology

- Patients with a history of cancer are at risk for obstruction. Colon cancer accounts for 25% to 40% of cases, followed by ovarian and gastric cancers.
- Nonmalignant obstructions include adhesions from previous operations, hernia, inflammatory bowel disease, fecal impaction, and bowel ischemia.
- Treatment of malignancy can cause obstruction, such as fibrosis from radiation therapy or neurotoxic effects from chemotherapy.
- Constipation occurs with palliative care and affects about 50% of patients admitted to hospice care.
- Obstructions can be caused by primary malignant neoplasms in any part of the bowel, abdomen, or pelvis or by metastases from many other sites.
- Risk factors include the following:
  - History of abdominal or pelvic malignancies
  - Previous abdominal surgery (i.e., potential for adhesions)
  - Inflammatory bowel disease
  - Herniations of the abdominal wall
  - Irradiation of the abdomen
  - Opioid use
  - Immobility
  - Chemotherapy drugs, particularly vinca alkaloids and thalidomide or its derivatives
  - Low fiber and fluid intake

Pathophysiology

- Mechanical bowel obstruction, whether in the large or small bowel, is the result of a physical block to the passage of intestinal contents.
- The bowel normally secretes approximately 6 to 8 L daily.
- Functional bowel obstruction results from a loss of propulsive peristalsis (e.g., paralytic ileus, postoperative adhesions).

- Winner and colleagues (2013) reported poor survival of patients with stage IV colon cancer who had bowel obstruction, regardless of treatment.

Signs and Symptoms

- Presenting symptoms depend on the site of the obstruction.
- Symptoms of obstruction include anorexia, nausea, vomiting, abdominal distention, abdominal fullness, early satiety, dyspepsia, diminished or absent bowel sounds, abdominal or pelvic cramping, pain, constipation or conversely liquid stool, and obstipation.
- Patients with early bowel obstruction may have paradoxical diarrhea as the bowel attempts to push contents past the obstruction.
- Dyspnea may accompany abdominal distention.

Cancers Associated with Disorder

- Ovarian
- Abdominal cancers
- All cancers have potential for bowel obstruction

Diagnostic Tests

- Computed tomography (CT) with contrast is the diagnostic test of choice.
- Abdominal radiography and positron emission tomography (PET) also are used.
- Studies include a complete blood cell count (CBC). An elevated white blood cell (WBC) count suggests strangulation, and an elevated hematocrit may point to dehydration.
- Electrolyte studies are done in cases of small bowel obstruction because acid-base disturbances are common due to vomiting and lack of fluid intake.

Differential Diagnosis

- Acute cholangitis
- Cholecystitis
- Cholelithiasis
- Constipation
- Diverticulitis
- Dysmenorrhea
- Endometriosis
- Inflammatory bowel disease

Treatment

Pharmacologic Management

- Octreotide inhibits the release of several GI hormones and reduces GI secretions.
- Antibiotics and antiemetics may be indicated.

355

- Electrolyte imbalances should be corrected.
- Role of corticosteroids in treating bowel obstruction is controversial, but they may be useful as adjuvant antiemetics.

Nonpharmacologic Management

- Immediate treatment is bowel rest and intravenous fluid replacement.
- Nasogastric (NG) tubes are useful for decompression and drainage. A rectal tube may be used to decompress the distal colon.
- Surgical intervention such as resection (i.e., removal of a portion of the bowel with or without the creation of an ostomy) may be necessary.
- Colorectal stents implanted with the use of endoscopy and fluoroscopy is an option for palliative treatment.

Patient Teaching

- Identify early signs and symptoms, especially for patients at risk.
- Instruct patients to notify providers about constipation unrelieved with current modalities.

Follow-up

- Provide a follow-up phone call following hospitalization to assess recovering bowel function.
- Continue a bowel regimen with clear instructions about what to do if constipation occurs—i.e., and how many days to wait before calling the provider
- Encourage patients to track bowel movements and notify providers if constipation occurs.

Bibliography

Alese, O. B., Kim, S., Chen, Z., Owonikoko, T. K., & El-Rayes, B. F. (2015). Management patterns and predictors of mortality among US patients with cancer hospitalized for malignant bowel obstruction. *Cancer, 121*(11), 1772–1778.

Andris, D. A., Krzyuda, E., Parrish, C. R., & Krenitsky, C. R. (2014). Gastrointestinal system. In S. M. Burns (Ed.), *AACN essentials of critical care nursing* (3rd ed.) (pp. 351–381). New York: McGraw-Hill.

Bosscher, M. R. F., van Leeuwen, B. L., & Hoekstra, H. J. (2014). Surgical emergencies in oncology. *Cancer Treatment Reviews, 40,* 1028–1036.

Ito, F., & Chang, A. E. (2014). Acute abdomen, bowel/biliary obstruction, and fistula. In J. E. Niederhuber, J. O. Armitage, J. H. Doroshow, M. B. Kastan, & J. E. Tepper (Eds.), *Ableoff's clinical oncology* (5th ed.) (pp. 694–704). Philadelphia: Elsevier/Saunders.

Longford, E., Scott, A., Fradsham, S., Jeffries, C., Ahmad, F., Holland, G., & Ferguson, H. (2015). Malignant bowel obstruction—a systematic literature review and evaluation of current practice. *BMJ Supportive & Palliative Care, 5*(1), 119–129.

Winner, M., Mooney, S. J., Hershman, D. L., Feingold, D. L., Allendorf, J. D., Wright, J. D., & Neugut, A. I. (2013). Management and outcomes of bowel obstruction in patients with stage IV colon cancer: A population-based cohort study. *Diseases of Colon and Rectum, 56*(7), 834–843.

Increased Intracranial Pressure

Definition

- Increased volume within the rigid cranium occupies space and increases pressure, disrupting normal brain activities and producing devastating effects.

Epidemiology

- Incidence is difficult to estimate in the oncology population. Primary brain tumors are associated with the highest risk of increased intracranial pressure (ICP) but make up less than 1.5% of new cancer diagnoses each year.
- The most common reason for increased ICP in the oncology population is metastatic disease. Approximately 20% to 40% of cancer patients develop metastatic disease to the brain. Melanoma, lung, breast, renal, and thyroid cancers have the highest incidence of brain metastases.
- Malignant cells from leukemias and lymphomas may invade the cerebrospinal fluid (CSF) and contribute to inflammation. The immunosuppressive therapies used for these hematologic malignancies may increase the risk of intracranial infection (e.g., meningitis, toxoplasmosis) or thrombocytopenia that can lead to ICP.
- Malignant tumor can obstruct outflow of CSF from the brain or cause local cerebral edema to develop, as can brain irradiation.
- Patients with an Ommaya reservoir, which is used to deliver chemotherapy medications directly into the CSF, may develop device-related obstruction, malposition, or infection that contributes to an increase in ICP.

Pathophysiology

- The adult skull is rigid, and its size is fixed.
- The three intracranial components are brain tissue, blood, and CSF.
- Increased volume inside the skull, whether from bleeding, injury, edema, primary or metastatic tumor, infection, or increased CSF production, increases pressure within the confined space of the skull.
- Initially, the body attempts to compensate by reducing blood or CSF volume in the skull, but response capabilities are limited. Pressure within the skull increases, and the patient experiences disruption of normal brain activities.
- Onset may be slow or rapid. Onset that occurs slowly allows the body to compensate more effectively, and symptoms may not be evident immediately.
- If unrecognized, ICP can progress to brain stem herniation and death.

Signs and Symptoms

- ICP may be initially difficult to detect in patients with slowly increasing intracranial volume.
- Signs and symptoms depend on the location of the pressure and the rate of increasing ICP.
- Altered mental status or level of consciousness is the most sensitive sign.
- Headache may worsen with bending over or Valsalva maneuvers.
- Patients may have nausea and vomiting.
- Focal changes depend on the location of pressure.
  - Changes in vision and pupil size
  - Speech changes such as slurring or inability to speak at a normal pace
  - Changes in handwriting and fine motor movements

- Memory loss
- Motor weakness
- Seizures may occur.
- The triad of hypertension, bradycardia, and respiratory depression is a late sign of brain stem compression and requires urgent intervention.
- Changes in vital signs should be monitored.
  - Widening pulse pressure in later stages
  - Decreased pulse with ongoing rise in ICP

Cancers Associated with Disorder

- Primary brain tumors
- Tumors that metastasize to the brain—see epidemiology on page 356
- Tumors with leptomeningeal (cerebral spinal fluid) metastases

Diagnostic Tests

- Contrast-enhanced magnetic resonance imaging (MRI) is preferred, but noncontrast computed tomography (CT) should be used in emergency situations when bleeding or hydrocephalus is suspected.
- Lumbar puncture is used to evaluate CSF if infection or malignant tumor cells are suspected.
- PET may be used as a complement to MRI or CT to determine cerebral blood flow to the brain.

Differential Diagnosis

- Acute nerve injury
- Blood dyscrasias
- Migraine headache
- Papilledema
- Stroke

Treatment

- Initial goal is to stabilize the patient and address emergent symptoms.
- If possible, definitive treatment of the underlying cause of ICP should be implemented.

Pharmacologic Management

- Steroids are used to reduce increased ICP related to edema due to brain tumors, cranial irradiation, or infection in the brain.
- Mannitol is an osmotic diuretic that is used to decrease cerebral edema.
- Hypertonic saline may be used to pull water into the intravascular space and away from the brain.
- Chemotherapy is primarily effective for chemotherapy-sensitive tumor types.
- Analgesics are used to relieve pain and sedate the patient, which can help to minimize increases in ICP.
- Anticonvulsants are used for patients experiencing or at risk for seizures.

Nonpharmacologic Management

- Surgical interventions
  - Resection or debulking of a primary brain tumor
  - Evacuation of a blood clot
  - Shunt placement to divert CSF
- Radiation therapy
  - Used for unresectable brain tumors or diffuse metastases
  - May cause edema with inflammatory reaction or necrosis that can contribute to increased ICP
- Hyperventilation
  - Used only in emergencies
  - Reduces carbon dioxide levels with subsequent cerebral vasoconstriction and drop in ICP
  - Short-term effect that can contribute to cerebral hypoxia
- Maintain blood pressure, fluid and electrolyte balance, and temperature in normal range to prevent exacerbation of ICP.
- Nursing interventions
  - Patient positioning: elevate head of the bed to at least 30 degrees to facilitate venous drainage from the head.
  - Maintain calm environment: avoid loud noises or bright lights.
  - Perform serial neurologic assessments to monitor changes in neurologic status and to assess treatment efficacy.
  - Maintain seizure precautions.
  - Treat or prevent symptoms that can increase ICP, such as coughing, vomiting, straining at stool with constipation, or pain.

Patient Teaching

- Emphasize early identification of signs and symptoms.
- Teach strategies to maximize safety in activities of daily living (ADLs) and ambulation.
- Medication management includes anticonvulsants, steroids, and analgesics.
- Interventions to minimize increased ICP
  - Elevate head of bed.
  - Maintain calm environment.
  - Avoid coughing, vomiting, and the Valsalva maneuver, including straining with bowel movements; use cough suppressants, antiemetics, and stool softeners if needed.
  - Avoid lifting heavy objects or bending down at the waist.
- Use measures to enhance adaptation and rehabilitation if neurologic deficits continue.

Follow-up

- Monitor signs and symptoms that suggest increased ICP during follow-up exams.
- Instruct patient and family to notify providers immediately with any signs or symptoms of increased ICP.

Bibliography

American Cancer Society. (2015). *Cancer facts and figures 2015.* Available at American Cancer Society (2015). Cancer facts and figures 2015 (accessed February 24, 2016).

Colton, K., Yang, S., Hu, P. F., Chen, H. H., Bonds, B., Scalea, T. M., & Stein, D. M. (2014). Intracranial pressure response after pharmacologic treatment of intracranial hypertension. *Journal of Trauma and Acute Care Surgery,* 77(1), 47–53.

Fields, M. (2014). Increased intracranial pressure. In C. H. Yarbro, D. Wujcik, & B. H. Gobel (Eds.), *Cancer symptom management* (4th ed.) (pp. 331–348). Burlington, MA: Jones & Bartlett.

Khan, U. A., Shanholtz, C. B., & McCurdy, M. T. (2014). Oncologic mechanical emergencies. *Emergency Medicine Clinics of North America, 32,* 495–508.

Lewis, M. A., Hendrickson, A. W., & Moynihan, T. J. (2011). Oncologic emergencies: Pathophysiology, presentation, diagnosis and treatment. *CA: Cancer Journal for Clinicians, 61,* 287–314.

Shelton, B. K., Ferrigno, C., & Skinner, J. (2013). Increased intracranial pressure. In M. Kaplan (Ed.), *Understanding and managing oncologic emergencies: A resource for nurses* (2nd ed.) (pp. 48–68). Pittsburgh, PA: Oncology Nursing Society.

Schimpf, M. M. (2012). Diagnosing increased intracranial pressure. *Journal of Trauma Nursing, 19*(3), 160–167.

Neoplastic Cardiac Tamponade

Definition

- Compression of the heart caused by accumulation of excessive fluid within the pericardial sac, resulting in decreased cardiac output.

Epidemiology

- The incidence of neoplastic cardiac tamponade is unknown. It may go undetected until there is a significant decrease in cardiac output.
- Approximately 20% of patients have metastatic disease to the pericardium at autopsy.

Pathophysiology

- The pericardium is a two-layered sac that encloses the heart and great vessels.
- The pericardial space is created between the two membranes that protect the heart (i.e., parietal and visceral) and normally contains a very small amount of fluid (10 to 50 mL) that serves as a lubricant.
- When cancer cells invade the pericardial space, pericardial fluid osmotically accumulates (i.e., pericardial effusion), increasing pressure and compressing the heart. To maintain cardiac output, the body attempts to compensate by increasing the heart rate and peripheral vasoconstriction.
- Onset may be slow or rapid. A slow onset may be tolerated for weeks because the pericardium can stretch to accommodate up to 2 L of fluid.

Signs and Symptoms

- Difficult to detect slowly accumulating effusions and may not be identified until fluid accumulation is significant
- Hoarseness, cough or hiccups, difficulty swallowing (i.e., compression of trachea, esophagus, and nerves)
- Dyspnea, orthopnea
- Anxiety and restlessness
- Muffled heart sounds
- Pericardial friction rub
- Increased jugular venous distention
- Decreased systolic blood pressure and increased diastolic pressure (i.e., narrowing of pulse pressure)
- Paradoxical pulse (i.e., decline in systolic blood pressure on inspiration)
- Other signs of decreased cardiac output: tachycardia, lightheadedness, peripheral cyanosis, oliguria, and shock

Cancers Associated with Disorder

- Tumors most often associated with pericardial metastasis are lung cancer, breast cancer, leukemia, Hodgkin disease, and melanoma.
- Primary tumors are rare and are usually mesotheliomas or sarcomas.
- Lung and breast cancers can spread by direct extension or lymphatic metastasis.
- Lymphomas and leukemias typically spread by hematogenous routes.
- Radiation therapy of 4000 cGy or greater to the mediastinum can lead to immediate or long-term complications.

Diagnostic Tests

- Routine chest radiographs initially reveal subtle changes and an enlarged pericardial silhouette.
- Electrocardiogram (ECG) findings may be nonspecific (e.g., sinus tachycardia).
- Echocardiography has a 96% accuracy.
- CT and MRI are noninvasive and reveal pleural effusion, masses, or pericardial thickening.
- Percutaneous pericardiocentesis is used only for large effusions or cardiac tamponade to help relieve symptoms and obtain fluid for evaluation.
  - Fluid is aspirated and assessed for type of effusion: transudate (i.e., low protein level, usually from a nonmalignant cause) or exudate (i.e., high protein level, usually from a malignant cause).
- Malignant cells are found in the pericardial fluid of approximately 60% of patients with cancer and effusions.

Differential Diagnosis

- Cardiogenic shock
- Pericarditis
- Pneumothorax
- Pulmonary embolism

Treatment

- Primary goal is to remove the fluid and relieve or prevent impending cardiac collapse.
- Degree of intervention is based on the underlying disease status, comorbid conditions, and previous treatment.

Pharmacologic Management

- Mild tamponade may respond to diuretics and steroids (usually temporary).
- Chemotherapy is primarily effective for chemotherapy-sensitive tumor types.
- Pericardial sclerosis is instillation of agents that cause irritation and subsequent fibrosis of the pericardial space; it has a 50% success rate.

Nonpharmacologic Management

- Surgical interventions
  - The pericardial window permits drainage of fluid into the pleural space and has a 90% response rate.
  - A pericardioperitoneal shunt may be used.

- Radiation therapy
  - Used successfully for radiosensitive tumors.
  - Cardiac tolerance is considered for radiation therapy (3500 to 4000 cGy).

Patient Teaching

- Emphasize early identification and reporting of signs and symptoms.
- Apply interventions to minimize severity of symptoms:
  - Elevate head of bed.
  - Provide oxygen.
  - Reduce energy expenditure.
  - Manage pain and dyspnea.
- Apply measures to enhance adaptation and rehabilitation.

Follow-up

- Monitor for signs and symptoms of fluid reaccumulation and decreased cardiac output.
- Instruct patient and family to notify providers for signs or symptoms of returning cardiac effusion.

Bibliography

Cope, D. G. (2014). Effusions. In C. H. Yarbro, D. Wujcik, & B. H. Gobel (Eds.), *Cancer symptom management* (4th ed.) (pp. 331–348). Burlington, MA: Jones & Bartlett.

Khan, U. A., Shanholtz, C. B., & McCurdy, M. T. (2014). Oncologic mechanical emergencies. *Emergency Medicine Clinics of North America, 32,* 495–508.

McCurdy, M. T., & Shanholtz, C. B. (2012). Oncologic emergencies. *Critical Care Medicine, 40,* 2212–2222.

Story, K. T. (2013). Cardiac tamponade. In M. Kaplan (Ed.), *Understanding and managing oncologic emergencies: A resource for nurses* (2nd ed.) (pp. 48–68). Pittsburgh, PA: Oncology Nursing Society.

Radiation Pneumonitis

Definition

- Radiation pneumonitis is a constellation of clinical, radiographic, and histologic findings reflecting acute toxicity due to inflammation of lung tissue exposed to radiation therapy.
- Incidence and severity are related to the following:
  - Volume of lung irradiated
  - Dose, rate, and quality of radiation therapy
  - Concomitant chemotherapy (e.g., bleomycin, paclitaxel)
  - History of previous radiation therapy
  - Baseline pulmonary function tests

Epidemiology

- Symptomatic injury may occur in up to 20% of cases and range from mild cough and dyspnea on exertion to respiratory failure.
- High-risk groups include the following:
  - Low pretreatment performance status
  - Comorbid lung disease
  - Smoking history
  - Low pulmonary function tests
  - Elderly patients (disease tends to be more severe)

Pathophysiology

- Radiation directly injures endothelial and epithelial cells, which results in alveolitis.
- Accumulation of inflammatory and immune cells takes place in the alveolar walls and spaces.
- Accumulation is thought to play a role in the development of pulmonary fibrosis or chronic inflammation and distorts the normal structures.
- Fibrosis is the repair process that follows; it thickens alveolar walls.
- Radiation pneumonitis usually occurs 2 to 9 months after radiation exposure but can evolve over months to years after initial damage.

Signs and Symptoms

- Dry cough is initially related to irritation of the main bronchus and decreased mucus production.
- One to 3 months after radiation therapy, symptoms may include dyspnea, productive cough, fever (usually low grade), and night sweats.
- More severe symptoms include acute respiratory distress with significant cough, dyspnea, hypoxia, fever, and tachycardia.

Cancers Associated with Disorder

- Radiation pneumonitis can be associated with any tumor type that is treated with radiation therapy alone to the chest and lung fields or in combination with chemotherapy.

Diagnostic Tests

- Chest radiographs may show diffuse haziness progressing to infiltrates within the irradiated area
- CT: effective diagnostic tool in this setting
- Pulmonary function tests
- Arterial blood gases (ABGs)
- CBC with differential count: elevated WBC count and increased sedimentation rate

Differential Diagnosis

- Diagnosis is not difficult when clear demarcation visualized and patient has a history of radiation therapy to the chest
- If the demarcation is unclear, differentials include ground-glass opacities or chronic airspace opacities

Treatment

- Prevention is the primary goal, including appropriate preassessment of underlying pulmonary impairment.
- Amifostine may be administered before radiation therapy to protect normal tissue and prevent damage; further studies are needed.

Pharmacologic Management

- Corticosteroids are the primary therapy.
- Antibiotics may be needed for a secondary infection.
- Bronchodilators and sedatives may be effective for relief.

Oncologic Emergencies ⑤

Nonpharmacologic Management

- Provide oxygen therapy.
- Monitor activities to minimize energy expenditure.
- Monitor adequate relief of symptoms.

Patient Teaching

- Identify critical symptoms or changes in status and report accordingly:
  - Chronic dry cough
  - Increased difficulty breathing
  - Skin changes
  - Use of accessory muscles
- Emphasize measures to minimize energy expenditure:
  - Frequent rest periods
  - Use of ready-made meals
  - Items used frequently within easy reach
- Ensure the patient understands and uses supportive therapies (e.g., morphine, oxygen, sedation).

Follow-up

- Ongoing palliative care visits to optimize supportive therapies and quality of life
- Assess efficacy and tolerance of steroid therapy that is commonly employed to reduce the severity of the disease
- Patients and families should be offered counseling or support group therapy due to the potential for disease chronicity

Bibliography

Demshar, R., Vanek, R., & Mazanec, P. (2011). Oncologic emergencies: New decade, new perspectives. *AACN Advanced Critical Care, 22,* 337–348.

Grewal, R. K., Rosenzweig, K. E., & Ginsberg, M. S. (2010). Thorax. In R. T. Hoppe, T. L. Phillips, & M. Roach (Eds.), *Leibel and Phillips textbook of radiation oncology* (3rd ed.) (pp. 362–377). Philadelphia: Elsevier/Saunders.

Sharma, N., Kim, E., & Machtay, M. (2014). Pulmonary complications of anticancer treatment. In J. E. Niederhuber, J. O. Armitage, J. H. Doroshow, M. B. Kastan, & J. E. Tepper (Eds.), *Ableoff's clinical oncology* (5th ed.) (pp. 845–857). Philadelphia: Elsevier/Saunders.

Wagner, H., Jr. (2012). Non-small cell lung cancer. In L. L. Gunderson, & J. E. Tepper (Eds.), *Clinical radiation oncology* (3rd ed.) (pp. 805–838). Philadelphia: Elsevier/Saunders.

Spinal Cord Compression

Definition

- Spinal cord compression is caused by direct injury to the spinal cord that leads to progressive motor and sensory deficits if untreated; motor weakness usually occurs before sensory loss.
- It can result from a tumor that compresses or compromises the spinal cord or invasion of the vertebrae, which subsequently collapse onto the spinal cord.

Epidemiology

- Malignant spinal cord compression can be caused by direct tumor compression of the spinal cord or pathologic vertebral body collapse.
- May be caused by metastases to the spinal column, leading to pain and potential collapse.
- A significant association exists with the ability to walk at diagnosis and recovery from compression.
- Occurs in 5% of oncology patient population
- Occurs in 20% of patient with metastases to the vertebral column
- Second most frequent neurologic complication of cancer

Pathophysiology

- The spinal cord is located within the epidural space in the spinal canal. Tumor may invade the epidural space and impinge on the cord or destroy vertebral bone, which collapses into the epidural space and compresses the cord.
- Compression of the cord produces edema and inflammation, leading to direct neural injury, vascular damage, and oxygen impairment.
- Level of cord involvement (e.g., cervical, thoracic, lumbar, sacral, cauda equina) determines the loss of function.
- Although not life-threatening, it represents a medical emergency. If untreated, it may progress to permanent paralysis.
- Rarely, primary tumors may arise in the spinal cord and cause compression.

Signs and Symptoms

- Depends on level of cord involvement
- Back pain: often the first symptom but significance may be unrecognized, can occur up to 6 months before diagnosis, and may be progressive
- Leg (one or both) weakness, with or without sensory loss
- Muscle atrophy in lower extremities
- Autonomic dysfunction (late effect): loss of bowel and bladder function, urinary hesitancy or urgency, impotence

Cancers Associated with Disorder

- Highest risk from metastases of solid tumors (e.g., lung, breast, prostate, kidney)
- Cancers of the lung, breast, and prostate account for 50% of cases
- Occurs with some hematologic malignancies (e.g., lymphomas, multiple myeloma)

Diagnostic Tests

- CBC with differential count and sedimentation rate to differentiate spinal cord compression from infection
- Chemistry profile, including calcium and liver function tests
- Imaging studies: plain radiographs, MRI, CT, and PET; plain films often used for vertebral blastic or lytic lesions, but contrast-enhanced MRI provides best definition of spinal lesions
- Lumbar punctures contraindicated because CSF removal may worsen spinal cord compression

Treatment

- Prompt diagnosis and treatment are crucial.
- Treatment is primarily palliation of symptoms and prevention of permanent disabilities.

Pharmacologic Management

- Corticosteroids
  - Reduce edema
  - Dose and duration based on patient response
- Pain management
- Chemotherapy
  - Indicated for chemotherapy-sensitive tumors (i.e., lymphoma or Hodgkin disease)
  - Adjuvant therapy in combination with radiation therapy or surgery
  - Bisphosphonates to reduce pain and skeletal complications from vertebral metastases

Nonpharmacologic Management

- Radiation therapy
  - Reduces symptoms
  - Initiated immediately after diagnosis
  - Usual course of 2 to 4 weeks
- Surgery
  - Surgical decompression is treatment of choice for patients whose tumors are not radiosensitive or for previously radiated sites.
  - Surgery is indicated with evidence of spinal instability or rapidly progressing loss of function.

Patient Teaching

- Early recognition of signs and symptoms
- Mobility, safety :
  Maximize environmental safety:
  - Side rails, low bed, items in easy reach
  - Eliminate throw rugs
  - Promote use of walker
- Skin integrity
- Pain management
- Bowel elimination regimen
- Coping strategies for potential motor and sensory limitations

Follow-up

- Monitor ongoing recovery in patients without deficits
- For patients with functional deficits and paraplegia
  - Referral to a rehabilitation center may be necessary to optimize functioning, depending on the patient's prognosis and ability to engage in therapy.
  - Assess family's ability to provide care for the disabled patient as needed.
  - Provide ongoing skin assessment, examining pressure points carefully.
  - Assess bowel and bladder care.
  - Assess comfort.

Bibliography

Kaplan, M. (2013). Spinal cord compression. In M. Kaplan (Ed.), *Understanding and managing oncologic emergencies: A resource for nurses* (2nd ed.) (pp. 337–383). Pittsburgh, PA: Oncology Nursing Society.

Khan, U. A., Shanholtz, C. B., & McCurdy, M. T. (2014). Oncologic mechanical emergencies. *Emergency Medicine Clinics of North America, 32,* 495–508.

Lewis, M. A., Hendrickson, A. W., & Moynihan, T. J. (2011). Oncologic emergencies: Pathophysiology, presentation, diagnosis and treatment. *CA: Journal for Clinicians, 61,* 287–314.

Stieber, V. W., & Siker, M. L. (2012). Spinal cord tumors. In L. L. Gunderson, & J. E. Tepper (Eds.), *Clinical Radiation Oncology* (3rd ed.) (pp. 511–528). Philadelphia: Elsevier/Saunders.

Superior Vena Cava Syndrome

Definition

- Superior vena cava (SVC) syndrome is a complex of symptoms and physical findings associated with compression or obstruction of the SVC.
  - Caused by extrinsic tumor or internal thrombus
  - Results in compromised venous drainage of the head, neck, and upper extremities

Epidemiology

- Between 75% and 85% of SVC syndrome cases have a malignant cause.
- About 80% of cases of neoplastic origin are related to lung cancer, most frequently small cell lung cancer, followed by non-Hodgkin lymphoma and metastatic tumors.
- Nonmalignant causes include central venous catheters and cardiac surgery.
- Risk factors include presence of central venous catheters and pacemakers and previous radiation therapy to the mediastinum

Pathophysiology

- The SVC is a thin-walled, low-pressure, major blood vessel.
  - Its primary function is to carry venous drainage from the head, upper extremities, and upper thorax to the heart.
  - The SVC is surrounded by rigid structures in the mediastinum and multiple lymph node chains.
  - It is easily compressed by direct tumor invasion, enlarged lymph nodes, or a thrombus within the vessel.
- Compression results in the following:
  - Increase in venous pressure in areas drained by the SVC
  - Decrease in cardiac output

Signs and Symptoms

- Progression of physical findings can be gradual and insidious or rapid and acute. Slower progression allows some collateral circulation to develop.
- Facial swelling
- Fine motor movements affected by swelling of neck, arms, and hands
- Neck and thoracic vein distention
- Dyspnea (most common)
- Nonproductive cough
- Cyanosis of the face and upper torso
- Late signs due to cerebral edema and airway compromise include the following:
  - Severe headache
  - Irritability
  - Visual disturbances
  - Change in level of consciousness

- Stridor, orthopnea, tachypnea
- Horner syndrome (i.e., ptosis, meiosis, and anhidrosis)
- Symptoms may be aggravated by lowering the head (e.g., bending down).

Cancers Associated with Disorder

- Lung cancer
- Lymphoma involving the mediastinum

Diagnostic Tests

- Radiographs (approximately 15% of patients have normal findings)
  - Superior mediastinal widening in approximately 66%
  - Pleural effusions in about 25%
  - Hilar mass in 12%
- CT with contrast
- Laboratory data
  - ABGs
  - Coagulation studies

Differential Diagnosis

- Cardiac tamponade
- Pneumonia, acute respiratory distress syndrome
- Chronic obstructive pulmonary disease
- Mediastinitis
- Thoracic aortic aneurysm

Treatment

- Early identification of clients at risk is essential.
- Goals are to provide rapid palliation or relief of symptoms and attempt to cure the underlying condition.

Pharmacologic Management

- Corticosteroids may reduce the inflammatory component and cerebral edema and improve venous blood flow.
- Chemotherapy for chemotherapy-sensitive tumors
- Fibrinolytic or anticoagulation therapy in appropriate situations
- Diuretics

Nonpharmacologic Management

- Radiation therapy
  - Therapy is indicated as urgent in cases of acute respiratory distress.
  - Many radiation fractionation protocols are effective.
- Removal of the central venous catheter combined with anticoagulation

- Percutaneous implantation of endovascular stents is associated with a high success rate and low morbidity.
- Supportive management
  - Oxygen therapy to relieve dyspnea
  - Anxiety reduction

Patient Teaching

- Emphasize early recognition and reporting of signs and symptoms:
  - Tight rings or watch
  - Swollen arms or fingers
  - Diminished fine motor movements
  - Headache, visual changes, or altered mental status due to cerebral edema
- Apply interventions to reduce symptoms of respiratory distress:
  - Elevate head of bed
  - Oxygen use
  - Anxiety management with morphine, antianxiety medications
- Use interventions to reduce symptoms of circulatory compromise:
  - Remove rings and restrictive clothing.
  - Avoid venipunctures or blood pressure measurement on upper extremities.
  - Monitor skin integrity.
  - Elevate upper arms to promote venous return.

Follow-up

- When SVCS is secondary to an internal thrombus, anticoagulation therapy and subsequent monitoring are indicated.
- If SVCS has a malignant cause, palliative or supportive care may be needed.

Bibliography

Kerber, A. S. (2010). Oncologic emergencies. In M. Baird & S. Bethel (Eds.), *Manual of critical care nursing* (6th ed.) (pp. 901–903). St. Louis: Elsevier Mosby.

Laskin, J., Cmelak, A. J., Meranze, S., Yee, J., & Johnson, D. H. (2014). Superior vena cava syndrome. In J. E. Niederhuber, J. O. Armitage, J. H. Doroshow, M. B. Kastan, & J. E. Tepper (Eds.), *Ableoff's clinical oncology* (5th ed.) (pp. 705–714). Philadelphia: Elsevier/Saunders.

Shelton, B. K. (2013). Superior vena cava syndrome. In M. Kaplan (Ed.), *Understanding and managing oncologic emergencies: A resource for nurses* (2nd ed.) (pp. 385–410). Pittsburgh, PA: Oncology Nursing Society.

Khan, U. A., Shanholtz, C. B., & McCurdy, M. T. (2014). Oncologic mechanical emergencies. *Emergency Medicine Clinics of North America, 32,* 495–508.

Lewis, M. A., Hendrickson, A. W., & Moynihan, T. J. (2011). Oncologic emergencies: Pathophysiology, presentation, diagnosis and treatment. *CA: Journal for Clinicians, 61,* 287–314.

Urologic Emergencies

Jennifer S. Webster

Cystitis

Definition

- Cystitis is a painful bladder disorder caused by diffuse inflammation of the bladder epithelium.
- The inflammatory lesion or process compromises the ability to store urine in the lower urinary tract.
- It is associated with cancer symptoms, treatment side effects, and disease sequelae.
- Hemorrhagic cystitis often arises from anticancer chemotherapy or radiation therapy for pelvic malignancies. Sudden onset of dysuria and hematuria most frequently results from use of the cytotoxic alkylating agents ifosfamide and cyclophosphamide.

Epidemiology

- In the individual with cancer, cystitis is most frequently related to the following:
  - Carcinoma of the bladder in 75% to 85% of patents with gross or microscopic hematuria
  - Irritable bladder symptoms in about 20% of cases
  - Drug-induced cystitis
- Unchanged drug is excreted in the urine and damages tissues.
- A metabolite, acrolein, of ifosamide and cyclophosphamide contributes to uric acid crystal formation that damages the bladder epithelium.
- Patients undergoing hematopoietic stem cell transplantation are at highest risk.
- Radiation-induced cystitis occurs after external beam radiation therapy and pelvic irradiation.

Pathophysiology

- The mucosal lining of the bladder is made of many layers of epithelial cells.
- Symptoms have several causes:
  - Tumor invasion
  - Infection
  - Chemotherapy
  - Radiation therapy
- Symptoms may be similar for different causes, but tumor invasion is usually more insidious and produces gross hematuria.
- In chemotherapy-induced cystitis, metabolites of cytotoxic drugs are excreted into the renal system and reside in the bladder for extended periods.
  - The metabolites may also form uric acid crystals, which damage the epithelial layers.

- Some symptoms are expected consequences of immune system stimulation and inflammatory reactions (e.g., bacillus Calmette-Guérin [BCG] used to treat superficial bladder cancer.).
- Radiation-induced cystitis is caused by external beam or interstitial irradiation to the pelvis.
- External beam radiation therapy can damage the urethra, impair blood flow, and induce fibrosis, stricture, or atrophy.

Signs and Symptoms

- Urinary frequency
- Mild burning to excruciating pain in the bladder, lower abdomen, perineum, or vagina
- Low back pain
- Urinary urgency
- May or may not have white blood cells (WBCs) or red blood cells (RBCs) in the urine

Cancers Associated with Disorder

- Bladder cancer or invasion of bladder by tumors in the pelvis
- Ovarian, cervical, uterine, rectal, prostate, or colon cancers
- Any tumor type treated with systemic cytotoxic drugs
  - Cyclophosphamide
  - Ifosfamide
  - Busulfan
- Intravesicular treatment with BCG

Diagnostic Tests

- Detailed urinalysis
  - Urine dipstick
  - pH
  - Microscopic analysis
- Urine culture (midstream or sterile specimen)
- Urine cytologic examination
- Intravenous pyelogram (IVP)
- Cystoscopy
- Renal and bladder ultrasonography

Differential Diagnosis

- Infectious: recurrent UTI, vaginitis
- Gynecologic: pelvic inflammatory disease, pelvic mass, endometriosis
- Urologic: overflow incontinence or bladder outlet obstruction, bladder cancer, chronic pelvic pain
- Neurologic: Parkinson disease, multiple sclerosis, spinal stenosis or tumor, cerebral vascular accident
- Other: Hernia, inflammatory bowel disease, diverticulitis, gastrointestinal malignancy, adhesions

Treatment

- Type of treatment is determined by the cause and severity of cystitis.
- Preventive strategies, particularly in immunocompromised patients, are essential.

Pharmacologic Management

- Antibiotics are used.
- IV hydration
- Systemic administration of thiols can prevent or ameliorate the bladder damage related to acrolein production; the most widely used is mercaptoethane sulfonate (MESNA).
- Symptomatic management of BCG-induced cystitis includes urinary system–specific analgesics or opioids and antispasmodics.

Nonpharmacologic Management

- Maintain oral hydration of at least 1500ml/day unless contraindicated. Avoid fluids with caffeine, alcohol or high acidity.
- Bladder irrigation for patients at highest risk of hemorrhagic cystitis (i.e., those receiving high doses of ifosfamide or cyclophosphamide). Irrigation dilutes acrolein and decreases contact time of uric acid crystals with the bladder lining. However, there is some question about its effectiveness (Gonella, di Pasquale, & Palese, 2015).
- Warm moist heat to lower back
- Warm baths

Patient Teaching

- Maintain hydration (at least 1500 mL daily).
- Encourage frequent bladder emptying.
- Create a voiding diary.
- Encourage patient to perform pelvic floor exercises (i.e., Kegel exercises) for urinary incontinence.
- Minimize foods or fluids known to promote acidic, concentrated urine.
- Avoid caffeine, alcohol, and carbonated beverages.
- Avoid bladder catheterization.

Follow-up

- Continue to monitor for signs and symptoms of infection
- Monitor for ongoing complications of cystitis as indicated
- Inform the patient to notify providers if symptoms arise

Bibliography

Gonella, S., di Pasquale, T., & Palese, A. (2015). Preventive measures for cyclophosphamide-related hemorrhagic cystitis in blood and bone marrow transplantation: An Italian multicenter retrospective study. *Clinical Journal of Oncology Nursing, 19*(1), E8–E14.

Schaeffer, A. J., & Schaeffer, E. T. (2012). Infections of the urinary tract. In A. J. Wein, L. R. Kavoussi, A. C. Novick, A. W. Partin, & C. A. Peters (Eds.), *Campbell-Walsh urology* (10th ed.) (pp. 257–326). Philadelphia: Elsevier/Saunders.

Yarbro, C. H., & Berry, D. L. (2014). Bladder disturbances. In C. H. Yarbro, D. Wujcik, & B. H. Gobel (Eds.), *Cancer symptom management* (4th ed.) (pp. 265–276). Burlington, MA: Jones & Bartlett.

Urinary Tract Infection

Definition

- In a lower urinary tract infection (UTI), the bladder epithelium undergoes inflammatory changes when colonized with an infectious agent.
- Bacteria are present in the urine (i.e., bacteriuria).
- UTIs can be symptomatic or asymptomatic.
- WBCs may be found in the urine (i.e., pyuria).

Epidemiology

- One of the most common conditions treated by physicians
- Highest rates among elderly, also the age group most likely to have cancer
  - 20% for women older than 65 years
  - 10% for men older than 65 years
- Most common bacteria: *Escherichia coli, Enterobacter,* and *Staphylococcus* species
- Most common infection acquired in the health care setting
- Men have increased protective factors:
  - Longer urethral length
  - Scrotum that provides a physical barrier
- Common causes of male dysuria:
  - Foreskin in early life
  - Prostate in middle and later life
- Women are at higher risk:
  - Shorter urethral length than men
  - Urethra exits close to vagina and rectum
- Common causes of female dysuria:
  - Use of spermicide vaginally or with condoms
  - Pregnancy
  - Estrogen deficiency in postmenopausal women
- Inefficient bladder emptying
- Catheterization of the urinary tract
- History of previous infections
- Immune deficiency disorders such as human immunodeficiency virus (HIV) infection, cancer, or diabetes mellitus
- Children and elders with constipation

Pathophysiology

- The urinary tract, adjacent to the bacteria-rich lower gastrointestinal tract, produces and stores urine. The periurethral area is typically colonized with gut and other flora, some capable of causing a UTI.
- Urination flushes bacteria from the urethral orifice. Periurethral pathogens occasionally enter the urethra and ascend, reaching the bladder and resulting in a UTI.
- UTIs can involve mucosal tissue (e.g., cystitis) or soft tissue (e.g., pyelonephritis, prostatitis).
- They may result in the spread of infection from the urinary tract to the bloodstream (i.e., urosepsis), with subsequent increased risk of death.
- In urethritis, inflammation and infection are limited to the urethra only or to the urethra and vagina in women;

infection is usually caused by a sexually transmitted pathogen.

- Acute pyelonephritis is an infection of the renal parenchyma and renal pelvis caused by ascending cystitis.

Signs and Symptoms

- Asymptomatic bacteriuria
  - Urine culture reveals significant growth of a pathogen, but the patient has no symptoms of a UTI.
- Symptomatic UTI
  - Bladder irritability
  - Dysuria
  - Urgency
  - Frequency
  - Fever
  - Strong or foul odor
  - Hematuria

Cancers Associated with Disorder

- Women with cancer have the highest risk.
- Not associated with specific malignancies

Diagnostic Tests

- Urine dipstick
  - Leukocyte esterase: finding indicates neutrophils in urine; results not valid in neutropenic patients
  - Protein
  - pH
- Urine culture
- Microscopic analysis

Differential Diagnosis

- Differentiation between UTI and bacteriuria
  - Pyuria alone versus inflammation
  - Bacteriuria without pyuria versus colonization
  - Pyuria versus bacteriuria versus nitrites versus infection

Treatment

Pharmacologic Management

- Antimicrobial therapy

Nonpharmacologic Management

- Maintain hydration.
- Avoid unnecessary catheterizations, use sterile technique when inserting, use evidence-based guidelines for indwelling catheters, and remove at the earliest opportunity.
- Use of alternative therapy is not supported by conclusive research.
  - The expected benefit of long-term adherence to blueberry or cranberry products may be overestimated.

Patient Teaching

- Emphasize identification and reporting of signs and symptoms.
- Ensure adequate fluid intake.
- Teach proper toileting techniques.

- Avoid bladder irritants that may induce acidic urine.
- Avoid catheterizations.

Follow-up

- Monitor for recurrence of signs and symptoms.
- Repeat urinalysis as needed during ambulatory visits.

Bibliography

Love, N., & Rodrigue, D. (2015). Catheter-associated urinary tract infection prevention in the oncology population: An evidence-based approach. *Clinical Journal of Oncology Nursing, 17,* 593–596.

Schaeffer, A. J., & Schaeffer, E. T. (2012). Infections of the urinary tract. In A. J. Wein, L. R. Kavoussi, A. C. Novick, A. W. Partin, & C. A. Peters (Eds.), *Campbell-Walsh urology* (10th ed.) (pp. 257–326). Philadelphia: Elsevier/Saunders.

Winkelman, C. (2013). Care of patients with urinary problems. In D. D. Ignatavicius, & M. L. Workman (Eds.), *Medical-surgical nursing: Patient-centered care* (7th ed.) (pp. 1489–1517). St. Louis: Elsevier/Saunders.

Yarbro, C. H., & Berry, D. L. (2014). Bladder disturbances. In C. H. Yarbro, D. Wujcik, & B. H. Gobel (Eds.), *Cancer symptom management* (4th ed.) (pp. 265–276). Burlington, MA: Jones & Bartlett.

Urinary Tract Obstruction

Definition

- A drop in urine outflow may indicate failure of the kidneys to filter blood and produce urine (i.e., oliguria or anuria).
- Urinary stasis or blockage of urine transport from upper to lower urinary tracts indicates an obstruction.
- Obstruction of the urinary tract may occur at multiple levels:
  - Ureter
  - Bladder
  - Urethra
- Obstruction blocks the urine flow, causing it to back up and damage one or both kidneys.
- Cancer can involve the urinary tract by direct extension, encasement, or invasion. Obstruction can also occur from metastases.

Epidemiology

- Many cases go undetected until there is a significant decrease in urinary output.
- Bladder outlet obstruction in men is most commonly caused by benign prostatitic hypertrophy (BPH).
- Cervical cancers cause most ureteral obstructions in women.
- Retroperitoneal fibrosis may result from radiation therapy.
- Risk factors include the following:
  - Ureteral stones
  - Bladder stones
- Urinary tract tumors
- Retroperitoneal fibrosis
- BPH (i.e., enlarged prostate)
- Inflammatory response to infection

Pathophysiology

- Urine is transported from the renal papilla to the bladder through the upper urinary tract to the lower urinary tract (i.e., bladder and urethra). Active transport depends on smooth muscle contractibility.

- Blockage causes an accumulation of urine and subsequent distention.
- Pressure builds directly on the tissue and causes structural damage.
- Tubular filtrate pressure may increase within the nephron because drainage in the urinary collecting system is impaired.
- Acute or chronic renal failure results.
- Renal failure with uremia and elevated serum potassium levels compromises cardiac function.

Signs and Symptoms

- Symptoms depend on whether the obstruction is acute or chronic, unilateral or bilateral, and complete or partial.
- Flank pain
  - Bilateral or unilateral
  - Intermittent or chronic
  - Moderate or severe
- Urinary tract infection
  - Fever
  - Difficulty or pain while urinating
  - Nausea or vomiting
  - Hypertension
  - Renal failure
  - Edema
  - Decreased urine output
  - Hematuria (i.e., microscopic or gross)

Cancers Associated with Disorder

- Tumors of nearby organs
  - Colon cancer
  - Cervical cancer
  - Uterine cancer

Diagnostic Tests

- Radiographic studies
  - Kidney, ureter, and bladder (KUB) study
  - Intravenous pyelogram (IVP)
  - Abdominal ultrasonography
  - Renal ultrasonography
  - Abdominal CT
- Laboratory studies
  - Complete blood cell count (CBC)
  - Blood urea nitrogen (BUN) and creatinine levels
  - Urinalysis

Differential Diagnosis

- Nephrolithiasis
- Prostatitis
- Diabetes mellitus

- Sickle cell anemia
- Priapism

Treatment

Pharmacologic Management

- Pain management
- Urine alkalinization to prevent stone formation
- Steroids
- Antibiotics to manage infections
- Chemotherapy

Nonpharmacologic Management

- Radiation therapy for management of invasive disease
- Extracorporeal shock wave lithotripsy (ESWL) for noninvasive stone management
- Surgery
  - Although temporary relief from the obstruction can be achieved without surgery, the cause of the obstruction must be removed and the urinary system repaired.
  - Stents in the ureter or in renal pelvis may provide short-term relief of symptoms. Nephrostomy tubes, which drain urine from the kidneys through the back, may be used to bypass the obstruction.
- Foley catheter to manage urethral obstruction

Patient Teaching

- Recognize and report early signs of urinary problems.
- Manage hypertension, and monitor blood pressure frequently.
- Maintain hydration.
- Minimize foods or fluids known to promote acidic, concentrated urine.
- Manage pain.
- Appropriately manage drainage tubes.

Follow-up

- Monitor urinary output, urinalysis as appropriate.
- Monitor renal function tests as appropriate.

Bibliography

Bosscher, M. R. F., van Leeuwen, B. L., & Hoekstra, H. J. (2014). Surgical emergencies in oncology. *Cancer Treatment Reviews, 40,* 1028–1036.

Kohn, I. J., & Weiss, J. P. (2014). Urologic emergencies. In P. M. Hanno, T. J. Guzzo, S. B. Malkowicz, & A. J. Wein (Eds.), *Penn clinical manual of oncology* (2nd ed.) (pp. 231–250). Philadelphia: Elsevier/Saunders.

Metro, M. J. (2014). Urethral stricture disease. In P. M. Hanno, T. J. Guzzo, S. B. Malkowicz, & A. J. Wein (Eds.), *Penn clinical manual of oncology* (2nd ed.) (pp. 284–300). Philadelphia: Elsevier/Saunders.

Nakada, S. Y., & Hsu, T. H. S. (2012). Management of upper urinary tract obstruction. In A. J. Wein, L. R. Kavoussi, A. C. Novick, A. W. Partin, & C. A. Peters (Eds.), *Campbell-Walsh urology* (10th ed.) (pp. 1122–1168). Philadelphia: Elsevier/Saunders.

Winkelman, C. (2013). Care of patients with urinary problems. In D. D. Ignatavicius, & M. L. Workman (Eds.), *Medical-surgical nursing: Patient-centered care* (7th ed.) (pp. 1489–1517). St. Louis: Elsevier/Saunders.

Metabolic Emergencies

Kristen W. Maloney

Adrenal Failure

Definition

- In adrenal failure, the adrenal gland is unable to produce adequate amounts of cortical hormones in response to physiologic demands.
- Glucocorticoids, which are required for the normal function of all cells, are normally secreted from the adrenal cortex in large quantities during times of physiologic stress to maintain homeostasis.
- Adrenal failure can be primary (i.e., Addison disease) or secondary and caused by a lack of adrenocorticotropic hormone (ACTH), also called *corticotropin* or *cosyntropin*.

Epidemiology

- Overall prevalence of adrenal insufficiency is 5 cases per 10,000 people.
- Prevalence of primary adrenal insufficiency is 93 to 140 cases per 1 million people.
- Prevalence of secondary adrenal insufficiency is 125 to 280 cases per 1 million people (mostly due to thalamic-pituitary tumors).

Pathophysiology

- The adrenal cortex produces cortisol that helps to regulate metabolism and the stress response and aldosterone that helps to control blood pressure.
- Adrenal failure results from destruction or dysfunction of the hypothalamic-pituitary-adrenal axis that regulates the hypothalamus, pituitary gland, and adrenal glands.
- Primary adrenal insufficiency or adrenal failure is caused by damage to the adrenal glands.
  - Most common causes: autoimmune adrenalitis and *Mycobacterium tuberculosis* infection
  - Less common causes: bilateral hemorrhage of the glands, malignancies, acquired immunodeficiency syndrome (AIDS), and fungal infections
  - Medication-related causes: anticoagulants, tyrosine kinase inhibitors, ketoconazole, fluconazole, etomidate, phenobarbital, phenytoin, and rifampin
- Secondary adrenal insufficiency or adrenal failure results from reduced secretion of corticotropin-releasing hormone (CRH) by the hypothalamus or ACTH by the pituitary gland.

- Most common cause: Abrupt discontinuation of long-term administration of glucocorticoids
- Less common causes: metastatic cancers to the brain or adrenals, pituitary infarction, surgery or radiation, and central nervous system disturbances (e.g., basilar skull fracture, infection)
- Medication-related causes: glucocorticoid therapy, fluticasone, megestrol acetate, medroxyprogesterone, ketorolac tromethamine, and opiates

Signs and Symptoms

- Ninety percent of both adrenal glands must be nonfunctioning before clinical symptoms are seen.
- Generalized symptoms
  - Fatigue and weakness
  - Hypotension
  - Nausea, vomiting, diarrhea, and abdominal pain
  - Tachycardia
  - Failure to thrive
  - Anorexia
  - Hyperpigmentation
  - Headache
- Electrolyte abnormalities associated with aldosterone deficiency
  - Hyperkalemia
  - Hyponatremia
- Electrolyte abnormalities associated with cortisol deficiency
  - Hypoglycemia
  - Hypercalcemia

Cancers Associated with Disorder

- Metastases to the adrenals or pituitary
- Solid cancers
  - Breast cancer
  - Malignant melanoma
  - Lung cancer
  - Colon cancer
  - Esophageal cancer
  - Rectal cancer
- Hematologic cancers
  - Non-Hodgkin lymphoma
    - Secondary involvement of the adrenal gland in 25% of patients
    - Diffuse, large B-cell lymphomas in 70% of cases
  - Primary adrenal lymphoma
    - Represents only 3% of extranodal lymphomas
    - Seen more often in males than females

Diagnostic Tests

- Low cortisol production is necessary for a diagnosis of adrenal insufficiency.
  - Cortisol level greater than 18 mcg/dL indicates normal adrenal function.
  - Cortisol level less than 3 mcg/dL indicates adrenal insufficiency.
  - Cortisol levels are evaluated in the morning, when serum cortisol levels are at their peak.
  - Cortisol circulates bound to albumin, and the level may be falsely low in patients with an albumin level less than 2.5 g/dL.
- ACTH stimulates production and release of cortisol from the adrenal gland cortex.
  - The ACTH level is elevated in primary adrenal insufficiency.
  - The ACTH level is low or normal in secondary adrenal insufficiency.
  - The ACTH stimulation test assesses adrenal insufficiency.
    - Draw a blood sample to determine the baseline cortisol level.
    - Administer 0.25 mg (250 mcg) of cosyntropin intravenously.
    - Draw samples for cortisol levels at 30 and 60 minutes after dosing.
    - Normal function is between 500 and 550 nmol/L, but the result depends on the assay used.
  - In primary adrenal insufficiency, no rise is seen in cortisol levels because the adrenal gland is dysfunctional.
  - In secondary adrenal insufficiency, a normal response is seen; a serum cortisol level of more than 18 mcg/dL at either time point is normal.
- Serum potassium level
  - Elevated in primary adrenal insufficiency
  - Normal in secondary adrenal insufficiency
- Serum sodium level is decreased.
- Serum glucose level is decreased.

Differential Diagnosis

- Primary adrenal failure
  - Autoimmune adrenalitis
  - Tuberculosis, histoplasmosis, or human immunodeficiency virus (HIV) infection
- Secondary adrenal failure
  - Pituitary adenomas

Treatment

- Treatment is prompt replacement of corticosteroids.
- Glucocorticoids are the main form of therapy for all forms of adrenal failure.
  - Hydrocortisone (10 to 12 mg/m²/day [15 to 30 mg/day]) divided in two to three doses per day, with most of the dose given in the morning to reflect normal body cortisol secretion
  - May require lower dose, particularly for secondary adrenal insufficiency
  - Smallest dose that improves symptoms is recommended.
  - Short half-life mimics normal cortisol circadian rhythm.
- Stress-dose steroids
  - For minor stress (e.g., fever, cold, surgery with local anesthesia), two to three times the usual daily dose.
  - For major stress (e.g., major surgery with anesthesia, trauma or disease requiring intensive care) dosing is controversial, but a significant increase in the dose is recommended, e.g., 150 mg/day intravenously over the first 24 hours and reduce to 100 mg/day intravenously.
  - Follow with switch to oral form and taper.
  - Consider this treatment for patients experiencing septic shock not resolved with fluid resuscitation and vasopressor agents.
- Mineralocorticoids are needed in addition to glucocorticoids for patients with primary adrenal insufficiency.
  - Required for patients with concomitant aldosterone deficiency resulting in persistent hyperkalemia
  - Fludrocortisone (0.05 to 0.2 mg/day) is given as a single dose in the morning, and the dose is adjusted according to symptoms.
  - Monitoring includes orthostatic blood pressure, serum sodium level, serum potassium level, and plasma renin concentration (PRC).
- Treatment with dehydroepiandrosterone (DHEA) remains controversial.

Patient Teaching

- The patient and caregiver should understand stress factors and recognize and report signs of a crisis.
- The patient should wear a medical alert bracelet or necklace stating the need for glucocorticoids in the event of an emergency.

Follow-up

- Consider an endocrinology consultation.
- Hydrocortisone may be needed during periods of stress.
- Monitor symptoms for signs of crisis.
- Provide emotional support to the patient during a crisis as needed.

Bibliography

Arlt, W. (2009). The approach to the adult with newly diagnosed adrenal insufficiency. *Journal of Clinical Endocrinology and Metabolism, 94*(4), 1059–1067.

Bornstein, S. R. (2009). Predisposing factors for adrenal insufficiency. *New England Journal of Medicine, 360*(22), 2328–2339.

Dasararaju, R., & Avery, R. A. (2013). Primary adrenal lymphoma with paraneoplastic syndrome. *North American Journal of Medical Sciences, 5*(12), 721–723.

Faulhaber, G. A., Borges, F. K., Ascoli, A. M., Seligman, R., & Furlanetto, T. W. (2011). Adrenal failure due to adrenal metastasis of lung cancer: A case report. *Case Reports in Oncological Medicine, 2011,* 326815.

Morton, P. G., & Fontaine, D. K. (Eds.). (2012). *Critical care nursing: A holistic approach* (10th ed.) Philadelphia: Lippincott, Williams & Wilkins.

Neary, N., & Nieman, L. (2010). Adrenal insufficiency: Etiology, diagnosis and treatment. *Current Opinion in Endocrinology, Diabetes, and Obesity, 17*(3), 217–223.

Suzuki, K., Ichikawa, T., Furuse, H., Tsuda, T., Tokui, K., Masaki, Y., & Tobe, K. (2015). Relationship of the urine cortisol level with the performance status of patients with lung cancer: A retrospective study. *Supportive Care in Cancer, 23*(7), 2129–2133.

Venkatesh, B., & Cohen, J. (2015). The utility of the corticotropin test to diagnose adrenal insufficiency in critical illness: An update. *Clinical Endocrinology, 83*(3), 289–297.

Zagkotsis, G. D., Malindretos, P. M., Markou, M. P., Koutroumbas, G. C., Makri, P. T., Kapsalas, D. V., & Syrganis, C. D. (2014). Adrenal insufficiency as the presenting feature in a patient with lung cancer. *Journal of Emergency Medicine, 46*(3), e91–e92.

Hypercalcemia of Malignancy

Definition

- Hypercalcemia of malignancy is an abnormally high level of calcium (i.e., serum calcium >11 mg/dL or ionized calcium >1.35 mmol/L).
- Rate of calcium mobilization from bone exceeds the renal threshold for calcium excretion.
- Two mechanisms can cause hypercalcemia: humoral hypercalcemia of malignancy (HHM) and local osteolytic hypercalcemia (LOH).

Epidemiology

- Hypercalcemia of malignancy occurs in 10% to 20% of all cancer patients.
- It is the most common oncologic emergency.

Pathophysiology

- Parathyroid hormone (PTH), 1,25-dihydroxyvitamin D (vitamin D), and calcitonin assist in regulation of calcium and bone metabolism.
- Stimulation of calcium resorption from bones and kidneys is supported by PTH.
- Vitamin D, which is released in response to low calcium levels, promotes absorption of calcium from dietary intake.
- Calcitonin decreases calcium levels in the body.
- Osteoblasts are cells that secrete an extracellular matrix for bone formation.
- Osteoclasts are large, multinucleate cells that absorb bone tissue during growth and healing. They breakdown tissue by releasing a proteolytic enzyme that dissolves the bone matrix and releases calcium into the extracellular space.
- LOH accounts for 20% of hypercalcemia of malignancy cases.
- Tumor cells infiltrating bone (i.e., bone metastasis) locally secrete cytokines that directly stimulate osteoclasts to resorb bone and inhibit osteoblasts, resulting in increased release of calcium into the extracellular fluid and the systemic circulation.
- HHM accounts for 80% of hypercalcemia of malignancy cases.
- Systemic cytokines secreted by tumor cells promote the release of calcium and phosphate from bone, increasing calcium resorption in the kidney.
- Parathyroid hormone–related protein (PTHrP) is the principal mediator of cancer-related hypercalcemia in patients with solid tumors. It acts similar to PTH and increases renal and bone resorption of calcium.
- Vitamin D–mediated hypercalcemia

- Vitamin D may be activated by certain lymphomas, increasing calcium absorption in the gut.
- Dehydration develops due to the effects of hypercalcemia and impairs renal excretion of calcium.

Signs and Symptoms

- Based on serum calcium levels, hypercalcemia of malignancy is categorized as mild, moderate, or severe.
- Most symptoms are seen in the gastrointestinal, neurologic, musculoskeletal, renal, and cardiovascular systems.
- Patients with mild hypercalcemia (10.5 to 11.5 mg/dL) may report the following symptoms:
  - Nausea, vomiting, abdominal cramping, and loss of appetite
  - Restlessness, difficulty concentrating, and confusion
  - Fatigue and generalized weakness
  - Excessive thirst (i.e., polydipsia), frequent urination (i.e., polyuria), and nocturia
- Patients with moderate hypercalcemia (11.5 to 13.5 mg/dL) may report the following as their calcium levels increase in addition to symptoms of mild hypercalcemia:
  - Constipation and increased bloating and abdominal pain
  - Psychosis and increased drowsiness
  - Increased weakness and bone pain
  - Feelings of dehydration
  - Palpitations and increasing anxiety (reflecting electrocardiographic [ECG] changes)
- Patients with severe hypercalcemia (>13.5 mg/dL) may experience the following symptoms in addition to those listed for mild and moderate hypercalcemia:
  - Ileus
  - Seizures and possible coma
  - Ataxia and pathologic fractures
  - Oliguria, renal insufficiency, and possible failure
  - Continued ECG changes and cardiac arrest

Cancers Associated with Disorder

- Greatest risk factors for hypercalcemia
  - Solid tumor diagnoses: breast, squamous cell lung, and prostate cancer
  - Hematologic cancer diagnoses: multiple myeloma and lymphoma

Diagnostic Tests

- Serum calcium level greater than 11 mg/dL
- Ionized serum calcium level greater than 1.35 mmol/L
- Serum albumin level is measured with calcium because calcium circulates bound to albumin.
  - Decreased albumin level may give a false-normal calcium value.
  - Corrected calcium level is the total serum calcium (mg/dL) + (4.0 − serum albumin [g/dL]) × 0.8.
- The PTH level is typically low, except in rare cases of a PTH-secreting tumor.
- A PTHrP level greater than 1 pmol/L is a specific indicator of malignancy.

Differential Diagnosis

- Primary or secondary hyperparathyroidism
- Renal failure
- Paget disease of bone
- Medications and supplements (e.g., thiazides, lithium, large doses of vitamins A or D)

Treatment

Pharmacologic Management

- Effective long-term management is treatment of the underlying disease.
- Continuing management requires pharmacologic measures to inhibit bone resorption and promote renal calcium excretion.
- Immediate goal is to restore fluid and electrolyte balance.
- Hydration is achieved with isotonic (0.9%) saline solution.
  - Rate of infusion depends on the severity of dehydration, level of serum calcium, and patient's ability to tolerate a high rate of infusion and large volume of fluid.
  - Hydration results in an approximately 2-mg/dL decrease in the serum calcium level.
  - Clinical improvement usually is seen within 24 hours, but the effect is temporary.
- Diuresis
  - A loop diuretic, such as 20 to 40 mg of furosemide, is given intravenously every 12 hours.
  - Diuresis enhances calcium excretion.
  - Thiazide diuretics are contraindicated due to inhibition of urinary excretion of calcium.
- Bisphosphonates and bone-modifying agents
  - They are used to prevent pathologic fracture, spinal cord compression, and hypercalcemia.
  - They inhibit normal and pathologic bone resorption by affecting osteoclasts and may inhibit adhesion of tumor cells to bone matrix.
  - All agents may cause osteonecrosis of the jaw.
  - They are administered intravenously because of poor oral absorption.
  - Zoledronic acid (4 mg given intravenously over 15 minutes every 3 to 4 weeks) has proved to be more effective than pamidronate.
  - Gallium nitrate is used when hypercalcemia recurs quickly after use of a bisphosphonate.
    - The dose is 200 mg/m^2/day given as a 5-day continuous infusion; 100 mg/m^2/day may be considered for patients with mild hypercalcemia and minimal symptoms.
    - It inhibits bone resorption and stimulates bone formation.
    - It inhibits tubular calcium resorption and PTH secretion.
    - The major complication is nephrotoxicity.
  - Calcitonin is given intramuscularly or subcutaneously in a dose of 4 to 8 IU/kg every 6 to 12 hours.
    - It inhibits osteoclast-mediated bone resorption.
    - Calcitonin promotes urinary calcium and sodium excretion.
    - It decreases the serum calcium level in 2 to 6 hours.
    - Resistance to effects develops within a few days of instituting therapy.
  - Denosumab is a monoclonal antibody approved for hypercalcemia in malignancy.
    - It is used after a failed response to bisphosphonate therapy.
    - It continues to be studied to refine its applications.
- Dialysis rapidly reduces the serum calcium level in patients who cannot tolerate aggressive hydration.

Patient Teaching

- Teach the patient and caregiver to recognize and report signs and symptoms of hypercalcemia.
- Discuss with the patient and caregiver how to maintain safety if the patient becomes confused.
- Educate the patient and caregiver about appropriate ways to maintain safe activity levels.
- The patient and caregiver are taught to take the patient's weight daily and monitor oral intake.

Follow-up

- Continue to monitor serum calcium levels and laboratory values related to renal function.
- Monitor fluid intake and output.
- Monitor for early signs and symptoms of hypercalcemia such as confusion and for fatigue and nausea, which can indicate recurrence.

Bibliography

Behl, D., Hendrickson, A. W., & Moynihan, T. J. (2010). Oncologic emergencies. *Critical Care Clinics, 26*(1), 181–205.

Clines, G. A. (2011). Mechanisms and treatment of hypercalcemia of malignancy. *Current Opinion in Endocrinology, Diabetes, and Obesity, 18*(6), 339–346.

Foulkes, M. (2010). Nursing management of common oncological emergencies. *Nursing Standard (Royal College of Nursing, Great Britain: 1987), 24*(41), 49–56, quiz 58.

Hu, M. I., Glezerman, I. G., Leboulleux, S., Insogna, K., Gucalp, R., Misiorowski, W., & Jain, R. K. (2014). Denosumab for treatment of hypercalcemia of malignancy. *Journal of Clinical Endocrinology and Metabolism, 99*(9), 3144–3152.

Kaplan, M. (2011). Hypercalcemia of malignancy. In C. H. Yarbro, D. Wujcik, & B. H. Gobel (Eds.), *Cancer nursing: Principles and practice* (7th ed.) (pp. 939–963). Sudbury, MA: Jones & Bartlett.

Legrand, S. B. (2011). Modern management of malignant hypercalcemia. *American Journal of Hospice & Palliative Care, 28*(7), 515–517.

Reagan, P., Pani, A., & Rosner, M. H. (2014). Approach to diagnosis and treatment of hypercalcemia in a patient with malignancy. *American Journal of Kidney Diseases, 63*(1), 141–147.

Hypoglycemia

Definition

- Hypoglycemia is an abnormal decrease in serum glucose levels.
- The diagnosis depends on three criteria (i.e., Whipple triad):
  - Signs and symptoms of hypoglycemia
  - Low plasma glucose concentration when the signs and symptoms occur
  - Resolution of signs and symptoms with treatment

- Glucose level of less than 40 mg/dL requires immediate treatment.
- Hypoglycemia can be mild to severe with various complications.
- Insulin-like growth factor, secreted by tumor cells, binds with insulin receptors, decreasing the blood glucose level.

Epidemiology

- Between 8% and 18% of patients with cancer have diabetes.
- As the number of cancer cases increases, especially among older adults, diabetes will become a significant comorbid condition.
- Of the patients with diabetes, 90% to 95% have type 2 diabetes.

Pathophysiology

- Normal brain function relies on a continuous supply of glucose in the circulation.
- The body maintains normal glucose levels through the following mechanisms:
  - Decreased insulin secretion when glucose levels decrease
  - Increased glucagon secretion
  - Increased epinephrine secretion
  - If those mechanisms fail, glucose levels continue to decline.
- Type 1 diabetes is an autoimmune disease in which pancreatic beta cells are destroyed, resulting in insufficient production or no production of insulin.
- Type 2 diabetes occurs when the body becomes resistant to insulin and the pancreas can no longer produce the amount of insulin needed to support the body's needs.
- Paraneoplastic syndrome, in which tumor cells secrete insulin-like growth factor 2 (IGF-2), may occur.
  - IGF-2 interacts with insulin receptors and IGF receptors, stimulating glucose uptake by muscle and fat and potentially by tumor cells while hepatic glucose output is suppressed.
  - IGF-2 may provide a survival signal for oncogene-induced abnormal cancer cell growth by increasing glucose consumption and use by the tumor and by inhibiting apoptosis.

Signs and Symptoms

- Symptoms of hypoglycemia are categorized as neuroglycopenic or neurogenic.
- Neuroglycopenic symptoms
  - Behavioral changes (e.g., fatigue, confusion)
  - Seizures
  - Loss of consciousness
  - Diaphoresis
  - Pallor
- Neurogenic symptoms
  - Palpitations
  - Tremor
  - Sweating
  - Hunger
  - Anxiety
  - Paresthesias

Cancers Associated with Disorder

- Insulin-like growth factors are involved in the following cancers:
  - Breast
  - Prostate
  - Colon
  - Lung
  - Head and neck squamous cell
- Non–islet cell tumors
- Mesenchymal tumors
- Hepatocellular carcinoma
- Fibrous pleural tumor

Diagnostic Tests

- Blood glucose levels are classified according to the National Cancer Institute (NCI) Common Terminology Criteria for Adverse Events (CTCAE):
  - Grade 1: less than 55 mg/dL (lower limit of normal [LLN])
  - Grade 2: less than 55-40 mg/dL
  - Grade 3: less than 40-30 mg/dL
  - Grade 4: less than 30 mg/dL
  - Grade 5: death
  - Level less than 40 mg/dL establishes severe hypoglycemia.
- Serum insulin level
  - Increased with an insulinoma (i.e., insulin-producing tumor of the pancreas)
  - Increased with exogenous insulin administration
  - Decreased with tumor-associated hypoglycemia
- Serum C peptide level
  - Increased with insulinoma
  - Decreased with tumor-associated hypoglycemia
  - Decreased with hypoglycemia from exogenous insulin administration

Differential Diagnosis

- Drug-induced hypoglycemia
- Surreptitious or therapeutic insulin administration
- Oral hypoglycemic agents
- Critical illness (e.g., infection, sepsis)
- Hormone deficiency
- Non–islet cell tumor
- Insufficient food intake or starvation
- Chronic liver disease
- Adrenal or pituitary failure

Treatment

- Treatment is based on the underlying cause.
  - If related to a malignancy, treating the cancer is the only effective method to correcting hypoglycemia long term.
  - Approximately 15 to 20 g of glucose can reverse hypoglycemia.
- If the patient can tolerate oral intake, supply carbohydrate (i.e., 4 to 6 oz. of fruit juice or 3 to 5 glucose tablets).

- If the patient cannot tolerate oral intake, glucagon (1 mg given subcutaneously or intramuscularly) is administered; may repeat one to two times as needed
- The glucose level should be checked 15 minutes after giving carbohydrate or glucagon.
- Severe hypoglycemia or coma requires immediate treatment.
  - Rapid intravenous push of 25 g of a 50% dextrose solution
  - Continuous intravenous infusion of glucose may be needed.
- Octreotide can be used to treat sulfonylurea-induced hypoglycemia.

Patient Teaching

- The patient and caregiver should be educated about the signs and symptoms of hypoglycemia.
- The patient should always carry the following for emergency use:
  - Glucose tablets, fruit juice, and a carbohydrate snack
  - A glucagon kit should be available and kept with the patient.
- The patient should report episodes of hypoglycemia to his or her provider.
- The patient should keep a diary of blood sugar trends.

Follow-up

- The glucose level should be monitored regularly.
- The underlying cause should be corrected if possible.

Bibliography

Cao, Y. (2014). VEGF-targeted cancer therapeutics—paradoxical effects in endocrine organs. *Nature Reviews. Endocrinology, 10*(9), 530–539.
Cancer Therapy Evaluation Program. (2010). *Common terminology criteria for adverse events (version 4.03)*. Washington, DC: National Institutes of Health and US Department of Health and Human Services.
Cryer, P. E., Axelrod, L., Grossman, A. B., Heller, S. R., Montori, V. M., Seaquist, E. R., & Endocrine Society. (2009). Evaluation and management of adult hypoglycemic disorders: An Endocrine Society clinical practice guideline. *Journal of Clinical Endocrinology and Metabolism, 94*(3), 709–728.
Gallagher, E. J., & LeRoith, D. (2010). The proliferating role of insulin and insulin-like growth factors in cancer. *Trends in Endocrinology and Metabolism, 21*(10), 610–618.
Leak, A., Davis, E. D., Houchin, L. B., & Mabrey, M. (2009). Diabetes management and self-care education for hospitalized patients with cancer. *Clinical Journal of Oncology Nursing, 13*(2), 205–210.
Maki, R. G. (2010). Small is beautiful: Insulin-like growth factors and their role in growth, development, and cancer. *Journal of Clinical Oncology, 28*(33), 4985–4995.
Morton, P. G., & Fontaine, D. K. (Eds.). (2012). *Critical care nursing: A holistic approach* (10th ed.) Philadelphia: Lippincott, Williams & Wilkins.
Murad, M. H., Coto-Yglesias, F., Wang, A. T., Sheidaee, N., Mullan, R. J., Elamin, M. B., & Montori, V. M. (2009). Clinical review: Drug-induced hypoglycemia: A systematic review. *Journal of Clinical Endocrinology and Metabolism, 94*(3), 741–745.
Rosenzweig, S. A., & Atreya, H. S. (2010). Defining the pathway to insulin-like growth factor system targeting in cancer. *Biochemical Pharmacology, 80*(8), 1115–1124.
Sorlini, M., Benini, F., Cravarezza, P., & Romanelli, G. (2010). Hypoglycemia, an atypical early sign of hepatocellular carcinoma. *Journal of Gastrointestinal Cancer, 41*(2), 209–211.

Syndrome of Inappropriate Antidiuretic Hormone

Definition

- Syndrome of inappropriate antidiuretic hormone (SIADH) secretion is an endocrine paraneoplastic syndrome in which inappropriate secretion of antidiuretic hormone (ADH) is produced by malignant cells or the posterior pituitary gland, resulting in water excess and dilutional hyponatremia.
- Malignant cells can synthesize, store, and release ADH independent of normal physiologic controls.
- Hyponatremia is classified as follows:
  - Mild: 125 to 135 mEq/L
  - Moderate: 115 to 125 mEq/L
  - Severe: less than 115 mEq/L (i.e., medical emergency)

Epidemiology

- SIADH occurs in 4% to 15% of hospitalized patients and is a common electrolyte disorder.
- It is often seen in patients with lung cancer:
  - In 10% to 15% of patients with small cell lung cancer
  - In 2% to 4% of patients with non–small cell lung cancer

Pathophysiology

- ADH is normally produced by the hypothalamus, stored in the posterior pituitary gland, and released in response to changes in plasma osmolality.
- The activated form of ADH is arginine vasopressin (AVP).
- Release of AVP causes renal tubules to resorb increased amounts of sodium and water. AVP is released in response to the following:
  - Plasma osmolality differences
  - Plasma volume changes
- SIADH is characterized by unregulated production of ADH.
  - Cancer cells can inappropriately synthesize and release ADH that is unregulated by negative feedback mechanisms.
  - Kidneys are stimulated to conserve water, leading to increased free water in the extracellular fluid and dilutional serum hyponatremia.
  - Kidneys excrete small amounts of concentrated urine with increased sodium osmolality.
- Increased free water is distributed through intracellular pathways, which can cause cerebral edema (i.e., water intoxication).
- Cerebral edema leads to disruption of neural function and may lead to death.

Signs and Symptoms

- Symptoms are primarily neurologic and gastrointestinal.
- The severity of symptoms is related to the degree of hyponatremia and rapidity of onset.

- Early manifestations:
  - Thirst
  - Anorexia
  - Nausea and vomiting
  - Weight gain without edema
  - Muscle cramps
  - Headache
  - Weakness
  - Lethargy and irritability
- More symptoms develop as the sodium level falls below 120 mg/dL (resulting from cerebral edema):
  - Hyporeflexia
  - Confusion and combativeness
  - Oliguria
- Symptoms of severe hyponatremia (<110 to 115 mg/dL):
  - Seizures
  - Coma
  - Death if hyponatremia is severe or rapid in onset

Cancers Associated with Disorder

- Solid cancers
  - Small cell and non–small cell lung cancers
  - Head and neck cancers
  - Duodenal and pancreatic cancers
  - Gynecologic cancers
  - Neuroblastoma
- Hematologic cancers
  - Lymphoma
  - Leukemia
- Chemotherapeutic agents associated with SIADH:
  - Vinca alkaloids (e.g., vincristine)
  - Platinum-based agents (e.g., cisplatin)
  - Alkylating agents (e.g., cyclophosphamide)
  - Methotrexate

Diagnostic Tests

- Serum sodium level (<130 mEq/L)
- Serum osmolality (<275 mOsm/kg)
- Urine sodium (>20 mEq/L)
- Urine osmolality greater than serum osmolality
- Decreased blood urea nitrogen (BUN) level
- Decreased creatinine level
- Elevated serum ADH level
- Decreased uric acid level
- Decreased albumin level

Differential Diagnosis

- Central nervous system
  - Infection
  - Trauma
  - Guillain-Barré syndrome
- Pulmonary system
  - Tuberculosis
  - Pneumonia
- Effects of chemotherapeutic agents and other drugs

- Antidepressants (e.g., tricyclic, selective serotonin reuptake inhibitors [SSRIs])
  - Opioids
  - Barbiturates
  - Nonsteroidal antiinflammatory drugs (NSAIDs)
- Renal failure
- HIV and AIDS

Treatment

- Goals include treatment of the underlying malignancy and management of hyponatremia.
- Monitoring serum sodium is essential because treatment is based on severity.
- Management of mild hyponatremia
  - Patient should be placed on fluid restriction (1000 mL/day).
  - Serial neurologic assessments should be performed.
  - Medication reconciliation should be performed.
- Management of moderate hyponatremia
  - Patient should be placed on fluid restriction (1000 mL/day).
  - Serial neurologic assessments should be performed.
  - Medication reconciliation should be performed.
  - Consider use of demeclocycline (300-600 mg twice daily initial dose; 300-450 mg twice daily maintenance dose).
    - Impairs effect of ADH on renal tubules
    - Facilitates free water excretion
    - Not used frequently due to potential side effects of hematologic changes, nephrotoxicity, photosensitivity, and nephrogenic diabetes insipidus
- Management of severe hyponatremia
  - Patient should be placed on fluid restriction (1000 mL/day).
  - Serial neurologic assessments should be performed.
  - Medication reconciliation should be performed.
  - Use of 3% saline solution
  - Severe symptoms: 100 mL of 3% NaCl infused intravenously over 10 minutes × 3 as needed
  - Mild to moderate symptoms: 3% NaCl infused at 0.5 to 2 mL/kg/h
    - Slow infusion prevents a rapid increase of sodium and pulmonary edema.
  - Use of a loop diuretic (e.g., furosemide)
    - Dose is 20 mg twice daily with hypertonic saline solution infusion.
    - It induces loss of free water.
- Untreated SIADH or too-rapid correction may result in severe neurologic impairment or death.
  - Osmotic demyelination syndrome can occur within 2 to 6 days of too-rapid correction.
  - Endothelial cells in the brain can be damaged from dehydration.
  - The blood-brain barrier can break down.
- If seizures result with too-rapid correction of sodium, dexamethasone (10-20 mg) and mannitol (50 g given intravenously) should be given immediately.

- Mild hypovolemic hyponatremia may be treated with isotonic (0.9%) saline solution given intravenously or, if tolerated, oral salt tablets, which may result in little or no net change in the sodium level.
- Recommend rate of correction is no more than 12 mEq/L/day over 2 to 3 days.

Patient Teaching

- The patient should monitor daily weights and report changes to the health care provider.
- Instruct the patient about the importance of fluid restriction. Explain the use of a chart to monitor fluid intake and output.
- Teach the patient and caregiver about the signs and symptoms of hyponatremia, including gastrointestinal and neurologic symptoms.

Follow-up

- Monitor the patient's weight.
- Record fluid intake and output.
- Monitor laboratory values, including levels of serum sodium, urine sodium, and urine osmolality.
- Monitor use of medications that may contribute to SIADH.
- Complete neurologic checks according to the severity of hyponatremia.

Bibliography

Behl, D., Hendrickson, A. W., & Moynihan, T. J. (2010). Oncologic emergencies. *Critical Care Clinics, 26*(1), 181–205.

Buffington, M. A., & Abreo, K. (2015). Hyponatremia: A review. *Journal of Intensive Care Medicine, 31*(4), 223–236.

Castillo, J. J., Vincent, M., & Justice, E. (2012). Diagnosis and management of hyponatremia in cancer patients. *Oncologist, 17*(6), 756–765.

Cope, D. G. (2013). Syndrome of inappropriate antidiuretic hormone secretion. In M. Kaplan (Ed.), *Understanding and managing oncologic emergencies: A resource for nurses.* Pittsburgh, PA: Oncology Nursing Society.

Esposito, P., Piotti, G., Bianzina, S., Malul, Y., & Dal Canton, A. (2011). The syndrome of inappropriate antidiuresis: Pathophysiology, clinical management and new therapeutic options. *Nephron Clinical Practice, 119*(1), c62–c73, discussion c73.

Gross, P. (2012). Clinical management of SIADH. *Therapeutic Advances in Endocrinology and Metabolism, 3*(2), 61–73.

Morton, P. G., & Fontaine, D. K. (Eds.). (2012). *Critical care nursing: A holistic approach* (10th ed.) Philadelphia: Lippincott, Williams & Wilkins.

Petereit, C., Zaba, O., Teber, I., Luders, H., & Grohe, C. (2013). A rapid and efficient way to manage hyponatremia in patients with SIADH and small cell lung cancer: Treatment with tolvaptan. *BMC Pulmonary Medicine, 13*, 55.

Sterns, R. H., Nigwekar, S. U., & Hix, J. K. (2009). The treatment of hyponatremia. *Seminars in Nephrology, 29*(3), 282–299.

Verbalis, J. G., Goldsmith, S. R., Greenberg, A., Korzelius, C., Schrier, R. W., Sterns, R. H., et al. (2013). Diagnosis, evaluation, and treatment of hyponatremia: expert panel recommendations. *American Journal of Medicine, 126*(10 Suppl 1), S1–42.

Tumor Lysis Syndrome

Definition

- Tumor lysis syndrome (TLS) is a spectrum of electrolyte abnormalities that can occur after the initiation of cytotoxic therapy that causes the breakdown of large numbers of malignant cells.

Epidemiology

- TLS severity depends on the following:
  - Tumors larger than 8 to 10 cm (e.g., abdominal mass, mediastinal mass)
  - Tumor cells with a high proliferation rate
  - Extensive lymph node involvement
  - Bulky tumors associated with lymphadenopathy or hepatosplenomegaly
- Elevated pretreatment lactate dehydrogenase (LDH) level
- Preexisting conditions
  - Chronic renal insufficiency
  - Oliguria
  - Dehydration
  - Hypotension
  - Ascites
  - Exposure to nephrotoxins (e.g., vancomycin, aminoglycosides)
- Between 5% and 20% of patients with TLS have serious complications that lead to death.

Pathophysiology

- Antineoplastic agents kill cells rapidly, increasing the cellular contents (i.e., potassium, phosphorus, and uric acid) released into the bloodstream.
- TLS results from inadequate excretion of the contents from the body and causes the following:
  - Hyperkalemia
  - Hyperuricemia
  - Hyperphosphatemia
  - Hypocalcemia
- The inability of the kidneys to clear the intracellular byproducts from the bloodstream can lead to life-threatening hemodynamic and renal complications:
  - Cardiac arrhythmias
  - Renal failure
  - Acute respiratory distress syndrome (ARDS)

Signs and Symptoms

- Caused by electrolyte abnormalities
- Most likely to occur 24 to 48 hours after starting chemotherapy treatment
- May last up to 7 days after therapy is completed
- Early signs
  - Weakness
  - Muscle cramps
  - Nausea, vomiting
  - Diarrhea
  - Lethargy
  - Paresthesias
- Late signs
  - Paralysis
  - Bradycardia
  - Hypotension

- Oliguria
- Edema
- Cardiac irritability
- Laryngospasm
- Flank pain
- Hematuria
- Crystalluria
- Tetany
- Renal failure
- Seizures
- Cardiac arrest

Cancers Associated with Disorder

- TLS most commonly occurs in hematologic cancers.
  - High-grade lymphomas (e.g., Burkitt lymphoma)
  - Acute leukemia (most commonly with acute lymphocytic leukemia)
- It is less common in solid cancers.
  - Breast cancer
  - Small cell lung cancer
  - Medulloblastoma
- Adenocarcinoma treatments associated with an increased risk of TLS
  - Chemotherapy
  - Immunotherapy (e.g., monoclonal antibodies)
  - Radiation therapy
  - Hormonal therapy
  - Corticosteroids

Diagnostic Tests

- Basic metabolic panel (e.g., electrolytes, renal function)
- Liver function test
- Urinalysis

Differential Diagnosis

- Acute nephrocalcinosis
- Acute renal failure

Treatment

- Identify persons at increased risk for TLS.
- Monitor laboratory data. Depending on the risk of TLS, samples may be drawn every 6 to 12 hours for analysis.
- Initiate preventative measures such as intravenous hydration:
  - Administer 24 to 48 hours before therapy to begins, and continue for up to 72 hours after therapy is completed.
  - Amount of hydration depends on the patient's age and comorbidities.
  - Normal saline solution or 5% dextrose in water (D_5W) is used as the hydration fluid before, during, and after treatment.
  - Excessive hydration is contraindicated for persons with poor cardiac status because it may lead to fluid overload.
  - Loop diuretics (e.g., furosemide) can be used to help decrease fluid retention and overload.
- Allopurinol is used to reduce the serum uric acid level.
  - It can be given orally or intravenously.

- Parenteral dosing 200 to 400 mg/m²/day in a single infusion or in divided infusions
- Oral dose of 600 to 800 mg should be given 24 to 48 hours before treatment.
- It blocks the enzyme xanthine oxidase and decreases the production of uric acid.
- Deposits of uric acid in the kidney are decreased.
- Rasburicase can be used instead of allopurinol or as prevention or initial therapy for TLS.
  - Dose is 0.2 mg/kg given intravenously over 30 minutes.
  - It is contraindicated for patients with a glucose-6-phosphate dehydrogenase (G6PD) deficiency.
- Hemodialysis is used when the level of potassium is greater than 6 mEq/L, uric acid is greater than 10 mEq/L, or phosphorus is greater than 10 mEq/L.
- Treat electrolyte abnormalities.
  - Manage mild hyperkalemia (i.e., potassium level less than 6.5 mEq/L).
    - Sodium polystyrene sulfonate (i.e., Kayexalate), given orally or by retention enema, can lower potassium levels.
    - Monitor dietary intake of potassium.
  - Manage severe hyperkalemia (i.e., potassium level greater than 6.5 mEq/L or ECG changes).
    - Calcium gluconate if ECG changes are apparent
    - Hypertonic glucose (e.g., 50% dextrose) given intravenously
    - Regular insulin
    - Sodium bicarbonate
    - Loop diuretics
  - Manage hyperphosphatemia.
    - Decreased phosphorus levels help to normalize calcium levels.
    - Give phosphate-binding, aluminum-containing antacids.
    - Consider hypertonic glucose and an insulin infusion.
    - Monitor dietary intake of phosphorus.
  - Manage hypocalcemia.
    - Treat only if symptomatic.
    - Calcium level is not corrected unless the patient is symptomatic or has a positive Chvostek or Trousseau sign.
    - Administer calcium gluconate.
  - Manage hyperuricemia.
    - Continue aggressive intravenous hydration.
    - Increase dose of allopurinol.
    - If maximum dose is reached, start rasburicase.

Patient Teaching

- The patient and caregiver should be able to describe the signs and symptoms of TLS and report them to the provider.
- The patient and caregiver should understand the purpose of frequent laboratory draws that can indicate electrolyte abnormalities.
- Encourage the patient to increase fluid intake before and after chemotherapy and monitor daily weight.

Oncologic Emergencies

5

- Provide dietary education about the intake of potassium- and phosphorus-rich foods.

Follow-up

- Continue to monitor for signs and symptoms of TLS.
- Monitor laboratory findings, and treat electrolyte imbalances as needed.
- Maintain monitoring of fluid intake and output.
- Assess daily weight.
- Continue to monitor cardiac function and assess ECG changes.

Bibliography

Howard, S. C., Jones, D. P., & Pui, C. H. (2011). The tumor lysis syndrome. *New England Journal of Medicine, 364*(19), 1844–1854.

Lopez-Olivo, M. A., Pratt, G., Palla, S. L., & Salahudeen, A. (2013). Rasburicase in tumor lysis syndrome of the adult: A systematic review and meta-analysis. *American Journal of Kidney Diseases, 62*(3), 481–492.

Lydon, G. (2011). Tumor lysis syndrome. In C. H. Yarbro, D. Wujcik, & B. H. Gobel (Eds.), *Cancer nursing: Principles and practice* (7th ed.). Sudbury, MA: Jones & Bartlett (2011).

Maie, K., Yokoyama, Y., Kurita, N., Minohara, H., Yanagimoto, S., Hasegawa, Y., & Chiba, S. (2014). Hypouricemic effect and safety of febuxostat used for prevention of tumor lysis syndrome. *Springerplus, 3*, 501.

Maloney, K., & Denno, M. (2011). Tumor lysis syndrome: Prevention and detection to enhance patient safety. *Clinical Journal of Oncology Nursing, 15*(6), 601–603.

Rasool, M., Malik, A., Qureshi, M. S., Ahmad, R., Manan, A., Asif, M., & Pushparaj, P. N. (2014). Development of tumor lysis syndrome (TLS): A potential risk factor in cancer patients receiving anticancer therapy. *Bioinformation, 10*(11), 703–707.

Vines, A. N., Shanholtz, C. B., & Thompson, J. L. (2010). Fixed-dose rasburicase 6 mg for hyperuricemia and tumor lysis syndrome in high-risk cancer patients. *Annals of Pharmacotherapy, 44*(10), 1529–1537.

Hematologic Emergencies

Jeanene "Gigi" Robison

Deep Vein Thrombosis

Definition

- Deep vein thrombosis (DVT), a type of venous thromboembolism (VTE), is partial or complete occlusion of blood flow in the deep veins caused by thrombus (clot) formation.

Epidemiology

- DVT is the most preventable cause of death among hospitalized or recently hospitalized patients.
- Two most common types are DVT of the lower extremities and pulmonary embolus.
- Persons with cancer have a much higher risk of having or developing DVT compared with those without cancer.
- DVT is the second leading cause of death of patients with cancer.
- DVT is a potentially fatal complication that primarily affects hospitalized patients.
  - Two million Americans are affected yearly.
  - Approximately 200,000 hospital visits are due to DVT.
  - About 50% of persons with DVT have symptoms; the other 50% are asymptomatic and do not receive treatment, which increases the risk of a significant complication.
- The risk of DVT is based on scoring of the Wells clinical prediction rule for diagnosing DVT:
  - Active cancer (score of 1), which can cause a hypercoagulable state
  - Paralysis, paresis, or plaster immobilization (score of 1)
  - Recently bedridden (score of 1)
  - Localized tenderness (score of 1)
  - Entire leg swelling (score of 1)
  - Calf swelling (score of 1)
  - Pitting edema in affected leg (score of 1)
  - Collateral superficial veins (score of 1)
  - Alternative diagnosis as likely as DVT (score of −2)
  - Clinical probability of DVT (low <0; intermediate 1 to 2; high ≥3)
- Other risk factors for the development of DVT
  - Surgery, especially lengthy surgical procedures
  - History of thrombotic events, especially DVT
  - Conditions in which local clotting takes place (e.g., phlebitis, trauma, inflammation)
  - Conditions that promote venous stasis:
    - Prolonged bed rest
    - Prolonged immobility resulting from pain, trauma, surgery, or paralysis

- Recent casting of a lower extremity (within 4 weeks)
- General debility
- Heart failure
- Infections related to gram-negative or gram-positive bacteria
- Hypercoagulable state (e.g., DIC)
- Peripheral vascular disease
- Medications such as antiestrogens (e.g., tamoxifen, raloxifene) and estrogen
- Medications that induce endothelial damage such as chemotherapy (especially adjuvant therapy for breast cancer), some vasopressor agents (e.g., dopamine), contrast medium, and high-dose antibiotics
- Burns or fractures that cause damage to the vessel
- Use of central venous catheters
- Antiphospholipid antibodies (associated with systemic lupus erythematosus [SLE])

Pathophysiology

- Patients with cancer have a higher incidence of DVT because clot formation is a common complication of malignancy.
  - Thrombus formation occurs in the cardiovascular system.
  - Embolus (i.e., thromboembolus), which is a traveling clot, may be formed when part of the thrombus is dislodged.
- Three mechanisms (i.e., Virchow triad) are integral to thrombus formation:
  - Abnormal blood flow because venous stasis predisposes to blood clot formation
    - Hyperviscosity due to high levels of plasma proteins, fibrinogen, white blood cells, or platelets
    - Immobilization or paralysis because venous stasis often occurs in the lower extremities, and pooling allows coagulation factors to accumulate and increases the chance of platelet aggregation and clot formation
    - External compression of the blood vessel, which is caused by the tumor and impedes blood flow (e.g., superior vena cava syndrome)
  - Breach of vascular integrity
    - Tumor invasion of the blood vessels
    - Proinflammatory cytokines (e.g., interleukin-1, interleukin-6, tumor necrosis factor-β), which are secreted by tumor, downregulate anticoagulation factors and create an environment for thrombus formation.

- Blood components
  - Procoagulant is secreted by tumor cells and induces a hypercoagulable state.
  - Tissue factor and cancer procoagulant can directly activate factor X, which initiates the clotting pathway.
  - Elevated levels of PAI-1 have been linked to an increased risk of DVT in persons with or without cancer.
- PE is a life-threatening complication of DVT.
  - When the blood clot is detached from the original source, the embolus travels with the blood flow.
  - A very large embolus may lodge in the main pulmonary artery, and smaller emboli pass to more distal branches of the pulmonary artery, causing partial or total occlusion of the vessel.

Signs and Symptoms

- Clinical manifestations
  - A dull ache, tight feeling, or frank pain in the calf, which is made worse with standing or walking and is made better with elevation
  - Localized tenderness or pain over the involved vein
  - Tender, palpable venous cord of the involved vein
  - Swollen calf or thigh by measurement; calf swelling of more than 3 cm in circumference in the symptomatic leg
  - Unilateral pitting edema in the involved extremity
  - Warmth and erythema of the involved extremity
  - Dilated superficial venous collateral vessels (nonvaricose)
  - Possible low-grade fever
- Assessment for the Homans sign as part of the physical examination
  - Calf pain is a positive sign and is produced by dorsiflexion of the foot with the knee bent in 30 degrees of flexion.
  - Positive results found for less than 50% of patients.
  - High incidence of false-positive results
  - Because the test for Homans sign may cause an embolism, it should not be performed if DVT is suspected.
- Signs and symptoms of PE may be the first indication of DVT and may include dyspnea, chest pain, tachypnea, tachycardia, and fever.

Cancers Associated with Disorder

- Small cell lung carcinoma (SCLC) and non–small cell lung cancer (NSCLC)
- Gastrointestinal: colorectal cancer, pancreatic tumors, and mucin-secreting tumors
- Ovarian and endometrial carcinoma
- Intracranial carcinoma
- APL, multiple myeloma, and myeloproliferative disorders
- Breast carcinoma
- Prostate and bladder carcinoma

Diagnostic Tests

- Laboratory tests
  - D-dimer
  - Blood assay detects blood clot fragments, which are produced by clot lysis.
  - It may be used with other diagnostic tests to rule out DVT.
  - A negative result has a high negative predictive value for DVT in patients without cancer, but a negative result does not reliably rule out DVT.
- Radiologic tests
  - Lower extremity venous ultrasonography is the initial test of choice for diagnosis of DVT.
  - Less accurate than venography
  - Low cost, noninvasive, highly sensitive, and specific for symptomatic DVT
  - Less sensitive and specific for detecting proximal and calf DVT for the high-risk postoperative patient who does not have symptoms
  - Doppler ultrasonography
  - Uses scanning and compression to detect thrombus by direct visualization or by interference when vein does not collapse during gentle compression
  - Impedance plethysmography to detect changes in blood volume that can occur with obstruction
- Contrast venography (i.e., phlebography)
  - Identifies DVT by infusing contrast material into the venous system by a catheter in the foot
  - A positive result is obstruction of the flow of dye within the vein, indicating a thrombus.
  - Not the first choice of diagnostic tests because it is expensive, invasive, and carries significant side effects resulting from hypersensitivity reactions to the contrast medium.
  - It is the gold standard for diagnosing DVT.
  - It is used when the diagnosis of DVT remains unclear after evaluation and initial testing.
- Magnetic resonance imaging (MRI)
  - May be alternative to venography
  - Especially useful for detecting thrombi in the pelvic vein
- Computed tomography (CT)
  - Spiral CT and CT angiography have been used to diagnose DVT.
- Radionuclide scintigraphy
  - Uses a variety of radiopharmaceuticals to detect DVT
  - Less reliable for calf DVT
  - Results do not differentiate intrinsic from extrinsic compression.
  - Expensive and not as reliable for recurrent DVT

Differential Diagnosis

- Calf muscle strain or tear
- Intramuscular hematoma
- Cellulitis, superficial phlebitis
- Obstruction of lymphatics by tumor, from irradiation or lymph node dissection
- Acute arterial occlusion
- Ruptured Baker cyst
- Chronic venous insufficiency
- Lymphangitis or fibrositis
- Kidney, liver, or heart disease (usually has bilateral edema)
- Hypoalbuminemia

Treatment

- Surgical placement of an inferior vena cava filter to prevent PE in recurrent DVT
  - An endoluminal filter is used to interrupt blood flow through the inferior cava vein.
  - Filters may not be beneficial and may increase the risk of recurrent DVT.
  - Treatment of choice in patients with contraindications for anticoagulant therapy

Pharmacologic Management

- Prevention
  - Acetylsalicylic acid (i.e., aspirin) may be administered on a daily basis.
  - Low-dose subcutaneous heparin may be administered for lower abdominal, pelvic, and lower extremity DVT.
  - Low-molecular-weight heparin (LMWH) may be administered for lower abdominal, pelvic, and hip or knee replacement operations
    - Enoxaparin (Lovenox)
    - Ardeparin (Normiflo)
    - Danaparoid (Orgaran)
    - Dalteparin (Fragmin)
  - Low-dose warfarin (Coumadin) may be administered to patients with a long-term indwelling central venous catheters.
- Anticoagulant therapy
  - Interrupts thrombosis
  - Allows the lytic system to dissolve the clot
  - Unfractionated heparin is the traditional standard for the initial treatment of DVT because of its rapid onset of action.
  - About 5 days of intravenous heparin is followed by a course of oral anticoagulants.
  - LMWH drugs are equally safe and effective for patients who are hemodynamically stable; they are used when patients are not candidates for warfarin therapy.
  - Enoxaparin and tinzaparin are approved in the United States for treatment of DVT with or without PE.
  - Vitamin K antagonists (e.g., warfarin) are oral agents that are used for long-term anticoagulation after PE occurs and for secondary prophylaxis.
  - These agents may be initiated concurrently with heparin:
- Thrombolytic therapy (e.g., streptokinase, recombinant tissue plasminogen activator [rtPA])
  - Promotes rapid resolution of emboli
  - Commonly not recommended for persons with DVT
  - May be used in persons with extensive obstruction of venous outflow

Nonpharmacologic Management

- Bed rest is indicated for the first 5 to 7 days with leg elevation for acute DVT.
- Mild analgesics and warm compresses may be used for the comfort of patients with acute DVT.
- Frequent leg exercises (i.e., range of motion [ROM] or isometric) if bedridden
  - Every 1 to 2 hours while awake to improve venous flow
  - Heel pumping and ankle circles for 10 to 12 repetitions
- Supplemental oxygen by nasal cannula may be administered to maintain a PaO_2 higher than 80 mm Hg in persons with acute DVT.
- Frequent ambulation, if tolerable, after 5 to 7 days of bed rest
- Antiembolic stockings or hose should be applied before surgery.
- Pneumatic compression stockings or devices may be used postoperatively to stimulate circulation and prevent DVT.
- Elevate the foot of the bed 15 to 20 inches with slight knee flexion; leg elevation should not exceed 45 degrees.
- Avoid popliteal pressure, which is produced by crossing the legs, placing pillows behind the knees, and elevation of the knee gatch.
- Do not massage the legs of persons with DVT.
- Regular position changes should be encouraged to prevent hypoventilation.
- Avoid smoking and caffeine to prevent vasoconstriction.

Patient Teaching

- Goals
  - Stimulate the patient's circulation.
  - Prevent additional DVTs, and resolve current clots.
  - Minimize or prevent respiratory compromise.
- Define DVT and describe the signs and symptoms of DVT.
- Explain the purpose of the laboratory and diagnostic tests, nursing care, and treatments.
- Encourage the patient to wear the pneumatic compression stockings or devices, as ordered.
- Teach the patient the rationale for ambulating as soon as possible after surgery.
- Encourage the patient to change position regularly, avoid sitting or standing for long periods, drink 8 to 10 glasses of fluid per day, avoid smoking and caffeine, and perform ROM or isometric exercises.
- Teach patients to avoid constrictive clothing or devices; to keep the legs elevated and straight; to move the toes, feet, and legs often; and to avoid pressure on the back of the knees (i.e., popliteal vessels) to prevent a clot from forming in the arms or legs.
- Teach the patient to take anticoagulant therapy at the same time every day.
- Teach the patient to avoid contact sports that could lead to serious injury.
- Teach the patient to use a soft toothbrush for oral care and use an electric razor.
- Teach the patient to maintain a diet consistent in the amount of vitamin K while on warfarin.
- The patient should report leg pain, bleeding, or signs of thrombophlebitis or PE.

Follow-up

- Continue to monitor for signs and symptoms of DVT.
- Monitor laboratory findings indicating continuation or resolution of DVT.
- Provide additional resources such as home equipment or assistance to address severe complications of DVT (e.g., PE).
- Monitor warfarin levels as indicated to keep the INR between 2.0 and 3.0.

Bibliography

Khorana, A. A. (2009). Cancer and thrombosis: Implications of published guidelines for clinical practice. *Annals of Oncology, 20,* 1619–1630.

Kuderer, N. M., Ortel, T. L., & Francis, C. W. (2009). Impact of venous thromboembolism and anticoagulation on cancer and cancer survival. *Journal of Clinical Oncology, 27,* 4902–4911.

Manasanch, E. E., & Lozier, J. N. (2013). Venous thromboembolism. In G. P. Rodgers & N. S. Young (Eds.), *The Bethesda handbook of clinical hematology* (3rd ed.) (pp. 311–327). Philadelphia: Lippincott Williams & Wilkins.

O'Leary, C., & Mack, L. (2013). Bleeding and thrombosis. In M. Kaplan (Ed.), *Understanding and managing oncological emergencies: A resource for nurses* (2nd ed.) (pp. 1–41). Pittsburgh, PA: Oncology Nursing Society.

Rodriguez, A. L. (2014). Bleeding and thrombotic complications. In C. Yarbro, D. Wujcik, & B. H. Gobel (Eds.), *Cancer symptom management* (4th ed.) (pp. 287–316). Sudbury, MA: Jones & Bartlett.

Turner Story, K. (2014). Deep vein thrombosis. In D. Camp-Sorrell & R. A. Hawkins (Eds.), *Clinical manual for the oncology advanced practice nurse* (3rd ed.) (pp. 349–361). Pittsburgh, PA: Oncology Nursing Society.

Disseminated Intravascular Coagulation

Definition

- Disseminated intravascular coagulation (DIC) is a systemic coagulation disorder.
- Widespread intravascular thrombosis can cause organ damage and the consumption of platelets and coagulation factors, which leads to hemorrhage.
- Two types of DIC
  - Acute DIC develops quickly and leads to excessive blood clotting in the small vessels and to serious bleeding.
  - Chronic DIC develops over weeks to months and causes excessive blood clotting without serious bleeding; cancer is the most common cause.

Epidemiology

- Chronic DIC is the most common coagulation disorder that occurs in cancer patients.
- DIC results from an underlying pathologic condition.
  - Sepsis or severe infections
    - Gram-negative or gram-positive bacterial infection (including rickettsial infection)
    - Viral infection (e.g., varicella, hepatitis, cytomegalovirus [CMV])
    - Parasitic infection
  - Septic or cardiogenic shock
  - Massive trauma or tissue injury
  - Placement of prosthetic devices such as an intraperitoneal shunt, LeVeen or Denver shunts, and aortic balloon assist devices

- Severe toxic or immunologic reactions such as a hemolytic transfusion reaction or transplant rejection
- Vascular disorders or stasis such as an abdominal aortic aneurysm, vasculitis, or grafts
- Microangiopathic hemolytic anemia (MAHA)
  - Thrombotic thrombocytopenic purpura (TTP)
  - Hemolytic uremic syndrome (HUS)
  - Malignant hypertension
- Hematologic diseases such as polycythemia vera and paroxysmal nocturnal hemoglobinuria
- Acute liver disease such as obstructive jaundice, acute hepatic failure, and intrahepatic or extrahepatic cholestasis
- Organ destruction such as acute pancreatitis and glomerulonephritis
- Metabolic acidosis
- Pregnancy and obstetric complications
- Fat embolism
- Heat stroke or malignant hyperthermia

Pathophysiology

- In a normal coagulation system, hemostasis is maintained by a balance between the processes of clot formation (i.e., thrombosis) and clot breakdown (i.e., fibrinolysis).
- In thrombus development, four pathologic mechanisms can occur simultaneously and stimulate a procoagulant state in DIC:
  - Enhanced generation of thrombin
    - Overwhelming thrombogenic stimulus such as infection, malignancy, or trauma
    - Triggers intrinsic or extrinsic pathway of the clotting cascade that leads to excessive circulating thrombin
    - Conversion of fibrinogen to fibrin
    - Activation of platelet activity and clotting factors
    - Results in multiple fibrin clots circulating in the bloodstream
    - Platelets trapped by excess fibrin clots
    - Leads to formation of microvascular and macrovascular fibrin thrombi (i.e., stationary blood clots)
  - Suppression of the anticoagulant pathways that tightly regulate thrombin
  - Suppression of the fibrinolytic system by high plasma levels of plasma activator inhibitor 1 (PAI-1)
  - Activation of proinflammatory cytokines (primarily interleukin-6 and tumor necrosis factor-α)
- When part of the thrombus is dislodged, an embolus (i.e., thromboembolus) is formed. The traveling clot can lead to diffuse microvascular obstruction and cause ischemia, impaired organ perfusion, and end-organ damage.
- Fibrinolysis
  - Normally, the fibrinolytic system is activated after clot formation to control how large the clot becomes and to reopen the healed blood vessel over time.
  - It can lead to bleeding and hemorrhaging.
  - Plasminogen is converted to plasmin by tissue plasminogen activator.
  - Plasmin release causes enzymatic lysis of the fibrin clot.

- Breakdown of fibrin clot causes release of fibrin-split products, also called fibrin-degradation products (FDPs).
- The fibrinolysis process may become uncontrolled.
  - FDPs are not effectively removed from circulation and accumulate in the bloodstream.
  - Accumulation contributes to bleeding that is observed in patients with DIC.
- Platelets and clotting factors are consumed at a rate greater than the body's ability to replace them during thrombosis, which leads to bleeding.

Signs and Symptoms

- Acute DIC symptoms
  - Bleeding often is the first obvious sign.
  - Clotting precedes bleeding and may have associated symptoms.
- Chronic DIC symptoms
  - Signs and symptoms may be absent.
  - Clotting may produce signs and symptoms.
- Signs and symptoms of bleeding (usually with acute DIC)
  - Skin and oral cavity symptoms
    - Pallor, sluggish capillary refill, and cool, clammy skin
    - Petechiae, purpura, and ecchymosis
    - Hematomas and epistaxis
    - Gingival or mucosal bleeding from the oral cavity
    - Acral cyanosis (i.e., generalized sweating with cold, mottled fingers and toes)
    - Bleeding ranging from oozing to frank hemorrhaging from any invasive site, including a wound, incision, injection site, and intravenous or central line
  - Respiratory symptoms
    - Shortness of breath, dyspnea, air hunger, hypoxia, and hemoptysis
    - Tachypnea
    - Abnormal lung sounds (e.g., crackles, rubs, wheezing), stridor, and accessory muscle use
  - Cardiovascular symptoms
    - Changes in vital signs: hypotension or tachycardia
    - Weak and thready pulse or narrow pulse pressure
    - Decreased peripheral pulses
    - Changes in color and temperature of extremities
    - Venous distention
    - Cardiac tamponade (e.g., muted heart sounds, hypotension, pulsus paradoxus, angina, palpitations)
  - Gastrointestinal symptoms
    - Hematemesis or coffee-ground emesis
    - Nausea, vomiting, anorexia, and weakness
    - Dysphagia
    - Abdominal tenderness, cramping, pain, or distention
    - Hyperactive or hypoactive bowel sounds
    - Diarrhea
    - Positive results for the guaiac stool test, frank blood in stool, or tarry stool
    - Hemorrhoids
  - Genitourinary and gynecologic symptoms
    - Hematuria (sometimes with a burning sensation), dysuria, frequency, and pain on urination
    - Decreased urinary output

- Renal failure
- Menorrhagia (e.g., heavily prolonged vaginal bleeding, suprapubic pain, cramping)
- Neurologic symptoms
  - Headache and vertigo
  - Mental status changes (e.g., restlessness, confusion, lethargy, obtundation, coma)
  - Changes in level of consciousness or pupil size and reactivity
  - Sensory or motor strength changes
  - Speech changes
  - Seizures
- Ocular symptoms
  - Scleral hemorrhage
  - Visual disturbances (e.g., blurring, diplopia, absent or altered fields of vision, nystagmus)
- Musculoskeletal symptoms
  - Warm, swollen, sore, or painful joints
  - Decreased mobility of joints (usually unilateral)
- Signs and symptoms of clotting
  - Cardiopulmonary symptoms (e.g., shortness of breath, chest pain with a pulmonary embolus)
  - Extremities (e.g., pain, warmth, swelling of extremity with deep vein thrombosis of the lower extremity)
  - Central nervous system (e.g., headache, speech changes, paralysis with stroke)
  - Renal compromise or failure with renal system clotting

Cancers Associated with Disorder

- Acute promyelocytic leukemia (APL), which is commonly associated with DIC
- Myeloproliferative diseases, including acute myelogenous leukemia (AML) and chronic myelogenous leukemia (CML)
- Lymphoproliferative diseases, including acute lymphoblastic leukemia (ALL), lymphomas (especially immunoblastic lymphoma and Hodgkin disease)
- Solid cancers such as mucin-secreting adenocarcinomas and prostate, lung, breast, stomach, biliary, colon, and ovarian cancers

Diagnostic Tests

- Primary laboratory tests for diagnosing DIC
  - Platelet count is usually decreased.
  - Fibrinogen level is usually decreased.
  - D-dimer assay (often combined with the FDP titer) value is increased.
  - FDP titer is increased.
- Coagulation tests (nonspecific in DIC)
  - Prothrombin time (PT) or international normalized ratio (INR) is usually prolonged or higher.
  - Activated partial thromboplastin time (aPTT) may be prolonged.
  - Thrombin time (TT) is usually prolonged.
- Laboratory tests to determine accelerated coagulation
  - Antithrombin III level is decreased.
  - Fibrinopeptide A level is increased.

- Prothrombin activation peptide level is increased.
- Thrombin-antithrombin complex concentration is increased.
- Laboratory tests to determine accelerated fibrinolysis
  - Plasminogen level is decreased.
  - α_2-Antiplasmin levels: decreased
- Laboratory tests to identify microvascular hemolysis
  - Numbers of schistocytes (i.e., RBC fragments) on a peripheral blood smear are increased in 25% to 50% of patients with DIC.
- Other tests to assist in diagnosis of DIC:
  - Hemoccult testing of stool, emesis, and nasogastric tube secretions
  - Urine dipstick testing for blood
  - Imaging studies are usually not indicated for DIC, except to identify an underlying cause.
    - Radiologic studies are used to assess internal bleeding or thrombosis.
    - Posteroanterior and lateral radiographs are used to rule out acute respiratory distress syndrome (ARDS).
    - Invasive studies should be preceded by administration of platelets and clotting factors and should be performed with caution due to the risk of bleeding.

Differential Diagnosis

- Massive blood loss
- Thrombotic microangiopathy (TMA)
- Heparin-induced thrombocytopenia (HIT)
- Vitamin K deficiency
- Sepsis, severe infection, or shock
- Malignancy or hematologic diseases
- Severe toxic or immunologic reaction
- Vascular disorders or stasis
- Acute liver disease or liver insufficiency
- Organ destruction or failure
- Pregnancy and obstetric complications
- ARDS

Treatment

- Treatment of the underlying or predisposing conditions causing DIC
- Support of the patient's hemodynamic status
- Management of the signs and symptoms related to bleeding or thrombosis
- For acute DIC, focus on oxygen and transfusion support for bleeding.
- For chronic DIC, focus on anticoagulants.

Pharmacologic Management

- Eliminate or treat the underlying condition to remove the trigger for DIC.
  - Administer chemotherapy if malignancy is the cause.
  - Administer antibiotics if infection is the cause.
  - Avoid medications that interfere with platelet function (e.g., nonsteroidal antiinflammatory drugs [NSAIDs], aspirin).

- Provide hemodynamic supportive care (usually for acute DIC and bleeding)
  - Administer fluid replacement to treat hypotension.
  - Use oxygen therapy to treat hypoxia.
  - Administer intravenous vasopressors (e.g., dopamine) to maintain blood pressure.
  - Administer diuretics or intravenous fluids to maintain central venous pressure.
- Use platelet transfusions.
  - Bleeding status of the patient determines the transfusion threshold.
  - For patients who are actively bleeding or at high risk of bleeding, the threshold for platelet transfusion is 50,000/mm^3.
  - Platelet transfusions may be indicated for patients who have a platelet count of 20,000/mm^3 with or without symptoms.
  - Target platelet count is 20,000 to 30,000/mm^3 for most patients with DIC or more than 50,000/mm^3 for patients who have intracranial or life-threatening hemorrhage.
- Use washed, packed red blood cells (RBCs).
  - Indicated if the patient has clinical symptoms of DIC or is actively bleeding and the hemoglobin level is less than 8 g/dL.
  - Goal is to maintain hemoglobin in range of 6 to 10 g/dL.
  - Washed, packed RBCs are preferred to whole blood because of fewer complications related to fluid overload and the immune response.
- Use fresh frozen plasma (FFP).
  - FFP contains all of the necessary coagulation factors and inhibitors.
  - FFP is used to replace factors that were depleted during active bleeding.
  - FFP should be given only to patients who are experiencing substantial bleeding and have prolonged PT and aPTT values.
  - There is no evidence that infusion of FFP stimulates the ongoing activation of coagulation.
- Use cryoprecipitate.
  - It contains fibrinogen, factor VIII, von Willebrand factor, factor XIII, and fibronectin.
  - It may correct severe fibrinogen deficiency that persists after FFP replacement.
  - Administer to patients with substantial active bleeding and severe hypofibrinogenemia (i.e., fibrinogen level that is consistently less than 80 to 100 mg/dL).
- Use prothrombin complex concentrate (PCC).
  - Consider PCC in actively bleeding patients if an FFP transfusion is not possible.
- Use intravenous or subcutaneous heparin.
  - Heparin is an anticoagulant that activates antithrombin and inhibits further thrombus formation.
  - It should be considered for patients with acute DIC who are bleeding despite ongoing appropriate treatment (e.g., blood product transfusions).

- It is commonly used in patients with chronic DIC in which thrombosis predominates (e.g., solid tumors).
- Consider only if a platelet count of 50,000/mm^3 or higher can be supported.
- If using unfractionated heparin, use a low-dose infusion (6 to 10 U/kg/hr) with no bolus dose.
- Contraindications include central nervous system disorders, diffuse gastrointestinal bleeding, open wounds, recent surgery (due to increased risk of hemorrhage), and obstetric complications that require surgical intervention.
- Do not administer to patients with APL because of the increased risk of death due to hemorrhage.
- Use fibrinolytic inhibitor medications.
  - They may be used to treat patients with excessive bleeding who have failed to respond to other treatments for DIC and when FDPs are thought to be inhibiting platelets.
  - Use ε-aminocaproic acid (Amicar) or tranexamic acid.
    - Antifibrinolytic agents inhibit the plasmin-plasminogen system.
    - The primary side effect is clotting, which can lead to organ failure from large vessel thrombosis.
    - They are rarely used to treat patients with DIC.
    - They may be considered for patients who have significant hemorrhage after transfusion of blood component therapy or for patients with strong fibrinolysis, such as those with APL and prostate cancer.
- Use the replacement product α$_2$-globulin.
  - It is derived from pooled human plasma and treated with heat to inactivate viruses.
  - Results of clinical trials are mixed, and additional studies are needed.
- Use of antithrombin III concentrates (AT III) is controversial.
  - They may be used to supplement low levels of AT III in cases of DIC.
- Use all-*trans* retinoic acid (ATRA), also known as *tretinoin therapy.*
  - ATRA causes the immature promyelocytes produced in APL to differentiate, which slows or stops the growth of the cancer cells.
  - The mortality rate for APL patients was substantially lower when using ATRA.
  - ATRA also has anticoagulant and antifibrinolytic effects.
  - Studies of APL patients with DIC who were treated with ATRA and tranexamic acid failed to show a reduction in bleeding, and the combination may result in severe thrombosis.
- Novel agents are used to treat DIC.
  - Recombinant tissue factor pathway inhibitor (rTFPI) inhibits the generation of thrombin from prothrombin, but it does not show an overall survival benefit.
  - Recombinant factor VII activated (rFVIIa) increases thrombin production to control ongoing hemorrhage in patients with DIC who are not responding to all other therapies. Further clinical studies are needed.
  - Recombinant human soluble thrombomodulin (rhTM) inhibits production of thrombin. Further clinical studies are needed.

Nonpharmacologic Management

- Monitor laboratory parameters (e.g., platelets, fibrinogen, PT, aPTT) every 6 hours for patients who are in the acute phase of DIC.
- Monitor hemodynamic signs and symptoms, vital signs, neurologic signs, and all sites of bleeding every 2 to 4 hours during the acute phase of DIC or as indicated.
- Monitor the amount of bleeding to determine the efficacy of therapeutic measures:
  - Count Peri-Pads.
  - Weigh affected dressings.
  - Measure bloody drainage.
- Monitor weights daily, and assess intake and output every 1 to 2 hours during the acute phase of DIC to check for dehydration or fluid overload.
- Measure abdominal girth every 4 hours if abdominal bleeding is suspected.
- Apply direct pressure or apply pressure dressings or sandbags to sites of active bleeding.
- Elevate sites of active bleeding if possible.

Patient Teaching

- Goals are to reverse the hypercoagulable state and maintain normal coagulation levels.
- Define DIC and differentiate between acute and chronic phases; describe the signs and symptoms of both.
- Explain the purpose of the laboratory tests, nursing care, and treatments for DIC.
- Teach patients self-care measures to maximize their safety:
  - Use an electric razor, not a straight-edged razor.
  - Maintain the bed in a low position with the side rails up.
  - Clear pathways in the room and hallway.
  - Minimize activities that could trigger bleeding; avoid contact sports and heavy lifting.
  - Take precautions against accidental bleeding because even minor scrapes or bumps can result in bleeding.
- Teach fall precautions if the patient is at risk for falls:
  - In the home, remove throw rugs and items that can obstruct the pathway.
  - Walk carefully and change positions gradually.
- Teach patients to avoid over-the-counter medications that may interfere with normal platelet function such as aspirin and NSAIDs (e.g., ibuprofen, naproxen sodium).
- Teach patients to minimize activities that contribute to development of additional clots and increase circulation in the lower extremities.
  - Avoid tight or restrictive clothing.
  - Use compression stockings to promote venous return.
  - Elevate legs when possible; do not sit with legs crossed or dangle feet on the side of the bed.
  - Do not use pillows under the knees or a knee gatch.
  - Instruct the patient to wiggle toes and feet and to rotate ankles, especially when in bed.
- Teach the patient and family to save urine, stool, and emesis for the nurse to check for blood.
- Teach the patient about critical signs and symptoms to report, such as bruising, red rash, headache, black stools, blood in

the urine or stools, and bleeding from the gums, nose, eyes, vagina, rectum, wound, or central venous catheter site.

Follow-up

- Patients in the acute phase of DIC often require hospitalization for close monitoring of signs and symptoms and laboratory results and for continuing treatment.
- Patients in the chronic phase of DIC may be carefully monitored in the outpatient setting.
  - Continue to monitor for signs and symptoms of DIC.
  - Monitor laboratory findings to determine whether DIC is continuing or resolving.
- Provide additional resources such as home equipment or assistance for severe complications of DIC (e.g., organ dysfunction) and activity limitations.
- Consult a hematologist if DIC is diagnosed during the initial evaluation or if bleeding continues despite therapy interventions.

Bibliography

Arruda, V. R., & High, K. A. (2012). Disseminated intravascular coagulation. In D. L. Longo, A. S. Fauci, D. L. Kasper, S. L. Hauser, J. L. Jameson, & J. Loscalzo (Eds.), *Harrison's principles of internal medicine* (18th ed.) (pp. 973–980). New York: McGraw-Hill Medical.

Becker, J. U., Kumar, A., Shaaban, H. S., & Wira, C. R. (2011). Disseminated intravascular coagulation in emergency medicine. Available at http://emedicine.medscape.com/article/779097-overview (accessed March 3, 2016).

Fogarty, P. F. (2013). Disorders of hemostasis II. In G. P. Rodgers, & N. S. Young (Eds.), *The Bethesda handbook of clinical hematology* (3rd ed.) (pp. 297–310). Philadelphia: Lippincott Williams & Wilkins.

Gobel, B. (2011). Disseminated intravascular coagulation. In C. H. Yarbro, D. Wujcik, & B. H. Gobel (Eds.), *Cancer nursing: Principles and practice* (7th ed.) (pp. 928–938). Burlington, MA: Jones & Bartlett.

Kaplan, M. (2013). Disseminated intravascular coagulation. In M. Kaplan (Ed.), *Understanding and managing oncological emergencies: A resource for nurses* (2nd ed.) (pp. 69–102). Pittsburgh, PA: Oncology Nursing Society.

Kitchens, C. S. (2009). Thrombocytopenia and thrombosis in disseminated intravascular coagulation (DIC). *Hematology, 1,* 240–246.

Kusuma, B., & Schulz, T. K. (2009). Acute disseminated intravascular coagulation. *Hospital Physician, 45*(3), 35–40.

Levi, M., Toh, C. H., Thachil, J., & Waton, H. G. (2009). Guidelines for the diagnosis and management of disseminated intravascular coagulation. *British Journal of Haematology, 145,* 24–33.

Maloney, K. W. (2015). Metabolic emergencies. In J. J. Itano, J. M. Brant, F. A. Conde, & M. G. Saria (Eds.), *Core curriculum for oncology nursing* (5th ed.) (pp. 478–494). St. Louis: Elsevier.

Venugopal, A. (2014). Disseminated intravascular coagulation. *Indian Journal of Anaesthesia, 58*(5), 603–608.

Wada, H., Thachil, J., di Nisio, M., Mathew, P., Kurosawa, S., Gando, S., & Toh, C. H. (2013). Guidance for diagnosis and treatment of disseminated intravascular coagulation from harmonization of the recommendations from three guidelines. *Journal of Thrombosis and Haemostasis, 11,* 761–767.

Walker, D. K. (2014). Disseminated intravascular coagulation. In D. Camp-Sorrell, & R. A. Hawkins (Eds.), *Clinical manual for the oncology advanced practice nurse* (3rd ed.) (pp. 1001–1010). Pittsburgh, PA: Oncology Nursing Society.

Hemolytic Uremic Syndrome

Definition

- HUS is a rare blood clotting disorder involving TMA, which is potentially life-threatening.
- Typical HUS, also referred to as diarrhea-associated HUS, is a syndrome of MAHA, thrombocytopenia, and acute renal failure, with a diarrhea prodrome caused by infection with Shiga toxin–producing bacteria (e.g., *Escherichia coli*).
- Atypical HUS is a syndrome of MAHA, thrombocytopenia, and acute renal failure without a diarrhea prodrome.

Epidemiology

- Typical HUS (90% to 95% of cases)
  - Most cases in previously healthy children (<5 years old); some adult cases
  - Usually epidemic
  - Usually occurs as a single episode
- Atypical HUS (5% to 10% of cases)
  - Manifests in early childhood; some cases in older adults
  - May be sporadic or familial
  - Children and adults often have recurrent episodes.
- Therapy-related HUS
  - May occur after recent (<200 days) hematopoietic stem cell transplantation (HSCT) or use of TMA-associated drugs (e.g., cyclosporine)
  - Incidence in patients with cancer estimated to be about 5%
  - Delayed and potentially fatal complication after HSCT
- Factors increasing the risk of HUS
  - Infections, particularly infections with the Shiga toxin–producing *E. coli* (STEC) and pneumococcal infection
  - Disorders of the complement system
  - Disorders interfering with the degradation of von Willebrand factor (VWF)
  - High-dose chemotherapy conditioning regimens (e.g., HSCT)
  - Graft rejection after HSCT
  - Chemotherapy regimens, especially with mitomycin C
  - Immunosuppressant drugs (e.g., cyclosporine, tacrolimus)
  - Immune disorders such as SLE and acquired immunodeficiency syndrome (AIDS)
  - Pregnancy, hemolysis, or HELLP syndrome (i.e., hemolysis, elevated liver enzymes, and low platelets)
  - Elevated levels of liver enzymes

Pathophysiology

- Typical HUS (diarrhea-positive HUS)
  - Frequently associated with diarrhea and acute renal failure
  - Caused by infections with Shiga toxin–producing *E. coli* (especially serotype O157:H7)
  - Shiga toxin–producing bacteria cause hemorrhagic enterocolitis manifested by abdominal pain and bloody diarrhea.
  - Bloody diarrhea occurs as a result of toxin-induced colonic epithelial cell injury. When the Shiga toxin enters the bloodstream, neutrophils and monocytes transport it to the kidneys.
  - Shiga toxin binds to and activates platelets. It promotes platelet aggregation by directly damaging renal endothelial cells or by other mechanisms.
  - Tissue factor is released, which renders the vessel wall prothrombotic.
  - Overall prognosis is good, and renal function usually recovers.

- Atypical HUS (diarrhea-negative HUS)
  - A chronic, often progressive disease
  - Not associated with the Shiga toxin or diarrhea
  - Commonly caused by dysregulation of the complement system, resulting in uncontrolled complement activation
  - Sporadic form triggered by complement disorders, disorders interfering with the degradation of VWF, pregnancy, *Streptococcus pneumoniae*, drugs (e.g., cyclosporine), and diseases (e.g., SLE, AIDS)
  - The familial form results from inherited mutations of genes (e.g., *CFH*, *DGKE*) that encode complement regulatory proteins (e.g., factor H, factor I, membrane cofactor protein) involved in the alternative pathway.
  - The familial form is rare but associated with a significant risk of morbidity and mortality.
  - The recurrent atypical HUS subgroup has a strong association with diseases of the complement system, and the prognosis is poor; acute renal failure and death occur in 54% of cases.
  - Patients often have end-stage renal disease and require a kidney transplant.
  - Patients in this subgroup commonly have severe arterial hypertension and require multidrug therapy.
- The trigger for HUS is endothelial damage.
  - Can be caused by defects in the complement system, which acts as a central defense of innate immunity
  - Endothelial damage leads to platelet aggregation, thrombocytopenia, and subsequent renal, neurologic, and pulmonary dysfunction.
  - Renal vasculature is primarily affected, often resulting in irreversible renal damage in patients with atypical HUS.
- TTP and HUS
  - Although TTP and HUS are distinct diseases with different causes and demographics, many patients are inaccurately diagnosed with "TTP-HUS disorder" on the basis of clinical and laboratory findings only.
  - Many clinical features of cancer-associated TTP and HUS overlap:
    - Localized microvascular thrombosis
    - MAHA
    - Thrombocytopenia
    - Neurologic or renal abnormalities
  - Several factors differentiate TTP from HUS:
    - Congenital TTP is caused by inherited deficiencies of the von Willebrand factor–cleaving metalloprotease ADAMTS13, and the classic form is caused by acquisition of antibodies to the protein. Secondary TTP may result from endothelial cell damage due to infection, drugs, or malignancy.
    - ADAMTS13 does not play a role in HUS.
    - A history of bone marrow transplantation (BMT) or Shiga toxin–associated hemorrhagic colitis suggests HUS.
    - The clinical presentation of TTP is dominated by hemorrhages and neurologic symptoms. Renal involvement (e.g., proteinuria, microscopic hematuria) is common, but oliguric acute renal failure is unusual.
    - In patients with HUS, acute renal impairment or failure is the dominant clinical feature.
    - For idiopathic TTP, plasma exchange is highly effective treatment, but for typical HUS, plasma exchange is usually ineffective.

Signs and Symptoms

- Typical HUS signs and symptoms
  - Intense abdominal pain
  - Diarrhea (often overtly bloody)
  - Renal insufficiency (i.e., oliguria) in all patients
  - Hypertension and swelling
  - Petechiae, easy bruising, or bleeding due to thrombocytopenia; occurs in 70% of patients and is absent or mild in 30%
  - MAHA
  - Shortness of breath, tachycardia, pale skin, or weakness that may correlate with the degree of anemia, which occurs in most patients
  - Neurologic symptoms resulting from cerebral edema or leukoencephalopathy
- Atypical HUS signs and symptoms
  - No symptoms of abdominal pain or overt bloody diarrhea
  - Renal impairment or failure (e.g., oliguria, anuria) in all patients
  - Hypertension and swelling
  - MAHA
  - Shortness of breath, tachycardia, pale skin, or weakness that may correlate with the degree of anemia, which occurs in most patients
  - Various degrees of petechiae, easy bruising, or bleeding due to thrombocytopenia
  - Neurologic symptoms such as seizures, loss of vision, loss of balance, confusion, and nystagmus
- Among bone marrow transplant recipients, onset of HUS typically occurs 30 to 875 days after the procedure and manifests with a triad of symptoms:
  - MAHA: hematuria and fatigue
  - Renal insufficiency with increased creatinine, reduced creatinine clearance, and fluid retention
  - Thrombocytopenia with increased bleeding or hemorrhaging

Cancers Associated with Disorder

- Adenocarcinomas, including gastric cancer, lung cancer, and breast cancer
- Lymphoma

Diagnostic Tests

- Diagnostic criteria for HUS
  - MAHA
  - Thrombocytopenia

- Acute renal failure
- Possible diarrhea
- Laboratory tests
  - Complete blood count (CBC) with a platelet count
    - Anemia, with an average hemoglobin of 7 to 9 g/dL
    - Thrombocytopenia with a platelet count less than 20,000 cells/mm^3
  - Diagnostic criteria for MAHA
    - Schistocytes in the peripheral blood smear (>1%, or >3 schistocytes per high-power microscopic field)
    - Positive markers for hemolytic anemia include an increased reticulocyte count, increased bilirubin level (mainly indirect reacting), and decreased serum haptoglobin levels. Increased levels of free plasma hemoglobin are seen in severe cases.
    - Elevated reticulocyte counts
  - Renal function test results, including blood urea nitrogen (BUN) and serum creatinine, are usually elevated.
  - Diarrhea assessment
    - Positive stool culture for *E. coli* (serotype O157:H7)
    - Positive for antibody to Shiga toxin
  - Comprehensive metabolic panel
    - Elevated lactate dehydrogenase (LDH) level due to hemolysis
    - Elevated electrolyte levels due to renal impairment
    - Elevated serum bilirubin level
  - Serum level of ADAMT[?]S13 is usually normal (≥67%) in persons with HUS.
  - Coombs test
    - Negative result: nonautoimmune, nondrug-induced hemolytic anemia
    - Positive result: autoimmune, drug-induced hemolytic anemia
  - Coagulation tests
    - Usually normal values for PT, aPTT, factor V, factor VIII, and fibrinogen
    - FDP level may be elevated.
    - Thrombin time may be prolonged.
  - Troponin T or troponin I levels to rule out cardiac involvement
  - Liver function tests to rule out liver involvement (usually normal)
  - Blood type and screen tests to prepare for provision of blood products
  - Hepatitis A, B, or C and human immunodeficiency virus (HIV) testing of blood products to exclude an underlying viral precipitant
  - Blood or urine cultures to identify infection as an underlying cause of HUS
  - Urinalysis, with proteinuria, microscopic hematuria, and granular or red cell casts as the most consistent findings
- Radiologic evaluation
  - Renal sonogram or renal angiogram
  - Intravenous pyelogram
  - CT of the abdomen to determine kidney involvement
  - CT of the chest, abdomen, and pelvis with or without tumor markers to assess for underlying malignancy
  - Electrocardiogram (ECG) or echocardiogram to document or monitor cardiac damage

Differential Diagnosis

- Classic or cancer-associated TTP
- MAHA
- Hematuria related to other diseases (e.g., infection, intrinsic kidney disease, benign prostatic hypertrophy)
- Hematuria related to medications (e.g., ifosfamide, high-dose cyclophosphamide, intravesical chemotherapy)
- Hematuria related to radiation therapy (e.g., pelvic irradiation, prostate seed implants)
- Systemic malignancy as a cause of thrombocytopenia and MAHA without signs of DIC
- Malignant hypertension as a cause thrombocytopenia, MAHA, renal failure, and severe neurologic abnormalities
- Autoimmune disorders may be indistinguishable from TTP (e.g., autoimmune hemolysis or Evans syndrome, acute scleroderma, lupus nephritis). Some patients have an autoimmune disorder (e.g., SLE, antiphospholipid antibody syndrome) and TTP.
- Systemic infection, typically viral (e.g., CMV, adenovirus, herpes simplex virus) or severe bacterial (e.g., meningococcus, pneumococcus) but may be fungal
- Vasculitis
- DIC
- HIT
- Drugs (e.g., quinine, simvastatin, interferon)
- Graft-versus-host disease (GVHD), veno-occlusive disease (VOD), diffuse alveolar hemorrhage (DAH), or CMV in persons undergoing BMT
- Pregnancy-associated conditions such as preeclampsia or HELLP syndrome can cause MAHA, thrombocytopenia, renal failure, and minor neurologic abnormalities.

Treatment

- Typical HUS (diarrhea-positive HUS)
  - Symptomatic treatment
    - Hemodialysis
    - Blood pressure control medications
    - Fluid management: Although persons with HUS may be dehydrated, fluids are given judiciously due to risk of kidney impairment.
    - Blood transfusions to treat anemia
  - Avoid antibiotics, antimotility agents, and opioids, which are associated worsening of disease
  - Avoid NSAIDs, which can decrease renal blood flow
- Atypical HUS (diarrhea-negative HUS)
  - Plasma exchanges, which benefit about one third of children, except for the subgroup with membrane cofactor protein mutations
  - Terminal complement inhibitor eculizumab

Pharmacologic Management

- Prevention
  - Vigorous pretransplantation parenteral or oral hydration
  - Continuous bladder irrigation with normal saline solution

- Management
  - Plasma exchange is less effective in HUS, with response rates of 20% to 30%, compared with response rates of 80% in classic TTP
  - Plasma infusion
    - Pathogen-reduced FFP is preferred.
    - Repetitive plasma infusions increase the risk of infection. Initially, the recommended volume is 60 to 65 mL/kg/week.
    - During maintenance, the recommended volume is 20 mL/kg/week.
  - Medication
    - For atypical HUS, treatment with eculizumab, a terminal complement inhibitor, has been successful.
    - For typical HUS, eculizumab may be effective in treating patients with diarrhea-positive HUS.
  - Cobalamin supplementation
  - Immunization program (including hepatitis A and B)
  - Discontinue administration of drugs that may be inducing the HUS (e.g., chemotherapy, immunosuppressants).
  - Platelet transfusions are contraindicated because they can worsen microvascular thrombi.

Nonpharmacologic Management

- Nephrology consultation to determine the most appropriate renal therapy
- Renal replacement therapy
  - May include peritoneal dialysis and hemodialysis
  - May be successful for patients with recurrent atypical HUS
  - Failure rate about 70% for renal transplantation complicated by recurrence of disease
  - Kidney transplantation not recommended for patients with soluble complement disorders
- Liver transplantation
  - Combined renal and liver transplantation is a logical form of treatment because factors H and I are synthesized in the liver.
  - Transplantation is not recommended for persons with complement disorders.

Patient Teaching

- Goals
  - Blood cell counts return to normal levels.
  - Symptoms (e.g., bleeding, renal abnormalities) subside.
- Define HUS, and describe its signs and symptoms.
- Explain the purpose of the laboratory tests, nursing care, and treatments for HUS.
- Encourage the patient to drink 8 to 10 glasses of fluid daily if kidney function is adequate.
- The patient should report increased bleeding, blood in the urine, and renal symptoms (e.g., decreased urine output, swelling in extremities).
- Provide patients with written material on HUS.
- Teach patients self-care measures to maximize their safety:
  - Use an electric razor, not a straight-edged razor.
  - Maintain the bed in a low position with the side rails up.
  - Clear pathways in the room and hallway.
  - Minimize activities that can trigger bleeding.
  - Avoid contact sports and lifting.
  - Take precautions against accidental bleeding because even minor scrapes or bumps can cause bleeding.
- Teach fall precautions if the patient remains at risk for falls.
  - In the home, remove throw rugs and items that can obstruct pathways.
  - Wear shoes that fit appropriately.
  - Walk carefully, and change positions gradually.
- Teach patients to avoid over-the-counter medications that may interfere with normal platelet function such as aspirin and NSAIDs (e.g., ibuprofen, naproxen sodium).
- Teach patients to minimize activities that contribute to development of additional clots and to increase circulation in the lower extremities:
  - Avoid tight or restrictive clothing.
  - Use compression stockings to promote venous return.
  - Elevate legs when possible.
  - Do not sit with legs crossed.
  - Do not dangle feet on the side of the bed.
  - Do not use pillows under the knees or a knee gatch.
- Instruct patients to wiggle toes and feet and to rotate ankles, especially when in bed.
- Teach the patient and family to save urine, stool, and emesis for the nurse to check for blood.
- Teach the patient about critical signs and symptoms and to report bruising, red rash, headache, black stools, blood in the urine or stools, and bleeding from the gums, nose, eyes, vagina, rectum, wound, or central venous catheter site.

Follow-up

- Continue to monitor for signs and symptoms of HUS.
- Monitor appropriate laboratory findings (especially platelet count and hemoglobin or hematocrit) to determine the continuation or resolution of HUS.
- Provide additional resources such as home equipment or assistance as needed.
- Monitor bone marrow transplant recipients treated with high-dose chemotherapy for potential long-term sequelae.

Bibliography

Gulleroglu, K., Fidan, K., Hancer, V. S., Bayrakci, U., Baskin, E., & Soylemezoglu, O. (2013). Neurological involvement in atypical hemolytic uremic syndrome and successful treatment with eculizumab. *Pediatric Nephrology, 28,* 827–830.

Legendre, C. M., Licht, C., Muus, P., Greenbaum, L. A., Babu, S., Bedrosian, C., & Loirat, C. (2013). Terminal complement inhibitor eculizumab in atypical hemolytic-uremic syndrome. *New England Journal of Medicine, 368,* 2169–2181.

Lemaire, M., Fremeaux-Bacchi, V., Schaefer, F., Choi, M., Tang, W. H., Le Quintrec, M., & Rioux-Leclerc, N. (2013). Recessive mutations in DGKE cause atypical hemolytic-uremic syndrome. *Nature Genetics, 45,* 531–536.

Loirat, C., & Fremeaux-Bacchi, V. (2011). Atypical hemolytic uremic syndrome. *Orphanet Journal of Rare Diseases, 6,* 60.

Mele, C., Remuzzi, G., & Noris, M. (2014). Hemolytic uremic syndrome. In P. Ronco & J. Floege (Eds.), *Seminars in immunopathology (36)4* (pp. 399–420).

Noel, P., & Jaben, E. A. (2013). Consultative hematology. In G. P. Rodgers & N. S. Young (Eds.), *The Bethesda handbook of clinical hematology* (3rd ed.) (pp. 389–404). Philadelphia: Lippincott Williams & Wilkins.

Punnoose, A. R., Lynm, C., & Golub, R. M. (2012). JAMA patient page: Hemolytic uremic syndrome. *Journal of the American Medical Association, 308*(18), 1934.

Rodriguez, A. L. (2014). Bleeding and thrombotic complications. In C. Yarbro, D. Wujcik, & B. H. Gobel (Eds.), *Cancer symptom management* (4th ed.) (pp. 287–316). Sudbury, MA: Jones & Bartlett.

Scully, M., Hunt, B. J., Benjamin, S., Liesner, R., Rose, P., Peyvandi, F., & Machin, S. J. (2012). Guidelines on the diagnosis and management of thrombotic thrombocytopenic purpura and other thrombotic microangiopathies. *British Journal of Haematology, 158,* 323–335.

Pulmonary Embolism

Definition

- Pulmonary embolism (PE) is partial or complete occlusion of blood flow in the pulmonary artery or one of its branches by an embolus.
- PE is a life-threatening complication of DVT.

Epidemiology

- DVT is the most preventable cause of death for hospitalized or recently hospitalized patients.
  - Approximately 10% of all hospital deaths are attributable to PE.
  - An estimated 100,000 cases of fatal PE occur yearly.
  - PE contributes to the deaths of another 100,000 patients in the United States.
- Two most common types of DVT
  - DVT of the lower extremities
  - PE
- In patients with cancer, DVT is the second leading cause of death.
- In the United States, the number of deaths attributed to PE is more than the number of deaths due to AIDS and breast cancer combined.
- Up to 80% of emboli are small and clinically undetectable because the pulmonary circulation has several sources of collateral flow.
- Pulmonary infarction occurs in 10% to 15% of cases, usually in persons with cardiopulmonary disease, and a high mortality rate is associated with large or multiple emboli.
- Increased risk for DVT is based on the 2014 National Comprehensive Cancer Network (NCCN) guidelines.
  - Individual risk factors
    - Obesity (body mass index ≥30 kg/m²)
    - Prior DVT or blood clotting disorders
    - Central venous access device or pacemaker
    - Associated diseases (e.g., cardiac disease, chronic renal disease, diabetes, acute infection) and immobilization
    - General surgery with any anesthesia or trauma
    - Use of erythropoietin
  - Myeloma-related risk factors
    - Diagnosis of myeloma
    - Hyperviscosity
  - Therapy with thalidomide or lenalidomide in combination with doxorubicin, multiagent chemotherapy, or high-dose dexamethasone (≥480 mg/month)
  - Alternative diagnosis as likely as DVT (score of −2)
  - Recommended prophylactic treatment is based on numbers and types of risk factors.
    - Score of 0 or 1, individual or myeloma risk factors: 81 to 325 mg of aspirin once daily.

- Score of 2 or more, individual or myeloma risk factors or for multiple myeloma treatment as outlined previously: LMWH (equivalent to 40 mg of enoxaparin once daily) or full-dose warfarin (i.e., target INR of 2 to 3)
- Other risk factors for PE
  - Cancer, which can cause a hypercoagulable state
    - Very high risk if the primary cancer site is the stomach or pancreas
    - High risk for lymphoma and gynecologic, bladder, testicular, and lung cancers
  - Blood viscosity determinants
  - Prechemotherapy platelet count of 350 × 10⁹/L or higher
    - Prechemotherapy leukocyte count higher than 11 × 10⁹/L
    - Heart rate greater than 100 beats per minute
  - Recent surgery or immobilization
  - Hemoptysis
  - Hypercoagulable state (e.g., DIC)
  - Conditions with local clotting such as phlebitis, trauma, and inflammation
  - Conditions that promote venous stasis such as prolonged bed rest; prolonged immobility resulting from pain, trauma, surgery, or paralysis; recent casting of a lower extremity (within 4 weeks); and general debility
  - Peripheral vascular disease
  - Medications such as antiestrogens (e.g., tamoxifen, raloxifene), estrogen, thalidomide, lenalidomide, and RBC growth factors (e.g., erythropoietin)
  - Medications that induce endothelial damage such as chemotherapy (especially adjuvant therapy for breast cancer), some vasopressor agents (e.g., dopamine), contrast medium, and high-dose antibiotics
  - Burns or fractures that cause vessel damage
  - Use of a central venous catheter
  - Antiphospholipid antibodies (associated with SLE)

Pathophysiology

- See DVT pathophysiology regarding clot formation.
- PE is a life-threatening complication of DVT.
  - When the blood clot is detached from the original source, the embolus travels with the blood flow.
  - The embolus may also be a fat globule, air, tumor, amniotic fluid, other tissue fragment, clumped bacteria, or a foreign body.
  - The embolism may migrate from a distal vein to the inferior vena cava, right atrium, right ventricle, and enter the pulmonary artery.
  - A very large embolus may lodge in the main pulmonary artery, and smaller emboli pass to more distal branches of the pulmonary artery.
  - When the embolus lodges in the pulmonary artery or one of its branches, it can cause partial or total occlusion of the vessel.
- PE may result from mechanical occlusion of a regional pulmonary artery.
  - Perfusion and ventilation changes occur in the section of lung supplied by the artery.
  - Lung volumes and compliance are usually reduced.

- Pulmonary shunting may cause hypoxia.
- Pulmonary artery pressure may become elevated.
- If the PE is massive, the right ventricle may be unable to generate enough pressure to maintain adequate cardiac output.
- Right ventricular failure can increase right arterial pressure, and cardiogenic shock can ensue.

Signs and Symptoms

- Clinical manifestations of PE depend on the size of the embolus and the patient's preexisting cardiopulmonary status.
- Up to 75% of PE cases have no initial observable symptoms. When emboli are small, there may be few or no symptoms.
- Consider a diagnosis of PE for patients who have the three most frequent signs:
  - Dyspnea (usually with a sudden onset) which can vary from mild to severe and from intermittent to progressive
  - Chest pain (often anginal type at onset) that worsens with deep breathing and later becomes pleuritic
  - Tachypnea (respiratory rate >24 breaths/min)
- Less frequent signs of PE
  - Cough, hemoptysis (usually a later symptom), and bloody sputum
  - Low-grade fever
  - Syncope
  - Diaphoresis
  - Nonpleuritic chest pain
  - Apprehension, anxiety, and restlessness
  - Respiratory crackles or rales, diminished breath sounds, and wheezing
  - Hypotension, tachycardia, cyanosis, and pleural rub
  - Back or abdominal pain, lower extremity pain, tenderness, or swelling
  - Thrombophlebitis symptoms: warmth, erythema, and palpable, cordlike veins
- Because it can be difficult to diagnose with tests, the clinical presentation is important in guiding management.
- Acute right ventricular failure, systemic hypotension, and sudden death may occur in patients with a massive PE.

Cancers Associated with Disorder

- SCLC, NSCLC
- Colorectal cancer, pancreatic tumors, and mucin-secreting gastrointestinal tumors
- Ovarian and endometrial carcinomas
- Intracranial carcinoma
- APL, multiple myeloma, and myeloproliferative disorders
- Breast carcinoma
- Prostate carcinoma
- Bladder carcinoma

Diagnostic Tests

- Laboratory tests
  - CBC with a platelet count
  - PT and aPTT
  - Liver and kidney function tests

- Radiologic workup
  - Chest radiograph
  - Elevation of a hemidiaphragm and pulmonary infiltrates are most commonly identified in patients with PE.
  - Findings are often determined to be abnormal, but they are frequently related to a history of chronic obstructive pulmonary disease (COPD) or cardiac disease rather than PE.
  - ECG
  - Tachycardia and nonspecific ST-T wave changes are most often observed but are not diagnostic for PE.
  - Computed tomography angiography (CTA)
    - CTA is used to assess for right ventricular enlargement or dysfunction.
    - If negative, evaluate for other causes.
    - If positive, initiate treatment for PE.
  - Pulmonary angiography
    - Angiography is rarely used unless coupled with clot extraction or thrombolytic therapy.
    - If negative, evaluate for other causes.
    - If positive, initiate treatment for PE.
  - Ventilation-perfusion ($\dot{V}/\dot{Q}$) lung scan
    - The scan is used if the patient has renal insufficiency or an uncorrectable allergy to contrast.
    - A normal scan rules out clinical PE; evaluate for other causes.
    - A low or intermediate result indicates a possible PE.
    - In conjunction with clinical signs, this test definitively indicates the need for immediate treatment of PE.

Differential Diagnosis

- Myocardial infarction, congestive heart failure, pericardial tamponade, or dissecting aortic aneurysm
- Infection (e.g., pneumonia, pneumonitis, pleuritis, pericarditis, endocarditis)
- Pneumothorax, pleural effusions (PE can lead to pleural effusions), pulmonary fibrosis, or COPD
- Superior vena cava syndrome
- Gastrointestinal abnormalities (e.g., esophageal rupture, ulcers, gastritis)
- Anxiety disorder with hyperventilation

Treatment

- Surgical placement of an inferior vena cava (IVC) filter to prevent PE in recurrent DVT is advocated for patients who have a contraindication to anticoagulants.
  - Procedure uses an endoluminal filter to interrupt blood flow through the inferior vena cava.
  - A retrievable filter is preferred.
- Thrombectomy or embolectomy (rare) is performed as a surgical procedure or as a catheter technique under radiographic guidance.
- Consider removal of the catheter for catheter-related DVT.

Pharmacologic Management

- Prevention
  - The goal is to prevent DVTs so PE does not occur.
  - For cancer patients with one or no individual/myeloma risk factors (NCCN, 2014) or for low-risk myeloma

patients, aspirin (81 to 325 mg) may be administered once daily.

- For patients with cancer and two or more individual or myeloma risk factors or who are receiving myeloma treatment (NCCN, 2014)
  - LMWH equivalent to 40 mg of enoxaparin once daily or
  - Full-dose warfarin (target INR of 2 to 3)
- Inpatient and outpatient prophylactic anticoagulation treatment (NCCN, 2014) includes the following:
  - LMWH: category 1 for inpatients includes 40 mg of enoxaparin (Lovenox) given subcutaneously daily or 5000 units of dalteparin (Fragmin) given subcutaneously daily.
  - Fondaparinux (Arixtra): category 1 for inpatients is 2.5 mg given subcutaneously daily.
  - Unfractionated heparin: category 1 for inpatients is 5000 units given subcutaneously every 8 to 12 hours.
  - Aspirin dose of 81 to 325 mg given once daily
  - Warfarin (Coumadin) adjusted to an INR of 2 to 3
- Management of PE
  - Anticoagulant therapy
    - Interrupts thrombosis and allows the lytic system to dissolve the clot
    - PE usually responds to treatment.
    - Unfractionated heparin is the traditional standard for initial treatment of PE because of its rapid onset of action.
    - Novel anticoagulant agents include the synthetic factor Xa inhibitors such as fondaparinux (Arixtra) and rivaroxaban (Xarelto).
    - Vitamin K antagonists (e.g., warfarin) are oral agents that are used for long-term anticoagulation after thromboembolism occurs and for secondary prophylaxis. Agents may be initiated concurrently with heparin.
  - Therapeutic anticoagulation treatment for venous thromboembolism constitutes acute management (NCCN, 2014).
    - LMWH (preferred): 1 mg/kg of enoxaparin (Lovenox) given subcutaneously every 12 hours or 200 units/kg of dalteparin (Fragmin) given subcutaneously daily.
    - Fondaparinux (Arixtra): 5 mg (patients <50 kg); 7.5 mg (patients 50 to 100 kg); or 10 mg (patients >100 kg) given subcutaneously daily.
    - Unfractionated heparin: 80 units/kg load given intravenously and then 18 units/kg per hour; target aPTT of 2 to 2.5 times the control value or per hospital standards.
    - Unfractionated heparin as a 333-U/kg load is given subcutaneously; a dose of 250 U/kg is then given every 12 hours.
  - Therapeutic anticoagulation treatment for venous thromboembolism constitutes chronic management (NCCN, 2014):
    - LMWH (category 1): preferred for the first 6 months as monotherapy without warfarin in patients with proximal DVT or PE and prevention of recurrent DVT in patients with advanced or metastatic cancer
    - Warfarin (2.5 to 5 mg every day initially; subsequent dosing based on INR value, with a target INR of 2 to 3)
  - Duration of anticoagulation (NCCN, 2014)
    - Minimum time of 3 months
    - Indefinite anticoagulation recommended for active cancer or persistent risk factors
    - For catheter-associated thrombosis, anticoagulate while the catheter is in place.

Nonpharmacologic Management

- Bed rest for the first 5 to 7 days with leg elevation for acute DVT and PE.
- Frequent leg exercises (i.e., ROM or isometric) if bedridden
  - Every 1 to 2 hours while awake to improve venous flow
  - Includes heel pumping and ankle circles for 10 to 12 repetitions
- Mild analgesics and warm compresses may be used for the comfort of persons with acute DVT and acute PE.
- Supplemental oxygen by nasal cannula may be administered to maintain a Pao_2 higher than 80 mm Hg in persons with acute DVT and acute PE.
- Frequent ambulation if tolerable after 5 to 7 days of bed rest
- Antiembolic stockings or hose should be applied before surgery.
- Pneumatic compression stockings or devices may be used postoperatively to stimulate circulation and prevent DVT and PE.
- Elevation of the foot of the bed by 15 to 20 inches with slight knee flexion. Leg elevation should not exceed 45 degrees.
- Avoid popliteal pressure, which is produced by crossing the legs, placing pillows behind the knees, and elevation of the knee gatch.
- Do not massage the legs of persons with DVT or PE.
- Regular position changes should be encouraged to prevent hypoventilation.
- Avoid smoking and caffeine to prevent vasoconstriction.
- Maintain adequate hydration.
- Do not perform the Homans test after DVT is diagnosed or the test result is positive.

Patient Teaching

- Goals
  - Stimulate the patient's circulation.
  - Prevent additional DVTs.
  - Avoid injury and bleeding while on anticoagulation therapy.
  - Prevent respiratory compromise.
  - Resolve PEs.
- Teach patients
  - To report signs and/ symptom of DVT
    - Leg pain or swelling
    - Other signs of subsequent or/ recurrent DVT
    - Signs of thrombophlebitis or PE

- To report bleeding if they are on anticoagulation therapy
- Purpose of laboratory and diagnostic tests, nursing care, and treatments for DVT
- Teach the patient ways to stimulate the circulation to prevent DVT.
  - Change position regularly,
  - Move the toes, feet, and legs often.
  - Avoid sitting or standing for long periods.
  - Avoid constrictive clothing or devices.
  - Perform ROM or isometric exercises.
  - Wear the pneumatic compression stockings or devices as ordered.
- Teach the patient other strategies to prevent DVT.
  - Ambulate soon after surgery.
  - Drink 8 to 10 glasses of fluid per day.
  - Avoid smoking and caffeine intake.
  - Keep the legs elevated and straight.
  - Avoid pressure on the back of the knees (i.e., popliteal area) to prevent a clot from forming.
- Teach the patient bleeding precautions and ways to avoid injury and bleeding while on anticoagulant therapy.
  - Avoid any contact sports that could lead to serious injury.
  - Use a soft toothbrush for oral care.
  - Avoid substances that can irritate the tissues of the mouth and gums such as hot or spicy foods, alcoholic beverages, and mouthwashes that contain alcohol.
  - Use an electric razor if there is a need to shave.
  - Avoid vigorous nose blowing; clean nares with a cotton swab or tissue.
  - To prevent nosebleeds, use saline nose drops and sprays and a small amount of moisturizing ointment (e.g., petroleum jelly) inside the nostrils.
  - Check the home for environmental hazards, and identify and remove bump and fall risks (e.g., throw rugs, clutter from rooms and pathways). Wear shoes or slippers to protect the feet.
- Teach the patient ways to prevent respiratory compromise.
  - Ambulate frequently.
  - Use incentive spirometry.
- Teach the patient how to administer medications and to understand the side effects.
  - Patients need to understand the blood count monitoring that is required for the medications.
  - Patients on warfarin need to take the medication at the same time every day.
  - Patients taking subcutaneously administered medications (e.g., LMWH) may need to know how to do so at home.
- Teach the patient on warfarin to maintain a diet consistent in the amount of vitamin K.
  - Foods that are high in vitamin K: green leafy vegetables (e.g., spinach, kale) and liver
  - Foods that contain small amounts of vitamin K: milk, meats, eggs, cereal, fruits, and vegetables
  - Recommended daily allowances of vitamin K are 80 μg/day for men and 65 μg/day for women.
  - Patients should not take supplemental vitamin K because it improves blood clotting.

Follow-up

- Continue to monitor for signs and symptoms of subsequent or recurrent DVT or PE.
- Monitor laboratory findings to determine the continuation or resolution of DVT or PE.
- Provide additional resources such as home equipment or assistance to address the severe complications of DVT (e.g., PE).
- Refer the patient for nutritional counseling about vitamin K in the diet if needed.

Bibliography

Büller, H. R., Prins, M. H., Lensing, A. W., Decousus, H., Jacobson, B. F., Minar, E., & Segers, A. (2012). Oral rivaroxaban for the treatment of symptomatic pulmonary embolism. *New England Journal of Medicine, 366*(14), 1287–1297.

Davies, M. (2014). Pulmonary embolism. In D. Camp-Sorrell & R. A. Hawkins (Eds.), *Clinical manual for the oncology advanced practice nurse* (3rd ed.) (pp. 273–280). Pittsburgh, PA: Oncology Nursing Society.

Institute for Clinical Systems Improvement. (2016). Venous thromboembolism diagnosis and treatment: Guideline summary. Available at https://www.icsi.org/guidelines__more/catalog_guidelines_and_more/catalog_guidelines/catalog_cardiovascular_guidelines/vte_treatment/ (accessed March 14, 2016).

Khorana, A. A. (2009). Cancer and thrombosis: Implications of published guidelines for clinical practice. *Annals of Oncology, 20*, 1619–1630.

Kuderer, N. M., Ortel, T. L., & Francis, C. W. (2009). Impact of venous thromboembolism and anticoagulation on cancer and cancer survival. *Journal of Clinical Oncology, 27*, 4902–4911.

Manasanch, E. E., & Lozier, J. N. (2013). Venous thromboembolism. In G. P. Rodgers & N. S. Young (Eds.), *The Bethesda handbook of clinical hematology* (3rd ed.) (pp. 311–327). Philadelphia: Lippincott Williams & Wilkins.

National Comprehensive Cancer Network. (2014). NCCN guidelines, version 1.2015. Deep or superficial vein thrombosis. Available at http://www.nccn.org/professionals/physician_gls/pdf/vte.pdf (accessed March 5, 2016).

O'Leary, C., & Mack, L. (2013). Bleeding and thrombosis. In M. Kaplan (Ed.), *Understanding and managing oncological emergencies: A resource for nurses* (2nd ed.) (pp. 1–41). Pittsburgh, PA: Oncology Nursing Society.

Sepsis

Definition

- Sepsis results from an overwhelming systemic infection that can lead to severe sepsis, septic shock, and multiple organ dysfunction syndrome (MODS).
- Diagnosis depends on documenting infection with two or more of the systemic inflammatory response syndrome (SIRS) criteria, including elevated temperature, heart rate, respiratory rate, and white blood cell count.

Epidemiology

- Sepsis is the 11th leading cause of death in the United States.
- Among patients who have had a febrile neutropenic event, 10% to 20% develop bacteremia or sepsis.
- Among cancer patients, the incidence of sepsis is approximately 25%, and the associated mortality rate is 28%.
- The incidence of severe sepsis is greater among patients with hematologic malignancies than those with solid tumors.

- Many microorganisms can cause sepsis.
  - Bacterial infections are the most common source of sepsis (45% to 50% of septic shock cases).
  - Viruses are rarely the main cause, but they may cause significant infectious complications in patients who are immunocompromised.
  - Fungal infections can result in severe morbidity and mortality for oncology patients.
  - Anaerobes and protozoa also can cause septic shock.
- Risk factors for infection
  - Neutropenia (absolute neutrophil count [ANC] <500 cells/mm^3)
  - Hematologic malignancies
  - High-dose chemotherapy, especially for patients undergoing BMT
  - Radiation therapy, especially total body irradiation
  - Febrile neutropenia and one or more high-risk factors (e.g., mucositis, diarrhea, clinical instability, advanced disease, overt organ dysfunction)
- Moderate risk of infection
  - Solid tumors
  - Neutropenia (ANC of 500 to 1000 cells/mm^3)
  - Standard-dose chemotherapy
  - Localized radiation therapy
  - Corticosteroids and immunosuppression therapy
  - Long intensive care stays
  - Age older than 65 years or younger than 1 year
  - Splenectomy
  - Breakdown of skin or mucous membranes
  - Invasive procedures or devices, including tunneled central venous catheters, indwelling urinary catheters, and feeding tubes
  - Antibiotic use
  - Protein-calorie malnutrition
  - Comorbid conditions such as diabetes or organ-related disease (e.g., renal, hepatic, cardiovascular, gastrointestinal, pulmonary)
- Lowest risk of infection
  - Neutropenia (ANC of 1000 to 1500 cells/mm^3)
  - Low-dose chemotherapy

Pathophysiology

- Mature neutrophils are the first line of defense against bacterial infection.
- Six phases of the septic shock cascade
  - Infection or bacteremia
    - Inflammatory response to invasion of host tissue by microorganisms
    - Viable bacteria (or fungi) in the bloodstream evidenced by positive blood cultures
  - SIRS or sepsis
    - Clinical evidence of systemic inflammatory response to invasion by microorganisms
    - Manifested by two or more of the following: temperature greater than 38° C (100.4° F) or less than 36° C (96.8° F), heart rate greater than 90 beats/min, respiratory rate greater than 20 breaths/min or Paco$_2$

less than 32 mm Hg, white blood cell (WBC) count greater than 12,000 cells/mm^3, WBC count less than 4000 cells/mm^3, or more than 10% immature (band) cells in the peripheral blood.
- *Sepsis* is a documented infection with two or more of the SIRS criteria.
- *Severe sepsis* is dysfunction of one or more organ systems.
- *Septic shock* is acute circulatory failure characterized by hypotension that does not respond to fluid hydration.
- MODS
  - Dysfunction of two or more organs
  - Immediate treatment required to maintain homeostasis
  - Can lead to death

Signs and Symptoms

- Signs and symptoms of infection may be subtle or absent, especially in neutropenic patients.
- SIRS or sepsis manifests with two or more of the following:
  - Elevated temperature
  - Elevated heart rate
  - Elevated respiratory rate
  - Elevated WBC count
- Sepsis signs and symptoms
  - Documented infection
  - Two or more of the SIRS criteria
  - Purulent drainage from a wound or site of a central venous catheter, which may not be seen in neutropenic patients, who are unable to exhibit signs of infection
- Severe sepsis signs and symptoms (affect one or more organ systems)
  - Hypotension (i.e., systolic blood pressure <90 mm Hg or reduction of >40 mm Hg from baseline), sinus tachycardia, or hypoperfusion
  - Tachypnea, hypoxia on room air, or decreased breath sounds
  - Dry, warm, flushed skin
  - Nausea, vomiting, or decreased gastrointestinal motility
  - Decreased urine output
  - Mental status changes, confusion, agitation, or chills
  - Lactic acidosis
- Septic shock signs and symptoms (with acute circulatory failure)
  - Hypotension, tachycardia, and arrhythmias
  - Shortness of breath, decreased breath sounds, crackles or wheezes, pulmonary edema, and ARDS
  - Cold, pale, clammy skin; decreased perfusion; acrocyanosis; and mottling
  - Stress ulcers, gastrointestinal bleeding, decreased motility, and jaundice
  - Oliguria, anuria, and acute renal failure
  - Obtundation and coma

Cancers Associated with Disorder

- Leukemia, especially acute leukemia and chronic lymphocytic leukemia
- Lymphoma (e.g., Hodgkin disease, non-Hodgkin lymphoma)
- Multiple myeloma

- Disease with bone marrow metastasis
- Solid tumors

Diagnostic Tests

- Temperature, heart rate, and respiratory rate
- Laboratory tests
  - CBC
  - Electrolyte levels
  - Liver function test
  - Renal function test
- Obtain the following at the first suspicion of sepsis:
  - Immediate blood cultures from two peripheral sites or from a peripheral site and a central venous access site if central venous access is in place
  - Urine culture and sensitivity and cultures of sputum, drainage, stool, wound, and central line site
- Laboratory tests
  - CBC to look for leukopenia or leukocytosis, thrombocytopenia, and anemia
  - Chemistry panel to assess electrolytes (increased glucose) and uric acid
  - Liver function test results are elevated.
  - Renal function test results show increased BUN and creatinine levels.
  - Coagulation study results show a prolonged PT or aPTT, decreased fibrinogen level, and increased FDP level.
  - Arterial blood gas (ABG) determinations show an increased lactic acid level.
- Imaging studies
  - Posteroanterior and lateral chest radiographs to rule out infection
  - Chest tomography (CT if chest radiographic results are suspicious)
  - Venogram or spiral chest CT to diagnose pulmonary embolism as source of fever
  - ECG or echocardiograms when a cardiac source of infection is suspected
  - Doppler ultrasound for diagnosing venous thrombosis as a source of fever
  - Lumbar puncture when neurologic infection is suspected
- Ongoing evaluation
  - Vital signs: temperature, heart rate, and respiratory rate
  - Strict intake and output measurements
  - Daily weights
  - Pulse oximetry and ABG determinations
  - Antibiotic levels, as indicated
  - CBC, chemistry panel, electrolytes, liver and renal function tests, and serum lactate level
  - Serologies and cultures for viral diseases

Differential Diagnosis

- Tumor-associated fever, especially in lymphoma, acute leukemia, chronic leukemia, multiple myeloma, solid tumors, and metastases to the liver or central nervous system
- Febrile response related to drug administration (e.g., amphotericin B, ganciclovir, interferons, interleukins) may occur at the start of therapy or 1 to 2 weeks later.

- Allergic reaction to drugs or blood products
- Nosocomial fever
- Early signs of septic shock

Treatment

- Early detection and treatment of sepsis and septic shock improves patient outcomes.
- Treat the underlying, predisposing conditions causing the infection.
- Support the patient's hemodynamic status.
- Manage the clinical manifestations of infection or sepsis.

Pharmacologic Management

- Prevention
  - Prophylactic antibiotics may be administered to neutropenic patients.
  - WBC growth factors (e.g., granulocyte colony-stimulating factor [G-CSF], granulocyte-macrophage colony-stimulating factor [GM-CSF]) may be administered to decrease the length of neutropenia and decrease the incidence of infection after chemotherapy administration.
- Management
  - Establish vascular access, and initiate aggressive fluid resuscitation.
  - Administer empiric antibiotics.
  - At the first suspicion of sepsis, blood cultures are obtained.
  - Broad-spectrum antibiotics, which cover common gram-negative and gram-positive organisms, should be administered immediately after obtaining blood cultures.
  - Empiric antifungal therapy
    - Initiated when the patient remains febrile for 5 to 7 days after the empiric antibiotic therapy is started
    - Amphotericin B is the drug of choice.
    - Antifungal agents, including nystatin, clotrimazole, fluconazole, and amphotericin B, are commonly administered prophylactically.
  - Antiviral agents (e.g., acyclovir, ganciclovir) and various formulations of immunoglobulin are used to prevent and treat viral infections.
  - Antipyretic therapy (primarily acetaminophen) is administered to decrease the patient's temperature and minimize the discomforts of fever (e.g., chills, seizures, delirium).
  - Fluid resuscitation
    - May be administered to manage hypotension or oliguria
    - Crystalloid solutions (e.g., normal saline solution, lactated Ringer solution) are used most commonly during the early phases of sepsis.
    - Colloid solutions (e.g., dextran, albumin, plasma protein fraction) are also used.
  - Vasopressors
    - Dopamine is the first-line therapy because of its vasopressor and inotropic effects.
    - Norepinephrine may be added for increased vasopressor support.
    - Dobutamine may be added for increased inotropic effects.

Nonpharmacologic Management

- Monitor vital signs every 4 hours or as clinically indicated.
- Monitor changes in laboratory values, and report significant changes, including organism growth in cultures and an increase in the WBC count.
- Assess signs and symptoms of infection, and obtain an order for a culture of suspicious sites.
- Monitor signs and symptoms of fluid overload, including rales, edema, and weight gain.
- Monitor intake and output every 4 to 8 hours or as clinically indicated.
- Monitor pulse oximetry and the patient's response to oxygen therapy.
- Use physical methods of controlling body temperature: tepid baths, sponging, cool washcloths, ice packs, cooling blankets, air conditioning, fans, and blankets during periods of chilling.
- Provide the patient with a high-calorie, high-protein diet to ensure proper nutrition.
- Encourage hydration (e.g., drinking 8 to 10 glasses of fluid/day).
- Implement strategies to prevent infection, including good hand hygiene and neutropenic precautions per institutional procedure.
- Implement strategies to manage sepsis or septic shock.
  - Administer antibiotics as ordered.
  - Monitor oxygen saturation, and administer oxygen as ordered.

Patient Teaching

- Goal is to protect the patient from infection and maintain a normal temperature.
- Define sepsis and septic shock, and describe their signs and symptoms.
- Explain the purpose of the laboratory tests (especially ANC), diagnostic tests, nursing care, and treatments for sepsis.
- Teach the patient and family to prevent infection with frequent hand washing and to keep the body clean by bathing daily and washing hands after using the bathroom.
- Teach the patient to brush the teeth at least twice daily and to floss once daily.
- Encourage the patient to drink 8 to 10 glasses of fluid per day.
- Teach the patient to avoid infection by avoiding large crowds, people who are sick, and infants, children, and adults who have been vaccinated within the past 3 weeks.
- Teach the patient to not clean up cat litter or clean up excreta from animals.
- Verify that the patient and family understand how to take the patient's temperature and provide additional teaching as needed.
- Teach the patient to turn, cough, and deep breathe to maintain optimal respiratory functioning.
- Teach the patient the rationale and schedule for oral prophylactic antibiotics or WBC growth factors if indicated.
- Teach the patient the rationale and schedule for having blood drawn for a CBC.
- The patient should report a temperature greater than 100.5° F and symptoms of infection such as redness, swelling, warmth, pain, or drainage.

Follow-up

- Continue to monitor for signs and symptoms of infection or sepsis.
- Monitor laboratory findings, especially CBC, to determine the continuation or resolution of sepsis.
- Provide additional resources such as home equipment or assistance as needed.

Bibliography

Angus, D. C., & van der Poll, T. (2013). Sepsis and septic shock. *New England Journal of Medicine, 369,* 840–851.

Dellinger, R. P., Levy, M. M., Rhodes, A., Annane, D., Gerlach, H., Opal, S. M., & Moreno, R. (2013). Surviving sepsis campaign: International guidelines for management of severe sepsis and septic shock, 2012. *Intensive Care Medicine, 39,* 165–228.

Gobel, B. H., Peterson, G. J., & Hoffner, B. (2013). Sepsis and septic shock. In M. Kaplan (Ed.), *Understanding and managing oncological emergencies: A resource for nurses* (2nd ed.) (pp. 287–335). Pittsburgh, PA: Oncology Nursing Society.

Kochanek, K. D., Xu, J., Murphy, S. L., Minino, A. M., & Kung, H. C. (2011). Deaths: Preliminary data for 2009 (vol. 59, no. 4). In *National vital statistics reports.* Hyattsville, MD: National Center for Health Statistics. Available at http://www.cdc.gov/nchs/data/nvsr59/nvsr59_04.pdf (accessed March 5, 2016).

Maloney, K. W. (2016). Metabolic emergencies. In J. J. Itano, J. M. Brant, F. A. Conde, & M. G. Saria (Eds.), *Core curriculum for oncology nursing* (5th ed.) (pp. 478–494). St. Louis: Elsevier.

Viviano, D. L. (2014). Shock. In D. Camp-Sorrell & R. A. Hawkins (Eds.), *Clinical manual for the oncology advanced practice nurse* (3rd ed.) (pp. 1361–1369). Pittsburgh, PA: Oncology Nursing Society.

Zhao, H., Heard, S. O., Mullen, M. T., Crawford, S., Goldberg, R. J., Frendl, G., & Lilly, C. M. (2012). An evaluation of the diagnostic accuracy of the 1991 American College of Chest Physicians/Society of Critical Care Medicine and the 2001 Society of Critical Care Medicine/European Society of Intensive Care Medicine/American College of Chest Physicians/American Thoracic Society/Surgical Infection Society sepsis definition. *Critical Care Medicine, 40*(6), 1700–1706.

Thrombotic Thrombocytopenic Purpura

Definition

- TTP is a blood clotting disorder that is rarely life-threatening. The VWF-rich microthrombi form in smaller blood vessels, resulting in hemolysis and thrombocytopenia.

Epidemiology

- The annual incidence of classic TTP is approximately 3 to 4 cases per 100,000 adults.
- The annual incidence of TTP is 1.9 to 6.4 cases per 100,000 children.
- Between 90% and 95% of patients with TTP are adults, and 5% to 10% are children.
- TTP has been described in patients 1 to 90 years old, and incidence peaks during the third decade.
- There is a slight female predominance, with a female-to-male ratio of 3 to 2.

- Without treatment, most persons with TTP rapidly deteriorate and die.
  - The mortality rate was 80% to 90% before plasma exchange was introduced.
  - The current mortality rate remains between 10% and 20% despite using plasma exchange.
- Risk factors
  - Autoimmune disorders such as SLE, antiphospholipid antibody syndrome, scleroderma, Wegener granulomatosis, and Sjögren syndrome
  - Inflammatory diseases and infection such as rheumatoid arthritis, polyarthritis, endocarditis, and sepsis
  - Malignancies such as lymphoma, BMT, HSCT, and advanced cancer with MAHA
  - Systemic disease such as malignant hypertension and systemic vasculitis
  - Chemotherapy drugs (e.g., gemcitabine, carmustine, mitomycin C, pentostatin), cyclosporine, iodine, oral contraceptives, statins, trimethoprim-sulfamethoxazole, vancomycin, and zoledronic acid
  - Hereditary predisposition (10%)
  - During pregnancy or the postpartum period

Pathophysiology

- TMAs may arise from factors that directly or indirectly cause platelet aggregation or endothelial cell damage, or both.
- Factors include toxins, cytokines, drugs, and deficiencies of the VWF-cleaving protease ADAMTS13.
- Microvascular thrombi and ischemia develop in involved organs.
- As RBCs encounter thrombotic obstruction and fibrin strands in the microvasculature, they are sheared, and hemolytic anemia results.
- Thrombocytopenia and bleeding result from the consumption of platelets.
- VWF is a carrier for factor VIII.
- Normally, ultralarge VWF multimers are synthesized in endothelial cells and megakaryocytes.
  - Endothelial cell injury activates the release of ultralarge VWF multimers into the blood.
  - In healthy persons, the ultralarge VWF multimers usually do not circulate because normal proteolysis by a plasma metalloproteinase (ADAMTS13) rapidly reduces them to smaller units after their release.
- The ADAMTS13 enzyme cleaves VWF, a large protein involved in blood clotting and essential in promoting homeostasis.
- In persons with TTP, cleavage of the unusually large VWF multimers is limited due to a deficiency of ADAMTS13.
  - With the failure of proteolysis, the large multimers accumulate in the patient's plasma.
  - The large multimers remain anchored to the endothelial cell surface, causing excessive aggregation of circulating platelets with small amounts of fibrin.
- Microthrombi formation is initiated where there is high shear stress (e.g., arterioles, capillaries), and MAHA results.
- Widespread microvascular thrombosis affects the brain and other organs.
- Three types of TTP: classic, secondary (cancer-associated), and congenital
  - Classic TTP (i.e., Moschcowitz syndrome) results from a deficiency of ADAMTS13 caused by antibodies directed against specific epitopes on the surface of the enzyme.
  - The acquired ADAMTS13 deficiency leads to an increase of ultralarge VWF multimers in the plasma.
  - Main features of classic TTP are fever, hemolytic anemia, thrombocytopenia, and neurologic and renal abnormalities.
  - The cause of secondary (cancer-associated) TTP is less well understood because ADAMTS13 activity is usually not as depressed as in classic TTP, and inhibitors cannot be detected.
  - In some cases, the cause appears to be endothelial cell damage, although the formation of thrombi resulting in vessel occlusion may not be essential in the pathogenesis.
  - Predisposing factors include cancer, BMT, drugs (e.g., antivirals, platelet aggregation inhibitors, immunosuppressants, estrogens), pregnancy, and HIV infection.
  - The manifestations of cancer-associated TTP are less pronounced, and many patients do not exhibit the full syndrome at diagnosis.
  - Congenital TTP (i.e., Upshaw Schulman syndrome) results from a deficiency of the ADAMTS13 enzyme caused by inherited frameshift and point mutations in the *ADAMTS13* gene.
  - Congenital deficiency of ADAMTS13 is an autosomal recessive disorder associated with the formation of platelet microthrombi in the small blood vessels.
  - Congenital TTP is a rare disorder.

Signs and Symptoms

- TTP is associated with various degrees of neurologic, renal, cardiac, abdominal, and constitutional symptoms.
- Patients diagnosed with classic TTP may have the full syndrome as a result of the widespread formation of microvascular thrombi and exhibit the following signs and symptoms:
  - Petechiae, easy bruising, or bleeding due to thrombocytopenia occurs in most patients, and symptoms are typically moderate to severe
  - Shortness of breath, tachycardia, pale skin, and weakness may correlate with the degree of anemia, which occurs in most patients.
  - Patients may have retinal and choroidal hemorrhaging, epistaxis, gingival bleeding, hematuria, menorrhagia, hemoptysis, or gastrointestinal bleeding.
  - Purpura occurs in more than 90% of cases.
- About 75% of patients have fever.

- Neurologic impairment occurs in about 66% of patients; it can be intermittent or variable.
  - Confusion or dizziness
  - Headache
  - Change in mental status (e.g., forgetfulness, trouble concentrating)
  - Paresis
  - Aphasia, dysarthria, and visual problems
- Major neurologic abnormalities occur in about 35% of patients.
  - Coma
  - Seizure
  - Stroke and focal abnormalities
  - Encephalopathy
- Renal impairment includes proteinuria and microscopic hematuria.
- Cardiac symptoms include chest pain, heart failure, hypotension, and dyspnea.
- Gastrointestinal symptoms include abdominal pain.
- Jaundice may result from hemolysis (i.e., MAHA) and hyperbilirubinemia.
- Cancer patients diagnosed with TTP have less pronounced signs and symptoms, which may include the following:
  - Signs and symptoms related to thrombocytopenia, anemia, and hemorrhaging as outlined for classic TTP
  - Neurologic symptoms as outlined for classic TTP
  - Fever (usually not seen at the onset but almost always occurs during the illness)
  - Renal involvement is common.
    - Proteinuria and microhematuria are the most consistent findings.
    - Decreased renal function occurs in 40% to 80% of patients.
  - Abdominal pain occurs in 10% to 30% of patients.
  - TTP has developed after clinical and laboratory demonstration of pancreatitis, raising the possibility that pancreatic inflammation triggered the onset of TTP.
  - Heart involvement occurs infrequently.
  - Lung involvement rarely includes alveolar and interstitial infiltrates.

Cancers Associated with Disorder

- Lymphoma
- Cancers being treated by BMT or HSCT
- Advanced cancers with MAHA

Diagnostic Tests

- Diagnostic criteria for TTP
  - MAHA and thrombocytopenia
  - With or without renal failure or neurologic abnormalities
  - Without another cause for TMA
- Laboratory tests
  - See hemolytic uremic syndrome
  - Reticulocyte counts are elevated.
  - Serum ADAMTS13 activity: normal levels are 67% or higher.
    - In persons with TTP, the level may be less than 5%, distinguishing TTP from HUS.

- It is appropriate to treat a person with a diagnosis of TTP who may have all of the clinical symptoms of TTP and a normal serum ADAMTS13 activity level.
- Renal function tests include an increased BUN and serum creatinine level for 40% to 80% of patients.
- Comprehensive metabolic panel
  - Elevated LDH level due to hemolysis
  - Elevated electrolyte levels due to renal impairment
  - Elevated serum bilirubin level
- Coombs test
  - Negative result: nonautoimmune, nondrug-induced hemolytic anemia
  - Positive result: autoimmune, drug-induced hemolytic anemia
- Coagulation tests
  - Usually normal values for PT, aPTT, factor V, factor VIII, and fibrinogen
  - FDP level may be elevated.
  - Thrombin time may be prolonged.
- Troponin T and troponin I to rule out cardiac involvement
- Liver function tests to rule out liver involvement (usually normal)
- Blood type and screen tests to prepare for provision of blood products
- Hepatitis A, B, and C and HIV testing of blood products to exclude an underlying viral precipitant
- Blood or urine cultures to identify infection as an underlying cause of TTP
- Urinalysis, with proteinuria, microscopic hematuria, and granular or red cell casts as the most consistent findings
- Radiologic evaluation
  - Renal sonogram or renal angiogram
  - Intravenous pyelogram
  - CT or MRI of the brain to determine neurologic involvement
  - CT of the chest, abdomen, and pelvis with or without tumor markers to assess for underlying malignancy
  - ECG or echocardiogram to document or monitor cardiac damage

Differential Diagnosis

- Differential diagnosis of TTP and HUS
  - Although TTP and HUS are distinct diseases with different causes and demographics, many patients are inaccurately diagnosed with "TTP-HUS disorder" on the basis of clinical and laboratory findings only.
- Many clinical features of TTP and HUS overlap.
  - Localized microvascular thrombosis
  - MAHA
  - Thrombocytopenia
  - Neurologic or renal abnormalities
- Several factors differentiate TTP from HUS.
  - Congenital TTP are caused by inherited deficiencies of the von Willebrand factor–cleaving metalloprotease ADAMTS13, and the classic form is caused

by acquisition of antibodies to the protein. Secondary TTP may result from endothelial cell damage by infection, drugs, or malignancy.
- ADAMTS13 does not play a role in HUS.
- A history of bone marrow transplantation (BMT) or Shiga toxin–associated hemorrhagic colitis suggests HUS.
- The clinical presentation of TTP is dominated by hemorrhages and neurologic symptoms. Renal involvement (e.g., proteinuria, microscopic hematuria) is common, but oliguric acute renal failure is unusual.
- In patients with HUS, acute renal impairment or failure is the dominant clinical feature.
- For classic TTP, plasma exchange is a highly effective treatment, but for typical HUS, plasma exchange is usually ineffective.
- ADAMTS13 deficiency sometimes does not lead to an accumulation of prothrombogenic, ultralarge VWF multimers in patients with TTP, pointing to other pathologic factors or concomitant abnormalities.
- Hematuria related to other diseases (e.g., infection, intrinsic kidney disease, benign prostatic hypertrophy), medications (e.g., ifosfamide, high-dose cyclophosphamide, intravesical chemotherapy), or radiation therapy (e.g., pelvic irradiation, prostate seed implants)
- Systemic malignancy can cause thrombocytopenia and MAHA without signs of DIC.
- Malignant hypertension can cause thrombocytopenia, MAHA, renal failure, and severe neurologic abnormalities.
- Autoimmune disorders may be indistinguishable from TTP (e.g., autoimmune hemolysis or Evans syndrome, acute scleroderma, lupus nephritis). Some patients may have an autoimmune disorder (e.g., SLE, antiphospholipid antibody syndrome) and TTP.
- Systemic infection, typically viral (e.g., CMV, adenovirus, herpes simplex virus) or severe bacterial (e.g., meningococcus, pneumococcus) but may be fungal
- Vasculitis
- DIC
- HIT
- Drug effects (e.g., quinine, simvastatin, interferon)
- GVHD, VOD, DAH, or CMV in persons undergoing BMT
- Pregnancy-associated conditions such as preeclampsia or HELLP syndrome can cause MAHA, thrombocytopenia, renal failure, and minor neurologic abnormalities.

Treatment
- An early diagnosis of TTP is crucial, but it may be difficult due to the lack of explicit diagnostic criteria.
- When the diagnosis is made, begin plasmapheresis as soon as possible.

Pharmacologic Management
- Prevention
  - Vigorous, parenteral or oral pretransplantation hydration before BMT or HSCT
  - Continuous bladder irrigations with normal saline solution

- Management
  - First-line therapy is plasmapheresis.
    - Most patients with an early diagnosis of TTP enter remission with this procedure.
    - Removes or reduces the circulating antibodies against ADAMTS13 and replenishes blood levels of the enzyme.
    - Reverses platelet consumption, which is responsible for thrombus formation and the symptoms associated with TTP.
    - FFP or cryoprecipitate-poor plasma more effective than albumin.
  - Second-line therapy is adjuvant immunotherapy (e.g., corticosteroids, intravenous immunoglobulin), which may be given with plasma exchange.
  - High-dose methylprednisolone (1000 mg/day for 3 days) or prednisone (1 mg/kg/day) is used with an oral proton pump inhibitor. The dose of prednisone varies and is titrated based on the platelet recovery.
    - Corticosteroids may suppress autoantibodies, inhibiting ADAMTS13 activity.
    - Potential benefit may be limited to the patient population with severe ADAMTS13 deficiency or those for whom the cause is unclear.
    - Potent immunosuppressive agents (e.g., rituximab, cyclosporine, vincristine, cyclophosphamide) may be added to plasma exchange and are usually administered for refractory TTP or chronic relapsing TTP.
  - Discontinue drugs that induce TTP.
    - For a patient undergoing allogeneic HSCT in whom TTP develops while on cyclosporine, a reasonable strategy is to discontinue cyclosporine.
    - However, removing the drug may not reverse the complication, and GVHD may worsen.
    - The recommendation is to discontinue cyclosporine and initiate tacrolimus.
  - Packed RBCs may be transfused based on the severity of anemia and amount of bleeding.
  - Platelet transfusions are usually not indicated to treat TTP due to the potential for generating platelet-rich microthrombi.
    - Platelet transfusion may be indicated for intracranial bleeding, which is documented by CT or MRI, or for life-threatening bleeding. Platelets may be transfused slowly.
    - Severe thrombocytopenia alone is not an appropriate indication for platelet transfusion in patients with classic TTP.
    - Complications associated with platelet transfusions in persons with TTP include development or progression of neurologic symptoms and acute renal failure.
  - To prevent thrombosis, antithrombotic agents (e.g., LMWH thromboprophylaxis, 75 mg of aspirin every other day) are recommended when the platelet count is more than 50,000/mm³.

Nonpharmacologic Management

- Splenectomy has a 50% success rate at best.
- A nephrology consultation is needed to determine the most appropriate renal therapy.
- Renal replacement therapy
  - May include peritoneal dialysis and hemodialysis (minority of patients with TTP)
  - May be successful treatment for patients with recurrent cancer-associated TTP

Patient Teaching

- Describe the goals of therapy: return of the patient's blood cell counts to normal levels and subsidence of symptoms (e.g., hemorrhagic, neurologic).
- Define TTP, and describe the signs and symptoms.
- Explain the purpose of the laboratory tests, nursing care, and treatments for TTP.
- Ask the patient to report symptoms such as bleeding and mental status changes.
- Teach patients self-care measures to maximize their safety:
  - Use an electric razor, not a straight-edged razor.
  - Maintain the bed in a low position with the side rails up.
  - Clear pathways in the room and hallway.
  - Minimize activities that could trigger bleeding.
  - Avoid contact sports and heavy lifting.
  - Take precautions against accidental bleeding because even minor scrapes or bumps could result in bleeding.
- Teach fall precautions if the patient is at risk for falls.
  - In the home, remove throw rugs and items that can obstruct pathways.
  - Wear shoes that fit appropriately.
  - Walk carefully and change positions gradually.
- Teach patients to avoid over-the-counter medications that may interfere with normal platelet function such as aspirin and NSAIDs (e.g., ibuprofen, naproxen sodium).
- Teach patients to minimize activities that contribute to the development of additional clots and increase circulation in the lower extremities.
  - Avoid tight or restrictive clothing.
  - Use compression stockings to promote venous return.
  - Elevate legs when possible.
  - Do not sit with legs crossed.
  - Do not dangle feet on the side of the bed.
  - Do not use pillows under the knees or a knee gatch.
  - Wiggle toes and feet and rotate ankles, especially when in bed.
- Teach the patient and family to observe and save urine, stool, and emesis for the nurse to check for blood.
- Teach the patient to report critical signs and symptoms such as bruising, red rash, headache, black stools, blood in the urine or stools, and bleeding from the gums, nose, eyes, vagina, rectum, wound, or central venous catheter site.

Follow-up

- Short-term follow-up
  - Monitor CBC on a daily basis during the acute phase to determine the continuation or resolution of TTP.
  - Monitor the patient once or twice each week until the hemoglobin, hematocrit, and platelet levels become stable.
  - After a remission occurs, patients gradually need fewer routine blood counts.
  - A platelet count is necessary when symptoms of any illness occur to diagnose a possible recurrence of TTP in a timely manner.
- Long-term follow-up
  - Monitor platelet counts frequently during the first year of initial treatment because patients often relapse during this time.
  - Provide additional resources such as home equipment or assistance as needed.

Bibliography

Adler, S., & Nast, C. C. (2013). Thrombotic thrombocytopenic purpura. In S. Gilbert (Ed.), *National Kidney Foundation primer on kidney diseases* (6th ed.) (p. 244). St. Louis: Elsevier Health Sciences.

Fairman, B. (2014). Thrombotic thrombocytopenic purpura. In D. Camp-Sorrell & R. A. Hawkins (Eds.), *Clinical manual for the oncology advanced practice nurse* (3rd ed.) (pp. 1053–1058). Pittsburgh, PA: Oncology Nursing Society.

Fogarty, P. F., & Dunbar, C. E. (2013). Thrombocytopenia. In G. P. Rodgers & N. S. Young (Eds.), *The Bethesda handbook of clinical hematology* (3rd ed.) (pp. 269–284). Philadelphia: Lippincott Williams & Wilkins.

Gauer, R. L., & Braun, M. M. (2012). Thrombocytopenia. *American Family Physician, 85*, 612–622.

George, J. N. (2010). How I treat patients with thrombotic thrombocytopenic purpura: 2010. *Blood, 116*(20), 4060–4069.

Hovinga, J. A., Vesely, S. K., Terrell, D. R., Lämmle, B., & George, J. N. (2010). Survival and relapse in patients with thrombotic thrombocytopenic purpura. *Blood, 115*, 1500–1511.

Maloney, K. W. (2016). Metabolic emergencies. In J. J. Itano, J. M. Brant, F. A. Conde, & M. G. Saria (Eds.), *Core curriculum for oncology nursing* (5th ed.) (pp. 478–494). St. Louis: Elsevier.

Noel, P., & Jaben, E. A. (2013). Consultative hematology. In G. P. Rodgers & N. S. Young (Eds.), *The Bethesda handbook of clinical hematology* (3rd ed.) (pp. 389–404). Philadelphia: Lippincott Williams & Wilkins.

Peyvandi, F., Palla, R., Lotta, L. A., Mackie, I., Scully, M. A., & Machin, S. J. (2010). ADAMTS-13 assays in thrombotic thrombocytopenic purpura. *Journal of Thrombosis and Haemostasis, 8*, 631–640.

Said, A., Haddad, R. Y., Stein, R., & Lerma, E. V. (2014). Thrombotic thrombocytopenic purpura. *Disease-A-Month, 60*(10), 500–504.

Saifan, C., Nasr, R., Mehta, S., Acharya, P. S., & El-Sayegh, S. (2012). Thrombotic thrombocytopenic purpura. *Journal of Blood Disorders & Transfusion, S3*(001), 1–5. http://dx.doi.org/10.4172/2155-9864.S3-001.

Scully, M. (2012). Rituximab in the treatment of TTP. *Hematology, 17*(s1), s22–s24.

Scully, M., Hunt, B. J., Benjamin, S., Liesner, R., Rose, P., Peyvandi, F., & Machin, S. J. (2012). Guidelines on the diagnosis and management of thrombotic thrombocytopenic purpura and other thrombotic microangiopathies. *British Journal of Haematology, 158*, 323–335.

Singhai, A. (2015). Thrombocytopenic purpura successfully treated with glucocorticoids. *Journal of Mahatma Gandhi Institute of Medical Sciences, 20*(1), 91–93.

Swisher, K. K., Terrell, D. R., Vesely, S. K., Kremer Hovinga, J. A., Lämmle, B., & George, J. N. (2009). Clinical outcomes after platelet transfusions in patients with thrombotic thrombocytopenic purpura. *Transfusion, 49*(5), 873–887.

Survivorship

Carrie Tompkins Stricker and Carrie Tilley

Introduction

Advances in cancer screening and treatment in the United States have produced almost 14.5 million cancer survivors as of January 1, 2014. This number is expected to approach 19 million by 2024 (DeSantis, Siegel, & Jemal, 2014).

The lifetime probability of developing cancer is 45% for men and 38% for women (National Cancer Institute [NCI], 2014). In the United States, one of two men and one of three women are expected to develop cancer (American Cancer Society [ACS], 2014). Among the people diagnosed with cancer, 68% are expected to be alive after 5 years, and survival rates continue to grow (Siegel, Naishadham, & Jemal, 2013).

With this growing number of cancer survivors comes health care delivery challenges. Cancer survivors require specialized care after the acute treatment period, and they continue to cope with the side effects of cancer treatment. Several studies have documented the numerous unmet medical and psychosocial needs and ongoing side effects experienced by cancer survivors (Hewitt, Bamundo, Day, & Harvey, 2007; Hewitt, Greenfield, & Stovall, 2006; Wu & Harden, 2015). Survivors must deal with persistent and emergent symptoms. A review of the literature concluded that one third of cancer survivors reported symptoms after treatment that were equivalent to those during treatment (Wu & Harden, 2015). Another study found that 92% of patients continued to experience symptoms a year after their cancer diagnosis (Shi et al., 2011). A third study showed that the symptom scores for breast cancer survivors 5 years out from treatment were not different from those undergoing active treatment (Murgić et al., 2012).

The tables in pages 400 and 401 list commonly reported symptoms of cancer survivors. The most common "severe problems" reported by cancer survivors in the ACS study of cancer survivors were being less physically able to have sexual intercourse and feeling fearful that the illness would return (Stein et al., 2006). The most frequently reported physical, emotional, and practical concerns reported in the LIVESTRONG survey of cancer survivors conducted in 2010 were energy, concentration, sexual functioning, fear of recurrence, grief and identity, and concerns about school (LIVESTRONG, 2011).

Beyond persistent symptoms, survivors are at risk for a broad array of long-term and late effects of treatment. They include recurrent and new cancers; increased morbidity and mortality from cardiovascular, skeletal, and other diseases; myriad physical effects such as lymphedema; and psychosocial distress that may affect work and social relationships (Hewitt et al., 2006; Stricker & Jacobs, 2008). However, these persistent and emergent issues are routinely underrecognized and undermanaged. The 2010 LIVESTRONG survey of approximately 3000 survivors found that among those who had emotional concerns (e.g., depression, fear of recurrence), only one half reported receiving care for their concerns. Among those with physical concerns (e.g., fatigue, pain), one third did not receive care for their concerns, and among those with practical concerns (e.g., financial issues, employment), almost 60% did not receive assistance (LIVESTRONG, 2011).

Many survivors do not receive recommended surveillance tests for cancer recurrence or for the late effects for which they are at increased risk. In one study, only 55.0% of 2297 colorectal cancer survivors received surveillance colonoscopies according to the recommended schedule (Salloum et al., 2012). In another study, 38% of older (≥65 years) breast cancer survivors did not receive annual mammography after diagnosis (Schapira, McAuliffe, & Nattinger, 2000). Studies have shown no more than one fourth of prostate cancer survivors at increased risk for bone loss and osteoporosis (i.e., late effects) undergo screening dual-energy x-ray absorptiometry (DEXA) scans (Tanvetyanon, 2005). In one small study of Hodgkin disease survivors who received mantle radiotherapy, 80% did not undergo recommended echocardiograms to monitor their increased risk of cardiotoxicity (Oeffinger et al., 2010).

In recognition of the growing number of survivors and their unmet posttreatment needs, the Institute of Medicine (IOM) issued in 2006 its seminal report on survivorship titled *From Cancer Patient to Cancer Survivor: Lost in Transition*. The consensus report identified gaps in comprehensive and coordinated care. It recommended providing cancer survivors with a personalized survivorship care plan (SCP) (Hewitt et al., 2006). The report was an urgent call to all those involved with cancer treatment to focus on improving the care delivered to patients after treatment.

CPILS Items with the Fraction of Individuals Who Rated the Problem as of Moderate or Severe Concern

Item	Description	Item Endorsement Rate (%)	Not a Problem (%)	Somewhat of a Problem (%)	A Severe Problem (%)
CPILS_D	Fatigue, loss of strength	96.99	34.5	52.7	12.8
CPILS_G	Eating difficulties	97.05	79.5	17.1	3.4
CPILS_U	Concerned about infection and crowd	97.13	75	20.8	4.2
CPILS_I	Diminished ability to concentrate	96.47	62.4	32.9	4.8
CPILS_J	Sleep difficulties	97.5	47.2	42.7	10.1
CPILS_E	Uncomfortable with changes in my physical appearance	97.13	59.9	32.7	7.5
CPILS_K	Feeling dependent	96.12	69.1	26.4	4.5
CPILS_W	Difficulty in returning to former roles	96.2	75.1	20.7	4.2
CPILS_DD	Continued major problems with my health	96.33	61.7	31.2	7.1
CP1LS_R	Feeling helpless	96.94	71.2	24.1	4.7
CPILS_Q	Feeling isolated	97.07	76.8	19.3	4
CPILS_S	Feeling vulnerable	96.37	62.2	32.6	5.2
CPILS_X	Problem communicating with spouse or partner"	92.18	80	16.1	3.9
CPILS_O	Feeling angry	96.86	70.1	24.9	4.9
CPILS_V	Problems with family/children	96.64	86.6	11.1	2.3
CPILS_N	Guilt feelings	96.7	78.5	17.6	3.9
CPILS_T	Being treated as different from others	96.76	86.7	11.6	1.8
CPILS_P	Having difficulties in making long-term plans	96.8	62.5	31	6.5
CPILS_H	Concern about being physically unable to have children	92.65	94.6	3.3	2
CPILS_BB	Difficulty in obtaining adequate insurance	96.02	81.3	12.6	6.1
CPILS_Y	Difficulty in meeting my medical expenses	96.78	74 7	18.8	6.5
CPILS_B	Job discrimination	93.04	91.6	5.8	2.6
CPILS_A	Not being able to change jobs for fear of losing my health insurance coverage	93.54	81.7	11.1	7.2
CPILS_AA	Being less able to provide for the financial needs of my family	95.01	72.9	19.6	7.5
CPILS_CC	Difficulties in pursuing the career of my choice	94.06	83 4	11.5	5.1
CPILS_Z	Feeling fearful that my illness will return	96 95	31.7	53.8	14 5
CPILS_C	Concern about relapsing	95.52	35.3	53.8	10.9
CPILS_M	Fear about the future	97.01	43	46.9	10.1
CPILS_F	Preoccupation with illness	96.55	62.9	32.2	4.9
CPILS_L	Less physically able to have sexual intercourse	97.45	52 7	30.1	17.2
CPILS_EE	Not able to get the information 1 need about cancer"	96.57	90.8	7.7	1.5

"These item were not in the original CPILS but added specifically forSCS-I.
From Zhao, L., Portier, K., Stein, K., Baker, F., (2009). Exploratory factor analysis of the cancer problems in living scale: a report from the American cancer society's studies of cancer survivors. *Journal of pain and symptom management, 37*(4), 676–686.

Evolution of Survivorship Care

Established in 1986, the National Coalition for Cancer Survivorship (NCCS) set out to redefine a *cancer victim* as a *cancer survivor*. Thirty years later, it is easy to see that they started a movement for what is now considered survivorship care. The NCCS worked with other patient advocacy groups to push legislation focused on quality cancer. By 1996, these efforts led to the formation of the NCI's Office of Cancer Survivorship. The Office of Cancer Survivorship's primary focus has become support of critical research on the long-term and late effects of cancer and its treatment on cancer survivors. Years later, the 2006 IOM report and 2014 American Society of Clinical Oncology (ASCO) report demanded focused care of cancer survivors after treatment.

In 2015, the growing momentum led to two major accreditation organizations (i.e., American College of Surgeons' Commission on Cancer [CoC] and the National Accreditation Program for Breast Centers [NAPBC]) adding survivorship care standards to their requirements. In the same year, the National Comprehensive Cancer Network (Ligibel & Denlinger, 2013) established survivorship guidelines that defined the standards for providing survivorship care. To incentivize centers to provide quality and cancer care, the Centers for Medicare and Medicaid Innovation (CMMI) launched the oncology-focused model (OCM) of payment in 2015 (see figure below).

What is Survivorship Care?

At some centers, *survivorship services* is the umbrella term for a range of comprehensive care services provided throughout the course of diagnosis, treatment, and after treatment. It is consistent with the NCCS definition that considers an individual a cancer survivor from the time of diagnosis through the balance of his or her life. However, the IOM report distinguished survivorship care (see figure in page 401) as being focused on the period after active treatment with the intent of cure (Hewitt et al., 2006), and this has become the most widely recognized definition of survivorship care. Mandates for survivorship care, such as the CoC's required delivery of SCPs (CoC, 2014), have adopted this definition by stating that required services apply to individuals after active treatment for curable malignancy.

Highest Reported Posttreatment Physical, Emotional, and Practical Concerns in the LIVESTRONG Survey of 2099 Cancer Survivors

PHYSICAL CONCERNS		EMOTIONAL CONCERNS		PRACTICAL CONCERNS	
Energy	59%	Fear of recurrence	80%	School	73%
Concentration	55%	Grief and identity	60%	Employment	45%
Sexual functioning	46%	Personal appearance	62%	Debt	27%
Neuropathy	42%	Family member risk	51%	Insurance	18%
Pain	34%	Sadness and depression	51%		
Lymphedema	23%	Personal relationships	31%		
Incontinence	22%	Social relationships	29%		

Data from LIVESTRONG. (2011). "I learned to live with it" is not good enough: Challenges reported by post-treatment cancer survivors in the LIVESTRONG survey. Available at http://images.livestrong.org/downloads/flatfiles/what-we-do/our-approach/reports/challenges/LSSurvivorSurveyReport_final.pdf (accessed March 4, 2016).

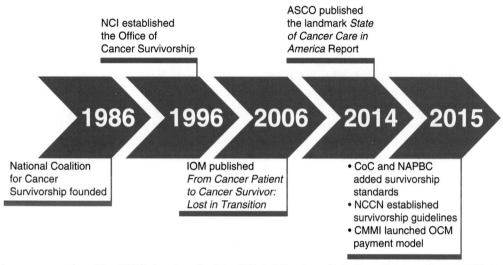

Key milestones in cancer survivorship. *ASCO*, American Society of Clinical Oncology; *CoC*, Commission on Cancer; *IOM*, Institute of Medicine; *NAPBC*, National Accreditation Program for Breast Centers; *NCCN*, National Comprehensive Cancer Network; *NCI*, National Cancer Institute.

The posttreatment follow-up care that is essential for cancer survivors who have completed their active cancer treatment includes a focus on the numerous long-term and late side effects and the potential risks that are unique to each survivor. Survivorship care is comprehensive, coordinated care that addresses the physical, emotional, spiritual, financial, psychosocial, and practical issues of each patient. Adapted from the 2006 IOM report, in their survivorship guidelines, the NCCN defined the standards for survivorship care as follows(Ligibel & Denlinger, 2013):

1. Prevention of new and recurrent cancers and other late effects
2. Surveillance for cancer spread, recurrence, or second cancers
3. Assessment of late psychosocial and physical effects
4. Intervention for consequences or cancer and treatment (e.g., medical, symptoms, psychological distress, financial and social concerns)
5. Coordination of care between primary care providers and specialists to ensure that all of the survivor's health needs are met

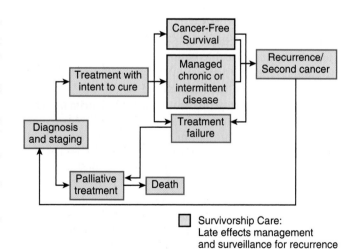

Survivorship care trajectory. (From Hewitt, M., Greenfield, S., & Stovall, E. [2006]. *From cancer patient to cancer survivor: Lost in transition.* Washington, DC: The National Academies Press.)

Models of Survivorship Care

A number of models of survivorship care delivery have been established, but there has been little evaluation to determine which models are most effective for which populations and outcomes. Models and systems for survivorship care have been well described (Landier, 2009; McCabe & Jacobs, 2008; Oeffinger & McCabe, 2006). A detailed description is beyond the scope of this chapter. Briefly, Landier (2009) described different systems of survivorship care, including the consultative system that involves single or multiple visits for assessment and management of survivorship concerns; the ongoing care system, consisting of ongoing care in long-term survivorship clinics or programs; and the integrated care system, previously described as the integration of survivorship care into care provided by the primary cancer care team.

Examples of the systems of survivorship care (i.e., consultative system, ongoing care system, and integrated care system) have been published (Stricker, Jacobs, & Miller, 2012). Models of care that predominantly belong to the classification of ongoing care systems also have been described (McCabe & Jacobs, 2008; Oeffinger & McCabe, 2006). Ongoing care survivorship clinics and programs can be further classified as nurse-led, multidisciplinary, and shared care models of care, depending on which providers staff the programs and on the degree to which care is coordinated or shared with clinicians in other disciplines and in other settings, especially primary care (McCabe & Jacobs, 2008).

Lost Between Primary Care and Oncology: Who is Responsible?

The call to focus on addressing gaps in care for posttreatment cancer survivors, including an emphasis on education about and management of late and long-term effects, comes in the setting of an expected shortage of oncologists (Erikson, Salsberg, Forte, Bruinooge, & Goldstein, 2007) and primary care physicians (U.S. Department of Health and Human Services, Health Resources and Services Administration, National Center for Workforce Analysis, 2013). Acknowledging the unmet needs of cancer survivors and the predicted shortage of oncologists and primary care physicians, ASCO addressed cancer survivorship care in its publication of *The State of Cancer Care in America* in 2014. In this first-ever report, ASCO (2014, 2015) emphasized the importance of and need for providing quality and coordinated cancer care.

Coordinated cancer care is easier said than done. When determining which practitioner is responsible for each piece of follow-up care for the cancer patient, miscommunication and confusion is commonly reported (Salz et al., 2012). Primary care providers and oncologists have been surveyed to determine which parts of survivorship care they think they are responsible for managing. Studies show both types of providers lack confidence in managing the late effects of cancer, lack knowledge in evidence-based screening recommendations, lack trust in each other to initiate screening tests, and disagree

about which provider is better suited to provided psychosocial support (Potosky & Han, 2011).

Ideas about who is best positioned to care for cancer survivors may vary from center to center, but the answer is likely to be the combined effort of many providers and cancer support staff (Earle & Neville, 2004). The consensus from ASCO focused on two conclusions: patients benefit from and should receive an SCP and the posttreatment care of cancer survivors should involve well-coordinated and communicated care to prevent the patient from getting "lost in transition" (Mayer et al., 2014).

Scope of a Survivorship Care Plan

An SCP is a personalized document containing a summary of the patient's treatment, implications of the diagnosis and treatment for follow-up care, and recommended health behaviors. The SCP should include evidenced-based screening and follow-up recommendations and symptom management interventions. It lists the potential late effects associated with the treatment, ongoing symptoms, and resources for the survivors, including referrals to appropriate specialists such as cancer rehabilitation and psychosocial care providers. Care plans should include clear directions for follow-up care, resources to address practical concerns (e.g., work, childcare, financial stress), and recommendations for lifestyle changes to help the survivor achieve health promotion goals aimed at reducing risk of other cancers and diseases (Mayer et al., 2014; Ligibel & Denlinger, 2013).

The care plan is intended to serve as a roadmap for cancer survivors. It shows them which providers they should see and when. It also allows providers to share detailed information about the patient's treatment, potential long-term risks associated with it, and the appropriate screening recommendations (Stricker & O'Brien, 2014).

Are Care Plans Required?

Accreditation and certification organizations, including the CoC, the NAPBC, and the ASCO Quality Oncology Practice Initiative (QOPI), require SCP delivery. Each of the organizations has specific requirements to achieve and maintain accreditation or certification. Although there are some variations in the certification requirements, most are quite similar.

In late 2014, ASCO released a consensus statement on survivorship care planning (Mayer et al., 2014), and the SCP requirements outlined in this document have been endorsed by the CoC as the minimum required to meet their accreditation standard. The committee that developed the consensus statement outlined key assumptions regarding SCPs that are summarized in the box below.

As of 2015, survivorship care planning was added to the requirements of other organizations. New value-based payment models were incorporated in the Centers for Medicare and Medicaid Services (CMS) Oncology Care Model. The CoC added SCP delivery to its list of requirements for accredited cancer centers. The NAPBC required accredited breast centers to provide care plans to 50% of patients who have completed active treatment for cancer within 6 months of completing treatment (NAPBC, 2014). Due to the new requirements, more and more cancer survivors are being provided with an SCP.

Key Assumptions About Survivorship Care Plans

- SCPs are a two-part tool: treatment summary and care plan.
- SCPs developed by ASCO are for patients completing active curative treatment, regardless of tumor type, and who have no active evidence of disease.
- SCPs should
  - Be simple, clear, and understandable
  - Identify who is responsible for outlined actions
  - Be shared with the patient and primary care provider and stored in the electronic medical record (EMR)
- SCPs do not replace
  - Discussions between the patient and oncology provider
  - The medical record

From Mayer, D. K., Gerstel, A., Leak, A. N., & Smith, S. K. (2012). Patient and provider preferences for survivorship care plans. *Journal of Oncology Practice,* 8(4), 80e-86e.

Survivorship Care Plans: Brief Evidence Review

Although the few randomized studies that have been conducted have had mixed outcomes, there is growing support from a variety of other studies for the value of care plan delivery (Stricker & O'Brien, 2014). Nonrandomized studies have shown that patients report finding care plans empowering, and they prefer a care plan with a clear layout with sections for follow-up care recommendations and surveillance guidelines (Mayer, Gerstel, Leak, & Smith, 2012). Patients have reported that care plans are useful to help change their lifestyle and health habits (Mayer et al., 2012). In a study of breast cancer survivors, 53% who received an SCP described the care plan as being "useful" or "very useful" (Buzaglo, Dougherty, Amsellem, & Golant, 2011). In another study that surveyed patients with a wider range of cancers, the patients reported that care plans were useful as a tool for communication (Marbach & Griffie, 2011).

Delivery of SCPs has been associated with an increase in perceived knowledge about survivorship care and care coordination (Siegel et al., 2013). In a study of 111 young adult cancer survivors who received a 1-page treatment summary and care plan, 95% reported valuing the information, and one third of those patients who had outside doctors shared the care plan with the other providers (Spain et al., 2012). Studies continue to measure outcomes and the value of delivering SCPs.

Randomized controlled trials (RCTs) have had mixed results. Four RCTs have examined the efficacy of using SCPs: two for breast cancer survivors (Grunfeld et al., 2011; Hershman et al., 2013) and two for gynecologic cancer survivors (Brothers, Easley, Salani, & Andersen, 2012; van de Poll-Franse et al., 2011). The largest of them was conducted in Canada and compared a standard oncologist discharge visit before transition to primary care with the same standard visit plus a nurse-delivered SCP for 408 breast cancer survivors (Grunfeld et al., 2011). There was no difference in cancer-specific distress (i.e., primary outcome) between the arms. However, methodologic flaws and questions related to the relevance of the population to U.S. cancer survivors have limited its application (Jefford, Schofield, & Emery, 2012; Stricker, Jacobs, & Palmer, 2012). A second study of breast cancer survivors ($N = 126$) showed no improvement in distress or concerns but did find decreased cancer-related worry among women receiving SCPs (Hershman et al., 2013). An RCT that enrolled 121 gynecologic cancer survivors revealed high ratings for care in both study arms, but it found no differences between women who did or did not receive SCPs (Brothers et al., 2012). A fourth RCT of SCPs provided by Dutch gynecologic oncology team members has been completed (van de Poll-Franse et al., 2013), and the trial showed no evidence of a benefit of SCPs on satisfaction with information and care. The patients receiving the SCPs reported receiving more information about their treatment. However the SCP group reported increased concerns, emotional impact, experienced symptoms, and the amount of cancer-related contact with the primary care physician. (Nicolaije et al., 2014).

Characteristics of Various Survivorship Care Plan Tools

Template	Data Entry	Configurable or Localized	Format	Other Considerations
American Society of Clinical Oncology (ASCO)	Manual	Manually	Word, Excel, some EMRs	www.asco.org
Journey Forward	Manual	No	Web based	CNExT tumor registry interface
LIVESTRONG Care Plan, Onco-life Care Plan	Manual	No	Downloadable program	Lengthy patient summary
Homegrown	Varies; some with partial automation	Yes	Varies, some built into EMR	High upfront costs; ongoing costs for maintenance of content and IT
Commercial (e.g., Carevive Care Planning System, Equicare CS)	Various degrees of automation	Yes	Varies	Higher degree of automation than other options; various levels of EMR and registry integration; various degrees of tailoring and content maintenance

EMR, Electronic medical record; *IT,* information technology

Nursing Role in Survivorship Care Plans

There is an enormous opportunity for oncology nurses and nurse practitioners who are already working as part of the treatment team to create and deliver care plans (Klemp, 2015). Understanding the diagnoses, having an active role in treatment, being able to identify the end of treatment, regularly assessing patient needs (e.g. rehabilitation, counseling, nutrition, practical issues, financial burden), and practicing care coordination as part of their everyday jobs position oncology nurses and nurse practitioners to create and deliver SCPs (Grant, Economou, & Ferrell, 2010). In addition to these qualifications, the ability of oncology nurses to access and recognize the learning needs of cancer survivors make them the ideal candidates to provide SCPs (Marbach & Griffie, 2011).

Care Plan Delivery: How to Get Started and Overcome Common Barriers

The most efficient and effective way to deliver a care plan is being tested at various centers. The IOM recommends providing a physical printed care plan to each patient and says that it should be accompanied by a review of the document by the patient with one of the primary providers of treatment (Hewitt et al., 2006).

Time constraints and underreimbursement are common barriers in creating and delivering care plans (Klemp, 2015). Designated nurses or clinicians often work with their clinical and reimbursement teams to evaluate coding and develop the most efficient process for care plan creation and delivery at each center. An initial step is deciding what method works best for an individual center. There are numerous models of survivorship care delivery (Klemp, 2015), and some of the most common models for delivering a care plan include the following:

- Dedicated survivorship clinic (i.e., physician- or nurse practitioner–led or with a multidisciplinary team)
- Follow-up SCP visit with a qualified provider
- Transition visit with an oncology nurse practitioner or physician's assistant that occurs before transitioning from an oncology center to a long-term follow-up clinic
- Regular follow-up visit with one of the principal providers
- Plan mailed to the patient with a follow-up phone discussion

Care plans can be generated using a computer program, a handmade template, embedded EMR templates, or a Web-based portal (Stricker & O'Brien, 2014). Each method has its advantages and disadvantages (see table above). To reduce the time needed to create a care plan, many cancer centers are building or purchasing electronic solutions. Some centers are using EMRs to create care plans. A with paper templates, using EMR templates can be time consuming and require extensive personnel and technologic resources to develop and maintain (Zabora, Bolte, Brethwaite, Weller, & Friedman, 2015). Information technology (IT) solutions should be carefully analyzed to ensure that all requirements required to maintain a specific accreditation are included. IT solutions should also be evaluated to ensure that the content (e.g., follow-up recommendations, surveillance plans, education about late effects) is kept up to date with the current guidelines and evidence-based care (Nicolajie, Ezendam, & Vos, 2015).

In an effort to identify key components of an SCP, ASCO has created a general care plan template and a handful of disease-specific care plan templates. With other clinical tools and resources, they can be found on the ASCO Web site (http://www.asco.org/practice-research/survivorship-care-clinical-tools-and-resources). Examples two survivorship care plans are listed 404 to 408.

Billings Clinic

Cancer Survivorship Care Plan

CARE TEAM

Primary Care Provider Stanford Jamieson, MD Jamieson Medical Associates	**Surgeon** Dr. Smith, MD Billings Clinic
Cancer Care Provider Michael Jones, MD Billings Clinic	**Nurse Practitioner / Nurse** Jennifer Kasper, RN, MSN Billings Clinic

DIAGNOSIS AND TREATMENT SUMMARY

DIAGNOSIS	11/2013 - Endometrioid; Ovarian cancer; Right ovaryNode negative; Pathologic Stage: Stage IC Biomarkers: CEA initial 600 (11/2013); CEA most recent 222 (03/2016);
SURGERY	12/2013: Primary Cancer Surgery = Unilateral salpingo-oophorectomy; Lymph node surgery = Lymph Node Dissection ;
CHEMOTHERAPY	12/2013 (start date): 06/2014 (end date): Carbo /Paclitaxel *(Other/Comment: Cycle every 3 weeks for 6 cycles)*
RADIATION THERAPY	Not received
HORMONAL THERAPY	Not received

PERSONAL AND FAMILIAL CANCER RISK ASSESSMENT

GENETIC TESTING HISTORY	Genetic tesing result: BRCA-2 postive
PAST CANCER HISTORY	No previous cancer
FAMILY CANCER HISTORY	Breast, Ovarian and/or Colorectal cancer in 1st or 2nd degree relatives: Yes

Follow-up Care and Surveillance

Ovarian Cancer Surveillance	YOUR ACTION ITEMS	
See your cancer care provider every 2-4 months for the first 2 years following completion of treatment; for years 3 through 5, you will be seen every 3- 6 months. After year 5, you will be seen annually	📅 Schedule:	Follow-up visit with your cancer care provider
	📄 Read:	*What Will Happen After Treatment for Ovarian Cancer?* Read online: https://url.carevive.com/1000227
Have your CA-125 or other cancer tumor markers checked at every visit if elevated at diagnosis, or as directed by your cancer care provider	📄 Read:	*Cancer Antigen 125.* Read online: https://url.carevive.com/1000228
You do not need to have routine tests such as CT/CAT scans, PET scans, and x-rays.	📞 Report:	*(to your cancer care provider)* Any of the following symptoms that either last more than 2 weeks or are severe at any time: new or unusual abdomen (belly) or pelvis pain, bloating, feeling full earlier than expected, difficulty in passing flatus (gas) or stool, unplanned weight loss, and/or worsening fatigue. Call the Billings Clinic GYN Oncology Navigator Deb Hofer, RN 406-435-7359 if you have these symptoms.
	📞 Report:	*(to your primary care provider)* Any other unusual or worrisome symptoms that last more than 2 weeks or are severe at any time, including vomiting, uncontrolled leakage of urine, blood in the urine, or unusual vaginal discharge. If these symptoms don't improve under the care of your primary care provider, call the Billings Clinic GYN Oncology Navigator Deb Hofer, RN 406-435-7359
Continue to see your primary care provider for all general health care recommended for someone your age, including cancer screening tests	📞 Report:	*(to your primary care provider)* Any other brand new, unusual, or worrisome symptoms that last more than 2 weeks or are severe at any time, including vomiting, uncontrolled leakage of urine, difficulty passing flatus (gas) or stool, or unusual vaginal discharge. If these symptoms don't improve under the care of your primary care provider, call the Billings Clinic GYN Oncology Navigator Deb Hofer, RN 406-435-7359
	📅 Schedule:	Follow up visit with your primary care provider. Call Billing's office staff or nurse navigator at (406) 435-7340 if you need help scheduling an appointment with a new primary care provider at Billings
	📄 Read:	*American Cancer Society Screening Guidelines for the Early Detection of Cancer.* Read online: https://url.carevive.com/1000226

Billings Clinic

Cancer Survivorship Care Plan

📧 Patient information

Patient: Cindy Survivorship
Date of birth: 10/13/1971
MRN/Alt ID: 33335555/-
Prepared on: 06/23/2016
Prepared by: Karen J. Hammelef

Possible Late Effects

Memory and Problems Concentrating	YOUR ACTION ITEMS
Up to 25% of cancer survivors report problems with memory and attention after chemotherapy. You may experience "brain fog" or "chemo brain." This can improve over time	**Schedule:** A visit with your primary care provider for a full physical and blood test to ensure there is no underlying cause of your memory problems **Report:** If your memory problems persist or get worse, ask your doctor for a referral to a neuropsychologist (brain specialist). They can perform tests and develop a plan to help improve your memory and concentration **Use:** Notebooks and calendars/planners to help keep you organized **Read:** *More about medications and health conditions that could be contributing to your problems with memory/concentration attention, thinking or memory problems.* Read online: http://www.cancer.net /navigating-cancer-care/side-effects /attention-thinking-or-memory-problems **Read:** *Improving Your Concentration: Three Key Steps.* Read online: https://url.carevive.com /1000168

Early (Premature) Menopause	YOUR ACTION ITEMS
Learn about the risk of your periods stopping early (known as premature menopause). This is due to the effect of cancer treatment on tissues and organs that make estrogen. Your personal risk depends on your age at time of treatment and your treatment type, length, and dose	**Read:** *Premature Menopause.* Read online: https://url.carevive.com/1000241

Another Cancer	YOUR ACTION ITEMS
There is a small risk of developing another cancer due to your cancer treatments. Many things can affect your risk for a second cancer, such as age, environmental exposures, genetics, smoking history, alcohol use, sun exposure and obesity	**Read:** *Understanding Your Risk of Secondary Malignancies.* Read online: https://url.carevive.com/1000235

Weight Gain	YOUR ACTION ITEMS
Weight gain is a common side effect of certain cancer treatments, including chemotherapy. Keeping a healthy weight can lower your chances of cancer returning	**Do:** Practice healthy eating habits and keep physically active (>150 minutes of mild to moderate physical activity per week). Start an exercise program, after approval by your health care provider, using endurance and resistance methods **Participate:** *Cancer center sponsored exercise program: YMCA LiveSTRONG Program.* Find online:https://url.carevive.com /2000157 **Schedule:** Consider appointment with a Billings Clinic oncology dietitian; Beth Hall, Kandis Wessel or Anna Harrower 406-238-2501 **Read:** *Managing Your Weight After a Cancer Diagnosis: A guide for patients and families.* Read online: https://url.carevive.com/1000290

Hearing Loss	YOUR ACTION ITEMS
Platinum chemotherapy can lead to a loss or reduction in your ability to hear. Report changes in your hearing or dizziness to your cancer doctor	**Read:** *Hearing Problems, Dizziness and Ototoxicity.* Read online: https://url.carevive.com/1000251

Reduced Kidney Function	YOUR ACTION ITEMS
Learn more about your slight risk of developing problems with kidney function due to platinum chemotherapy	**Schedule:** Annual checkups as directed with your oncologist (cancer care doctor), nephrologist (kidney doctor), or primary care for kidney function screening tests including serum creatinine and urine albumin

Bowel Obstruction	YOUR ACTION ITEMS
Learn about your possible risk of developing a bowel obstruction after treatment of your cancer; know which signs or symptoms to report	**Report:** *(To your cancer care team)* Abdominal pain, vomiting, and/or difficulty with or inability to pass flatus (gas) or stool. Call Billings' nurse line at (406) 435-7340 if you experience these symptoms **Read:** *Bowel Obstruction.* Read online: https://url.carevive.com/1000250

Legs and Lower Body Lymphedema	YOUR ACTION ITEMS
Swelling of the legs or lower body may be a symptom of lymphedema. This is caused by surgery and/or radiation therapy that interrupts the circulation of fluid in these areas. Learn ways to reduce your risk of lymphedema including practicing good skin care, avoiding tight clothing, exercising, and maintaining an ideal body weight	**Report:** New onset swelling, heaviness, fullness, aching, and/or tightness of fit of clothing in your leg(s), pelvis, or buttocks to our office. These are possibly early signs of lymphedema. Call Billings' nurse line at (406) 435-7340 if you experience these symptoms **Participate:** *Cancer center sponsored exercise program: YMCA LiveSTRONG Program* **Read:** *Understanding Lymphedema.* Read online: https://url.carevive.com/1000191

Billings Clinic

Cancer Survivorship Care Plan

📠 Patient information

Patient: Cindy Survivorship
Date of birth: 10/13/1971
MRN/Alt ID: 33335555/-
Prepared on: 06/23/2016
Prepared by: Karen J. Hammelef

Sexual Concerns

Many people experience changes in sexual function and intimacy from cancer treatment. Find resources to help you manage your sexual health concerns

YOUR ACTION ITEMS

Schedule: An appointment with your gynecologist or a urologist to evaluate persistent physical sexual problems

Consider: Meeting with an American Association of Sexuality Educators, Counselors and Therapists (ASSECT) certified therapist. Visit http://www.assect.org or call (202) 449-1099 for more information or to find a provider

Read: *Sexuality.* Read online: http://www.cancer.gov/about-cancer/coping/self-image

Numbness and Tingling of Hands and Feet

Numbness and tingling of the hands and feet (peripheral neuropathy) occurs from damage to nerve cells. This can be caused by cancer treatment such as chemotherapy or radiation therapy and medical conditions such as diabetes

YOUR ACTION ITEMS

Schedule: An appointment with your cancer care provider or primary care provider to discuss ongoing peripheral neuropathy that is interfering with your quality of life

Record: Keep a pain diary and record daily

Do: Take precautions to avoid falls and injury to your hands and feet. *If your feet are involved:* Wear supportive shoes, examine your feet daily for injuries and use handrails and extra caution when walking as you are at an increased risk for falling. *If your hands are involved:* Wear oven mitts, garden gloves and use a thermometer to check water temperatures

Do: *(with your cancer care doctor)* Talk about your symptoms and how they are affecting your daily activities. There are treatments available to help reduce your symptoms and your risk of injury and falls

Read: *Peripheral Neuropathy Caused by Chemotherapy.* Read online: https://url.carevive.com/1000212

Possible Emotional/Practical Late Effects

Financial Strain

Financial strain is commonly reported after cancer treatment and can have long-term implications for you and your family. It is important for you to ask for help to find ways to lessen the burden

YOUR ACTION ITEMS

Contact: Financial counselor or social worker if you are having financial problems related to your cancer diagnosis or treatment, Jennifer Finn LCSW, OSW-C (406) 238-2501, Maggie Hirsch or Laurie Slavin

Find: Support at http://www.patientadvocate.org/ or http://www.cancer.net/navigating-cancer-care/financial-considerations/financial-resources

Read: *How to Find a Professional Financial Counselor Sensitive to Cancer Issues: Financial Guidance for Cancer Survivors and Their Families.* Read online: http://www.cancer.org/acs/groups/content/@editorial/documents/document/acsq-020181.pdf

Work and Parenting Challenges

Work and parenting challenges are commonly experienced by cancer survivors. It is important to discuss any challenges you are experiencing so that you can gain access to available support and legal advice

YOUR ACTION ITEMS

Contact: An oncology social worker, Jennifer Finn LCSW, OSW-C (406) 238-2501

Contact: The Cancer Legal Resource Center at (866) THE-CLRC and/or the Patient Advocate Foundation at (800) 532-5274

Read: *Cancer and Careers.* Read online: http://www.cancerandcareers.org

Read: *About parenting while living with cancer online at:* http://www.cancer.net/coping-with-cancer/talking-with-family-and-friends/parenting-while-living-with-cancer

Fear of Recurrence

Know that fear of cancer returning (recurrence) is common after cancer treatment

YOUR ACTION ITEMS

Report: *(to your primary care provider)* If fear of recurrence interferes with your ability to function or your quality of life. Being informed and finding ways to reduce your stress can help you cope with this fear. Consider working with a mental health professional if this persists

Read: *Living with Uncertainty: The Fear of Cancer Recurrence.* Read online: https://url.carevive.com/1000239

Depression and Anxiety

Depression and anxiety are common after cancer treatment and can, if left untreated, negatively affect your quality of life. Know the symptoms of depression/anxiety and ask for help if you are experiencing them

YOUR ACTION ITEMS

Report: *(To your primary care provider and oncology care providers)* Persistent feelings of sadness, anxiety or worry, feeling blue or down, loss of interest or pleasure in daily activities, especially if it interferes with your ability to function or your quality of life

Participate: In peer support programs online at: http://www.cancerhopenetwork.org/

Schedule: Appointment with mental health professional or oncology social worker if needed, contact Jennifer Finn LCSW, OSW-C (406) 238-2501

Read: *Anxiety, Fear and Depression.* Read online: http://www.cancer.org/acs/groups/cid/documents/webcontent/002816-pdf.pdf

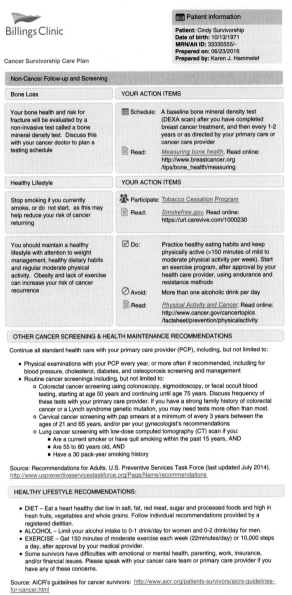

Courtesy of Carevive and Billings Clinic

Future of Cancer Survivorship: Opportunity for Nurses

The IOM's recommendation to deliver SCPs to all cancer survivors provides an important opportunity for oncology nurses to educate their patients and lead efforts to establish a process for survivorship care and care plan delivery. As with cancer treatment, it is essential to stay up to date on survivorship care through ongoing education. The courses are focused on the latest in survivorship care:

1. Cancer Survivorship E-Learning Series for Primary Care Providers: a program of the National Cancer Survivorship Resource Center (http://gwcehp.learnercommunity.com/elearning-series)
2. Cancer Survivorship in Primary Care: resources for primary care providers (http://cancerpcp.org)
3. Cancer Survivorship Training, Inc.: resources for health care professionals (www.cancersurvivorshiptraining.com)

References

American Society of Clinical Oncology. (2014). *The state of cancer care in America: 2014.* Available at http://www.asco.org/search/site/2014%20state%20of%20cancer%20care for 2014 (accessed March 4, 2016).

American Society of Clinical Oncology. (2015). *The state of cancer care in America: 2015.* Available at http://www.asco.org/sites/www.asco.org/files/2015ascostateofcancercare.pdf (accessed March 4, 2016).

American Cancer Society. (2014). *Lifetime risk of developing or dying from cancer.* Available at http://www.cancer.org/cancer/cancerbasics/lifetime-probability-of-developing-or-dying-from-cancer (accessed March 4, 2016).

Brothers, B. M., Easley, A., Salani, R., & Andersen, B. L. (2012). Do survivorship care plans impact patient evaluations of care? A randomized evaluation with gynecologic oncology patients. *Gynecologic Oncology, 129*(3), 554–558.

Buzaglo, J., Dougherty, K., Amsellem, M., & Golant, M. (2011). *Patient experience with survivorship care plans: Findings from an online registry of breast cancer survivors.* Chicago, IL: Abstract presented at the ASCO annual meeting. June 2011.

Commission on Cancer. (2014). *Accreditation committee clarifications for standard 3.3 survivorship care plan.* Available at https://www.facs.org/publications/newsletters/coc-source/special-source/standard33 (accessed March 4, 2016).

DeSantis, C., Siegel, R., & Jemal, A. (2014). *Cancer treatment & survivorship facts & figures 2014-2015*. American Cancer Society. Available at http://www.cancer.org/acs/groups/content/@research/documents/document/acspc-042801.pdf (accessed March 4, 2016).

Earle, C. C., & Neville, B. A. (2004). Underuse of necessary care among cancer survivors. *Cancer, 101*(8), 1712–1719.

Erikson, C., Salsberg, E., Forte, G., Bruinooge, S., & Goldstein, M. (2007). Future supply and demand for oncologists: Challenges to assuring access to oncology services. *Journal of Oncology Practice, 3*, 79–86.

Grant, M. E., Economou, D., & Ferrell, B. R. (2010). Oncology nurse participation in survivorship care. *Clinical Journal of Oncology Nursing, 14*(6), 709–715.

Grunfeld, E., Julian, J. A., Pond, G., Maunsell, E., Coyle, D., Folkes, A., & Levine, M. N. (2011). Evaluating survivorship care plans: Results of a randomized, clinical trial of patients with breast cancer. *Journal of Clinical Oncology, 29*(36), 4755–4762.

Hershman, D. L., Greenlee, H., Awad, D., Kalinksy, K., Maurer, M., Kranwinkel, G., & Crew, K. D. (2013). Randomized controlled trial of a clinic-based survivorship intervention following adjuvant therapy in breast cancer survivors. *Breast Cancer Research and Treatment, 138*(3), 795–806.

Hewitt, M. E., Bamundo, A., Day, R., & Harvey, C. (2007). Perspectives on post-treatment cancer care: Qualitative research with survivors, nurses, and physicians. *Journal of Clinical Oncology, 25*(16), 2270–2273.

Hewitt, M., Greenfield, S., & Stovall, E. (2006). *From cancer patient to cancer survivor: Lost in transition. Institute of Medicine*. Washington, DC: The National Academies Press.

Jefford, M., Schofield, P., & Emery, J. (2012). Improving survivorship care. *Journal of Clinical Oncology, 30*(12), 1391–1392.

Klemp, J. R. (2015). Survivorship care planning: One size does not fit all. *Seminars in Oncology Nursing, 13*(1), 67–72.

Landier, W. (2009). Survivorship care: Essential components and models of delivery. *Oncology (Williston Park), 23*(4 suppl), 46–53.

Ligibel, J. A., & Denlinger, C. S. (2013). New NCCN guidelines for survivorship care. *Journal of the National Comprehensive Cancer Network, 11*(5), 640–644.

LIVESTRONG. (2011). *"I learned to live with it" is not good enough: Challenges reported by post-treatment cancer survivors in the LIVESTRONG surveys*. Available at http://images.livestrong.org/downloads/flatfiles/what-we-do/our-approach/reports/challenges/LSSurvivorSurveyReport_final.pdf (accessed March 4, 2016).

Marbach, T. J., & Griffie, J. (2011). Patient preferences concerning treatment plans, survivorship care plans, education, and support services. *Oncology Nursing Forum, 38*(3), 335–342.

Mayer, D. K., Gerstel, A., Leak, A. N., & Smith, S. K. (2012). Patient and provider preferences for survivorship care plans. *Journal of Oncology Practice, 8*(4), 80e–86e.

Mayer, D. K., Nekhlyudov, L., Snyder, C. F., Merrill, J. K., Wollins, D. S., & Shulman, L. N. (2014). American Society of Clinical Oncology clinical expert statement on cancer survivorship care planning. *Journal of Oncology Practice, 10*(6), 345–351.

McCabe, M. S., & Jacobs, L. (2008). Survivorship care: Models and programs. *Seminars in Oncology Nursing, 24*(3), 202–207.

Murgić, C., Soldić, C., Vrljić, D., Samija, I., Kirac, I., Bolanca, A., & Kusić, Z. (2012). Quality of life of Croatian breast cancer patients receiving adjuvant treatment: Comparison to long-term breast cancer survivors. *Collegium Antropologicum, 36*(4), 1335–1341.

National Accreditation Program for Breast Centers. (2014). *NAPBC standards manual, 2014 edition: standard 2.20, Breast cancer survivorship care*. Available at https://www.facs.org/~/media/files/quality%20programs/napbc/2014%20napbc%20standards%20manual.ashx (accessed March 4, 2016).

National Cancer Institute. (2014). *Lifetime risk (percent) of being diagnosed with cancer by site and race/ethnicity, 2009-2011 (Tables 1.15 through 1.17). SEER Cancer Statistics Review, 1975-2011*. Available at http://seer.cancer.gov/csr/1975_2011/results_merged/topic_lifetime_risk_diagnosis.pdf (accessed March 4, 2016).

Nicolaije, K. A., Ezendam, N. P., Vos, M. C., Pijnenborg, J. M., van de Poll-Franse, L. V., & Kruitwagen, R. F. (2014). Oncology providers' evaluation of the use of an automatically generated cancer survivorship care plan: Longitudinal results from the ROGY Care trial. *Journal of Cancer Survivorship, 8*(2), 248–259.

Nicolaije, K. A., Ezendam, N. P., & Vos, M. C. (2015). Impact of an Automatically Generated Cancer Survivorship Care Plan on Patient-Reported Outcomes in Routine Clinical Practice: Longitudinal Outcomes of a Pragmatic, Cluster Randomized Trial. *Journal of Clinical Oncology, 34*(13).

Oeffinger, K. C., Hudson, M. M., Mertens, A. C., Smith, S. M., Mitby, P. A., Eshelman-Kent, D. A., & Robison, L. L. (2010). Increasing rates of breast cancer and cardiac surveillance among high-risk survivors of childhood Hodgkin lymphoma following a mailed, one-page survivorship care plan. *Pediatric Blood & Cancer, 56*(5), 818–824.

Oeffinger, K. C., & McCabe, M. S. (2006). Models for delivering survivorship care. *Journal of Clinical Oncology, 24*(32), 5117–5124.

Potosky, A., & Han, P. K. (2011). Differences between primary care physicians' and oncologists' knowledge, attitudes and practices regarding the care of cancer survivors. *Journal of General Internal Medicine, 26*(12), 1403–1410.

Salloum, R. G., Hornbrook, M. C., Fishman, P. A., Ritzwoller, D. P., O'Keeffe Rossetti, M. C., & Elston Lafata, J. (2012). Adherence to surveillance care guidelines after breast and colorectal cancer treatment with curative intent. *Cancer, 118*(22), 5644–5651.

Salz, T., Oeffinger, K. C., Lewis, P. R., Williams, R. L., Rhyne, R. L., & Yeazel, M. W. (2012). Primary care providers' needs and preferences for information about colorectal cancer survivorship care. *Journal of the American Board of Family Medicine, 25*(5), 635–651.

Schapira, M. M., McAuliffe, T. L., & Nattinger, A. B. (2000). Underutilization of mammography in older breast cancer survivors. *Medical Care, 38*(3), 281–289.

Shi, Q., Smith, T. G., Michonski, J. D., Stein, K. D., Kaw, C., & Cleeland, C. S. (2011). Symptom burden in cancer survivors 1 year after diagnosis: A report from the American Cancer Society's Studies of Cancer Survivors. *Cancer, 117*(12), 2779–2790.

Siegel, R., Naishadham, D., & Jemal, A. (2013). Cancer statistics, 2013. *CA: Cancer Journal for Clinicians, 63*(1), 11–30.

Spain, P. D., Oeffinger, K. C., Candela, J., McCabe, M., Ma, A., & Tonorezos, E. S. (2012). Response to a treatment summary and care plan among adult survivors of pediatric and young adult cancer. *Journal of Oncology Practice, 8*(3), 196–202.

Stein, K., Smith, T., Kim, Y., Mehta, C., Stafford, J., Spillers, R., & Baker, F. (2006). The American Cancer Society's Studies of Cancer Survivors: The largest, most diverse investigation of long-term cancer survivors so far. *American Journal of Nursing, 106*(3), 83–85.

Stricker, C. T., & Jacobs, L. A. (2008). Physical late effects in adult cancer survivors. *Oncology (Williston Park), 22*, 33.

Stricker, C. T., Jacobs, L. A., & Miller, K. (2012). Cancer survivorship care planning. In K. Miller (Ed.), *Excellence in cancer survivorship care* (pp. 86–104). Santa Barbara, PA: Praeger Press.

Stricker, C. T., Jacobs, L. A., & Palmer, S. C. (2012). Survivorship care plans: An argument for evidence over common sense. *Journal of Clinical Oncology, 30*, 1392–1393.

Stricker, C. T., & O'Brien, M. (2014). Implementing the Commission on Cancer standards: Survivorship care plans. *Clinical Journal of Oncology Nursing, 18*(suppl 1), 15–22.

Tanvetyanon, T. (2005). Physician practices of bone density testing and drug prescribing to prevent or treat osteoporosis during androgen deprivation therapy. *Cancer, 103*(2), 237–241.

U.S. Department of Health and Human Services, Health Resources and Services Administration, National Center for Health Workforce Analysis. (2013). *Projecting the supply and demand for primary care practitioners through 2020*. Rockville, MD: U.S. Department of Health and Human Services. Available at http://bhpr.hrsa.gov/healthworkforce/supplydemand/usworkforce/primarycare/ (accessed March 4, 2016).

van de Poll-Franse, L. V., Nicolaije, K. A., Vos, M. C., Pijnenborg, J. M., Boll, D., Husson, O., & Kruitwagen, R. F. (2011). The impact of a cancer Survivorship Care Plan on gynecological cancer patient and health care provider reported outcomes (ROGY Care): study protocol for a pragmatic cluster randomized controlled trial. *Trials, 12*, 256.

Wu, H., & Harden, J. (2015). Symptom burden and quality of life in survivorship: A review of the literature. *Cancer Nursing, 38*(1), E29–E54.

Zabora, J. R., Bolte, S., Brethwaite, D., Weller, S., & Friedman, C. (2015). The challenges of the integration of cancer survivorship care plans with electronic medical records. *Seminars in Oncology Nursing, 31*(1), 73–78.

Palliative Care and End-of-Life Issues

6

Palliative Care

Debra E. Heidrich

Introduction

Health care professionals usually are not as comfortable dealing with issues related to death and dying as they are with supporting the patient through curative treatment. Knowledge and skill in providing physical and emotional comfort to dying patients and their families are essential in providing optimal care to persons with advanced, progressive diseases. Palliative care is a relatively new but growing specialty that focuses on promoting the best possible quality of life (QOL) for patients facing life-threatening illness through optimal management of physical, psychosocial, emotional, and spiritual symptoms. This specialty grew out of the hospice movement and is continuing to evolve as more palliative care teams are integrated into health care systems, more palliative care content is taught in schools of medicine and nursing, and more research is conducted to support an evidence base for palliative interventions.

Definition

Palliative care is a philosophy of care and a highly organized system for delivering care. The goal of palliative care is to prevent and relieve suffering and to support the best possible QOL for patients and their families, regardless of the stage of the disease or the need for other therapies (National Consensus Project for Quality Palliative Care [NCP], 2013). Palliative care expands the traditional disease model of medical treatment to include the goals of enhancing QOL for the patient and family, optimizing function, assisting with decision making, and providing opportunities for personal growth. It can be delivered concurrently with life-prolonging care or as the main focus of care. Palliative care is distinguished from routine symptom management by the following:

- The interdisciplinary approach
- Focus on physical, emotional, social, and spiritual needs
- Inclusion of the family in the unit of care

The box below and on page 411 summarizes the practice guidelines outlined by the NCP (2013).

Clinical Practice Guidelines for Quality Palliative Care

1. Structure and processes of care
   1.1. A comprehensive and timely interdisciplinary assessment of the patient and family forms the basis of the plan of care.
   1.2. The care plan is based on the identified and expressed preferences, values, goals, and needs of the patient and family and is developed with professional guidance and support for patient-family decision making. Family is defined by the patient.
   1.3. An interdisciplinary team provides services to the patient and family consistent with the care plan. In addition to chaplains, nurses, physicians, and social workers, other therapeutic professionals who provide palliative care services to patients and families may include child-life specialists, nursing assistants, nutritionists, occupational therapists, recreational therapists, respiratory therapists, pharmacists, physical therapists, massage therapists, art and music therapists, psychologists, and speech and language pathologists.
   1.4. The palliative care program is encouraged to use appropriately trained and supervised volunteers to the extent feasible.
   1.5. Support for education, training, and professional development is available to the interdisciplinary team.
   1.6. In its commitment to quality assessment and performance improvement, the palliative care program develops, implements, and maintains an ongoing data-driven process that reflects the complexity of the organization and focuses on palliative care outcomes.
   1.7. The palliative care program recognizes the emotional impact of the provision of palliative care on the team providing care to patients with serious or life-threatening illnesses and their families.
   1.8. Community resources ensure continuity of the highest quality palliative care across the care continuum.
   1.9. The physical environment in which care is provided meets the preferences, needs, and circumstances of the patient and family to the extent possible.
2. Physical aspects of care
   2.1. The interdisciplinary team assesses and manages pain or other physical symptoms and their effects based on the best available evidence.
   2.2. The assessment and management of symptoms and side effects are contextualized according to the disease status.
3. Psychological and psychiatric aspects of care
   3.1. The interdisciplinary team assesses and addresses psychological and psychiatric aspects of care based on the best available evidence to maximize patient and family coping and quality of life.
   3.2. A core component of the palliative care program is a grief and bereavement program available to patients and families based on assessment of needs.
4. Social aspects of care
   4.1. The interdisciplinary team assesses and addresses the social aspects of care to meet patient-family needs, promote patient-family goals, and maximize patient-family strengths and well-being.
   4.2. A comprehensive, person-centered interdisciplinary assessment (as described in domain 1, guideline 1.1 of the NCP guidelines) identifies the social strengths, needs, and goals of each patient and family.
5. Spiritual, religious, and existential aspects of care
   5.1. The interdisciplinary team assesses and addresses spiritual, religious, and existential dimensions of care.
   5.2. A spiritual assessment process, including a spiritual screening, history questions, and a full spiritual assessment as indicated, is performed. This assessment identifies religious

Clinical Practice Guidelines for Quality Palliative Care—cont'd

or spiritual/existential background, preferences, and related beliefs, rituals, and practices of the patient and family, as well as symptoms such as spiritual distress or pain, guilt, resentment, despair, and hopelessness.

5.3. The palliative care service facilitates religious, spiritual, and cultural rituals or practices as desired by patient and family, especially at and after the time of death.

6. Cultural aspects of care

6.1. The palliative care program serves each patient, family, and community in a culturally and linguistically appropriate manner.

6.2. The palliative care program strives to enhance its cultural and linguistic competence.

7. Care of the patient at the end of life

7.1. The interdisciplinary team identifies, communicates, and manages the signs and symptoms of patients at the end of life to meet the physical, psychosocial, spiritual, social, and cultural needs of patients and families.

7.2. The interdisciplinary team assesses and, in collaboration with the patient and family, develops, documents, and implements a care plan to address preventative and immediate

treatment of actual or potential symptoms and the patient and family preferences for site of care, attendance of family and community members at the beside, and desire for other treatments and procedures.

7.3. Respectful postdeath care is delivered in a respectful manner that honors the patient, family culture, and religious practices.

7.4. An immediate bereavement plan is activated after death.

8. Ethical and legal aspects of care

8.1. The patient or surrogate's goals, preferences, and choices are respected within the limits of acceptable state and federal law, current accepted standards of medical care, and professional standards of practice. Person-centered goals, preferences, and choices form the basis for the plan of care.

8.2. The palliative care program identifies, acknowledges, and addresses the complex ethical issues arising in care of people with serious or life-threatening illnesses.

8.3. The provision of palliative care occurs in accordance with professional, state, and federal laws, regulations, and current accepted standards of care.

Data from National Consensus Project for Quality Palliative Care. (2013). *Clinical practice guidelines for quality palliative care* (3rd ed.). Available at http://www.nationalconsensusproject.org/NCP_Clinical_Practice_Guidelines_3rd_Edition.pdf (accessed March 4, 2016).

Palliative care should be initiated at the diagnosis of a life-threatening or chronic, progressive illness and continued throughout the course of the illness across all care settings. As illustrated in the figure in the next column, palliative care is started along with life-prolonging therapies at the initial diagnosis of a life-threatening illness. As the disease progresses, there is greater emphasis on palliative interventions than life-prolonging interventions. Hospice care is part of the palliative care continuum when the emphasis is no longer on life prolongation but primarily on comfort. In the United States, this is often defined as the last 6 months of life and is based on the eligibility requirements for hospice benefits under Medicare.

Palliative Care in Persons with Cancer

Every cancer patient needs palliative care starting at the time of diagnosis and continuing throughout treatment, follow-up care, and the end of life (National Cancer Institute, 2010). The expertise of the palliative care interdisciplinary team can be especially helpful in four key areas (Ramchandran & von Roenn, 2013):

- Advanced disease with a prognosis of less than 1 year
- Significant symptom burden from the disease or from treatment
- Significant social or psychological distress
- Poor functional status

Models of Palliative Care Delivery

Palliative care services are most effective when integrated into the care setting. Various models are used to facilitate access to the expertise of the palliative care team and include one or some combination of the following:

- Internal consultation team in an acute or rehabilitation hospital, nursing home, or free-standing inpatient hospice
- External consultation team in an acute or rehabilitation hospital, nursing home, or free-standing inpatient hospice

- Dedicated inpatient unit in an acute or rehabilitation hospital, nursing home, or free-standing inpatient hospice
- Hospital- or private practice–based outpatient palliative care practice or clinic
- Hospice- or private practice–based palliative care in the home care setting

Hospice and Palliative Care

The figure below illustrates that hospice care is part of the palliative care continuum when life-prolonging therapies are no longer providing benefit. The focus of care is on comfort and quality of living by affirming life and viewing dying as a normal process. Services provided by the hospice interdisciplinary team include pain and symptom management, psychosocial and spiritual support, assistance and support with direct caregiving, and bereavement care for the patient and family. The practice guidelines outlined by the NCP (2013) (see box on page 412) also apply to the organized, comprehensive services available through hospice programs.

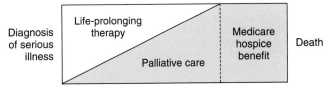

Palliative care's place in the course of illness. (From National Consensus Project for Quality Palliative Care. [2013]. *Clinical practice guidelines for quality palliative care* [3rd ed.]. Pittsburgh, PA).

Medicare, some state Medicaid programs, and some private insurance companies require that patients have a prognosis of 6 months or less to be eligible for hospice services. However, the median length of stay in hospice programs in 2013 was only 18.5 days (National Hospice and Palliative Care Organization, 2014). Barriers that interfere with initial and timely referrals to hospice programs include the following (Friedman, Harwood, & Shields, 2002):

- Discomfort in discussing end-of-life care issues by patients, family members, and health care professionals
- Difficulty in determining a prognosis of 6 months or less
- Lack of information or misinformation about hospice care by patients, family members, and health care providers
- Real or perceived requirement to discontinue life-prolonging therapies to receive hospice services

The Hospice Medicare Benefit

Eligibility Criteria (Required of the Patient)
- Have Medicare Part A
- Be certified as having a terminal diagnosis with a prognosis of 6 months or less by a physician
- Accept palliative care (for comfort) instead of care to cure the illness
- Choose hospice care instead of other Medicare-covered treatments for the terminal illness and related conditions
- Enroll in a Medicare-approved hospice program

Services Covered (All Services for the Terminal Illness)
- Physician services
- Nursing care
- Medical equipment
- Medical supplies
- Prescription drugs
- Hospice aide and homemaker services
- Physical and occupational therapy
- Speech-language pathology services
- Social work services
- Dietary counseling
- Grief and loss counseling for the patient and family
- Short-term inpatient care (for pain and symptom management)
- Short-term respite care
- Any other Medicare-covered services needed to manage the terminal illness and related conditions, as recommended by the hospice team

Services Not Covered
- Treatment intended to cure the terminal illness and/or related conditions
- Prescription drugs (except for symptom control or pain relief)
- Care from any provider that is not arranged by the hospice medical team
- Room and board
- Care in an emergency room, inpatient facility care, or ambulance transportation that is not arranged by the hospice team or is unrelated to the terminal illness and related conditions

Benefit Period
- There are two 90-day periods followed by an unlimited number of 60-day periods.
- At the start of each period of care, the hospice medical director or other hospice doctor must recertify that the patient is terminally ill.

Payment for Service
- Hospice programs are paid a per diem rate to provide all the services, and there is no deductible.
- The patient may be required to pay a copayment of up to $5 per prescription for outpatient prescription drugs for pain and symptom management.
- The patient may be required to pay 5% of the Medicare-approved amount for inpatient respite care.

From Centers for Medicare and Medicaid Services. (2016). Medicare hospice benefits. CMS Product No. 02154. Baltimore, MD: U.S. Department of Health and Human Services. Available at https://www.medicare.gov/Pubs/pdf/02154.pdf (accessed March 4, 2016).

Eligibility requirements and an outline of the services provided under the Medicare hospice benefit are listed in the box to the left. Hospices receive a per diem rate from Medicare to pay for all services related to the terminal illness. Traditional Medicare coverage remains in place for services related to problems other than the identified terminal illness. Many private insurance companies have hospice benefits that are similar to those provided under Medicare.

The services from hospice programs are much more comprehensive than can be provided under a traditional home care insurance benefit, giving the patient and family more physical, clinical, psychosocial, emotional, and spiritual support over a longer period of time than is available under other benefits. Patients whose residence is a long-term care facility receive these same benefits in addition to the services provided by the facility.

Services not paid for under the Medicare hospice benefit include the following:
- Treatment or medications intended to cure the terminal illness rather than for symptom control
- Care from any provider or in any facility that is not arranged by the hospice team
- Room and board

Because Medicare does not pay for room and board at nursing homes, patients who qualify for skilled care in a long-term care facility may have less out-of-pocket expense by using their "skilled days" before enrolling in a hospice program. This is unfortunate because many of these patients and families could benefit from the expertise and support of the hospice team during this difficult time. Palliative care teams in long-term care facilities, when available, can address the symptom management and support needs of this population of patients.

References

Friedman, B., Harwood, K., & Shields, M. (2002). Barriers and enablers to hospice referrals: An expert overview. *Journal of Palliative Medicine, 5*, 73–81.

National Cancer Institute. (2010). *Palliative care in cancer.* Available at http://www.cancer.gov/cancertopics/advanced-cancer/care-choices/palliative-care-fact-sheet (accessed March 4, 2016).

National Consensus Project for Quality Palliative Care (NCP). (2013). *Clinical practice guidelines for quality palliative care* (3rd ed.). Available http://www.nationalconsensusproject.org/NCP_Clinical_Practice_Guidelines_3rd_Edition.pdf (accessed March 4, 2016).

National Hospice and Palliative Care Organization. (2014). *NHPCO's facts and figures: Hospice care in America.* Available at http://www.nhpco.org/sites/default/files/public/Statistics_Research/2014_Facts_Figures.pdf (accessed March 4, 2016).

Ramchandran, K. J., & von Roenn, J. H. (2013). What is the role for palliative care in patients with advanced cancer? In N. E. Goldstein, & R. S. Morrison (Eds.), *Evidence-based practice of palliative medicine* (pp. 276–280). Philadelphia: Elsevier.

Bibliography

Ferrell, B., Coyle, N., & Paice, J. A. (2015). *Oxford textbook of palliative nursing* (4th ed.). New York: Oxford University Press.

Goldstein, N. E., & Morrison, R. S. (2013). *Evidence-based practice of palliative medicine.* Philadelphia: Elsevier Saunders.

Final Hours

Mary Murphy and Trechia Gross

Introduction

Patients in the final hours and days before death may experience a variety of emotional, psychosocial, spiritual, and physical symptoms. Patients, families, health care workers, and physicians may misdiagnose or refuse to identify the signs and symptoms of imminent death. Barriers include the diagnosis, age, religion, and moral beliefs, along with denial and apprehension about discussing the dying process or ongoing treatment options.

Failure to identify a patient's terminal state may lead to inappropriate diagnostic testing, futile treatment, and mismanagement of end-of-life symptoms that would be better managed with palliative or hospice care. Estimation of a short-term prognosis may be complex because of the diagnosis, disease trajectory, and care provider's emotional value system. An honest conversation about functional decline and prognosis is needed to allow the patient and family to identify their goals of care (Feliu et al., 2011).

Similar physical and psychosocial characteristics are seen during the final weeks, days, and hours of a patient's life. The period is often divided into two major categories: the preactive phase and active phase of dying. The following symptoms are seen during the preactive phase, which is 7 to 14 days before death (Matzo, 2011):

- Increased weakness
- Need for assistance with activities of daily living increasing to total care needs
- Bed-to-chair or bed-bound status
- Increased sleeping
- Disorientation, confusion, or episodes of near-death awareness
- Decreasing food and fluid intake
- Fever
- Incontinence or bowel or bladder retention
- Swallowing difficulty, including a need to discontinue or alter the route of medication
- Restlessness, agitation, withdrawal, loss of bowel and bladder control, withdrawal from family and friends, fear of the dying process, or asking when it will happen
- Increased spiritual needs, visions of deceased friends and family members (Callanan & Kenny, 1992).
- Family and caregiver fatigue

The following symptoms are seen during the active phase, which is 2 to 3 days before death:

- Altered vital signs
  - Lowered blood pressure
  - Lowered or elevated temperature
  - Abnormal respiratory pattern (e.g., apnea, Cheyne-Stokes breathing)
  - Heart rate (i.e., faded, muffled, or rapid)

- Decreased level of consciousness
- Terminal respiratory congestion
- Cool, dusky, or mottled skin
- Decreased responsiveness to external stimuli
- Limited oral intake
- Restlessness, agitation, staring, disconnectedness, viewing of environment from a distance (symptoms vary according to the person and time of the event, but some patients experience last-minute surges of energy)
- Crying out, moaning, whimpering when touched
- Pain
- Urinary or bowel incontinence (Hui et.al, 2014).

Nursing Considerations Before Death

Discuss the following issues with the patient or family members:

- Review advance directives and durable power of attorney for health care (DPOA-HC) status and code status.
- Review with the patient and family the DPOA for financial issues.
- Review wishes about the desire for an autopsy and cremation or burial. Offer resources for funeral plans and phone numbers.
- Check the family's need to be present at the time of death, and obtain list of family members to call. Obtain information on how far from center the family is located to determine if the request can be achieved.
- Review goals of care such as palliation or active treatment.
- Address hydration and feeding concerns.
- Review signs and symptoms of the terminal phase.
- Review treatment and medication modalities to relieve symptoms. Avoid the use of medical jargon. Offer open, honest, and supportive concern.
- Provide a supportive environment in which to deliver bad news.
- Be aware of rituals, traditions, and rites that may be important to care or related to religious or cultural beliefs.
- Support storytelling and journaling.
- Identify what support is available at the time of death and in the days following.
- Address unfinished business, goals, or family concerns.
- Check for potential posttraumatic stress disorder (PTSD) concerns (Boyd, 2011).
- Coach families in distress to accomplish four tasks (Byock, 1997):
  - Ask for forgiveness
  - Say thank you
  - Say I love you
  - Say good-bye

Palliative Therapy Options for End-of-Life Patients

Pain Management

- Use observation scales (e.g., Universal Pain Assessment tool, Pain Assessment in Advanced Dementia [PAINAD]) that are appropriate to the level of alertness and current situation and are approved at the facility where the staff members are working.
- Never discontinue opioids or benzodiazepines.
- Seek alternative routes as needed.

Dyspnea

- Use oxygen for support.
- Elevate the head of the bed.
- Suction mildly as needed.
- Use benzodiazepines and low-dose opioids.

Dehydration

- Provide mouth and lip care.
- Offer sips of fluids as appropriate.
- Use hypodermoclysis if appropriate and the staff members know how to do the procedure.
- Discuss food and fluid issues.

Incontinence

- Provide skin care.
- Use a Foley catheter (assess for bladder distention).
- Use incontinence barriers.
- Provide manual impaction removal with the use of a suppository only if the patient has distention and discomfort.

Confusion and Agitation

- Use benzodiazepines and phenothiazines.

Respiratory Congestion or Death Rattle

- Suction only if necessary.
- Elevate the head of the bed.
- Manage medications:
  - Hyoscyamine (Levsin)
  - Atropine
  - Scopolamine

Physical Care

- Provide mouth care.
- Continue turning and positioning for comfort.
- Provide skin care.
- Provide safety.
- Provide emotional care.
- Provide a quiet environment or sounds that are comforting (e.g., tapes, voices).
- Engage in story telling (i.e., past pleasant events).

- Call the patient by name.
- Explain who is in the room, and state who you are and what you will be doing.

Special Considerations

- Increased preparation is needed for some diagnoses and expected symptoms:
  - Hemorrhage
  - Seizures
  - Severe and uncontrolled terminal agitation
  - Children or younger patients
  - PTSD
  - Management of severe symptoms e.g., pain, nausea, vomiting, dyspnea, obstructed airway (Ferrell, Coyle, & Paice, 2015)

Nursing Care After Death

- Clarify who needs to be present or notified before the body is removed.
- Determine whether any ritual (e.g., poem, prayer) should take place.
- Remove personal items (e.g., rings, hair).
- Offer support services based on individual or family religious values and support systems.
- Prepare the body.
- Say final good-byes (Olausson & Ferrell, 2013).

Last-Minute Concerns

- No one can predict the time of death, which may be associated with symptoms, significant events in the patient's life (e.g., birthdays, holidays, anniversaries), or other events that are outside of everyone's control.

Bibliography

Boyd, D., Merkh, K., Rutledge, D., & Randall, V. (2011). Nurses' perceptions and experiences with end-of-life communication and care. *Oncology Nursing Forum*, 38(3), 229–239.

Byock, I. (1997). *Dying well: The prospects for growth at end-of-life.* New York: Riverhead Books.

Callanan, M., & Kenny, P. (1992). *Final gifts: Understanding the special awareness needs and communications of the dying.* New York: Bantam Books.

Feliu, J., Jiménez-Gordo, A. M., Madero, R., Rodriguez-Aizcorbe, J. R., Espinosa, E., Castro, J., & González-Barón, M. (2011). Development and validation of a prognostic nomogram for terminally ill cancer patients. *Journal of the National Cancer Institute*, 103, 1613.

Ferrell, B. Coyle, N. & Paice, J. (2015). Care of the Imminently Dying. New York: Oxford University Press.

Hui, D., dos Santos, R., Chisholm, G., Bansal, S., Silva, T. B., Kilgore, K., & Bruera, E. (2014). Clinical signs of impending death in cancer patients. *The Oncologist*, 19, 681.

Matzo, M. L. (2010). Peri-death nursing care. In M. L. Matzo, & D. W. Sherman (Eds.), *Palliative care nursing: Quality care to the end of life* (3rd ed.). New York: Springer Publishing Company.

Olusson, J., & Ferrell, B. (2013). Care of the body after death. *Clinical Journal Oncology Nursing*, 17(6), 647–51.

Loss, Grief, and Bereavement

Debra E. Heidrich

Introduction

People with cancer and their family members experience multiple losses throughout the cancer experience, including body image changes, loss of control over time and schedules, loss of the ability to fulfill usual roles at work or home, and the ultimate loss of life. Grief is a normal and expected reaction to these losses. Oncology nurses play an important role in supporting individuals through the normal grieving process and in identifying individuals who may require additional support for complicated grief.

Definition

Several terms are used when discussing grief and bereavement (Corless, 2015; Rando, 1984).
- *Loss:* The absence of an object, position, ability, or attribute
- *Grief:* The psychological, social, and somatic responses to loss
- *Anticipatory grief:* The psychological, social, and somatic responses to an anticipated loss
- *Mourning:* The outward and active expression of grief through participation in various death and bereavement rituals that vary by culture
- *Bereavement:* The state of having suffered a loss or the period of time during which grief and mourning occur; the first year after a loss is usually the most difficult
- *Complicated grief:* A disturbance in the normal grief process

  Many factors affect grief and bereavement:
- Support systems (e.g., children, organizations, family)
- Previous experiences
- Suddenness of the event
- Coping mechanisms
- Relation to and significance of the person or event
- Knowledge and understanding
- Timing of the event
- Life sequence of the event
- Concurrent stresses
- Rituals and expectations
- Religion, spirituality, and culture
- Boundaries
- Financial burden or support
- Events from diagnosis to death
- Role in the family and community
- Personal value system (e.g., body image, self-concept)
- Role in the family (i.e., internal or external)
- Perception of the loss, esteem, or identity
- Future goals (i.e., what will not be)

Normal Manifestations of Grief

Manifestations of grief include social, physical, and cognitive-emotional reactions, which can vary widely from one individual to another. There is no right way to grieve.

Social Manifestations
- Restlessness and inability to sit still
- Feeling uncomfortable around other people or social withdrawal
- Feeling of not wanting to be alone
- Lack of ability to initiate and maintain organized patterns of activity

Physical Manifestations
- Anorexia and weight loss or overeating and weight gain
- Heart palpitations, nervousness, tension, or panic
- Shortness of breath
- Tightness in the throat
- Inability to sleep
- Lack of energy and feelings of physical exhaustion
- Headaches, muscular aches, and gastrointestinal distress

Cognitive-Emotional Manifestations
- Sadness and crying
- Forgetfulness or difficulty concentrating
- Feelings of anger or guilt
- Mood swings
- Sense of helplessness
- Yearning for the deceased
- Dreams of the deceased

Grief Theories

Grief theories provide a framework to help explain an individual's response to grief and the process of adjusting to a loss. The following three theories show the evolution of our understanding of the grief process.
1. *Stages of grief:* Denial, anger, bargaining, depression, and acceptance (Kübler-Ross, 1969)
2. *Tasks of grief work:* Accept reality of loss, experience the pain of the loss, adjust to the environment without the deceased person, and withdraw emotionally from the deceased by forming an ongoing relationship with the memories of the deceased in a way that allows the individual to continue with life (Worden, 2002):
3. *Dual-process model of coping with bereavement:* Understanding the dynamic nature of grief as involving oscillation between loss-oriented coping (i.e., working through

the loss) and restoration-oriented coping (i.e., mastering new tasks, reorganizing life, and developing a new identity) (Stroebe & Schut, 2010)

Complicated Grief

- *Prolonged grief:* Persistent and severe yearning for the deceased beyond 6 to 12 months after the loss (Bryant, 2013). Prolonged grief disorder is recognized as a mental disorder causing significant distress and disability, and it is included in the *Diagnostic and Statistical Manual of Mental Disorders,* 5th ed. (DSM-V)(American Psychiatric Association, 2013; Bryant, 2013).
- *Disenfranchised grief:* Grief that occurs when the loss cannot be openly acknowledged. Examples of disenfranchised grief include the death of a person in a nonsanctioned relationship (e.g., extramarital affair, homosexual partner), loss from miscarriage or abortion, or the loss of the essence of the individual before the actual death, such as with severe dementia.

Support and Counseling

- Provide a safe, accepting environment that allows expression of feelings, thoughts, and emotions.
- Provide education about the manifestations of grief to validate that the feelings, thoughts, and emotions the individual is experiencing are normal and expected.

- Encourage the patient and family to express feelings and reconcile difficult relationships while the patient has the mental and physical capacity to participate in conversations.
- Support individuals to participate in mourning practices that are meaningful to them.
- Facilitate referrals to social workers and chaplains as appropriate.
- Facilitate referrals to bereavement counselors and support programs.
- Assess for signs of complicated grief and facilitate referrals to psychological or psychiatric specialists as appropriate.

References

American Psychiatric Association. (2013). *Diagnostic and statistical manual of mental disorders* (5th ed.). Washington, DC: American Psychiatric Association.

Bryant, R. A. (2013). Is pathological grief lasting more than 12 months grief or depression? *Current Opinion in Psychiatry, 26,* 41–46.

Corless, I. B. (2015). Bereavement. In B. R. Ferrell, N. Coyle, & J. A. Paice (Eds.), *Oxford textbook of palliative nursing* (4th ed.) (pp. 487–499). New York: Oxford University Press.

Kübler-Ross, E. (1969). *On death and dying.* New York: Macmillan.

Rando, T. (1984). *Grief, dying, and death: Clinical interventions for caregivers.* Champaign, IL: Research Press Company.

Stroebe, M., & Schut, H. (2010). The dual process model of coping with bereavement: A decade on. *Omega, 61,* 273–389.

Worden, J. W. (2002). *Grief counseling and grief therapy: A handbook for the mental health practitioner* (3rd ed.). New York: Springer.

Communication

Lisa Kennedy Sheldon

Communication Skills

Communication skills are the foundation of patient-centered cancer care. The skills are especially important for oncology clinicians, who must regularly adjust their approach to meet the physiologic and psychosocial needs of patients. Timely communication is also needed among multidisciplinary oncology team members, primary care providers, and specialists in palliative and end-of-life care.

Effective communication in cancer care links specific clinician behaviors with patient outcomes (de Haes & Bensing, 2009; Street, Makoul, Arora, & Epstein, 2009). For example, when clinicians provide information to patients, the desired outcome is increased patient autonomy and decision making, but too much information may increase patient uncertainty (de Haes & Bensing, 2009). Communication by clinicians requires a balance between delivering factual information about managing the disease and compassionately talking with patients about their concerns (Eggly, Albrecht, Kelly, Prigerson, Sheldon, & Studts, 2009). According to Epstein and Street (2007), patient-clinician communication has six main functions in cancer care:

1. Fostering healing relationships
2. Exchanging information
3. Responding to emotions
4. Managing uncertainty
5. Making decisions
6. Enabling patient self-management

Communication between people occurs verbally and nonverbally (e.g., body posture, facial expressions). Oncology clinicians use verbal and nonverbal skills to promote trust and openness with patients and provide an atmosphere in which patients are comfortable asking questions and sharing concerns. Clinicians must tailor communication to the individual patient by incorporating his or her values, beliefs, culture, ethnicity, and preferred method of communicating and by including the patient's family members and social network. Clinicians can promote communication by using effective verbal and nonverbal behaviors (see table in the next column).

Patients' nonverbal behaviors often indicate their concerns, which may include symptoms such as pain or dyspnea, attitudes such as friendliness or dominance, and personality characteristics such as shyness (Mast, Klockner, & Hall, 2010). Nonverbal cues from patients often contain essential information about their condition and concerns that enhance verbal information. For example, a subdued demeanor with lack of eye contact may indicate deeper emotions. Information from verbal and nonverbal cues provides a more comprehensive picture of the patient that can help to direct assessment and interventions.

Behaviors by Oncology Clinicians That Promote or Inhibit Communication

Behaviors That Promote Communication	Behaviors That Inhibit Communication
Body posture, such as facing the patient, closer distance (as culturally appropriate), leaning forward	Greater distance, blocking with the computer, crossed arms
Direct eye gaze (as culturally appropriate)	Looking away or at a chart or computer screen
Pauses and listening	Interrupting the patient, speaking faster, dominating the conversation content
More expression in voice and face, nodding	Greater distance, less expression, loud voice
Smiling	Less or no smiling
Open-ended questions	Dominating conversation, limiting questions
Soliciting the patient's expectations and preferences	Telling the patient options without asking about preferences
Use of emotional probes and questions about concerns	Providing factual information and directing the focus of the conversation
Promoting partnership, building with the patient	Providing information and prescribing treatment

In oncology care, communicating with patients and families occurs in two areas:

1. Information about diagnosis, treatment, and symptom management
2. Psychosocial and emotional responses to the disease, treatment, symptoms, and prognosis.

Information Sharing

Sharing information by oncology clinicians is essential for making decisions, setting realistic goals, and preparing for the end of life. As specialists in cancer care, clinicians must interpret and clearly share information in words that are appropriate for patients' language and literacy levels. For example, for clinicians, a *positive biopsy result* means that evidence of disease has been found, but the term may be misinterpreted as a good finding or absence of disease by people not in health care professions.

Information can be shared verbally in a conversation and then reinforced with written material, videos, or Internet resources. Confirmation is an important step to ensure patients have the information they need to make decisions and for self-management. To check that the patient has understood the message, the clinician may say, "Tell me what you know about your diagnosis" or "Tell me what you understand about what I have said so far." These open-ended statements allow patients to describe their level of understanding in their own words, and they provide a foundation for the next steps in the conversation.

Psychosocial and Emotional Responses

Oncology clinicians care for people adjusting to changes in health and adapting to illness. By virtue of the time spent with patients, nurses often hear patients' psychosocial concerns. This is especially true at vulnerable points in the course of a cancer illness, when patients and families are prone to more anxiety and fear. Oncology clinicians have an obligation to assess patient concerns at these vulnerable points and during routine care (see box below).

Vulnerable Points

1. Waiting for diagnostic and genetic test results
2. Giving the diagnosis
3. When discussing prognosis, survival, and treatment effectiveness
4. When the disease recurs or progresses, the treatment fails, or the disease metastasizes
5. When new symptoms or severe side effects occur
6. When stopping active treatment and transitioning to palliative care or during do not resuscitate discussions
7. Sudden, unexpected death

Discussions occurring at these vulnerable points are also called *bad news conversations*. The SPIKES protocol can provide structure for the delivery of difficult information (Baile, Buckman, Lenzi, Globera, Bealea, & Kudelkabet, 2000).

S (setting): Use privacy and quietness, include all parties who need to be there, and prevent distractions.

P (perception): Assess what the patient and family know and their perceptions of the situation first. Ask open-ended questions such as the following:

"What is your understanding of why your family member is in the hospital?"

"What have you been told about your illness?"

"How do you feel the treatment has been working?"

I (invitation or information): Ask directly how much and what kind of information the patient and family wish to know.

K (knowledge): Communicate the bad news honestly while being direct and caring, provide information in small segments, and check for comprehension.

E (empathy): Acknowledge and validate the emotions and reactions; use active listening.

S (summarize and strategize): Review what was said; ensure and verify comprehension; and present plan for further intervention, treatment, palliation, or hospice.

Assessment of Psychosocial Concerns

The Institute of Medicine (IOM) emphasized psychosocial care for patients in its report: *Cancer Care for the Whole Patient: Meeting Psychosocial Health Needs* (IOM, 2007). Accreditation standards by the American College of Surgeons Commission on Cancer (2016) include assessment of psychosocial concerns of people with a diagnosis of cancer and a referral pathway for those with significant distress.

Psychosocial assessment requires tools that measure concerns and detect significant distress. For example, the National Comprehensive Cancer Network (NCCN) has been advocating for screening of distress since 1999 and created a tool, the distress thermometer, for use in clinical practice. It contains a visual scale of 0 (no distress) to 10 (extreme distress) displayed on a thermometer. If a patient scores 4 or higher on the scale, referrals and interventions are warranted to address specific concerns. The tool also has 38 items for practical, family, emotional, spiritual or religious, or physical problems. Because of the simplicity of the tool, oncology nurses can administer it and refer to the primary oncology team for distress levels of 4 or higher or unrelieved physical symptoms. More specific tools are available for assessing specific conditions such as the Patient Health Questionnaire (PHQ-9) for depression (Spitzer, Korenke, & Williams, 1999) (see box below).

Assessment of concerns requires referral and treatment options

---

Measures of Distress, Anxiety, Depression, Fear, and Worry

- National Comprehensive Cancer Network (NCCN) distress thermometer
- Hospital Anxiety and Depression Scale (HADS)
- State Trait Anxiety Inventory (STAI)
- Center for Epidemiologic Studies depression (CES-D)

- Beck Depression Inventory
- Structured clinical interview
- Functional Assessment of Cancer Treatment (FACT)
- Worry scale
- Fear questionnaire
- Padua inventory

---

for people with significant psychosocial problems. To treat psychosocial problems such as anxiety and depression, the Oncology Nursing Society Putting Evidence into Practice (PEP) program was one of the first initiatives to review the literature and compile levels of evidence for translation of evidence to clinical practice. The PEP Web sites for anxiety (http://www.ons.org/Research/PEP/Anxiety) and depression (http://www.ons.org/Research/PEP/Depression) contain information on the levels of evidence and a compilation of current tools useful in measuring these conditions. The NCCN (2013) also developed evidence-based guidelines to assess and manage distress associated with cancer.

Specific aspects of communication between patients and clinicians may improve assessment and detection of psychosocial concerns. For example, patients are more descriptive about their concerns if a clinician initiates the conversation (Heyn, Finset, & Ruland, 2013). In another study, patients who expressed their concerns more often and those expressing more explicit emotion were more likely to have their concerns assessed and treated (Sheldon, Blonquist, Hilaire, Hong, & Berry, 2015). Nurses can play an active role in initiating discussions about psychosocial concerns and encourage their patients to speak clearly and frequently about their concerns, allowing the oncology team to meet their needs.

Responding to Emotions

Interventions to patient verbal responses are based on evidence-based strategies and clinician experience. Systematic reviews of the literature by nurses such as the PEP have revealed effective interventions for anxiety (Sheldon, Swanson, Dolce, Marsh, & Summers, 2008) and sadness in depression (Fulcher, Badger, Gunter, Marrs, & Reese, 2009). One common concern of oncology clinicians is how to react to the negative emotional responses of patients, which may be potent expressions of anger or profound sadness. Some of the most effective strategies for clinicians include nonverbal skills such as availability, presence, respect, listening, eye contact, and touch as appropriate. However, strong emotions from patients may also prompt emotional responses in clinicians and impede therapeutic communication. Specific communication skills may be useful in addressing emotion during conversations with patients. The NURSE mnemonic is can be applied in these situations (Kaplan, 2010) (see box below).

NURSE Mnemonic for Responding to Emotion

N: Name the emotion or feeling expressed by the patient.
  "What I said made you sad."
U: Understand or acknowledge the emotional reaction as reasonable.
  "Given what you have been through, it is understandable that you would be scared."
R: Respect the patient's abilities and challenges.
  "You have been through a lot and keep fighting."
S: Supportive statements demonstrate that the clinician is prepared to help the patient.
  "I am here to help you; let me know what you need."
E: Ask the patient to elaborate the emotion.
  "Tell me more about how being sad affects you."

The NURSE mnemonic is a guide to provide structure during emotionally laden conversations. The clinician does not have to agree with the patient's response but demonstrates understanding, respect, and support. These therapeutic responses express respect and appreciation for the patient's abilities to cope with difficult situations.

Uncertainty

Living after a cancer diagnosis means learning strategies to live with uncertainty. The patient may fear recurrence, uncontrolled symptoms such as pain, or a potentially shortened life. An unpredictable future may create a pervasive sense of uncertainty that results in chronic anxiety and decreased pleasure in the present. The intensity, duration, and extent of these feelings differentiate normal from abnormal responses. Assessment of general distress is a first step in understanding the extent of the patient's concerns. Patients often offer hints rather than directly expressing their fears, especially at points of vulnerability (see Vulnerable Points box on page 418).

Transition to Palliative Care

Conversations at the time of transition from active, curative treatment to palliative care are often difficult for the patient and family (see Communication Skills at the Transition to Palliative Care box in the next column). Although palliative care involving symptom management is a vital component of all cancer care, patients often see palliative care as a less aggressive, not curative part of their care. They may ask about the meaning of palliative care and the difference between it and hospice care.

It is important to understand the patient's knowledge about and preferences for care. The clinician should ask for permission from the patient to discuss her or his condition. For example, the clinician may inquire, "Tell me what you know about your illness." When patients are not receptive to having a discussion about their illness, the next question becomes, "With whom would you like me to talk?" It is important to explore the patient's usual decision-making practices, such as consulting with family or clergy:

- How do you make decisions?
- Whom do you include in making decisions?
- If you cannot make decisions, who will make them for you?

Communication Skills at the Transition to Palliative Care

- Recognize patient cues and the clinical situation.
- Establish the patient and family or caregiver's understanding of disease progression.
- Discuss patient values, priorities, preferences, and goals.
- Respond to emotions (i.e., NURSE pneumonic).
- Negotiate the shift in care goals.
- Promote understanding of transitions.
- Address the family or caregiver's concerns.
- Refer the patient for services.
- Plan the next steps, and close the discussion.

When the focus changes from aggressive care to palliative, hospice, and end-of-life care, patients and families need a meeting to discuss and decide on the next steps. The efforts of oncology clinicians focus on excellent symptom management and maintenance of quality of life (Tulsky, 2005). A family meeting may help to honor patient requests and facilitate informed choices. Communication during a family meeting is structured to establish patient and family goals (see box below).

Family Meetings

- Clearly state the agenda.
- Make partnership statements.
- Check the patient and family or caregiver's understanding of the situation.
- Reinforce the patient's level of decision making, and give permission to ask questions.
- Clarify, empathize, and normalize.
- Validate, respect, summarize, and offer help.
- Make partnership statements.
- Ask open questions.
- Summarize, check understanding, and plan the next steps.

Special communication strategies are needed to address complex issues. Clinicians need to respectfully frame messages when discussing issues such as do-not-resuscitate orders. The table on page 420 provides some communication strategies to avoid and suggestions for more sensitive approaches to these discussions with the patient and family.

Transition to Hospice Care: Communication Mistakes and Solutions

Statements to Avoid	Statements to Try
There is nothing more to be done.	Although we cannot shrink the cancer, we can improve quality of life.
If your heart stops, would you want us to do everything? They would pound on your chest and put in a breathing tube.	What do you know about cardiopulmonary resuscitation? It will not prolong your life and may increase your suffering.
He has failed third-line chemotherapy.	The treatment did not work. The cancer is very aggressive (i.e., the patient is not a failure).
If we discuss hospice and end-of-life care, he will give up hope.	The discussion may allow him to feel prepared and supported.
His cancer has advanced or progressed. He is in denial.	Where do you see things going? What is your understanding of your condition?

Caring for the Clinician

Many situations in cancer care provoke strong reactions in patients and clinicians. These human responses require acknowledgment and reflection so that they do not stifle other experiences and relationships. For clinicians, job stress can lead to burnout and lack of satisfaction with clinical care. Specific training in communication skills, self-awareness of emotional responses, and distinct strategies to handle stress in cancer care can reduce burnout (Goldstein, Concato, Fried, Kasl, Johnson-Hurzeler, & Bradley, 2004; Taylor, Graham, Potts, Richards, & Ramirez, 2005). Self-care strategies for handling stress include the following:

- Journaling
- Support groups for debriefing and grieving
- Self-reflection exercises
- Training in self-awareness of emotional responses to patient care
- Mindfulness training and meditation

Conclusion

Communication among patients, families, and oncology clinicians is essential for creating healing environments that improve the treatment of the disease and symptoms and promote quality of life. Effective communication comprises sharing information and addressing psychosocial needs. Verbal and nonverbal forms of communication provide information about the patient's needs and responses to care. This information enlightens treatment of the disease, palliation of symptoms, and care at the end of life. Compassionate communication requires an understanding of the patient's preferences, beliefs, and psychosocial and emotional needs.

Clinicians also experience stressful and emotional situations arising in cancer care and can benefit from training in effective communication skills. Ultimately, combining the art and science of communication improves the delivery of cancer care and enhances the well-being of all people.

References

American College of Surgeons Commission on Cancer. (2016). *Cancer program standards: Ensuring patient-centered care.* Available at http://www.facs.org/cancer/coc/programstandards2012.html (accessed March 12, 2016).

Baile, W. B., Buckman, R., Lenzi, R., Globera, G., Bealea, E. A., & Kudelkab, A. P. (2000). *SPIKES: A six-step protocol for delivering bad news: Application to the patient with cancer.* Available at http://theoncologist.alphamedpress.org/content/5/4/302 (accessed March 12, 2016).

de Haes, H., & Bensing, J. (2009). Endpoints in communication research: Proposing a framework of functions and outcomes. *Patient Education and Counseling, 74,* 287–294.

Eggly, S. S., Albrecht, T. L., Kelly, K., Prigerson, H. G., Sheldon, L. K., & Studts, J. (2009). The role of the clinician in cancer clinical communication. *Journal of Health Communication, 14*(1), 66–75.

Epstein, R. M., & Street, R. L. (2007). *Patient-centered communication in cancer care: Promoting healing and reducing suffering.* Bethesda, MD: National Cancer Institute.

Heyn, L., Finset, A., & Ruland, C. M. (2013). Talking about feelings and worries in cancer consultations. *Cancer Nursing, 36*(2), E20–E30.

Fulcher, C. D., Badger, T., Gunter, A. K., Marrs, J. A., & Reese, J. M. (2009). Putting evidence into practice: Interventions for depression. *Clinical Journal of Oncology Nursing, 12*(1), 131–140.

Goldstein, N. E., Concato, J., Fried, T. R., Kasl, S. V., Johnson-Hurzeler, R., & Bradley, E. H. (2004). Factors associated with caregiver burden among caregivers of terminally ill patients with cancer. *Journal of Palliative Care, 20,* 38–43.

Institute of Medicine (IOM). (2007). *Cancer care for the whole patient: Meeting psychosocial health needs.* Washington, DC: National Academies Press.

Kaplan, M. (2010). SPIKES: A framework for breaking bad news to patients with cancer. *Clinical Journal of Oncology Nursing, 14*(4), 514–516.

Mast, M. S., Klockner, C., & Hall, J. A. (2010). Gender, power and nonverbal communication. In D. W. Kissane, B. D. Bultz, P. M. Butow, & I. G. Finaly (Eds.), *Handbook of communication in oncology and palliative care* (p. 63). New York: Oxford University Press.

National Comprehensive Care Network (NCCN). (2013). *Distress guidelines.* version 2.2013. Available at http://www.nccn.org/professionals/physician_gls/pdf/distress.pdf (accessed March 12, 2016).

Sheldon, L. K., Blonquist, T. M., Hilaire, D. M., Hong, F., & Berry, D. L. (2015). Patient cues and symptoms of psychosocial distress: What predicts assessment and treatment of distress by oncology clinicians? *Psycho-oncology, 24*(9), 1020–1027.

Sheldon, L. K., Swanson, S., Dolce, A., Marsh, K., & Summers, J. (2008). Putting evidence into practice: Evidence-based interventions for anxiety. *Clinical Journal of Oncology Nursing, 12,* 789–797.

Spitzer, R. L., Korenke, K., & Williams, J. B. (1999). Validation and utility of a self-report version of PRIME-MD: The PHQ primary care study. *Journal of the American Medical Association, 282*(18), 1737–1744.

Street, R. L., Makoul, G., Arora, N. K., & Epstein, R. M. (2009). How does communication heal? Pathways linking clinician-patient communication with health outcomes. *Patient Education and Counseling, 74,* 295–301.

Taylor, C., Graham, J., Potts, H. W., Richards, M. A., & Ramirez, A. J. (2005). Changes in mental health un UK hospital consultants since the mid-1990s. *Lancet, 366*(9487), 742–744.

Tulsky, J. A. (2005). Beyond advance directives: Importance of communication skills at the end of life. *Journal of the American Medical Association, 294,* 359–365.

Cultural Considerations

Joanne Itano

Definition of Culture

Culture comprises the values, beliefs, norms, and practices of a particular group that are learned and shared. It guides thinking, decisions, and actions in a patterned way (Leininger, 1991) and includes the following:

- Country of origin, length or location of current residence, and reasons for migration
- Communication, including native language, willingness to share personal thoughts or feelings, use of touch and by whom, meaning of eye contact, time orientation, and format of names
- Family roles, including who is the decision maker, caregiver, or spokesperson; gender-related roles; and role of the extended family
- Workforce issues, including current employment, economic impact of illness, and educational preparation
- Biologic differences, including skin color, physical attributes, differences in incidence of illnesses, and variations in drug metabolism
- Therapy-compromising behaviors such as use of alcohol, tobacco, and recreational drugs and participation in health promotion and safety practices
- Nutrition, including the meaning of food, types of foods eaten, food rituals, and dietary practices
- Pregnancy and childbearing practices
- Death rituals
- Spirituality, including identifying with a formal religion or cult, meaning of life, use of prayer or meditation, and relationship between spiritual beliefs and health practices
- Health care practices, including practices that impact health promotion and prevention practices, who is responsible for health care, beliefs about the meaning of illness and health, barriers to health care, and beliefs about acceptance of treatments, drugs, blood transfusions, and loss of organs
- Health care practitioners, including the role of traditional and folk practitioners; age, gender, and race of the health care provider; and acceptance of care by the patient and family (Purnell, 2012)

Providing Culturally Competent Care

Culturally competent care is a process, not an end point, in which the nurse works to provide care within the cultural context of the patient, family, or community. It includes the following:

- Awareness of the nurse's background and its influence on patient care
- Knowledge of the patient's culture and how it affects health care practices
- Accepting and respecting cultural differences and their impact on health care delivery

- Awareness that the beliefs of health care providers and patients may differ and may affect care
- Avoidance of judgmental acts and beliefs
- Openness to diverse cultural encounters
- Adaptation of care to be congruent with cultural needs (Andrews & Boyle, 2012; Purnell, 2012)

Assessment Model

The assessment model is delineated by the acronym CONFHER:

- **C** (communication): What language does the patient speak? What words does the patient use for common health terms (e.g., pain, fever)?
- **O** (orientation): What cultural group does the patient identify with? What are the values that influence the patient? How long has the patient been in the United States?
- **N** (nutrition): What are the patient's food preferences? Are there food taboos? Are there concerns about artificial nutrition and hydration?
- **F** (family relationships): How is the family defined, and who is in the family? Who is the decision maker in the family? What are the roles of the men, women, and children?
- **H** (health beliefs): What are the beliefs about health and illness? Are there conflicts with Western medicine? Who is consulted about health concerns? What does illness mean to the culture? What beliefs may interfere with delivery of care?
- **E** (education): What is the patient's learning style and education level? What is the patient's occupation?
- **R** (religion): What are the patient's religious beliefs? Do the beliefs have an impact on health care and illness (Fong, 1985)?

Barriers to Cultural Competence

- Ethnocentrism: using one's customs or values to judge others
  - The nurse's cultural background
  - The culture of Western health care
- Stereotyping: making assumptions that an individual reflects all characteristics associated with a group
  - Assuming, for instance, a Latino patient has limited English proficiency and arranging for an interpreter before confirming this
  - Assuming an Asian male patient is stoic about pain and will not ask for pain medication (Berman, Snyder, & Frandsen, 2015)

Cancer Disparities

Cancer incidence and mortality rates are different among the four major minority groups in the United States. Cancers in these minorities are detected at a later stage compared with non-Hispanic whites.

National Standards for Culturally and Linguistically Appropriate Services

The National Standards for Culturally and Linguistically Appropriate Services (CLAS) in health care aim to improve health care quality and advance health equity by establishing a framework for organizations to serve the nation's increasingly diverse communities.

Principal Standard

- Provide effective, equitable, understandable, and respectful quality care and services that are responsive to diverse cultural health beliefs and practices, preferred languages, health literacy, and other communication needs.

Governance, Leadership, and Workforce

- Advance and sustain organizational governance and leadership that promote CLAS and health equity through policy, practices, and allocated resources.
- Recruit, promote, and support a culturally and linguistically diverse governance, leadership, and workforce that are responsive to the population in the service area.
- Educate and train governance, leadership, and the workforce in culturally and linguistically appropriate policies and practices on an ongoing basis.

Communication and Language Assistance

- Offer language assistance to individuals who have limited English proficiency or other communication needs at no cost to them to facilitate timely access to all health care and services.
- Inform all individuals of the availability of language assistance services clearly and in their preferred language, verbally and in writing.
- Ensure the competence of individuals providing language assis-

tance, recognizing that the use of untrained individuals or minors as interpreters should be avoided.
- Provide easy-to-understand print and multimedia materials and signage in the languages commonly used by the populations in the service area.

Engagement, Continuous Improvement, and Accountability

- Establish culturally and linguistically appropriate goals, policies, and management accountability, and infuse them throughout the organization's planning and operations.
- Conduct ongoing assessments of the organization's CLAS-related activities and integrate CLAS-related measures into assessment measurement and continuous quality improvement activities.
- Collect and maintain accurate and reliable demographic data to monitor and evaluate the impact of CLAS on health equity and outcomes and to inform service delivery.
- Conduct regular assessments of community health assets and needs, and use the results to plan and implement services that respond to the cultural and linguistic diversity of populations in the service area.
- Partner with the community to design, implement, and evaluate policies, practices, and services to ensure cultural and linguistic appropriateness.
- Create conflict- and grievance-resolution processes that are culturally and linguistically appropriate to identify, prevent, and resolve conflicts or complaints.
- Communicate the organization's progress in implementing and sustaining CLAS to all stakeholders, constituents, and the general public.

From U.S. Department of Health and Human Services Office of Minority Health, The national CLAS standards. Available at http://minorityhealth.hhs.gov/omh/browse.aspx?lvl=2&lvlid=53 (accessed March 13, 2016).

- Blacks
  - Black men and women are more likely to die of cancer than any other racial or ethnic group.
  - Death rate for cancer among blacks is 29% higher for men and 14% higher for women compared with non-Hispanic whites.
  - Incidence and death rates are higher for black males compared with non-Hispanic whites for every cancer type except kidney cancer.
- Hispanics
  - They have the lowest rates of tobacco-related cancers because of low rates of smoking.
  - They have the highest rate for cancers associated with infection, including cancers of the liver (i.e., hepatitis B infection), stomach (i.e., *Helicobacter pylori*), and uterine cervix (i.e., human papillomavirus), depending on countries of origin.
- Asian and Pacific Islanders
  - They have the lowest overall cancer incidence and mortality rates.
  - They have the highest rates for cancers of the liver and stomach, similar to Hispanics.
- American Indians and Alaska Natives
  - They have the highest kidney cancer incidence and mortality rates, likely due to the prevalence of smoking, obesity, and hypertension (American Cancer Society, 2015).

Strategies for Promoting Cultural Competence in the Organization

In 2013, the Office of Minority Health updated the National Standards for Culturally and Linguistically Appropriate Services (CLAS) in health care, which were directed at health care organizations (see box above).

References

American Cancer Society. (2015). *Cancer facts & figures 2015.* Atlanta: American Cancer Society.

Andrews, M. M., & Boyle, J. S. (2012). *Transcultural concepts in nursing care* (6th ed.). Philadelphia: Wolters Kluwer.

Berman, A., Snyder, S. J., & Frandsen, G. (2015). *Fundamentals of nursing, concepts, process and practice.* Boston: Pearson.

Fong, C. M. (1985). Ethnicity and nursing practice. *Topics in Clinical Nursing, 7*(3), 1–10.

Leininger, M. (1991). Transcultural nursing: The study and practice. *Imprint, 38,* 55–66.

Purnell, L. (2012). *Transcultural health care: A culturally competent approach* (4th ed.). Philadelphia: F. A. Davis.

U.S. Department of Health and Human Services Office of Minority Health. The national CLAS standards. http://minorityhealth.hhs.gov/omh/browse.aspx?lvl=2&lvlid=53 (accessed March 13, 2016).

Ethical Considerations

Lisa Balster

Introduction

Ethical considerations play a major role in oncology nursing practice and in excellent patient and family care. In 2001, the American Nurses Association (ANA) established a framework for nursing practice, which includes the following:

1. Practice with unconditional compassion and respect.
2. Have commitment to the patient, whether an individual, family, or group.
3. Promote and advocate for health and safety.
4. Take responsibility for providing optimal care (and recognizing what is beyond the scope of practice).
5. Respect self and others, preserving integrity, safety, and professional growth.
6. Take responsibility for a healthy work environment.
7. Contribute to professional practice, education, and administration.
8. Collaborate in community efforts to meet health care needs.
9. Take responsibility for articulating nursing values to shape policy and practice.

Ethics is derived from the Greek term *ethos*, meaning "customs, conduct, or character." It involves the study of how a person determines right and wrong. Analytical thinking and reasoning must be employed when faced with complex choices, and the benefits and risks of each choice should be thoroughly articulated and communicated.

Ethical dilemmas arise when conflicting values are associated with decision options, and it is essential to carefully weigh each option before a decision is made. In the event of an ethical dilemma, an organizational ethics committee can be consulted to weigh risks and benefits according to ethical principles.

Key Ethical Theories

- *Ethical relativism:* Morality is understood in the context of culture.
- *Feminist theory:* Feminist ethics attempt to revise traditional ethics to the extent the system depreciates or devalues women's moral experience. The philosophy is also concerned with decisions in the context of how the patient, family, others who depend on one another, and the community may be affected.
- *Deontology:* Ethical decisions are those for which the intentions are good; the good intention is the primary value rather than the outcome.
- *Utilitarianism:* The philosophy supports what is best for the majority. The value of the decision is based on usefulness; the outcome is the primary value rather than the intention.

Key Ethical Principles

- *Fidelity:* Duty to alleviate suffering and commitment to caring for others
- *Respect for persons:* Unconditional positive regard for others (includes truth telling, also known as veracity)
- *Autonomy:* Self-determination, which is based on effective informed consent
- *Nonmaleficence:* Avoiding harm; the core of the medical oath and nursing ethics
- *Beneficence:* Doing good (i.e., implies that nurses are competent to provide good care); core principle of patient advocacy
- *Human rights:* Basic rights and freedom from arbitrary interference or restriction that are based on moral principles and thought to belong to all persons; includes maintaining confidentiality and respecting diversity
- *Justice:* Fairness related to equal distribution of resources in the context of a benefit-burden analysis
- *Paternalism:* Health care professionals in positions of authority make decisions about diagnosis, prognosis, and treatment based partly on their own beliefs and restrict the freedom and responsibilities of those subordinate to them.

Framework for Ethical Decision Making

- Gather and document relevant data.
- Assess the social and interpersonal dynamics of the issue at hand.
- Determine the ethical issue apart from other dimensions (e.g., legal, institutional, medical).
- Identify relevant assumptions, beliefs, and values of all stakeholders.
- Determine core values of the issue at hand.
- Determine whether conflicts exist related to these values (i.e., ethical dilemmas).
- Identify ethically acceptable options and their consequences.
- Provide options and make choices.
- Support choices.
- Evaluate the outcome, and assess for process improvements.

Effective Informed Consent

- Informed consent depends on an ethical and legal commitment to explain the risks, benefits, and alternatives needed to make a decision.
- Patient understanding must be ensured.
- Patient participation is important and is verified by asking questions and clarifying meanings (e.g., surgical consent, blood transfusion consent, research participation).

Requirements for Effective Informed Consent

- Adequate decision-making capacity (i.e., decision maker able to weigh benefits and risks)
- Adequate time for thorough discussion of benefits and risks of each option
- Inclusion of the family and others in the discussion at the patient's request
- Lack of coercion
- Provision of a surrogate decision maker, including the following:
  - Health care power of attorney (HCPOA) (i.e., substituted judgment)
  - Next-of-kin (i.e., substituted judgment)
  - Guardianship
  - Physician acting in the best interest of the patient (if the patient lacks capacity and has no other surrogate)
- Accurate documentation of the discussion
- Agreement of the patient or decision maker to the treatment plan

Elements of Decision-Making Capacity

- Ability to understand information regarding medical treatment options and consequences of choices
- Ability to evaluate the information, comparing benefits and risks of each option
- Ability to communicate a choice that remains consistent over time (i.e., new information may cause a different choice to be made)
- Lack of any of the previous criteria constitutes a lack of decision-making capacity.

Barriers to Ethical Decision Making and Effective Informed Consent

- Language and other communication barriers
- Culture and religious beliefs (if discussion is refused because of these influences)
- Lack of adequate time to discuss all options (i.e., benefits versus risks)
- Altered capacity (i.e., physical, mental, or emotional)
- Confirmation bias (i.e., staff tendency to easily go along with a decision if it aligns with their own values regardless of established informed consent)
- Coercion
- Literacy
- Legal disputes
- Staff negligence to provide or establish all criteria in the "Requirements for an Effective Informed Consent" section

Factors That May Impair Decisional Capacity

Patients with cancer may have impaired decision-making capacity temporarily or permanently. The following situations require frequent monitoring to find a time when the patient has optimal decisional capacity:

- Cognitive impairment
- Delirium
- Weakness
- Depression or anxiety
- Uncontrolled pain and symptoms
- Grief
- Sleep deprivation
- Medications

Common Ethical Issues in Oncology

- Life-sustaining treatments, especially at the end of life
- Treatment choices in the context of quality-of-life goals
- Artificial nutrition or hydration
- Medical futility
- Palliative sedation at the end of life
- Family requests to withhold information from the patient
- Assisted suicide and euthanasia
- Ethical decisions for children (When do they have decisional capacity?)
- Moral distress of professional staff and others (i.e., moral distress can exist when the right course of action is known but people are unable to take it for any reason)
- Impact of moral distress of others on the patient
- Clinical trials and research

Role of the Nurse in Ethical Decision Making

- Provide education and support the health care team in explaining options, benefits, and risks.
- Offer support to the patient and family as they consider options.
- Facilitate communication of all involved parties.
- Serve as an advocate for the patient.
- Serve as a witness according to the guidelines of the organization.
- Provide thorough and accurate documentation of discussions, questions, responses, and choices.
- Evaluate complex cases.

Ethical Support for Nursing

- Administrative policies and leadership staff
- Ethics committee
- Nurse Practice Act
- ANA code of ethics with interpretive guidelines
- Peer support
- Bioethics networks (state or local community)

Bibliography

Arnold, R. M., Berkowitz, K. A., Dubler, N. N., Dudzinski, D., Fox, E., Frolic, A., Glover, J. J., Kipnis, K., Natali, A. M., Nelson, W. A., Rorty, M. V., Schyve, P. M., Skeel, J. D., & Tarzian, A. J. (2011). *Core competencies for healthcare ethics consultation* (2nd ed.) (pp. 22–33). Chicago: American Society for Bioethics and Humanities.

Calman, K. (2010). Ethical issues. In G. Hanks, N. Cherny, N. Christakis, M. Fallon, S. Kaasa, & R. K. Portenoy (Eds.), *Oxford textbook of palliative medicine* (4th ed.) (pp. 277–280). New York: Oxford Palliative Press.

Derse, A. R. (2013). Decision-making capacity. In D. M. Hester & T. Schonfeld (Eds.), *Guidance for healthcare ethics committees* (2nd ed.) (pp. 56–57). New York: Cambridge University Press.

Fowler, M. D. (2010). *Guide to the code of ethics for nurses: Interpretation and application*. Washington, DC: American Nursing Association, p. 143.

Horton, R., & Brody, H. (2013). Informed consent, shared decision-making, and the ethics committee. In D. M. Hester & T. Schonfeld (Eds.), *Guidance for healthcare ethics committees* (2nd ed.) (pp. 48–54). New York: Cambridge University Press.

Pojman, L. P. (2010). *Ethical theory: Classical and contemporary readings* (5th ed.) (pp. 15–37). Florence, KY: Cengage Learning.

Tattersall, M. H. (2010). Truth telling and consent. In G. Hanks, N. Cherny, N. Christakis, M. Fallon, S. Kaasa, & R. K. Portenoy (Eds.), *Oxford textbook of palliative medicine* (4th ed.) (pp. 290–295). New York: Cambridge University Press.

Quality and Safety

Julie Ponto

Quality and Safety in Oncology

Quality programs and initiatives in oncology help to ensure that individuals with cancer and their families receive care that is based on evidence and aligns with national and, in some cases, international standards. Quality and safety are closely related concepts in oncology because of unique treatment modalities that can pose safety concerns. For example, hazardous drugs and radiation therapies are key elements in oncology practice that require unique safety standards. Safety systems and procedures are designed to ensure that patients, families, and health care workers are not harmed. This chapter outlines several programs, initiatives, and standards that promote quality and safety in settings where cancer care is delivered.

Cancer Treatment–Specific Quality and Safety Information

Chemotherapy

The American Society of Clinical Oncology (ASCO) and Oncology Nursing Society (ONS) produced the Chemotherapy Administration Safety Standards Including Standards for the Safe Administration and Management of Oral Chemotherapy (http://www.instituteforquality.org/sites/instituteforquality.org/files/oral_standards_jop_article.pdf) describing the safe use of parenteral chemotherapy in the outpatient setting.

- Originally published in 2009, the protocol outlined 31 chemotherapy safety standards related to staffing, preparation and administration of chemotherapy, monitoring, and other principles of safe practice
- The ASCO/ONS chemotherapy safety standards were revised in 2012 to incorporate inpatient settings and in 2013 to include oral chemotherapy.
- The revised list has 36 standards address staffing, chemotherapy planning, chemotherapy ordering and prescribing, drug preparation, patient consent and education, chemotherapy administration, patient monitoring and assessment, and other principles of safe practice.

Radiation Therapy

The American Society for Radiation Oncology (ASTRO) (https://www.astro.org/) offers several guidelines and safety programs for radiation oncology clinicians.

- The Target Safely Campaign (https://www.astro.org/Clinical-Practice/Patient-Safety/Target-Safely/Index.aspx) is a multipronged initiative addressing practice, regulatory, patient, and professional safety and quality issues related to the safe administration of radiation therapy.
- The Radiation Oncology Incident Learning System (RO-ILS) (https://www.astro.org/Clinical-Practice/Patient-Safety/ROILS/Index.aspx) is a secure and nonpunitive system of tracking radiation-related incidents for the purpose of shared learning and safety and quality improvement within the field of radiation oncology.
- ASTRO practice guidelines and best practice statements (https://www.astro.org/Clinical-Practice/Best-Practices/Index.aspx) are topical, evidence-based guidelines and best practice statements related to the use of radiotherapy for specific cancer diagnoses.
- Quality assurance white papers (https://www.astro.org/Clinical-Practice/White-Papers/Index.aspx) are five articles that explain the roles and responsibilities of the radiation oncology team, describe practices to promote safety and prevent disastrous errors, and outline quality assurance methods for specific radiotherapy protocols:
  - Image-guided radiation therapy (IGRT)
  - Intensity-modulated radiation therapy (IMRT)
  - Stereotactic radiosurgery and stereotactic body radiation therapy (SRS/SBRT)
  - Peer review
  - High-dose-rate (HDR) brachytherapy
- The ASTRO Accreditation Program for Excellence (APEx) (https://www.astro.org/Practice-Management/Practice-Accreditation/Index.aspx) is a voluntary certification program for radiation oncology practices.
  - Standards of practice for certification are based on practice guidelines.
  - White papers focus on five aspects of safe and high-quality radiation oncology practice:
    - The process of care
    - The radiation oncology team
    - Safety
    - Quality management
    - Patient-centered care
  - An on-site survey is conducted by a medical physicist and radiation oncologist or other radiation oncology personnel. Successful practices receive APEx certification for 4 years.

Surgery

The American College of Surgeons (ACOS) offers programs on quality and safety to optimize the standards of surgical care and ethical practice.

- The ACOS Commission on Cancer (CoC) (https://www.facs.org/quality-programs/cancer/coc) develops cancer care standards and offers an accreditation program in oncology.
  - The CoC accreditation program focuses on five elements: clinical services, cancer committee, cancer conferences, quality improvement, and a cancer registry and database.
  - Eligibility requirements for accreditation include programmatic structural elements (e.g., facility accreditation, cancer committee authority, cancer conference policy, oncology nurse leadership, cancer registry) and services (e.g., diagnostic imaging, radiation oncology, systemic therapy, clinical trial information, psychosocial support, rehabilitation, nutrition).
  - Applicants submit evidence of meeting the accreditation standards and receive an on-site survey demonstrating compliance with all standards. Full accreditation is awarded in 3-year accreditation cycles.
- The National Cancer Data Base (NCDB) (https://www.facs.org/quality-programs/cancer/ncdb/about) in a joint effort with the American Cancer Society (ACS) receives data from CoC-accredited cancer programs.
  - Data are used to analyze cancer trends, create benchmarks, and inform quality improvement efforts.
  - Data reflect hospital (e.g., type of accredited program), patient (e.g., age, diagnosis, gender, race or ethnicity, income, insurance status), and treatment (e.g., surgery, chemotherapy, radiation therapy) quality indicators.

Oncology Professional Organizations' Initiatives on Quality and Safety

Oncology Nursing Society Quality and Safety Initiatives

- ONS Quality Improvement Registry (www.ons.org/practice-resources/quality-improvement-registry)
  - The registry identifies 14 quality measures related to care of patients receiving intravenous chemotherapy in the ambulatory setting or the first year of posttreatment care for survivors of breast cancer.
  - The registry fulfills the Center for Medicare and Medicaid (CMS) Physician Quality Reporting System (PQRS) requirements.
- The Red Flags in Caring for Cancer Survivors Report (https://www.ons.org/practice-resources/standards-reports/red-flags) identifies barriers and omissions in caring for cancer survivors, the effects of cancer treatment, and management guidelines for common physical and psychological side effects (Oncology Nursing Society, 2014).
- Role-Specific Core Competencies (https://www.ons.org/practice-resources/competencies)
  - The ONS publications on role-specific competencies describe the required skills and responsibilities of nurses in many oncology nursing roles:
    - Oncology nurse navigator
    - Oncology clinical trials nurse
    - Oncology nurse practitioner
    - Oncology clinical nurse specialist
    - Leadership
  - Competency articles can be used to determine expected behaviors of oncology nurses, establish consistent role responsibilities, and develop job descriptions for newly created oncology roles.
- The ONS, sometimes in conjunction with the Oncology Nursing Certification Corporation (ONCC), offers a variety of educational programs and online courses aimed at improving nursing knowledge and resulting in higher quality cancer care (https://www.ons.org/education/courses-articles?combine=&field_ilna_hours_ilna_tid=All&page=10
  - ONS Chemotherapy Basics Course
  - ONS/ONCC Chemotherapy Biotherapy Certificate Course
  - ONS Chemotherapy for Non-Oncology Conditions
  - ONS Chemotherapy in Non-Oncology Settings
  - ONS/ONCC Radiation Therapy Certificate Course

American Society of Clinical Oncology Quality and Safety Initiatives

- ASCO Institute for Quality (http://www.instituteforquality.org/)
  - Developed to promote quality, value, and accountability in cancer care
  - Provides information and resources related to ASCO's quality initiatives
- Cancer-LinQ (http://cancerlinq.org/) is a health information technology initiative that aggregates and analyzes quality data to promote rapid learning and improve patient outcomes.
- Quality Oncology Practice Initiative (QOPI) (http://qopi.asco.org/)
  - The cancer care quality initiative provides an opportunity for oncology practices to submit data on multiple quality measures (e.g., core, symptoms, breast, colorectal, end of life). Participants receive quality reports and can compare quality measure results with other de-identified practices.
  - Practice improvement resources are available for care at the end of life, chemotherapy administration, family history and genetic testing or counseling, supportive care, and treatment (http://www.instituteforquality.org/practice-improvement-resources).
  - The QOPI Web site provides information and resources (e.g., publications) regarding the ASCO/ONS Chemotherapy Administration Safety Standards.
- QOPI Certification Program (QCP) (http://qopi.asco.org/certification.html) is a certification program for outpatient oncology practices.
  - The practice applies for certification, submits evidence of meeting select ASCO/ONS Chemotherapy Administration Safety Standards, and receives an on-site survey.
  - Practices that successfully meet the standards receive a 3-year QOPI certification.
- ASCO clinical practice guidelines (http://www.instituteforquality.org/practice-guidelines) are published for many aspects of oncology practice, such as assays and predictive markers; prevention, screening, treatment, and follow-up of specific cancers; and supportive care.

- Informed consent for chemotherapy administration (http://www.instituteforquality.org/informed-consent-chemotherapy-administration) provides recommendations for the process of informed consent for chemotherapy and an informed consent template.
- The ASCO and European Society for Medical Oncology (ASCO-ESMO) Consensus Statement on Quality Cancer Care (http://www.asco.org/sites/default/files/consensus_statement.pdf) reflects the international consensus regarding 10 goals of quality cancer care (ASCO-ESMO, 2006):
  - Access to information
  - Privacy, confidentiality, and dignity
  - Access to medical records
  - Prevention services
  - Nondiscrimination
  - Consent to treatment and choice
  - Multidisciplinary cancer care
  - Innovative cancer care
  - Survivorship care planning
  - Pain management, supportive care, and palliative care
- ASCO chemotherapy treatment plans and summaries http://stage.asco.org/quality-guidelines/chemotherapy-treatment-plan-and-summaries)
  - Numerous treatment plan and summary templates describe documentation components before and after chemotherapy.
  - Templates are intended to improve communication among oncology clinicians, other care providers, and patients for better coordination of care.
  - Templates are available for chemotherapy, cancer treatment, lymphoma, and breast, colon, non–small cell lung, and small cell lung cancers.
  - Additional treatment plans and summaries are in development.

General Health Care Quality and Safety Initiatives

The Joint Commission

The Joint Commission (TJC), formerly called the Joint Commission on Accreditation of Healthcare Organizations (JCAHO), accredits more than 21,000 health care organizations and certifies many quality and safety programs (http://www.jointcommission.org/certification/certification_main.aspx).

- Although TJC does not offer a general certification program in oncology, an oncology practice can apply for certification in specific areas of cancer care (e.g., breast cancer, colorectal cancer, leukemia, lymphoma) in the Disease-Specific Care Certification Program.
  - Performance measurement and improvement indices include the following:
    - Creating an organized, comprehensive approach to performance improvement
    - Using comparative data to evaluate processes and patient outcomes
    - Evaluating participant's perception of care quality
    - Maintaining data quality and integrity
  - Because no TJC-prescribed performance measures in oncology exist, a practice selects four performance measures from existing clinical practice guidelines to implement.
- TJC offers an Advanced Certification Program for Palliative Care for hospital inpatient programs (http://www.jointcommission.org/certification/palliative_care.aspx).
  - To be eligible for certification, a hospital must do the following:
    - Follow an organized approach supported by an interdisciplinary team of health professionals
    - Use standardized clinical practice guidelines or evidence-based practice
    - Have the ability to direct the clinical management of patients and coordinate care
    - Provide a full range of palliative care services to hospitalized patients 24 hours per day, 7 days per week, with on-site or on-call staff
    - Use performance measurement to improve quality over time
  - The Advanced Certification Program for Palliative Care does not prescribe quality measures but requires palliative care programs to collect and analyze data on at least four performance measures that are evidence based, relevant, valid, and reliable.
- National Patient Safety Goals (NPSGs) (http://www.jointcommission.org/standards_information/npsgs.aspx)
  - Each year, TJC identifies key patient safety goals organized into programs or settings of care (e.g., ambulatory health care, critical access hospital, home care, hospital, long-term care).
  - NPSGs are developed and updated by a multidisciplinary team of experts, including nurses, physicians, pharmacists, risk managers, clinical engineers, and others who identify emerging safety issues in health care.

Institute of Medicine

The Institute of Medicine (IOM) produced a report called "Delivering High-Quality Cancer Care: Charting a New Course for a System in Crisis" (http://iom.edu/~/media/Files/Report%20Files/2013/Quality-Cancer-Care/qualitycancercare_slides2.pdf)

- The IOM report identified the significant patient care and workforce issues confronting the United States in regard to the growing number of individuals with cancer, particularly older adults. Recommendations from the report address care coordination, cost, research, technology, competencies of the cancer workforce, end-of-life care, and reduction of disparities.
- A specific recommendation is development of a national quality reporting program for cancer care, establishment of a public reporting system, identification of meaningful quality measures, and development of a national reporting infrastructure.

Quality and Safety Education in Nursing

Begun in 2005 as collaboration among the Robert Wood Johnson Foundation, American Association of Colleges of Nursing (ACCN), and the University of North Carolina, the

Quality and Safety Education in Nursing (QSEN) initiative (www.qsen.org) was created to improve quality and safety education in prelicensure through graduate nursing education.

- Six competencies comprise the QSEN initiative: patient-centered care, teamwork and collaboration, evidence-based practice, quality improvement, safety, and informatics. The quality improvement and safety competencies reflect knowledge, skills, and attitudes required of nurses and are categorized by level of education.
- Numerous resources are available for staff education and development, including literature reviews, learning modules, videos, and webinars.

Occupational Safety and Health Administration

The Occupational Safety and Health Administration (OSHA) (http://www.jointcommission.org/certification/certification_main.aspx) develops and monitors workplace standards.

- OSHA provides education and training, and it enforces rules and regulations related to workplace safety issues, including the administration of hazardous drugs and ionizing radiation.
- OSHA maintains a large database of workplace safety issues with search and query functionality.

National Institute for Occupational Safety and Health

The National Institute for Occupational Safety and Health (NIOSH) (http://www.cdc.gov/niosh/) is the U.S. agency responsible for conducting research and making recommendations for the prevention of work-related injury and illness.

- NIOSH updated the list of antineoplastic and other hazardous drugs to reflect the plethora of new chemotherapy drugs in 2014. The report called "Preventing Occupational Exposure to Antineoplastic and Other Hazardous Drugs in Health Care Settings" (http://www.cdc.gov/niosh/docs/2004-165/pdfs/2004-165.pdf) is a useful reference for recommendations on antineoplastic and other hazardous drug preparations, including their transport, administration, and disposal.
  - No recommended exposure limits are established for hazardous drugs.
  - Factors affecting workplace exposure include drug handling (i.e., preparation, administration, or disposal), amount of drug prepared, frequency and duration of drug handling, potential for absorption, use of ventilated cabinets, personal protective equipment, and work practices.
- Detailed recommendations in the report include assessing hazards in the workplace, handling drugs safely, and using and maintaining equipment properly (see box in the next column.).

NIOSH Recommendations for Administering Hazardous Drugs

1. Administer drugs safely by using protective medical devices (e.g. needleless systems, closed systems) and techniques (e.g., priming of IV tubing by pharmacy personnel inside a ventilated cabinet, inline priming with nondrug solutions).
2. Wear PPE (including double gloves, goggles, and protective gowns) for all activities associated with drug administration, such as opening the outer bag, assembling the delivery system, delivering the drug to the patient, and disposing of all equipment used to administer drugs.
3. Attach drug administration sets to the IV bag, and prime them before adding the drug to the bag.
4. Never remove tubing from an IV bag containing a hazardous drug.
5. Do not disconnect tubing at other points in the system until the tubing has been thoroughly flushed.
6. Remove the IV bag and tubing intact when possible.
7. Place disposable items directly into a yellow chemotherapy waste container and close the lid.
8. Remove outer gloves and gowns, and bag them for disposal in the yellow chemotherapy waste container at the site of drug administration.
9. Double bag the chemotherapy waste before removing inner gloves.
10. Consider double bagging all contaminated equipment.
11. Wash hands with soap and water before leaving the drug administration site.

IV, Intravenous; *NIOSH*, National Institute for Occupational Safety and Health; *PPE*, personal protective equipment.
From Department of Health and Human Services, Centers for Disease Control and Prevention. (2004). *NIOSH alert: Preventing occupational exposure to antineoplastic and other hazardous drugs in health care settings.* Publication number 2004-165. Available at http://www.cdc.gov/niosh/docs/2004-165/pdfs/2004-165.pdf (accessed March 14, 2016).

Bibliography

American Society of Clinical Oncology–European Society for Medical Oncology. (2006). ASCO-EMSO consensus statement on quality cancer care. *Journal of Clinical Oncology, 24,* 3498–3499.

Institute of Medicine. (2013). *Delivering high-quality cancer care: Charting a new course for a system in crisis.* Washington, DC: National Academies Press.

Jacobson, J. O., Polovich, M., Gilmore, T., Schulmeister, L., Esper, P., LeFebvre, K. B., & Neuss, M. N. (2012). Revisions to the 2009 American Society of Clinical Oncology/Oncology Nursing Society chemotherapy administration safety standards: Expanding the scope to include inpatient settings. *Journal of Oncology Practice, 8,* 2–6.

Oncology Nursing Society. (2014). *Red flags in caring for cancer survivors.* Pittsburgh, PA: Oncology Nursing Society.

Neuss, M. N., Jacobson, J. O., Polovich, M., McNiff, K., Esper, P., Gilmore, T. R., & Jacobson, J. O. (2013). 2013 Updated American Society of Clinical Oncology/Oncology Nursing Society chemotherapy administration safety standards including standards for the safe administration and management of oral chemotherapy. *Journal of Oncology Practice, 9,* 5s–13s.

Polovich, M., Whitford, J. M., & Olsen, M. (2014). *Chemotherapy and biotherapy guidelines and recommendations for practice* (4th ed.). Pittsburgh, PA: Oncology Nursing Society.

Evidence-Based Practice

Diane G. Cope

Definition

- Evidence-based practice (EBP) is the purposeful use of current evidence for making decisions about the care of a patient.
- EBP integrates the best evidence with clinical expertise and the patient's desires, values, and needs to facilitate clinical decision making.

Goals of Evidence-Based Practice

- EBP provides the highest quality of care to patients and families.
- EBP provides practicing nurses with the best and most current evidence.
- EBP resolves problems in the clinical setting.
- EBP reduces variations in nursing care.
- EBP promotes effective nursing interventions.
- EBP assists with efficient and effective decision making.

Five Steps of Evidence-Based Practice

- Step 1: Ask a searchable clinical question.
- Step 2: Find the best evidence to answer the question.
- Step 3: Critically appraise the evidence.
- Step 4: Apply the evidence with clinical expertise, taking the patient's wants and needs into consideration.
- Step 5: Evaluate the effectiveness and efficiency of the process.

Step 1: Ask a Searchable Clinical Question

- Use the PICOT format.
- The PICOT variables provide a framework for searching electronic databases for the most relevant articles to address the clinical question:

  P: patient population of interest
  I: intervention or area of interest
  C: comparison intervention or group
  O: outcome
  T: time

Step 2: Find the Best Evidence to Answer the Question

- Consider scheduling a meeting with a science librarian.
- Identify key searchable words or phrases from the clinical question.
- Combine searches using the Boolean connector *AND*.
- Select relevant databases to search for the evidence:
  - Cochrane Database of Systematic Reviews (www.cochrane.org)
  - Database of Abstracts of Reviews of Effects
  - PubMed/Medline (www.ncbi.nlm.nih.gov/pubmed)
  - Cumulative Index to Nursing and Allied Health Literature (CINAHL) (www.ebscohost.com/cinahl)
  - National Guideline Clearinghouse (www.guideline.gov)

Step 3: Critically Appraise the Evidence

- Research is systematically examined to appraise its trustworthiness, value, and relevance in a particular context.
- Strong evidence fulfills the requirements of three criteria:
  - *Quality*: randomized, controlled trials (RCTs) to avoid selection bias
  - *Validity*: outcomes that are large and statistically significant
  - *Size*: trials with large numbers of patients
- Levels of evidence (i.e., hierarchy of evidence) (see table below) are assigned to studies based on the methodologic quality of their design, validity, and applicability to patient care, factors that determine the grade (i.e., strength) of the recommendation.
  - Many scales for levels of evidence exist, and they can use three to seven levels.
  - Although standardized definitions of the levels of evidence are lacking, systematic reviews or meta-analyses of RCTs and EBP guidelines are considered the strongest level of evidence, and expert opinions are considered the weakest level of evidence to guide practice decisions.
- High levels of evidence may not exist for all clinical questions.

Hierarchy of Evidence

Evidence Level	Type of Evidence*	Type of Evidence†
I	Randomized, controlled trial (RCT) Meta-analysis of RCTs	Systematic review or meta-analysis
II	Quasi-experimental study	RCT
III	Nonexperimental study Qualitative study Meta-synthesis	Controlled trial without randomization
IV		Case-control or cohort study
V		Descriptive study Systematic review of qualitative or descriptive studies
VI		Descriptive study Qualitative study
VII		Opinion or consensus

*Using the system of Dearholt, S. L., & Dang, D. (2012). *Johns Hopkins nursing evidence based practice model and guidelines*. Indianapolis, IN: Sigma Theta Tau International.
†Using the system of Melnyk, B. M., & Fineout-Overholt, E. (Eds.). (2011). *Evidence-based practice in nursing and healthcare: A guide to best practice*. Philadelphia: Lippincott Williams & Wilkins.

- Types of studies
  - *Systematic review:* An article in which the authors have systematically searched for, appraised, and summarized all of the medical literature for a specific topic
  - *Meta-analysis:* A systematic review that uses quantitative methods to combine and reanalyze results from the combined studies to summarize results based on the pool of studies
  - *RCT:* Study that includes patients randomized to an experimental group or a control group of those not receiving the intervention. The groups are evaluated over time for the variables or outcomes of interest.
  - *Quasi-experimental study:* An interventional study in which subjects are not randomly assigned to treatment groups or a control group
  - *Nonexperimental study:* A study in which data are collected without introducing an intervention, usually descriptive in nature
  - *Cohort study:* Research that identifies two groups (i.e., cohorts) of patients (i.e., one group that received the exposure or intervention and one that did not), with the cohorts followed to examine the outcomes
  - *Case-control study:* Research that identifies patients who have the outcome of interest (i.e., cases) and persons without the same outcome (i.e., controls) to determine the exposure of interest
  - *Descriptive study:* Research that examines individual characteristics or circumstances and the frequency in which they occur in a population
  - *Qualitative study:* A study of phenomena that are difficult or impossible to quantify mathematically that is performed by collection of narrative data that is analyzed for cross-cutting themes
  - *Expert opinion:* Handbooks, encyclopedias, textbooks, and clinical experience of respected authorities

Step 4: Apply the Evidence with Clinical Expertise, Taking the Patient's Wants and Needs into Consideration

- Applies the evidence to the patient or family, or both
- Incorporates clinical knowledge gained over time
- Incorporates the patient's unique situation, desires, and values

Step 5: Evaluate the Effectiveness and Efficiency of the Process

- After implementation, evaluation is performed to determine whether the practice resulted in positive outcomes.
- Outcome measurement
  - How are outcomes measured?
  - Who performs the measurement?
  - Do instruments exist for measurement of the outcomes?

Oncology Nursing Society Putting Evidence into Practice

The Oncology Nursing Society (ONS) coordinates Putting Evidence into Practice (PEP) projects that summarize evidence-based interventions for the care of patients.

- Systematic reviews that are conducted by oncology nurses cover a wide array of topics.
- Categories of assessment
  - *Recommended for practice:* interventions for which effectiveness has been established
  - *Likely to be effective:* interventions for which evidence is less well established
  - *Benefits balanced with harms:* clinicians advised to consider the risk-benefit ratio
  - *Effectiveness not established:* insufficient data are available or data may not be of adequate quality to determine the effectiveness of an intervention
  - *Effectiveness unlikely:* effectiveness of an intervention is less well established
  - *Not recommended for practice:* ineffectiveness or harm demonstrated
  - *Expert opinion:* intervention appears consistent with sound clinical practice

Relevance of Evidence-Based Practice to Nursing Practice

- Nursing practice should be based on science rather than tradition.
- EBP improves patient outcomes.
- EBP decreases unnecessary procedures.
- EBP empowers nursing through sound knowledge.

Bibliography

Dearholt, S. L., & Dang, D. (2012). *Johns Hopkins nursing evidence based practice model and guidelines.* Indianapolis, IN: Sigma Theta Tau International.

Melnyk, B. M., & Fineout-Overholt, E. (2011). *Evidence-based practice in nursing and healthcare: A guide to best practice.* Philadelphia: Lippincott Williams & Wilkins.

Melnyk, B. M., Fineout-Overholt, E., & Stillwell, S. B. (2010a). Evidence-based practice: Step by step: The seven steps of evidence-based practice. *American Journal of Nursing, 110*(1), 51–53.

Melnyk, B. M., Fineout-Overholt, E., & Stillwell, S. B. (2010b). Evidence-based practice: Step by step: Igniting a spirit of inquiry. *American Journal of Nursing, 109*(11), 49–52.

Melnyk, B. M., Fineout-Overholt, E., & Stillwell, S. B. (2010c). Evidence-based practice: Step by step: Critical appraisal of the evidence, part III. *American Journal of Nursing, 110*(11), 43–51.

Mitchell, S. A., & Friese, C. R. (2015). *ONS PEP weighting system overview.* Available at https://www.ons.org/practice-resources/pep (accessed March 23, 2016).

Polit, D. F., & Beck, C. T. (2012). *Nursing research: Generating and assessing evidence for nursing practice.* Philadelphia: Lippincott Williams & Wilkins.

Stevens, K. (2013). The impact of evidence-based practice in nursing and the next big ideas. *Online Journal of Issues in Nursing, 18*(2), 4.

Stillwell, S. B., Fineout-Overholt, E., & Melnyk, B. M. (2010). Evidence-based practice: Step by step: Asking the clinical question: A key step in evidence-based practice. *American Journal of Nursing, 110*(3), 58–61.

Patient Navigation

Karyl Blaseg

Introduction

Patient navigation is typically credited to the foundational work led by Dr. Harold P. Freeman in the 1990s with low-income women diagnosed with breast cancer in Harlem, New York. Dr. Freeman created the nation's first navigation program in response to concerns identified regarding health care disparities among vulnerable populations, including low-income and racial/ethnic minority groups (Freeman & Rodriguez, 2011). The program provided a framework to ensure available access to timely care and support systems to help eliminate financial, social, and cultural barriers to care. As a result of the navigation interventions delivered, significant shifts were noted in terms of earlier stage at diagnosis and improved survival. These demonstrated successes in Harlem, New York, led to widespread national attention regarding the important role patient navigation can play in improving cancer outcomes and reducing health care disparities. Over the past 10 years, funds from multiple sources, including private foundations, community organizations, and local, state, and federal governments, have been allocated to advance the efforts of navigation and further expand adoption of the service with the overall intent of reducing health care disparities.

Definitions of Patient Navigation

C-Change, a collaborative organization involving cancer leaders from public, private, and not-for-profit groups, is frequently cited as providing the first definition of navigation in 2005 as "individualized assistance offered to patients, families, and caregivers to help overcome health care system barriers and facilitate timely access to quality medical and psychosocial care." Other organizations have adopted and embraced this definition of patient navigation, including the American College of Surgeons Commission on Cancer (2012), who revised their cancer program standards to include a component related to patient navigation services.

The Oncology Nursing Society, Association of Oncology Social Work, and National Association of Social Workers (2010) issued a joint position statement that used the C-Change definition of patient navigation as the basis for their work. However, attention was given to the specific verbiage of "quality *medical* and psychosocial care," and modifications were incorporated to instead read "quality *health* and psychosocial care."

Models of Patient Navigation

The first navigation program created by Dr. Freeman consisted predominantly of two interventions: access to free- and low-cost mammography services paired with individualized assistance in obtaining timely diagnosis and initiation of treatment. His program engaged community members in cancer outreach efforts who were deemed to be successful because of their inherent knowledge of and sensitivity to the community's cultural and language barriers.

As additional navigation programs have been implemented, various models and adaptations have evolved. Over the past 20 years, Dr. Freeman has identified and vetted nine core principles of patient navigation (Freeman & Rodriguez, 2011, p. 3542):

1. Patient navigation is a patient-centric health care service delivery model.
2. Patient navigation serves to virtually integrate a fragmented health care system for the individual patient.
3. The core function of patient navigation is the elimination of barriers to timely care across all segments of the health care continuum.
4. Patient navigation should be defined with a clear scope of practice that distinguishes the roles and responsibilities of the navigator from that of all other providers.
5. Delivery of patient navigation services should be cost-effective and commensurate with the training and skills necessary to navigate an individual through a particular phase of the care continuum.
6. The determination of who should navigate should be determined by the level of skills required at a given phase of navigation.
7. In a given system of care, there is the need to define the point at which navigation begins and the point at which navigation ends.
8. There is a need to navigate patients across disconnected systems of care, such as primary care sites and tertiary care sites.
9. Patient navigation systems require coordination.

Various navigation models, along with key characteristics and potential program advantages, are outlined in the table on page 432.

A key concept regarding the various models of navigation is that those deemed to be most effective have been specifically designed to meet the needs of a defined population and an

Examples of Patient Navigation Models

	Community	Professional
Community/Lay Navigation vs Professional Navigation		
Characteristics	Non–health care professional • Typically a member of the community served • May or may not be a cancer survivor	Health care professional • RN most commonly • Social worker • Other (e.g., APRN, mammography technician) Paid employee, full- or part-time Typically embedded within a health care system
Advantages	Volunteer or paid employee, full- or part-time May or may not be embedded within a health care system Lower program costs Keen awareness of financial, social, and cultural barriers Great potential for cultural diversity	Professional scope of practice allowing for greater patient education and supportive care Good working knowledge of complex health care systems
Site-Specific Navigation vs Setting-Specific Navigation		
	Site-Specific	**Setting-Specific**
Characteristics	Professional or community/lay navigator Dedicated to single or multiple types of cancers	Professional or community/lay navigator Focused on a single aspect of care, such as • Outreach/prevention/screening • Mammography diagnostic center • Inpatient unit • Survivorship care
Advantages	Commonly embedded within health care system Focused on timely coordination of multidisciplinary care Professional scope of practice allowing for greater patient education and supportive care Clinical expertise regarding specific types of cancers and national care guidelines Good working knowledge of complex health care systems	Narrow scope of responsibilities, which may facilitate hard-wiring of specific processes
Mixed Model Navigation		
Characteristics	Combination of one or more of the above models	
Advantages	Potential for more cost-effective utilization of resources Potential for greater diversity Recognition for the positive attributes of both professional and community/lay navigators	

individual cancer program. A common notion among experienced navigators and program administrators is that "one size does *not* fit all" when it comes to navigation programs and interventions. Rather, thoughtful assessment and program planning are essential to create a program that can best meet the needs of one's community.

Roles, Responsibilities, and Core Competencies

Specific roles and responsibilities of patient navigators vary according to the particular navigation model created, the defined start and end points for navigation, and the extent of services provided. Despite this variability, core fundamental roles can be identified among navigators. These include identification and resolution of barriers to care, coordination of timely access to care, facilitation of open communication and collaboration, and provision of emotional support.

In 2010, the Oncology Nursing Society (ONS) launched a role delineation study for oncology nurse navigators to better understand the core responsibilities and job functions of this emerging specialty. A total of 330 nurses participated in the role delineation study. Data obtained from participants helped identify knowledge, tasks, and skills specific to the oncology nurse navigator role, as outlined in the box in the next column.

Competence has largely been associated with the knowledge, skills, and attitudes required to fulfill a specific role. A clearly defined competency framework is essential to

Nurse Navigator Role's Top Tasks, Knowledge Areas, and Skills

Tasks
- Provide emotional and educational support for patients.
- Practice according to professional and legal standards.
- Advocate on behalf of the patient.
- Demonstrate ethical principles in practice.
- Orient patients to the cancer care system.
- Receive and respond to new patient referrals.
- Pursue continuing education opportunities related to oncology and navigation.
- Collaborate with physicians and other health care providers.
- Empower patients to self-advocate.
- Assist patients to make informed decisions.
- Provide education or referrals for coping with the diagnosis.
- Identify patients with a new diagnosis of cancer.

Knowledge Areas
- Confidentiality and informed consent
- Advocacy
- Symptom management
- Ethical principles
- Quality of life
- Goal of treatment
- Therapeutic options
- Evidence-based practice guidelines
- Professional scope of practice
- Legal and professional guidelines

Skills
- Communication
- Problem solving
- Critical thinking
- Multitasking
- Collaboration
- Time management
- Advocacy

establishing the role expectations and responsibilities for a patient navigator. The National Coalition of Oncology Nurse Navigators (NCONN) developed the first set of core competencies for patient navigation. These competencies, originally defined in 2009 and revised in 2013, focused on five broad categories, including professional, legal, and ethical nursing practice; health promotion and health education; management and leadership; advocacy; and personal effectiveness and professional development (Francz & Simpson, 2013). Similar efforts were undertaken by an ONS project team with four broad categories of core navigation competencies defined as education, professionalism, coordination of care, and communication (Oncology Nursing Society, 2013).

Considerations for Building a Successful Navigation Program

Program Preparations

Those with the vision to create a successful patient navigation program should not operate in an isolated manner; rather, they must engage the support of administrative leadership and key stakeholders including providers, patients, other staff, and local community organizations. The desire to develop a navigation program may be prompted by an accreditation standard or funding requirement of an external agency. However, even if that is the impetus, it is important to take the time to conduct a thorough community and cancer-program needs assessment to clearly identify and understand existing needs for which navigation services can effectively address and positively impact patient care. A robust needs assessment might include information from local community health reports, local and state cancer registries, the Centers for Disease Control and Prevention and National Cancer Institute databases, and the American Cancer Society Cancer Facts and Figures data to identify any concerning trends in access to care, stage at diagnosis, and increasing rates of incidence or mortality. Also, key pieces of information can be gleaned through community focus groups with patients, families, and caregivers affected by cancer to learn firsthand the barriers and challenges experienced when seeking cancer care and any gaps in the health care delivery system.

Once the needs assessment has been completed and analyzed, the structure of the navigation program can be developed along with identified goals and objectives. Key considerations when establishing the program framework include clearly identifying the start and end points for navigation interventions, aligning the program with organizational priorities, and setting realistic program goals and objectives. Objectives direct the focus of a program and should be used to break down large, long-term goals into manageable and achievable pieces. Once goals and objectives have been determined, measures should be identified to assess program performance and processes and the achievement of defined objectives. Most sustainable and successful patient navigation programs have been established over time by starting small and building incrementally through continuous process improvements and program expansion as objectives are achieved and positive outcomes demonstrated.

Job descriptions should be established and should clearly define position requirements that are reflective of program needs along with key roles and responsibilities. Along with the creation of job descriptions, high-level process maps should be outlined to clearly identify the scope of responsibilities, system bottlenecks, and where patient navigation attention might initially be focused. Standard operating procedures (SOPs) should be documented. SOPs set role expectations by outlining the specific steps associated with various responsibilities and tasks required of the patient navigator. These documents should be reviewed on an established schedule (i.e., annually or biennially) and updated to reflect process and role changes.

Successful Onboarding

The importance of hiring the right person and providing meaningful orientation and training for a patient navigation program cannot be overemphasized. Consideration must first be given to the specific navigation model to be implemented and whether this would best be suited for a professional or a community/lay navigator. Further thought should then be given to specific qualities and characteristics of the desired candidate, including cultural competence, superb communication skills, thorough familiarity with disease processes, sound knowledge of resources, and demonstrated leadership skills. An orientation checklist provides a structured "roadmap" for the orientation process and helps to direct the patient navigator in obtaining a broad understanding and solid knowledge base of the organization's systems, processes, and overall culture.

Aside from orientation to the specific organization and role expectations, a number of navigation training programs as well as online program resources and toolkits are available for those just getting started in the role. Some examples follow.
- Training Programs
  - Patient Navigator Training Collaborative: http://www.patientnavigatortraining.org
  - EduCare: http://www.educareinc.com
  - The George Washington Cancer Institute: http://smhs.gwu.edu/gwci/patient-care/patient-navigation
  - Harold P. Freeman Patient Navigation Institute: http://www.hpfreemanpni.org
  - Northwest Georgia Regional Cancer Coalition Cancer Navigator Program: http://www.cancernavigatorprogram.org
  - Smith Center for Healing and the Arts: http://www.smithcenter.org
  - Sonoma State University: http://www.sonoma.edu/exed/health-navigator/
- Program Development Resources
  - Association of Community Cancer Centers: Patient Navigation Resources and Tools for the Multidisciplinary Team: https://www.accc-cancer.org/resources/PatientNavigation-Tools.asp

- The Boston Medical Center Patient Navigation Toolkit: http://www.avonfoundation.org/assets/bmc-patient-navigation-toolkit-vol-2.pdf
- Patient Navigation in Cancer Care (Pfizer, Inc.): http://www.patientnavigation.com

Program Expansion

The Navigation Assessment Tool was developed in 2011 by members of the National Cancer Institute Community Cancer Centers Program (NCCCP) as a tool to assess the growth potential of both new and existing patient navigation programs. This document was developed by consensus and structured in a matrix format with 16 identified core measures that are important elements in building a strong navigation program, each with up to five levels of maturity. The intent of this tool was to provide an institutional self-assessment of the maturity of individual programs and to offer a structure to systematically expand the depth and breadth of patient navigation services provided. Swanson, Strusowski, Mack, and DeGroot (2012) outlined the 16 core measures of the Navigation Assessment Tool as follows:

1. Key stakeholders
2. Community partnerships
3. Acuity system/patient risk factors
4. Quality improvement measures
5. Marketing of the navigation program
6. Percentage of patients offered patient navigation
7. Continuum of navigation
8. Support services available and used by the navigation team
9. Tools for reporting navigator statistics
10. Financial assessment
11. Focus on disparities
12. Navigator responsibilities
13. Patient identification process
14. Navigator training
15. Engagement with clinical trials
16. Multidisciplinary care/conference involvement

Outcomes and Performance Measures

The literature on patient navigation is rapidly expanding, with evidence showing the positive impact navigation has on improving not only clinical outcomes but also the overall patient experience. Despite some common outcome themes that have emerged (e.g., screening access, time to diagnostic resolution and treatment, satisfaction levels, health care costs and resource utilization, access to community-based resources), concern exists with regard to inconsistencies in reporting outcomes as well as program variations, making it challenging to compare outcomes and advance the scientific evidence related to patient navigation.

In response to these concerns, the American Cancer Society organized the National Patient Navigation Leadership Summit in 2010 with the intent of establishing a national consensus on core program metrics and outcome measures related to patient navigation across the cancer continuum. The Leadership Summit was attended by 115 participants from more than 65

organizations (Esparza & Calhoun, 2011). A compilation of the articles pertaining to patient navigation outcome metrics was published in the August 2011 supplement of *Cancer*. Some of the interesting findings that warrant further review of individual articles within the supplement are highlighted as follows:

- Battaglia, Burhansstipanov, Murrell, Dwyer, and Caron (2011) delineated common constructs along with associated data elements and outcome measures pertaining to screening, diagnostic, and process metrics.
- Guadagnolo, Dohan, and Raich (2011) defined domains along with metrics and suggested quality benchmarks for core patient navigation metrics during the diagnosis and early treatment of cancer. They further identified patient-reported outcome domains with associated measurement scales.
- Pratt-Chapman, Simon, Patterson, Risendal, and Patierno (2011) shared potential health care utilization and patient-reported outcomes related to survivorship navigation along with specific navigation activities and provided suggestions on how to measure each.
- Hauser et al. (2011) summarized domains along with associated outcomes pertaining to navigation in palliative care.
- Fiscella et al. (2011) outlined patient-reported outcome measures according to phase of the cancer continuum, domain, metric, strengths of measure, limitations of measure, and languages available.
- Whitley et al. (2011) categorized fixed and variable costs associated with patient navigation programs and costs related to employment, training, and supervision.

Future of Navigation

Patient navigation has demonstrated significant strides over the past 20 years and has documented the positive impact supportive systems can have on reducing the financial, social, and cultural burdens of cancer while improving clinical outcomes. Initiatives related to patient navigation continue to build momentum through focused efforts and widespread adoption as organizations increasingly recognize these benefits. The role of patient navigation appears to be a consistent and core element of Accountable Care and Medical Home initiatives introduced across the country. The future truly holds endless possibilities for patient navigation and the need to ensure continuity of care across the health care continuum.

References

American College of Surgeons. Commission on Cancer. (2012). *Cancer program standards 2012: Ensuring patient-centered care v1.2.1*. Chicago, IL: American College of Surgeons.

Battaglia, T. A., Burhansstipanov, L., Murrell, S. S., Dwyer, A. J., & Caron, S. E. (2011). Assessing the impact of patient navigation: Prevention and early detection metrics. *Cancer, 117*(Suppl. 15), 3553–3564.

Brown, C. G., Cantril, C., McMullen, L., Barkley, D. L., Dietz, M., Murphy, C. M., & Fabrey, L. J. (2012). Oncology nurse navigator role delineation study: An Oncology Nursing Society report. *Clinical Journal of Oncology Nursing, 16*(6), 581–585.

Esparza, A., & Calhoun, E. (2011). Measuring the impact and potential of patient navigation. *Cancer, 117*(Suppl. 15), 3535–3536.

Fiscella, K., Ransom, S., Jean-Pierre, P., Cella, D., Stein, K., Bauer, J. E., & Walsh, K. (2011). Patient-reported outcome measures suitable to assessment of patient navigation. *Cancer, 117*(Suppl. 15), 3603–3617.

Francz, S. L., & Simpson, K. D. (2013). Oncology nurse navigators: A snapshot of their educational background, compensation, and day-to-day roles and responsibilities. *Oncology Issues, 28*(1), 36–43.

Freeman, H. P., & Rodriguez, R. I. (2011). History and principles of patient navigation. *Cancer, 117*(Suppl. 15), 3539–3542.

Guadagnolo, B. A., Dohan, D., & Raich, P. (2011). Metrics for evaluating patient navigation during cancer diagnosis and treatment. *Cancer, 117*(Suppl. 15), 3565–3574.

Hauser, J., Sileo, M., Araneta, N., Kirk, R., Martinez, J., Finn, K., & Harney, C. (2011). Navigation and palliative care. *Cancer, 117*(Suppl. 15), 3585–3591.

Oncology Nursing Society. (2013). *Oncology Nurse Navigator Core Competencies*. Pittsburgh, PA: Oncology Nursing Society.

Oncology Nursing Society, Association of Oncology Social Work, & National Association of Social Workers. (2010). Oncology Nursing Society, the Association of Oncology Social Worker, and the National Association of Social Workers joint position on the role of oncology nursing and oncology social work in patient navigation. *Oncology Nursing Forum, 37*, 251–252.

Pratt-Chapman, M., Simon, M. A., Patterson, A. K., Risendal, B. C., & Patierno, S. (2011). Survivorship navigation outcome measures: A report from the ACS patient navigation working group on survivorship navigation. *Cancer, 117*(Suppl. 15), 3575–3584.

Swanson, J. R., Strusowski, P., Mack, N., & DeGroot, J. (2012). Growing a navigation program: Using the NCCCP Navigation Assessment Tool. *Oncology Issues, 27*(4), 36–45.

Whitley, E., Valverde, P., Wells, K., Williams, L., Teschner, T., & Shih, Y. C. (2011). Establishing common cost measures to evaluate the economic value of patient navigation programs. *Cancer, 117*(Suppl. 15), 3616–3623.

Patient Education

Leah A. Scaramuzzo

Patient education is an important part of almost every nursing intervention. It involves more than just telling patients to take their medications. Rather, it encompasses skill building and helping patients learn when, how, and even why to make changes. Patient education requires a baseline needs assessment of the patient and caregiver in order to comprehensively address needs adequately (see table on page 437). Understanding and overcoming educational, ethnic, cultural, and spiritual barriers should also be incorporated into the education plan. Ultimately, the process should build patient knowledge and skills and enable patients and their caretakers to participate actively in their care and contribute to positive outcomes. Education that patients can understand will contribute greatly to their satisfaction with care and increase the quality of their lives.

What are the Challenges of Providing Patient Education?

- Shorter hospitalizations and therefore less time to teach
- Ambulatory clinic visits with limited time allocated for patient education
- Increased complexity of care at home and need for more comprehensive education
- Patients' seeking information from at least one other source besides the physician
- Information on the Internet that may be misleading, subject to interpretation, or clearly incorrect
- Literacy level or difficulty interpreting and retaining information
- Anxiety, physical symptoms, or medications that may affect concentration and recollection

Need for Varied Teaching Methods

Although many clinicians believe they have given adequate instruction or information during a patient visit, they may fail to realize that patients do not retain everything they are told while in the examination room, clinic, or hospital. Patients retain:

- 20% of what they hear
- 30% of what they see
- 50% of what they see and hear
- 70% of what they see, hear, and say
- 90% of what they see, hear, say, and do

Content needs to be reinforced by various learning methods. Combining different methods—written materials, verbal instruction, demonstration, and patient participation—during the learning process makes it more likely that patients will retain the information provided.

Outcomes of Patient Education

- Promote communication between patient and health care provider
- Reduce uncertainty
- Encourage participation in decision making
- Increase adherence to plan of care
- Maximize self-care skills
- Increase ability to cope with health status
- Promote healthy lifestyles and behaviors
- Increase empowerment and autonomy
- Reduce health care expenditures

Mandates and Standards for Patient Education

- American Hospital Association (AHA)—*A Patient's Bill of Rights*
- The Federal Plain Language Guidelines—*The Plain Language Action and Information Network (PLAIN)*: a community of federal employees dedicated to the idea that citizens deserve clear communications from government
- National Health Education Standards—*The Joint Committee on National Health Education Standards*: written expectations for what students should know and be able to do by grades 2, 5, 8, and 12 to promote personal, caregiver, and community health. These standards provide a framework for curriculum development, selection, instruction, and student assessment in health education.
- National Culturally and Linguistically Appropriate Services (CLAS) Standards—*Department of Health and Human Services, Office of Minority Health*: helps organizations address cultural and language differences between people who provide information and services and the people they serve. The principal standard is to provide effective, equitable, understandable, and respectful quality care and services that are responsive to diverse cultural health beliefs, practices, preferred languages, health literacy, and other communication needs.
- The Joint Commission
- Centers for Medicare and Medicaid Services (CMS) Electronic Health Record Incentive Program—Meaningful Use requirement
- American Society of Clinical Oncology/Oncology Nursing Society Chemotherapy Administration Safety Standards Including Standards for the Safe Administration and Management of Oral Chemotherapy
- U.S. News & World Report's ranking of leading cancer hospitals: includes patient education as part of excellent health care

Role of the Nurse in Patient Education

Definition	Roles
To determine the patient's knowledge base and his or her need to know: • Assess learning barriers and best means to learn. • Assess preference for brief or plentiful information.	Identify the potential learner: • Patient, caregiver, spouse, significant other Identify barriers than may influence learning outcomes: • Physical • Sensory (vision/hearing) • Emotional, readiness to learn • Denial of need to learn • Cultural, religious • Cognitive • Literacy level, educational level • Special learning needs • Speech • Financial concerns • Language (non–English speaking) • Anxiety Identify preferred learning method: • Reading • Pictures • Video • Listening • Demonstration
To develop and strategize the best means to educate the patient/caregiver	Identify expressed educational needs/concerns: • Diagnosis–disease process, plan of care and treatment options • Procedures, preoperative and postoperative teaching • Medical equipment and skills • Pain management • Cancer treatments and side effect management • Medications • Nutrition, drug/food interactions • Community resources, coping strategies, advance directives • Activity • Personal hygiene • Speech and hearing evaluations • Discharge planning • Other areas as identified by the patient/caregiver
To prioritize and execute teaching content to ensure that the learner's needs are met and self-care activities vital to ongoing physical and psychological well-being are taught.	Establish an environment that encourages patients and families to ask questions, learn, and participate: • Provide respect • Offer privacy • Establish eye contact • Listen attentively • If possible, sit with patient/caregiver Mutually determine goals and time frame Methods of teaching: • Explanation • Demonstration • Written • Audio/visual • Settings • Telephone
To determine whether the content has been learned	Verbalize understanding via the teach-back method: • Ask patient to explain in his or her own words the information shared. • Example: "Share with me what you will explain to your wife about your medicines for nausea and vomiting and how you will take them." Identify need for further information or reinforcement

Education Theory

- *Behavioral Learning Theory:* Learning is based on observable behaviors (e.g., relaxation)
- *Cognitive Learning Theory:* Internal processes lead to learning (example: creation of mnemonic for symptoms to call the physician)
- *Social Learning Theory:* Learning takes place based on watching and imitating others
- *Motivational Learning Theory:* Learning results from personal cues (e.g., "I want to be here for my children, so I have to quit smoking")
- *Adult Learning Theory:* Uses approaches that are problem-based, collaborative, and less didactic; the six principles of adult learners are
  1. They are internally motivated and self-directed
  2. They bring life experiences and knowledge to learning experiences
  3. They are goal oriented.
  4. They are relevancy oriented.
  5. They are practical.
  6. They like to be respected.

Learner Barriers to Education
- Lack of emotional readiness
  - Anxiety, support system, motivation
  - Risk-taking behaviors
  - Frame of mind in accordance with Maslow's hierarchy of feeds (e.g., if basic needs are not met, learning cannot occur)
- Lack of experimental readiness
  - Level of aspiration
  - Past coping mechanisms
  - Cultural background
  - Locus of control, assertiveness
- Limited cognitive ability
  - Extent to which information can be processed
  - Behavioral objectives + Cognitive ability = Learning
  - Knowledge versus Competence
  - Competency validation
  - Health literacy + Activation = Health outcomes

Barriers to Providing Effective Patient Education
- Lack of awareness regarding the patient's level of health literacy
- Lack of time to talk with patients and answer questions
- Accurate simplification of complex scientific information
- A view that simplifying information means "dumbing it down"
- Concerns about offending skilled readers
- Staff turnover and need for periodic training
- Lack of staff buy-in or interest

Health Education Goals
- Inform and instruct
- Empower
- Prevent problems and complications
- Enhance quality of life
- Supplement information given verbally

Health Literacy

Definition

Health literacy is the ability to obtain, process, understand, and act on health care information. Examples include

- Reading consent forms and medicine labels
- Understanding written and oral information
- Acting on procedures and instructions

Health Literacy in the United States

- The health of 90 million people may be at risk because of difficulty understanding and acting on health information.
- Literacy skills are a stronger predictor of an individual's health status than age, income, employment status, education level, or racial/ethnic group.
- One out of five American adults reads at the 5th grade level or below.
- The average American reads at the 8th to 9th grade level, yet most health care materials are written above the 10th grade level.
- More than 66% of adults in America age 60 and older have inadequate or marginal literacy skills.
- According to the Center for Health Care Strategies, a disproportionate number of minority group members and immigrants have limited literacy (e.g., 50% of Hispanics, 40% of Blacks, 33% of Asians).

High-Risk Groups

- Elderly individuals
- Minority group members
- Immigrants
- Poor people
- Homeless people
- Prisoners
- People with limited education

Possible Results of Low Health Literacy

- Poor health outcomes such as higher rates of hospitalization, less frequent use of preventive services, higher health care costs
- Poor patient adherence with medications including oral therapy
- Medication or treatment errors
- Poor self-care management strategies
- Difficulty navigating the health care system

Indirect Indicators of Reading Problems

- Mouthing words
- Pointing to text as it is read
- Complaints of poor eyesight or wrong glasses

Health Education Materials

Advantages of Printed Educational Materials

- Consistency of message content
- Flexibility of delivery
- Portability and reusability
- Low cost to produce and update
- Permanence of information
- Reinforcement verbal instructions

Goals of Patient Education Materials

Patient education materials should ensure patient and caregiver ability to do the following:

- Read prescription bottles and appointment slips
- Understand informed consents and discharge instructions
- Follow diagnostic test instructions
- Read health education materials
- Complete health insurance applications

Outcomes of Providing Understandable Health Care Instructions

- Improved treatment adherence
- Decreased return visits to the hospital
- Improved health outcomes

Developing Written Materials

- Define target audience: involve audience in planning and writing. Ensure material is relevant and appropriate for the patient's literacy level, age, sex, and culture.
- Identify key points of the material to impart.
- Determine the tone: aim for a friendly and conversational tone.
- Ascertain readability: ensure material is easy to read and understand; have more than one person review it.
- Use common words; give examples to explain uncommon words.
- Use short sentences.
- Include interaction, if possible.
- Place key information first.
- Use headers.
- Use serif type and lowercase lettering.
- Use 12- to 14-point fonts.
- Avoid using capital letters.

Content and Organization

- Content should be verified by experts.
- The purpose of the material should be clear to the audience.
- Present only the most important information.
- New information should be related to what the audience already knows.
- Retention of information is lower when the content is unfamiliar.
- Organize content to convey the meaning of the material and to motivate the learner.
- Examples should be limited to those that the audience can understand and relate to.
- Summarize points throughout the text.

Organizing Principles

- Use short titles that convey meaning clearly.
- Include a table of contents.
- Repeat important information in bulleted lists.

- Keep related ideas together; present only one idea per paragraph.
- State the main idea in the first sentence of the paragraph.
- Keep sentences short and simple.

Appropriate Language and Format
- Language should not exceed 6th grade reading level.
- Limit sentences to one idea.
- Avoid complicated medical terms, acronyms, and words of three or more syllables.
- If a medical term must be used, define it clearly and provide a glossary of terms.
- Consider linguistic capabilities and possible limitations of the target audience.
- Use large print for those with visual problems.
- Keep the tone reader-friendly.
- Address patients' needs and questions in terms that reassure rather than frighten.
- Use positive phrases such as "Avoid smoking" instead of "Do not smoke."
- Use a clear, concise, and friendly format if patients are anxious or nervous.

Motivational Principles
- Focus on what audience should know or do.
- Use the active voice.
- Use questions as headings.

Linguistic Principles
- Use one- and two-syllable words.
- Use words that are easily understood by the target audience.
- Avoid multiple clauses and double negatives.
- Define unfamiliar terms.
- Use contractions.

Plain Language. Plain language is a strategy for making written and oral information easier to understand. For example:
- Original sentence: "It is now well established that the substance currently under investigation is effective for the duration of a minimum of 4 hours."
- Revised to: "The tablet being tested works for at least 4 hours."

Strategies for Developing Culturally Appropriate Materials
- Be familiar with beliefs and values if addressing a specific group of patients.
- If language barriers exist, provide information in patients' native language.
- Include the audience's beliefs and values.
- Collaborate with community organizations.
- Choose words that show respect.
- Use graphics, pictures, and examples.
- Field-test materials, and involve the target audience in development.

Tone
- Be reader-friendly.
- Address patients' needs.

- Capture and hold readers' attention.
- Be realistic but reassuring.
- Tell the truth.
- Avoid negatives.

Formatting Educational Materials
- Write simple, catchy titles.
- Keep the page layout simple.
- Use an unjustified righthand margin.
- Use Times New Roman font for easier reading.
- Use bulleted lists; number bullets and lists if there is an order.
- Title each list or table.
- Use black ink on light-colored paper that is heavy, dull-coated, and matte.
- Make liberal use of white space to help rest the eyes.
- Present some material in tables, diagrams, drawings, and photographs.

Readability Statistics
- Assesses the reading difficulty of printed material.
- Reading statistics formulas should not be the sole basis for evaluating reading materials; context and other factors must also be considered.
- Most common instruments are the following:
  - Flesch-Kincaid grade level scale
  - Fry graph
  - FOG scale (Gunning FOG formula)
  - SMOG index
  - Readability assessment tools are available at http://www.readabilityformulas.com/free-readability-formula-tests.php

Tools for Assessing Health Literacy
- Reading Recognition Tests
- Suitability Assessment of Materials (SAM)
- Wide Range Achievement Test (WRAT)
- Slosson Oral Reading Test
- Rapid Estimate of Adult Literacy in Medicine (REALM)
- Medical Achievement Reading Test
- Peabody Individual Achievement Test
- Test of Functional Health Literacy in Adults (TOFHLA)

Using Technology in Patient Education
- The World Wide Web
  - More than 50% of Americans use it to obtain health information
  - Viewers can watch videos of procedures, ask questions, or receive information
  - Online health seekers use the Web to
    - Search for health information
    - Research a diagnosis or prescription
    - Prepare for surgery or how to best recover
    - Get online tips from other patients and caregivers about symptom management
    - Keep caregivers and friends informed of a loved one's condition
  - Nurses play an important role in teaching patients how to evaluate information (see table on page 440)

How to Evaluate Health Information on the Internet

Question	Criteria
Who	
Who runs the site?	• Should be easily found on every major page of the site.
Who pays for the site?	• Does it sell advertising or is it sponsored by a drug company? (".org" and ".gov" sites are unbiased and reliable; ".com" sites are businesses that may promote their sales)
	• Is there an editorial board? (if so, may be more reliable)
Who chooses and reviews the information?	• Do the reviewers have professional or scientific qualifications? (will increase reliability)
What	
What is the purpose of the site?	• Look at the "About This Site" link
What information is provided or claimed?	
Is it unbiased?	• Is it too good to be true?
	• Are sources or references listed?
	• Can the information be verified on another site?
	• What amount of information is given?
	• What personal information does the site collect, and why?
	• Are topics covered completely, or are links given for more information?
Where	
Where was the site developed?	• Government agencies ".gov"
	• Colleges and universities ".edu"
	• Institutions and organizations ".org" or ".net"
	• Commercial sites ".com"
When	
When was the site published, reviewed, and updated?	• Medical information must be current
	• Even if the information has not changed, date of review should be noted on site
How	
How does the site look?	• Is it easy to use?
	• Is the spelling and grammar correct?
	• Do the links work?
How does the site interact with visitors?	• Can you contact someone with questions or feedback?

- Social Media
  - Communication format for people with similar interests to share information
    - Blogs, wikis, Facebook, Twitter, YouTube
  - Used to educate, empower, send messages, and gather information on public perceptions about health
  - Potential risks: may market/show unhealthy behaviors such as smoking
- Webcasts and Webinars
  - Mechanisms to deliver presentations with audio and/or video
  - Webcasts allow for participant interaction
  - Useful when trying to reach learners in broad geographic locations
  - Risk: can be frustrating for learner and instructor if not able to communicate

- E-Mail
  - Inexpensive and quick way to communicate with patients
  - Allows patients time to gather thoughts and retain written information from clinician's response
  - Risk: need to ensure privacy for patient's computer and health care organization (Health Insurance Portability and Accountability Act [HIPAA])
- Online chats
  - Online conversation in real time
  - Useful for ongoing education or information exchange
  - Benefits patients who are homebound or isolated
  - Risk: fast pace; may be difficult to keep up with conversation

Professional Resources: Patient Education

- The Joint Commission "Speak Up Initiatives": http://www.jointcommission.org/speakup.aspx
- Agency for Healthcare Research and Quality (AHRQ): Health Literacy Universal Precautions Toolkit: http://www.ahrq.gov/professionals/quality-patient-safety/quality-resources/tools/literacy-toolkit/
- National Patient Safety Foundation—provider and patient information about health literacy: http://www.npsf.org/?page=askme3
- National Institutes of Health: Clear Communication—defines health literacy, states health literacy objectives in and links to more information: http://www.nih.gov/clearcommunication/healthliteracy.htm
- Fox Chase Cancer Center: Educating Families and Communities: http://www.fccc.edu/prevention/hchd/resources/index.html
- Health Literacy Studies—this site is designed for professionals in health and education who are interested in health literacy: http://www.hsph.harvard.edu/healthliteracy/
- Health on the Net Foundation (HON)—promotes and guides the deployment of useful and reliable online health information: http://www.hon.ch/
- MedinePlus: http://www.nlm.nih.gov/medlineplus/etr.html
- Medical Library Association focusing on health information literacy: http://www.mlanet.org/p/cm/ld/fid=396
- AHRQ's Patient Education Materials Assessment Tool (PEMAT) and User's Guide—provides a systematic method to evaluate and compare the understandability and actionability of patient education materials: http://www.ahrq.gov/pemat/
- AHRQ (Agency for Healthcare Research and Quality): http://pharmacyhealthliteracy.ahrq.gov/sites/PharmHealthLiteracy/default.aspx
- Plain Language Action and Information Network (PLAIN)—a community of federal employees from many different agencies and specialties: PlainLanguage.gov
- Project to Review and Improve Study Materials (PRISM) at the Group Health Center for Health Studies—a resource that shows research teams how to create consent forms and other patient materials in plain language: https://www.grouphealthresearch.org/about-us/capabilities/research-communications/prism/

- Centers for Disease Control and Prevention—tips for creating easy-to-read print materials your audience will want to read and use: http://www.cdc.gov/healthliteracy/pdf/Simply_Put.pdf

Patient Resources: Cancer Patient Education

- The Cancer Patient Education Network: http://www.cancerpatienteducation.org/
- National Cancer Institute: http://www.cancer.gov
- American Cancer Society: http://www.cancer.org
- Association of Cancer Online Resources: http://acor.org/
- Cancer Care: http://www.cancercare.org
- Oncolink: http://www.oncolink.org
- Navigating Cancer and Blood Disorders: https://www.navigatingcancer.com/
- Cancer.Net: http://www.cancer.net
- Leukemia and Lymphoma Society: https://www.lls.org/support-resources
- National Comprehensive Cancer Network (NCCN): http://www.nccn.org/patients/guidelines/

Bibliography

Bastable, S. B. (Ed.). (2013). *Nurse as educator: Principles of teaching and learning for nursing practice* (4th ed.). Burlington, MA: Jones & Bartlett.

Doak, C. C., Doak, L. G., & Root, J. H. (1996). The literacy problem. In C. C. Doak, L. G. Doak, & J. H. Root (Eds.), *Teaching patients with low literacy skills* (2nd ed.). Philadelphia: J.B. Lippincott.

Finkelman, A., & Kenner, C. (2009). *Teaching IOM: Implications of the Institute of Medicine reports for nursing education* (2nd ed.). Silver Spring, MD: American Nurses Association.

Tamura-Lis, W. (2013). Teach-Back for quality education and patient safety. *Urol Nurs, 33*(6), 267–271, 298.

Institute of Medicine. (2004). *Health literacy: A prescription to end confusion.* Washington, DC: Institute of Medicine, Board on Neuroscience and Behavioral Health, Committee on Health Literacy. Available at https://iom.nationalacademies.org/Reports/2004/Health-Literacy-A-Prescription-to-End-Confusion.aspx (accessed March 11, 2016).

Sand-Jecklin, K., Murray, B., Summers, B., & Watson, J. (2010, July 23). Educating nursing students about health literacy: From the classroom to the patient bedside. *OJIN: The Online Journal of Issues in Nursing, 15*(3).

Note: Pages followed by *b*, *t*, or *f* refer to boxes, tables, or figures, respectively.